ENT Diseases: Diagnosis and Treatment during Pregnancy and Lactation

Cemal Cingi • Halil Erdem Özel
Nuray Bayar Muluk

Editors

ENT Diseases: Diagnosis and Treatment during Pregnancy and Lactation

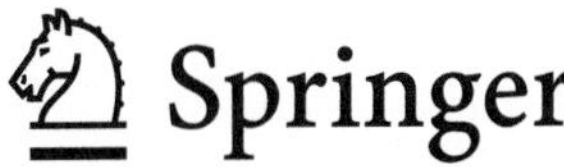 Springer

Editors
Cemal Cingi
Department of Otorhinolaryngology
Faculty of Medicine, Eskişehir Osmangazi
University
Eskisehir, Turkey

Nuray Bayar Muluk
Department of Otorhinolaryngology
Faculty of Medicine, Kırıkkale University
Kırıkkale, Turkey

Halil Erdem Özel
Department of Otorhinolaryngology
Derince Training and Research Hospital
Faculty of Medicine, Health Sciences
University
Kocaeli, Turkey

ISBN 978-3-031-05305-4   ISBN 978-3-031-05303-0   (eBook)
https://doi.org/10.1007/978-3-031-05303-0

This Springer imprint is published by the registered company Springer Nature Switzerland AG
The registered company address is: Gewerbestrasse 11, 6330 Cham, Switzerland

Preface

The formation of a new and completely unique human being through the combination of genes from the parents is surely Nature's greatest miracle. Male pride leads many cultures to grant the father a leading role in procreation, but, biologically speaking, his contribution to pregnancy is over in a matter of minutes, whereas for the mother, the next 9 months are a time of vast changes as she literally builds a new human being within her body and prepares to accept her lifetime role as caregiver. Even once the child is delivered, the mother's body still miraculously produces all the sustenance a baby needs in the form of milk. *Mother* Nature indeed!

In physiological terms, both pregnancy and the postpartum period are special and complex periods in a patient's life. ENT disorders are highly prevalent throughout the lifecycle, but when they occur in pregnant patients or nursing mothers, they call for special care in treatment. Without a deep knowledge of this period in a patient's life, it is all too easy for an ENT practitioner inadvertently to harm both the mother and her developing child. For this reason, we decided to write the book you are now holding, *ENT Diseases: Diagnosis and Treatment During Pregnancy and Lactation.*

My sincerest thanks go to Mrs. Nuray Bayar Muluk, my co-author, whose patience and diligent industry have, once again, brought another major project to fruition. It is an honour and a pleasure to be able to collaborate with her.

I also owe a great debt of gratitude to Mr. Halil Erdem Özel for his great diligence and meticulous sensitivity as an authority on ENT matters. As the storm of COVID 19 raged, he remained steadfast in his efforts to write, even after both he and all his family were struck down by the disease.

It is our hope and wish that the current volume of 73 chapters, representing, as it does, a collaboration between 170 authors in 30 different countries, will prove a go-to reference for all clinicians who encounter ENT disorders in their work. Perhaps, too, it may serve as a source of reliable information for the growing numbers of pregnant and postpartum patients who, these days, seek out their own information online prior to getting an ENT opinion!

"God who gives life also gives sustenance."
But loving mothers and growing babies still need our protection and support...

Eskişehir, Turkey   Cemal Cingi
1 July, 2022

Preface

Clinical management of pregnant or breastfeeding mothers and their offspring presents unique challenges because of the way management directly impacts both maternal and child health. It necessitates the joint evaluation of two people who are vital to each other's welfare. Scientific knowledge in this challenging field has many limitations and is based, for the most part, on animal models and observations in humans. Accordingly, conjecture and probability often take the place of definite facts. Thus, not only the management of patients during pregnancy and lactation is a real challenge, but also the task of gathering and writing down reliable information for hard-pressed clinicians to consult. This book provides much-needed specific guidance on the management of ENT and lower respiratory tract diseases during pregnancy and the post-partum period. Additionally, it serves to inform clinicians about physiological changes in pregnancy and the post-partum period. A number of chapters that complete the picture or offer a different perspective on the core topics have also been included.

The first germ of an idea for this book was planted during my period of obligatory state service in a secondary care hospital in the initial years after I completed residency training. I observed that a significant portion of those attending outpatient clinics are women who are either pregnant, post-partum, or with a suspected pregnancy. The fact that these patients primarily attend regional primary or secondary healthcare centres may mean this important group of patients is rarely encountered in tertiary centres responsible for residency training. As a result, young specialists may lack adequate experience of ENT conditions in pregnant and post-partum women and their offspring. Furthermore, there are only limited recommendations, even in major ENT textbooks, regarding management in pregnancy and the post-partum period. I am confident that this book will contribute to filling an important knowledge gap and will become one of the key resources in this area.

Cemal Cingi, one of the editors of this book, is an exceptional scientist and clinician who has always cared deeply about the ideas of younger colleagues and supported them in projects. Precisely because of Prof. Cingi's reputation, it was to him that I presented my idea for this volume, when it first came to me as a young ENT specialist. The first stages in writing coincided with a time when COVID-19 had begun to spread rapidly. Prof. Cingi's support in the form of wise counsel and superlative organisational skills meant writing the book became a major boost to my morale, at an otherwise very trying time when I, my wife, and many other colleagues were ourselves suffering from COVID-19, and has ensured the book will attract a wide readership amongst clinicians. Another editor, Nuray Bayar Muluk, through her devoted contributions, has brought the project to fruition, despite her own health problems. Many sincere thanks are due to the editors of the book.

For such a challenging subject, the authors have been at pains to take all the scientific data into detailed consideration, by conducting a thorough review of the evidence base before writing their chapters. Without their invaluable efforts, this book would not have been possible. I am grateful to all the authors for their diligence and industry. The meticulous attention of the publisher was vital to ensure the book could reach its current form. I also owe an immense debt of gratitude to our patients, who, as always, are our greatest teachers. I am delighted to present this book to our readers, whose suggestions and criticisms are welcome for future editions.

I dedicate this book to my dear wife, son, mother, and also to my beloved father, whose recent death was unexpected by any of us.

Derince, Kocaeli, Turkey																Halil Erdem Özel
23 April, 2022

Contents

Part V   Laryngology

**Part VI   Head and Neck Neoplasms and Surgery During
Pregnancy and the Postpartum Period**

**Part VII   Lower Airway Diseases During Pregnancy and the
Postpartum Period**

List of Contributors

Mustafa Acar The Acar Ear, Nose, and Throat Diseases and Surgery Clinic, Eskişehir, Turkey

Latif Akan Department of Otolaryngology Head and Neck Surgery, Dışkapı Yıldırım Beyazıt Training and Research Hospital, University of Health Sciences Turkey, Ankara, Turkey

Fatih Alper Akcan Department of Otorhinolaryngology, Düzce University, Faculty of Medicine, Düzce, Turkey

Fatma Tokgoz Akyil Ministry of Health, Yedikule Chest Diseases and Thoracic Surgery Training and Research Hospital, Istanbul, Turkey

Bahar Alagöz ENT Department, Ordu State Hospital, Ordu, Turkey

Nezar Y. Albar Internal Medicine and Endocrinology, First Clinic, International Medical Center, Jeddah, Saudi Arabia

Melike Aloğlu Department of Pulmonology, Ankara Atatürk Hospital for Chest Diseases and Chest Surgery, Ankara, Turkey

Nurcan Altaş Faculty of Dentistry, Periodontology Department, Istanbul Medipol University, Istanbul, Turkey

Nitin R. Ankle Department of ENT and Head-Neck Surgery, KLE Academy of Higher Education and Research, (KAHER), J. N. Medical College, Belagavi, Karnataka, India

Nevra Güllü Arslan Department of Pulmonology, Samsun Training and Research Hospital, Samsun, Turkey

Deniz Avcı Department of Otorhinolaryngology, Nevsehir State Hospital, Nevşehir, Turkey

Asena Aydin Department of Chest Diseases, Inegol State Hospital, Bursa, Turkey

Sevilay Aynacı Department of Otorhynolaryngology, Eskisehir City Hospital, Eskisehir, Turkey

Muhammet Ayral Medical Faculty, Otorhinolaryngology Department, Dicle University, Diyarbakır, Turkey

Bartu Badak Department of General Surgery, Eskisehir Osmangazi University, Eskisehir, Turkey

Kemal Koray Bal Faculty of Medicine, Department of Otorhinolaryngology, Mersin University, Mersin, Turkey

Hacer Baran Faculty of Medicine, Department of Otolaryngology—Head and Neck Surgery, İstanbul Dr. Lütfi Kırdar Research and Training Hospital, Health Sciences University, İstanbul, Turkey

Duygu Ayhan Başer Department of Family Medicine, Faculty of Medicine, Hacettepe University, Ankara, Turkey

Şeyma Başlılar Department of Pulmonology, Ümraniye Training and Research and Hospital, İstanbul, Turkey

Ferit Bayakır Department of Otolaryngology—Head and Neck Surgery, İnegol State Hospital, Bursa, Turkey

Nuray Bayar Muluk Department of Otorhinolaryngology, Faculty of Medicine, Kırıkkale University, Kırıkkale, Turkey

Ömer Bayir Department of Otolaryngology Head and Neck Surgery, Dışkapı Yıldırım Beyazıt Training and Research Hospital, University of Health Sciences Turkey, Ankara, Turkey

Müzeyyen Yıldırım Baylan Medical Faculty, Otorhinolaryngology Department, Dicle University, Diyarbakır, Turkey

Ali Bayram Department of Otorhinolaryngology, Kayseri City Hospital, Kayseri, Turkey

Jeffrey C. Bedrosian Rhinology and Skull Base Surgery, Specialty Physician Associates, St. Luke's Medical Center, Bethlehem, PA, USA

Luisa Maria Bellussi University of Siena—ENT Clinic, Siena, Italy

Nagihan Bilal Faculty of Medicine, Department of Otorhinolaryngology, Kahramanmaras Sutcu Imam University, Kahramanmaraş, Turkey

Sebla Çalışkan Faculty of Medicine, Department of Otorhinolaryngology, Derince Training and Research Hospital, Health Sciences University, Kocaeli, Turkey

Derya Cebeci Department of Otorhinolaryngology, Şanlıurfa Viranşehir State Hospital, Şanlıurfa, Turkey

Işıl Taylan Cebi Faculty of Medicine, Department of Otorhinolaryngology, İstanbul Haseki Research and Training Hospital, Health Sciences University, İstanbul, Turkey

İrem Kaya Cebioğlu Faculty of Health Sciences, Department of Nutrition and Dietetics, Yeditepe University, Istanbul, Turkey

Erdogan Cetinkaya Department of Pulmonology, Yedikule Chest Diseases and Thoracic Surgery Training and Research Hospital, University of Health Sciences, Istanbul, Turkey

Dennis Chua Department of Otorhinolaryngology, Mount Elizabeth Hospital, ENT Surgeons Medical Centre, 3 Mount Elizabeth, Singapore

Can Cemal Cingi Faculty of Communication Sciences, Communication Design and Management Department, Anadolu University, Eskisehir, Turkey

Güle Çınar Medical Faculty, Infectious Diseases and Clinical Microbiology Department, Ankara University, Ankara, Turkey

Cemal Cingi Department of Otorhinolaryngology, Faculty of Medicine, Eskisehir Osmangazi University, Eskisehir, Turkey

Gülce Cingi Private Nutrition and Dietetics Clinic, Istanbul, Turkey

Eugenio De Corso Department Head and Neck Surgery, Institute of Otorhinolaryngology, Catholic University of Sacred Heart, Rome, Italy

İbrahim Çukurova Section of Otorhinolaryngology, Tepecik Training and Research Hospital, İzmir Faculty of Medicine, University of Health Sciences, İzmir, Turkey

Sinem Daşlı Faculty of Medicine, Department of Otorhinolaryngology, Derince Research and Training Hospital, Health Sciences University, Kocaeli, Turkey

Baris Demirkol Department of Pulmonology, Basaksehir Cam and Sakura City Hospital, University of Health Sciences, Istanbul, Turkey

Ilter Denizoglu Vocology Centre, Izmir, Turkey

Khassan M. Diab Federal State Budgetary Institution, Scientific and Clinical Center of Otorhinolaryngology of the Medico-Biological Agency, and Ministry of Health, Pirogov Russian National Research Medical University, Moscow, Russia

Ozlem Sengoren Dikis Department of Chest Diseases, School of Medicine, Mugla Sitki Kocman University, Mugla, Turkey

Muhammet Dilber The Dilber Ear, Nose, and Throat Diseases and Surgery Clinic, İstanbul, Turkey

Alper Dilci Division of Otorhinolaryngology, Head and Neck Surgery, Usak University Faculty of Medicine, Usak, Turkey

Murat Doğan Department of Otorhinolaryngology, Private Acıbadem Kayseri Hospital, Kayseri, Turkey

Yusuf Dundar Department of Otolaryngology—Head and Neck Surgery, Health Sciences Center, Texas Tech University, Lubbock, TX, USA

Sena Genç Elden Department of Otorhinolaryngology, Pamukova State Hospital, Pamukova, Sakarya, Turkey

Duygu Erdem Department of Otorhinolaryngology, Medical School, Zonguldak Bülent Ecevit University, Zonguldak, Turkey

Tuba Erdoğan Division of Immunology and Allergy, Department of Internal Medicine, Baskent University School of Medicine, Ankara, Turkey

Dilek Eroğlu Department of Foreign Languages, School of Foreign Languages, Anadolu University, Eskisehir, Turkey

Erhan Eroğlu Faculty of Communication Sciences, Communication Design and Management Department, Anadolu University, Eskisehir, Turkey

Başat Fethallah Department of Otorhinolaryngology, Samsun Gazi State Hospital, Samsun, Turkey

Cem Fıçıcıoğlu Acıbadem Health Group, Graduate School of Health Sciences, Acıbadem Mehmet Ali Aydınlar University, İstanbul, Turkey

Gülden Genç Faculty of Medicine, Department of Radiology, Derince Research and Training Hospital, Health Sciences University, Kocaeli, Turkey

Sebahat Genç Medical Faculty, Department of Pulmonology, Muğla Sıtkı Koçman University, Muğla, Turkey

Selahattin Genç Department of Otorhinolaryngology, Health Sciences University, Faculty of Medicine, Derince Training and Research Hospital, Kocaeli, Turkey

Samet Genez Faculty of Medicine, Department of Radiology, Derince Research and Training Hospital, Health Sciences University, Kocaeli, Turkey

Klara Van Gool Department of Otorhinolaryngology, Head & Neck Surgery, University Hospital Antwerp, Antwerp, Belgium

Aylin Gül Department of Otorihinolaryngology, Medical Park Gaziantep Hospital, Gaziantep, Turkey

Emrah Gülmez Department of Otorihinolaryngology, Fethi Sekin City Hospital, Health Sciences University, Elazığ, Turkey

Şule Gül Ministry of Health, Yedikule Chest Diseases and Thoracic Surgery Training and Research Hospital, Istanbul, Turkey

Ramazan Gündoğdu Department of Otorhinolaryngology, Derince Training and Research Hospital, Faculty of Medicine, Health Sciences University, Kocaeli, Turkey

Alp Gurbet Faculty of Medicine, Department of Anesthesiology and Reanimation, Uludağ University, Bursa, Turkey

Hande Gurbuz Faculty of Medicine, Department of Anaesthesiology and Reanimation, Bursa Yuksek Ihtisas Research and Training Hospital, Health Sciences University, Bursa, Turkey

Faculty of Medicine, Department of Anatomy, Kocaeli University, İzmit, Turkey

Özer Erdem Gür Department of Otorhinolaryngology, Antalya Training and Research Hospital, Antalya, Turkey

Mehmet Güven Department of Otorhinolaryngology, Sakarya University Faculty of Medicine, Serdivan, Sakarya, Turkey

Sheng-Po Hao Department of Otorhinolaryngology, Shin Kong Wu Ho-Su Memorial Hospital and Fu Jen Catholic University, Taipei, Taiwan

İbrahim Hıra Department of Otorhinolaryngology, Ankara Şereflikoçhisar State Hospital, Ankara, Turkey

Ömer Hızlı Department of Otolaryngology—Head and Neck Surgery, Giresun Research and Training Hospital, Giresun, Turkey

Leman İnanç Faculty of Medicine, Department of Psychiatry, İzmir Bakırçay University, İzmir, Turkey

Sefa İnce Department of Gynaecology and Obstetrics, Erzurum Regional Training and Research Hospital, Erzurum, Turkey

Kamil Janeczek Department of Pulmonary Diseases and Children Rheumatology, Medical University of Lublin, Lublin, Poland

Ljiljana Jovancevic Faculty of Medicine, Department of Otorhinolaryngology, Head and Neck Surgery, Clinical Centre of Vojvodina, University of Novi Sad, Novi Sad, Serbia

Yunus Kantekin Department of Otorhinolaryngology, Kayseri City Hospital, Kayseri, Turkey

Abdullah Karataş Faculty of Medicine, Department of Otorhinolaryngology, İstanbul Haseki Research and Training Hospital, Health Sciences University, İstanbul, Turkey

Sergei Karpischenko Department of Otorhinolaryngology, The First Pavlov State Medical University of Saint Petersburg, Saint Petersburg, Russia

Ulugbek Khasanov Department of Otorhinolaryngology and Stomatology, Tashkent Medical Academy, Tashkent, Uzbekistan

Saffet Kılıçaslan Department of Otorhinolaryngology, Düzce Ataturk State Hospital, Düzce, Turkey

Rahmi Kılıç Faculty of Medicine, Department of Otolaryngology—Head and Neck Surgery, Ankara Research and Training Hospital, Health Sciences University, Ankara, Turkey

Vildan Kılıç Yılmaz Faculty of Medicine, Department of Anesthesiology and Reanimation (Algology), Derince Research and Training Hospital, Health Sciences University, Kocaeli, Turkey

Derya Kocakaya Medical Faculty, Department of Pulmonology, Marmara University, İstanbul, Turkey

Iordanis Konstantinidis Academic Medical Faculty, Second Academic Department of Otorhinolaryngology, Aristotle University of Thessaloniki, Thessaloníki, Greece

Gabriela Kopacheva-Barsova Faculty of Medicine, Cyril and Methodius University of Skopje, Skopje, Republic of Macedonia

Hakan Korkmaz Department of Otolaryngology Head and Neck Surgery, Dışkapı Yıldırım Beyazıt Training and Research Hospital, University of Health Sciences Turkey, Ankara, Turkey

Erdem Köroğlu Faculty of Medicine, Department of Otorhinolaryngology, Derince Training and Research Hospital, Health Sciences University, Kocaeli, Turkey

Hüseyin Köseoğlu Faculty of Medicine, Department of Gastroenterology, Hitit University, Çorum, Turkey

Gözde Orhan Kubat Faculty of Medicine, Department of Otorhinolaryngology, Alaattin Keykubat University, Alanya, Turkey

Nurcan Yurtsever Kum Department of Otorhinolaryngology, Ankara City Hospital, Ankara, Turkey

Yücel Kurt Section of Otorhinolaryngology, Ministry of Health, Finike State Hospital, Finike, Antalya, Turkey

Andrey Lopatin Policlinic №1, Medical Department, Business Administration of the President of Russian Federation, Moscow, Russia

Annina Lyly Skin and Allergy Hospital, Helsinki University Hospital, Inflammation Centre, University of Helsinki, Helsinki, Finland

Department of Otorhinolaryngology-Head and Neck Surgery, Helsinki University Hospital, University of Helsinki, Helsinki, Finland

Felicia Manole Faculty of Medicine and Pharmacy, Department of Otorhinolaryngology, University of Oradea, Oradea, Bihor, Romania

Masaany Binti Mansor Department of Otolaryngology—Head and Neck Surgery, Universiti Teknologi MARA Selangor Branch, Sungai Buloh Campus, Sungai Buloh, Selangor, Malaysia

Fevzi Meşe Department of Otorhynolaryngology, Private Batman World Hospital, Batman, Turkey

Mario Milkov Faculty of Medicine, Department of Otorhinolaryngology, Varna University, Varna, Bulgaria

Ugur Muşabak Division of Immunology and Allergy, Department of Internal Medicine, Baskent University School of Medicine, Ankara, Turkey

Hesham Negm Faculty of Medicine, Department of Otorhinolaryngology, Cairo University, Cairo, Egypt

Pamela Nguyen Department of Radiology, Irving Medical Center, Columbia University, New York, NY, USA

Tam Nguyen Department of Otolaryngology—Head and Neck Surgery, Health Sciences Center, Texas Tech University, Lubbock, TX, USA

Marcel Noujeim American Board of Oral and Maxillofacial Radiology, Advanced Imaging Diagnostics, San Antonio, TX, USA

Fatma Ceyda Akın Öçal Department of Otorhinolaryngology, Gülhane Training and Research Hospital, University of Health Sciences, Ankara, Turkey

Ramazan Öçal Faculty of Medicine, Department of Otolaryngology, Head and Neck Surgery, Ankara Research and Training Hospital, Health Sciences University, Ankara, Turkey

Sabri Berkem Ökten Acıbadem Health Group, İstanbul, Turkey

Fatih Öner Otorhinolaryngology Section, Erzurum Regional Training and Research Hospital, Erzurum, Turkey

Talih Özdaş Faculty of Medicine, Department of Otorihinolaryngology, Adana City Training and Research Hospital, Health Sciences University, Adana, Turkey

Fatih Özdoğan Faculty of Medicine, Department of Otorhinolaryngology, Derince Training and Research Hospital, Health Sciences University, Ankara, Turkey

Berna Özel Private Dental Center, Trabzon, Turkey

Halil Erdem Özel Department of Otorhinolaryngology, Derince Training and Research Hospital, Faculty of Medicine, Health Sciences University, Kocaeli, Turkey

Mehmet Birol Özel Faculty of Dentistry, Department of Orthodontics, Kocaeli University, Kocaeli, Turkey

Selcan Arslan Özel Derince Training and Research Hospital Clinical Microbiology and Infectious Diseases Department Derince, Derince, Kocaeli, Turkey

Gül Soylu Özler Faculty of Medicine, Department of Otorhinolaryngology, Mustafa Kemal University, Antakya, Turkey

Atakan Özturan Department of Otorhynolaryngology, Eskisehir City Hospital, Eskisehir, Turkey

Murat Öztürk Faculty of Medicine, Department of Otorhinolaryngology, Kocaeli University, Kocaeli, Turkey

Nilüfer Aylin Acet Öztürk Medical Faculty, Department of Pulmonology, Uludağ University, Bursa, Turkey

Desiderio Passali Department of Medical, Surgical and Neuroscience Sciences, and Department of Otorhinolaryngology, Univerity of Siena, Siena, Italy

Francesco Maria Passali Department of Clinical Sciences and Translational Medicine, University Tor Vergata, Rome, Italy

Giulio Cesare Passali Department of Otorhinolaryngology, Catholic University of Sacred Heart, Rome, Italy

Emmanuel P. Prokopakis Department of Otorhinolaryngology, University of Crete School of Medicine, Heraklio, Crete, Greece

Marwan Al Qunaee Division of Otolaryngology, Head and Neck Surgery, Saint Paul's Sinus Center, University of British Columbia, Vancouver, BC, Canada

William Reisacher, MD Department of Otolaryngology—Head and Neck Surgery, Weill Cornell Medical College/New York-Presbyterian Hospital, New York, NY, USA

Ali Seyed Resuli Faculty of Medicine, Department of Otorhinolaryngology, İstanbul Yeni Yüzyıl University, İstanbul, Turkey

Chae-Seo Rhee Department of Otorhinolaryngology, Head and Neck Surgery, College of Medicine, Seoul National University, Seoul, South Korea

Michael Rudenko Section of Pediatric Allergy and Immunology, The London Allergy and Immunology Centre, London, UK

Bayram Şahin Department of Otorhinolaryngology, Head and Neck Surgery, Derince Training and Research Hospital, Kocaeli Health Sciences University, Kocaeli, Turkey

Caner Şahin Faculty of Medicine, Department of Otorhinolaryngology, Alaattin Keykubat University, Alanya, Turkey

Özlem Naciye Şahin Faculty of Medicine, Department of Pediatrics, Acıbadem Mehmet Ali Aydınlar University, İstanbul, Turkey

Öner Sakallıoğlu Department of Otorihinolaryngology, Fethi Sekin City Hospital, Health Sciences University, Elazığ, Turkey

Mustafa Salış Department of General Surgery, Eskisehir Osmangazi University, Eskisehir, Turkey

Suela Sallavaci Department of Otorhinolaryngology, University Hospital Centre "Mother Teresa", Tirana, Albania

Nergis Salman Department of Otorhinolaryngology, Private Saygı Hospital, İstanbul, Turkey

K. Tolga Saracoglu Faculty of Medicine, Department of Anaesthesiology and Reanimation, Lütfi Kırdar Kartal Research and Training Hospital, Health Sciences University, İstanbul, Turkey

Codrut Sarafoleanu ENT&HNS Department, Sfanta Maria Clinical Hospital, University of Medicine and Pharmacy "Carol Davila", Bucharest, Romania

Alper Sarı Faculty of Medicine, Department of Internal Medicine, Afyon University of Health Sciences, Afyon, Turkey

Tuğba Sarı Medical Faculty, Infectious Diseases and Clinical Microbiology Department, Pamukkale University, Denizli, Turkey

Glenis Scadding Consultant Allergist & Rhinologist, RNENT Hospital, University College Hospital, London, UK

Bert Schmelzer Ziekenhuis Netwerk Antwerpen (ZNA), Section of Otorhinolaryngology, Head and Neck Surgery, Antwerpen, Belgium

Umut Seki Faculty of Dentistry, Department of Oral and Maxillofacial Radiology, Kocaeli University, Kocaeli, Turkey

Adin Selçuk Faculty of Medicine, Department of Otorhinolaryngology, Medical Park Göztepe Hospital, Bahçeşehir University, Istanbul, Turkey

Omer Tarik Selcuk Faculty of Medicine, Department of Otolaryngology—Head and Neck Surgery, Antalya Research and Training Hospital, Health Sciences University, Antalya, Turkey

Ümit Başar Semiz Faculty of Humanities and Social Sciences, Department of Psychiatry, İstanbul Sabahattin Zaim University, Istanbul, Turkey

Rezarta Taga Senirli Faculty of Medicine, Department of Otolaryngology—Head and Neck Surgery, Antalya Research and Training Hospital, Health Sciences University, Antalya, Turkey

Sultan Şevik Eliçora Department of Otorhinolaryngology, Medical School, Zonguldak Bülent Ecevit University, Zonguldak, Turkey

Mesut Sezikli Faculty of Medicine, Department of Gastroenterology, Hitit University, Çorum, Turkey

Tania Sih LIM—Laboratory of Medical Investigations, ISOM (International Society of Otitis Media), Medical School, University of São Paulo (FMUSP), São Paulo, Brazil

E. Alper Sinanoglu Faculty of Dentistry, Department of Oral and Maxillofacial Radiology, Kocaeli University, Kocaeli, Turkey

Bilal Sizer Department of Otorihinolaryngology, Istanbul Arel University Faculty of Medicine, Istanbul, Turkey

Szymon Skoczyński Faculty of Medical Sciences in Katowice, Department of Pneumonology, Medical University of Silesia, Katowice, Poland

Gordon Soo Department of Otorhinolaryngology, Head and Neck Surgery, The Chinese University of Hong Kong, Hong Kong Special Administrative Region, Hong Kong, China

Harun Soyalıç Faculty of Medicine, Department of Otorhinolaryngology, Head and Neck Surgery, Ahi Evran University, Kırşehir, Turkey

Michael B. Soyka Department of Otorhinolaryngology, Head and Neck Surgery, University Hospital and University of Zurich, Zurich, Switzerland

Slobodan Spremo Faculty of Medicine, Department for Otorhinolaryngology, University Clinic Center Banja Luka, University of Banja Luka, Banja Luka, Bosnia and Herzegovina

Georg Mathias Sprinzl Department of Otorhinolaryngology, Head and Neck Surgery, University Clinic St. Poelten, St. Poelten, Austria

Özge Oral Tapan Medical Faculty, Department of Pulmonology, Muğla Sıtkı Koçman University, Muğla, Turkey

Emel Çadallı Tatar Otolaryngology Department, Dışkapı Yıldırım Beyazıt Research and Training Hospital, University of Health Sciences, Ankara, Turkey

Ömer Can Topaloğlu Department of Endocrinology, Derince Training and Research Hospital, Kocaeli Health Sciences University, Kocaeli, Turkey

Hulya Topcu Faculty of Medicine, Department of Anaesthesiology and Reanimation, Erol Olçok Research and Training Hospital, Hitit University, Çorum, Turkey

Sanna Toppila-Salmi Skin and Allergy Hospital, University of Helsinki and Helsinki University Hospital, Helsinki, Finland

Serdar Ferit Toprak Medical Faculty, Otorhinolaryngology Department, Dicle University, Diyarbakır, Turkey

Vedat Topsakal Department of Otorhinolaryngology, Head and Neck Surgery, Vrije Universiteit Brussel (VUB), University Hospital UZ Brussel, Brussels Health Campus, Brussels, Belgium

Gökhan Toptaş Otolaryngology Department, Dışkapı Yıldırım Beyazıt Research and Training Hospital, University of Health Sciences, Ankara, Turkey

Elvan Evrim Ünsal Tuna Faculty of Medicine, Department of Otorhinolaryngology, Ankara City Training and Research Hospital, Health Sciences University, Ankara, Turkey

Onur Tunca Faculty of Medicine, Department of Internal Medicine, Afyon University of Health Sciences, Afyon, Turkey

Sevinc Sarinc Ulasli Department of Chest Diseases, School of Medicine, Hacettepe University, Ankara, Turkey

Gaye Ulubay Faculty of Medicine, Department of Chest Diseases, Baskent University, Ankara, Turkey

Mehmet Atilla Uysal Ministry of Health, Yedikule Chest Diseases and Thoracic Surgery Training and Research Hospital, Istanbul, Turkey

Esra Uzaslan Medical Faculty, Department of Pulmonology, Uludağ University, Bursa, Turkey

Rahul Varman Department of Otolaryngology-Head and Neck Surgery, Health Sciences Center, Texas Tech University, Lubbock, TX, USA

Elif Hilal Vural Faculty of Medicine, Department of Medical Pharmacology, Lokman Hekim University, Ankara, Turkey

Ismail Mert Vural Gülhane Pharmacy Faculty, Department of Pharmacology, Health Sciences University, Ankara, Turkey

Volker Wenzel Department of Anaesthesiology, Klinikum Friedrichshafen, Intensive Care Medicine, Emergency Medicine and Pain Therapy, Bodensee Campus Medicine, Friedrichshafen, Germany

Necdet Fatih Yaşar Department of General Surgery, Eskisehir Osmangazi University, Eskisehir, Turkey

Dilara Tütüncü Yavuz Department of Otorhinolaryngology, Istanbul Sisli Hamidiye Etfal Training and Research Hospital, Istanbul, Turkey

Atılay Yaylacı Faculty of Medicine, Department of Otorhinolaryngology, Kocaeli University, Kocaeli, Turkey

Gökçe Aksoy Yıldırım Department of Otorhinolaryngology, Bozyaka Training and Research Hospital, University of Health Sciences, Izmir, Turkey

Fusun Yıldız Department of Pulmonology, Cyprus International University, Nicosia, Cyprus

Yavuz Fuat Yılmaz Department of Otorhinolaryngology, Gülhane Training and Research Hospital, University of Health Sciences, Ankara, Turkey

Nevreste Didem Sonbay Yılmaz Department of Otorhinolaryngology, Antalya Training and Research Hospital, Antalya, Turkey

Zeynep Çukurova Yılmaz Faculty of Dentistry, Oral and Maxillofacial Surgery Department, Istanbul Medipol University, Istanbul, Turkey

Arzu Yorgancıoğlu Medical Faculty, Department of Pulmonology, Celal Bayar University, Manisa, Turkey

Physiological Changes During Pregnancy and the Postpartum Period

Maternal Physiology During Pregnancy

Sabri Berkem Ökten and Cem Fıçıcıoğlu

1.1 Introduction

Pregnancy is a "physiologic" period that extends beyond normal physiology. Numerous changes take place from anatomy to biochemistry, psychology to physiology. Knowing these changes is crucial for the right diagnosis and treatment as they can exacerbate an existing disorder, cause a new disorder, or just could be misinterpreted as pathologic. In order to tailor the right approach to pregnant patients, healthcare professionals should know every aspect of the adaptations of this period.

1.2 Hematological Changes

1.2.1 Blood Volume

The blood volume increases during pregnancy in order to provide the necessary elements and nutrients for the fetal and placental growth and to meet the needs of the expanded uterus. It also provides protection against impaired venous blood return related to maternal position (erect and supine positions) during pregnancy and compensation for the postpartum blood loss. Blood volume increases gradually

S. B. Ökten (✉)
Acıbadem Health Group, İstanbul, Turkey
e-mail: berkemokten@gmail.com

C. Fıçıcıoğlu
Acıbadem Health Group, Acıbadem Mehmet Ali Aydınlar University, Graduate School of Health Sciences, İstanbul, Turkey
e-mail: cemficicioglu@gmail.com

© The Author(s), under exclusive license to Springer Nature Switzerland AG 2022
C. Cingi et al. (eds.), *ENT Diseases: Diagnosis and Treatment during Pregnancy and Lactation*, https://doi.org/10.1007/978-3-031-05303-0_1

throughout pregnancy. It shows an increase of about 15% in the first trimester and then with the most rapid increase at mid-trimester especially until 32–34 weeks of gestation with an average of 40–45% above nonpregnant state. Then, it shows a slight increase and plateau at the last weeks of gestation [1, 2].

The spleen enlarges in size up to 50% throughout pregnancy [3]. The certain reason of this splenomegaly is unknown, yet it might be due to the increase in blood volume and hemodynamic changes.

1.2.2 Red Blood Cells

The expansion in the blood volume involves an increase in plasma volume along with red cell and white cell volumes. However, red cell volume shows relatively less increase (15–20%) than plasma volume (40–50%) which causes a dilutional anemia known as the "physiological anemia of pregnancy" [4]. This decrease in the blood viscosity provides a better placental perfusion while reducing the cardiac work [5].

During pregnancy, due to a higher metabolic oxygen requirement, moderate bone marrow erythroid hyperplasia develops, and reticulocyte count increases as a result of elevated maternal plasma erythropoietin level. Erythrocyte volume rises about 450 mL at term compared to nonpregnant state [6].

1.2.3 Iron Supplementation

At term, the average hemoglobin concentration is 12.5 g/dL. Hemoglobin level below 11 g/dL indicates maternal anemia, and its main reason is iron deficiency, not hypervolemia. The prevalence of anemia among pregnant women is as high as 41.8% [7] worldwide, whereas with the adequate iron supplementation, this rate can be reduced to 6% [8].

As the fetus and placenta grow and the maternal circulating erythrocyte volume increases, the need of iron supplementation becomes more crucial especially at the second half of pregnancy. Total iron amount required throughout pregnancy is about 1000 mg. During this period, approximately 300 mg iron is needed for feto-placental unit and 500 mg for expanded maternal red blood cell mass, whereas 200 mg of iron is excreted from the body mostly through the gastrointestinal tract. Since each erythrocyte contains 1.1 mg of iron, in order to ensure the required erythrocyte volume expansion (450 mL during pregnancy as mentioned before), 6–7 mg daily iron intake is needed especially at the second half of the pregnancy [9]. It's usually hard to obtain this amount of iron from diet, and iron supplementation is needed to keep hemoglobin and hematocrit levels balanced with the increasing plasma volume. Even in non-anemic pregnant women, daily oral 30–60 mg iron and additional 400 mcg folic acid supplementation are recommended to support increased red blood cell production and prevent maternal anemia [10].

1.2.4 Immunological Changes

Immunologic alterations play a crucial role to maintain a healthy pregnancy. A transplanted organ would be rejected without powerful immune-suppressive agents, whereas a semi-allogeneic fetus that carries also paternal antigens is protected from an attack by maternal immune response. This tolerative relationship at maternal-fetal site still has a lot of questions to answer.

Yet, there is a special adaptation at this particular site. Normally, every cell of the body expresses major histocompatibility complex (MHC) molecule that labels the cell as an acquaintance to the own immune system. As the immune system recognizes its own cells, it doesn't attack them. MHC class Ia composes most of these molecules in the body, and they are usually specific to the individual, not compatible between unrelated individuals. The adaptation takes place at maternal-fetal site during pregnancy as the trophoblast cells express a special MHC called "human leukocyte antigen (HLA) class Ib." What makes it special is that it is a "compatible for all" molecule that keeps the maternal natural killer cells located in the decidua dormant as it provides a recognition and so keeps the "foreign" fetus safe from a host attack [11].

T-helper (TH) 1-mediated immunity is suppressed during pregnancy along with T-cytotoxic (TC) 1 cells which lead to a decrease in the secretions of interleukin (IL)-2, interferon-α, and tumor necrosis factor (TNF) -β, whereas TH 2 and TC 2 cells are upregulated and cause an increase in the secretions of IL-4, IL-6, IL-10, and IL-13. This mechanism is thought to be an important factor for maintenance of the pregnancy as imbalance at TH-1/TH-2 ratio is highly related with recurrent spontaneous abortions [12].

Some cell-mediated autoimmune diseases related to TH-1 cytokines such as rheumatoid arthritis and Hashimoto thyroiditis show remission due to suppression of TH-1 cells during pregnancy, whereas the upregulation of TH-2 cytokines during pregnancy may flare the symptoms of autoimmune diseases related with humoral immunity such as systemic lupus erythematosus [13].

1.2.5 White Blood Cells and Inflammatory Markers

Leukocyte count shows an increase during pregnancy with the upper values about 15,000/μL. Leukocytosis during pregnancy is considered to be a result of physiologic stress caused by pregnant state [14]. During labor and the postpartum period, levels can rise up to 25,000/μL [15].

During first and second trimesters, the lymphocyte count decreases and then shows an increase at the third trimester [16]. The monocyte/lymphocyte ratio increases, while eosinophil and basophil counts do not change significantly during pregnancy [17].

During pregnancy, many tests related to inflammation are not reliable. C-reactive protein, leukocyte alkaline phosphatase, erythrocyte sedimentation rate (ESR), and complement factor C3 and C4 levels increase in pregnant women compared to nonpregnant state [18–21]. Elevated plasma globulins and fibrinogen levels are responsible for the increase in ESR. Procalcitonin, a marker which increases during bacterial infections or nonspecific inflammatory diseases, also shows an increase at the last trimester and a few days after delivery [22].

1.2.6 Coagulation and Fibrinolysis

Pregnancy is a state in which coagulation and fibrinolysis are amplified yet hemostasis still remains balanced [23].

As the platelet activity and consumption rise during pregnancy, a relatively hypercoagulable state occurs [24]. A slight decline at platelet count may be observed mostly due to increased consumption of platelets along with gestational hemodilution [25]. Gestational thrombocytopenia refers to platelet count between 70,000 and 150,000/mm^3 without a history of prepregnancy thrombocytopenia. This mild and asymptomatic condition occurs in about 8% of all pregnancies and resolves mostly by the first month after delivery [26].

Fibrinogen and coagulation factors II, VII, VIII, X, and XII increase, while factors XI and XIII decrease during pregnancy [27]. Fibrinogen levels nearly double throughout the pregnancy (300 mg/dL prepregnancy levels may rise up to 600 mg/dL at term) with an average of 450 mg/dL at term [28].

Other factors that contribute to relatively hypercoagulable state by increased levels during pregnancy are von Willebrand factor, plasminogen activator inhibitor types 1 and 2 (PAI-1 and PAI-2), and thrombin cleavage products [29, 30]. The excess fibrin is removed by fibrinolytic system, and tissue plasminogen activator (tPA) takes place in this system by converting plasminogen into plasmin which in turn degrades fibrin and causes D-dimer formation. Especially in the third trimester of pregnancy, it should be kept in mind that D-dimer concentration increases as its diagnostic value decreases for conditions like venous thromboembolism (VTE) [31].

Against the procoagulant effects of factors Va and VIIIa, activated protein C together with protein S and factor V plays a neutralizing anticoagulant role. An increasing resistance develops against activated protein C throughout pregnancy which is related to a decrease in protein S levels and an increase in factor VIII concentrations [32]. Antithrombin levels also decrease about 13% from midpregnancy until term [33].

As a result, even though both systems—coagulation and fibrinolysis—show increase during pregnancy, it's a relatively more hypercoagulable period. Women at this period are 4–5 times more likely to develop VTE or pulmonary embolism than women who are not pregnant [34].

1.3 Cardiovascular System Changes

Cardiovascular and hemodynamic changes during pregnancy have a crucial role in meeting the needs of the growing fetus but at the same time in maintaining the integrity of maternal cardiovascular functions.

As the uterus grows throughout the pregnancy, it elevates the diaphragm and so pushes the heart to left-upward position while causing the heart to rotate on its long axis. Along with increased plasma volume, the heart shows enlargement in myocardial mass and intracardiac volume. At term, left ventricle mass expands 18–22% to ensure the adequate blood supply to mother and fetus [35]. The reason of this expansion is the increased preload due to increased plasma volume between gestational weeks 10 and 20.

One of the major changes during pregnancy is the 30–40% increase in cardiac output. This increase can even be 20% more in multifetal pregnancies compared to singletons [36]. On 24th week of gestation, cardiac output reaches its maximum level [37]. This increase is associated with increased stroke volume and heart rate along with reduced systemic vascular resistance. Heart rate shows 10–15 beats/min increase at term which starts by the second trimester [38]. Uterine size and maternal position also affect cardiac output. Especially at the further weeks of gestation, maternal supine position can reduce the cardiac filling by causing aortocaval compression which directly affects cardiac function. Supine hypotensive syndrome develops in approximately 10% of term pregnancies and is characterized by hypotension, bradycardia, and syncope [39]. In the supine position, the pressure on the inferior vena cava along with femoral and pelvic veins increases which in turn slows down the circulation and causes frequently seen edema which may predispose the development of varicose veins in the legs and vulva and hemorrhoids and even deep-vein thrombosis. As the mother changes her supine position to lateral recumbent position (laying to her side), elevated venous pressure returns to normal [40].

During normal pregnancy systemic vascular resistance, systolic, and diastolic blood pressures decrease about 20%, 8%, and 2.0% respectively [41]. Hormones which take a role in blood pressure maintenance with their elevated levels are renin, angiotensin II (AII), prostacyclin (PGI_2), atrial natriuretic peptide (ANP), brain natriuretic peptide (BNP), nitric oxide (NO), estradiol (E2), and progesterone (P).

Sinus tachycardia or benign dysrhythmias, depression at ST segments and flattened T waves, left axis deviation, and left ventricular hypertrophy are among normal electrocardiogram findings of parturient. Systolic murmur of tricuspid valve or mitral regurgitation and presence of third or fourth heart sound are the frequent auscultation findings.

Briefly, cardiovascular and hemodynamic changes during pregnancy include increased cardiac output, heart rate, and stroke volume and decreased systemic and pulmonary vascular resistance and blood pressure.

1.4 Endocrine System Changes

Thyroid gland shows physiological enlargement and an increase in vascularization during pregnancy. The mean thyroid volume increases from 12 to 15 mL throughout gestation [42]. As the human chorionic gonadotropin (HCG) increases during the first trimester, it stimulates the thyroid gland due to its alpha subunit's resemblance with thyroid-stimulating hormone (TSH) [43]. Parallel with this increase in α-HCG, serum TSH decreases during first trimester [44].

High estrogen levels stimulate hepatic synthesis of thyroid-binding globulin (TBG), which in turn causes a rise in total serum thyroxine (T4) and triiodothyronine (T3) levels [45]. Free T3 and T4 levels are controversial during pregnancy. Some studies report no change or even an increase, whereas some report a slight decrease, yet in general, compared to nonpregnant women, free-hormone concentrations tend to be lower at term pregnancy [46, 47]. Interestingly, Glinoer et al. reported that T4 and T3 secretions are not similar for all pregnant women [42].

Iodine need is increased. The increased renal clearance of iodide along with the fetal requirements is responsible for this increase which causes a relative iodine-deficient state. Especially in regions where the iodine intake is low, goiter is commonly observed during pregnancy and may manifest as high TSH and low T4 levels [48].

The pituitary gland enlarges by 136% during pregnancy [49]. Hypertrophy and hyperplasia of lactotroph cells stimulated by high estrogen levels are responsible for this growth [50]. Parallel to this growth, prolactin levels may increase up to more than 200 ng/mL at term [51].

Antidiuretic hormone (vasopressin) level doesn't change during pregnancy.

Somatotrophs are suppressed because of the placental secretion of growth hormone which becomes detectable at sixth week of gestation [52].

Adrenocorticotropic hormone (ACTH), cortisol (both free and total), and urinary free cortisol levels increase throughout gestation reaching to the highest level during labor [53]. Aldosterone level increases during pregnancy as well.

More et al. reported that during pregnancy, all of bone turnover markers increase, and even 12 months after birth they fail to reach baseline levels [54]. Fetal growth and lactation require calcium which is probably provided from the maternal skeleton. After the first trimester, parathyroid hormone plasma concentrations show an increase throughout pregnancy [55]. Calcitonin also favors the fetus as its level decreases during pregnancy [56].

1.5   Metabolic Changes

Throughout the pregnancy, maternal metabolism shows crucial changes in order to meet the needs of the growing fetus and placenta. Compared with the nonpregnant state, metabolic rate increases 20% during pregnancy [57]. The approximate total weight gain in pregnancy is 12 kg [58]. Fetus, placenta, and amniotic fluid comprise about 35% of this weight gain, while the rest is due to expanded blood and extravascular fluid volumes, fat tissues, enlarged breast, and uterine tissues of the mother [59].

1.5.1   Glucose Metabolism

Pregnancy is characterized by hyperinsulinemia, postprandial hyperglycemia, and fasting hypoglycemia. Unlike second and third trimesters, in early pregnancy, insulin secretion and sensitivity increase as the insulin-secreting pancreatic beta cells become hyperplastic. A progressive insulin resistance starts after first trimester with the increase of hormones such as human placental lactogen, placental growth hormone, cortisol, prolactin, and progesterone [60]. This mild physiological diabetogenic state is important to spare the required maternal glucose for the fetal development [61]. Mild fasting hypoglycemia is seen during pregnancy; even basal insulin levels are higher compared to nonpregnant women. Fetal consumption of glucose, increased storage of tissue glycogen, and increased peripheral glucose use are the reasons of fasting hypoglycemia [62]. During pregnancy, maternal glucose is preferentially spared for fetal use even in hypoglycemic state which switches the energy source to lipids instead of glucose. Free fatty acid, triglyceride, and cholesterol levels increase due to lipolysis during fasting state. Due to these alterations, pregnant women are more prone to experience ketonemia if the fasting is prolonged.

In susceptible women who can't meet the needed insulin production, the insulin resistance may progress to gestational diabetes.

1.5.2   Lipid Metabolism

Pregnancy is characterized by maternal hyperlipidemia mostly induced by emerging insulin resistance and high levels of estrogen.

Triglyceride, very low-density lipoprotein (VLDL), low-density lipoprotein (LDL), and high-density lipoprotein (HDL) cholesterol show increased levels compared to nonpregnant state. At term, LDL and HDL cholesterol levels are 50% and 15% higher than nonpregnant state, respectively [63].

First two trimesters of pregnancy form the anabolic phase. During this period, maternal tissue deposits lipids mainly by increased lipid synthesis and food intake [64]. The catabolic phase starts with the third trimester which is characterized with a high adipose tissue lipolytic activity. Triglyceride uptake to adipose tissue from circulation is reduced by the decreased activity of lipoprotein lipase which provides energy for the mother while sparing the glucose for the fetus if needed. LDL cholesterol is critical for placental steroidogenesis, while fatty acids have an important role in organogenesis [65].

1.5.3   Protein Metabolism

As protein is required in development of the fetus, placenta, enlarging uterus, and breasts and expanding maternal blood volume (plasma proteins and hemoglobin), increased intake is needed during pregnancy. Amino acids are actively transported across the placenta to maintain fetal growth. Urinary nitrogen excretion is reduced as this nitrogen retention is important for fetal tissue formation.

1.6   Ear, Nose, and Throat Changes

Physiologic, endocrinologic, and metabolic changes during pregnancy affect every organ system and, thus, the ear, nose, and throat as well. As mentioned before, pregnancy is associated with increased oxygen consumption, expanded blood volume, and increased cardiac output. Especially at the last trimester, with the increased intravascular and extravascular fluid volume and enlarged uterus which makes compression to adjacent organs and vessels, occurrence of boggy mucus membranes and extremity edema can be observed [66].

Estrogen and progesterone levels also increase especially at the last trimester, which affect mucosal surfaces of the nose, gingiva, and larynx. During pregnancy, a relative immunosuppression occurs due to hematologic, immunologic, and hormonal alterations as well, which in turn might lead to reactivation of some latent viral infections [66]. Although the pregnancy-related ear, nose, and throat symptoms are mostly minor and transient, otolaryngologist should be familiar with these symptoms in order to manage and reassure the patient.

1.6.1 Ear Changes

A prospective study conducted with 82 pregnant women reported that the most common auditory complaint was tinnitus (33%) followed by pressure in the ear (24%), hearing reduction (18%), otalgia (5%), and secretion in the ear (2%). In the same study, tinnitus rate was 11% for nonpregnant control group [67].

Due to increased mucosal edema at upper respiratory airway (nasopharynx, larynx), the eustachian tube (ET) may get obstructed which in turn leads to plugged sensation in the ears with muffled sounds and eventually to serous otitis media [66, 68]. Other than obstruction, another reason for ET dysfunction may be patulous tube which is normally related to fat tissue loss around cartilaginous portion of ET due to rapid weight loss [69]. However, during pregnancy it's mostly related with inadequate weight gain especially during the third trimester [70]. Intermittent autophony and roaring sensation are the common symptoms which can be exacerbated with the upright position, exercise, and the use of decongestants. Supine position, high humidity (steam inhalation), and Muller and Valsalva maneuvers alleviate the symptoms [71]. Patulous tube is a transient condition and the symptoms resolve after delivery [72].

Low-frequency sensorineural hearing loss might be observed during pregnancy. Decreased level of hearing increases gradually throughout pregnancy for the frequencies below 500 Hz, whereas there is no significant change for the frequencies above this level. This condition occurs probably due to hormonal changes, yet it never reaches a pathologic level. This clinically not significant hearing loss returns to normal at postpartum period [73]. Sudden hearing loss is uncommon during pregnancy. However, pregnancy-related hypercoagulable state, preeclampsia, and hypertension may cause a microembolus that interrupts the blood supply of the inner ear [66]. Another underlying cause might be virus related. If no etiological factor is found, systemic corticosteroids (category C) can be used during second and third trimesters, if necessary [74].

Pregnancy can also exacerbate the symptoms of already existing Meniere's disease due to fluid retention followed by endolymphatic hydrops. As the serum osmotic pressure decreases during pregnancy, the vertigo attacks may occur more often, which is related to inner ear involvement. Hormonal changes (increase in estrogen and progesterone levels) are another probable reason for vertigo [66]. Conservative treatment is recommended with vestibular suppressants and antiemetics during pregnancy. The combination of pyridoxine (vitamin B6) and dimenhydrinate is a safe option to choose during pregnancy (category B) [75]. Meclizine is also a safe alternative [66]. Diuretics should be avoided because of their hypotensive, hypovolemic, and cardiac output-lowering effects which lead to placental hypoperfusion.

The relationship between pregnancy and otosclerosis is controversial. In patients with already existing otosclerosis, pregnancy seems to be related with deterioration of hearing loss [76]. Estrogen is blamed for the relationship between pregnancy and otosclerosis as it ossifies the oto-spongeotic lesions by stimulating otosclerotic foci [77]. Besides, estrogen receptors were found on otosclerotic cells of which the specific regulatory mechanisms are not well known yet [78]. On the other hand, Lippy et al. found no significant relationship between pregnancy and otosclerosis [79]. Hearing aid can be used during pregnancy, and stapedectomy can be performed after delivery, if needed. Sodium fluoride is contraindicated because of its adverse fetal effects [66].

1.6.2 Nasal Changes

Hyperemia and edema of the nasal mucosa are induced with pregnancy. Many pregnant women experience nasal congestion of which many theories have been proposed to explain the mechanisms underlying for these nasal mucosal changes. Increased estrogen levels are blamed to cause increased vasodilatation and gland secretion through vasoactive intestinal peptide and cholinergic action [80–82]. Another study attributed these changes to nasal epithelial cells' H1 receptor expression increase caused by increased sex hormone levels [83]. However, the evidence supporting these "increased estrogen and/or progesterone levels mediated mucosal changes" assertion is limited [84]. Placental growth factor is believed to be another factor related to nasal mucosal changes during pregnancy as it induces nasal mucosal growth [85, 86]. Increased tissue fluid retention and plasma volume during pregnancy also contribute to nasal congestion [87].

Philpott et al. followed 18 pregnant women from their first trimester until postpartum period and evaluated the changes of nasal airway throughout pregnancy by anterior rhinoscopy, peak inspiratory nasal flow, acoustic rhinometry, anterior rhinomanometry, and mucociliary clearance time measurements and reported that there is no significant decrease in combined intranasal volume during pregnancy, yet there is a decrease in nasal resistance as the gestational age increases [88]. Another study conducted with 85 pregnant women by Demir et al. reported a significant decrease in minimal cross-sectional area at third trimester when compared with first trimester. In the same study, authors observed no significant difference between total nasal resistance and subjective reports of nasal congestion between trimesters and even when compared with nonpregnant controls [89].

Pregnancy rhinitis is defined as nasal congestion that arises during pregnancy and involves at least the last 6 weeks of pregnancy without presence of any known allergic cause or respiratory tract infection and resolves completely within 2 weeks at postpartum period [90]. It may begin at any trimester and involves about 22–39% of all pregnancies [91, 92]. It has been suggested that this condition might be a result of pregnancy-induced sensitization to allergens in women with already existing subclinical allergy. In a study, women with pregnancy rhinitis exhibited increased IgE levels against house dust mites without an increase in allergic symptoms [93]. As this might be a possible reason of pregnancy rhinitis, allergen avoidance is an important preventive step.

Saline nasal spray or nasal irrigation use is a safe and first step intervention for pregnant women with rhinitis symptoms [94]. In mild cases, sodium cromoglycate sprays may also be used safely in every trimester [95]. Glucocorticoid nasal spray use is another safe treatment option of which the safety evidence is mostly gathered from women who used glucocorticoid inhalers (contain higher doses than nasal sprays) for asthma during pregnancy [96]. Two studies that investigated the safety of intranasal glucocorticoid use during pregnancy and gathered data from over 140,000 pregnant women of which 2502 of them were exposed to these drugs during their first trimester reported no increased major congenital malformation nor spontaneous abortion rate [97, 98]. In the study conducted by Berard et al., triamcinolone use during first trimester showed a potential risk on fetal respiratory system (adjusted odds ratio [OR] = 2.71 [95% CI 1.11–6.64]) based on a few number of cases (two of them had abnormalities in the trachea and bronchus, two of them had unspecified congenital malformations of the respiratory tract, one had congenital malformation of the larynx and one had choanal atresia). Although most of the intranasal glucocorticoids show safe profile during pregnancy, budesonide is the only category B classified medication by the US Food and Drug Administration (FDA) among them. In a randomized controlled trial, Ellegard et al. reported that fluticasone showed no additional benefit compared with placebo in the treatment of pregnancy rhinitis [99].

Among oral antihistamines, second-generation agents are more preferable since they have less cholinergic side effects and are less sedative. Chlorpheniramine can be the drug of choice among first-generation antihistamines as it has been used for a long time and has shown no adverse effect when used during pregnancy [100]. Loratadine and cetirizine (both 10 mg once daily) may be used safely if needed since both have reassuring data in the literature regarding their use during pregnancy and both are pregnancy category B medications [101, 102].

Smell disturbance is also studied in pregnant women, yet the scientific evidence is inconclusive regarding this topic. Gilbert and Wysocki analyzed data gathered from 13,610 pregnant women who participated in National Geographic Smell Survey and reported an increased smell intensity without hyperacuity during pregnancy [103]. In another study, the University of Pennsylvania Smell Identification Test was performed to 100 nonsmoking women in 3 different groups: pregnant, postpartum, and women with no pregnancy history. Pregnant group showed higher self-rated olfactory sensitivity, yet the objective assessment showed no difference from nonpregnant group, and the study concluded that the effect of pregnancy on olfaction is small and inconsistent [104].

Epistaxis is also common during gestation and observed approximately in 20% of pregnant women [105]. It's most probably due to increased vascularity and vascular engorgement in the nasal mucosa caused by hormonal changes. Conservative approach is the first step in acute epistaxis treatment, while silver nitrate cautery may be used in chronic or recurrent epistaxis [106]. A rare disorder, pyogenic granuloma which is mostly observed in the oral cavity, may sometimes occur in nasal mucosa during pregnancy. It is believed to occur due to nasal mucosal glandular hyperplasia induced by increased sex hormones [107]. It's mostly asymptomatic and resolves after delivery. Although it's rare, it should be kept in mind in massive nose bleedings as it may require surgical excision [108].

1.6.3 Throat Changes

Especially during the third trimester, dysphonia may occur due to nasal obstruction, altered breathing support, and laryngopharyngeal reflux (LPR). The prevalence of vocal fatigue increases at term with a decrease in the maximum phonation time compared to immediate postpartum period [109]. Oral and laryngeal dryness may occur due to continuous mouth breathing caused by pregnancy rhinitis, as the humidifying effect of nasal breathing would be bypassed [110]. Another reason of dysphonia during pregnancy is LPR as an extension of gastroesophageal reflux (GER) which is reported in up to 80% of pregnancies [111]. The relaxative effects of progesterone on esophageal sphincter along with displacement of the stomach and esophageal sphincter by the compressive effect of gradually enlarging uterus are responsible for GER during pregnancy [112]. Along with dysphonia, throat clearing, globus, and dysphagia may occur due to LPR during gestation [113]. Losing excess weight, eating smaller meals, elevating the head of the bed, avoiding lying down just after a meal, and avoidance of products that trigger reflux like fatty and fried foods, onion, spices, caffeine, alcohol, and tobacco are among some of the lifestyle changes and dietary modifications to prevent GER. In severe cases when the symptoms cannot be relieved despite these conservative precautions, proton pump inhibitors (PPI), H2 antagonists, and liquid alginate may be used as most studies and meta-analysis regarding the use of these drugs during pregnancy showed no increased risk for major congenital birth defects, spontaneous abortions, or preterm delivery [114–116].

Laryngopathia gravidarum is a highly rare disorder which shows resemblance with angioedema of the larynx. Macroscopically, patchy and localized edema is observed on the larynx and epiglottis, whereas microscopical evaluation exhibits edematous submucosa with normal surface epithelium and mucus glands [117]. It may cause hoarseness, cough, dysphonia, and nonfebrile sore throat. The pathogenesis is still not well known, yet the most probable reason seems to be the effect of the hormonal change on laryngeal mucosa during pregnancy, as the symptoms rapidly resolve at postpartum period.

1.7 Respiratory System Changes

As the uterus grows throughout the pregnancy, it elevates the diaphragm about 4 cm [118]. Chest circumference shows an increase of about 6 cm, whereas subcostal angle widens from 68.5° to 103.5°, while the transverse diameter of the thorax increases about 2 cm [119]. Also, the increasing levels of relaxin and progesterone hormones during pregnancy cause relaxation of the ligaments connecting the sternum to the ribs [120]. Despite all these changes, residual lung volume decreases by the 4 cm elevation of the diaphragm, yet by their compensation, no significant reduction (unchanged or decreases only by <5%) occurs in total lung capacity (TLC). Total pulmonary resistance decreases whereas airway conductance increases probably due to progesterone. Lung compliance is unchanged during pregnancy [118].

Pulmonary function alterations are as below.

Vital capacity is unchanged, which is the maximum volume expired after inspiration with a maximal capacity [118].

The functional residual capacity (FRC) is the total of residual volume (RV) and expiratory reserve volume (ERV). As the uterus grows throughout the pregnancy, due to diaphragmatic elevation it causes, RV and ERV both decrease, therefore causing a reduction in FRC about 10–25%. Residual volume is the remaining volume after a maximal expiration and shows a reduction of about 20–25% which corresponds to 200–400 mL during pregnancy. ERV is decreased about 15–20% (200–300 mL) which is the remaining volume that can be forcefully expired from the lungs after tidal end-expiratory level (expiration point during normal breathing) [118].

Total lung capacity (TLC) consists of FRC, and inspiratory capacity (IC) is mostly unchanged or decreased about just 5% at term because of the compensatory mechanisms mentioned above. IC increases about 5–10% (200–350 mL) which is the maximum volume that can be inhaled from FRC [118].

Forced vital capacity (FVC) is the volume forcibly exhaled after a full inspiration, in other words the remaining volume when RV is subtracted from TLC. Forced expiratory volume measured with spirometry at the first second of forceful expiration after a full inspiration (FEV1) along with FVC is used as lung function test. FVC, FEV1, FEV1/FVC, and peak expiratory flow rate (PEFR) mostly remain unchanged during pregnancy, which means pregnancy doesn't cause abnormal spirometry parameters [121].

Tidal volume shows 30–50% (500–700 mL) increase during pregnancy. Respiratory rate also increases about 1–2 breaths/min. Both these elevations cause a 20–50% (7.5–10.5 L/min) increase in resting minute ventilation (the amount of gas exchange through the lungs in 1 min) [122]. Compensated respiratory alkalosis and low expiratory reserve volume are among the reasons of this increased maternal respiratory drive (increased minute ventilation) [123]. Also, increased progesterone concentrations during pregnancy show a stimulatory effect on respiration [124].

Oxygen consumption increases by 20% in singletons, whereas it increases about 30% in multifetal pregnancies [125]. Total hemoglobin mass and the total oxygen-carrying capacity increase during pregnancy, which in turn cause diminished maternal arteriovenous oxygen difference.

Especially after 30th week of gestation, a dyspnea-like feeling arises and occurs in about 60–70% of pregnant women [126]. This common state of "awareness of a desire to breath" is a physiological dyspnea, paradoxically caused by lower levels of $PaCO_2$. Along with the increased tidal volume, progesterone plays an important role where it acts centrally and increases the sensitivity of the chemoreflex response to CO_2 by lowering down its threshold [127].

As a result of respiratory adaptations during pregnancy, PaO_2 increases while $PaCO_2$ decreases in the maternal circulation [128]. This state facilitates the oxygen transfer from mother to fetus and likewise carbon dioxide transfer from fetus to mother. This "lower $PaCO_2$" state of maternal circulation causes respiratory alkalosis. To compensate the maternal pH change caused by respiratory alkalosis, bicarbonate excretion increases during pregnancy [129]. Women with insulin-dependent diabetes show increased susceptibility to diabetic ketoacidosis complications during their pregnancies since the buffering capacity decreases along with this pregnancy-related lowered bicarbonate levels (18–21 mmol/L) [130]. Another advantage of this "lower levels of bicarbonate" is that it reduces the maternal hemoglobin affinity to oxygen (due to maternal oxygen dissociation curve shift to the right), thus facilitating the release of O_2 from maternal hemoglobin to the fetus [131].

1.8 Gastrointestinal System Changes

Anatomic and hormonal changes during pregnancy have broad effects on the gastrointestinal system (GIS) as well. Most common GIS-related problems are nausea, vomiting, and heartburn. Nausea and vomiting mostly complicate the early weeks of gestation (peak between 8 and 12 gestational weeks) with an incidence of about 66% and decline gradually thereafter [132]. The exact pathophysiology of nausea and vomiting is still not well understood, but the hormonal changes such as increasing levels of human chorionic gonadotropin, estrogen, and progesterone during pregnancy are considered to be responsible [133].

1.8.1 Oral Cavity

Elevated estrogen and progesterone levels during pregnancy increase vascular permeability while decreasing immune resistance which in turn predispose to gingival hyperplasia and gingivitis [134]. The increasing salivary estrogen level contributes to gingivitis also by causing a proliferative and desquamative effect on oral mucosa that provides a suitable environment for the bacterial growth [135]. Pregnant women should be more cautious about their oral hygiene to reduce the effects of pregnancy-mediated oral inflammatory changes and prevent caries. Increased gingival probing depths, tooth mobility, and pyogenic granuloma incidence are other pregnancy-related conditions. Pyogenic granuloma (granuloma gravidarum, pregnancy tumor) is a benign, hyperplastic, vascular, and rapid-growing tumoral lesion which occurs on mucosal surfaces [136]. Gingival tissue is the most common site, yet rarely it also can occur on different sites like the tongue, buccal mucosa, or lips [137]. During the first 20 weeks of gestation, about 2% of women develop intraoral pyogenic granuloma [138] in which some of them do not require any treatment, whereas highly vascular and large ones may require surgical excision.

1.8.2 Gastrointestinal Tract

Despite total acid production decreases during pregnancy, incidence of reflux increases. As the uterus grows gradually, it pushes and displaces the lower esophageal sphincter along with the stomach. When this high mechanical compression is combined with the relaxative effect of the progesterone (which increases throughout the pregnancy as well) on the lower esophageal sphincter, the incidence of heartburn (pyrosis) reaches up to 80% at term [112].

Gastric emptying time remains unchanged. It may be prolonged only during labor and especially with administration of analgesics by any route [139]. Gastrointestinal motility and food absorption decrease during pregnancy because of increased progesterone levels [140]. It appears that along with progesterone, elevated estrogen levels also play a role in slowing down the gastrointestinal motility [141]. According to experimental evidence, estrogen conducts its gastrointestinal motility modulation effect by enhancing the nitric oxide release from noncholinergic and noradrenergic nerves [142].

Due to the common episodes of constipation during pregnancy and venous compression caused by enlarged uterus, hemorrhoids are observed frequently [143].

1.8.3 Liver

Hepatic arterial and portal venous circulations increase throughout the pregnancy, yet hepatic size remains unchanged [144]. Serum alanine transaminase (ALT), aspartate transaminase (AST), gamma-glutamyltransferase (GGT), and bilirubin levels are usually unchanged or show a slight decrease during normal pregnancy compared to nonpregnant state [145, 146]. Because of the additional placental production, total alkaline phosphatase shows an increase about two folds during pregnancy [145]. Albumin concentration shows a decline throughout pregnancy due to pregnancy-related plasma expansion. The normal value of 4.2 g/dL may decrease to 3.1 g/dL at term [146]. Also, cholesterol and triglyceride levels increase during pregnancy [135].

1.8.4 Gallbladder

Gallbladder contraction is regulated by cholecystokinin-mediated smooth muscle stimulation. Elevated levels of progesterone during pregnancy inhibit this stimulation and cause an impaired contractility. The increased residual volume followed by impaired emptying of the bladder leads to bile stasis and thus gallstone formation. Gallbladder sludge or stone incidence increases with pregnancy and shows strong relation with higher parity in women [147].

1.9 Renal System Changes

Kidneys enlarge about 1–1.5 cm in size, and physiologic hydronephrosis is observed in approximately 80% of women. Advancing mechanical compression to ureters throughout the pregnancy leads to a dilatation at kidney pelvis and calyceal system. The urinary tract infection risk is 40% higher during pregnancy due to urinary stasis caused by the dilatation of the collecting system [148].

The decrease in the oncotic pressure and protein concentration due to hypervolemia-related hemodilution, along with increased renal plasma flow, causes an increase in glomerular filtration rate (GFR) during pregnancy [149, 150]. GFR increases about 50%, whereas renal plasma flow increases 50–80%. Increased level of relaxin also contributes to the increase in GFR and renal plasma flow by its renal vasodilatation effect via nitric oxide production [150]. Increased GFR causes a slight decline in plasma blood urea nitrogen (BUN) and creatinine concentrations. The normal range of nonpregnant levels may indicate an abnormal kidney function during pregnancy. Reabsorption of sodium from tubules increases. Renal excretions of amino acids and water-soluble vitamins increase [151]. Glycosuria occurs due to impaired resorptive capacity of the tubules along with increased GFR. Even glycosuria might be physiologic; when detected, an evaluation for diabetes should be performed [152]. Proteinuria is also considered physiologic at levels below 300 mg/day [150]. Some drugs' serum concentration can be lower during pregnancy due to expanded blood volume and increased GFR.

1.10 Reproductive Tract Changes

Starting from a size of a pear with approximately only 10 mL of cavity, the uterus shows the most prominent change among other organs during pregnancy, reaching to a capacity that may accommodate 5 L or even more (20 L). The 50 g weighted organ at nonpregnant state enlarges gradually throughout pregnancy and weights approximately 1100 g at term. Stretching and hypertrophy of the muscle cells are responsible for this enlargement. After first trimester, the uterus extends beyond the pelvis and becomes adjacent to the abdominal wall, gradually displaces the intestines superolaterally, and finally may reach even up to the liver. At supine position the enlarged uterus compresses at vertebral column and adjacent great vessels, whereas the abdominal wall supports it while standing. The uterine enlargement comes with an increase in blood flow as well.

Increased levels of estrogen, progesterone, and relaxin hormones are secreted by ovaries to maintain a healthy pregnancy. Ovulation stops due to the pituitary inhibition caused by increased progesterone and estrogen levels. Corpus luteum, which is responsible for the secretion of these hormones at early gestation, shows its maximal function at sixth to seventh weeks of gestation and gradually degenerates after tenth week. Vascularity of both ovaries increases throughout pregnancy. The capacity of ovarian veins increases about 60 folds at 36th week of gestation compared to nonpregnant state [153]. Fallopian tube musculature exhibits a slight hypertrophy whereas the epithelium flattens.

At about fourth week of gestation, the cervix softens, and the color of it starts to get bluish due to the increased vascularity and edema. Cervical glands proliferate throughout pregnancy, and the endocervical columnar epithelium extends to the ectocervix, which is called ectropion. Compared to the uterus, the cervix is less muscular. Collagen fibers and a matrix rich in proteoglycans mostly form its connective tissue [154]. The cellular component undergoes proliferation and hyperplasia as the collagen gets reorganized and consolidated. This collagen-rich structure supports the growing fetus and hence maintains pregnancy until term. The rearrangement of these cells by complex interactions provides dilatation during delivery and repair at postpartum period [155].

As seen in the cervix, the vagina also gets a deep blue, violet color due to increased vascularization, and it's called Chadwick sign. Increased cervical secretions cause a discharge which is mostly odorless, transparent or white, and mucous. The lactic acid production is increased due to glycogen energy store metabolism by *Lactobacillus acidophilus* which makes the pH acidic (3.5–6). Epithelial thickening, loosening of connective tissue, and hypertrophy of muscle cells are the adaptation of vaginal wall during pregnancy for the delivery.

1.11 Mammary Tissue Changes

Pregnancy is a period where mammary tissue goes through many changes as it gets prepared to nourish the baby. Breast tenderness, nipple sensitivity, and paresthesia are commonly seen as early pregnancy signs caused by increased blood flow. Breasts grow in size while the veins get more prominent under the skin. A rare condition characterized by incapacitating, diffuse, and extreme enlargement of one or both breasts during pregnancy is called gestational gigantomastia, which may require surgical reduction at postpartum period [156].

Nipples become more pigmented, plumper, larger, and more erectile. From about 16th week of pregnancy, colostrum—a yellowish, thick fluid—is produced by the breasts and can be discharged from the nipples with a gentle massage. The areola gradually becomes darker and enlarged. Montgomery glands are responsible for lubrication of the areola during breastfeeding. These sebaceous glands dispersed around the areola become hypertrophic and more prominent during pregnancy and sometimes might swell due to a blockage like an acne.

1.12   Musculoskeletal Changes

Musculoskeletal symptoms are common during pregnancy. As the uterus grows, the changing center of gravity causes lordosis. Parallel with this postural change, mechanical strain on the back and sacroiliac joints increases. The mechanical stress on the joints increases especially at the third trimester in which the weight gain is maximum. Maternal weight gain during pregnancy is so important that a 20% increase in the weight means a 100% increase in the force on the joints [157]. All these mechanical and postural alterations cause lower back pain in about 50–80% of pregnant women [158, 159].

Ligamentous laxity and joint hypermobility occur during pregnancy which is essential in symphysis pubis widening during delivery. This laxity in the ligamentous structures is thought to be a result of the increasing relaxin hormone (a peptide hormone which is secreted by corpus luteum and placenta and associated with collagen remodeling) levels during pregnancy [160]. However, this relationship between relaxin and joint laxity is controversial since no correlation between levels of hormone and laxity was observed in different studies [161, 162].

The water retention especially at the third trimester may cause soft tissue edema in the lower limbs and thus joint effusion and nerve entrapment. The growing uterus stretches abdominal muscles, and the width between rectus abdominis muscles increases parallel to the gestational age which may cause diastasis recti at term.

1.13   Skin Changes

Increased pigmentation of the skin is observed in approximately 90% of pregnant women [163]. Hyperpigmentation occurs mostly in localized areas. It's still not fully understood why some particular areas are prone to increased pigmentation. It might be due to the difference of melanocyte density of those regions which get stimulated by elevated pregnancy-related hormones. The increased estrogen and progesterone levels may play a role in stimulation of melanocytic activity [164]. Another possible reason is the plasma level elevation of α-melanocyte-stimulating hormone (MSH), yet this increase occurs in late gestation which doesn't correlate with the early onset of hyperpigmentation during pregnancy [165]. Other common skin areas which exhibit hyperpigmentation are the neck, nipples, areola, axillae, perineum, and inner thighs.

The most common site of hyperpigmentation is the linea alba—midline of the abdomen that extends from the xiphoid process to the symphysis pubis—which is darkened during pregnancy and then called as linea nigra. Another pigmentation change during pregnancy which causes most cosmetic complaints is melasma (mask of pregnancy or chloasma) [164]. Melasma may show up as centrofacial (forehead, upper lip, nose, cheeks, and chin), malar (cheeks and nose), or mandibular (ramus of the mandible) [166]. Recent scars are also prone to become more pigmented during pregnancy. Hyperpigmentation regresses and most areas become less pigmented at postpartum period, yet some do not resolve completely. Protection from sunlight is an important part of preventive treatment [167].

In the second half of pregnancy, the growing uterus stretches abdominal skin gradually which causes connective tissue changes on the skin. They begin as pinkish linear patches and progress to hypopigmented, slightly depressed linear wrinkles. These changes occur also in other regions like breasts and thighs which are called striae gravidarum or stretch marks. The etiology of striae gravidarum is unknown, but young maternal age, family history, and large weight gain during pregnancy appear to be associated risk factors. There is no preventive step or definitive treatment for this condition [168].

Proliferation of blood vessels along with vascular distention and instability occurs most probably due to hyper-estrogenic state of pregnancy. Spider angiomas are common, and they appear as reddish extensions which radiate outward from a central red spot slightly beneath the skin and occur mostly on the face, neck, upper chest, and arms. Vasomotor instability (fascial flushing, hot/cold sensations) due to increased cutaneous blood flow and purpura caused by increased hydrostatic pressure and capillary fragility are commonly observed during pregnancy [169].

References

1. Pritchard JA. Changes in the blood volume during pregnancy and delivery. Anesthesiology. 1965;26:393–9.
2. Lund CJ, Donovan JC. Blood volume during pregnancy. Significance of plasma and red cell volumes. Am J Obstet Gynecol. 1967;98(3):394–403.
3. Maymon R, Zimerman AL, Strauss S, Gayer G. Maternal spleen size throughout normal pregnancy. Semin Ultrasound CT MR. 2007;28(1):64–6.
4. Ueland K. Maternal cardiovascular dynamics. VII. Intrapartum blood volume changes. Am J Obstet Gynecol. 1976;126(6):671–7.
5. Stephansson O, Dickman PW, Johansson A, Cnattingius S. Maternal hemoglobin concentration during pregnancy and risk of stillbirth. JAMA. 2000;284(20):2611–7.
6. Pritchard JA, Adams RH. Erythrocyte production and destruction during pregnancy. Am J Obstet Gynecol. 1960;79:750–7.
7. McLean E, Cogswell M, Egli I, Wojdyla D, de Benoist B. Worldwide prevalence of anaemia, WHO Vitamin and Mineral Nutrition Information System, 1993–2005. Public Health Nutr. 2009;12(4):444–54.
8. ACOG practice bulletin no. 95: anemia in pregnancy. Obstet Gynecol 2008;112(1):201–207.
9. Pritchard J, Scott D. Iron demands during pregnancy. In: Iron deficiency-pathogenesis: clinical aspects and therapy. London: Academic; 1970. p. 173–82.
10. WHO. Recommendations on antenatal care for a positive pregnancy experience. Geneva: World Health Organization; 2016.
11. Djurisic S, Hviid TVF. HLA class Ib molecules and immune cells in pregnancy and preeclampsia. Front Immunol. 2014;5:652.
12. Michimata T, Sakai M, Miyazaki S, Ogasawara MS, Suzumori K, Aoki K, et al. Decrease of T-helper 2 and T-cytotoxic 2 cells at implantation sites occurs in unexplained recurrent spontaneous abortion with normal chromosomal content. Hum Reprod. 2003;18(7):1523–8.

13. Wilder RL. Hormones, pregnancy, and autoimmune diseases. Ann N Y Acad Sci. 1998;840(1):45–50.
14. Fleming AF. Hematological changes in pregnancy. Clin Obstet Gynecol. 1975;2(2):269–83.
15. Taylor DJ, Phillips P, Lind T. Puerperal haematological indices. Br J Obstet Gynaecol. 1981;88(6):601–6.
16. Chandra S, Tripathi AK, Mishra S, Amzarul M, Vaish AK. Physiological changes in hematological parameters during pregnancy. Indian J Hematol Blood Transfus. 2012;28(3):144–6.
17. Edelstam G, Löwbeer C, Kral G, Gustafsson SA, Venge P. New reference values for routine blood samples and human neutrophilic lipocalin during third-trimester pregnancy. Scand J Clin Lab Invest. 2001;61(8):583–92.
18. Anderson BL, Mendez-Figueroa H, Dahlke JD, Raker C, Hillier SL, Cu-Uvin S. Pregnancy-induced changes in immune protection of the genital tract: defining normal. Am J Obstet Gynecol. 2013;208(4):321.e1–9.
19. Watts DH, Krohn MA, Wener MH, Eschenbach DA. C-reactive protein in normal pregnancy. Obstet Gynecol. 1991;77(2):176–80.
20. Gallery ED, Raftos J, Gyory AZ, Wells JV. A prospective study of serum complement (C3 and C4) levels in normal human pregnancy: effect of the development of pregnancy-associated hypertension. Aust N Z J Med. 1981;11(3):243–5.
21. Richani K, Soto E, Romero R, Espinoza J, Chaiworapongsa T, Nien JK, et al. Normal pregnancy is characterized by systemic activation of the complement system. J Matern Neonatal Med. 2005;17(4):239–45.
22. Thornburg LL, Queenan R, Brandt-Griffith B, Pressman EK. Procalcitonin for prediction of chorioamnionitis in preterm premature rupture of membranes. J Matern Neonatal Med. 2016;29(13):2056–61.
23. Kenny LC, Mccrae KR, Cunningham FG. Platelets, coagulation, and the liver. In: Taylor RN, Roberts JM, Cunningham FG, Lindheimer MDBT-CHD in P (Fourth E, editors). Chesley's hypertensive disorders in pregnancy [internet]. San Diego: Academic; 2015. p. 379–396.
24. Valera M-C, Parant O, Vayssiere C, Arnal J-F, Payrastre B. Physiologic and pathologic changes of platelets in pregnancy. Platelets. 2010;21(8):587–95.
25. Matthews JH, Benjamin S, Gill DS, Smith NA. Pregnancy-associated thrombocytopenia: definition, incidence and natural history. Acta Haematol. 1990;84(1):24–9.
26. Burrows RF, Kelton JG. Incidentally detected thrombocytopenia in healthy mothers and their infants. N Engl J Med. 1988;319(3):142–5.
27. Hellgren M. Hemostasis during normal pregnancy and puerperium. Semin Thromb Hemost. 2003;29(2):125–30.
28. Uchikova EH, Ledjev II. Changes in haemostasis during normal pregnancy. Eur J Obstet Gynecol Reprod Biol. 2005;119(2):185–8.
29. Ku D-HW, Arkel YS, Paidas MP, Lockwood CJ. Circulating levels of inflammatory cytokines (IL-1 beta and TNF-alpha), resistance to activated protein C, thrombin and fibrin generation in uncomplicated pregnancies. Thromb Haemost. 2003;90(6):1074–9.
30. Hui C, Lili M, Libin C, Rui Z, Fang G, Ling G, et al. Changes in coagulation and hemodynamics during pregnancy: a prospective longitudinal study of 58 cases. Arch Gynecol Obstet. 2012;285(5):1231–6.
31. Kline JA, Williams GW, Hernandez-Nino J. D-dimer concentrations in normal pregnancy: new diagnostic thresholds are needed. Clin Chem. 2005;51(5):825–9.
32. Walker MC, Garner PR, Keely EJ, Rock GA, Reis MD. Changes in activated protein C resistance during normal pregnancy. Am J Obstet Gynecol. 1997;177(1):162–9.
33. James AH, Rhee E, Thames B, Philipp CS. Characterization of antithrombin levels in pregnancy. Thromb Res. 2014;134(3):648–51.
34. Heit JA, Kobbervig CE, James AH, Petterson TM, Bailey KR, Melton LJ 3rd. Trends in the incidence of venous thromboembolism during pregnancy or postpartum: a 30-year population-based study. Ann Intern Med. 2005;143(10):697–706.
35. Stewart RD, Nelson DB, Matulevicius SA, Morgan JL, McIntire DD, Drazner MH, et al. Cardiac magnetic resonance imaging to assess the impact of maternal habitus on cardiac remodeling during pregnancy. Am J Obstet Gynecol. 2016;214(5):640.e1–6.

36. Ghi T, degli Esposti D, Montaguti E, Rosticci M, Tancredi S, Youssef A, et al. Maternal cardiac evaluation during uncomplicated twin pregnancy with emphasis on the diastolic function. Am J Obstet Gynecol. 2015;213(3):376.e1–8.
37. Mashini IS, Albazzaz SJ, Fadel HE, Abdulla AM, Hadi HA, Harp R, et al. Serial noninvasive evaluation of cardiovascular hemodynamics during pregnancy. Am J Obstet Gynecol. 1987;156(5):1208–13.
38. Nelson DB, Stewart RD, Matulevicius SA, Morgan JL, McIntire DD, Drazner M, et al. The effects of maternal position and habitus on maternal cardiovascular parameters as measured by cardiac magnetic resonance. Am J Perinatol. 2015;32(14):1318–23.
39. Howard BK, Goodson JH, Mengert WF. Supine hypotensive syndrome in late pregnancy. Obstet Gynecol. 1953;1(4):371–7.
40. McLennan CE. Antecubital and femoral venous pressure in normal and toxemic pregnancy. Am J Obstet Gynecol [Internet]. 1943;45(4):568–591.
41. Clark SL, Cotton DB, Lee W, Bishop C, Hill T, Southwick J, et al. Central hemodynamic assessment of normal term pregnancy. Am J Obstet Gynecol. 1989;161(6 Pt 1):1439–42.
42. Glinoer D, Nayer PDE, Bourdoux P, Lemone M, Robyn C, Steirteghem AVAN, et al. Regulation of maternal thyroid during pregnancy. J Clin Endocrinol Metab. 1990;71(2):276–87.
43. Soldin OP, Tractenberg RE, Hollowell JG, Jonklaas J, Janicic N, Soldin SJ. Trimester-specific changes in maternal thyroid hormone, thyrotropin, and thyroglobulin concentrations during gestation: trends and associations across trimesters in iodine sufficiency. Thyroid. 2004;14(12):1084–90.
44. Glinoer D. The regulation of thyroid function in pregnancy: pathways of endocrine adaptation from physiology to pathology. Endocr Rev. 1997;18(3):404–33.
45. Kurtz A, Dwyer K, Ekins R. Serum free thyroxine in pregnancy. Br Med J. 1979;2:550–1.
46. Hopton MR, Ashwell K, Scott IV, Harrop JS. Serum free thyroxine concentration and free thyroid hormone indices in normal pregnancy. Clin Endocrinol. 1983;18(4):431–7.
47. Boss AM, Kingstone D. Further observations on serum free thyroxine concentrations during pregnancy. Br Med J (Clin Res Ed). 1981;283(6291):584.
48. Casey BM, Leveno KJ. Thyroid disease in pregnancy. Obstet Gynecol. 2006;108(5):1283–92.
49. Gonzalez JG, Elizondo G, Saldivar D, Nanez H, Todd LE, Villarreal JZ. Pituitary gland growth during normal pregnancy: an in vivo study using magnetic resonance imaging. Am J Med. 1988;85(2):217–20.
50. Laway BA, Mir SA. Pregnancy and pituitary disorders: challenges in diagnosis and management. Indian J Endocrinol Metab. 2013;17(6):996–1004.
51. Rigg LA, Lein A, Yen SS. Pattern of increase in circulating prolactin levels during human gestation. Am J Obstet Gynecol. 1977;129(4):454–6.
52. Pérez-Ibave DC, Rodríguez-Sánchez IP, de Lourdes Garza-Rodríguez M, Barrera-Saldaña HA. Extrapituitary growth hormone synthesis in humans. Growth Hormon IGF Res. 2014;24(2–3):47–53.
53. Carr BR, Parker CRJ, Madden JD, MacDonald PC, Porter JC. Maternal plasma adrenocorticotropin and cortisol relationships throughout human pregnancy. Am J Obstet Gynecol. 1981;139(4):416–22.
54. More C, Bhattoa HP, Bettembuk P, Balogh A. The effects of pregnancy and lactation on hormonal status and biochemical markers of bone turnover. Eur J Obstet Gynecol Reprod Biol. 2003;106(2):209–13.
55. Pitkin RM, Reynolds WA, Williams GA, Hargis GK. Calcium metabolism in normal pregnancy: a longitudinal study. Am J Obstet Gynecol. 1979;133(7):781–90.
56. Møller UK, Streym S, Mosekilde L, Heickendorff L, Flyvbjerg A, Frystyk J, et al. Changes in calcitropic hormones, bone markers and insulin-like growth factor I (IGF-I) during pregnancy and postpartum: a controlled cohort study. Osteoporos Int. 2013;24(4):1307–20.
57. Berggren EK, Presley L, Amini SB, Hauguel-de Mouzon S, Catalano PM. Are the metabolic changes of pregnancy reversible in the first year postpartum? Diabetologia. 2015;58(7):1561–8.

58. Jebeile H, Mijatovic J, Louie JCY, Prvan T, Brand-Miller JC. A systematic review and metaanalysis of energy intake and weight gain in pregnancy. Am J Obstet Gynecol. 2016;214(4):465–83.
59. Pitkin RM. Nutritional support in obstetrics and gynecology. Clin Obstet Gynecol. 1976;19(3):489–513.
60. Newbern D, Freemark M. Placental hormones and the control of maternal metabolism and fetal growth. Curr Opin Endocrinol Diabetes Obes. 2011;18(6):409–16.
61. Handwerger S, Freemark M. The roles of placental growth hormone and placental lactogen in the regulation of human fetal growth and development. J Pediatr Endocrinol Metab. 2000;13(4):343–56.
62. Brizzi P, Tonolo G, Esposito F, Puddu L, Dessole S, Maioli M, et al. Lipoprotein metabolism during normal pregnancy. Am J Obstet Gynecol. 1999;181(2):430–4.
63. Soma-Pillay P, Nelson-Piercy C, Tolppanen H, Mebazaa A. Physiological changes in pregnancy. Cardiovasc J Afr. 2016;27(2):89–94.
64. Herrera E, Ortega-Senovilla H. Lipid metabolism during pregnancy and its implications for fetal growth. Curr Pharm Biotechnol. 2014;15(1):24–31.
65. Mennitti LV, Oliveira JL, Morais CA, Estadella D, Oyama LM, Oller do Nascimento CM, et al. Type of fatty acids in maternal diets during pregnancy and/or lactation and metabolic consequences of the offspring. J Nutr Biochem. 2015;26(2):99–111.
66. Torsiglieri AJJ, Tom LW, Keane WM, Atkins JPJ. Otolaryngologic manifestations of pregnancy. Otolaryngol Head Neck Surg. 1990;102(3):293–7.
67. da Silva Schmidt PM, da Trindade Flores F, Rossi AG, da Silveira AF. Hearing and vestibular complaints during pregnancy. Braz J Otorhinolaryngol. 2010;76(1):29–33.
68. Izci B, Vennelle M, Liston WA, Dundas KC, Calder AA, Douglas NJ. Sleep-disordered breathing and upper airway size in pregnancy and post-partum. Eur Respir J. 2006;27(2):321–7.
69. Miller JB. Patulous eustachian tubes in pregnancy. West J Surg Obstet Gynecol. 1962;70:156–9.
70. Shiny Sherlie V, Varghese A. ENT changes of pregnancy and its management. Indian J Otolaryngol Head Neck Surg. 2014;66(Suppl 1):6–9.
71. Derkay CS. Eustachian tube and nasal function during pregnancy: a prospective study. Otolaryngol Head Neck Surg. 1988;99(6):558–66.
72. Weissman A, Nir D, Shenhav R, Zimmer EZ, Joachims ZH, Danino J. Eustachian tube function during pregnancy. Clin Otolaryngol Allied Sci. 1993;18(3):212–4.
73. Sennaroglu G, Belgin E. Audiological findings in pregnancy. J Laryngol Otol. 2001;115(8):617–21.
74. Ambro BT, Scheid SC, Pribitkin EA. Prescribing guidelines for ENT medications during pregnancy. Ear Nose Throat J. 2003;82(8):565–8.
75. Vlastarakos PV, Nikolopoulos TP, Manolopoulos L, Ferekidis E, Kreatsas G. Treating common ear problems in pregnancy: what is safe? Eur Arch Otorhinolaryngol. 2008;265(2):139–45.
76. Rudic M, Keogh I, Wagner R, Wilkinson E, Kiros N, Ferrary E, et al. The pathophysiology of otosclerosis: review of current research. Hear Res. 2015;330(Pt A):51–6.
77. Walsh TE. The effect of pregnancy on the deafness of otosclerosis. Trans Am Acad Ophthalmol Otolaryngol. 1954;58(3):420–3; discussion 423–6.
78. Imauchi Y, Lainé P, Sterkers O, Ferrary E, Bozorg GA. Effect of 17 beta-estradiol on diastrophic dysplasia sulfate transporter activity in otosclerotic bone cell cultures and SaOS-2 cells. Acta Otolaryngol. 2004;124(8):890–5.
79. Lippy WH, Berenholz LP, Schuring AG, Burkey JM. Does pregnancy affect otosclerosis? Laryngoscope. 2005;115(10):1833–6.
80. Mabry RL. Rhinitis of pregnancy. South Med J. 1986;79(8):965–71.
81. Incaudo GA, Takach P. The diagnosis and treatment of allergic rhinitis during pregnancy and lactation. Immunol Allergy Clin North Am. 2006;26(1):137–54.
82. Nappi C, Di Spiezio SA, Guerra G, Di Carlo C, Bifulco G, Acunzo G, et al. Comparison of intranasal and transdermal estradiol on nasal mucosa in postmenopausal women. Menopause. 2004;11(4):447–55.

83. Hamano N, Terada N, Maesako K, Ikeda T, Fukuda S, Wakita J, et al. Expression of histamine receptors in nasal epithelial cells and endothelial cells—the effects of sex hormones. Int Arch Allergy Immunol. 1998;115(3):220–7.

84. Ellegård EK, Karlsson NG, Ellegård LH. Rhinitis in the menstrual cycle, pregnancy, and some endocrine disorders. Clin Allergy Immunol. 2007;19:305–21.

85. Ellegård EK. Clinical and pathogenetic characteristics of pregnancy rhinitis. Clin Rev Allergy Immunol. 2004;26(3):149–59.

86. Ellegård E, Oscarsson J, Bougoussa M, Igout A, Hennen G, Edén S, et al. Serum level of placental growth hormone is raised in pregnancy rhinitis. Arch Otolaryngol Head Neck Surg. 1998;124(4):439–43.

87. Goldstein G, Govindaraj S. Rhinologic issues in pregnancy. Allergy Rhinol (Providence). 2012;3(1):e13–5.

88. Philpott CM, Conboy P, Al-Azzawi F, Murty G. Nasal physiological changes during pregnancy. Clin Otolaryngol Allied Sci. 2004;29(4):343–51.

89. Demir UL, Demir BC, Oztosun E, Uyaniklar OO, Ocakoglu G. The effects of pregnancy on nasal physiology. Int Forum Allergy Rhinol. 2015;5(2):162–6.

90. Ellegård E, Karlsson G. Nasal congestion during pregnancy. Clin Otolaryngol Allied Sci. 1999;24(4):307–11.

91. Ellegård E, Hellgren M, Torén K, Karlsson G. The incidence of pregnancy rhinitis. Gynecol Obstet Invest. 2000;49(2):98–101.

92. Dzieciolowska-Baran E, Teul-Swiniarska I, Gawlikowska-Sroka A, Poziomkowska-Gesicka I, Zietek Z. Rhinitis as a cause of respiratory disorders during pregnancy. Adv Exp Med Biol. 2013;755:213–20.

93. Ellegård E, Karlsson G. IgE-mediated reactions and hyperreactivity in pregnancy rhinitis. Arch Otolaryngol Head Neck Surg. 1999;125(10):1121–5.

94. Garavello W, Somigliana E, Acaia B, Gaini L, Pignataro L, Gaini RM. Nasal lavage in pregnant women with seasonal allergic rhinitis: a randomized study. Int Arch Allergy Immunol. 2010;151(2):137–41.

95. Schatz M, Zeiger RS, Harden K, Hoffman CC, Chilingar L, Petitti D. The safety of asthma and allergy medications during pregnancy. J Allergy Clin Immunol. 1997;100(3):301–6.

96. Busse WW. NAEPP expert panel report: managing asthma during pregnancy: recommendations for pharmacologic treatment—2004 update. J Allergy Clin Immunol. 2005;115(1):34–46.

97. Bérard A, Sheehy O, Kurzinger M-L, Juhaeri J. Intranasal triamcinolone use during pregnancy and the risk of adverse pregnancy outcomes. J Allergy Clin Immunol. 2016;138(1):97–104.e7.

98. Namazy JA, Schatz M. The safety of intranasal steroids during pregnancy: a good start. J Allergy Clin Immunol. 2016;138:105–6.

99. Ellegård EK, Hellgren M, Karlsson NG. Fluticasone propionate aqueous nasal spray in pregnancy rhinitis. Clin Otolaryngol Allied Sci. 2001;26(5):394–400.

100. Schatz M, Petitti D. Antihistamines and pregnancy. Ann Allergy Asthma Immunol. 1997;78:157–9.

101. Gilbert C, Mazzotta P, Loebstein R, Koren G. Fetal safety of drugs used in the treatment of allergic rhinitis: a critical review. Drug Saf. 2005;28(8):707–19.

102. Källén B. Use of antihistamine drugs in early pregnancy and delivery outcome. J Matern Neonatal Med. 2002;11(3):146–52.

103. Gilbert AN, Wysocki CJ. Quantitative assessment of olfactory experience during pregnancy. Psychosom Med. 1991;53(6):693–700.

104. Cameron EL. Measures of human olfactory perception during pregnancy. Chem Senses. 2007;32(8):775–82.

105. Dugan-Kim M, Connell S, Stika C, Wong CA, Gossett DR. Epistaxis of pregnancy and association with postpartum hemorrhage. Obstet Gynecol. 2009;114(6):1322–5.

106. Kumar R, Hayhurst KL, Robson AK. Ear, nose, and throat manifestations during pregnancy. Otolaryngol Head Neck Surg. 2011;145(2):188–98.

107. Park YW. Nasal granuloma gravidarum. Otolaryngol Head Neck Surg. 2002;126(5):591–2.

108. Zarrinneshan AAZ, Zapanta PE, Wall SJ. Nasal pyogenic granuloma. Otolaryngol Head Neck Surg. 2007;136(1):130–1.
109. Hamdan A-L, Mahfoud L, Sibai A, Seoud M. Effect of pregnancy on the speaking voice. J Voice. 2009;23(4):490–3.
110. Sivasankar M, Fisher KV. Oral breathing increases Pth and vocal effort by superficial drying of vocal fold mucosa. J Voice. 2002;16(2):172–81.
111. Ali RAR, Egan LJ. Gastroesophageal reflux disease in pregnancy. Best Pract Res Clin Gastroenterol. 2007;21(5):793–806.
112. Richter JE. Gastroesophageal reflux disease during pregnancy. Gastroenterol Clin North Am. 2003;32(1):235–61.
113. Koufman JA, Aviv JE, Casiano RR, Shaw GY. Laryngopharyngeal reflux: position statement of the committee on speech, voice, and swallowing disorders of the American Academy of Otolaryngology-Head and Neck Surgery. Otolaryngol Head Neck Surg. 2002;127(1):32–5.
114. Gill SK, O'Brien L, Einarson TR, Koren G. The safety of proton pump inhibitors (PPIs) in pregnancy: a meta-analysis. Am J Gastroenterol. 2009;104(6):1541–5; quiz 1540, 1546.
115. Gill SK, O'Brien L, Koren G. The safety of histamine 2 (H2) blockers in pregnancy: a meta-analysis. Dig Dis Sci. 2009;54(9):1835–8.
116. McGlashan JA, Johnstone LM, Sykes J, Strugala V, Dettmar PW. The value of a liquid alginate suspension (Gaviscon advance) in the management of laryngopharyngeal reflux. Eur Arch Otorhinolaryngol. 2009;266(2):243–51.
117. Bhatia PL, Singh MS, Jha BK. Laryngopathia gravidarum. Ear Nose Throat J. 1981;60(9):408–12.
118. Hegewald MJ, Crapo RO. Respiratory physiology in pregnancy. Clin Chest Med. 2011;32(1):1–13.
119. Weinberger SE, Weiss ST, Cohen WR, Weiss JW, Johnson TS. Pregnancy and the lung. Am Rev Respir Dis. 1980;121(3):559–81.
120. Goldsmith LT, Weiss G, Steinetz BG. Relaxin and its role in pregnancy. Endocrinol Metab Clin North Am. 1995;24(1):171–86.
121. Milne JA, Mills RJ, Howie AD, Pack AI. Large airways function during normal pregnancy. Br J Obstet Gynaecol. 1977;84(6):448–51.
122. Rees GB, Broughton Pipkin F, Symonds EM, Patrick JM. A longitudinal study of respiratory changes in normal human pregnancy with cross-sectional data on subjects with pregnancy-induced hypertension. Am J Obstet Gynecol. 1990;162(3):826–30.
123. Heenan AP, Wolfe LA. Plasma osmolality and the strong ion difference predict respiratory adaptations in pregnant and nonpregnant women. Can J Physiol Pharmacol. 2003;81(9):839–47.
124. Bayliss DA, Millhorn DE. Central neural mechanisms of progesterone action: application to the respiratory system. J Appl Physiol. 1992;73(2):393–404.
125. Ajjimaporn A, Somprasit C, Chaunchaiyakul R. A cross-sectional study of resting cardio-respiratory and metabolic changes in pregnant women. J Phys Ther Sci. 2014;26(5):779–82.
126. Contreras G, Gutiérrez M, Beroíza T, Fantín A, Oddó H, Villarroel L, et al. Ventilatory drive and respiratory muscle function in pregnancy. Am Rev Respir Dis. 1991;144(4):837–41.
127. Jensen D, Wolfe LA, Slatkovska L, Webb KA, Davies GAL, O'Donnell DE. Effects of human pregnancy on the ventilatory chemoreflex response to carbon dioxide. Am J Physiol Regul Integr Comp Physiol. 2005;288(5):R1369–75.
128. Templeton A, Kelman GR. Maternal blood-gases, PAo2–Pao2), hysiological shunt and VD/VT in normal pregnancy. Br J Anaesth 1976;48(10):1001–1004.
129. Prowse CM, Gaensler EA. Respiratory and acid-base changes during pregnancy. Anesthesiology. 1965;26:381–92.
130. Tan EK, Tan EL. Alterations in physiology and anatomy during pregnancy. Best Pract Res Clin Obstet Gynaecol. 2013;27(6):791–802.
131. Tsai CH, de Leeuw NK. Changes in 2,3-diphosphoglycerate during pregnancy and puerperium in normal women and in beta-thalassemia heterozygous women. Am J Obstet Gynecol. 1982;142(5):520–3.

132. Sherman PW, Flaxman SM. Nausea and vomiting of pregnancy in an evolutionary perspective. Am J Obstet Gynecol. 2002;186(5 Suppl Understanding):S190–7.
133. Lee NM, Saha S. Nausea and vomiting of pregnancy. Gastroenterol Clin North Am. 2011;40(2):309–34, vii.
134. Soory M. Hormonal factors in periodontal disease. Dent Update. 2000;27(8):380–3.
135. Suresh L, Radfar L. Pregnancy and lactation. Oral Surg Oral Med Oral Pathol Oral Radiol Endod. 2004;97(6):672–82.
136. Aldulaimi S, Saenz A. A bleeding oral mass in a pregnant woman. JAMA. 2017;318(3):293–4.
137. Arunmozhi U, Priya RS, Kadhiresan R, Sujatha G, Shamsudeen-Ss SM. A large pregnancy tumor of tongue—a case report. J Clin Diagn Res. 2016;10:ZD10–2.
138. Kroumpouzos G, Cohen LM. Dermatoses of pregnancy. J Am Acad Dermatol. 2001;45(1):1–22.
139. Carp H, Jayaram A, Stoll M. Ultrasound examination of the stomach contents of parturients. Anesth Analg. 1992;74(5):683–7.
140. Baron TH, Ramirez B, Richter JE. Gastrointestinal motility disorders during pregnancy. Ann Intern Med. 1993;118(5):366–75.
141. Hogan AM, Collins D, Baird AW, Winter DC. Estrogen and its role in gastrointestinal health and disease. Int J Color Dis. 2009;24(12):1367–75.
142. Shah S, Nathan L, Singh R, Fu YS, Chaudhuri G. E2 and not P4 increases NO release from NANC nerves of the gastrointestinal tract: implications in pregnancy. Am J Physiol Regul Integr Comp Physiol. 2001;280(5):R1546–54.
143. Shin GH, Toto EL, Schey R. Pregnancy and postpartum bowel changes: constipation and fecal incontinence. Am J Gastroenterol. 2015;110(4):521–9; quiz 530.
144. Clapp JF 3rd, Stepanchak W, Tomaselli J, Kortan M, Faneslow S. Portal vein blood flow-effects of pregnancy, gravity, and exercise. Am J Obstet Gynecol. 2000;183(1):167–72.
145. Cattozzo G, Calonaci A, Albeni C, Guerra E, Franzini M, Ghezzi F, et al. Reference values for alanine aminotransferase, α-amylase, aspartate aminotransferase, γ-glutamyltransferase and lactate dehydrogenase measured according to the IFCC standardization during uncomplicated pregnancy. Clin Chem Lab Med. 2013;51:e239–41.
146. Elliott JR, O'Kell RT. Normal clinical chemical values for pregnant women at term. Clin Chem. 1971;17(3):156–7.
147. Ko CW, Beresford SAA, Schulte SJ, Matsumoto AM, Lee SP. Incidence, natural history, and risk factors for biliary sludge and stones during pregnancy. Hepatology. 2005;41(2):359–65.
148. Cheung KL, Lafayette RA. Renal physiology of pregnancy. Adv Chronic Kidney Dis. 2013;20(3):209–14.
149. Conrad KP, Davison JM. The renal circulation in normal pregnancy and preeclampsia: is there a place for relaxin? Am J Physiol Renal Physiol. 2014;306(10):F1121–35.
150. Odutayo A, Hladunewich M. Obstetric nephrology: renal hemodynamic and metabolic physiology in normal pregnancy. Clin J Am Soc Nephrol. 2012;7(12):2073–80.
151. Shibata K, Fukuwatari T, Sasaki S, Sano M, Suzuki K, Hiratsuka C, et al. Urinary excretion levels of water-soluble vitamins in pregnant and lactating women in Japan. J Nutr Sci Vitaminol (Tokyo). 2013;59(3):178–86.
152. Chesley LC. Renal function during pregnancy. Mod Trends Hum Reprod Physiol. 1963;15:205–14.
153. Hodgkinson CP. Physiology of the ovarian veins during pregnancy. Obstet Gynecol. 1953;1(1):26–37.
154. Aubard Y, Chinchilla AM, Dubayle G, Cantaloube M, Gana J, Baudet J. The cervix uteri in pregnancy. J Gynecol Obstet Biol Reprod (Paris). 1998;27(8):755–64.
155. Ludmir J, Sehdev HM. Anatomy and physiology of the uterine cervix. Clin Obstet Gynecol. 2000;43(3):433–9.
156. Mangla M, Singla D. Gestational gigantomastia: a systematic review of case reports. J Midlife Health. 2017;8(1):40–4.
157. Ritchie JR. Orthopedic considerations during pregnancy. Clin Obstet Gynecol. 2003;46(2):456–66.

158. Wang S-M, Dezinno P, Maranets I, Berman MR, Caldwell-Andrews AA, Kain ZN. Low back pain during pregnancy: prevalence, risk factors, and outcomes. Obstet Gynecol. 2004;104(1):65–70.
159. Mogren IM, Pohjanen AI. Low back pain and pelvic pain during pregnancy: prevalence and risk factors. Spine (Phila Pa 1976). 2005;30(8):983–91.
160. Owens K, Pearson A, Mason G. Pubic symphysis separation. Fetal Matern Med Rev. 2002;13(2):141.
161. Marnach ML, Ramin KD, Ramsey PS, Song S-W, Stensland JJ, An K-N. Characterization of the relationship between joint laxity and maternal hormones in pregnancy. Obstet Gynecol. 2003;101(2):331–5.
162. Aldabe D, Ribeiro DC, Milosavljevic S, Dawn BM. Pregnancy-related pelvic girdle pain and its relationship with relaxin levels during pregnancy: a systematic review. Eur Spine J. 2012;21(9):1769–76.
163. Martin AG, Leal-Khouri S. Physiologic skin changes associated with pregnancy. Int J Dermatol. 1992;31(6):375–8.
164. Geraghty LN, Pomeranz MK. Physiologic changes and dermatoses of pregnancy. Int J Dermatol. 2011;50(7):771–82.
165. Clark D, Thody AJ, Shuster S, Bowers H. Immunoreactive alpha-MSH in human plasma in pregnancy. Nature. 1978;273(5658):163–4.
166. Sanchez NP, Pathak MA, Sato S, Fitzpatrick TB, Sanchez JL, Mihm MCJ. Melasma: a clinical, light microscopic, ultrastructural, and immunofluorescence study. J Am Acad Dermatol. 1981;4(6):698–710.
167. Elling SV, Powell FC. Physiological changes in the skin during pregnancy. Clin Dermatol. 1997;15(1):35–43.
168. Korgavkar K, Wang F. Stretch marks during pregnancy: a review of topical prevention. Br J Dermatol. 2015;172(3):606–15.
169. Parmley T, O'Brien TJ. Skin changes during pregnancy. Clin Obstet Gynecol. 1990;33(4):713–7.

Physiological Changes During the Postpartum Period: General Overview

Sefa İnce and Nezar Y. Albar

2.1 Introduction

The puerperium is the period beginning when the placenta is delivered and lasting for several weeks (generally 6) thereafter. At a point 6 weeks following delivery, the majority of the physiological alterations affecting the woman during pregnancy, labour and delivery have reverted, and the physiological state thereafter resembles that of a non-pregnant woman [1].

2.2 Physiological Changes During the Postpartum Period

2.2.1 Physiological Changes in the Organs of Reproduction and the Perineum

2.2.1.1 Uterus

The uterine mass at term (excluding the foetus, placenta, amniotic fluid, etc.) is in the region of 1 kg. During the puerperium, this mass falls to between 50 and 100 g [1].

In the immediate aftermath of delivery, the fundus of the uterus may be palpated. It lies at the level of the mother's umbilicus. Over the following 2 weeks, the uterus keeps getting smaller and losing mass, so that it eventually lies within the pelvis

S. İnce (✉)
Department of Gynaecology and Obstetrics, Erzurum Regional Training and Research Hospital, Erzurum, Turkey
e-mail: drsefaince@gmail.com

N. Y. Albar
Internal Medicine and Endocrinology, First Clinic, International Medical Center, Jeddah, Saudi Arabia
e-mail: drnezaralbar@icloud.com

C. Cingi et al. (eds.), *ENT Diseases: Diagnosis and Treatment during Pregnancy and Lactation*, https://doi.org/10.1007/978-3-031-05303-0_2

proper. The uterus resumes its non-pregnant state gradually, a process lasting several weeks. After reverting to a non-pregnant state, the uterus is still bigger than it was before pregnancy occurred [1].

There is a swift regeneration of the endometrium, with glandular endometrium apparent by day 7. By day 16, the endometrium has recoated the entire uterus, with the exception of where the placenta had been [1].

There are a series of alterations affecting the site within the uterus previously occupied by the placenta. Straight after the foetus is delivered, the smooth muscle surrounding the arteries contracts, as does the myometrium, and this squeezes the vessels shut, preventing further blood loss. This process is termed physiological suture formation. There is a 50% reduction in the magnitude of the placental bed. It is these alterations in the bed of the placenta that account for the volume and type of lochia observed [1].

Once delivery has occurred, there is an extensive discharge of red-coloured blood from the uterus up to the point when the arterial bed begins to contract. Once contraction begins, there is a swift reduction in the volume of discharge via the vagina (i.e. lochia). The bloody discharge is termed lochia rubra, and it may continue for variable lengths of time. The red colour begins to assume an increasingly brownish tinge, and becomes more and more watery. This type of discharge is lochia serosa. The gradual change from lochia serosa to lochia alba (smaller volume, less coloured, finally becoming yellow) progresses over several weeks [2]. The exact duration of lochia is variable, but the mean duration is around 5 weeks [3].

How much discharge and what colour it is may differ significantly from woman to woman. Lochia is still observed at 6 weeks post delivery in 15% of mothers. In many cases, the haemorrhage may be greater from a week to a fortnight after birth, resulting from the eschar covering the placental site being sloughed off. This is the point at which a delayed postpartum bleed is most likely to be seen [1].

2.2.1.2 Cervix

The cervix is another structure which undergoes a swift reversion to the non-pregnant state, albeit it differs from the exact state it was in before any pregnancy occurred. Before a week has elapsed following delivery, the external os has closed to the extent that a finger may no longer be placed in the canal [1].

2.2.1.3 Vagina

The vagina also undergoes reversion to a non-pregnant state, but its size is increased compared with before pregnancy. The pregnant vagina has a greater than usual blood supply and is more oedematous. Both these changes revert to the non-pregnant state by the third week. If women are not lactating, the vaginal rugae are reformed. A cytological smear taken from the vagina during this period has atrophic appearances. The atrophic appearances disappear sometime between the sixth and tenth week. If the mother is breastfeeding, the level of oestrogen remains low and thus atrophy persists in these cases [1].

2.2.1.4 Ovaries

The extent to which the ovaries begin functioning as usual once more differs considerably between women, with lactation playing a key role. Breastfeeding mothers have a cessation in their menses and do not ovulate for longer than non-breastfeeding mothers. In a mother who is not nursing, ovulation is known to occur even on the 27th day postpartum. The majority of women do experience menses by the 12th week postpartum, and the average time for this to occur is between the seventh and ninth week after delivery [1].

For women who are nursing an infant, how menstruation recommences varies to a large extent, with numerous factors involved, such as the amount of milk the infant is taking and the frequency of feeds, in addition to whether breast milk is supplemented by artificial baby milk. Lactation suppresses the usual function of the ovaries by causing hyperprolactinaemia. However, between 50 and 75% of lactating women have resumed menstruation by the 36th week postpartum [1].

2.2.1.5 Perineum

There is often stretching and injury to the perineal region during the process of childbirth, and it may have been torn or cut. The vulva is generally oedematous and engorged following delivery, but resolution usually occurs within the space of 1–2 weeks. By the time of the sixth week postpartum, the musculature usually possesses a nearly normal level of tone with further improvement as months progress. Whether the musculature is able to regain fully its original tone depends on how much trauma to muscular, neural and connective tissue was sustained in childbirth [1].

2.2.2 Physiological Adaptation in the Reproductory System

The term involution refers to the process by which the organs of the reproductive system revert back to the usual non-pregnant state. As soon as delivery occurs, the uterus and, in particular, the site of the previous placenta undergo a swift process of contraction to achieve haemostasis. When the uterus contracts in such a rapid way, the mother may experience abdominodynia or cramping. Following delivery, the uterine mass is 1 kg, and it possesses a high degree of tone and is firm to the touch. One week later, its mass has reduced to 500 g, and at the sixth week postpartum, the mass is even less at around 50 g. The first stage in uterine shrinkage occurs due to a reduction in the size of the myometrium. The cells get smaller and remain contracted to prevent further haemorrhage. The second stage in shrinking comes about because the vasculature undergoes autolysis and a degree of infarction [4–7]. As the levels of oestrogen and progesterone fall, enzymes capable of proteolysis, such as uterine collagenase, become active, promoting autolysis [8]. There is fibrosis and hyaline degeneration in the intimal and elastic layers of the wall of arteries supplying the uterus, and this produces infarcted regions. Autolysed cell fragments are scavenged by histiocytes. The endometrial base and surface undergo necrosis and are shed [9]. A new endometrial lining is generally regenerated after a fortnight or 3 weeks [4, 10].

There is a discharge of these tissues via the vagina, which is referred to as lochia. The initial lochia rubra is red and is formed from blood, decidual tissue, shed endometrium and mucus. It is discharged for up to 4 days. In the next stage, from the fifth to the ninth day, the lochia is brownish or somewhat yellow and made up of blood, mucus and white cells. The final stage of lochia is whitish and consists principally of mucus. It may be seen from the tenth to the fourteenth postpartum day. In some cases, lochia may still be observed on the fifth week after delivery. If lochia rubra lasts for more than 7 days, this may be because the uterus has insufficiently involuted following delivery. If lochia is associated with a bad smell or there are substantial-sized tissue fragments or thrombus in the discharge, or if lochia fails to occur, infection should be suspected [11–13]. In the initial period following delivery, the cervix and vagina may be swollen and bruised and thus may require longer to recover from birth trauma [14].

As the ovaries return to their usual role, the vaginal rugae reform, a development that typically has already happened by week 3 after delivery, unless the mother is lactating. The epithelial lining of the vagina has an atrophic appearance on cytology during the puerperium, but afterwards (from week 6 up to week 10) after labour, this atrophy resolves. If the mother is nursing, the atrophic appearances persist for longer, since the low oestrogen levels which caused it persist during lactation. The perineum may well be swollen and may tear during labour or be damaged by an episiotomy, and this can lead to pain and discomfort immediately after delivery [4, 15, 16].

2.2.3 Physiological Changes in Breasts

The breasts undergo physiological adaptations during the entire period the woman is pregnant. Even at only the 16th week of the pregnancy, the breasts may be capable of secreting milk, i.e. lactogenesis has already occurred by this point. Placental production of progesterone results in a high plasma concentration, which then stimulates the mature alveolar cells within the mammary glands to secrete milk in small quantities. Once the placenta has been delivered, progesterone levels fall precipitously, and this activates the synthesis of milk and the filling up (engorgement) of the mother's breast following delivery. From the first to around the fourth postpartum day, the breasts secrete a liquid termed colostrum. Colostrum contains a high level of protein and contains protective antibodies which help to defend the neonate against infection. Colostrum has already been formed in the mammary glands before the baby's suckling causes it to be released. Initially, control of milk synthesis is under endocrine control, but this process then becomes autocrine-directed, insofar as release of milk by the breast triggers fresh production. In the first week postpartum, the milk changes in composition, such that it supplies the entire nutritional requirements of the newborn. During the whole period for which lactation occurs, the composition of milk keeps maturing in line with the developing nutritional needs of the infant [1].

During lactation there is a continuous synthesis and release of milk in adequate quantities. For this process to remain operative, milk needs to be regularly taken (emptied) from the breast, an action which stimulates prolactin secretion by the adenohypophysis. The process also depends on the nipple receiving stimulation by the infant suckling, which activates release of oxytocin from the neurohypophysis. There is a contractile response of the myoepithelial cells within the mammary gland to high levels of oxytocin. This contraction propels milk into the lumen of the alveolus and forward into the ducts, which eventually discharge their contents from the nipple. If the mother does not release the milk, milk builds up inside the lumen of the mammary alveoli, and there is an increased pressure within the breast. Distension caused by accumulated milk prevents the vascular supply from reaching the alveoli, and this then interferes with the milk production process. Furthermore, the accumulation of milk causes a rise in a signalling molecule, the Feedback Inhibitor of Lactation (FIL) which causes the level of prolactin to fall. Once breastfeeding halts, the breast involutes and returns to its resting state within the space of between 2 and 3 weeks [1].

2.2.4 Physiological Changes: Lactation

Following delivery, the mammary glands produce even more colostrum. Colostrum contains abundant protein, vitamins and antibodies, together with humoral factors, such as lactoferrin. The humoral factors and immunoglobulins are important in neonatal immune defence against pathogens [17]. Mammogenesis is the physiological adaptation of the mammary gland to enable lactation. It commences during pregnancy. The cells of the ducts, lobules and alveoli increase in size and in number [18]. However, during pregnancy, the existence of elevated plasma concentrations of oestrogen and progesterone renders the mammary gland unable to respond to prolactin. With the precipitous fall in oestrogen and progesterone after delivery, the breast starts to secrete milk in response to stimulation by prolactin. Lactogenesis (milk production) begins 3–4 days after delivery. When the nipple is stimulated by suckling, there are afferent impulses carried by the sensory nerves of the thorax towards the hypothalamic paraventricular and supraoptic nuclei. These nuclei then stimulate the neurohypophysis to manufacture and release oxytocin, a hormone which causes myoepithelial cells to contract, propelling milk into and along the mammary ducts, a process termed galactokinesis. Other terms used to describe the response to oxytocin are milk ejection and let-down. There are a number of ways in which galactokinesis may fail to occur, in particular if the woman is in pain or is suffering from anxiety, low mood or depressive disorder, or the breasts are over-engorged. Prolactin is essential to keeping the mammary gland functioning efficiently and continuously to produce milk, i.e. performing galactopoiesis. The breasts normally release between half a litre and 800 mL milk daily in a healthy mother. For this volume of galactopoiesis, the mother must have available 700 kcal each day. Pregnant women may store up to 5 kg of additional adipose tissue whilst pregnant, and this store may be used up if the woman fails to consume adequate calories. A frequent complication during breastfeeding is the development of sore nipples or mastitis [4, 19, 20].

2.3 Physiological Changes in the Endocrine System

When a woman recommences menstruation following childbirth varies, with breastfeeding playing a key role. Women who do not nurse their infants generally begin menstruating between 6 and 8 weeks after delivery. The number of anovulatory cycles is influenced by how often the infant feeds and how much milk is consumed. This effect is mediated through the highly elevated plasma prolactin concentration seen following suckling [19]. In the presence of high levels of prolactin, the ovary does not respond to follicle-stimulating hormone (FSH). Furthermore, prolactin also prevents secretion of luteinising hormone (LH). Thus, elevated prolactin levels suppress gonadotropin release. Breastfeeding acts as a naturally occurring contraceptive in breastfeeding women for the initial months after childbirth. However, menstruation typically re-establishes itself around 4–5 months after delivery, albeit it may be as much as 2 years delayed. Even if there is no shedding of menses, egg release may still occur and thus pregnancy is possible [20–22]. Mothers who are not nursing will require contraception starting 3 weeks after delivery, whilst those who are nursing will require contraception starting 3 months after childbirth [23]. Immediately after delivery, there is a sudden drop in the plasma concentration of human chorionic gonadotropin. This hormone mimics the action of thyroid-stimulating hormone (TSH). The result is that the thyroid undergoes enlargement during pregnancy. Following delivery, the thyroid involutes and is back to its non-pregnant state in functional terms by 4 weeks after delivery, and in size terms by 12 weeks after delivery [24, 25]. The placenta secretes insulinase, corticotropin-releasing hormone and human placental lactogen, which produce insulin resistance in pregnant women, i.e. pregnancy induces a diabetes-like state [26]. Once birth occurs, the woman's insulin resistance rapidly decreases, and the diabetogenic effect is lost by the second or third day postpartum [27]. If the mother suffers from obesity, the insulin resistance may persist for longer, up to 15 or 16 weeks after giving birth [4, 28].

2.4 Physiological Changes in Fluid Balance

During pregnancy, fluid moves from the extravascular to intravascular compartment. This equates to an increase in total body water of between 6 and 8 L, caused by retention of 950 mEq sodium, under control of the renin-angiotensin-aldosterone system [29]. Following delivery there is a 50% elevation in the circulating atrial natriuretic peptide, with inhibition of aldosterone, angiotensin II and vasopressin. This leads the kidneys to lose sodium. There is a large amount of urine passed for 2 weeks following delivery, with a daily urine volume passed of 3 L not being unusual. This increased urinary output usually correlates with the extent of increase in total body water whilst the woman was pregnant. At a point 8 weeks after delivery, the glomerular filtration rate should be as it was in the pre-pregnant state [30]. Sometimes there is lactose detectable in the urine of nursing mothers 3 or 4 days after breastfeeding begins [4, 31].

2.5 Physiological Changes in the Haematological System

There may be an initial fall in the mother's haematocrit if the delivery resulted in substantial haemorrhage, but this returns to normal as the woman passes increasing volumes of urine and the blood begins to be more concentrated [32]. The haematocrit should be normal 3–5 days after delivery, following the reduction in circulating volume. The haemoglobin level varies somewhat after childbirth, reflecting inter-compartmental movement of fluid. Research which examined serial haemoglobin measurements in women following delivery has shown that haemoglobin does not return to its pre-pregnancy levels until between 4 and 6 months after delivery [33]. The stress surrounding giving birth may result in a raised white cell count (around 25,000 cells per cubic mm). This leucocytosis resolves in 4 weeks or less after delivery [34]. The low platelet count related to pregnancy is rectified within 4–10 days following childbirth, as new thrombocytes are manufactured to replace those consumed whilst the baby was being delivered [35, 36]. Whilst the woman is pregnant, there is a steady rise in the levels of fibrinogen; factors VII, VIII, X and XII; and von Willebrand factor, and ristocetin-induced platelet aggregation increases. This pro-thrombotic state is a protective reflex which makes massive haemorrhage during delivery less likely [36]. Shortly after delivery the level of fibrinogen remains elevated, whilst the thrombocyte count also returns to the basal value. However, tissue plasminogen activity does not increase towards normal at this stage, so the pro-thrombotic state persists. However, the haemostatic parameters do return to normal in the months following delivery, with clotting values being unexceptional when measured around 8–12 weeks after delivery [4, 37, 38].

2.6 Physiological Changes in the Cardiovascular System

During pregnancy, there are raised plasma concentrations of progesterone and relaxin, manufactured by the corpus luteum and placenta. These hormones cause the systemic vessels to dilate, and the systemic vascular resistance (SVR) therefore keeps falling. The SVR is between 35 and 40% less in pregnant women, but this returns to its basal level 2 weeks after delivery. The systemic tension falls by between 5 and 10 mmHg in pregnant women, with this effect more noticeable on the diastolic than systolic value. In the final trimester of pregnancy, the blood pressure begins to go up again, and it is back to its basal value 16 weeks after delivery [39]. The cardiac rate steadily rises as the pregnancy progresses, settling at 10–20 beats per minute above the pre-pregnant rate. This effect has disappeared by 6 weeks after delivery [4, 40]. In pregnant women the ventricles change shape, with the left ventricle becoming thicker and having a mass some 28–52% above the pre-pregnant value. Some of the recently published research in this area indicates that there may also be a 40% increase in the size and weight of the right ventricle, too. At a point 4 weeks after delivery, this normal change has reverted back to the size, and mass that existed before pregnancy occurred [41, 42]. Neither the contractile strength of the heart nor the ventricular ejection fraction alter significantly during pregnancy or postpartum [4, 40].

References

1. Kansky C. Normal and abnormal puerperium. In: Isaacs C, editor. Medscape. 2016. https://emedicine.medscape.com/article/260187-overview#a2. Accessed online 21 Apr 2021.
2. Oppenheimer LW, Sherriff EA, Goodman JD. The duration of lochia. Br J Obstet Gynaecol. 1986;93(7):754–7.
3. Sherman D, Lurie S, Frenkel E. Characteristics of normal lochia. Am J Perinatol. 1999;16(8):399–402.
4. Chauhan G, Tadi P. Physiology, postpartum changes. [Updated 2020 Dec 8]. In: StatPearls [Internet]. Treasure Island: StatPearls Publishing; 2021. https://www.ncbi.nlm.nih.gov/books/NBK555904/.
5. Negishi H, Kishida T, Yamada H, Hirayama E, Mikuni M, Fujimoto S. Changes in uterine size after vaginal delivery and cesarean section determined by vaginal sonography in the puerperium. Arch Gynecol Obstet. 1999;263(1–2):13–6.
6. Mulic-Lutvica A, Bekuretsion M, Bakos O, Axelsson O. Ultrasonic evaluation of the uterus and uterine cavity after normal, vaginal delivery. Ultrasound Obstet Gynecol. 2001;18(5):491–8. https://doi.org/10.1046/j.0960-7692.2001.00561.x.
7. Sokol ER, Casele H, Haney EI. Ultrasound examination of the postpartum uterus: what is normal? J Matern Fetal Neonatal Med. 2004;15(2):95–9. https://doi.org/10.1080/14767050310001650798.
8. Cyganek A, Wyczalkowska-Tomasik A, Jarmuzek P, Grzechocinska B, Jabiry-Zieniewicz Z, Paczek L, Wielgos M. Activity of proteolytic enzymes and level of cystatin C in the Peripartum period. Biomed Res Int. 2016;2016:7065821. https://doi.org/10.1155/2016/7065821. Epub 2016 Jan 20.
9. Anderson WR, Davis J. Placental site involution. Am J Obstet Gynecol. 1968;102(1):23–33. https://doi.org/10.1016/0002-9378(68)90428-6.
10. Sharman A. Post-partum regeneration of the human endometrium. J Anat. 1953;87(1):1–10.
11. Sherman D, Lurie S, Frenkel E, Kurzweil Y, Bukovsky I, Arieli S. Characteristics of normal lochia. Am J Perinatol. 1999;16(8):399–402. https://doi.org/10.1055/s-1999-6818.
12. Oppenheimer LW, Sherriff EA, Goodman JD, Shah D, James CE. The duration of lochia. Br J Obstet Gynaecol. 1986;93(7):754–7.
13. Chi C, Bapir M, Lee CA, Kadir RA. Puerperal loss (lochia) in women with or without inherited bleeding disorders. Am J Obstet Gynecol. 2010;203(1):56.e1–5. https://doi.org/10.1016/j.ajog.2010.02.042. Epub 2010 Apr 24.
14. McLaren HC. The involution of the cervix. Br Med J. 1952;1(4754):347–52. https://doi.org/10.1136/bmj.1.4754.347.
15. Christianson LM, Bovbjerg VE, McDavitt EC, Hullfish KL. Risk factors for perineal injury during delivery. Am J Obstet Gynecol. 2003;189(1):255–60. https://doi.org/10.1067/mob.2003.547.
16. Albers L, Garcia J, Renfrew M, McCandlish R, Elbourne D. Distribution of genital tract trauma in childbirth and related postnatal pain. Birth. 1999;26(1):11–7. https://doi.org/10.1046/j.1523-536x.1999.00011.x. PMID: 10352050.

17. Thapa BR. Health factors in colostrum. Indian J Pediatr. 2005;72(7):579–81. https://doi. org/10.1007/BF02724182. PMID: 16077241.
18. Lamote I, Meyer E, Massart-Leën AM, Burvenich C. Sex steroids and growth factors in the regulation of mammary gland proliferation, differentiation, and involution. Steroids. 2004;69(3):145–59. https://doi.org/10.1016/j.steroids.2003.12.008. PMID: 15072917.
19. Crowley WR. Neuroendocrine regulation of lactation and milk production. Compr Physiol. 2015;5(1):255–91. https://doi.org/10.1002/cphy.c140029. PMID: 25589271.
20. The World Health Organization multinational study of breast-feeding and lactational amenorrhea. II. Factors associated with the length of amenorrhea. World Health Organization task force on methods for the natural regulation of fertility. Fertil Steril. 1998;70(3):461–71. https:// doi.org/10.1016/s0015-0282(98)00191-5. PMID: 9757874.
21. Campbell OM, Gray RH. Characteristics and determinants of postpartum ovarian function in women in the United States. Am J Obstet Gynecol. 1993;169(1):55–60. https://doi. org/10.1016/0002-9378(93)90131-2. PMID: 8333476.
22. Campino C, Ampuero S, Díaz S, Serón-Ferré M. Prolactin bioactivity and the duration of lactational amenorrhea. J Clin Endocrinol Metab. 1994;79(4):970–4. https://doi.org/10.1210/ jcem.79.4.7962307. PMID: 7962307.
23. Jackson E, Glasier A. Return of ovulation and menses in postpartum nonlactating women: a systematic review. Obstet Gynecol. 2011;117(3):657–62. https://doi.org/10.1097/ AOG.0b013e31820ce18c. PMID: 21343770.
24. Gaberšček S, Osolnik J, Zaletel K, Pirnat E, Hojker S. An advantageous role of spectral Doppler sonography in the evaluation of thyroid dysfunction during the postpartum period. J Ultrasound Med. 2016;35(7):1429–36. https://doi.org/10.7863/ultra.15.07033. Epub 2016 May 20. PMID: 27208199.
25. Stagnaro-Green A, Abalovich M, Alexander E, Azizi F, Mestman J, Negro R, Nixon A, Pearce EN, Soldin OP, Sullivan S, Wiersinga W, American Thyroid Association Taskforce on Thyroid Disease During Pregnancy and Postpartum. Guidelines of the American Thyroid Association for the diagnosis and management of thyroid disease during pregnancy and postpartum. Thyroid. 2011;21(10):1081–125. https://doi.org/10.1089/thy.2011.0087. Epub 2011 Jul 25. PMID: 21787128; PMCID: PMC3472679.
26. Sonagra AD, Biradar SM, Dattatreya K, Jayaprakash Murthy DS. Normal pregnancy—a state of insulin resistance. J Clin Diagn Res. 2014;8(11):CC01–3. https://doi.org/10.7860/ JCDR/2014/10068.5081. Epub 2014 Nov 20. PMID: 25584208; PMCID: PMC4290225.
27. Ryan EA, O'Sullivan MJ, Skyler JS. Insulin action during pregnancy. Studies with the euglycemic clamp technique. Diabetes. 1985;34(4):380–9. https://doi.org/10.2337/diab.34.4.380. PMID: 3882502.
28. Sivan E, Chen X, Homko CJ, Reece EA, Boden G. Longitudinal study of carbohydrate metabolism in healthy obese pregnant women. Diabetes Care. 1997;20(9):1470–5. https://doi. org/10.2337/diacare.20.9.1470. PMID: 9283800.
29. Ogueh O, Clough A, Hancock M, Johnson MR. A longitudinal study of the control of renal and uterine hemodynamic changes of pregnancy. Hypertens Pregnancy. 2011;30(3):243–59. https://doi.org/10.3109/10641955.2010.484079. PMID: 21740248.
30. Cheung KL, Lafayette RA. Renal physiology of pregnancy. Adv Chronic Kidney Dis. 2013;20(3):209–14. https://doi.org/10.1053/j.ackd.2013.01.012. PMID: 23928384; PMCID: PMC4089195.
31. Andria M, Vargiu N. La lattosuria in gravidanza ed in puerperio [Lactosuria in pregnancy and the puerperium]. Minerva Ginecol. 1968;20(9):773–6. Italian. PMID: 5738768.
32. Nicol B, Croughan-Minihane M, Kilpatrick SJ. Lack of value of routine postpartum hematocrit determination after vaginal delivery. Obstet Gynecol. 1997;90(4 Pt 1):514–8. https://doi. org/10.1016/s0029-7844(97)00354-2. PMID: 9380307.
33. Taylor DJ, Lind T. Red cell mass during and after normal pregnancy. Br J Obstet Gynaecol. 1979;86(5):364–70. https://doi.org/10.1111/j.1471-0528.1979.tb10611.x. PMID: 465384.
34. Chandra S, Tripathi AK, Mishra S, Amzarul M, Vaish AK. Physiological changes in hematological parameters during pregnancy. Indian J Hematol Blood Transfus. 2012;28(3):144–6.

https://doi.org/10.1007/s12288-012-0175-6. Epub 2012 Jul 15. PMID: 23997449; PMCID: PMC3422383.

35. Shehata N, Burrows R, Kelton JG. Gestational thrombocytopenia. Clin Obstet Gynecol. 1999;42(2):327–34. https://doi.org/10.1097/00003081-199906000-00017. PMID: 10370851.

36. Clark P, Brennand J, Conkie JA, McCall F, Greer IA, Walker ID. Activated protein C sensitivity, protein C, protein S and coagulation in normal pregnancy. Thromb Haemost. 1998;79(6):1166–70. PMID: 9657443.

37. de Boer K, ten Cate JW, Sturk A, Borm JJ, Treffers PE. Enhanced thrombin generation in normal and hypertensive pregnancy. Am J Obstet Gynecol. 1989;160(1):95–100. https://doi.org/10.1016/0002-9378(89)90096-3. PMID: 2521425.

38. Eichinger S. D-dimer testing in pregnancy. Pathophysiol Haemost Thromb. 2003–2004;33(5–6):327–9. https://doi.org/10.1159/000083822. PMID: 15692237.

39. Nama V, Antonios TF, Onwude J, Manyonda IT. Mid-trimester blood pressure drop in normal pregnancy: myth or reality? J Hypertens. 2011;29(4):763–8. https://doi.org/10.1097/HJH.0b013e328342cb02. PMID: 21178781.

40. Grindheim G, Estensen ME, Langesaeter E, Rosseland LA, Toska K. Changes in blood pressure during healthy pregnancy: a longitudinal cohort study. J Hypertens. 2012;30(2):342–50. https://doi.org/10.1097/HJH.0b013e32834f0b1c. PMID: 22179091.

41. Umar S, Nadadur R, Iorga A, Amjedi M, Matori H, Eghbali M. Cardiac structural and hemodynamic changes associated with physiological heart hypertrophy of pregnancy are reversed postpartum. J Appl Physiol (1985). 2012;113(8):1253–9. https://doi.org/10.1152/japplphysiol.00549.2012. Epub 2012 Aug 23. PMID: 22923507; PMCID: PMC3472485.

42. Hill JA, Olson EN. Cardiac plasticity. N Engl J Med. 2008;358(13):1370–80. https://doi.org/10.1056/NEJMra072139. PMID: 18367740.

Immune System and Pregnancy

Ugur Muşabak and Tuba Erdoğan

3.1 Introduction

Pregnancy is a physiological process that is necessary for the maintenance of living lineage [1]. The average pregnancy period calculated for women with regular cycles of 28 days corresponds to 280 days or 40 weeks. Whole pregnancy period is divided into three equal trimesters of 3 months each. The success of pregnancy depends on the stages of fertilization, embryo implantation, decidualization and placentation successfully taken place in the first trimester [2, 3]. A healthy pregnancy, in which all periods successfully completed, results in a successful parturition. In the contrary case, female infertility occurs, characterized by implantation failure and/or recurrent miscarriages [3].

Pregnancy genetically resembles to semi-haplotype-compatible solid organ transplants [4]. Half of the genes of embryo comes from the mother and half from the father. Because of this, tissue antigens of the foetus are half compatible with the mother. The antigens referred to herein are human leukocyte antigens (HLA) [5]. These antigens are mainly responsible for adaptive immune responses against foreign antigens. Theoretically, it might be expected that foetus is rejected by the mother's immune system due to foreign tissue antigens coming from the father [6]. However, instead of the rejection of foetus, immune tolerance is developed by the mother's immune system and the placenta [7]. With another point of view, while the life of foetus is maintained by the immune tolerance developed naturally in the maternal womb, the survival of the organ in the solid organ transplantations depends on the success of the immunosuppressive treatment regimens given to the patients.

U. Muşabak (✉) · T. Erdoğan
Division of Immunology and Allergy, Department of Internal Medicine, Baskent University School of Medicine, Ankara, Turkey
e-mail: umusabak@hotmail.com; tubacantc@gmail.com

© The Author(s), under exclusive license to Springer Nature Switzerland AG 2022

C. Cingi et al. (eds.), *ENT Diseases: Diagnosis and Treatment during Pregnancy and Lactation*, https://doi.org/10.1007/978-3-031-05303-0_3

While the traditional view is that the placenta is thought to form a barrier between mother and foetus, recent studies show that foetal or placental components in both mice and humans are widely spread in the maternal bloodstream and accumulate in maternal tissues [7]. Since foreign foetal antigens originating from the father can reach the mother, we are faced with the question of how it is possible that the mother does not develop an immune response and the pregnancy continues. In this article, the immune tolerance mechanisms required for a successful pregnancy will be described in light of the current literature. However, to understand this issue better, some basic knowledges on the pregnancy physiology will also be reminded during the reviewing of the pregnancy immunology.

3.2   Endometrium and Menstrual Cycle

The main cellular components of endometrium are epithelial cells, mesenchymal stromal cells, immune cells and endothelial cells [8, 9]. While single-layer epithelial cells lay the inner surface of the uterus, the epithelial cells invaginated into the stroma form branched tubular glands. Endometrial stroma arising from mesenchymal cells consists of connective tissue and extracellular matrix that supports other neighbouring structures. Endothelial cells participate in the structure of spiral arteries that carry the nutrients and oxygen to the foetus. Adaptive changes also occur in the endometrium, while hormonal changes occur during the menstrual cycle. While the upper layer of the endometrium (functional layer) is shed by menstrual bleeding, the lower layer (basal layer) is responsible for the renewal of the shed layer [9].

The menstrual cycle in humans is approximately 28 days (Fig. 3.1) [10]. Menstrual bleeding occurs between the 0th and 4th day of the cycle. The 5th–13th day of the cycle is called as the follicular phase. In this period, the glandular and vascular structures increase in the endometrium with the influence of oestrogen (E2) hormone. Epidermal growth factor (EGF), transforming growth factor alpha (TGFα), fibroblast growth factor 9 (FGF9) and vascular endothelial growth factor (VEGF) are the other factors affecting the endometrium in the follicular phase [11, 12]. Ovulation occurs on the 14th day of the cycle by the LH peak; then, the luteal phase comes between the 15th–28th day of the cycle. In this period, the endometrium has optimal conditions for implantation with the influence of progesterone (P4). In the luteal phase, together with E2 and P4, the effect of C-X-C motif chemokine ligand 10 (CXCL10), interferon gamma-induced protein 10 (IP-10); C-X-C motif chemokine ligand 11 (CXCL11), interferon-inducible T cell alpha chemoattractant (I-TAC); and interleukin (IL)-15 increases especially decidual NK (dNK) cells and T cells in the endometrium pre-decidual changes which occur in the functional layer [13].

The level of endometrial receptivity is the highest between the 20th and 24th days of cycle which is called as window of implantation (WOI) [12, 14]. If the blastocyst implantation occurs during this time, P4 secretion from the corpus luteum

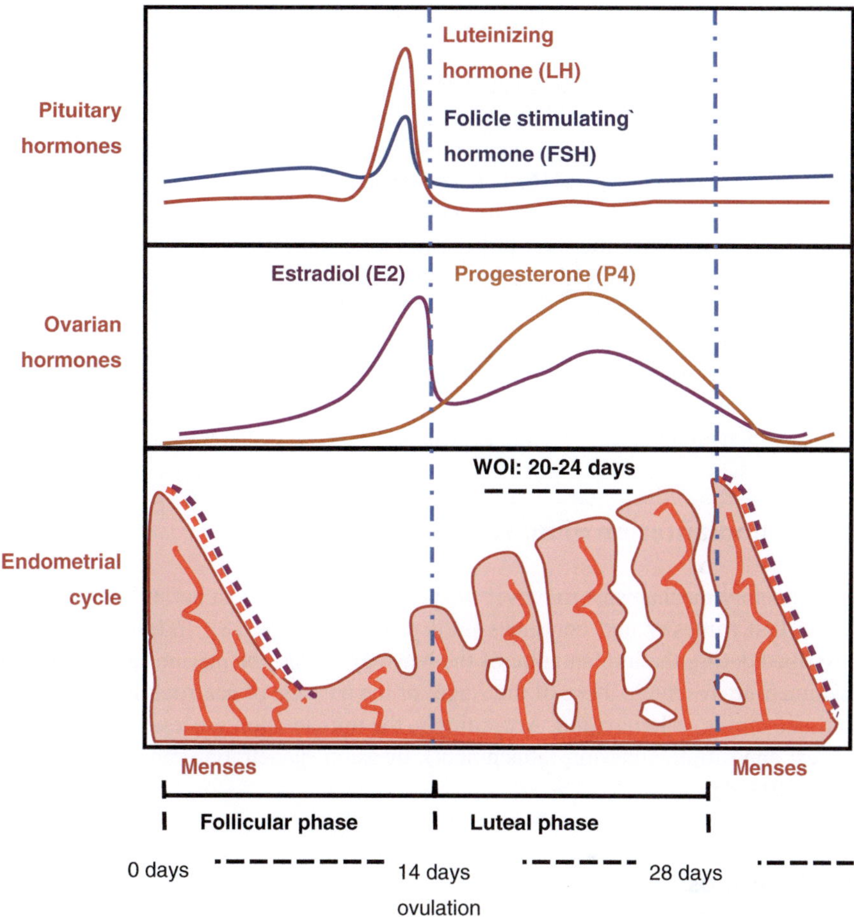

Fig. 3.1 The menstrual cycle

and pre-decidual changes persists in the functional layer of the endometrium. The process after WOI occurs between the 23rd and 28th days of the cycle, in which the endometrial glands and spiral arteries become more prominent. In the same period, immune cells responsible for immunomodulation also continue to accumulate in the stroma. These cells and the various mediators secreted by them are the important factors that determine the success of pregnancy. If blastocyst implantation does not occur, P4 level declines due to luteolysis and the cycle ends with menstrual bleeding [9].

The hormone profile and immune tolerance required for a successful pregnancy appear to be disadvantageous in terms of susceptibility to sexually transmitted infections. However, foetomaternal interface (FMI) is in a dynamic change that adapts to new conditions and various microbial threats [15].

3.3   Fertilization and Blastocyst Formation

The fusion of female and male gametes (oocyte, sperm) in the fallopian tubes is called fertilization [14]. A diploid unicellular zygote is created by this process. The zygote divides consecutively to form a cluster of cells called as morula (postconceptional first and second days) [16, 17]. The cluster of dividing cells moves from the fallopian tubes into the uterine cavity with the help of ciliary motility (postconceptional third day). Once the morula becomes a blastocyst (postconceptional fourth and fifth days), it is now ready for implantation into the endometrium (postconceptional sixth and seventh day). While the embryo develops from the inner cell mass of the blastocyst, placenta develops from the outer layer of the blastocyst which consists of the trophoblast cells (trophectoderm) (Fig. 3.2a). The placenta plays a crucial role in transporting the nutrients and oxygen from the maternal blood to the foetus, which are necessary for the growth and survival of the foetus.

3.4   Implantation of Blastocyst

Inflammatory mechanisms rule over the process that starts just before implantation in the first trimester and continues until placentation [9, 18]. Indeed, the stages described during the implantation of the blastocyst from the uterine cavity into the endometrium resemble those of the stages of the passage of neutrophils from blood to tissue during inflammation. Accordingly, the implantation process has four main stages: apposition, adhesion (attachment), invasion (penetration) and placentation (Fig. 3.2) [14].

3.4.1   Apposition

Apposition is the stage where the blastocyst first encounters with the endometrium (Fig. 3.2a). In this stage, the cytokines and chemokines [IL-6, IL-8, IL-15, tumour necrosis factor alpha (TNFα), granulocyte-macrophage colony-stimulating factor (GM-CSF), chemokine (C-X-C motif) ligand 1 (CXCL1), GRO1 oncogene (GROα); chemokine (C-C motif) ligands 4 (CCL4), macrophage inflammatory protein-1β (MIP-1β)] secreted from endometrial stromal cells at the implantation site create a pro-inflammatory micro-environment and weaken the mucin layer (mucin-1: MUC-1) covering the intrauterine cavity [18, 19]. MUC-1, which is an antiadhesion molecule secreted in the apical surface of the endometrial epithelium in the midluteal phase in dependence on P4 [14]. The role of MUC-1 in the apposition stage is preventing the implantation of blastocyst in the wrong place over the luminal epithelium.

The pro-inflammatory micro-environment also stimulates the expression of an adhesion molecule, L-selectin, which slows the movement of the blastocyst on the endometrial epithelium. The ligand of L-selectin is expressed on the pinopods appearing on the apical surface of luminal epithelium during WOI [20]. Pinopods

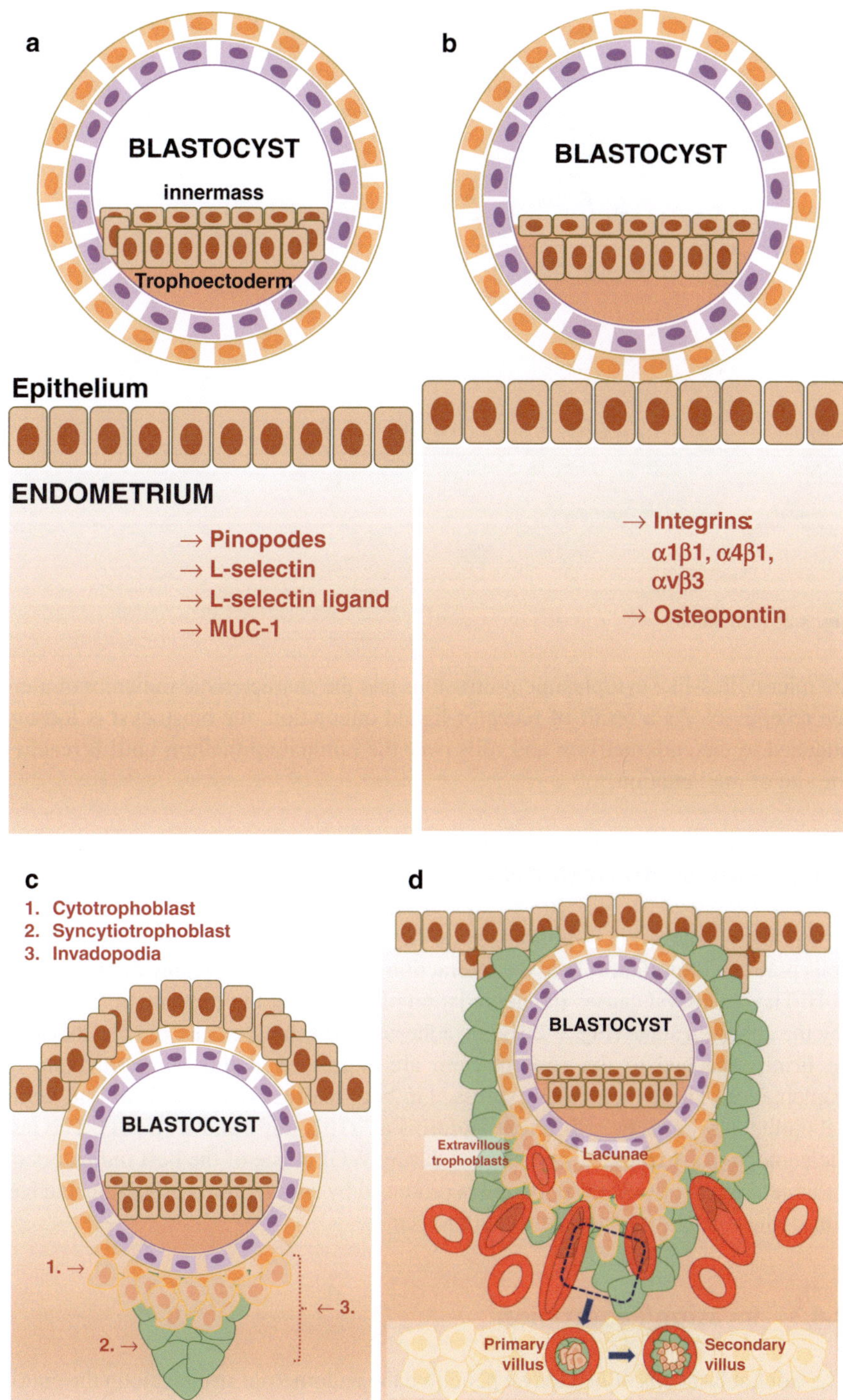

Fig. 3.2 Blastocyst implantation. (**a**) Apposition, (**b**) Adhesion, (**c**) Invasion, (**d**) Placentation, (**e**) Decidualisation and immune regulation

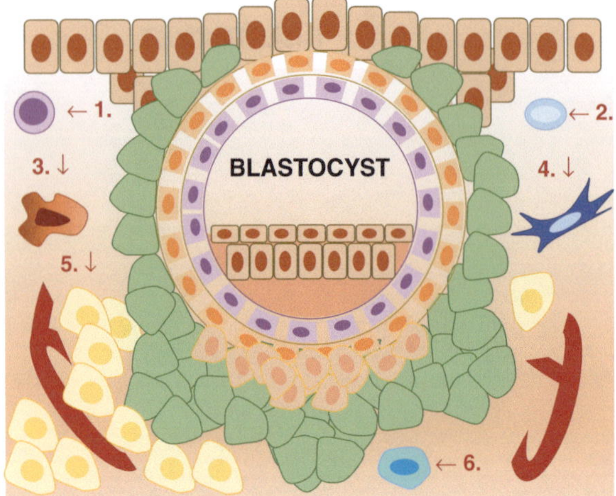

Fig. 3.2 (continued)

are microvillus-like cytoplasmic protrusions and the characteristic indicator of uterine receptivity. As a result of receptor-ligand interaction, the blastocyst is loosely attached to the endometrium and rolls over the luminal epithelium until it reaches the site of implantation.

3.4.2 Adhesion/Attachment

In this stage, leukaemia inhibitory factor (LIF) produced by endometrial epithelial cells plays an important role in the interaction between endometrium and blastocyst [14]. The blastocyst causes the degradation of MUC-1 at the implantation site during the adhesion stage (Fig. 3.2b). The adhesion molecules, ensure the blastocyst to be firmly attached to the endometrium are expressed at this stage, mediate to implantation. These molecules expressed in both blastocyst trophoblasts and luminal epithelium have three different isoforms as $\alpha1\beta1$, $\alpha4\beta1$ and $\alpha V\beta$ [21]. The last molecule, $\alpha v\beta3$, expressed in pinopods during WOI is one of the best indicators of endometrial receptivity. Osteopontin is produced by endometrial epithelium and has a bridging role between the adhesion molecules.

3.4.3 Invasion/Penetration

The trophoblast cells of blastocyst penetrate the endometrial stroma along the endometrial epithelium during the invasion stage (Fig. 3.2c). At the beginning of this process, the invadopodia formed by trophoblast cells migrate through the spaces between adjacent endometrial epithelial cells and reach the basement membrane beneath the epithelial cells [14]. Then, the basement membrane and the extracellular matrix (ECM) are destructed by activated gelatinases (matrix metalloproteinases: MMPs), allowing trophoblasts to reach the stroma [21]. The interaction between selectin and its ligand expressed on the trophoblasts and stromal cells plays a role in the invasion of trophoblasts into the decidua. Once the blastocyst is completely embedded in the endometrium, the implantation site is covered with a fibrin layer. While the pro-inflammatory micro-environment enables trophoblasts to invade the endometrium, trophoblasts secrete chemokines [chemokine (C-C motif) ligands 2 (CCL2), monocyte chemotactic protein-1 (MCP1); C-X-C motif chemokine ligand 12 (CXCL12), stromal cell-derived factor 1 (SDF-1); C-X-C motif chemokine ligand 8 (CXCL8), interleukin-8 (IL-8)] that make the implantation site attractive to immune cells [22].

3.4.4 Placentation

The proliferating trophoblast cells differentiate into outer syncytiotrophoblast and inner cytotrophoblast (postconceptional eighth day) [16, 17]. In the endometrium, the fluid-filled lacunae separated by trabeculae are formed and give the syncytiotrophoblasts a sponge-like appearance (postconceptional 12th day) (Fig. 3.2d) [15, 23]. After the superficial decidual capillaries are surrounded by syncytiotrophoblasts, the lacunae are filled with maternal blood by trophoblast invasion. At the end of this process, as a single and interconnected system, maternal sinusoids result. After the primary villi develop, maternal sinusoids form the intervillous spaces. The proliferating cytotrophoblasts into the trabeculae of the syncytiotrophoblast form the chorionic primary villi (postconceptional 13th day). While secondary villi are formed after the extra-embryonic mesoblast grows into the primary villus (postconceptional 16th day), tertiary villi are formed after the mesoblast differentiates into connective tissue and foetal capillaries (postconceptional 21st day). These vessels connect with the embryonic blood vessels. Thus, the chorionic plate (chorion frondosum), which is the foetal part of the placenta, is formed from the villi, trophoblasts and intervillous spaces [24].

On the other hand, cytotrophoblasts express a high level of adhesion molecules called e-cadherin at the beginning of their differentiation and restrict trophoblast invasion [25]. During the ongoing process, extra-villous trophoblasts grow, and the expression of e-cadherins decreases to facilitate the trophoblast invasion into the decidua, myometrium and uterine vessels. The extra-villous cytotrophoblasts differentiate into interstitial and endovascular trophoblasts. While the first type trophoblasts accumulate around the spiral arteries and prepare them for endovascular trophoblast invasion, the second type trophoblasts enter the lumen of the spiral arteries and spread along the vessels. Thus, the basal plate (decidua basalis), which is the maternal part of the placenta, is formed from the cytotrophoblast (embryonic tissue), and decidua basalis (maternal tissue) [24].

Foetomaternal interface is formed where the foetal and maternal tissues are in contact with each other [14]. Herein, the exchange of nutrients, gases and wastes between mother and foetus is provided by the foetomaternal blood circulation. Ultimately, the placenta functions as an immunomodulatory organ regulating immune responses both at the site of implantation and in the systemic circulation.

3.4.5 Decidualization and Immune Regulation

Once the blastocyst locates under the luminal epithelium, the stromal cells surrounding the blastocyst differentiate into the decidualized cells (Fig. 3.2e) [14, 15]. In midluteal phase, the fibroblast-like stromal cells in the endometrium transform into the round epithelium-like decidual cells because of the effect of P4. This process, which is called pre-decidualization, is necessary for the maintenance of a successful pregnancy. During the decidualization process, not only size of the cells increases, but also the number of cells also gradually increases. Decidual cells demonstrate the characteristics of epithelioid cells in terms of the properties of their cytoplasm, nuclei and the organelles [26]. Accordingly, ECM proteins such as laminin, type IV collagen, fibronectin and heparan sulphate proteoglycans are synthesized by decidual cells. There are the junctions between adjacent decidual cells that allow the trophoblasts to spread and are not as tight as the desmosome [25].

Through the controlled trophoblast invasion, the first contact between the embryo and the mother is provided, but this event does not harm the mother [14]. While the decidua provides a micro-environment that stimulates trophoblast invasion, it limits the aggressive invasion of trophoblast cells by forming a dense ECM [27]. In the first stage, ECM degradation required for trophoblast invasion occurs via MMPs secreted by trophoblasts and stromal cells. In ongoing process, the effects of MMPs are inhibited by tissue inhibitor metalloproteinases (TIMPs) and transforming growth factor beta (TGFβ) secreted from the stromal cells. Herein, the main inhibitor is especially TIMP-3 that is secreted under the influence of P4.

As the foetus grows, it protrudes from the uterine wall into the cavity. In this stage, decidua is divided into three layers as decidua basalis, decidua parietalis and decidua capsularis according to foetus position in the uterine cavity [17]. As the pregnancy progresses, while the decidua basalis forms the discoid placenta with the chorion frondosum (FMI), the remaining parts of the decidua (parietalis capsularis) undergo degeneration [24].

The other important events influencing the success of pregnancy during decidualization are angiogenesis, vascular remodelling and accumulation of immune cells [14, 15]. The immune cells such as dNK, T cells, B cells, dendritic cells and macrophages, surrounding the endometrial glands and vessels, play immunomodulatory roles during the decidualization stage and prevent the rejection of embryo (Fig. 3.2e).

3.5   Hormonal Factors in the Implantation

All the changes and transformations which take place in the endometrium are under the influence of human chorionic gonadotropin (hCG) and the balance between ovarian hormones E2 and P4 [14, 15]. hCG binds to a receptor called luteinizing hormone/choriogonadotropin receptor (LHCGR), which is common with the LH receptor. While the nuclear receptors to which ovarian hormones bind increase in the stromal cells during implantation, they decrease in the epithelial cells of endometrium.

hCG secreted from mainly syncytiotrophoblast stimulates the important signals that increase endometrial receptivity [10, 28]. hCG supports the pregnancy by keeping the corpus luteum alive. In other words, it acts as LH agonist by binding to the LH receptor (LHCGR). hCG contributes to decidualization by stimulating the synthesis and secretion of the enzymes [prostaglandin E synthase (PGES), cyclooxygenase 2 (COX2)] that control prostaglandin E2 (PGE2) production in the endometrial epithelial cells and leading to an increase in c-AMP level in the stromal cells [14].

In addition, hCG triggers the pathways that protect the endometrial stroma against apoptosis and drive it to decidualization [14, 28]. In this way, the Notch pathway plays an important role in the decidualization process [14]. The signalling molecules of this pathway consist of four transmembrane receptors (Notch1 to Notch4) that can bind to transmembrane ligands (Delta-like or Jagged-like) on neighbouring cells. In the endometrium, while the Notch1–3 molecules are expressed in epithelial and stromal cells, their ligands are primarily expressed on epithelial cells. Notch1 expression is enhanced by hCG and P4 [29]. The interaction between Notch1 and its target molecule alpha-smooth muscle actin (αSMA) protects stromal cells from apoptosis and promotes decidualization. Forkhead box protein O1 (FOXO1), the other target molecule of Notch1, independently increases IGFBP-1 and prolactin (PRL) expression in decidual cells. These molecules are good indicators of decidualization. The other secretory molecules produced in the decidual cells include IL-11, EGF, heparin-binding epidermal growth factor (HB-EGF), activin A and neuropeptides.

In the decidualization process, P4 acts by binding to its nuclear receptor (progesterone receptor A: PGR-A). PGR-A is the dominant isoform in the stromal cells. The genes (decidualization associated) whose synthesis is regulated by P4 are homeobox A10 (HOXO10), FOXO1, bone morphogenetic protein 2 (BMP2), WNT, Krueppel-like factor 9 (KLF9) and FK506-binding protein (FK-BP52) [29–31].

On the other hand, hCG regulates the functions of endometrium and decidual immune cells to synthesize and secretes various factors that support implantation, trophoblast invasion, angiogenesis and tissue remodelling. Accordingly, while hCG leads increase in expression of galectin-3 (GAL3), macrophage migration inhibitory factor (MIF) and VEGF in decidua decrease in expression of PRL, insulin-like growth factor-binding protein-1 (IGFBP-1), macrophage colony-stimulating factor (M-CSF) and TIMPs [32]. Meanwhile, the synthesis of the trophoblasts is also increased by hCG. In addition, hCG allows the uterus to adapt to the growing foetus and suppresses myometrial contractions.

3.6 Cytokines in the Implantation

Implantation is a mild inflammatory process that is under the control of certain cytokines [14, 15]. These cytokines play a role in initiating the inflammatory process, binding the blastocyst to the endometrium, remodelling endometrial tissue, developing immune tolerance against the embryo and formation of the placenta. The cytokines that have pro-inflammatory properties and involved in the implantation are mainly LIF, IL-6 and IL-1β.

LIF: LIF is produced by the endometrium and blastocyst and regulates the growth and development of the embryo [33]. However, this cytokine primarily acts on both receptive endometrium and stroma and contributes the implantation and decidualization processes by increasing the production of various cytokines and PGE2. This cytokine, as well as mediating the interaction between blastocyst and endometrial pinopods, plays a role in the development of trophoblasts and placenta [14, 20]. Finally, LIF stimulates the recruitment of immune cells involved in the implantation and decidualization process.

IL-1β: IL-1β is secreted at the highest level by cytotrophoblasts in the first trimester of pregnancy [14]. This cytokine stimulates COX2 synthesis in stromal cells [18]. In the presence of E2 and P4, IL-1β together with COX2 and PGE2 contributes to the decidualization process by increasing the cyclic adenosine monophosphate (cAMP) level in stromal cells. As a result, IGFBP-1 expression increases in decidual cells. In the stromal cells, IL-1β also stimulates the stromal cells for MMP3 synthesis in inactive form. As a result of the activation of this precursor molecule, ECM is disrupted, and the changes occur in the cytoskeletal structure of the stromal cells.

IL-6: IL-6 is mainly produced by endometrial epithelium and stromal cells [14]. Its level is the highest in the midluteal phase, but gradually declines towards late secretory phase. The high level of IL-6, especially in WOI, indicates that this cytokine has a crucial role in the pre-implantation period [34].

3.7 The Composition of Immune Cells in Decidua

Foetomaternal interface consisting of trophoblasts and maternal decidua is a specialized tissue that provides nutrition and oxygenation of the foetus and protects it from the maternal immune system so as not to be reject because of its semi-allogenic feature [4, 6, 7]. The studies show that the immune cells at the FMI develop immune tolerance against the foetus rather than an immune response. Immune tolerance to foetus is achieved by decidual immune cells and peripheral tolerance mechanisms of gravida. It has been reported that uterine microbiota also affects immune tolerance mechanisms during pregnancy [35].

In the decidua, the main cell types are decidualized endometrial stromal cells, as well as haematopoietic immune cells (Fig. 3.2e) [36]. The composition and functions of immune cells present some differences according to pregnancy period for successful formation and maintenance of pregnancy. In especially implantation process, these cells have immune-tolerant phenotypes of the NK cells, macrophages, dendritic cells, T cells and B cells, and provide a micro-environment conducive to foetal growth [36]. The essential factors determining the distribution of immune cells and their immunophenotypes are various cytokines, chemokines and angiogenic factors secreted from the cellular components of decidual micro-environment under the influence of sex hormones and hCG [32].

dNK cells: The NK cells are specialized for killing the cells either infected with virus or transformed to tumour [36]. The functions of NK cells are regulated by receptors with activator and inhibitory properties expressed on their surface [37]. The numbers, immunophenotypes and functions of NK cells in the circulating peripheral blood are different from decidual NK cells [38]. While the ratio of NK cells is between 5 and 10% of all lymphocytes in peripheral blood, this ratio increases to 70–90% in decidua during pregnancy. Most of the NK cells in peripheral blood (pNK) have cytotoxic properties, and CD56 expression level is low (CD56^{dim}) on their surface. However, most of the decidual NK cells have immunomodulatory properties, and CD56 expression level is high (CD56^{bright}) on their surface [39]. In other words, 90% of pNK cells is CD16$^+$CD56^{dim} and has cytotoxic capability, while 80% of dNK cells is CD16$^-$CD56^{bright} and has an immunomodulatory capability. There is a higher level of killer-cell immunoglobulin-like receptors (KIRs), CD94/NKG2A (NKG2 receptors dimerized with CD94 molecule) and C-X-C chemokine receptor type 6 (CXCR6: CD186) expression in dNK cells compared to those of pNK cells. After NKG2A receptor binds to HLA-C and HLA-E ligands, they generate inhibitory signals in target cells.

The dNK cells begin to increase in the midluteal phase in the endometrium and become the dominant cell population during implantation period in the early pregnancy. Besides the immunomodulatory cytokines [TGFβ, interferon gamma (IFNγ), TNFα, GM-CSF, IL-4, IL-5, IL-10, IL-13, etc.] for implantation, they secrete some angiogenic factors for angiogenesis and vascular remodelling [CXCL10 (IP-10), angiopoietin-2 (Ang-2), placental growth factor (PLGF), EGF, VEGF] [39]. In addition, the dNK cells produce the chemokines that can attract both granulocytes and T cells, such as IL-8, C-C motif chemokine ligand 5 (CCL5), regulated upon activation, normal T cell expressed and secreted (RANTES); chemokine (C-C motif) ligands 3 (CCL3), macrophage inflammatory protein 1α (MIP-1α); and CXCL12 (SDF-1) and chemokine (C-C motif) ligands 4 (CCL4), macrophage inflammatory protein-1β (MIP-1β). In the decidua, IFNγ arising from the dNK cells stimulates CD14$^+$ cells to synthesize a molecule called indoleamine 2,3-dioxygenase (IDO) that plays a key role in placental development [39, 40]. It has been shown experimentally that regulatory T cells (Tregs) responsible for immune tolerance to foetus are differentiated from the unpolarized T cells co-cultured with dNK cells and CD14+ cells. In addition, while the dNK cells suppress the activation and proliferation of T cells by secreting immunomodulatory molecules such as galectin-1 and glycodelin-A, they support the development of tolerant immunophenotypes such as Th2 and Treg [41].

The cytotoxicity of dNK cells is low despite their cytotoxic granule content. The interaction of dNK cells with HLA-E and HLA-G molecules expressed in trophoblasts suppresses their cytotoxic activity [39]. On the other hand, the soluble HLA-G (sHLA-G) molecule stimulates cellular ageing signals by binding to the KIR2DL4 ligand commonly expressed in NK cells [40]. Accordingly, while the cytotoxicity of NK cells decreases, their secretion profile changes in favour of angiogenesis and vascular remodelling in decidua. Thus, the cytokines comprising IL-1β, IL-6, IL-8 and urokinase plasminogen activator receptor (uPAR) constitute the senescence-associated secretion phenotype (SASP) [42].

The dNK cell cytotoxicity may increase in an inflammatory micro-environment. For example, cytomegalovirus (CMV)-infected cells activate the dNK cells via NKG2C/D/E receptors, giving them cytotoxic properties [43]. Additionally, while dNKs are stimulated with different pathogen-associated molecular patterns (PAMPs), they produce different amounts of inflammatory cytokines such as IFNγ, IL-6 and TNFα [44]. While toll-like receptor (TLR)3 or TLR9 stimulation with PAMPs most strongly increases cytokine synthesis in dNK cells, TLR2, TLR3 and TLR9 stimulation increases the production in favour of TNFα. These findings support that dNK cells develop a balanced inflammatory response to microbial stimuli.

Dendritic cells: Maternal dendritic cells are professional antigen-presenting cells and act as a bridge between innate and adaptive immunity [36]. The maternal dendritic cells are 1–2% of the immune cells in the decidua. Although the migration capability of maternal dendritic cells in the decidua to secondary lymphoid organs is low, foetal antigens can be transferred to secondary lymphoid organs by foetomaternal circulation [45]. Herein, the foetal antigens released from trophoblasts by apoptosis transform the dendritic cells into tolerogenic immunophenotype. The presentation of processed foetal antigens by dendritic cells "in the presence of retinoic acid, TGFβ and IDO" stimulates Treg development from unpolarized CD4+ T cells (helper T cell 0: Th 0). Either central or peripherally induced Tregs prevent the miscarriages by suppressing the effector T cells located at the FMI. After the priming of naive T cells by dendritic cells, effector or memory T cells that have anergic (CD4+) or hypofunctional (CD8+) features also differentiate [46]. Meanwhile, T cells reactive to foetal antigens undergo apoptosis and are deleted.

T cells: The maternal T cells, most of which are CD8+ T cells and Tregs, constitute 3–10% of the immune cells in the decidua [36]. While the Th1 cells (CXCR3+CCR4−CCR6−) are higher in decidua than peripheral blood (maternal) in the first trimester, Th2 and Th17 cells are lower [47]. It has been suggested that these cells play a role in CD8+ T cell activation. Although Th1 cells in the decidua produce high levels of IFNγ, the main source of this cytokine is dNK cells. After a successful implantation process, foetal growth and development accelerate in the second trimester. At this stage, the gravida, placenta and foetus are symbiotic. The inflammatory environment completes its task and leaves its place to the anti-inflammatory environment [36]. Then, the Th1/Th2 balance increases in favour of Th2. The effector T (Teff) cells sensitive to foetal antigens are inhibited by the cytokines (IL-10, TGFβ, IL-35) secreted from Tregs and IDO secreted from M2 phenotype macrophages.

The Th17 cell population is also found in the decidua, and these cells multiply during pregnancy, although not as much as Treg cells [36]. While Th17 cells, which have a pro-inflammatory phenotype, act as a defence against microbial infections at the FMI, the Tregs also regulate the functions of these cells. The alterations in Th17/Treg ratio in decidua have been shown to be associated with spontaneous abortions, pre-eclampsia and preterm labour [48].

γδT cells are a subgroup of T cells whose role in pregnancy is not sufficiently known. These cells make up 5–10% of circulating T cells in adult peripheral blood and form a bridge between innate and adaptive immunity [49]. There is a difference between the phenotypes of these cells between decidua parietalis and basalis. While more than 50% of cells express Vδ1 in the former, more than 90% of cells express Vδ2 in the latter. It has been shown that an increase in the ratio of Vδ2/Vδ1 in decidua is associated with the risk of early pregnancy loss.

Macrophages: The macrophages are divided into two subgroups according to their inflammatory and anti-inflammatory properties. The decidual macrophages, most of them are in the M2 subgroup, constitute 20–25% of the immune cells in the decidua [36, 50]. They play a role in tissue regeneration during trophoblast invasion and placental development. Due to their high phagocytic capacity, decidual macrophages effectively remove the cells that undergo apoptosis and are damaged. In this way, the encounter of the paternal antigens with the maternal immune system is minimized, and a harmful immune response against the embryo is prevented.

Bregs: The regulatory B cells (Bregs), a rare cell population in decidua, provide a tolerogenic micro-environment herein by secreting IL-10 and TGF [49]. In addition, these cells inhibit the maturation of immature dendritic cells, and keep them tolerogenic.

iNKT cells: Although the human studies are inadequate, the experimental studies shown that invariant natural killer T cell (iNKT) cells are involved in maternal immune tolerance mechanisms [49]. These cells are activated by stimulation with glycolipids presented by a nonclassical MHC complex, CD1d. On the one hand, the ability to produce cytokines with both inflammatory and anti-inflammatory properties and, on the other hand, their cytotoxic capability through fas/fasL interaction make iNKT cells as a powerful effector cell population.

ILC3: It has been shown that there are two types of type 3 innate lymphoid cells (ILC3) in the decidua in the first trimester in humans, one of which produces IL-22 and IL-8 and the other produces TNFα and IL-17A [49]. There are also ILC1 cells that produce IFNγ in the decidua. Therefore, it has been suggested that these cells contribute to the recruitment of neutrophils to the decidua and have roles in the microbial defence. However, their role in foetomaternal tolerance has not been investigated in detail yet.

3.8 Microbiota

Maternal microbiota contributes to the development of a tolerogenic, anti-inflammatory environment in the second trimester of pregnancy [36]. The trophoblast cells express TLRs and nod-like receptors (NLRs) that can detect commensal bacterial products and bind to them. When TLR4 expressed on the surface of trophoblast cells is stimulated by lipopolysaccharide (LPS), the pathway that triggers type I IFN (IFNα, IFNβ) production is activated instead of NFκB-mediated inflammatory response. Type I IFNs trigger apoptosis in the active T cells and increase the production of immunosuppressive molecules such as IL-10, PDL1 and IDO. Type I IFNs protect the foetus against rejection through their antiviral and anti-inflammatory effects. Some viral infections such as influenza A counteract the production of type I IFNs provided by the commensal microbiota and their immunomodulatory effects. In this case, the response of trophoblast cells to commensal bacteria may shift from a state of tolerance to a cytokine storm that promotes premature birth.

3.9 Delivery

In the third trimester, there is a switch to an inflammatory and Th1-type immune state, which is necessary for labour and delivery [36]. Immediately after foetal development is complete, a pro-inflammatory environment is required for delivery [36, 51]. This happens when surfactant-A protein secreted from foetal lungs and damage-associated molecular patterns (DAMPs) (high mobility group box 1: HMGB1) produced as a result of stress activates nuclear factor kappa B (NFκB) pathway via TLR4. The entry of macrophages into the myometrium and subsequent release of pro-inflammatory cytokines are crucial to stimulate contraction of the uterus, separation of the placenta and the birth of the baby [51].

3.10 Conclusions

The immune system plays an active role as in coordination with endocrine changes in the pregnancy process that starts with implantation and continues until birth. Healthy progression of pregnancy and labour take place under the condition in which natural immunomodulation mechanisms work in favour of inflammation or immune tolerance specific to the period of pregnancy. Qualitative or quantitative insufficiencies in these mechanisms result in early pregnancy loss, implantation failure, preterm birth, pre-eclampsia and ultimately infertility. For this reason, the full explanation of the immune mechanisms during pregnancy will shed light on the studies conducted for the treatment of these adverse pregnancy outcomes. However, it is possible to carry out human studies on pregnancy to some extent due to ethical rules. Therefore, emphasis should be placed on in vivo and in vitro experimental studies rather than human studies. On the other hand, explaining the naturally developing immune tolerance mechanisms against semi-haplotype-compatible semi-allograph (foetus) will also pave the way for important discoveries in the treatment of allergic and immunological diseases and in tumour and transplantation immunology.

References

1. Sawin SW, Morgan MA. Dating of pregnancy by trimesters: a review and reappraisal. Obstet Gynecol Surv. 1996;51:261–4.
2. Mor G, Cardenas I, Abrahams V, Guller S. Inflammation and pregnancy: the role of the immune system at the implantation site. Ann N Y Acad Sci. 2011;1221:80–7.
3. Laird S, Tuckerman E, Li TC. Cytokine expression in the endometrium of women with implantation failure and recurrent miscarriage. Reprod Biomed Online. 2006;13:13–23.
4. Ober C. HLA and pregnancy: the paradox of the fetal allograft. Am J Hum Genet. 1998;62:1–5.
5. Turner D. The human leucocyte antigen (HLA) system. Vox Sang. 2004;87:87–90.
6. Hunt JS, Orr HT. HLA and maternal-fetal recognition. FASEB J. 1992;6:2344–8.
7. Adams K, Yan Z, Stevens A, Nelson JL. The changing maternal "self" hypothesis: a mechanism for maternal tolerance of the fetus. Placenta. 2007;28:378–82.
8. Campo H, Murphy A, Yildiz S, Woodruff T, Cervelló I, Kim JJ. Microphysiological modeling of the human endometrium. Tissue Eng Part A. 2020;26:759–68.
9. Maybin JA, Critchley HOD. Menstrual physiology: implications for endometrial pathology and beyond. Hum Reprod Update. 2015;21:748–61.
10. Kayisli U, Guzeloglu-Kayisli O, Arici A. Endocrine-immune interactions in human endometrium. Ann N Y Acad Sci. 2004;1034:50–63.
11. Ejskjær K, Sørensen B, Poulsen S, Mogensen O, Forman A, Nexø E. Expression of the epidermal growth factor system in human endometrium during the menstrual cycle. Mol Hum Reprod. 2005;11:543–51.
12. Jabbour HN, Kelly RW, Fraser HM, Critchley HOD. Endocrine regulation of menstruation. Endocr Rev. 2006;27:17–46.
13. Santoni A, Carlino C, Gismondi A. Uterine NK cell development, migration and function. Reprod Biomed Online. 2008;16:202–10.
14. Ochoa-Bernal MA, Fazleabas AT. Physiologic events of embryo implantation and decidualization in human and non-human primates. Int J Mol Sci. 2020;21:1973.
15. Robertson SA, Petroff MG, Hunt JSJ. Knobil and Neill's physiology of reproduction. 4th ed. Immunology of pregnancy. Oxford; 2015. p. 1835–1874.
16. Coticchio G, Lagalla C, Sturmey R, Pennetta F, Borini A. The enigmatic morula: mechanisms of development, cell fate determination, self-correction and implications for ART. Hum Rerod Update. 2019;25:422–38.
17. Mundy DC, Vilchez G. Overview of the normal development of the human embryo and fetus. In: The diagnosis and management of the acute abdomen in pregnancy. Springer; 2018. p. 25–39.
18. Castro-Rendon W, Castro-Alvarez J, Guzman-Martinez C, Bueno-Sanchez JC. Blastocyst-endometrium interaction: intertwining a cytokine network. Braz J Med Biol Res. 2006;39:1373–85.
19. Simón C, Caballero-Campo P, García-Velasco JA, Pellicer A. Potential implications of chemokines in reproductive function: an attractive idea. J Reprod Immunol. 1998;38:169–93.
20. Quinn KE, Matson BC, Wetendorf M, Caron KM. Pinopodes: recent advancements, current perspectives, and future directions. Mol Cell Endocrinol. 2020;501:110644.
21. Kimber SJ, Spanswick C. Blastocyst implantation: the adhesion cascade. In: Seminars in cell & developmental biology. Elsevier; 2000. p. 77–92.
22. Kayisli UA, Mahutte NG, Arici A. Uterine chemokines in reproductive physiology and pathology. Am J Reprod Immunol. 2002;47:213–21.

23. Ernst LM, Ruchelli ED, Carreon CK, Huff DS. Color atlas of human fetal and neonatal histology. Springer Nature; 2019.
24. Sneddon SF. Embryology of the foetal membranes and placenta. In: Clinical embryology. Springer; 2019. p. 31–38.
25. Adu-Gyamfi EA, Czika A, Gorleku PN, Ullah A, Panhwar Z, Ruan L-L, Ding Y-B, Wang YX. The involvement of cell adhesion molecules, tight junctions, and gap junctions in human placentation. Reprod Sci. 2021;28:305–20.
26. Pan-Castillo B, Gazze SA, Thomas S, Lucas C, Margarit L, Gonzalez D, Francis LW, Conlan RS. Morphophysical dynamics of human endometrial cells during decidualization. Nanomedicine. 2018;14:2235–45.
27. Burrows TD, King A, Loke YW. Trophoblast migration during human placental implantation. Hum Reprod Update. 1996;2:307–21.
28. Silva JF, Serakides R. Intrauterine trophoblast migration: a comparative view of humans and rodents. Cell Adhes Migr. 2016;10:88–110.
29. Afshar Y, Miele L, Fazleabas AT. Notch1 is regulated by chorionic gonadotropin and progesterone in endometrial stromal cells and modulates decidualization in primates. Endocrinology. 2012;153:2884–96.
30. Okada H, Tsuzuki T, Murata H. Decidualization of the human endometrium. Reprod Med Biol. 2018;17:220–7.
31. Large MJ, DeMayo FJ. The regulation of embryo implantation and endometrial decidualization by progesterone receptor signaling. Mol Cell Endocrinol. 2012;358:155–65.
32. Schumacher A, Zenclussen AC. Human chorionic gonadotropin-mediated immune responses that facilitate embryo implantation and placentation. Front Immunol. 2019;10:2896.
33. Aghajanova L. Leukemia inhibitory factor and human embryo implantation. Ann N Y Acad Sci. 2004;1034:176–83.
34. Tabibzadeh S, Kong Q, Babaknia A, May LT. Progressive rise in the expression of interleukin-6 in human endometrium during menstrual cycle is initiated during the implantation window. Hum Reprod. 1995;10:2793–9.
35. Agostinis C, Mangogna A, Bossi F, Ricci G, Kishore U, Bulla R. Uterine immunity and microbiota: a shifting paradigm. Front Immunol. 2019;10:2387.
36. Mor G, Aldo P, Alvero AB. The unique immunological and microbial aspects of pregnancy. Nat Rev Immunol. 2017;17:469–82.
37. Moffett A, Colucci F. Co-evolution of NK receptors and HLA ligands in humans is driven by reproduction. Immunol Rev. 2015;267:283–97.
38. Tohma YA, Musabak U, Gunakan E, Akilli H, Onalan G, Zeyneloglu HB. The role of analysis of NK cell subsets in peripheral blood and uterine lavage samples in evaluation of patients with recurrent implantation failure. J Gynecol Obstet Hum Reprod. 2020;49:101793.
39. Jabrane-Ferrat N. Features of human decidual NK cells in healthy pregnancy and during viral infection. Front Immunol. 2019;10:1397.
40. Vacca P, Cantoni C, Vitale M, Prato C, Canegallo F, Fenoglio D, Ragni N, Moretta L, Mingari MC. Crosstalk between decidual NK and CD14+ myelomonocytic cells results in induction of Tregs and immunosuppression. Proc Natl Acad Sci U S A. 2010;107:11918–23.
41. Dixit A, Karande AA. Glycodelin A and galectin-1: role in foetal tolerance. J Reprod Health Med. 2016;2:S1–8.
42. Rajagopalan S. HLA-G-mediated NK cell senescence promotes vascular remodeling: implications for reproduction. Cell Mol Immunol. 2014;11:460–6.
43. Siewiera J, El Costa H, Tabiasco J, Berrebi A, Cartron G, Bouteiller P, Jabrane-Ferrat N. Human cytomegalovirus infection elicits new decidual natural killer cell effector functions. PLoS Pathog. 2013;9:e1003257.
44. Duriez M, Quillay H, Madec Y, El Costa H, Cannou C, Marlin R, De Truchis C, Rahmati M, Barré-Sinoussi F, Nugeyre M-T. Human decidual macrophages and NK cells differentially express Toll-like receptors and display distinct cytokine profiles upon TLR stimulation. Front Microbiol. 2014;5:316.

45. Taglauer ES, Waldorf KMA, Petroff MG. The hidden maternal-fetal interface: events involving the lymphoid organs in maternal-fetal tolerance. Int J Dev Biol. 2010;54:421.
46. Porrett PM. Biologic mechanisms and clinical consequences of pregnancy alloimmunization. Am J Transplant. 2018;18:1059–67.
47. Feyaerts D, Benner M, van Cranenbroek B, van der Heijden OW, Joosten I, van der Molen RG. Human uterine lymphocytes acquire a more experienced and tolerogenic phenotype during pregnancy. Sci Rep. 2017;7:2884.
48. Figueiredo AS, Schumacher A. The T helper type 17/regulatory T cell paradigm in pregnancy. Immunology. 2016;148:13–21.
49. Erkers T, Stikvoort A, Uhlin M. Lymphocytes in placental tissues: immune regulation and translational possibilities for immunotherapy. Stem Cells Int. 2017;2017:5738371.
50. Yao Y, Xu X-H, Jin L. Macrophage polarization in physiological and pathological pregnancy. Front Immunol. 2019;10:792.
51. Wright JR. Immunoregulatory functions of surfactant proteins. Nat Rev Immunol. 2005;2005:58–68.

Gülden Genç, Samet Genez, and Pamela Nguyen

4.1 Introduction

The use of diagnostic imaging methods in pregnant and breastfeeding women has increased considerably in recent years. As there is no ionizing radiation exposure associated with ultrasonography (US), it has been used safely for many years in pregnant women (Fig. 4.1). In some cases, computed tomography (CT) and magnetic resonance imaging (MRI) may be required to make a final diagnosis, and this situation may also require an injection of intravenous contrast agents. If pregnant and lactating women are not sufficiently informed about the safety of these imaging modalities, they may be concerned about having these diagnostic tests and continuing to breastfeed. In this chapter, the potential risks to the fetus or infant associated with maternal exposure to radiation, high magnetic field, or iodinated and gadolinium-based contrast media during pregnancy or breastfeeding will be evaluated.

4.2 Ultrasonography

US is an imaging method that uses high-frequency sound waves to characterize tissue. It is generally the first-line method for imaging the anatomical structures and soft tissue lesions in the head and neck region (Figs. 4.2 and 4.3). US can be used in

G. Genç (✉) · S. Genez
Faculty of Medicine, Derince Research and Training Hospital, Department of Radiology,
Health Sciences University, Kocaeli, Turkey
e-mail: drmggenc@yahoo.com; sametgenez@hotmail.com

P. Nguyen
Department of Radiology, Columbia University, Irving Medical Center, New York, NY, USA
e-mail: pamelanguyen09@gmail.com

© The Author(s), under exclusive license to Springer Nature
Switzerland AG 2022
C. Cingi et al. (eds.), *ENT Diseases: Diagnosis and Treatment during Pregnancy
and Lactation*, https://doi.org/10.1007/978-3-031-05303-0_4

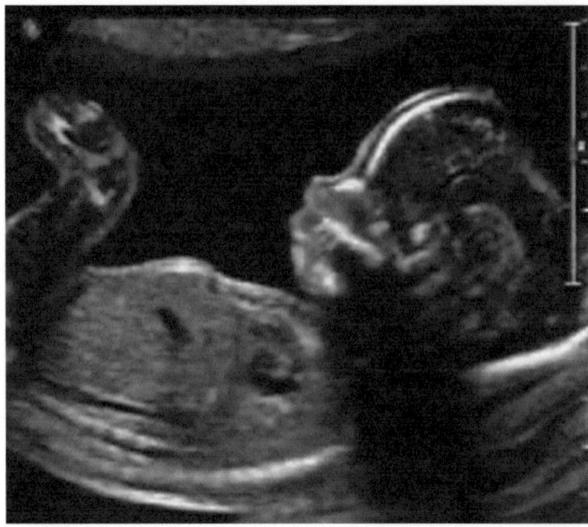

Fig. 4.1 Obstetrical ultrasound: US image of 24+ week gestation; lack of any ionizing radiation makes US the optimal imaging modality for pregnancy

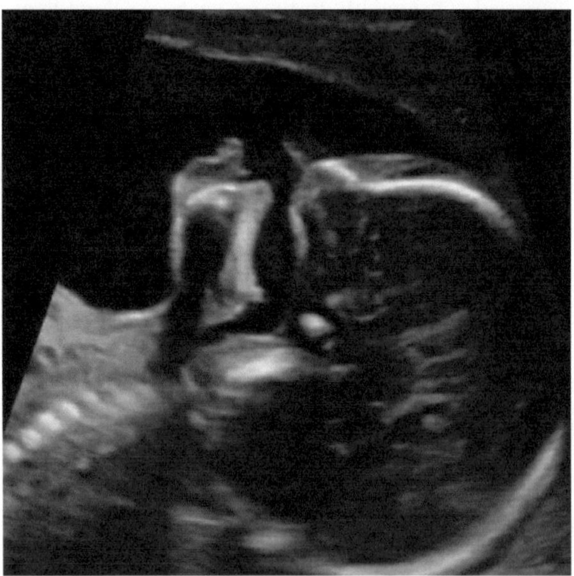

Fig. 4.2 Focus US image of head and neck showing cleft lip and palate defect in a fetus

the evaluation of thyroid and salivary gland diseases, soft tissue tumors, lymphadenopathy, cervical infections, and abscesses in the head and neck region. Also, if clinically indicated, fine needle aspiration or core needle biopsy can be performed to diagnose these lesions under ultrasound guidance. Animal studies show that direct exposure to ultrasound may have several adverse effects on the fetus; the reason for such a risk is due to the increase in heat generated by high-frequency sound waves in the tissue. While the temperature increase in the tissue is the least in grayscale ultrasonography, it is at the highest level in color Doppler and spectral

Fig. 4.3 US image in coronal plane showing cleft lip defect in fetus

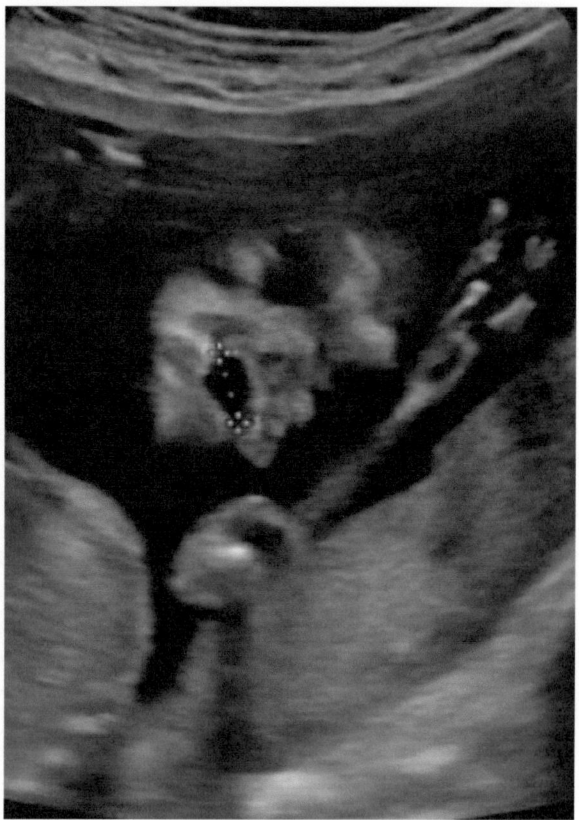

Doppler examination. The increase in temperature may cause reversible or irreversible cavitation in the tissue and consequently genetic damage to the fetus [1, 2]; however, no documented adverse fetal effects have been reported for diagnostic ultrasound procedures so far [3, 4]. Additionally, there is no such increased risk in head and neck imaging of pregnant women as the fetus is not directly exposed to high-frequency sound waves.

4.3 Magnetic Resonance Imaging

In clinical practice, MRI is a great imaging method because it does not use ionizing radiation and has a high soft tissue resolution. Theoretically, the negative effects of MR imaging on the fetus are teratogenic and biological. Potential risks are defect in cell migration in the first trimester due to high magnetic field, tissue heating due to radiofrequency pulse, and hearing damage due to high-frequency acoustic noise [5]. The energy produced by the radiofrequency pulse is measured using a specific absorption rate. In animal studies, it has been shown that heat generated due to the high specific absorption rate causes malformations. Due to the serious increase in

SAR values, MRI with magnetic field strengths above 1.5 T is not recommended for pregnant women [6]. The FDA has determined the highest SAR limit that the patient can be exposed to in body MRI as 4 W/kg. However, even at this energy level, the fetal effect is negligible due to absorption in the maternal tissues [7], and it has not been reported that there are any adverse effects of MR imaging in pregnant women and fetuses [8]. According to the American College of Radiology (ACR) guidelines, MRI can be performed in any period of pregnancy in case medical benefits are weighed against the unknown potential risk [9]. However, the ICNIRP recommends elective MR imaging after the first trimester because of its potential risks.

4.4 Ionizing Radiation

Natural background radiation rate exposed by a pregnant woman during pregnancy is approximately 2.3 msv, and the average fetal dose is 0.5–1 msv because of attenuation through the maternal tissues [10].

The biological effects of ionizing radiation exposure on the fetus occur in two ways: deterministic and stochastic effects. The deterministic effects occur when a large number of cells are damaged due to high radiation doses. Congenital malformations, cognitive impairments, growth and mental retardation, and even death may result from such exposure. Stochastic effects of ionizing radiation occur at any radiation dose as a result of mutation in a single cell and are associated with childhood cancers [11].

Various imaging techniques associated with fetal radiation exposure are shown in Table 4.1. Week of gestation and radiation dose are the most important parameters determining the effect of radiation on the fetus. During the preimplantation and preorganogenesis stages in the first weeks of pregnancy, a fetal radiation dose above

Table 4.1 Fetal radiation doses in some of the imaging techniques

Imaging technique	Fetal dose (mGy)
Cervical spine X-ray	<0.001
Head or neck CT	0.001–0.01
Chest radiography	0.0005–0.01
Abdominal X-ray	0.1–3.0
Lumbar spine X-ray	1.0–10
Chest CT or CT pulmonary angiography	0.01–0.66
Perfusion scintigraphy	0.1–0.5
Technetium-99m bone scintigraphy	4–5
Pulmonary DSA	0.5
Abdominal CT	1.3–35
Pelvic CT	10–50
^{18}F PET/CT	10–50

CT computed tomography, *PET* positron emission tomography, *DSA* digital subtraction angiography

50 mGy may cause the failure of blastocyst implantation and spontaneous abortus. However, if the embryo survives, the radiation dose probably does not cause harmful effects in the child, since the embryonic cells are omnipotent. Therefore, this period of pregnancy is called the "all or none period" [12, 13]. The embryo is more sensitive to the teratogenic effects of radiation between 8 and 15 weeks of gestation due to neuronal development and cell migration [14]. If the fetus is exposed to a radiation dose of less than 50 mGy, the teratogenic and carcinogenic risk is likely to be negligible [15]. It is unlikely to reach these radiation levels even after abdominopelvic CT imaging in which the fetus is directly in the field of view (FOV). In any case, imaging should be performed if the potential benefits outweigh the amount of risk, and ALARA (as low as reasonably achievable) principles should be taken into consideration especially in methods involving ionizing radiation (Figs. 4.4, 4.5, and 4.6).

4.5 Computed Tomography and Angiography

Head and neck CT is the most effective method for imaging pregnant trauma patients [16]. Fetal radiation dose is highest with direct exposure to X-rays, such as abdominopelvic CT imaging. In head and neck CT, the dose levels are very low as the fetus is exposed to scattered radiation rather than direct exposure. Therefore, a

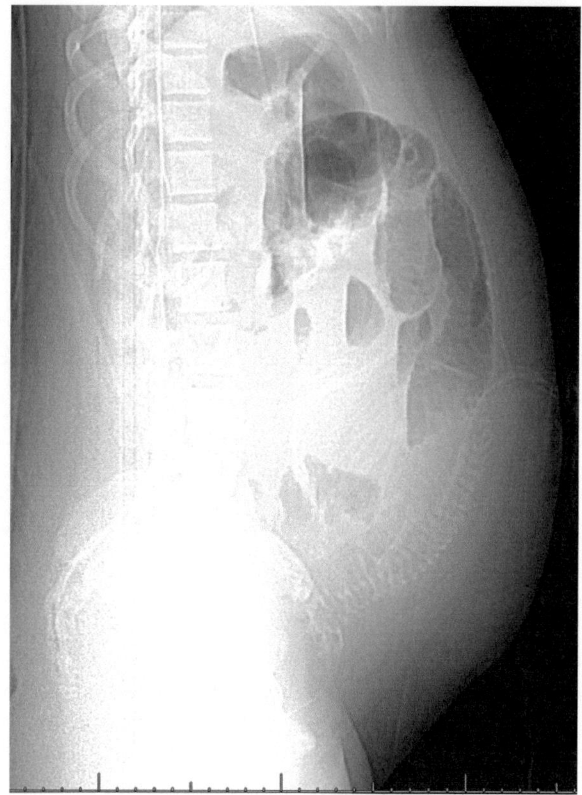

Fig. 4.4 CT scan performed on 21+ week pregnant patient with symptoms of bowel obstruction. *Lateral scout image from an abdominal CT scan on a pregnant patient who had sx of acute bowel obstruction; clinical team determined the risk of radiation exposure to patient worth the benefit given the declining clinical status of the patient. Performed with patient consent; image shows visible mineralized spine of the fetus*

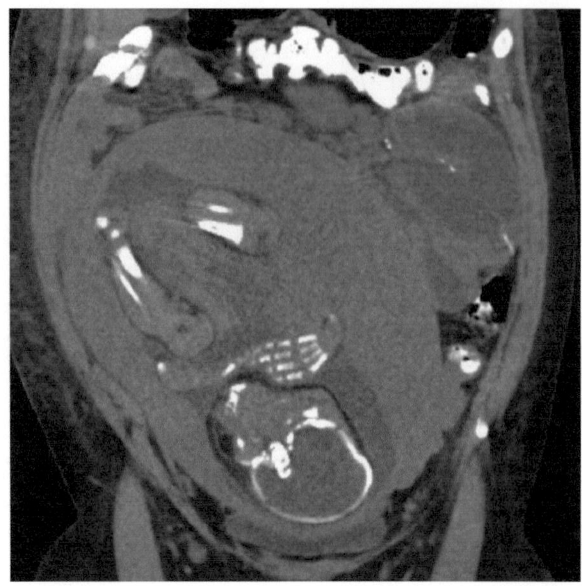

Fig. 4.5 CT scan on 21+ week pregnant patient. Coronal reformat image of abdominal CT scan performed on pregnant patient showing presence of the fetus (same patient as in Fig. 4.4)

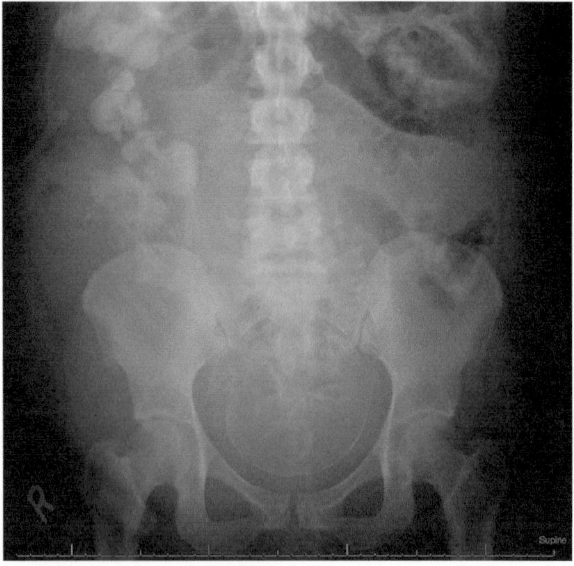

Fig. 4.6 Abdominal radiograph performed on 24+ week pregnant patient for sx of bowel obstruction

head and neck CT scan can be performed safely in any trimester of pregnancy when indicated. However, the ALARA principles should always be considered since the stochastic effects of radiation on the fetus are not dose-dependent. Therefore, dose reduction techniques should be preferred instead of standard protocols in pregnant patients. Although abdominal shielding is frequently used for chest X-ray during pregnancy (Fig. 4.7), it does not provide significant dose reduction in head and neck

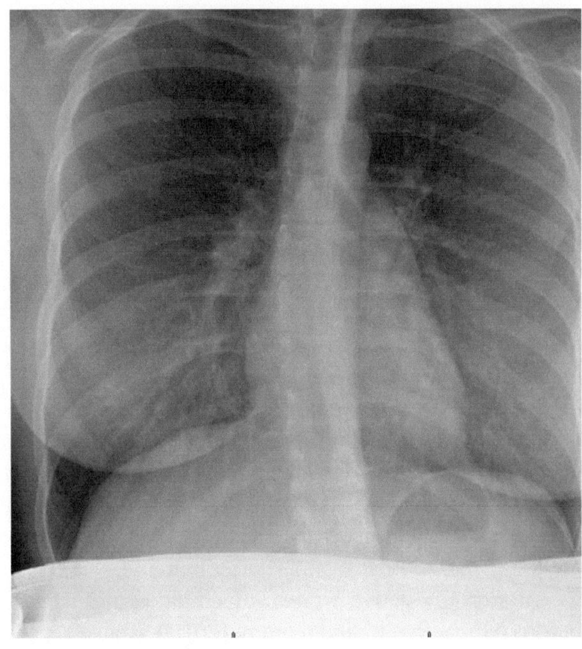

Fig. 4.7 Chest radiograph performed on pregnant patient using abdominal shield. Chest X-ray image showing the radio-opaque abdominal shield used to reduce radiation exposure to fetus

Table 4.2 CT dose reduction techniques in pregnancy

Monitor CT protocols and the resulting dose
Decrease kilovoltage for small patients
Decrease mAS and use automatic tube current modulation
Increase pitch
Try to keep the fetus out of the field of view
Try to perform single-phase imaging
Use oral barium sulfate solution for internal shielding

CT, since fetal exposure is mostly dependent on scattered radiation. However oral barium sulfate solution before the procedure may be effective in preventing internal scattered radiation. Table 4.2 shows the dose reduction techniques in CT. The clinician should inform the radiologist and radiology technician before imaging and request the application of dose reduction techniques.

Post-traumatic vascular injuries in the head and neck region are a life-threatening emergency. Vascular injuries can be seen in 3–20% of head and neck injuries [17]. Although conventional angiography is accepted as the gold standard in the diagnosis of these injuries, computed tomography angiography (CTA) is generally the first preferred imaging method because of its easy accessibility and high diagnostic value as conventional angiography. As it is mentioned in the CT imaging, the dose exposure is very low in the angiographic examination of this region as the fetus is not directly exposed to X-rays. ALARA principles should be taken into consideration, and dose reduction methods should be used in this examination too. The FOV and the exposure time should be reduced as much as possible.

4.6 Nuclear Medicine

Nuclear medicine imaging techniques play an important role in the diagnosis and treatment of head and neck cancer.

In nuclear medicine procedures, fetal risks are associated with ionizing radiation, as with imaging techniques using X-ray. The fetus is exposed to ionizing radiation due to the transport of radiopharmaceuticals through the placenta or via radioactive material accumulated in the maternal organs. The physical and biochemical properties of the radioisotope are the most important factors that determine fetal exposure. After the use of radiopharmaceuticals excreted by the kidneys, it is recommended that the patient should increase fluid intake and urinate frequently to reduce fetal exposure.

Since radioactive iodine (I-131) crosses through the placenta, it causes permanent damage to the fetal thyroid gland, especially if it is used after 10–12 weeks of gestation [18, 19]. The American College of Obstetricians and Gynecologists (ACOG) recommends delaying radioactive iodine therapy until the postpartum period and using iodine 123 (^{123}I) or ^{99m}Tc in diagnostic thyroid examination, due to the lower radiation dose and shorter half-life.

All sexually active women of childbearing age should have a pregnancy test before radioactive iodine therapy [20]. It is also recommended to use an effective contraceptive method for 3 months to 1 year to prevent problems in the fetus after this treatment [21].

PET/CT may be indicated in head and neck cancers for staging, early detection of recurrent disease, and treatment strategies. The use of PET imaging in pregnant women is controversial due to ionizing radiation and fetal uptake of radiopharmaceuticals. According to the current data, although the fetal radiation dose obtained from 18F-FDG PET studies is the highest in the first trimester, it is well below the dangerous limit when all periods of pregnancy are considered [22, 23]. For this reason, screening should not be interrupted due to the concern that the fetus will be exposed to high radiation. When available, PET/MR imaging should be the preferred option for PET imaging of pregnant patients [23].

The breastfed infant may be exposed to radiation due to the excretion of radiopharmaceuticals into milk. The recommended breastfeeding interruptions for different radiopharmaceuticals may vary depending on the half-lives of these drugs. Additionally, excretion rates of the same compound may vary between patients. During this time, the mother can express and store the milk until the radioactive effect disappears. Or, she can perform these procedures before taking the radioactive material to continue feeding the baby during the interruption.

4.7 Use of Contrast Media During Pregnancy and Lactation

Intravenous iodinated contrast media is known to cross the human placenta and reach fetal circulation. The reason for concern about the use of iodinated contrast media is related to the possibility that iodine uptake may cause fetal hypothyroidism [24]. The US Food and Drug Administration classifies iodinated contrast media as pregnancy risk category B drugs. This means that animal studies show no fetal risk, but there are no controlled studies in pregnant women and they should only be used after the potential risk-benefit ratio has been evaluated [25]. However, if the mother was administered iodinated contrast media during pregnancy, thyroid hormone levels of the infant should be checked immediately after birth [24].

Gadolinium-based contrast agents are classified as pregnancy category C and have been shown to have teratogenic effects when administered at high doses in animal studies. In a recent study, it was found that, the risk of congenital anomaly in the fetus did not increase after the use of gadolinium-based contrast material during pregnancy [8]. However, in the same study, an increase was observed in still-births and neonatal deaths in pregnant women who received gadolinium-based contrast agents, especially in the first trimester. In addition, neurological, inflammatory, and infiltrative skin diseases were found at a higher rate. Therefore, as with iodinated contrast agents, the ACR recommends the use of gadolinium-based contrast agents only if the potential benefits clearly outweigh the risks. Before the use of any contrast agent in pregnant women, sufficient information should be provided, and informed consent should be obtained.

It is known that less than 1% of iodinated and gadolinium-based contrast agents excrete into breast milk, and less than 1% of contrast material in breast milk enters the baby's circulation. The ACR and ACOG recommend that the mother continue breastfeeding after administration of contrast agents. Despite this, if the mother is still concerned about breastfeeding, she can express and discard breast milk for 24 h [5, 26].

References

1. Torloni MR, Vedmedovska N, Merialdi M, et al. Safety of ultrasonography in pregnancy: WHO systematic review of the literature and meta-analysis. Ultrasound Obstet Gynecol. 2009;33(5):599–608.
2. Barnett SB, Ter Haar GR, Ziskin MC, Rott HD, Duck FA, Maeda K. International recommendations and guidelines for the safe use of diagnostic ultrasound in medicine. Ultrasound Med Biol. 2000;26(3):355–66.
3. Committee opinion no. 723: guidelines for diagnostic imaging during pregnancy and lactation. Obstet Gynecol. 2017;130(4):e210–e216. https://doi.org/10.1097/AOG.0000000000002355. Erratum in: Obstet Gynecol 2018 Sep;132(3):786. PMID: 28937575.
4. Stratmeyer ME. Effects on animals. In; Stewart HF, editor. An overview of ultrasound: theory, measurement, medical applications, and biological effects
5. De Wilde JP, Rivers AW, Price DL. A review of the current use of magnetic resonance imaging in pregnancy and safety implications for the fetus. Prog Biophys Mol Biol. 2005;87:335–53.
6. Ciet P, Litmanovich DE. MR safety issues particular to women. Magn Reson Imaging Clin N Am. 2015;23(1):59–67.
7. Pahade JK, Litmanovich D, Pedrosa I, Romero J, Bankier AA, Boiselle PM. Quality initiatives: imaging pregnant patients with suspected pulmonary embolism: what the radiologist needs to know. Radiographics. 2009;29(3):639–54. https://doi.org/10.1148/rg.293085226. Epub 2009 Mar 30. PMID: 19270072.

8. Ray JG, Vermeulen MJ, Bharatha A, et al. Association between MRI exposure during pregnancy and fetal and childhood outcomes. JAMA. 2016;316:952–61.

9. Kanal E, Barkovich AJ, Bell C, Borgstede JP, Bradley WG, Froelich JW, et al. ACR guidance document on MR safe practices: 2013. J Magn Reson Imaging. 2013;37:501–30.

10. Wang PI, Chong ST, Kielar AZ, et al. Imaging of pregnant and lactating patients. I. Evidence-based review and recommendations. AJR Am J Roentgenol. 2012;198(4):778–92.

11. Wall BF, Meara JR, Muirhead CR, Bury RF, Murray M. Protection of pregnant patients during diagnostic medical exposures to ionizing radiation: advice from the Health Protection Agency, the Royal College of Radiologists, and the College of Radiographers. Documents of the Health Protection Agency: radiation, chemical and environmental hazards. United Kingdom; 2009.

12. Brent RL. Saving lives and changing family histories: appropriate counseling of pregnant women and men and women of reproductive age, concerning the risk of diagnostic radiation exposures during and before pregnancy. Am J Obstet Gynecol. 2009;200:4–24.

13. De Santis M, Di Gianantonio E, Straface G, et al. Ionizing radiations in pregnancy and teratogenesis: a review of literature. Reprod Toxicol. 2005;20:323–9.

14. Tremblay E, Thérasse E, Thomassin-Naggara I, Trop I. Quality initiatives: guidelines for use of medical imaging during pregnancy and lactation. Radiographics. 2012;32(3):897–911.

15. McCollough CH, Schueler BA, Atwell TD, et al. Radiation exposure and pregnancy: when should we be concerned? Radiographics. 2007;27(4):909–17; discussion 917–918.

16. Tirada N, Dreizin D, Khati NJ, Akin EA, Zeman RK. Imaging pregnant and lactating patients. Radiographics. 2015;35(6):1751–65. https://doi.org/10.1148/rg.2015150031. PMID: 26466183.

17. Ssenyonga PK, Le Feuvre D, Taylor A. Head and neck neurovascular trauma: clinical and angiographic correlation. Interv Neuroradiol. 2015;21:108–13.

18. Berg GE, Nyström EH, Jacobsson L, et al. Radioiodine treatment of hyperthyroidism in a pregnant woman. J Nucl Med. 1998;39(2):357–61.

19. Stoffer SS, Hamburger JI. Inadvertent 131I therapy for hyperthyroidism in the first trimester of pregnancy. J Nucl Med. 1976;17(02):146–9.

20. America College of Radiology. ACR standard for the performance of therapy with unsealed radionuclide sources. In: Standards 1999–2000. Reston: American College of Radiology; 1999. p. 265–70.

21. Schlumberger M, De Vathaire F, Ceccarelli C, et al. Exposure to radioactive iodine-131 for scintigraphy or therapy does not preclude pregnancy in thyroid cancer patients. J Nucl Med. 1996;37(4):606–12.

22. Takalkar AM, Khandelwal A, Lokitz S, Lilien DL, Stabin MG. 18F-FDG PET in pregnancy and fetal radiation dose estimates. J Nucl Med. 2011;52:1035–40.

23. Zanotti-Fregonara P, Laforest R, Wallis JW. Fetal radiation dose from 18F- FDG in pregnant patients imaged with PET, PET/CT, and PET/MR. J Nucl Med. 2015;56:1218–22.

24. Patel SJ, Reede DL, Katz DS, Subramaniam R, Amorosa JK. Imaging the pregnant patient for nonobstetric conditions: algorithms and radiation dose considerations. Radiographics. 2007;27(6):1705–22.

25. Webb JA, Thomsen HS, Morcos SK. The use of iodinated and gadolinium contrast media during pregnancy and lactation. Members of contrast media safety Committee of European Society of Urogenital Radiology (ESUR). Eur Radiol. 2005;15:1234–40.

26. American College of Radiology. ACR manual on contrast media: version 9. Reston: American College of Radiology; 2013.

Treatment of Respiratory Infections in Pregnant Patients: Overview

5

Şeyma Başlılar, Derya Kocakaya, and Arzu Yorgancıoğlu

5.1 Introduction

It is reported that antibiotics represent almost 80% of the drugs prescribed to pregnant women and that between 1 in 5 and 1 in 4 pregnant women are administered antibiotic pharmacotherapy [1–3]. In pregnant women, the most frequently occurring infections are urinary tract infections (UTIs) (cystitis and pyelonephritis), venereal infections and the upper respiratory tract infections (URTIs) [1].

Maternal use of antibiotics has been linked to adverse effects on the weight of the child, both in the short and longer term. It was recently reported by one study that in utero exposure to antimicrobial pharmacotherapy, as reported by the mother, resulted in lower birth weight. On average the infant weighed around 138 g less than expected, after other factors were controlled for [4]. Another recent study has also noted a link between foetal exposure to antibiotics and the child subsequently becoming obese, albeit these data did not indicate which class of agents was involved [5]. There have also been separate studies examining any association between foetal exposure to antibiotics and neurological disorders, such as epilepsy and cerebral palsy, or allergic disorders, such as allergic eczema and asthma. In some studies, a correlation has been found, whilst in others no such correlation appeared [6–8].

Ş. Başlılar (✉)
Department of Pulmonology, Ümraniye Training and Research and Hospital, İstanbul, Turkey
e-mail: seymabaslilar@yahoo.com

D. Kocakaya
Department of Pulmonology, Marmara University, Medical Faculty, İstanbul, Turkey
e-mail: drderyagun@gmail.com

A. Yorgancıoğlu
Department of Pulmonology, Celal Bayar University, Medical Faculty, Manisa, Turkey
e-mail: arzuyo@hotmail.com

C. Cingi et al. (eds.), *ENT Diseases: Diagnosis and Treatment during Pregnancy and Lactation*, https://doi.org/10.1007/978-3-031-05303-0_5

5.2 FDA Pregnancy Categories

The US FDA is undertaking work with two principal aims in mind: the first is to increase the evidence base and evidential quality concerning the safety of drugs when used in pregnant women, whilst the second aim is to ensure this information is widely known and understood. A key component in these initiatives is to ensure that labelling of drugs reflects safety information. In the USA, the labelling of medications is regulated at a federal level, and thus alterations in labelling must also be agreed at this level. The lengthy process by which the stakeholders were consulted prior to any changes in labelling policy began in September 1997 [9].

At present, medications that undergo systemic absorption are obliged to carry a warning about their use in pregnant women. This part of the labelling includes an explication of any known teratogenicity and consequences for reproductive function and pregnancy. All pharmacological agents fall under one of five categories, denoted by the letters A to D and X. This classification is based on the balance of possible benefit vs risk of harm to the foetus or woman (21 Code of Federal Regulations 201.57(f)) [10]. It is envisaged that the latest style of labelling will contain three sections, namely:

1. *Clinical considerations*, which will relate the findings of the FDA regarding risk to how the agent is used clinically
2. *Summary risk assessment*, in which the key evidence from animal and human studies is outlined
3. *Discussion*, which explains further details about the evidence currently in existence [11]

Since the current categorisation of agents as class A–D or X fails to capture the complexity of the evidence base and the difficulties faced clinically, it has been suggested this system may need to be abandoned [9].

Alongside the initiative to develop a better system of product labelling for pregnancy use, the FDA has instigated an initiative aiming to ensure that the evidence submitted by pharmaceutical manufacturers is of maximum quality and to ensure that any data received on use in animals or humans can be interpreted in the most effective way. In a number of cases, there are guidelines produced to direct the initiatives [9].

5.3 Current FDA Classification Scheme

5.3.1 Category A

Agents in this class have evidence from sufficient, methodologically sound trials to show that the agent does not pose a risk to the foetus when used in the initial trimester, nor do data indicate a risk when used at a later stage in the pregnancy [12].

5.3.2   Category B

Experimental data from animal models indicate no apparent foetal teratogenicity, but there is inadequate knowledge at present from methodologically sound studies in pregnant humans [12].

5.3.3   Category C

Teratogenicity has been demonstrated in research utilising animal models, but there is inadequate knowledge at present from methodologically sound studies in pregnant humans. Nonetheless, in some situations the benefit from use may outweigh the risk in pregnancy [12].

5.3.4   Category D

There is a known risk to the foetus, established on the basis of either specific studies involving pregnant women or from pharmacovigilance data. There may be situations in which the benefit from the use of the agent is such as to outweigh the known risk to the foetus [12].

5.3.5   Category X

Data obtained from studies of use in pregnant animals or humans indicate specific foetal anomalies occur, with or without pharmacovigilance data indicating the same. In these agents the risk is sufficiently great to outweigh any possible benefit from the use of the agent [12].

5.4   Antibiotic Groups

5.4.1   Penicillins

The penicillins and the agents subsequently developed by modification of them are the class of antibiotic in most frequent use in pregnant women [1, 2]. The agent of choice in a woman with colonisation by group B Streptococci is still penicillin administered intravenously, with ampicillin the suggested second choice [13]. The penicillins are easily able to traverse the placental barrier; however, those agents in this class which are highly protein-bound, e.g. the penicillins with activity against Staphylococci (with the exception of methicillin), reach lower levels in the foetal circulation than those agents which are less protein-bound, such as penicillin G or ampicillin [14]. In pregnancy, the maternal plasma volume and renal clearance both go up, and the consequence of these changes is that the plasma concentrations may fall by up to half, necessitating an upward adjustment in the dose and dosing frequency [15].

Evidence has accumulated over a lengthy period to confirm that penicillins are safe in use. The strongest safety evidence is for the original molecule, penicillin, and its amino derivatives (ampicillin and amoxicillin) [16]. The entire range of penicillins and related drugs, including co-amoxiclav and sulbactam, which inhibit beta-lactamase activity by bacteria, is classified by the FDA as category B agents [17]. If a pregnant woman is detected with *Treponema pallidum* infection, first she should be desensitised and then administered penicillin.

5.4.2 Cephalosporins and Cephamycins

The cephalosporins, like the penicillins, have been administered to pregnant patients for a long time [1]. This class of antibiotic is still the agent of choice in many infections in pregnant patients, usually where patients have an allergy to penicillin or are unable to take it. The serum concentration of cephalosporins is lower in pregnant women since they have an enhanced renal clearance. This calls for adjustment in the dose and dose interval [18].

The cephalosporins and cephamycins as a class fall under FDA category B [17]. Research utilising data from a system belonging to the Michigan Medicaid organisation has shown that ceftriaxone may be linked to heart anomalies in the foetus [17]. In pregnant women who have an infection with *Neisseria gonorrhoeae*, ceftriaxone remains the first-line agent [19]. Caution needs to be exercised when administering ceftriaxone to women at the end of pregnancy as it is associated with neonatal jaundice and potential brain damage. The more recently developed cephalosporins, e.g. ceftaroline, ceftolozane-tazobactam and ceftazidime-avibactam, also fall under FDA category B. This categorisation should be interpreted carefully, since there is little evidence in the literature regarding safety in pregnant patients [20].

5.4.3 Carbapenems

The carbapenems suffer from the scarcity of evidence regarding their use in pregnant women. The FDA considers ertapenem, meropenem and doripenem as category B, but imipenem-cilastatin a category C medication [17]. As with other antibiotics, the plasma concentration in pregnant women may be lower than in non-pregnant individuals [17]. The use of carbapenems in pregnant patients is best limited to bacterial infections by penicillin- and cephalosporin-resistant organisms and where other options are few.

5.4.4 Glycopeptides and Lipoglycopeptides

Vancomycin is a glycopeptide. The FDA considers it a category B medication, and it is considered appropriate to use in pregnancy when a severe infection with a Gram-positive bacterial species develops, especially in the mid or last trimester [17]. Vancomycin enters many tissues of the body. There is 55% protein binding. Elimination mostly occurs via renal filtration. These pharmacokinetic parameters may be different in pregnant women [20]. Vancomycin is capable of traversing the placental barrier, and it has been detected in blood of the umbilical cord after it was given intravenously to the mother [16, 21]. Although there is little high-quality evidence available, some authors state that this agent may be safely used in pregnant patients. One report concerned the administration of vancomycin in ten cases where the patient was pregnant and infected by methicillin-resistant *S. aureus* (MRSA) [22]. The antibiotic was given for a minimum of 1 week, and all the women were in the mid or last trimester. There were no teratogenic consequences, such as auditory impairment and renal toxicity. In cases where the course of vancomycin lasted for 13 or 28 days, there were also no congenital abnormalities observed, nor any harm to the mother [21]. However, since evidence is lacking for the consequences of vancomycin given in the initial trimester, caution should be exercised if a case occurs at this point in a pregnancy [20]. Rats and rabbits have been used to test for teratogenicity, with no teratogenic consequences observed even when the dose was the equivalent of up to five times the highest human dose [17, 20]. Oral administration of vancomycin leads to low levels in the systemic circulation, and it is thought this will not lead to harmful effects to the mother or foetus [16, 17].

5.4.5 Macrolides and Ketolides

The data concerning how safe it is to use macrolide antibiotics in pregnant women exhibit considerable variety [23]. Macrolides are mostly unbound to protein in the circulation, have a high volume of distribution and are metabolised by the liver. The physiological changes brought about by pregnancy should not alter their action to any great extent [20]. The first reported association between foetal erythromycin exposure and congenital anomalies of the circulatory system was in 2003. This association has not been found in studies undertaken since 2003, and the agent remains under category B of the FDA classification [24, 25]. One study, which employed a retrospective cohort design, examined any cases of congenital defects, pyloric stenosis or intussusception to see whether macrolide exposure had occurred in utero [23]. There were 1033 cases where a pregnant woman was administered a macrolide antibiotic (namely, erythromycin, azithromycin, clarithromycin or roxithromycin). In none of these cases did exposure to the drug correlate with any significant congenital defect in the foetus. In cases where the drug was given in the final trimester, there was no association with pyloric stenosis or intussusception, either [23]. A review which examined pregnancies over a period of 15 years in which erythromycin was administered to the mother did note that there was a persistent association with anomalies of the circulatory system (risk estimate 1.70; 95% CI 1.26–2.39) [24]. In the majority of cases, the defects were of mild degree. Where cases of congenital cardiac disease or pyloric stenosis were identified, the foetus was not more likely to have been exposed to macrolide antibiotics [25]. Nonetheless, the decision to treat a pregnant woman with any preparation containing erythromycin should be informed by a risk-benefit analysis and only taken when the benefit clearly exceeds the risk. In general, azithromycin is thought safe to employ in pregnant women, and its FDA categorisation is class B [17]. Animal studies where a dose between double and quadruple the dose in humans was employed found no teratogenicity in rats or mice [26]. When pregnant women who had taken azithromycin were compared with those taking other antimicrobials or agents known not to cause defects, the groups did not differ in terms of the frequency of major congenital defects [27]. Research into clarithromycin, however, as with erythromycin, has drawn conflicting conclusions. This agent is FDA category C. Different studies in which rats were exposed in utero to clarithromycin in the initial trimester have confusingly found both no evidence of congenital anomaly and a somewhat low but increased rate of heart defects [26]. Studies of teratogenicity in mice found cleft palate occurred, and in monkeys foetal growth restriction was detected [26]. Clinical studies, which also encompassed a trial with a prospective design and incorporated controls, have concluded that major congenital defects do not occur at a raised frequency in pregnancies where there was exposure to clarithromycin [15, 28, 29]. Despite this complicated picture, the general consensus is that azithromycin may be safely employed in pregnant women, whereas clarithromycin is best used cautiously, and only where the benefit clearly exceeds potential harm.

5.4.6 Fluoroquinolones

Despite the FDA having classified the fluoroquinolones as category C agents, there is a general contraindication to employing these agents in pregnant women [17]. The fluoroquinolones distribute throughout the tissues, and there are differences between particular compounds in how they are eliminated [20]. The degree to which they are protein-bound varies from 20 to 50% [20]. Fluoroquinolones are potentially safe in early pregnancy, but the results of animal testing, which indicated teratogenic potential, prevent their being recommended [16, 30, 31]. The data imply that fluoroquinolone exposure may cause harm to the foetal kidneys, heart and brain/spinal cord [32, 33]. Animals exposed to these agents have defective osseous and cartilaginous development [17]. However, there are inconsistencies in the evidence and more research is called for. A recently published review of the literature on the teratogenicity of fluoroquinolones came to the conclusion that the teratogenic potential in animals may differ from that in humans, and cited weaknesses in the trial data involving human subjects, such as a lack of methodological rigour, low numbers of participants and the existence of confounders. These criticisms, however, do not amount to a recommendation that fluoroquinolones be used in pregnancy, unless exceptionally [31]. The state of current knowledge is such as to indicate that fluoroquinolone use is only advisable where no other agent can be relied upon [17, 31].

5.4.7   Miscellaneous Antibiotics

5.4.7.1 Clindamycin
Clindamycin is an antibiotic of lincosamide type which is capable of traversing the placental barrier. The FDA classifies it as a class B agent [17]. This agent undergoes distribution into the majority of tissue compartments. There is 92–94% protein binding [20]. Elimination is complex, with 10% via the kidneys in active form and a further 3.6% via the faeces is also active. The remaining portion of excreted metabolites are inactive [20]. Research involving 647 neonates who underwent exposure to clindamycin in the initial trimester of pregnancy failed to associate exposure with teratogenic consequences [17]. There are few data available for the use of clindamycin by mouth in the later stages of gestation. However, evidence does show that clindamycin used within the vagina is not advisable in pregnancy due to the high level of systemic absorption (which may reach 30%), low efficacy and the raised potential for negative pregnancy outcomes (infection of the newborn and a low birth weight) [17, 19]. Using clindamycin at an advanced stage of gestation (up to the 32nd week of pregnancy) has an association with adverse pregnancy outcomes. Accordingly, the Centers for Disease Control and Prevention of Sexually Transmitted Diseases Treatment Guidelines advocate against administering clindamycin vaginally in the second half of pregnancy [19, 34].

5.4.7.2 Metronidazole
Despite its being classified by the FDA as a class B agent, metronidazole is contraindicated in pregnant women who are within the initial trimester [17]. A number of studies have found an association between the use of metronidazole for the indication of either infection with *Trichomonas vaginalis* without symptoms or raised foetal fibronectin and increased risk of premature delivery [35, 36]. However, multivariate analysis did not find any correlation between maternal use of metronidazole at any stage of gestation and premature delivery, low birth weight or congenital anomaly [37]. Metronidazole should only be administered vaginally to pregnant women very cautiously, as it has been hypothesised that this practice results in congenital hydrocephalus [38]. Guidelines continue to advocate that metronidazole be used to treat pregnant women with bacterial vaginosis or infection due to *T. vaginalis*. It is worth noting that the safety of repeated administration of metronidazole has not yet been established and it has not been definitively demonstrated that these interventions can prevent premature delivery [19].

References

1. Heikkila AM. Antibiotics in pregnancy—a prospective cohort study on the policy of antibiotic prescription. Ann Med. 1993;5:467–71.
2. Santos F, Oraichi D, Berard A. Prevalence and predictors of anti-infective use during pregnancy. Pharmacoepidemiol Drug Saf. 2010;4:418–27.
3. de Jonge L, Bos HJ, van Langen IM, de Jong-van den Berg LT, Bakker MK. Antibiotics prescribed before, during and after pregnancy in the Netherlands: a drug utilization study. Pharmacoepidemiol Drug Saf. 2014;1:60–8.
4. Vidal AC, Murphy SK, Murtha AP, et al. Associations between antibiotic exposure during pregnancy, birth weight and aberrant methylation at imprinted genes among offspring. Int J Obes. 2013;7:907–13.
5. Mueller NT, Whyatt R, Hoepner L, et al. Prenatal exposure to antibiotics, cesarean section and risk of childhood obesity. Int J Obes. 2015;39:665–70.
6. Lapin B, Piorkowski J, Ownby D, et al. Relationship between prenatal antibiotic use and asthma in at-risk children. Ann Allergy Asthma Immunol. 2015;3:203–7.
7. Stensballe LG, Simonsen J, Jensen SM, Bonnelykke K, Bisgaard H. Use of antibiotics during pregnancy increases the risk of asthma in early childhood. J Pediatr. 2013;4:832–8.e3.
8. Thomas M, Price D. Prenatal antibiotic exposure and subsequent atopy. Am J Respir Crit Care Med. 2003;11:1578; author reply 78–9.
9. Weiss SR. Prescription medication use in pregnancy. Medscape. 2000. https://www.medscape.com/viewarticle/408598_3. Accessed online 21 Apr 2021.
10. Weiss SR, Cooke CE, Bradley LR, Manson JM. A pharmacist's guide to pregnancy registry studies. J Am Pharm Assoc. 1999;39:830–4.
11. Kweder SL. Medicines and pregnancy, labeling and beyond. Presented to the Pregnancy Labeling Subcommittee of the Advisory Committee for Reproductive Health Drugs. Washington, DC. March 28–29, 2000. http://www.fda.gov/ohrms/dockets/ac/00/slides/3601s1a.PPT.
12. Content and format of labeling for human prescription drug and biological products; Requirements for pregnancy and lactation labeling (Federal Register/Vol. 73, No. 104/ Thursday, May 29, 2008).
13. Centers for Disease Control and Prevention. Prevention of perinatal group B streptococcal disease. MMWR Recomm Rep. 2010;59(RR-10):3–23.
14. Pacifici GM, Nottoli R. Placental transfer of drugs administered to the mother. Clin Pharmacokinet. 1995;3:235–69.
15. Einarson A, Shuhaiber S, Koren G. Effects of antibacterials on the unborn child: what is known and how should this influence prescribing. Paediatr Drugs. 2001;11:803–16.
16. Lamont HF, Blogg HJ, Lamont RF. Safety of antimicrobial treatment during pregnancy: a current review of resistance, immunomodulation and teratogenicity. Expert Opin Drug Saf. 2014;12:1569–81.
17. Briggs GGFR. Drugs in pregnancy and lactation. Baltimore: Lippincot Williams & Wilkins; 2014.
18. Chow AW, Jewesson PJ. Pharmacokinetics and safety of antimicrobial agents during pregnancy. Rev Infect Dis. 1985;3:287–313.
19. Centers for Disease Control and Prevention. Update to CDC's sexually transmitted diseases treatment guidelines. http://www.cdc.gov/mmwr/preview/mmwrhtml/rr6403a1.htm. Accessed 6 July 2015.
20. United States National Library of Medicine. DailyMed. http://dailymed.nlm.nih.gov/dailymed/index.cfm. Accessed 27 Apr 2015.
21. Adam MP, Polifka JE, Friedman JM. Evolving knowledge of the teratogenicity of medications in human pregnancy. Am J Med Genet. 2011;157C(3):175–82.
22. Reyes MP, Ostrea EM Jr, Cabinian AE, Schmitt C, Rintelmann W. Vancomycin during pregnancy: does it cause hearing loss or nephrotoxicity in the infant? Am J Obstet Gynecol. 1989;4:977–81.

23. Bahat Dinur A, Koren G, Matok I, et al. Fetal safety of macrolides. Antimicrob Agents Chemother. 2013;7:3307–11.
24. Kallen B, Danielsson BR. Fetal safety of erythromycin. An update of Swedish data. Eur J Clin Pharmacol. 2014;3:355–60.
25. Lin KJ, Mitchell AA, Yau WP, Louik C, Hernandez-Diaz S. Safety of macrolides during pregnancy. Am J Obstet Gynecol. 2013;3:221.e1–8.
26. Amsden GW. Erythromycin, clarithromycin, and azithromycin: are the differences real? Clin Ther. 1996;1:56–72; discussion 55.
27. Sarkar M, Woodland C, Koren G, Einarson AR. Pregnancy outcome following gestational exposure to azithromycin. BMC Pregnancy Childbirth. 2006;18:1–5.
28. Drinkard CR, Shatin D, Clouse J. Postmarketing surveillance of medications and pregnancy outcomes: clarithromycin and birth malformations. Pharmacoepidemiol Drug Saf. 2000;7:549–56.
29. Einarson A, Phillips E, Mawji F, et al. A prospective controlled multicentre study of clarithromycin in pregnancy. Am J Perinatol. 1998;9:523–5.
30. Harbison AF, Polly DM, Musselman ME. Antiinfective therapy for pregnant or lactating patients in the emergency department. Am J Health Syst Pharm. 2015;3:189–97.
31. Yefet E, Salim R, Chazan B, Akel H, Romano S, Nachum Z. The safety of quinolones in pregnancy. Obstet Gynecol Surv. 2014;11:681–94.
32. Crider KS, Cleves MA, Reefhuis J, Berry RJ, Hobbs CA, Hu DJ. Antibacterial medication use during pregnancy and risk of birth defects: National Birth Defects Prevention Study. Arch Pediatr Adolesc Med. 2009;11:978–85.
33. Guinto VT, De Guia B, Festin MR, Dowswell T. Different antibiotic regimens for treating asymptomatic bacteriuria in pregnancy. Cochrane Database Syst Rev. 2010;9:CD007855.
34. Joesoef MR, Hillier SL, Wiknjosastro G, et al. Intravaginal clindamycin treatment for bacterial vaginosis: effects on preterm delivery and low birth weight. Am J Obstet Gynecol. 1995;5:1527–31.
35. Ramsey PS, Andrews WW. Biochemical predictors of preterm labor: fetal fibronectin and salivary estriol. Clin Perinatol. 2003;4:701–33.
36. Klebanoff MA, Carey JC, Hauth JC, et al. Failure of metronidazole to prevent preterm delivery among pregnant women with asymptomatic *Trichomonas vaginalis* infection. N Engl J Med. 2001;7:487–93.
37. Koss CA, Baras DC, Lane SD, et al. Investigation of metronidazole use during pregnancy and adverse birth outcomes. Antimicrob Agents Chemother. 2012;9:4800–5.
38. Kazy Z, Puho E, Czeizel AE. Teratogenic potential of vaginal metronidazole treatment during pregnancy. Eur J Obstet Gynecol Reprod Biol. 2005;2:174–8.

The Variations in Communication During Pregnancy and the Postpartum Period

6

Can Cemal Cingi, Dilek Eroğlu, and Erhan Eroğlu

6.1 Introduction

It has been appreciated for many years that healthcare practitioners need to communicate effectively, and communication in healthcare as a whole has accordingly attracted considerable research. Recently published research in the area of healthcare communication includes a study on the part communication plays in taking decisions [1, 2], as well as a study exploring the effect communication has on how safe and effective healthcare interventions are [3]. Researchers have also examined how communication enables the types of care in maternity services that incorporate respect [4]. Communication skills are taught throughout the training of doctors, nurses and midwives in several countries, including the UK and the USA, as well as several other countries in Europe [5–8]. To be granted a licence to practise a healthcare profession, some countries mandate evidence of the ability to communicate well in verbal, non-verbal and written form. This is, for example, the case in the UK, as outlined in the 'UK Standards for Pre-Registration Education' [9]. Yet, whilst there is undoubtedly agreement that communication is key, there exists no unique way to judge the effectiveness of communication, whether in maternity services or in healthcare generally [1].

There is support on a worldwide scale for increasing the involvement of midwives in maternity care, and this may lead to communicative styles that put the

C. C. Cingi (✉) · E. Eroğlu
Faculty of Communication Sciences, Communication Design and Management Department,
Anadolu University, Eskisehir, Turkey
e-mail: ccc@anadolu.edu.tr; eeroglu@anadolu.edu.tr

D. Eroğlu
Department of Foreign Languages, Anadolu University, School of Foreign Languages,
Eskisehir, Turkey
e-mail: dteroglu@anadolu.edu.tr

C. Cingi et al. (eds.), *ENT Diseases: Diagnosis and Treatment during Pregnancy and Lactation*, https://doi.org/10.1007/978-3-031-05303-0_6

mother centre stage [10]. It has been noted that women desire information of the highest quality, consistency and for professionals involved in their care to communicate effectively with each other [11]. There has been an effort to improve communication, but pregnant mothers still frequently report that doctors fail to communicate in an effective way with the mother whilst she is in labour and giving birth, leaving the patient feeling she has no control over what is happening and that nobody is paying attention to her wishes [12–14]. If a woman perceives the maternity care she has received as suboptimal and lacking respect, including during the birth itself, she may be more prone to developing post-traumatic stress disorder following birth [15], may not bond as well with her baby [16] and may feel dissatisfied with the experience of birth and entertain negative perceptions towards it [17]. If this type of problem is not solved, there is a risk that pregnant women will avoid maternity services when giving birth, which is an especially dangerous development in those settings where resources are more limited and effective maternity care is essential to ensuring that both mother and baby remain healthy [18, 19].

6.2 Birth and Communication

Women's satisfaction with how doctors communicated with them during labour has been studied by Bashour and colleagues [20], who canvassed women's opinions a fortnight after they had given birth. Crofts et al. [21] investigated communicative aspects in various clinical scenarios, asking for the women's opinions immediately after the scenario. The questions focused on how well healthcare staff communicated, how respectful the communication was and the level of safety.

The main outcome measure in the study by Bashour et al. was the degree to which the women were satisfied with the experience of giving birth [20]. There was both a control group and an intervention group, where healthcare practitioners were provided with additional communication training. Satisfaction was rated on a scale from 1 to 5, with 5 indicating the highest level of satisfaction. The intervention group rated the experience on average as 3.23 (with a standard deviation of 0.72), whilst the controls gave an average score of 3.42 (SD = 0.73). These results indicate no difference statistically between the groups; indeed the confidence intervals for the mean difference between groups crossed zero. The researchers found no significant differences in specific elements of communication, either, such as whether a doctor introduced him- or herself prior to examining a patient, whether greetings were used and whether a doctor looked at the patient whilst speaking.

Although being an effective communicator is considered a key competency for those working in maternity services to acquire, precisely what this competency consists of has so far never been fully delineated. Nicholls and Webb [22] conducted a systematic review of 33 different studies, displaying a high degree of heterogeneity in method adopted, and concluded that a good midwife was one who possessed a good level of communicative ability. Nicholls and Webb subsequently carried out research using the Delphi method to investigate the attitudes of patients, midwives and trainers of midwives towards what constituted good midwifery practice. They discovered that being skilled in communication was commonly considered of great importance [23]. Communicative excellence is stated repeatedly to be a vital element in high-quality maternity services by various official bodies and key policy documents, such as the WHO Quality of Care Framework for Maternal and Newborn Health [24] and the Lancet Framework for Quality Maternal and Newborn Care [25]. Only in this way can women be treated with adequate respect and their experience of giving birth be improved, amongst other desired outcomes.

Research into the wishes and requirements of women giving birth has shown that the expectation was for sensitivity, kindness and a caring attitude to be the norm, with women being afraid of witnessing instead distance, insensitivity or rudeness [26, 27]. A recent qualitative study aims to put together the opinions from a variety of professions involved in providing maternity care to women and the women themselves and come up with common ideas on how to develop maternity services affording dignity to women. The research gathered the findings from 67 studies carried out in 32 countries, representing the entire range of average income [28]. Concepts that emerged in the search for maternity services offering dignity were the need for communicative efficiency, as demonstrated in conversations with the mothers, the need to be alert to non-verbal communicative cues, honesty, provision of interpreting services where there was a linguistic or cultural gap to be bridged and the need for staff to be empathic. The perceived need for such practices is evident from this study and applies across multiple settings. The study could not, however, comment on how frequently these ideals were achieved or what healthcare workers can do to ensure they meet such expectations. There are, nonetheless, data showing that inappropriate ways of managing the labour and birth process did lead to a higher risk of illness or death in both mother and child [17] and that a previously poor experience of giving birth may lead women in some countries to avoid giving birth in a particular maternity setting [29, 30].

6.3 Communication with Women and Healthcare Providers at Birth and Postpartum

Data are unfortunately lacking which can support evidence-based practice aiming to improve communication between mothers-to-be and their care providers in the phases of giving birth and postpartum. If there are to be clear protocols on how to make communication effective and able to ensure a good-quality, safe maternity service is available, there is a need for rigorous studies that take into account mothers' choices, the location of any facilities, the professionals supplying care and other details of the maternity service [1].

There is a need to overcome any shortcomings in communicative practice at the level of individuals, healthcare units and the healthcare system as a whole for maternity outcomes to offer greater benefit to women. Some limitations, such as work intensity, may occur in every facility, whereas other limitations may arise from sociocultural factors (such as the status of women) that are particular to specific countries. Further studies are called for to address how women envisage communication to be most effective during childbirth, where the mothers and their relatives feel efforts should be concentrated, the methods of assessment to be employed and when the ideal time is to carry out assessments of communicative efficiency [1].

6.4 Communication with Disabled Women Giving Birth

There are multiple examples of women with disabilities who have been able to bear healthy children [31]. Despite these successes, there are also numerous reports indicating that disabled women struggle to access adequate maternity care [32]. A study involving 410 women with a physical disability living in South Korea indicated that they had high rates of terminations, spontaneous abortion and caesarian section and rarely used contraception [33]. There are particular chronic conditions which have an association with poor outcomes from pregnancy. Examples include rheumatoid arthritis and schizophrenia [34]. It has been noted that mothers who suffer from schizophrenia have an 11.8% risk of giving birth to a child of low weight, compared with a background rate of 6.8% [35].

It has been proposed [31] that an approach in which healthcare practitioners concentrate on a woman's abilities rather than disabilities is more conducive to a healthy pregnancy and birth of a healthy child. Accordingly, communication in care settings should aim to provide women with empowerment. However, qualitative studies [36, 37] indicate that disabled women encountering maternity services do not receive a service addressing their requirements. Disabled women complain of a lack of visibility within healthcare settings, with issues that go beyond the clinical to involve sociopolitical aspects, too. Accessibility involves more than simply being physically reachable, they state [38]. Given the fact that a disability throws up unforeseen difficulties on a day-to-day basis, women in this position feel the need for maternity care that coheres to a careful plan and assists in reducing these kinds of events [39].

The UK NICE Antenatal Care Guidelines at present recommend that any woman who finds herself pregnant should be in contact with maternity care services at the earliest opportunity. There is a general problem with the accessibility of healthcare for disabled individuals [40]. The small body of research in existence that examines disabled mothers is skewed towards the effects of disability itself, rather than on the ability of such individuals to successfully reproduce [41].

One study [42] examined how pregnancy as an experience in 197 women with auditory or visual impairment differed from pregnancy in those with no such disability. There were no significant differences between the groups in terms of age, ethnic origin, language used at home or previous births. Women in both groups had very similar experiences during antenatal care and similar feelings about the care received, in particular how communication occurred and how decisions were taken. The antenatal care was rated as good by 94% of the disabled women. Furthermore, during labour and parturition, these similarities persisted. The key difference noted was that previous acquaintance with staff involved in their care at this stage was more common in the group with the sensory disabilities (33% vs 23%).

In a different study [42], however, differences were observed. A pregnant woman suffering from a learning disability (LD) had a lower likelihood of having consulted a healthcare practitioner by the 12th week of pregnancy (85% vs 95%). However, those with a learning disability and those without had the same number of antenatal check-ups, ultrasound imaging appointments and antenatal screening. The other area of difference was in how care was perceived. Only 64% of the women with LD reported always being able to comprehend what they were being told (compared to 84% of those without LD), only 63% (compared to 74%) reported involvement in decision-making, and only 58% felt a midwife always responded to a request for assistance, compared with 73% of those without LD. Despite the fact that the women with LD rated a number of aspects of maternity care as deficient, their overall assessments of maternity care indicated a high level of satisfaction, with 93% rating the service as 'good' or better.

There were more frequent calls on antenatal maternity services by physically disabled women, those with a mental health disability and women with multiple disabilities. It was noted that a physically disabled woman's preferences about where to give birth and the progress of labour were less frequently taken into consideration. With the exception of those whose disability involved mental health, the women with disabilities had a greater likelihood of already knowing the staff who attended their birth. Women with an LD expressed a lower sense of satisfaction with the level of support and communicative style both before and during the birth [42].

Some Norwegian research examined the experience of 21 physically disabled women in pregnancy. The study examined social aspects and drew the conclusion that a negative approach by healthcare professionals and inexperience and a lack of knowledge about disability were factors in stopping these women from accessing appropriate care from maternity services [43].

References

1. Chang YS, Coxon K, Portela AG, Furuta M, Bick D. Interventions to support effective communication between maternity care staff and women in labour: a mixed-methods systematic review. Midwifery. 2018;59:4–16. https://doi.org/10.1016/j.midw.2017.12.014.
2. Ames HMR, Glenton C, Lewin S. Parents' and informal caregivers' views and experiences of communication about routine childhood vaccination: a synthesis of qualitative evidence. Cochrane Database Syst Rev. 2017;2:CD011787.
3. Doyle C, Lennox L, Bell D. A systematic review of evidence on the links between patient experience and clinical safety and effectiveness. BMJ Open. 2013;3:e001570.
4. Vogel J, Bohren M, Tunçalp Ö, Oladapo O, Gülmezoglu A. Promoting respect and preventing mistreatment during childbirth. BJOG Int J Obstet Gynaecol. 2016;123:671–4.
5. Deveugele M, Derese A, De Maess-chalck S, Willems S, Van Driel M, De Maeseneer J. Teaching communication skills to medical students, a challenge in the curriculum? Patient Educ Couns. 2005;58:265–70.
6. Butler M, Fraser D, Murphy R. What are the essential competencies required of a midwife at the point of registration? Midwifery. 2008;24:260–9.

7. Bosse HM, Nickel M, Huwendiek S, Jünger J, Schultz JH, Nikendei C. Peer role-play and standardised patients in communication training: a comparative study on the student perspective on acceptability, realism, and perceived effect. BMC Med Educ. 2010;10:27.

8. King A, Hoppe RB. "Best practice" for patient-centered communication: a narrative review. J Grad Med Educ. 2013;5:385–93.

9. Nursing and Midwifery Council. The code. Professional standards of practice and behaviour for nurses and midwives. London: NMC; 2015.

10. Homer CS, Friberg IK, Dias MA, ten Hoope-Bender P, Sandall J, Speciale AM, Bartlett L. The projected effect of scaling up midwifery. Lancet. 2014;384:1164–57.

11. National Maternity Review, better births: improving outcomes of maternity services in England. A five year forward view for maternity care, 2016. https://www.england.nhs.uk/wp-content/uploads/2016/02/national-maternity-review-report.pdf. Accessed 18 Aug 2020.

12. Green JM, Baston HA. Feeling in control during labor: concepts, correlates, and consequences. Birth. 2003;30:235–47.

13. Care Quality Commission. National findings from the 2013 survey of women's experiences of maternity care. Newcastle Upon Tyne: Care Quality Commission; 2013.

14. Alderdice F, Hamilton K, McNeill J, Lynn F, Curran R, Redshaw M. Birth NI: a survey of women's experience of maternity care in Northern Ireland. Belfast: School of Nursing and Midwifery, Queen's University of Belfast; 2016. http://www.qub.ac.uk/schools/SchoolofNursingandMidwifery/FileStore/Filetoupload,670193,en.pdf?platform=hootsuite. Accessed 18 Aug 2020.

15. Ayers S, Bond R, Bertullies S, Wijma K. The aetiology of post-traumatic stress following childbirth: a meta-analysis and theoretical framework. Psychol Med. 2016;46:1121–34.

16. Hauck Y, Fenwick J, Downie J, Butt J. The influence of childbirth expectations of Western Australian women's perceptions of their birth experience. Midwifery. 2007;23:235–47.

17. Mannava P, Durrant K, Fisher J, Chersich M, Luchters S. Attitudes and behaviours of maternal health care providers in interactions with clients: a systematic review. Glob Health. 2015;11:36.

18. Bohren MA, Hunter EC, Munthe-Kaas HM, Souza JP, Vogel JP, Gülmezoglu AM. Facilitators and barriers to facility-based delivery in low- and middle-income countries: a qualitative evidence synthesis. Reprod Health. 2014;11:71.

19. Bohren MA, Vogel JP, Hunter EC, Lutsiv O, Makh SK, Souza JP, Aguiar C, Saraiva CF, Diniz AL, Tunçalp Ö, Javadi D, Oladapo OT, Khosla R, Hindin MJ, Gülmezoglu AM. The mistreatment of women during childbirth in health facilities globally: a mixed-methods systematic review. PLoS Med. 2015;12:e1001847.

20. Bashour HN, Kanaan M, Kharouf MH, Abdulsalam AA, Tabbaa MA, Cheikha SA. The effect of training doctors in communication skills on women's satisfaction with doctor–woman relationship during labour and delivery: a stepped wedge cluster randomised trial in Damascus. BMJ Open. 2013;3:e002674.

21. Crofts JF, Bartlett C, Ellis D, Donald F, Winter CJ, Hunt LP, Draycott TJ. Patient-actor perception of care: a comparison of obstetric emergency training using manikins and patient-actors. Qual Safety Health Care. 2008;17:20–4.

22. Nicholls L, Webb C. What makes a good midwife? An integrative review of methodologically-diverse research. J Adv Nurs. 2006;56:414–29.

23. Nicholls L, Skirton H, Webb C. Establishing perceptions of a good midwife: a Delphi study. Br J Midwifery. 2011;19:230–6.

24. World Health Organization (WHO). Standards for improving quality of maternal and newborn care in healthcare facilities. Geneva: World Health Organization; 2016.

25. Renfrew MJ, McFadden A, Bastos MH, Campbell J, Channon AA, Cheung NF, Silva DRAD, Downe S, Kennedy HP, Malata A, McCormick F, Wick L, Declercq E. Midwifery and quality care: findings from a new evidence-informed framework for maternal and newborn care. Lancet. 2014;384:1129–45.

26. White Ribbon Alliance. Respectful maternity care: the universal rights of childbearing women. Washington, DC: White Ribbon Alliance; 2012. Accessed 18 Aug 2020.

27. Downe S, Finlayson K, Oladapo OT, Bonet M, Gülmezoglu AM. What matters to women during childbirth: a systematic qualitative review. PLoS One. 2018;13(4):e0194906.
28. Shakibazadeh E, Namadian M, Bohren MA, Vogel JP, Rashidian A, Nogueira Pileggi V, Madeira S, Leathersich S, Tunçalp Ö, Oladapo OT, Souza JP, Gülmezoglu AM. Respectful care during childbirth in health facilities globally: a qualitative evidence synthesis. BJOG. 2018;125(8):932–42.
29. Kumbani L, Bjune G, Chirwa E, Malata A, Odland J. Why some women fail to give birth at health facilities: a qualitative study of women's perceptions of perinatal care from rural southern Malawi. Reprod Health. 2013;10:9.
30. Moyer CA, Adongo PB, Aborigo RA, Hodgson A, Engmann CM. 'They treat you like you are not a human being': maltreatment during labour and delivery in rural northern Ghana. Midwifery. 2014;30:262–8.
31. Smeltzer CS. Pregnancy in women with physical disabilities. J Obstet Gynecol Neonatal Nurs. 2007;36:88–96.
32. Coyle CP, Santiago MC. Healthcare utilization among women with physical disabilities. Medscape Women Health. 2002;7(4):2.
33. Lee LO, Heykyung OH. A wise wife and good mother: reproductive health and maternity among women with disability in South Korea. Sex Disabil. 2005;23(3):121–44.
34. Lin HC, Chen YH, Lee HC. Prenatal care and adverse pregnancy outcomes among women with schizophrenia; a national population-based study in Taiwan. J Clin Psychiatry. 2009;70(9):1297–303.
35. Lin HC, Lee HC. The relation between maternal schizophrenia and low birth weight is modified by parental age. Can J Psychiatr. 2010;55(6):377–85.
36. Lipson JG, Rogers JG. Pregnancy, birth, and disability: women's health care experiences. Health Care Women Int. 2000;21:11–26.
37. Prilleltensky O. A ramp to motherhood: the experiences of mothers with physical disabilities. Sex Disabil. 2003;21(1):21–47.
38. Gill C, Kerotoski MA, Turk NMA. Becoming visible: personal health experiences of women with disabilities. In: Krotoski DM, editor. Women with physical disabilities: achieving and maintaining health and wellbeing. Baltimore: Pall H. Brookes; 1996. p. 5–15.
39. Signore C, Spong CY, Krotoski D, Shinowara NL, Blackwell SC. Pregnancy in women with physical disabilities. Obstet Gynecol. 2011;117:935–47.
40. Hanson KW, Neuman P, Dutwin D, Kasper JD. Uncovering the health challenges facing people with disabilities: the role of health insurance. Health Affairs—Web Exclusive. p. 552–565. http://content.healthaffairs.org/content/early/2003/11/19/hlthaff.w3.552.full.pdf+html.
41. Thierry JM. Promoting the health and wellness of women with disabilities. J Womens Health. 1998;7:505–7.
42. Redshaw M, Malouf R, Gao H, et al. Women with disability: the experience of maternity care during pregnancy, labour and birth and the postnatal period. BMC Pregnancy Childbirth. 2013;13:174. https://doi.org/10.1186/1471-2393-13-174.
43. Grue L, Tafjord-Laerum KT. Doing motherhood: some experiences of mothers with physical disabilities. Disabil Soc. 2002;17(6):671–83.

Effect of Pregnancy on the Upper Respiratory Tract and Chest Wall

7

Sena Genç Elden, Mehmet Güven, and Suela Sallavaci

7.1   Introduction

Physiological and anatomical changes that occur during pregnancy cause significant differences in respiratory physiology. Knowing these completely physiological changes is of great importance in the evaluation of pathological events that may occur during pregnancy. In addition, when completely normal respiratory physiology changes are perceived as signs of disease, it may lead to the application of many unnecessary diagnostic procedures. In addition, it should not be forgotten that the physiology of pregnancy and the anatomical changes caused by pregnancy may exacerbate some diseases.

The physiology of pregnancy is characterized by hormonal, cardiovascular, respiratory, and muscular-skeletal changes that are associated with the modification of both the morphology and function of several organ systems. Both biochemical and mechanical pathways affect the anatomy and regulate the physiology of the respiratory system during normal pregnancy [1].

Pregnancy affects the respiratory system through two pathways, chemical and mechanical. The former includes increased levels of progesterone and relaxin which

S. G. Elden (✉)
Department of Otorhinolaryngology, Pamukova State Hospital, Pamukova, Sakarya, Turkey
e-mail: ssenagenc@gmail.com

M. Güven
Department of Otorhinolaryngology, Sakarya University Faculty of Medicine,
Serdivan, Sakarya, Turkey
e-mail: guvenmehmet28@yahoo.com

S. Sallavaci
Department of Otorhinolaryngology, University Hospital Centre "Mother Teresa",
Tirana, Albania
e-mail: sallavacis@gmail.com

C. Cingi et al. (eds.), *ENT Diseases: Diagnosis and Treatment during Pregnancy and Lactation*, https://doi.org/10.1007/978-3-031-05303-0_7

induces collagen loss, with consequent relaxation of ligaments and cartilage. These factors progressively influence the geometry and the dimensions of the chest wall in terms of increasing subcostal angle as well as thoracic and abdominal perimeters [1]. Estrogen is responsible for nasal mucous membrane changes. Estrogens increase the hyaluronic acid component, leading to tissue hydration and edema. In addition, estrogen regulates the development of hyperplastic and hypersecretory mucus glands [2]. Because of these changes in the upper respiratory tract, patients prefer mouth breathing.

Due to hormonal changes and increase in intra-abdominal volume, normal pregnancy may have a mechanical and functional impact on respiratory functioning. The percentage of pregnant women who complain of dyspnea varies from 50% before the 20th week of pregnancy to 76% past the 31st week of pregnancy [3].

Hyperemia, hypersecretion, mucosal edema, and fragility in the airway mucosa are present from the beginning of pregnancy and reach a maximum especially in the first trimester. These changes often lead to changes in tone of voice with nasal obstruction, epistaxis, and coughing attacks and become more pronounced especially when the individual lies on her back.

In this section, the physiological changes caused by pregnancy on the respiratory system and their effects on respiratory functions are evaluated in the light of the literature. Table 7.1 summarizes the effect of pregnancy on the upper airway, lung, and chest wall.

Table 7.1 The effect of pregnancy on the upper airway, lung, and chest wall

Upper airway changes	
Mucosal edema	• Increased resistance to flow • Mean pharyngeal cross-sectional area is smaller • Oropharyngeal junction size is smaller • Increase in sleep disorders
Lung and chest wall changes	
Anatomical changes	• The diaphragm is pushed up by 4 cm • Diaphragmatic excursion increases by about 2 cm • Rib cage expands: subcostal angle of the ribs at the xiphoidal level increases from 68.5° at the beginning of pregnancy to 103.5° at term • Anatomical dead space increases
Lung volumes	• Tidal volume increases • Respiratory rate increases • Minute volume increases • TLC decreases • IC decreases • FRC decreases • ERV decreases • Chest wall compliance decreases • Lung compliance remains the same
Ventilation and gas exchange	• $PaCO_2$ decreases • PaO_2 increases • Respiratory alkalosis

TLC total lung capacity, *IC* inspiratory capacity, *FRC* functional residual capacity, *ERV* expiratory reserve volume, *PaCO₂* partial pressure of carbon dioxide, *PaO₂* partial pressure of oxygen

7.2   Upper Airway Changes in Pregnancy

In pregnancy, the physiological changes potentially predisposing to increased resistance and reduced cross-sectional area of the upper airways include the following: weight gain; a decreased functional residual capacity (FRC) due to mass displacement of the diaphragm; pharyngeal edema of pregnancy; and, possibly, the effect of sleep deprivation or fragmentation on pharyngeal dilator muscle activity and upper airway collapsibility [4]. Functional residual capacity is decreased by 15–25% in pregnancy due to increased abdominal mass raising the diaphragm [5]. In turn, the decreased functional residual capacity and tracheal shortening can produce upper airway narrowing.

In addition to prepregnancy BMI and gestational weight gain, fat deposition that infiltrates pharyngeal muscle tissue or soft tissue deposition in the neck and around upper airway may cause upper airway narrowing in pregnancy [4]. This finding was supported by studies showing that the cross-sectional area of the pharynx increased and the diaphragm lowered and increased FRC with weight loss [6, 7]. Pien et al. showed a decrease in neck size in postpartum and confirmed that the neck circumference increased during pregnancy [8]. In another study, it was shown that pregnant women suffering from snoring have a small oropharynx and abnormal oropharyngeal anatomy [9].

Using acoustic reflectance measurements, oropharyngeal junction size is smaller in the seated position, and mean pharyngeal cross-sectional area is smaller in the supine, lateral, and seated position in pregnant women compared with nonpregnant controls [10]. Mean pharyngeal cross-sectional area increases significantly postpartum compared with intrapartum, but it is not clear when or whether these changes return to preconception size.

7.2.1   Nasal Physiological Changes

There are many proposed theories to explain the association between nasal physiological changes and pregnancy; these include effects of sex hormones via enhanced expression of H1 receptors on nasal epithelial cells, shift of increased plasma volume to extracellular space, the influence of estrogen via increased gland secretion, and vasodilation via both vasoactive intestinal peptide and cholinergic action. Placental growth factor was suggested to induce overgrowth of nasal mucosa, which eventually leads to obstruction of the nasal airway. Smoking and previous atopy were the only identifiable risk factors in the pathogenesis of nasal congestion during pregnancy. However, there is still considerable controversy regarding the diagnosis, classification, etiopathogenesis, and treatment of this clinical entity [11].

The nasal and respiratory tract mucosa become edematous and hyperemic because of the increased estrogen and increased blood volume of pregnancy [12]. All of these result in nasal congestion often called rhinitis of pregnancy. The clinical definition of rhinitis of pregnancy is "nasal congestion present during the last 6 or more weeks of pregnancy without other signs of respiratory tract infection and with no known allergic cause, disappearing completely within 2 weeks after delivery." The incidence of rhinitis of pregnancy has been reported to be between 18 and 42% [10]. These symptoms resolve within 48 h following delivery [12].

It is very important to inform every pregnant woman before medical treatment for pregnancy rhinitis. Pregnant women with nasal congestion may be recommended to lie down with their head elevated with a 45° inclination and physical exercise due to its decongestant effect. The pregnant can wash the nose with physiological saline solution, thus reducing the amount of secretion and removing the crusts. Nasal decongestants give good temporary relief in pregnancy rhinitis. But because the condition does not resolve in a few days, like a common cold do, pregnant women who have nasal symptoms tend to use them for prolonged periods of time. This results in the additional condition of rhinitis medicamentosa, which does not resolve spontaneously after delivery. Rebound swelling of the mucosa increases nasal congestion when the decongestive effect of the drug has disappeared. To alleviate this symptom, patients gradually use larger doses of the vasoconstrictor more frequently. Therefore, it is recommended not to use them as much as possible. Although nasal corticosteroids are not as effective as decongestants, they can be used as another option. Published data show that the currently available inhaled steroids used at clinically relevant doses do not impair intrauterine growth [13, 14].

It is well known that nasal congestion increases when the subject is in the supine position, especially in patients who suffer from rhinitis, and that nasal congestion may result in snoring. The Mallampati score, which indicates the airway patency, has been shown to increase during pregnancy [15]. For this reason, there is an increase in sleep disorders during pregnancy. Snoring is common during pregnancy, and may have negative effects, such as maternal hypertension, preeclampsia, intrauterine growth retardation, and lower Apgar scores [5].

Prolonged nasal congestion can predispose to sinusitis, and continuous mouth breathing can cause dry mouth and tooth decay [13]. Because the upper airways are more edematous and friable, the pregnant patient is more prone to nosebleeds and to bleeding with manipulation [12, 16]. Therefore, procedures such as laryngoscopy and intubation should be performed carefully, using sufficient lubricant for minimize trauma.

7.3 Lung and Chest Wall Mechanics in Pregnancy

The thorax undergoes significant structural changes in pregnancy: The subcostal angle of the rib cage and the circumference of the lower chest wall increase and the diaphragm moves up [10]. These changes are necessary to accommodate the enlarging uterus and increasing maternal weight, but the changes occur early in pregnancy before the uterus is significantly enlarged. By examining chest roentgenograms, Thomson and Cohen documented a 4 cm maximal increase in the level of the diaphragm during pregnancy along with a 2.1 cm maximal increase in the transverse diameter of the chest. In the same study, the subcostal angle was found to increase progressively from an average of 68.5° in early pregnancy to 103.5° in late pregnancy [17].

Diaphragmatic elevation and altered configuration of the thorax appear to be the major factors that affect alterations in lung volume during pregnancy. The consensus of many studies is that lung volumes mostly are well preserved in pregnancy [18]. Although elevation of the diaphragm should decrease the volume in the lungs in the resting state, i.e., the functional residual capacity (FRC), inspiratory movement of the diaphragm and thoracic musculature are unimpaired, and vital capacity (VC) should be unchanged.

Hyperventilation observed in pregnant women is probably caused by the ventilatory stimulating effect of progesterone. Tidal volume (TV) and minute ventilation increase, while functional residual capacity (FRC) and expiratory reserve volume (ERV) decrease. There have not been any definitive reports on changes in vital capacity (VC) during pregnancy [3].

The decreased chest wall compliance is the result of the enlarging uterus increasing the abdominal pressure, because the reduction in FRC is correlated with the increase in end-expiratory abdominal pressure, but not end-expiratory pleural pressure [18].

It has been found that FEV1 during pregnancy is directly proportional to the infant's birth weight, but it is inversely proportional to intrauterine growth retardation, gestational hypertension, and preterm birth in asthmatic women. Suboptimal respiratory system function may be expected in the course of uncomplicated pregnancy as well as in pregnant women who are pregestationally overweight, who experience excessive weight gain during pregnancy, or who smoke cigarettes. Pregestational obesity and excessive weight gain during pregnancy are both recognized as being associated with increased risk of maternal complications during pregnancy [3].

7.4   Respiratory Muscle Function

There is no significant change in respiratory muscle strength during pregnancy despite the cephalad displacement of the diaphragm and changes in the chest wall configuration. Despite the upward displacement of the diaphragm by the gravid uterus, diaphragm excursion actually increases by 2 cm compared with the nonpregnant state. Increased diaphragmatic excursion and preserved respiratory muscle strength are important adaptations, given the increase in tidal volume and minute ventilation that accompanies pregnancy [10].

7.5   Effect of Pregnancy on Ventilation and Gas Exchange

Resting minute ventilation increases during pregnancy [18]. Because the dead space/tidal volume ratio remains normal during pregnancy, the increased tidal volume leads to increased alveolar ventilation [19]. Typically, resting minute ventilation is increased about 30% during pregnancy compared with the postpartum value. In part, the increase in minute ventilation is caused by an increase in metabolic rate and carbon dioxide (CO_2) production. This trend was mirrored by the fall in capillary PCO_2 [18].

The end-expiratory volume, functional residual capacity (FRC), and irreducible residual volume (RV) have consistently been shown to decrease steadily from early in gestation [20]. The kidney excretes excess bicarbonate to compensate for the respiratory alkalosis, and maintains a serum bicarbonate level of about 15–20 mEq/L to preserve a normal arterial pH. The respiratory alkalosis causes a rightward shift in the oxyhemoglobin dissociation curve that aids oxygen transfer across the placenta [21].

There is general agreement that the main cause of the increased respiratory drive that causes the hyperpnea of pregnancy is the elevation of serum progesterone, a direct respiratory stimulant. It is debated whether progesterone acts directly on the respiratory center or with an increase in the gain of chemoreceptors [22]. Studies have shown that when progesterone is administered to nonpregnant persons, it increases minute ventilation, CO_2 chemosensitivity, and airway obstruction pressure [23]. The increase in chemosensitivity occurs early in pregnancy and remains constant up until delivery. Shortly after delivery, the respiratory drive returns to normal with the decrease in progesterone levels and the reduction in metabolic and mechanical loads that were induced by pregnancy [18].

References

1. LoMauro A, Aliverti A, Frykholm P, et al. Adaptation of lung, chest wall, and respiratory muscles during pregnancy: preparing for birth. J Appl Physiol. 2019;127(6):1640–50.
2. Paparella MM, Shumrick DA, Gluckman JL, et al. Otolaryngology. Philadelphia: WB Saunders; 1991. p. 1892–3.
3. Hirnle L, Lysenko L, Gerber H, et al. Respiratory function in pregnant women. In: Mieczyslaw P, editor. Neurobiology of respiration. Dordrecht: Springer; 2013. p. 153–60.
4. Izci B, Vennelle M, Liston WA, et al. Sleep-disordered breathing and upper airway size in pregnancy and post-partum. Eur Respir J. 2006;27(2):321–7.
5. Izci B, Riha RL, Martin SE, et al. The upper airway in pregnancy and pre-eclampsia. Am J Respir Crit Care Med. 2003;167(2):137–40.
6. Hoffstein V, Zamel N, Phillipson EA. Lung volume dependence of pharyngeal cross-sectional area in patients with obstructive sleep apnea. Am Rev Respir Dis. 1984;130(2):175–8.
7. Welch KC, Foster GD, Ritter CT, et al. A novel volumetric magnetic resonance imaging paradigm to study upper airway anatomy. Sleep. 2002;25(5):530–40.
8. Pien GW, Pack AI, Schwab RJ. Changes in neck size during pregnancy. Am J Respir Crit Care Med. 2003;167:601A.
9. Guilleminault C, Kreutzer M, Chang JL. Pregnancy, sleep disordered breathing and treatment with nasal continuous positive airway pressure. Sleep Med. 2004;5(1):43–51.
10. Hegewald MJ, Crapo RO. Respiratory physiology in pregnancy. Clin Chest Med. 2011;32(1):1–13.
11. Demir UL, Demir BC, Oztosun E, et al. The effects of pregnancy on nasal physiology. In: Kennedy DW, editor. International forum of allergy & rhinology, vol. 5. Amsterdam: The Netherlands; 2015. p. 162–6.
12. Hill CC, Pickinpaugh J. Physiologic changes in pregnancy. Surg Clin North Am. 2008;88(2):391–401.
13. Ellegård EK. Pregnancy rhinitis. Immunology and allergy. Clinics. 2006;26(1):119–35.

14. Namazy JA, Schatz M. Update in the treatment of asthma during pregnancy. Clin Rev Allergy Immunol. 2004;26(3):139–48.
15. Pilkington S, Carli F, Dakin MJ, et al. Increase in Mallampati score during pregnancy. Br J Anaesth. 1995;74(6):638–42.
16. Camann WR, Ostheimer GW. Physiological adaptations during pregnancy. Int Anesthesiol Clin. 1990;28(1):2–10.
17. Weinberger SE, Weiss ST, Cohen WR, et al. Pregnancy and the lung. Am Rev Respir Dis. 1980;121(3):559–81.
18. Wise RA, Polito AJ, Krishnan V. Respiratory physiologic changes in pregnancy. Immunol Allergy Clin North Am. 2006;26(1):1–12.
19. Templeton AA, Kelman GR. Maternal blood-gases, (PAO2—PaO2), physiological shunt and VD/VT in normal pregnancy. Br J Anaesth. 1976;48(10):1001–4.
20. Milne JA. The respiratory response to pregnancy. Postgrad Med J. 1979;55(643):318–24.
21. Tsai CH, de Leeuw NK. Changes in 2, 3-diphosphoglyeerate during pregnancy and puerperium in normal women and in β-thalassemia heterozygous women. Am J Obstet Gynecol. 1982;142(5):520–3.
22. Skatrud JB, Dempsey JA, Kaiser DG. Ventilatory response to medroxyprogesterone acetate in normal subjects: time course and mechanism. J Appl Physiol. 1978;44(6):939–44.
23. Schoene RB, Pierson DJ, Lakshminarayan S, et al. Effect of medroxyprogesterone acetate on respiratory drives and occlusion pressure. Clin Respir Physiol. 1980;16(5):645–53.

## Part II

General Otolaryngology During Pregnancy and the Postpartum Period

ENT Emergencies During Pregnancy

8

Muhammet Ayral, Müzeyyen Yıldırım Baylan, and Dennis Chua

8.1 Introduction

Otorhinolaryngological (ENT) emergencies can affect individuals of all age groups. ENT emergencies are of high importance due to the vital organs located in the head and neck region. The approach to the pregnant patient is of higher importance due to the presence of two living individuals. Otorhinolaryngological emergencies may occur due to various metabolic, endocrinological, and physiological changes during pregnancy. For the management of these emergencies, physicians must be familiar with all medical evidence and guidelines. The emergency treatment of most pregnant patients requires a multidisciplinary approach involving obstetricians and anesthesiologists in addition to otorhinolaryngologists. A treatment or intervention should be implemented after obtaining maternal informed consent regarding the possible effects on the mother and fetus. In this section, we tried to summarize how physicians should approach pregnant patients presenting with ENT emergencies.

8.2 Epistaxis

Epistaxis is a common problem during pregnancy due to increased vascularization of the nasal mucosa. It has a prevalence of 20.3% in pregnant women, with a prevalence of 6.2% in non-pregnant individuals [1]. Large-volume epistaxis is

M. Ayral (✉) · M. Y. Baylan
Medical Faculty, Otorhinolaryngology Department, Dicle University, Diyarbakır, Turkey
e-mail: drayral@hotmail.com; muzeyyenyldrm@hotmail.com

D. Chua
ENT Surgeons Medical Centre, Department of Otorhinolaryngology, Mount Elizabeth Hospital, 3 Mount Elizabeth, Singapore
e-mail: dennis.chua.yk@gmail.com

C. Cingi et al. (eds.), *ENT Diseases: Diagnosis and Treatment during Pregnancy and Lactation*, https://doi.org/10.1007/978-3-031-05303-0_8

rare for women without pre-existing risk factors or conditions (such as the use of anticoagulant treatments or blood coagulation disorders) [2]. Fortunately, the majority of epistaxis cases are self-limiting and can be managed with simple first aid measures or nasal packing. Although severe epistaxis episodes are less frequently reported, they can reach a life-threatening level [3–5]. A surgical intervention may sometimes be required to treat severe and prolonged non-localized epistaxis.

In the general population, epistaxis is accelerated by both local and systemic factors. Pregnant patients may develop several additional disorders that further predispose to epistaxis. Hormonal changes during pregnancy can affect nasal physiology. It has been hypothesized that estrogen increases the production of acetylcholine, thus causing a mucosal edema through a direct cholinergic effect. Patients become most symptomatic during the third trimester of pregnancy, when estrogen levels peak. Nasal vascular occlusion is also affected by increased plasma volume and tissue fluid retention [6, 7].

Estrogens can also have indirect effects on the vascular wall by regulating NO signaling pathway (i.e., VEGF, VEGFR-2) [8]. It is thought that increasing estrogen levels during pregnancy may increase vascularization of the nasal mucosa, with a resulting prolongation in bleeding time [9, 10]. Moreover, in severe epistaxis, progesterone may mask blood loss due to cardiovascular compensation in the absence of coagulation disorders or organic nasal abnormalities (polyps) [7]. Even the placenta contributes to the risk of epistaxis by secreting placental growth hormone, which has systemic vasodilatory effects. It has been reported that immunological changes may lead to nasal hypersensitivity [9]. Indirect hormonal effects include vascular inflammatory and immunological changes that may predispose to nasal hypersensitivity and thus problems such as nasal granuloma gravidarum [7]. Pregnancy granulomas are considered to be a hormone-dependent, fast-growing, benign fibrovascular tumor, which rarely occurs in about 2–5% of pregnant women, histologically resembling a pyogenic granuloma or lobular capillary hemangioma, and does not cause large amounts of bleeding during pregnancy [11–13]. These lesions typically occur after birth, but become a potential source of epistaxis during pregnancy and usually regress after pregnancy. However, they can cause a significant amount of epistaxis. Surgical excision is the best treatment option, if there are significant symptoms of epistaxis and obstruction or concerns about a possible malignancy [11–13]. In addition to hormonal changes, hypertension, HELLP syndrome, and gestational thrombocytopenia may also play a role in the etiology of pregnancy-related epistaxis. HELLP syndrome refers to a condition characterized by the progression of thrombocytopenia, hemolysis, increase in liver enzyme levels, and a decrease in thrombocyte count [14]. It is a disease that requires urgent delivery as it can be very fatal for both mother and fetus. Therefore, HELLP syndrome in mothers with thrombocytopenia should be differentially diagnosed by liver function tests and peripheral blood smear [15, 16]. As with essential hypertension, hypertensive conditions during pregnancy can also precipitate epistaxis. Gestational hypertension is defined as a persistent hypertension or a temporary increase in blood pressure (above 140/90 mmHg) in the second half of pregnancy.

Gestational thrombocytopenia is a common hematological problem encountered by obstetricians and hematologists in approximately 10% of all pregnancies. The majority of patients have a gestational thrombocytopenia (GT) characterized by mild thrombocytopenia, requiring no treatment and not associated with the risk of maternal or fetal bleeding. Despite the high frequency of GT, there is no known specific underlying mechanism, which can complicate the distinction from other causes of thrombocytopenia [17, 18].

8.2.1 Treatment

Mild epistaxis can usually stop spontaneously without the need for an intervention. Prophylactic measures such as damp and saline nasal sprays can help. The indications for nasal packing and management are the same as for non-pregnant patients.

Severe epistaxis has a more limited treatment option in pregnant women compared to non-pregnant women. Acute blood loss can be life-threatening for both mother and fetus. Hospitalization is mandatory in case of severe bleeding. The first-line treatment of severe epistaxis may always include intravenous administration of tranexamic acid, silver nitrate cauterization and bipolar cauterization, or anterior packing with materials such as Merocel, Rapid Rhino, etc. Bismuth iodoform paraffin paste (BIPP) and soaked strip gauze are contraindicated during pregnancy [2, 8]. If conservative treatment fails, two radical treatments should be considered: surgical vascular ligation and termination of pregnancy [2].

There are a limited number of prophylactic antibiotics for nasal packing that can be used in pregnant women, but it is known that penicillin, cephalosporin, and erythromycin are safe for use in pregnant women [19]. In addition, postnasal packing, which is often considered when anterior nasal packing fails, is a difficult choice for pregnant women. Severe posterior epistaxis that is not well-controlled with conservative treatment options in pregnant women also poses an important problem for clinicians. Rebleeding may occur after posterior nasal packing, which is also associated with known complications such as adhesions, ocular cellulitis, sinusitis, toxic shock syndrome, and hypoxia. The obstruction in the posterior nasal cavity may cause a great stress to the patient and further increase the fetal stress [20]. Early consideration of surgery under general anesthesia, including sphenoid artery ligation, is thought to be a good treatment strategy [21]. Although endoscopic sphenoidal artery ligation requires general anesthesia, it has a high success rate of around 90% and a low complication rate compared to posterior nasal packing. Compared to the former methods, including external carotid artery ligation and internal mandibular artery ligation, endoscopic sphenoidal artery ligation is associated with less collateral bleeding and circulation, resulting in lower frequency of rebleeding and shorter hospital stay. It has the advantage of low morbidity rates [22, 23]. However, pregnant women who are subjected to surgery and anesthesia during pregnancy are known to have the risk of preterm delivery and spontaneous abortion. In addition, the absence of any fetal abnormalities should be ensured by an ultrasonographic examination immediately after the operation [21].

Pregnancy requires special consideration because of the risk of general anesthesia. The effects of intravenous and inhaled anesthetics on the fetus are not fully understood, but it is known that there is an increased risk of preterm labor, especially in the first two trimesters of pregnancy. The use of local anesthetic and topical vasoconstrictor nasal preparations may be considered, but systemic absorption should be used with caution because it may cause a decrease in uterine blood flow [24]. Although radiological embolization may be considered in some cases, it is recommended only if absolutely necessary in current guidelines, due to the as yet unknown effects of intravenous contrast on the fetus, which could result in a potential fetal loss [21].

As a result, epistaxis is a common problem in pregnancy, and at least one in five women will have two or more epistaxis episodes during pregnancy. Accordingly, a multidisciplinary approach is required that includes obstetricians, otolaryngologists, and obstetric anesthesiologists.

8.3 Bell's Palsy

8.3.1 Epidemiology

Idiopathic facial palsy, first described by British surgeon Sir Charles Bell, is a sudden-onset, unilateral, partial, or full facial paralysis that develops due to various factors. It is the most common cause of facial nerve palsy, with an estimated incidence of 11–40/100,000 [25]. Both genders are affected equally, with an average age of onset of 40 years [26].

Some studies have reported that pregnant women are at a 2–4 times higher risk, especially in the third trimester and in the first 2 weeks postpartum [26–33]. Because the underlying mechanism of Bell's palsy is partially known, the reason for its increased risk is also unclear. Perineural edema, hypercoagulation causing thrombosis in the vasa nervorum, and relative immunosuppression during pregnancy have been suggested as potential etiological factors [34]. Also, it has recently been associated with the herpes simplex virus (HSV) [35]. In pregnant women, physiological and pathophysiological conditions and immunosuppressive conditions such as puerperium; susceptibility to viral infections, especially HSV; hypercoagulation state; hypertension and preeclampsia; increase in total body water; changes in estrogen and progesterone levels; and increased cortisol levels may explain the higher frequency of facial paralysis during pregnancy [36].

In a study involving a high number of participants, the annual incidence of Bell's palsy was 43.4 in the patient group including 100,000 pregnant women (15–49 years old), while it was higher (80.2) in 100,000 non-pregnant women (15–49 years old) in the control group. In addition, the annual incidence or overall prevalence of Bell's palsy in the patient group of pregnant women was about half that of the control group. It has been stated that pregnancy cannot be considered as a possible risk factor for Bell's paralysis [37].

8.3.2   Physiopathology

Bell's palsy occurs through the same mechanism in pregnant and non-pregnant women. However, pregnant women are typically considered to have a more severe course and a worse prognosis [30, 38, 39]. Although most patients regain normal or near-normal functions, pregnant women are more likely to develop full facial paralysis, which results in incomplete resolution. The reason for the incomplete recovery is either the delay in the treatment of pregnant women or the facial paralysis during pregnancy is more severe. It is not clear whether the risk of recurrence is higher in pregnant women compared to non-pregnant women [40].

8.3.3   Diagnosis

Patients with Bell's palsy typically develop facial weakness within 1–2 days. They may report leakage of fluids or food from the affected side of the mouth, failure to close the eyelid, or difficulty speaking. The first key to evaluating the patient is to determine whether the facial weakness is peripheral or centrally caused. In peripheral facial palsy, there is weakness of all muscles of facial expression and inability to raise the eyebrow, a larger palpebral fissure, and a flattened nasolabial fold. The patient cannot inflate his cheek or whistle, and experiences a pulling in the mouth toward the unaffected side while smiling or showing his/her teeth [41].

8.3.4   Treatment

Some clinicians have been hesitant to treat women with steroids during pregnancy due to concerns about maternal and fetal side effects. Stopping or delaying treatment in this way may partly explain the worse prognosis in pregnant women reported in the literature.

Treatment recommendations for Bell's palsy during pregnancy are the same as for non-pregnant patients.

There is strong evidence to support treatment with steroids. Some authors recommend the use of steroids alone, while others recommend the use of steroids in combination with antivirals. Because Bell's palsy has a worse prognosis in pregnant women than in non-pregnant women, early treatment with steroids is highly recommended. It is recommended to use the lowest effective glucocorticoid dose during pregnancy. A short course of oral glucocorticoids is recommended for all patients with incipient Bell's palsy, ideally starting within 3 days of onset of symptoms. There are variations in the doses and regimens studied. In the largest randomized trial, patients were treated with 60 mg of oral "prednisolone" daily for 5 days, followed by a 5-day taper at 10 mg per day. There is high-quality evidence from randomized studies that early initiation of glucocorticoids improves outcomes in patients with Bell's palsy. Two large randomized studies have shown that antivirals alone have no added benefit to steroids [25, 42]. In addition, in an evidence-based guideline published in 2012 [43], the American Academy of Neurology recommends treating Bell's palsy with corticosteroids alone within 3–7 days after symptom onset. In another randomized controlled trial in 2012, prednisolone treatment resulted in higher cure rates regardless of the initial severity of the disease. Regardless of the degree of paralysis, it is recommended to consider prednisolone treatment in all patients [44]. The recommendation indicated no significant benefit of antiviral therapy and did not support the addition of antiviral therapy.

It remains unclear whether antiviral therapy provides additional benefit to glucocorticoids in patients with new-onset Bell's palsy. In a Cochrane review in 2015, antiviral agents were associated with a greater risk reduction when administered in combination with corticosteroids compared to corticosteroids alone [45]. In addition, a double-blind randomized clinical trial in 2016 reported that the combination of steroids and antivirals increased the likelihood of recovery from moderate to complete acute Bell's palsy [46]. Concomitant administration of oral valaciclovir or acyclovir with glucocorticoids is recommended in patients with House-Brackmann (HB) grade IV or higher, considered to be severe facial palsy. Antiviral therapy alone (without glucocorticoids) is not recommended. The recommended antiviral regimen in patients with severe Bell's palsy includes the use of 1000 mg valaciclovir three times a day for a week [42]. Nucleoside analogs, including valaciclovir and famciclovir, are classified as pregnancy category B and pose a very low risk to the mother or fetus [42].

All patients with Bell's palsy should be evaluated for complete eyelid closure.

Eye care is the least controversial and is of important in terms of preventing ocular complications such as corneal erosion. Eye care usually consists of the use of preservative-free artificial tears, a thicker ointment to apply during sleep, and possibly a taping, patch, or moisture chamber.

Long-term use of systemic steroids during pregnancy is not without risks. Maternal and fetal risks of prednisone can be defined during pregnancy. Risks of systemic steroid treatment for the pregnant patient include worsening of peptic ulcer disease, acute psychosis, fluid retention, exacerbation of diabetes control, increased risk of infections, and osteoporosis if used over a long period of time [47].

Risks to the fetus include adrenal suppression, low birth weight, and an increased risk of cleft palate, especially when used in the first trimester [48, 49]. Data from various publications show that repeated steroid treatments during pregnancy are associated with low birth weight and low head circumference in newborns [50–52].

Early evidence suggested an increased risk of cleft palate in fetuses exposed to glucocorticoids during the first trimester of pregnancy [48]. Contrary to these observations, a cohort study including 832,636 live births did not detect an increase in orofacial clefts in 51,973 infants exposed to glucocorticoids during the first trimester of pregnancy compared to infants who were not exposed [49]. Available data suggest that exposure to glucocorticoids in early pregnancy is unlikely to increase the risk of cleft palate. Prednisone and prednisolone have a limited effect on the fetus as they are converted into an inactive form by the placenta. The large amount of data obtained over time did not show an identifiable or demonstrable increased risk of birth defects in women who used corticosteroids during pregnancy [48].

To avoid these risks, it is recommended to use the lowest possible glucocorticoid dose to control disease activity during pregnancy [50, 51]. A detailed discussion should be made about the potential risks and benefits of high-dose glucocorticoids during pregnancy.

Facial nerve decompression during pregnancy has been reported very rarely and is not recommended.

8.4 Sudden Sensorineural Hearing Loss

Sudden sensorineural hearing loss (SSNHL) is an emergency otological condition, typically defined as sensorineural hearing loss of >30 dB at three consecutive frequencies in a pure tone audiogram over a 72-h period [53]. The exact pathophysiology of SSNHL has not yet been clearly explained in most cases [54, 55]. There are several hypotheses for the etiology of SSNHL in pregnancy, all of which are based on physiological changes occurring in the maternal body.

Pregnancy is a unique condition for women and is characterized by a series of physiological changes in all body systems including the hearing system [56]. It has been shown that hormonal, metabolic, and emotional changes caused by pregnancy are associated with various audiometric phenotypes in pregnant/postpartum women [57, 58]. Although there are suggested potential mechanisms linking pregnancy with SSNHL, little evidence has been reported to address this association [59, 60]. Estrogen and progesterone are the main pregnancy hormones. During pregnancy, there is a significant increase in the production of estrogen and progesterone hormones. High estrogen concentration causes an electrolyte imbalance, resulting in an increase in extracellular fluid volume. Moreover, there may be a deterioration in the chemical composition of the inner ear and an affection in the cochlea similar to that of Ménière's disease, resulting in SSHNL. Other researchers reported a hypercoagulable state with an increase in factors other than factor XI during pregnancy. This increases the risk of thromboembolism, which can lead to vascular occlusion in the cochlear microcirculation through microembolism, which can eventually induce SSNHL [56, 60–62]. However, evidence of thromboembolic occlusion in the cochlea causing SSNHL has not yet been clearly explained. Considering that the cochlea is mainly affected by the last arterial supply from the anterior lower cerebellar artery [63], it is not known whether gestational hypercoagulation affects thrombotic arterial occlusion in the cochlea.

The reported global incidence of SSNHL ranges from 5 to 20 per 100,000 people [53, 54]. A population-based study in Taiwan covering data from 2000 to 2009 revealed an incidence of 2.71 SSNHL per 100,000 pregnancies, which is lower than in the general female population [64]. In the South Korean study, the estimated annual SSNHL incidence during pregnancy was 19.5 per 100,000 pregnant women. The rate of SSNHL in the postpartum period was 37.9 per 100,000 women, comparable to the rate of 36.3 per 100,000 women in the control group [65].

It has been reported that most pregnant patients are exposed to SSNHL in the third trimester and older pregnant women are at higher risk than younger ones.

Early intervention has been identified as a beneficial prognostic factor for SSNHL [66]. Although 32–65% of non-pregnant SSNHL patients usually have spontaneous recovery in the first 2 weeks, the natural course of sudden hearing loss in pregnant women has not yet been established [67].

8.4.1 Treatments

Treatment of SSNHL in a pregnant woman is challenging due to limited clinical data and treatment options. Otologists are faced with a dilemma as pregnant patients may refuse treatment for fear of potential harmful side effects on the fetus. SSNHL tends to resolve spontaneously. However, the natural course of this clinical problem during pregnancy has not yet been determined, which necessitates medical therapy.

There are several treatment options for SSNHL. Systemic or topical administration of steroids and hyperbaric oxygen (HBO) therapy are the most commonly recommended treatments for SSNHL [68]. Other treatment modalities such as antivirals, thrombolytics, vasodilators, vasoactive agents, and antioxidants are not recommended. Previous studies have reported improvement of SSNHL in some pregnant patients after a few days or after birth without any treatment [69–71].

Wang and Young [70] reported a remarkable improvement in hearing in six pregnant patients with SSNHL with treatment with intravenous dextran-40. The mechanism of dextran-40 is to lower blood viscosity, increase microcirculation, and theoretically decrease cochlear hypoxia. From this study, there is a significant difference in hearing recovery between the dextran-40 group and the control group. Unfortunately, some side effects (e.g., coagulopathy, acute renal failure, and non-cardiogenic pulmonary edema) have been reported with the use of dextran-40 as SSNHL therapy. However, no significant side effect of dextran-40 has been detected when used as a treatment for SSNHL in pregnant women [70]. Therefore, the therapeutic benefits of dextran-40 in pregnant patients and their fetuses likely outweigh its potential risks [72].

Systemic and localized steroid therapy has been the mainstream for SSNHL for decades in the non-pregnant population [68, 73–78]. Systemic corticosteroids however are not recommended for use in the first trimester due to its potential teratogenicity [79]. Systemic corticosteroids are generally considered safe to use during the third trimester [80]. Zeng [71] and Zhang [81] showed that oral prednisone use provided an improvement in pregnant patients with SSNHL. There were no apparent harmful side effects in mothers and babies after follow-up for several years.

Intratympanic corticosteroids is an option for patients with SSNHL, especially in those who have contraindications to or refuse to use systemic corticosteroids [77, 82]. This therapy is also recommended by some otologist as an initial treatment for severe and profound SSNHL [83]. Injection of intratympanic corticosteroids is more efficacious compared to systemic administration of corticosteroids because it provides much higher therapeutic steroid effects in the affected ear, and also minimizes the side effects of systemic corticosteroid concentrations [77, 82, 83]. Dexamethasone and methylprednisolone have been used in intratympanic injection, but methylprednisolone (US FDA category B) may be a more suitable option for pregnant patients compared to dexamethasone (US FDA category C). Many studies have shown that pregnant patients with SSNHL can achieve complete or partial recovery after intratympanic corticosteroid injection without any side effects [72, 73, 84].

Hyperbaric oxygen therapy often acts as an adjunct therapy for SSNHL. Because the safety of short-term exposure to a hyperoxic atmosphere has been confirmed by studies in the literature, some physicians use it as the sole treatment for SSNHL in pregnant patients [85]. However, there is no strong evidence to support the efficacy of hyperbaric oxygen therapy for SSNHL in pregnancy.

8.5 Maxillofacial Trauma

Maxillofacial injuries should only be treated after the obstetric condition has been managed. The most common fractures are those of the mandible and the orbito-zygomatic-maxillary complex. Treatment of maxillofacial trauma in the pregnant patient is not significantly different from that in other patients: Maternal and fetal stability should be evaluated. The need for fetal monitoring should be determined. When the ability of the airway to maintain itself is in doubt, precise control of the airway by intubation or tracheotomy may be required. After stabilization of the patient's condition, maxillofacial examinations can be performed [86].

First and foremost, it must be determined whether the patient is in a nonurgent, urgent, or life-threatening situation. Elective or routine oral and maxillofacial surgical procedures are considered "relative contraindications" in pregnant women and should be delayed until after delivery [87]. More serious or *life-threatening* conditions require prompt diagnosis and treatment. Fractures of facial bones (nose, zygoma, maxilla, mandible) can be open (combined from the skin or oral cavity) or closed, simple or comminuted, and displaced or non-displaced. Open and comminuted fractures are more urgent to treat and are most likely to become infected, especially if not fixed immediately.

Nasal fractures can usually be treated with manipulation and closed nasal under local anesthesia. Isolated, non-displaced alveolar fractures with loosened jaw or lower jaw teeth can also be fixed with dental arch rods under local anesthesia. Some open and comminuted facial fractures will require open reduction and internal fixation. Selected maxillary and most mandible fractures can be fixed with transoral incisions. Displaced zygomatic and periorbital fractures may require cutaneous incisions for reduction/fixation. Nasal fractures that require open reduction can often be repaired with the same type of transfection incision used for rhinoplasty. Rigid internal fixation plates used in maxillary and mandibular fracture stabilization often eliminate the need for intermaxillary fixation (interconnection of the upper and lower teeth). Antibiotics are usually indicated preoperatively for compound fractures, and analgesics are usually required for the first week following injury [88]. The pregnant patient and fetus will be closely monitored during this period of time.

The therapeutic point to consider is that due to the increased abdominopelvic mass, there is the potential for significant compression of the inferior vena cava by the fetus when the pregnant patient is placed in the supine position. The important point to be considered during treatment is that due to the increased abdominopelvic mass, there is the potential for significant compression of the inferior vena cava by the fetus when the pregnant patient is placed in the supine position. Supine hypotension syndrome is clinically characterized by hypotension, syncope, and bradycardia. Although a patient does not show symptoms of supine hypotension syndrome, there is still the potential for a significant disruption in uteroplacental flow when the patient is placed in the supine position. To prevent or alleviate supine hypotension, the pregnant patient should sit to the left at an angle of 5°–15° (in a position where the right hip rises up to 10–12 cm) [89–91].

8.6 Deep Neck Infections

Deep neck infections (DNI) are serious bacterial infections in the potential cavities and facial planes of the neck. They can spread in these facial planes from the skull base to the mediastinum. Although there has been a decrease in the frequency and morbidity and mortality rates of such severe infections since the introduction of antibiotic treatments, they can still cause serious complications and have a mortal course [92–94].

Early diagnosis is essential for effective treatment of such severe infections, which is even more important due to potential life-threatening conditions for the pregnant patient and the fetus. Most authors suggest that an abscess in the head and neck area should be treated promptly with an incision and drainage. Untreated or poorly treated infections are likely to spread in the potential cavities and facial planes of the neck [95]. The most common etiologies are odontogenic (35–42%) and pharyngotonsillar infections. Oral health problems and odontogenic infections present various difficulties in pregnant women. Pregnancy is a relative contraindication to dental surgery. However, in emergency situations, the procedure can be done safely with the selection of appropriate antibiotherapy, the use of appropriate local anesthetic agents, and the right technical knowledge [96]. When treatment is avoided, serious complications can occur for both the mother and the fetus [97]. In conclusion, when deep neck infections reach deep anatomical cavities, they should be treated aggressively with surgical drainage and correct antibiotic therapy, using a multidisciplinary approach by a team including obstetricians, infectious diseases specialists, and otolaryngologists.

References

1. Dugan-Kim M, Connell S, Stika C, Wong CA, Gossett DR. Epistaxis of pregnancy and association with postpartum hemorrhage. Obstet Gynecol. 2009;114(6):1322–5.
2. Piccioni MG, et al. Management of severe epistaxis during pregnancy: a case report and review of the literature. Case Rep Obstet Gynecol. 2019;2019:5825309.
3. Cornthwaite K, Varadharajan K, Oyarzabal M, Watson H. Management of prolonged epistaxis in pregnancy: case report. J Laryngol Otol. 2013;127(8):811–3.

4. Braithwaite JM, Encomides DL. Severe recurrent epistaxis causing antepartum fetal distress. Int J Obstet Gynecol. 1995;50(2):197–8.
5. Cooley SM, Geary M, O'Connell MP, Keane DP. Hypovolaemic shock secondary to epistaxis in pregnancy. J Obest Gynecol. 2002;22(2):229–30.
6. Vlastarakos PV, et al. Treating common problems of the nose and throat in pregnancy: what is safe? Eur Arch Otorhinolaryngol. 2008;265(5):499–508.
7. Goldstein G, Govindaraj S. Rhinologic issues in pregnancy. Allergy Rhinol. 2012;3(1):e13–5.
8. Crunkhorn REM, Mitchell-Innes A, Mufazzar J. Torrential epistaxis in the third trimester: a management conundrum. BMJ Case Rep. 2014;2014:bcr2014203892.
9. Sobol S, Frenkiel S, Nachtigal D, Wiener D, Teblum C. Clinical manifestations of sinonasal pathology during pregnancy. J Otolaryngol. 2001;30:24–8.
10. Osol G, Ko NL, Mandalà M. Plasticity of the maternal vasculature during pregnancy. Annu Rev Physiol. 2019;81:89–111.
11. Jones JE, Nguyen A, Tabaee A. Pyogenic granuloma (pregnancy tumor) of the nasal cavity. A case report. J Reprod Med. 2000;45:749–53.
12. Kapella M, Panosetti E, Rombaux P, Delos M, Weynand B. Lobular capillary haemangioma of the nasal cavity: observation of three specific cases. Acta Otorhinolaryngol Belg. 2001;55:241–6.
13. Choudhary S, MacKinnon CA, Morrissey GP, Tan ST. A case of giant nasal pyogenic granuloma gravidarum. J Craniofac Surg. 2005;16:319–2.
14. Sibai BM. Diagnosis, controversies, and management of the syndrome of hemolysis, elevated liver enzymes, and low platelet count. Obstet Gynecol. 2004;103(5 Pt 1):981–91.
15. Garg R, Nath MP, Bhalla AP, Kumar A. Disseminated intravascular coagulation complicating HELLP syndrome: perioperative management. BMJ Case Rep. 2009;2009:bcr10.2008.1027.
16. Geary M. The HELLP syndrome. Br J Obstet Gynaecol. 1997;104:887–91.
17. Fogerty AE. Thrombocytopenia in pregnancy: mechanisms and management. Transfus Med Rev. 2018;32(4):225–9.
18. McCrae KR. Thrombocytopenia in pregnancy. In: Michelson AD, editor. Platelets. New York: Elsevier; 2006. p. 925–33.
19. Crider KS, Cleves MA, Reefhuis J, Berry RJ, Hobbs CA, Hu DJ. Antibacterial medication use during pregnancy and risk of birth defects: National Birth Defects Prevention Study. Arch Pediatr Adolesc Med. 2009;163:978–85.
20. Braithwaite JM, Economides DL. Severe recurrent epistaxis causing antepartum fetal distress. Int J Gynecol Obstet. 1995;50(2):197–8.
21. Kang H, et al. A case of severe epistaxis during pregnancy treated by sphenopalatine artery ligation. Korean J Otorhinolaryngol Head Neck Surg. 2016;59(5):392–5.
22. Schwartzbauer HR, Shete M, Tami TA. Endoscopic anatomy of the sphenopalatine and posterior nasal arteries: implications for the endoscopic management of epistaxis. Am J Rhinol. 2003;17(1):63–6.
23. Christmas DA, Yanagisawa E, Pastrano JA. Transnasal endoscopic ligation of the sphenopalatine artery. Ear Nose Throat J. 1998;77(7):524–5.
24. Leicht CH. Anesthesia for the pregnant patient undergoing nonobstetric surgery. Anesthesiol Clin N Am. 1990;8:140.
25. Sullivan FM, Swan IR, Donnan PT. Early treatment with prednisolone or acyclovir in Bell's palsy. N Engl J Med. 2007;357:1598–607.
26. Baugh RF, Basura GJ, Ishii LE, et al. Clinical practice guideline: Bell's palsy. Otolaryngol Head Neck Surg. 2013;149:S1.
27. Ferreira MA, Lavori M, deCarvalho GM, Guimarães AC, Silva VG, Paschoal JR. Facial palsy and pregnancy: management and treatment. Rev Bras Ginecol Obstet. 2013;35:368–72.
28. Shmorgun D, Chan WS, Ray JG. Association between Bell's palsy in pregnancy and pre-eclampsia. QJM. 2002;95:359–62.
29. Hilsinger RL Jr, Adour KK, Doty HE. Idiopathic facial paralysis, pregnancy, and the menstrual cycle. Ann Otol Rhinol Laryngol. 1975;84:433.
30. Gillman GS, Schaitkin BM, May M, Klein SR. Bell's palsy in pregnancy: a study of recovery outcomes. Otolaryngol Head Neck Surg. 2002;126:26–30.

31. Pope TH Jr, Kenan PD. Bell's palsy in pregnancy. Arch Otolaryngol. 1969;89:830–4.
32. Hussain A, et al. Bell's facial nerve palsy in pregnancy: a clinical review. J Obstet Gynaecol. 2017;37(4):409–15.
33. Vrabec JT, Isaacson B, Van Hook JW. Bell's palsy and pregnancy. Otolaryngol Head Neck Surg. 2007;137:858.
34. De Diego-Sastre JI, Prim-Espada MP, Fernandez-Garcia F. The epidemiology of Bell's palsy. Rev Neurol. 2005;41:287–90.
35. Murakami S, Mizobuchi M, Nakashiro Y, et al. Bell palsy and herpes simplex virus: identification of viral DNA in endoneurial fluid and muscle. Ann Intern Med. 1996;124(1 Pt 1):27–30.
36. Falco NA, Eriksson E. Idiopathic facial palsy in pregnancy and the puerperium. Surg Gynecol Obstet. 1989;169:337–40.
37. Choi HG, Hong SK, Park SK, Kim HJ, Chang J. Pregnancy does not increase the risk of Bell's palsy: a national cohort study. Otol Neurotol. 2020;41(1):e111–7.
38. Edwards CE. Bell's palsy in the last trimester of pregnancy and the puerperium. Am J Obstet Gynecol. 1964;89:274–6.
39. Kunze M, Arndt S, Zimmer A, Földi M, Hanjalic-Beck A, Echternach M, et al. Idiopathic facial palsy during pregnancy. HNO. 2012;60:98–101.
40. Deshpande AD. Recurrent Bell's palsy in pregnancy. J Laryngol Otol. 1990;104:713–4. [Google Scholar].
41. Reich SG. Bell's palsy. Continuum. 2017;23(2):447–66.
42. Engström M, Berg T, Stjernquist-Desatnik A, et al. Prednisolone and valaciclovir in Bell's palsy: a randomised, double-blind, placebo-controlled, multicentre trial. Lancet Neurol. 2008;7:993.
43. Gronseth GS, Paduga R, American Academy of Neurology. Evidence-based guideline update: steroids and antivirals for bell palsy: report of the guideline development Subcommittee of the American Academy of Neurology. Neurology. 2012;79:2209.
44. Axelsson S, Berg T, Jonsson L, Engström M, Kanerva M, Stjernquist-Desatnik A. Bell's palsy—the effect of prednisolone and/or valaciclovir versus placebo in relation to baseline severity in a randomised controlled trial. Clin Otolaryngol. 2012;37(4):283–90.
45. Gagyor I, Madhok VB, Daly F, et al. Antiviral treatment for Bell's palsy (idiopathic facial paralysis). Cochrane Database Syst Rev. 2015;9:CD001869.
46. Khedr EM, Badry R, Ali AM, Abo El-Fetoh N, El-Hammady DH, Ghandour AM, Abdel-Haleem A. Steroid/antiviral for the treatment of Bell's palsy: double blind randomized clinical trial. Restor Neurol Neurosci. 2016;34(6):897–905. https://doi.org/10.3233/RNN-150605. PMID: 27689547.
47. Lockwood CJ, Radunovic N, Nastic D, et al. Corticotropin-releasing hormone and related pituitary-adrenal axis hormones in fetal and maternal blood during the second half of pregnancy. J Perinat Med. 1996;24:243.
48. Park-Wyllie L, Mazzotta P, Pastuszak A, Moretti ME, Beique L, Hunnisett L, et al. Birth defects after maternal exposure to corticosteroids: prospective cohort study and meta-analysis of epidemiological studies. Teratology. 2000;62:385–92.
49. Hviid A, Mølgaard-Nielsen D. Corticosteroid use during pregnancy and risk of orofacial clefts. CMAJ. 2011;183:796.
50. Wapner RK, Sorokin Y, Thom EA, et al. Single versus weekly courses of antenatal corticosteroids: evaluation of safety and efficacy. Am J Obstet Gynecol. 2006;195:633–42.
51. Crowther CA, Haslam RR, Hiller JE, et al. Neonatal respiratory distress syndrome after repeat exposure to antenatal corticosteroids: a randomised controlled trial. Lancet. 2006;367:1913–9.
52. Lockshin MD, Sammaritano LR. Corticosteroids during pregnancy. Scand J Rheumatol Suppl. 1998;107:136–8.
53. Rauch SD. Idiopathic sudden sensorineural hearing loss. N Engl J Med. 2008;359:833–40.
54. Kim SY, Sim S, Kim HJ, Choi HG. Sudden sensory neural hearing loss is not predictive of myocardial infarction: a longitudinal follow-up study using a national sample cohort. Sci Rep. 2018;8:946.

55. Oh JH, Park K, Lee SJ, Shin YR, Choung YH. Bilateral versus unilateral sudden sensorineural hearing loss. Otolaryngol Head Neck Surg. 2007;136:87–91.
56. Carlin A, Alfirevic Z. Physiological changes of pregnancy and monitoring. Best Pract Res Clin Obstet Gynaecol. 2008;22:801–23.
57. Yannone ME. Hormonal changes in pregnancy. MCV/Q. 1972;8:43–51.
58. Haas JS, Jackson RA, Fuentes-Afflick E, et al. Changes in the health status of women during and after pregnancy. J Gen Intern Med. 2005;20:45–51.
59. Glover V. Maternal stress or anxiety in pregnancy and emotional development of the child. Br J Psychiatry. 1997;171:105–6.
60. Goh AY, Hussain SS. Sudden hearing loss and pregnancy: a review. J Laryngol Otol. 2012;126:337–9.
61. Ashok Murthy V, Krishna K. Hearing loss in pregnancy. Indian J Otolaryngol Head Neck Surg. 2013;65:1–2.
62. Al-Mana D, Ceranic B, Djahanbakhch O, Luxon LM. Hormones and the auditory system: a review of physiology and pathophysiology. Neuroscience. 2008;153:881–900.
63. Asai Y, Umemura K, Kohno Y, Uematsu T, Nakashima M. An animal model for hearing disturbance due to inner-ear ischemia: photochemically induced thrombotic occlusion of the rat anterior inferior cerebellar artery. Eur Arch Otorhinolaryngol. 1993;250:292–6.
64. Yen TT, Lin CH, Shiao JY, Liang KL. Pregnancy is not a risk factor for idiopathic sudden sensorineural hearing loss: a nationwide population-based study. Acta Otolaryngol. 2016;136:446–50.
65. Lee S-Y, et al. Pregnancy does not increase the risk of sudden sensorineural hearing loss: a national cohort study. Laryngoscope. 2020;130(4):E237–42.
66. Lyu Y-L, et al. Intratympanic dexamethasone injection for sudden sensorineural hearing loss in pregnancy. World J Clin Cases. 2020;8(18):4051.
67. Chandrasekhar SS, Tsai Do BS, Schwartz SR, Bontempo LJ, Faucett EA, Finestone SA, Hollingsworth DB, Kelley DM, Kmucha ST, Moonis G, Poling GL, Roberts JK, Stachler RJ, Zeitler DM, Corrigan MD, Nnacheta LC, Satterfield L. Clinical practice guideline: sudden hearing loss (update). Otolaryngol Head Neck Surg. 2019;161:S1–S45.
68. Stachler RJ, Chandrasekhar SS, Archer SM, et al. Clinical practice guideline: sudden hearing loss. Otolaryngol Head Neck Surg. 2012;146:S1–S35.
69. Hou ZQ, Wang QJ. A new disease: pregnancy-induced sudden sensorineural hearing loss? Acta Otolaryngol. 2011;131:779–86.
70. Wang YP, Young YH. Experience in the treatment of sudden deafness during pregnancy. Acta Otolaryngol. 2006;126:271–6.
71. Zeng XL, He JC, Li P, et al. Sudden sensorineural hearing loss during pregnancy: a 21 cases report. Chin J Otol Chinese. 2014;12:207–10, in Chinese.
72. Xu M, Jiang Q, Tang H. Sudden sensorineural hearing loss during pregnancy: clinical characteristics, management and outcome. Acta Otolaryngol. 2019;139:38–41.
73. Dazhi S, Juan X, Li Y, et al. Clinical characteristics and prognosis of sudden sensorineural hearing loss during pregnancy. J Audiol Speech Pathol. 2019;27:156–9.
74. Lee JB, Choi SJ, Park K, Park HY, Choo OS, Choung YH. The efficiency of intratympanic dexamethasone injection as a sequential treatment after initial systemic steroid therapy for sudden sensorineural hearing loss. Eur Arch Otorhinolaryngol. 2011;268:833–9.
75. Ng JH, Ho RC, Cheong CS, Ng A, Yuen HW, Ngo RY. Intratympanic steroids as a salvage treatment for sudden sensorineural hearing loss? A meta-analysis. Eur Arch Otorhinolaryngol. 2015;272:2777–82.
76. Schreiber BE, Agrup C, Haskard DO, et al. Sudden sensorineural hearing loss. Lancet. 2010;375:1203–11.
77. Rauch SD, Halpin CF, Antonelli PJ, et al. Oral vs intratympanic corticosteroid therapy for idiopathic sudden sensorineural hearing loss: a randomized trial. JAMA. 2011;305:2071–9.
78. Canlon B, Erichsen S, Nemlander E, et al. Alterations in the intrauterine environment by glucocorticoids modifies the developmental programme of the auditory system. Eur J Neurosci. 2003;17:2035–41.

79. Vlastarakos PV, Nikolopoulos TP, Manolopoulos L, et al. Treating common ear problems in pregnancy: what is safe? Eur Arch Otorhinolaryngol. 2008;265:139–45.
80. Ambro BT, Scheid SC, Pribitkin EA. Prescribing guidelines for ENT medications during pregnancy. Ear Nose Throat J. 2003;82:565–8.
81. Zhang Q. Clinical diagnosis and treatment of 7 cases of neurosensory deafness during pregnancy. Neural Injury Funct Reconstruct. 2015;10:322–4, in Chinese.
82. Plontke SK, Lowenheim H, Mertens J, et al. Randomized, double blind, placebo controlled trial on the safety and efficacy of continuous intratympanic dexamethasone delivered via a round window catheter for severe to profound sudden idiopathic sensorineural hearing loss Xie and Wu 11 after failure of systemic therapy. Laryngoscope. 2009;119:359–69.
83. Demirhan H, Gokduman AR, Hamit B, et al. Contribution of intratympanic steroids in the primary treatment of sudden hearing loss. Acta Otolaryngol. 2018;138:648–51.
84. Fu Y, Jing J, Ren T, et al. Intratympanic dexamethasone for managing pregnant women with sudden hearing loss. J Int Med Res. 2019;47:377–82.
85. Van Hoesen KB, et al. Should hyperbaric oxygen be used to treat the pregnant patient for acute carbon monoxide poisoning?: a case report and literature review. JAMA. 1989;261(7):1039–43.
86. Sadr-Eshkevari P, et al. Oral and maxillofacial surgery for the pregnant patient. In: Non-obstetric surgery during pregnancy. Cham: Springer; 2019. p. 237–52.
87. Jo C, Jo J. Preoperative considerations for the pregnant patient. In: Bagheri SC, editor. Clinical review of oral and maxillofacial surgery: a case-based approach. 2nd ed. Elsevier/Mosby: St. Louis; 2014. p. 69–72.
88. O'Connor RC, Shakib K, Brennan PA. Recent advances in the management of oral and maxillofacial trauma. Br J Oral Maxillofac Surg. 2015;53:913.
89. Turner M, Aziz SR. Management of the pregnant oral and maxillofacial surgery patient. J Oral Maxillofac Surg. 2002;60:1479–88.
90. Suresh L, Radfar L. Pregnancy and lactation. Oral Surg Oral Med Oral Pathol Oral Radiol Endod. 2004;97(6):672–8210.
91. Duvekot JJ, Peeters LL. Maternal cardiovascular hemodynamic adaptation to pregnancy. Obstet Gynecol Surv. 1994;49(Suppl):S1–S14.
92. Beck HJ, Salassa JR, McCaffrey TV, et al. Life-threatening soft-tissue infections of the neck. Laryngoscope. 1984;94:354–62.
93. Marioni G, Staffieri A, Parisi S, et al. Rational diagnostic and therapeutic management of deep neck infections: analysis of 233 consecutive cases. Ann Otol Rhinol Laryngol. 2010;119:181–7.
94. Velhonoja J, Lääveri M, Soukka T, Irjala H, Kinnunen I. Deep neck space infections: an upward trend and changing characteristics. Eur Arch Otorhinolaryngol. 2020;277(3):863–72.
95. Parhiscar A, Har-El G. Deep neck abscess: a retrospective review of 210 cases. Ann Otol Rhinol Laryngol. 2001;110:1051–4.
96. Mylonas I. Antibiotic chemotherapy during pregnancy and lactation period: aspects for consideration. Arch Gynecol Obstet. 2011;283:7–18.
97. Dalla Torre D, Burtscher D, Höfer D, Kloss FR. Odontogenic deep neck space infection as life-threatening condition in pregnancy. Aust Dent J. 2014;59(3):375–8.

Postpartum ENT Emergencies

Serdar Ferit Toprak, Müzeyyen Yıldırım Baylan,
and Nitin R. Ankle

9.1 Introduction

Many ear, nose and throat (ENT) emergencies occur during postpartum period. Most of these emergencies are benign; however, there are certain ENT disorders that are critical and require immediate intervention. Several studies have been published that have improved the knowledge of the pathophysiology of these conditions and helped us define appropriate investigations and management for these conditions.

9.2 Postpartum Thyroiditis

Dysfunction of the thyroid gland in a previously euthyroid female diagnosed 12 months after pregnancy is termed as postpartum thyroiditis. Some of these cases have been reported to occur after miscarriage, but majority occur after a period of pregnancy. The natural history of postpartum thyroiditis is triphasic. The three phases which include initial thyrotoxic phase followed by a hypothyroid phase and then a euthyroid phase all these occur within 12 months [1]. 25–40% of these patients have the three classic phases, while 20–30% have only the thyrotoxic

S. F. Toprak (✉) · M. Y. Baylan
Medical Faculty, Otorhinolaryngology Department, Dicle University, Diyarbakır, Turkey
e-mail: serdarferit@yahoo.com; muzeyyenyldrm@hotmail.com

N. R. Ankle
Department of ENT and Head-Neck Surgery, KLE Academy of Higher Education and Research (KAHER), J. N. Medical College, Belagavi, Karnataka, India
e-mail: drnitinankale@gmail.com

C. Cingi et al. (eds.), *ENT Diseases: Diagnosis and Treatment during Pregnancy and Lactation*, https://doi.org/10.1007/978-3-031-05303-0_9

phase and 40% have only hypothyroid phase [1–3]. The initial thyrotoxic phase starts within 2–6 months after delivery, the median time of onset is around 13 weeks, and this phase is mostly asymptomatic. The duration of this is 2–3 months. Some symptoms like fatigue, intolerance to heat, palpitations and nervousness are common in the thyrotoxic phase [4]. The second phase, the hypothyroid phase, starts 3–12 months after delivery; the median onset time was found to be 19 weeks and is usually symptomatic with patients complaining of intolerance to cold, dryness of the skin, easy fatiguability and difficulty concentrating [4]. On examination, most of the women in this phase have small and painless enlargement of the thyroid gland. Some studies have also explored the role of this postpartum thyroiditis in the development of postpartum depression. The treatment for this condition is similar to disorders like silent thyroiditis, but there is a need for extra precautions when treating breastfeeding women. During the thyrotoxic phase, beta-blockers are used to relieve symptoms, but mild symptoms require no treatment. L-T4 can be used if necessary to treat symptoms in the hypothyroid phase. TSH levels should be checked at regular intervals, at every 1–2 months for a duration of 12 months postpartum [4]. Postpartum thyroiditis often tends to end up in hypothyroidism for long durations of time, especially in high-risk groups of women. In these cases, the patient will have to be continued on L-T4 even if they are breastfeeding. The decision to discontinue L-T4 needs to be discussed with the patient taking into consideration personal situations like women who are considering a second pregnancy within a year, in which case hypothyroidism can be detrimental to the continuation of pregnancy as well as to foetal development. Prevention of postpartum thyroiditis using supplements has been studied by performing controlled trials that were randomised. Two of these trials tried the administration of iodine or L-T4 either during or after pregnancy in women who had anti-TPO antibodies; these failed to cause a decrease in the risk of development of postpartum thyroiditis [5, 6]. Another trial attempted to administer selenium to women who had anti-TPO antibodies during and after pregnancy, and was successful in reducing the rate of development of thyroiditis; 50% of women on the placebo developed thyroiditis, whereas only 29% of those treated with selenium developed thyroiditis [7]. They also noted a decrease in the rate of development of permanent hypothyroidism in the long term from 20% to just 12% after administration of selenium. Even so, the new ATA guidelines do not recommend the prescription of selenium in high-risk women until there are more studies with regard to its efficacy and safety [4]. A high recurrence rate of about 70% in subsequent pregnancies was noted in anti-TPO-positive women recovering from postpartum thyroiditis [1, 4]. Persistence of a hypothyroid phase was seen in about 15–50% of these women in the long term [8, 9]. Thirty-eight percent of 700 women in a study conducted 12 years ago had hypothyroidism [8]. The risk for the development of permanent hypothyroidism is seen to be higher in women with certain parameters such as high anti-TPO antibody titres, hypoechogenicity on ultrasound and high TSH levels in the sixth month after delivery [8, 9]. Keeping these in mind, it is important that TSH levels be checked yearly for all women with a history of postpartum thyroiditis, and continued indefinitely [4].

9.3 Epistaxis

At least 60% of the general population have had a history of nasal bleed [10]. Some of these people will have recurrent or habitual history of nasal bleeding. These individuals have been found to have an increased risk of impaired haemostasis [11–15], and therefore obtaining the history of episodes of nasal bleed can help identify patients with an increased risk of intraoperative bleeding [16, 17]. Obstetricians believe that pregnant women are at a higher risk of developing epistaxis, and this has been attributed to increased incidence of rhinitis in patients due to vascular occlusion and development of mucosal oedema during pregnancy as a result of high oestrogen during pregnancy [18]. This theory has not been proven by research as of yet. The exact prevalence of epistaxis in pregnancy is also not known.

9.4 Hereditary Angioedema

This disorder is characterised by recurrent episodes of non-pitting oedema. This oedema tends to be localised and well-defined, but can affect any region of the human body. Sometimes, it can cause pain, especially in regions like extremities, face, torso, throat and internal organs of the abdomen. A high mortality rate is seen in cases with laryngeal involvement [19, 20]. Patients with hereditary angioedema also have urinary tract infections, spontaneous abortions and preterm labour. Heartburn and rheumatic symptoms are also noted more commonly [21].

The role of oestrogen in HAE has been discussed. It has been reported that increased attacks during menstruation with oral contraceptives cause more frequent and severe attacks. Both CI-inhibitory activity and mean values of antigen titres were significantly reduced in normal women using oral contraceptives compared to those who did not. Angioedema attacks not due to a lack of C1 inhibitor and that are oestrogen induced and familial have also been described [22, 23]. The treatment of HAE can be divided into prophylactic treatment, either short or long term, and the treatment of an acute attack. There is no role or benefit in treatment with adrenaline, antihistamine agents or corticosteroids in patients with HAE. Replacement therapy is the main treatment of an acute episode and has also been used to treat other protein deficiencies like haemophilia and hypogammaglobulinaemia. Fresh-frozen plasma infusion has also been shown to improve the disease even though theoretically it could worsen the attack. It has also been shown that the C1 inhibitor concentrate is safe and effective in resolving acute episodes. Intravenously administered in doses of 500–1000 units, oedema starts to recover within 2 h, and within 24 h complete remission is noted [22, 23].

9.5 Vertigo

Postpartum women often complain of dizziness and imbalance [24, 25]. Delivery seems to cause superior semicircular canal-like symptoms. At the time of normal vaginal delivery, there is a rise in the intracranial pressure. This rise in intracranial pressure can compress an exposed semicircular canal labyrinth due to a thin or dehiscent bone covering it.

Minor [26] reported a series of surgical repairs for a series of semicircular canal dehiscence from 1995 to 2004, in 20 patients a craniotomy into the middle cranial fossa and SSCD repair were performed, and 9 of these were occluded and 11 reappeared [26].

In 89% of the patients, vestibular symptoms resolved completely, after duct obstruction, whereas in 64% of the patients, the symptoms resolved after resurfacing [26].

Mikulec et al. [27] presented ten patients with separation obstruction, and one patient had reclosure. There was no improvement in the symptoms of the patient who underwent reroofing, but this patient also had bilateral opening [27].

Vestibular symptoms were improved in all ten patients with obstruction, and postoperatively hearing improved in four out of five patients with conductive hearing loss preoperatively.

Minor et al. [26] also reported a patient who had postoperative improvement of 20 dB in air conduction threshold after resurfacing a dissected superior duct.

9.6   Laryngeal Oedema

A caesarean section is often an emergency procedure and frequently requires general anaesthesia, women who undergo emergency caesarean section have a high risk for airway complications, and it is important to pay attention towards airway management.

There needs to be a recognition of the risk of pulmonary aspiration in these patients, and hence proper airway management is essential [28].

There are several national surveys about airway complications during anaesthesia like confidential Investigations on Maternal Death in the United Kingdom [29].

Cormack and Lehane have established an optimal laryngoscopy method for tracheal intubation [30] and also gave the first algorithm for management of difficult airway [31].

In order to prevent pulmonary aspiration and to minimise the administration of drugs required for anaesthesia to the foetus during emergency caesarean sections done under general anaesthesia, it is vital to intubate the patient immediately after the induction of anaesthesia.

The effects of the injected drugs should be short, so that in case tracheal intubation fails, it is possible to awaken the patient.

It is indicated to also have rapid initiation of anaesthesia; in the 1950s and 1960s, the method of aesthesia included preoxygenation, application of pressure over the cricoid cartilage and usage of thiamylal or thiopentone for induction of general anaesthesia. The airway is first protected using a cuffed endotracheal tube prior to initiation of manual ventilation. This traditional method has remained unchanged, but it has evolved since the mid-1980s; however, the fundamental protocol of minimising the duration of airway protection from aspiration and allowing for rapid awakening in the case of failure of tracheal intubation.

9.7 Bell's Palsy

The seventh cranial nerve, or the facial nerve, is primarily a motor nerve that additionally contains a small sensory component known as Wrisberg's nervus intermedius. The facial nerve can suffer various injuries and insults as it exits from the pons and passes through the facial canal which extends till the stylo-mastoid foramen, from where the nerve innervates the facial muscles. Trauma secondary to surgery, vascular pathologies, infections and autoimmune causes are considered the possible mechanisms of Bell's palsy. No association was observed between the female menstrual cycle and the occurrence of Bell's palsy [32], but in pregnant women the rise in steroid hormones has been considered as the cause of Bell's palsy [33].

Other aetiological factors include herpes simplex virus infection noted in 79% of patients with Bell's palsy. Interestingly, Herpes zoster virus is said to play an aetiological role in peripheral facial paralysis ('zoster sine herpete') even without skin rashes. In pregnant women, immunosuppression is considered the aetiology of viral reactivation. Herpes simplex or herpes zoster virus reactivated from cranial ganglia required treatment with acyclovir and prednisone [34].

References

1. Lazarus JH. The continuing saga of postpartum thyroiditis. J Clin Endocrinol Metab. 2011;96:614–6.
2. Kita M, Goulis DG, Avramides A. Post-partum thyroiditis in a Mediterranean population: a prospective study of a large cohort of thyroid antibody positive women at the time of delivery. J Endocrinol Invest. 2002;25:513–9.
3. Lucas A, Pizarro E, Granada ML, et al. Postpartum thyroiditis: epidemiology and clinical evolution in a nonselected population. Thyroid. 2000;10:71–7.
4. Stagnaro-Green A, Abalovich M, Alexander E, American Thyroid Association Taskforce on Thyroid Disease During Pregnancy and Postpartum, et al. Guidelines of the American Thyroid Association for the diagnosis and management of thyroid disease during pregnancy and postpartum. Thyroid. 2011;21(10):1081–125.
5. Nøhr SB, Jørgensen A, Pedersen KM, et al. Postpartum thyroid dysfunction in pregnant thyroid peroxidase antibody-positive women living in an area with mild to moderate iodine deficiency: is iodine supplementation safe? J Clin Endocrinol Metab. 2000;85:3191–8.
6. Kämpe O, Jansson R, Karlsson FA. Effects of L-thyroxine and iodide on the development of autoimmune postpartum thyroiditis. J Clin Endocrinol Metab. 1990;70:1014–8.
7. Negro R, Greco G, Mangieri T, et al. The influence of selenium supplementation on postpartum thyroid status in pregnant women with thyroid peroxidase autoantibodies. J Clin Endocrinol Metab. 2007;92:1263–8.
8. Stuckey BG, Kent GN, Ward LC, et al. Postpartum thyroid dysfunction and the long-term risk of hypothyroidism: results from a 12-year follow-up study of women with and without postpartum thyroid dysfunction. Clin Endocrinol. 2010;73:389–95.

9. Stagnaro-Green A, Schwartz A, Gismondi R, et al. High rate of persistent hypothyroidism in a large-scale prospective study of postpartum thyroiditis in southern Italy. J Clin Endocrinol Metab. 2011;96:652–7.

10. Kucik C, Clenney T. Management of epistaxis. Am Fam Physician. 2005;71:305–11.

11. Beran M, Petruson B, Stigendal L. Haemostatic disorders in habitual nose-bleeders. J Laryngol Otol. 1987;101:1020–8.

12. Parkin JD, Smith IL, O'Neill AI, Ibrahim KM, Butcher LA. Mild bleeding disorders. A clinical and laboratory study. Med J Aust. 1992;156:614–7.

13. Thaha M, Nilssen E, Holland S, Love G, White PS. Routine coagulation screening in the management of emergency admission for epistaxis—is it necessary? J Laryngol Otol. 2000;114:38–40.

14. Dizdar O, Onal IK, Ozakin E, Karakiliç E, Karadag O, Kalyoncu U, et al. Research for bleeding tendency in patients presenting with significant epistaxis. Blood Coagul Fibrinolysis. 2007;18:41–3.

15. Jones GL, Browning S, Phillipps J. The value of coagulation profiles in epistaxis management. Int J Clin Pract. 2003;57:577–8.

16. Barash P, Cullen B, Stoelting R. Clinical anesthesia. 3rd ed. Philadelphia: Lippincott Williams & Wilkins; 2006.

17. Dunn P. Clinical anesthesia procedures of the Massachusetts General Hospital. 3rd ed. Philadelphia: Lippincott Williams & Wilkins; 2007.

18. Sobol S, Frenkiel S, Nachtigal D, Wiener D, Teblum C. Clinical manifestations of sinonasal pathology during pregnancy. J Otolaryngol. 2001;30:24–8.

19. Dennehy JJ. Hereditary angioneurotic oedema. Report of a large kindred with defect in C' 1 esterase inhibitor and review of the literature. Ann Intern Med. 1970;73:55–9.

20. Winnewisser J, Rossi M, Spath P, Burgi H. Type I hereditary angio-oedema. Variability of clinical presentation and course within two large kindreds. J Intern Med. 1997;241:39–46.

21. Nielsen EW, Gran JT, Straume B, Mellbye OJ, Johansen HT, Mollnes TE. Hereditary angio-oedema: new clinical observations and autoimmune, screening, complement and kallikrein-kinin analyses. J Intern Med. 1996;239:119–30.

22. Pickering RJ, Kelly JR, Good RA, Gewurtz H. Replacement therapy in hereditary angioedema. Successful treatment of two patients with fresh frozen plasma. Lancet. 1969;1:326–30.

23. Sim TC, Grant JA. Hereditary angioedema: its diagnostic and management perspectives. Am J Med. 1990;88:656–64.

24. Gjerdingen DK, Froberg DG, Chaloner KM, et al. Changes in women's physical health during the first postpartum year. Arch Fam Med. 1993;2:277Y83.

25. Streubel SO, Cremer PD, Carey JP, et al. Vestibular-evoked myogenic potentials in the diagnosis of superior canal dehiscence syndrome. Acta Otolaryngol Suppl. 2001;545:41Y9.

26. Minor LB. Clinical manifestations of superior semicircular canal dehiscence. Laryngoscope. 2005;115:1717Y27.

27. Mikulec AA, Poe DS, McKenna MJ. Operative management of superior semicircular canal dehiscence. Laryngoscope. 2005;115:501Y7.

28. Asai T, Shingu K. Should Mendelson's syndrome be renamed? Anaesthesia. 2001;56:398–9.

29. Report on confidential enquiries into maternal deaths in the UK 1988–1990. Department of Health. London: HMSO; 1994. p. 80–96.

30. Cormack RS, Lehane J. Difficult tracheal intubation in obstetrics. Anaesthesia. 1984;39:1105–10.

31. Tunstall ME. Failed intubation in the parturient. Can J Anaesth. 1989;36:611–3.

32. Peitersen E. Bell's palsy: the spontaneous course of 2,500 peripheral facial nerve palsies of different etiologies. Acta Otolaryngol Suppl. 2002;122:4–30.

33. Hilsinger RL Jr, Adour KK, Doty HE. Idiopathic facial paralysis, pregnancy, and the menstrual cycle. Ann Otol Rhinol Laryngol. 1975;84:433–42.

34. Adour KK, Ruboyianes JM, Trent CS, VonDoersten PG, Quesenberry CP, Byl FM, Hitchcock T. Bell's palsy treatment with acyclovir and prednisone compared with prednisone alone: a double-blind, randomized, controlled trial. Ann Otol Rhinol Laryngol. 1996;105:371–8.

Use of Antibiotics During Pregnancy and the Postpartum Period

10

Selcan Arslan Özel, Güle Çınar, and Georg Mathias Sprinzl

10.1 Introduction

Pregnant women and fetuses are the weakest groups in terms of safety and efficacy of drugs. Although more than 89% of women in United States of America (USA) use at least one prescription or nonprescription drug during pregnancy, there is no human pregnancy data in 70% of the medications approved in the United States between 2000 and 2010 [1].

During pregnancy, all systems in the body undergo significant adaptive changes, and metabolic conditions are quite different from those in the nonpregnant period. These changes are mainly due to the effects of hormones. Detailed pharmacological information is needed to determine therapeutic treatment strategies during pregnancy. It is necessary to understand both the physiology of pregnancy and the pregnancy-specific pharmacology of different agents. Clinical studies have shown that there are numerous changes in pregnancy that affect the pharmacological properties of drugs [2].

S. A. Özel (✉)
Derince Training and Research Hospital Clinical Microbiology and Infectious Diseases Department Derince, Derince, Kocaeli, Turkey
e-mail: selcandr@yahoo.com

G. Çınar
Medical Faculty, Infectious Diseases and Clinical Microbiology Department,
Ankara University, Ankara, Turkey
e-mail: gbinjune@gmail.com

G. M. Sprinzl
Department of Otorhinolaryngology, Head and Neck Surgery, University Clinic St. Poelten,
St. Poelten, Austria
e-mail: georg.sprinzl@gmail.com

© The Author(s), under exclusive license to Springer Nature Switzerland AG 2022

C. Cingi et al. (eds.), *ENT Diseases: Diagnosis and Treatment during Pregnancy and Lactation*, https://doi.org/10.1007/978-3-031-05303-0_10

The postpartum period, also known as the puerperium and the "fourth trimester," defines the time after delivery when maternal physiological changes about pregnancy return to the nonpregnant conditions. Numerous disorders and complications may occur in the immediate postpartum period or after discharge from the birth facility. The end is less defined, but is generally considered to be 6–8 weeks after birth because the effects of pregnancy on many systems have largely returned to the prepregnancy conditions by this time. However, not all organ systems return to baseline during this time, and return to baseline is not necessarily linear over time. For this reason, the American College of Obstetricians and Gynecologists considers postpartum care to extend up to 12 weeks after delivery [2]. Some researchers have thought that up to 12 months after birth, women experience the postpartum period.

10.2 Drug Absorption

Drug absorption is generally defined as bioavailability, the fraction, or percentage of a drug that reaches the systemic circulation without degradation by any means. Intravascular drugs' bioavailability is 100% because they are given directly into the bloodstream. However, most drugs are given intravenously and expected to effect systematically. Therefore, absorption and bioavailability are prerequisites for the pharmacological action of a drug.

Delays in absorption or loss of medication can cause changes in desired effects and side effects. Intramuscular and subcutaneous administration may delay the maximum concentration of the drug, but is not very effective on bioavailability. The greatest variability in drug absorption is seen when a drug is given per oral. Oral bioavailability is affected by gastric pH, food, intestinal transit time, metabolism, and transport processes.

During pregnancy, the motility of the gastrointestinal tract decreases under the influence of hormone metabolism, which delays ejaculation, so the drug remains in the gastrointestinal tract for a long time, which increases drug absorption. Nausea and vomiting in early pregnancy can lessen the proportion of oral medication. Therefore, medication should be taken in the period when nausea is the least. While gastric acid production decreases during pregnancy, mucus secretion increases, resulting in an increase in gastric pH. These changes increase the ionization of weak acids (e.g., aspirin) and may decrease their absorption. It can increase the absorption of weak bases (e.g., caffeine) primarily by nonionizing. Also, reduced bowel movements and gastric acid discharge during pregnancy can change drug absorption and oral bioavailability. Despite the varying gastrointestinal tract during pregnancy, the bioavailability and therapeutic effect of an orally administered drug have a minimal effect, particularly with repeated doses of drugs. In addition, poor blood flow to the lower extremities due to changes in hemodynamics during late pregnancy will affect the absorption of drugs by subcutaneous or intramuscular injection. Therefore, intravenous injection should be used for rapid response [2].

10.3   Drug Distribution

Distribution represents the reversible transferation of a drug between several sites after it reaches the systemic circulation. The volume of distribution (Vd) is utilized to define how well a systemic dose of drug is distributed in organism. Vd is substantial for determining the loading dose of drug required to achieve therapeutic concentration. The blood volume in pregnancy increases until the 32–34th weeks of gestation from the beginning of pregnancy. Plasma volume increases by around 50%; serum albumin and alpha 1 acid glycoprotein concentrations reduce by 31% and 19%, respectively, in late pregnancy [2]. This results in decreased plasma protein binding and increased free drug concentrations. There is an increase of about 33% in cardiac output during pregnancy. For this reason, the required amount of medication is higher in pregnant women than in nonpregnant women. Increased extracellular volume and total body fluid will increase the volume of distribution for hydrophilic drugs, leading to lower plasma concentrations. Also, mother's body fat increases by about 4 kg and increases the volume of distribution for lipophilic drugs [3].

10.4   Drug Metabolism

The mechanisms underlying modifications in drug metabolism in a pregnant woman are well understood. However, physiological changes are probably accountable for the changes reported in drug metabolism during pregnancy.

Drug metabolism includes the modification of a drug chemically by specific enzymes. Hepatic drug metabolism involves phase 1 (oxidation, reduction, or hydrolysis) reactions that add more polar or reactive moieties to drug molecules, followed by phase 2 (conjugation) reactions in which small, polar, ionizable groups such as sulfate and glucuronic acid are enzymatically added to the molecule [3].

Oxidative phase 1 reactions are mostly performed by the cytochrome p450 (CYP) enzymes which vary in substrate specificity. Among the 18 CYP enzyme groups discovered in humans to date, enzymes in three CYP groups (CYP1, CYP2, and CYP3) are in charge of phase 1 reactions mostly. CYP3A (CYP3A4 and CYP3A5) and CYP2C (CYP2C8, CYP2C9, CYP2C18, and CYP2C19) are the richest ones in the liver and constitute 30% and 20% of the total CYP family, respectively. Other forms make minor contributions to hepatic CYP expression: CYP1A2 (13%), CYP2E1 (7%), CYP2A6 (4%), CYP2D6 (2%), and CYP2B6 (0.4%) [3].

While a significant increase occurs in the activities of some drug-metabolizing enzymes during pregnancy, a significant decrease occurs in some of them. CYP3A4, CYP2A6, CYP2D6, and CYP2C9 activities all increase during pregnancy. In contrast, some CYP isoforms are known to have decreased activity during pregnancy. CYP1A2 and CYP2C19 activities gradually decrease later in pregnancy. It is thought that changes in hepatic CYP activity during pregnancy occur when high concentrations of female hormones activate nuclear receptors and affect the expression of hepatic drug metabolism enzymes. Estradiol increases CYP2A6, CYP2B6, and CYP3A4 expression and decreases CYP1A2 expression in human hepatocytes [4].

Glucuronidation mediated by UDP-glucuronyltransferases (UGTs) is the main route of phase 2 reactions. The UGT1A and UGT2B subfamily is primarily liable for hepatic glucuronidation of drugs. UGT isoforms expressed in the liver contain UGT1A1, UGT1A3, UGT1A4, UGT1A6, UGT1A9, UGT2B4, UGT2B7, and UGT2B15. Estradiol regulates UGT1A4 expression by ERα activation, and progesterone regulates UGT1A1 expression by PXR activation. The activity of phase 2 enzymes, including UGTs, changes during pregnancy and shows a twofold rise in UGT1A4 activity in the first and second trimesters and a threefold rise in the third trimester [2].

As the activities of UGT1A4, UGT2B7, CYP2A6, CYP2C9, CYP2D6, and CYP3A4 increase during pregnancy, the elimination of drugs metabolized by these enzymes increases, while CYP1A2 and CYP2C19 activities decrease, so the elimination of drugs metabolized by these enzymes decreases [3].

During gravidity, hepatic blood flow rises by 60%, potentially influencing liver excretion of drugs with a high hepatic extraction rate. During pregnancy, high estrogen levels cause bile to accumulate in the liver and slow down metabolism [3].

10.5 Drug Excretion

In the first trimester of pregnancy, renal blood flow increases by 35%, and glomerular filtration rate increases by 50%. This condition continues at these high levels throughout pregnancy. Renal excretion of drugs that do not change during pregnancy increases due to the increase in glomerular filtration rate and possibly increased renal secretion by carriers. It is observed that the activity of several renal transporters such as organic cation transporter and P-glycoprotein increases during pregnancy. The increase in total body fluid and plasma volume during pregnancy has a significant effect on the distribution of the drug in the body. As the plasma volume increases, the amount of serum albumin per unit volume decreases. Therefore, hypoalbuminemia is common in pregnant women. Drug deficit is frequently experienced in drugs excreted from the kidneys of pregnant women [5].

There is no effective drug that has no side effects. In case of pregnancy, all drugs should be avoided as much as possible in the first trimester, but if it is necessary, care should be taken especially in drug selection. The number of pregnant women using drugs has more than doubled in the last 30 years. Antibiotics constitute 80% of all drugs prescribed during pregnancy [5–7].

That was suggested that exposure to antibiotics in fetal/neonatal life affects both the mother's and the child's intestinal microbiota, as well as the negative and long-term effects of the mother's vaginal microbiota and the development of allergic diseases. Antibiotic use during pregnancy is usually prescribed for preterm labor, intrapartum fever, and cesarean section. Apart from this, it is generally prescribed for community-acquired infections (respiratory, urinary tract, ear, nose, and throat infections, etc.) [8].

It is predicted that only 10% of the existing drugs have adequate data on secure and efficient use during pregnancy. An increased risk of cerebral palsy in preterm babies born to women receiving antibiotic therapy has been reported in a large randomized controlled trial. Antibiotic use in gravidity has been correlated with a rising in asthma and epilepsy and an obesity risk in children [9–11].

Drug use and possible side effects during pregnancy are classified by the Food and Drug Administration (FDA). These risk categories are often not given by the manufacturers. In this case, the risk category is defined retrospectively in feedbacks that occur after the use of the drug. If the manufacturer company has made a risk statement, the phrase "m" is used next to the expression of the risk category of the drug (e.g., Bm) [12].

The FDA has divided the drugs into five groups in terms of their effects on the baby during pregnancy.

Category A: There aren't found any adverse effects on the fetus in studies conducted on humans. There are very few drugs included in this group.

Category B: No adverse effects on animal fetuses were found in animal studies, but studies in humans are not available.

Category C: Studies in animals and/or humans are insufficient. Or, adverse effects were detected in animal experiments, but there is no human data. Drugs in this group can be used if it is believed that they will bring more benefit to the patient than harm.

Category D: The drugs in this group have had a negative effect on the human fetus. The drugs in this group are drugs that can be used if they must be used, if not used, if the mother or fetus will be harmed, and if the profit/loss ratio is in favor of profit.

Category X: The drugs in this group have also found negative effects on the human fetus. However, when the drugs in this group are used during pregnancy, they are drugs whose profit/loss ratio always favors the loss. Therefore, it should never be used during pregnancy.

10.5.1 Penicillins

B-lactam antibiotics are the oldest class of antibiotics used to treat infections. Penicillins are the most commonly used antibiotics during pregnancy. B-lactam antibiotics pass into the extravascular fluid by passive diffusion. To achieve adequate concentrations in the extravascular fluid, the plasma concentration must exceed the minimum inhibitory concentration (MIC) value by severalfold. In pregnant women, it is recommended to shorten the dosage interval or increase the dosage of the drug to compensate for the decreased plasma concentration due to accelerated elimination and increased plasma volume [13].

For penicillin group drugs, the FDA gives category B. In addition, other maternal side effects such as nausea, diarrhea, hypersensitivity reactions, central nervous system irritability, and phlebitis can be seen in this group of drugs [12].

Phenoxymethylpenicillin (penicillin V) is the most commonly used antibiotic during pregnancy. It is known to be safe during pregnancy and cross the placenta. Its concentration is lower in pregnant women due to its rapid elimination [13].

Aminopenicillins (ampicillin, amoxicillin) are also drugs that can be used safely during pregnancy. Since the gastrointestinal absorption of amoxicillin is much better, amoxicillin should be preferred in oral applications and ampicillin in parenteral applications. Ampicillin is a good option in urinary tract infections due to its effectiveness on enterococci. However, there may be resistance in diseases caused by *Escherichia coli* [13].

10.5.2 Cephalosporins

Cephalosporins are drugs that specifically affect bacterial cells without affecting human cells. For this reason, it is thought that it can be used safely in all periods of pregnancy [14]. Although there are insufficient studies on their use and safety in pregnancy, the FDA gave it category B due to the lack of negative reports on embryo toxicity [12].

10.5.3 Carbapenems

Imipenem is a preferred antibiotic in severe infections. It is used in combination with cilastatin, a dipeptidase inhibitor, to prevent nephrotoxicity. The FDA gives category C because the data on its use in pregnancy are not sufficient [12, 13].

10.5.4 Fluoroquinolones

There are not enough studies about their use in pregnancy. It has a high affinity for cartilage and has been reported to cause acute arthropathy in weight-bearing joints in young animals in laboratory animal studies. It is not recommended for use in pregnancy. The FDA provides category C [12, 15].

Analysis of human studies has not reported that exposure to fluoroquinolones (ciprofloxacin) during the first trimester increases the frequency of congenital anomalies or the risk of musculoskeletal disorders. However, quinolones are contraindicated during pregnancy and up to adolescence [12, 15].

10.5.5 Macrolides

Erythromycin, azithromycin, and clarithromycin are in this group. According to most antibiotics, erythromycin passes through the placenta minimal. Although erythromycin is not the first choice drug in the treatment of syphilis during pregnancy, it is recommended in pregnant women with penicillin allergy. The estolate salt of erythromycin can induce hepatotoxicity in pregnant women. Hepatic transaminases are increased in approximately 10% of pregnant women who used this form in the first 3 months. Therefore, erythromycin estolate is contraindicated in pregnancy [12, 15].

The FDA provides category B for erythromycin and azithromycin and category C for clarithromycin [12].

10.5.6 Aminoglycosides

Streptomycin, gentamicin, amikacin, tobramycin, kanamycin, and netilmicin are in this group. It should be kept in mind that aminoglycosides may cause ototoxicity and nephrotoxicity in the fetus and pregnant women [16].

The most frequently aminoglycoside which is used in pregnant women is gentamicin. Although congenital anomalies and neonatal ototoxic and nephrotoxic effects have not been reported due to gentamicin exposure, 26 first trimester gentamicin exposures have been analyzed retrospectively and 1 newborn (4%) with dilated renal pelvis with no caliectasis consistent with bilateral hydronephrosis has been reported, and that newborn died 4 h after birth [17]. But the mother of the baby received an antimicrobial combination which consists of ciprofloxacin, gentamicin, and methenamine. The combination was used 7–10 days for urinary tract infection treatment. It is not clear whether it is a direct effect of gentamicin or not. In a case series of six gentamicin usage in the second and third trimesters, there weren't any birth defects or fetal/neonatal adverse effect outcomes reported [18]. The FDA admits aminoglycosides as category C [12].

10.5.7 Sulfonamides and Trimethoprim

Sulfonamides are preferred mainly in the treatment of urinary tract infections in gravidity. They are found teratogenic in some animal species, but not connection in humans, and it is thought that there is currently no teratogenic risk. Therefore, the FDA gives it category B. When sulfonamides are given just before birth (after 32 weeks), they are replaced by bilirubin and bound to albumin. Therefore, it has been reported that it may cause hyperbilirubinemia and kernicterus in newborns [12, 19].

Trimethoprim, a folic acid antagonist, is often used in combination with sulfamethoxazole. However, its use in the first trimester is not recommended because it is associated with structural defects such as cardiovascular defects and neural tube. The FDA provides category C [12, 15, 20].

Considerable relationships between prenatal TMP-SMX exposure and gravidity and fetal/neonatal outcomes are seen in some studies. In a cohort of 7039 TMP-SMX exposures in first trimester, increased risk of spontaneous abortion has been reported (OR 3.5, 95% CI 2.3–5.6) [21].

10.5.8 Tetracyclines

These broad-spectrum antibiotics cross the placenta, chelate with calcium, and accumulate in the developing bones and teeth of the fetus. Around the 14th week of pregnancy, milk teeth begin to mineralize and continue until 2–3 months after birth. Tetracyclines are more likely to stain permanent teeth yellow-brown when given after 24 weeks. Therefore, all tetracyclines are used in all gestational periods, especially in the calcification phase of the hard tissue; they are contraindicated after the 20th week of pregnancy. The FDA gives category D [15].

In a population-based case-control study comparing 164 pregnancies exposed to doxycycline in the first trimester with 124,469 unexposed pregnancies, exposed infants were found to have a two- to three-fold higher likelihood of cardiovascular birth defects (heart and circulatory system birth defects) compared to those who were not exposed (OR 2.4%, 95% CI 1.2–4.7) [22].

10.5.9 Azteronam

It is the only example of the monobactam antibiotic group that can be used clinically. Lots of studies have come to a conclusion that aztreonam usage during pregnancy is safe. Conversely, studies conducted in the first trimester of pregnancy are insufficient. For this reason, teratogenicity potency of aztreonam has not been fully determined. The FDA provides category B [15].

10.5.10 Lincosamides

Clindamycin plasma concentrations during pregnancy are like nonpregnant women. In 647 babies with clindamycin exposure in the first trimester, there weren't found any rise in teratogenic risk. Clindamycin and lincomycin are in category B by the FDA [15].

10.5.11 Linezolid

There aren't any well-designed studies in pregnancy. That's why it should only be used during pregnancy if the potential benefit to the fetus outweighs the potential harm. The FDA provides the linezolid as category C [15].

10.5.12 Metronidazole

It is an antibiotic used in the treatment of infections caused by *Trichomonas vaginalis* and anaerobic microorganisms. Its usage in pregnant women is controversial, because of its mutagenic and carcinogenic effects in bacteria and animals. It seems to be contraindicated in the first trimester of pregnancy. It can be used in the second and third trimesters if remaining treatments fail. The FDA provides category B [12, 15].

10.5.13 Nitrofurantoin

It is used primarily in urinary tract infections during pregnancy. There is not enough information about its teratogenicity. The FDA provides category B [12].

10.5.14 Rifampicin

Rifampicin is regarded as safe by the CDC for pregnant tuberculosis patients' treatment as the same as other first-line antituberculosis agents. Although there is an increased ototoxicity risk in infants, no teratogenic effects have been reported, except for those due to streptomycin. The FDA provides category C [12, 15].

10.5.15 Vancomycin

Vancomycin administration has been associated with bradycardia induction in fetus. Ototoxicity has been reported in newborns who have in utero vancomycin exposure. Hearing loss improved after 3–12 months. In addition, red man syndrome may occur, which is characterized by the release of excess histamine after injection of the drug and causes intense uterine contraction; preterm delivery has been connected with vancomycin treatment. Thus, although vancomycin usage is beneficial in the second and third trimesters of pregnancy, the practice is limited in this regard. While standard dose doesn't pose a threat to the fetus, the FDA categorized it in category C [15].

References

1. Ke AB, Greupink R, Abduljalil K. Drug dosing in pregnant women: challenges and opportunities in using physiologically based pharmacokinetic modelling and simulations. CPT Pharmacometrics Syst Pharmacol. 2018;7(2):103–10.
2. Feghali M, Venkataramanan R, Caritis S. Pharmacokinetics of drugs in pregnancy. In: Seminars in perinatology. Elsevier; 2015.
3. Jeong H. Altered drug metabolism during pregnancy; hormonal regulation of drug-metabolizing enzymes. Expert Opin Drug Metab Toxicol. 2010;6(6):689–99.
4. Tasnif Y, Morado J, Hebert M. Pregnancy related pharmacokinetic changes. Clin Pharmacol Therap. 2016;100(1):53–62.
5. Nakajima K. Establishing evidence for appropriate drug use during pregnancy and lactation. Yakugaku Zasshși. 2019;139(4):565–70.
6. Alsaleh R, Gari S, Gari M. The awareness of pregnant patient about effect of antibiotics in pregnancy. J Microsc Ultrastruct. 2019;7(2):72.
7. Bookstaver PB, Bland CM, Griffin B, Sover KR, Eiland LS, McLaughlin M. A review of antibiotic use in pregnancy. Pharmacotherapy. 2015;35(11):1052–62.
8. Tejada B. Antibiotic use and misuse during pregnancy and delivery: benefits and risks. Int J Environ Res Public Health. 2014;11(8):7993–8009.

 9. Kenyon S, Pike K, Jones D, Brocklehurst P, Marlow N, Salt A, et al. Childhood outcomes after prescription of antibiotics to pregnant women with spontaneous preterm labour: 7-year follow up of the ORACLE II trial. Lancet. 2008;372(9646):1319–27.
10. Mueller NT, Whyatt R, Hoepner L, Oberfield S, Dominguez-Bello MG, Widen E, et al. Prenatal exposure to antibiotics, cesarean section and risk of childhood obesity. Int J Obes. 2015;39(4):665.
11. Lapin B, Piorkowski J, Ownby D, Freels S, Chavez N, Hernandez E, et al. Relationship between prenatal antibiotic use and asthma in at-risk. Ann Allergy Asthma Immunol. 2015;114(3):203–7.
12. Mungan MT. Gebelikte antibiyotik kullanımı. J Clin Obstet Gynecol. 2001;11(6):451–60.
13. Zorlu CG, Ari EŞ. Gebelerde Antibiyotik kullanımı ve Paraziter İnfestasyonların Tedavisi. J Clin Obstet Gynecol. 2006;16(1):17–32.
14. İnci M, Davarcı M. Gebelikte görülen üriner sistem enfeksiyonları ve tedavisi. Turk Urol Sem. 2011;2:124–6.
15. Bafios J-E, Cruz N, Farre M. Use of antibiotics in pregnant patients in the intensive care unit. In: Infectious diseases in critical care. Springer; 2007. p. 168–82.
16. Sargın S, Arpalı E. İdrar yolu enfeksiyonları. In: Anafarta K, Yaman M, editors. Campbell Üroloji 8, p. 515–602.
17. Yaris F, Kadioglu M, Kesim M, et al. Urinary tract infections in unplanned pregnancies and fetal outcome. Eur J Contracept Reprod Health Care. 2004;9:141–6.
18. Prasanna M, Singh K. Early burn wound excision in "major" burns with "pregnancy": a preliminary report. Burns. 1996;22:234–7.
19. Czeizel AE, Rockenbauer M, Sorensen HT, Olsen J. The teratogenic risk of trimethoprim-sulfonamides: a population based case-control study. Reprod Toxicol. 2001;15(6):637–46.
20. Lee M, Bozzo P, Einarson A, Koren G. Urinary tract infections in pregnancy. Can Fam Physician. 2008;54(6):853–4.
21. Muanda FT, Sheehy O, Berard A. Use of trimethoprim-sulfamethoxazole during pregnancy and risk of spontaneous abortion: a nested case control study. Br J Clin Pharmacol. 2018;84:1198–205.
22. Muanda FT, Sheehy O, Berard A. Use of antibiotics during pregnancy and the risk of major congenital malformations: a population based cohort study. Br J Clin Pharmacol. 2017;83:2557–71.

Use of Corticosteroid During Pregnancy and the Postpartum Period

11

Ramazan Öçal, Rahmi Kılıç, and Cemal Cingi

11.1 Introduction

Beyond all physiological states, pregnancy is the one that leads to most dramatic changes in the human body. Changes in the female body initiate with the beginning moment of pregnancy. Various factors as the hormonal effects, fetal growth in the uterus, and physical adaptation of the mother's body are the causes of these changes.

Until the discovery of the relationship between defects at birth and rubella infection in the first trimester in 1941, doctors believed the uterus was protecting the growing fetus from the environment. The drug effect on developing fetuses was finally acknowledged in the 1960s, when the effect of thalidomide on congenital extremity defects was determined. A total of 1.2 billion drug prescriptions are written each year; in a questionnaire which pregnant women participated, 86% of them used medication during pregnancy [1]. Over-the-counter medicines and herbal medicines are usually used upon an advice from a doctor, nurse, or a certified nurse-midwife.

Teratogenesis due to medicine consumption is a problem for both the doctor and the patient. Knowledge of the whole risk underlying the congenital malformations which is seen in 2–4% of all newborns are crucial. Environmental teratogens as radiation, infections, and chemical and pharmaceutical agents are the underlying

R. Öçal (✉) · R. Kılıç
Faculty of Medicine, Department of Otolaryngology, Head and Neck Surgery, Health Sciences University, Ankara Research and Training Hospital, Ankara, Turkey
e-mail: drramazanocal@gmail.com; drkilic@gmail.com

C. Cingi
Medical Faculty, Department of Otorhinolaryngology, Eskisehir Osmangazi University, Eskisehir, Turkey
e-mail: ccing@gmail.com

125

C. Cingi et al. (eds.), *ENT Diseases: Diagnosis and Treatment during Pregnancy and Lactation*, https://doi.org/10.1007/978-3-031-05303-0_11

causes of 10% of congenital malformations. Additionally, genetics affects the sensitivity of the mother and fetus to the environmental activity. Drugs are thought to cause only 1–5% of all malformations related with environmental factors [2].

Pregnant women and their care providers are frequently faced with the decision-making about drug use during pregnancy. The critical issue in this process is to cure the medical problem without extremely damaging both the mother and the fetus.

Both in pediatric and adult patient groups, steroids are one of the commonly used drugs. During pregnancy, the use of glucocorticoids as betamethasone, dexamethasone, and prednisone may be indicated. These agents are used for their anti-inflammatory or immune-suppressive effects [3].

11.2 Corticosteroid and Pregnancy

In pregnancy the most sensitive period in terms of drug use is the organogenesis period which covers the 18–21st and 56–60th days. In this period the cellular division is intense; since differentiation of tissue and organ systems is observed, this period is stated as the most vulnerable period of the fetus to teratogenic effects [4].

During pregnancy some physiological changes that affect the pharmacokinetics of drugs occur. Gastrointestinal motility decreases and the intestinal passage prolongs. This causes an increase in the absorption of slowly absorbed drugs. The decreased plasma albumin rates alter the kinetics of drugs that normally bind to albumin. The increased plasma and extracellular fluid volume change the concentrations of compounds and eventually affect their transfer. Renal perfusion increases though in the advanced stages of gestation, it is affected by the body's new conformation. On the contrary the hepatic perfusion does not change significantly.

Drugs and other environmental agents that lead to anomalies in fetal growth and development are called teratogens [5]. When planning drug use, first, the potential teratogenic effect, next if the teratogenic effect occurs; and its effects on the fetal organs, fetal growth, and newborn and in long term on the child must be seriously considered [6]. This is because the drug and its metabolites can pass through the fetus by the placenta. The placenta is an organ that enables the exchange of nutrients, gasses, and various metabolites [7]. A nonpolar, fat-soluble, nonprotein-bound matter with low molecular mass can easily pass the placenta [8].

The American Food and Drug Administration has developed a pregnancy risk category listed from A to X for drug use in pregnancy.

Category A includes drugs that are safe to use during pregnancy, while category X includes drugs that are absolutely contraindicated for use during pregnancy. This classification does not fully reflect the real situation regarding drug use and risks in pregnancy because of several reasons. The FDA frequently uses date obtained from animal experiments, and new studies are not conducted due to the cost; also the existing data is not updated [9].

Any drug used during pregnancy causes doubts about not only because of the possible fetal and maternal risks in short term but also because of their possible outcomes years after exposure on the child. In spite of the lack of studies in the field, the complications due to extended use of antenatal steroids are a source of concern. In premature babies, harmful developmental effects due to long-term daily dexamethasone treatment have been shown [10]. However, Doyle et al. have studied the results of children with a birth weight lower than 1501 g in which some received steroid treatment. These children were evaluated again after 14 years, and children who received steroid treatment were taller and had better cognitive functions. The study showed that corticosteroids do not cause significant unfavorable effects [11].

The use of corticosteroids during pregnancy was found to be related with increased maternal and neonatal infection risk, decreased neonatal birth weight and brain dimensions, maternal and fetal adrenal suppression, psychomotor retardation, and behavioral problems. The data about the before mentioned is not certain; however, until new data is gathered from upcoming clinical trials, the present suggestion is not using repetitive corticosteroid cures routinely [12–14]. There is an increasing concern about using repetitive doses of betamethasone (without dose reduction) which may cause low birth weight and decreased fetal skull dimensions which has developmental, intellectual, and behavioral outcomes itself [10].

Results about the possible damage of antenatal exposure to CS on the fetus are controversial. Although there are reports that CS exposure in an early period may increase the rates of cleft palate and cleft lip, the risk is quite low. In a meta-analysis that Park-Wyllie et al. conducted, no significant increase in terms of major congenital anomalies was detected [15]. A cohort study in Denmark done by Bay Bjorn et al. indicated that CS exposure in an early period was not associated with congenital anomalies or cleft palate [16]. In general CS treatment seems safe. However, even though the risk is very low, the mother should be informed about the cleft palate and lip anomaly especially when CS administration is done in the first trimester.

There are conflicting reports on whether there is a relationship between CS use during pregnancy and prematurity and low birth weight [17]. In a prospective study by Park-Wyllie et al., 184 women using CS during pregnancy and 188 women who did not use it were compared, and it was found that the frequency of prematurity and low birth weight was higher in the group using CS [15]. On the other hand, a study conducted by Norgard et al. in Denmark with 900 children born to mothers diagnosed with Crohn's disease showed that there was no relationship between CS use during pregnancy and prematurity, low birth weight, and congenital abnormalities [18].

In a study in which infants exposed to dexamethasone in the early period were examined neuropsychiatrically at the age of 7–17 years, it was reported that these children had weaker verbal memory, decreased self-esteem, and increased social anxiety [9]. No neuropsychiatric disorder was observed in the babies of anti-Ro-positive pregnant women who were exposed to high-dose (average 186 mg) dexamethasone since 18th and 32nd weeks of gestation due to congenital heart block [19]. Although some of the studies on this subject have found a relationship between dexamethasone exposure and neuropsychiatric development, it has been claimed that the presence of anti-Ro antibodies may cause some neuropsychiatric disorders. In the light of these findings, betamethasone is recommended to be used during pregnancy when necessary [20]. Kelly et al. reported that the use of dexamethasone in cases with anti-Ro-positive congenital heart block is ineffective on neuropsychiatric development [21]. Although it has been claimed that exposure to in utero betamethasone increases the cardiovascular risk of the baby in advanced ages, it has been reported that this risk does not increase in 30 years of follow-up [22]. In conclusion, although many studies have shown that in utero exposure of CS with fluoride has negative consequences on neuropsychiatric development, the opposite is also stated in other publications. There is no clearly proven data. Although dexamethasone has been claimed to have fewer side effects in this regard, there are similar results with dexamethasone. When necessary, both drugs can be used during pregnancy.

Zeng and Zang achieved satisfactory results in the treatment of sudden hearing loss with oral prednisone treatment in pregnant women, and in long-term follow-up, they did not face any problems in both the mother and the infant [23, 24].

In SNHL if patients have a contraindication or if they refuse CS treatment, increasingly, intratympanic CS has been started to be used [25, 26]. Thus, the harmful adverse effects of systemic CS treatment are precluded.

Dexamethasone and methylprednisolone are the preferred agents in intratympanic treatments, and since the pregnancy category of methylprednisolone is B and that of dexamethasone is C, it would be more appropriate to prefer methylprednisolone in pregnant women. Beclomethasone (FDA category C) stands out as the preferred inhaled corticosteroid during pregnancy [27]. Inhaled corticosteroids have minimal systemic effects, but have been reported to cause adrenal suppression. High doses of corticosteroids can cause life-threatening side effects. These are fluid retention, electrolyte imbalance, hyperglycemia, weight gain, peptic ulcers, increased susceptibility to infections, osteoporosis, electrolyte imbalances, muscle wasting, psychosis, striae, thinning of the skin, impaired wound healing, ecchymoses, acne, hirsutism, cataracts, and fat accumulation.

Steroids may lead to an increase in blood sugar levels in a diabetic mother. In order to prevent excessively high maternal glucose levels, alert monitoring and possibly intravenous infusion of insulin are required. High maternal blood sugar may have a faster effect on the fetus than prolonged exposure, resulting in growth disturbances. When a fetus encounters excessive glucose levels, the effort required to metabolize this excess glucose may result in hypoxia in the fetus.

The risk of peptic ulcer increases when steroids are given concomitantly with salicylates or nonsteroidal anti-inflammatory drugs such as indomethacin. Steroids also increase the clearance of salicylates by reducing blood levels. There may be a decrease in potassium, T3, and T4. People on long-term steroid use may experience capillary fragility and thinning of the skin due to reduced protein of the skin and vascular walls. Wound healing may be disrupted due to decreased fibroblast proliferation and collagen accumulation.

11.3   Corticosteroid and Lactation

In 1930–1960 a breastfeeding refusal flare was recognized in the USA. By 1972, only 20% of newborns were breastfed, and at the same time, it was found out that breastfeeding times were also decreased. Later, there was an increase in breastfeeding, and 50% of the mothers started breastfeeding before they were discharged from the hospital. This increase has led to concerns about the safety and potential toxicity of drugs excreted in breast milk. While prescribing drugs, the profit-loss ratio should be taken into account in breastfeeding women, as in pregnancy. Although there are no studies on the use of betamethasone or dexamethasone during lactation, the molecular weights of both are low enough to pass into breast milk.

Prednisone and prednisolone can be detected in breast milk. It is considered safe to use prednisone at doses less than 20 mg/day during breastfeeding. The American Academy of Pediatrics considers prednisone to be suitable during breastfeeding, but others recommend that breastfeeding should be delayed for at least 4 h if high doses are required [28].

When prednisolone is taken orally, less than 0.1% can pass into milk, which corresponds to less than 10% of infant cortisol production. At these levels, CS exposure is considered to be ineffective on infant development [29]. The time for CS to reach the maximum level in milk is in the second hour. Nevertheless, if high-dose CS treatment is required for a long time, it should be taken 3–4 h before breastfeeding to minimize the infant's exposure to CS [30]. The use of CS can increase the risk of maternal hypertension, hyperglycemia, and osteoporosis. One should also not ignore other classic side effects. Since these already create an increased risk for the mother and fetus during pregnancy, it is necessary to be careful in these aspects while using CS. If the aim is to treat the pregnant, prednisolone or methyl prednisolone should be preferred; if the aim is to treat the fetus, then dexamethasone or betamethasone should be preferred.

11.4   Conclusion

During the 40 weeks of pregnancy, the woman is in a psychological and physical change. The changes seen are a result of the increase in the needs of the mother for the preparation of the birth and the growth of the fetus.

CSs work by decreasing inflammation and immune response, altering microvascular circulation. When the fetus is exposed to high-dose CSs, it affects the metabolic and endocrine balance of various fetal organs [31].

The decision to use any steroid is influenced by whether the drug is given for maternal benefit or fetal benefit. General principles of teratogenicity include dosage, duration of exposure, delivery route, and gestational age at exposure. The fetus is most susceptible during 4–10 weeks after the last menstrual period, but it is possible for the transplacental passage of drugs to affect the fetus at other times during pregnancy.

References

1. Larimore WL, Petrie KA. Drug use during pregnancy and lactation. Prim Care. 2000;27(1):35–53.
2. Wendel PJ. Asthma in pregnancy. Obstet Gynecol Clin North Am. 2001;28(3):537–51.
3. Coustan DR, Mochizuki TK. Handbook for prescribing medications during pregnancy. 3rd ed. Philadelphia: Lippincott-Raven; 1998.
4. Syme MR, Paxton JW, Keelan JA. Drug transfer and metabolism by the human placenta. Clin Pharmacokinet. 2004;43:487–514.
5. Kayaalp SO. Rasyonel Tedavi Yönünden Tıbbi Farmakoloji. Ankara: Pelikan Yayıncılık; 2012.
6. Duman M, Kalyoncu Nİ. Gebelikte ilac seçimi ve teratojenite bilgi servisleri. Türkiye Klinikleri J Surg Med Sci. 2006;2:62–8.
7. Nagi AH. Placenta examination and pathology. Biomedica. 2011;27:81–9.
8. Conley JM, Richards SM. Teratogenesis. In: Jorgensen S, editor. Ecotoxicology. San Diego: Academic; 2008. p. 3528.
9. Krause ML, Amin S, Mako A. Use of DMARDs and biologics during pregnancy and lactation in rheumatoid arthritis: what the rheumatologist needs to know. Ther Adv Musculoskelet Dis. 2014;6(5):169–84.
10. French NP, Hagan R, Evans SF, Godfrey M, Newnham NP. Repeated antenatal corticosteroids: size at birth and subsequent development. Am J Obstet Gynecol. 1999;180(1 Pt 1):114–21.
11. Doyle LW, Ford GW, Rickards AL, et al. Antenatal corticosteroids and outcome at 14 years of age in children with birth weight less than 1501 grams. Pediatrics. 2000;106(1):E2.
12. Bloom SL, Sheffield JS, McIntire DD, Leveno KJ. Antenatal dexamethasone and decreased birth weight. Obstet Gynecol. 2001;97(4):485–90.
13. Goldenberg RL, Wright LL. Repeated courses of antenatal corticosteroids. Obstet Gynecol. 2001;97(2):316–7.
14. Guinn DA, Atkinson MW, Sullivan L, et al. Single vs weekly courses of antenatal corticosteroids for women at risk of preterm delivery: a randomized controlled trial. JAMA. 2001;286(13):1581–7.
15. Park-Wyllie L, Mazzotta P, Pastuszak A, et al. Birth defects after maternal exposure to corticosteroids: prospective cohort study and meta-analysis of epidemiological studies. Teratology. 2000;62:385–39.
16. Bay Bjorn A, Ehrenstein V, Holmager Hundborg H, et al. Use of corticosteroids in early pregnancy is not associated with risk of oral clefts and other congenital malformations in offspring. Am J Ther. 2014;21(2):73–80.
17. Ostensen M, Forger F. Management of RA medications in pregnant patients. Nat Rev Rheumatol. 2009;5:382–90.
18. Norgard B, Pedersen L, Christensen L, Sorensen H. Therapeutic drug use in women with Crohn's disease and birth outcomes: a Danish nationwide cohort study. Am J Gastroenterol. 2007;102:1406–13.
19. Hirvikoski T, Nordenström A, Lindholm T, et al. Cognitive functions in children at risk for congenital adrenal hyperplasia treated prenatally with dexamethasone. J Clin Endocrinol Metab. 2007;92:542–8.
20. Brucato A, Astori MG, Cimaz R, et al. Normal neuro psychological development in children with congenital complete heart block who may or may not be exposed to high dose dexamethasone in utero. Ann Rheum Dis. 2006;65:1422–6.
21. Kelly EN, Sananes R, Chiu-Man C, Silverman ED, Jaeggi E. Prenatal anti-Ro antibody exposure, congenital complete atrioventricular heart block, and high-dose steroid therapy: impact on neurocognitive outcome in school-age children. Arthritis Rheumatol. 2014;66(8):2290–6.
22. Dalziel SR, Walker NK, Parag V, et al. Cardiovascular risk factors after antenatal exposure to betamethasone: 30-year follow-up of a randomised controlled trial. Lancet. 2005;365:1856–62.
23. Zeng XL, He JC, Li P, et al. Sudden sensorineural hearing loss during pregnancy: a 21 cases report. Chin J Otol Chinese. 2014;12:207–10, in Chinese.

24. Zhang Q. Clinical diagnosis and treatment of 7 cases of neurosensory deafness during pregnancy. In: Neural injury and functional reconstruction, vol. 10. 2015. p. 322–324, in Chinese.
25. Rauch SD, Halpin CF, Antonelli PJ, et al. Oral vs intratympanic corticosteroid therapy for idiopathic sudden sensorineural hearing loss: a randomized trial. JAMA. 2011;305:2071–9.
26. Plontke SK, Lowenheim H, Mertens J, et al. Randomized, double blind, placebo controlled trial on the safety and efficacy of continuous intratympanic dexamethasone delivered via around window catheter for severe to profound sudden idiopathic sensorineural hearing loss after failure of systemic therapy. Laryngoscope. 2009;119:359–69.
27. Aaronson DW. Medical-legal aspects of prescribing during pregnancy. Immunol Allergy Clin North Am. 2000;20(4):699–714.
28. Briggs GG, Freeman RK, Yaffe SJ. Drugs in pregnancy and lactation. 6th ed. Philadelphia: Lippincott Williams & Wilkins; 2002.
29. Greenberger PA. Pharmacokinetics of prednisolone transfer to breastmilk. Clin Pharmacol Ther. 1993;53:324–8.
30. Østensen M, Motta M. Therapy insight: the use of antirheumatic drugs during nursing. Nat Clin Pract Rheumatol. 2007;3(7):400–6.
31. Canlon B, Erichsen S, Nemlander E, et al. Alterations in the intrauterine environment by glucocorticoids modifies the developmental programme of the auditory system. Eur J Neurosci. 2003;17:2035–41.

Erdem Köroğlu, Gül Soylu Özler,
and Iordanis Konstantinidis

12.1 Introduction

Treatment selection choices during pregnancy should be based on the US Food and Drug Administration (FDA) risk categories. The FDA categorized drugs as A, B, C, D, and X based on animal and human studies. Category D and category X drugs should be avoided during pregnancy, whereas category A and category B drugs are safe to use. Category C drugs should be considered case by case as there are no adequate studies on humans, but animal studies have shown the adverse effects on fetus.

Topical therapies are used often alone or in addition to other treatments in otorhinolaryngology. The use of medications during pregnancy involves additional risks. The most important advantage of topical treatments is that they have less systemic side effects and they can be used more safely in pregnant women compared to their systemic forms. In this section, topical treatments will be discussed according to the regions of their application during pregnancy and postpartum period.

E. Köroğlu (✉)
Faculty of Medicine, Derince Training and Research Hospital, Department of Otorhinolaryngology, Health Sciences University, İzmit, Turkey
e-mail: erdemkoroglu1907@gmail.com

G. S. Özler
Faculty of Medicine, Department of Otorhinolaryngology, Mustafa Kemal University, Antakya, Turkey
e-mail: soylugul@yahoo.com

I. Konstantinidis
Academic Medical Faculty, Second Academic Department of Otorhinolaryngology, Aristotle University of Thessaloniki, Thessaloníki, Greece
e-mail: jordan_orl@hotmail.com

C. Cingi et al. (eds.), *ENT Diseases: Diagnosis and Treatment during Pregnancy and Lactation*, https://doi.org/10.1007/978-3-031-05303-0_12

12.2 Topical Ear Drugs (Or Drops)?

Otitis externa is an inflammatory process of the external auditory canal and auricle. The spectrum of disease can vary from a simple dermatitis of the external auditory canal to osteomyelitis of the skull base. It is common in people living at humid environment, swimmers, those with narrow ear canals, use of hearing aids, and after local trauma [1]. Topical eardrops are the treatment of choice for this condition [2]. Topical preparations alone may be sufficient for the treatment of mild and moderate cases, while in severe cases they are used together with systemic antibiotics. Debris and cerumen should be cleared from the external ear before topical therapy is applied. If the patient has a tympanic membrane perforation, it is useful to do this procedure under a microscope. An otowick can be inserted if the swelling of external auditory canal is severe.

In addition to external otitis, topical drugs are used in the management of ear discharge in chronic and acute suppurative otitis media. Topical ear medications are basically divided into four groups: antibiotics, glucocorticoids, antiseptics, and acidifying solutions.

12.2.1 Antibiotics

The main advantage of a topical treatment is that it can be delivered to an infected tissue at a very high concentration [3]. Common topical antibiotic drops used are aminoglycosides (neomycin, gentamicin, tobramycin), polymyxins (polymyxin B), and quinolones (ciprofloxacin, ofloxacin). The local treatment should be effective against *Pseudomonas aeruginosa* and *Staphylococcus aureus*, which are the most common microbial causative agents. If culture is possible, then treatment should be selected according to drug resistance results. Neomycin is effective against both *P. aeruginosa* and staphylococci, but it is likely to cause contact dermatitis and has an ototoxic effect. Gentamicin and tobramycin can be applied locally, but they also have ototoxic effects especially in cases with tympanic membrane perforation. Polymyxin is only effective against *P. aeruginosa* [4]. Quinolone group antibiotics are frequently preferred because of their broad-spectrum, antimicrobial effect, lack of potential ototoxic effect, and less risk of allergic reactions. A Cochrane database of systematic reviews revealed that there was no difference between quinolone group antibiotics and non-quinolone antibiotics in terms of clinical effects [5].

Aminoglycosides other than gentamicin are contraindicated during pregnancy due to their teratogenic effects. No congenital anomaly, neonatal ototoxic effect, and nephrotoxic effect have been reported due to intrauterine exposure to gentamicin. Therefore, the US FDA labeled gentamicin in pregnancy as category C and the rest of aminoglycosides as category D. Although topical aminoglycosides do not have a significant systemic absorption, they are not the first choice in pregnant women. If an aminoglycoside has to be used, then gentamicin is preferred. Negligible amounts of aminoglycosides are excreted into breast milk. Maternal use of eardrops containing gentamicin poses little or no risk for the nursing baby [6].

There are limited data about the use of topical polymyxin B in pregnancy. Also, animal studies have not been reported.

Because of poor absorption after topical application, polymyxin B is considered low risk at pregnancy and lactation period [7].

Systemic quinolones are not preferred in pregnant and breastfeeding women due to their side effects. Quinolones can cross the human placenta, and they can be found in the amniotic fluid at low concentrations [8]. Systemic effects to ciprofloxacin after topical application are negligible. Therefore, it is thought that it has no harmful effects on pregnant women. Systemic ciprofloxacin taken in the postpartum period is excreted into breast milk. After oral intake, breastfeeding should be avoided for 3–4 h in order to reduce its concentration in human milk. The calcium in breast milk generally has a protective role in preventing or reducing infant absorption of quinolones. Topical use may pose a negligible risk to newborns during the postpartum period.

12.2.2 Glucocorticoids

Glucocorticoid drops are given alone or in addition to other preparations as they decrease the inflammation and edema of the external auditory canal. Topical steroids used to treat external otitis may include prednisolone, dexamethasone, and hydrocortisone.

There are insufficient data on the use of dexamethasone in pregnant women. It is categorized in group C. The potential risk for humans is unknown. Dexamethasone should be used during pregnancy only if the potential benefit outweighs the potential fetal risk.

Systemically administered corticosteroids pass into human milk in amounts that may affect the nursing infant and may cause impaired growth, inhibition of physiological corticosteroid production, or undesirable side effects. When used topically, systemic absorption is low. A decision must be taken as to whether to stop breastfeeding or to stop systemic corticosteroid treatment considering the risks and benefits on a case-by-case basis.

12.2.3 Antiseptics and Acidifying Solutions

The most important defense mechanism of the ear canal is the skin pH. External auditory canal pH environment which is normally acidic presents changes during infection becoming more alkaline. Therefore, acidifying agents can be used to lower the pH of the ear canal environment inhibiting the bacterial growth. *P. aeruginosa* and *S. aureus* do not grow in an environment with a pH lower than 6 [9]. In a Cochrane analysis, antibiotics and antiseptic agents yielded equally good clinical results, and no difference was found between single agent or combination with corticosteroids [5].

Various topical antiseptics, such as acetic acid, boric acid, hydrogen peroxide, chlorhexidine, aluminum acetate, silver nitrate, and N-chlorotaurine, can be used in the treatment of external otitis and chronic suppurative otitis media [10–13].

Boric acid and acetic acid, which are the most preferred antiseptics, are categorized in group C. Minimal systemic absorption is expected from maternal use of these solutions. Therefore, they can be preferable choices in pregnant or breastfeeding women. Since boric acid is not excreted with milk, it can be the first choice for breastfeeding women. Its weak fungistatic and bacteriostatic action makes it a very good mild disinfectant in concentrations of up to 5%.

12.3 Topical Nasal Drugs

Nasal obstruction is a common problem during pregnancy. In addition to hormonal effects, the clinical condition can be challenging in the presence of concomitant other forms of rhinitis and rhinosinusitis. Nasal symptoms can have a significant negative impact on the quality of life as evidenced by disturbed sleep patterns, daytime fatigue, and the emotional changes of the pregnant woman that can eventually harm the fetus [14, 15].

Inferior turbinate enlargement is one of the most important causes of nasal congestion in pregnancy. In the medical treatment of inferior turbinate hypertrophy, intranasal steroid sprays are the frequently used treatment option because they reduce soft tissue volume due to their anti-inflammatory effects. The most commonly used surgical methods are turbinate lateralization, turbinoplasty, turbinate partial resection, and radiofrequency ablation [16].

Topical nasal medications are basically divided into four groups: corticosteroid, decongestants, antihistamines, and saline lavages.

12.3.1 Intranasal Corticosteroid

Intranasal corticosteroids (INCSs) are potent anti-inflammatory drugs that are used in allergic rhinitis and chronic rhinosinusitis with or without nasal polyps [17, 18]. Due to their anti-inflammatory effects, they have inhibitory effects on both the early and late phases of allergic rhinitis. Therefore, improvement in all nasal symptoms of allergic rhinitis such as nasal discharge, postnasal drip, blockage, and itching has been noted after this kind of treatment [19]. They can be used safely in the general population considering minimal local side effects such as nose bleedings, dryness, itching, and burning sensation [20]. They do not cause mucosal atrophy in longterm use, but very rarely they can cause septal perforation. However, they do not cause significant suppression on the hypothalamo-pituitary axis as in systemic use.

Due to insufficient human studies, the FDA did not include any INCS in category A during pregnancy [21]. Almost all of these drugs are in category C for pregnancy. The only medication included in category B is budesonide. It was previously in category C and upgraded to category B after a large study from Sweden

[22]. In this study, 28 newborns out of 2230 from pregnant women who used intranasal budesonide had cardiovascular defects, a number that was not statistically significant.

Systemic bioavailability differs between INCS agents (Table 12.1). Fetal exposure risk increases in those with high systemic bioavailability. In second-generation INCS (fluticasone furoate, mometasone, fluticasone propionate), systemic bioactivity is less than 1% due to its pharmacokinetic characteristics, while this rate is higher in old agents (triamcinolone acetonide, flunisolide, beclomethasone) [19].

Intranasal triamcinolone has high systemic bioavailability (46%) and is associated with congenital respiratory defects [23]. Therefore, it is not recommended for use during pregnancy. Although congenital malformations are not observed after use of intranasal beclomethasone, it is not recommended because of its high systemic bioavailability (44%) [23].

Due to the relatively high systemic bioavailability of intranasal budesonide (31%), it may increase the chance of fetal exposure [24]. Although many clinicians use budesonide as the first choice as it belongs in category B regarding safety, there are also publications that recommend INCSs such as fluticasone furoate and mometasone furoate, which are safer due to their very low systemic bioavailability (<0.1%) [19]. All these modern INCSs (budesonide, fluticasone, and mometasone) seem safe for treatment of rhinosinusitis and rhinitis during pregnancy.

12.3.2 Intranasal Decongestants

Nasal decongestants are drugs that cause contraction of blood vessels in the nasal mucosa, thereby reducing the swelling of the nasal mucosa. Sympathomimetic amines (phenylpropanolamine, phenylephrine) and imidazolines (naphazoline, oxymetazoline, xylometazoline) are the two main categories of nasal decongestants. All of these drugs belong to category C during pregnancy. Their use should be limited to 5–7 days since it may cause serious side effects such as rhinitis medicamentosa.

Phenylephrine is in the short-acting group and used to immediately treat nasal congestion and sinus pressure. A case-control study showed an association between phenylephrine use during pregnancy and the occurrence of congenital malformations [15]. However, subsequent studies could not confirm such correlation [14].

Xylometazoline and oxymetazoline are the most commonly used nasal decongestants and are members of the long-acting group. There has been a risk of

Table 12.1 Systemic bioavailability of INCS

INCS	Systemic bioavailability (%)
Triamcinolone	46
Beclomethasone	44
Budesonide	31
Fluticasone propionate/furoate	0.4–0.5
Mometasone furoate	<0.1

tracheoesophageal fistula associated with exposure to imidazoline derivatives during the first trimester [25]. This association was not observed during second or third trimester exposure. Pyloric stenosis has been also reported from imidazoline derivatives specifically xylometazoline, during first trimester [25]. In general oxymetazoline spray can be used with caution after the first trimester. However, it is not recommended for use during labor.

12.3.3 Intranasal Antihistamines

There are currently two intranasal antihistamines that have been approved by the FDA: olopatadine hydrochloride and azelastine hydrochloride [26]. Intranasal antihistamines are more effective on nasal obstruction and have a faster action and less systemic side effects. Therefore, they are commonly used for mild and moderate allergic and nonallergic rhinitis.

Intranasal antihistamines should be avoided during pregnancy [27]. They have been associated with developmental toxicity in animals, and there are no adequate data in humans. There are also no available data about azelastine and olopatadine and their presence in human milk and their effects on a breastfed infant.

12.3.4 Saline Lavages

Saline nasal irrigation is one of the most common treatment modalities of sinonasal diseases. It acts directly on nasal mucosa removing thick mucus, allergens, and air pollutants. In clinical practice two forms are mainly used: (1) hypertonic solution with over 0.9% weigh per volume of sodium chloride and (2) isotonic solution. Hypertonic solutions are more beneficial than isotonic solutions in the immediate improvement of symptoms [28]. They reduce mucosal edema decreasing the intracellular watery content through osmotic process. In addition, the hypertonic solution improves mucociliary function due to excessive hydration.

Considering that the majority of drugs cross the placenta, caution should always be taken when administering medication to a pregnant woman especially during the first trimester when organogenesis occurs [29]. Nasal rinsing with isotonic and hypertonic solutions can be used as a simple alternative to medical treatment in sinonasal diseases during pregnancy. In addition, nasal irrigation with hypertonic saline is an effective option in the treatment of pregnant women with seasonal allergic rhinitis [30]. This approach seems particularly safe as no harmful effects on the fetus are expected.

12.4 Other Topical Drugs

Topical drugs are also used in the oral cavity and skin diseases at ENT practice. It is known that antiseptic mouth rinses (like chlorhexidine gluconate, sanguinarine extract, cetylpyridinium chloride, hexetidine, etc.) are clinically effective when used as supplements in the treatment of periodontal diseases. Mouthwash rinses during pregnancy have been shown to improve gum health [31]. In addition, it was observed that there was no change in gestational age and a reduced rate of premature rupture of membranes occurred [31]. Chlorhexidine is the most preferred mouthwash as it belongs to category B during pregnancy. However, it should be noted that there are not adequate studies performed in humans with chlorhexidine.

Topical corticosteroids are also common drugs used for treating mucosal lesion of the oral cavity. Steroids such as clobetasol propionate should not be used for oral local application during pregnancy [32]. In addition, these drugs should not be used during breastfeeding. In general topical corticosteroids with mild to moderate potency should be preferred during pregnancy.

Pregnant women may need topical steroids that are the most commonly used medicines for skin conditions. Atopic dermatitis is the disease in which topical steroids are most commonly used. In the Cochrane study published in 2015, no relationship was found between maternal use of topical steroids of different potencies and types and birth defects, preterm births, or low Apgar score [33].

Epistaxis is a common problem during pregnancy, due to increased nasal mucosa vascularity. The prevalence in pregnant women is 20.3%, and often local application of decongestants and antiseptic ointments is required. Decongestants' use has been already discussed in the management of nasal obstruction. A classic example of nasal ointment prescribed after nose bleeds is mupirocin.

Mupirocin ointment falls into category B in Australia (TGA AU) but in US FDA has not been assigned. There is a lack of well-designed studies in humans with mupirocin ointment. In animal studies with pregnant animals receiving this medication, the babies did not show any related to mupirocin medical issues.

References

1. Hajioff D, MacKeith S. Otitis externa. BMJ Clin Evid. 2015;2015:0510.
2. Llor C, McNulty CAM, Butler CC. Ordering and interpreting ear swabs in otitis externa. BMJ. 2014;349:g5259.
3. Rosenfeld RM, Schwartz SR, Cannon CR, et al. Clinical practice guideline: acute otitis externa. Otolaryngol Head Neck Surg. 2014;150(1 Suppl):S1–S24.
4. Sander R. Otitis externa: a practical guide to treatment and prevention. Otitis Externa. 2001;63:10.
5. Kaushik V, Malik T, Saeed SR. Interventions for acute otitis externa. Cochrane Database Syst Rev. 2010;1:CD004740.
6. Niebyl JR. Use of antibiotics for ear, nose, and throat disorders in pregnancy and lactation. Am J Otolaryngol. 1992;13:187–92.
7. Leachman SA, Reed BR. The use of dermatologic drugs in pregnancy and lactation. Dermatol Clin. 2006;24:167–97, vi.
8. Ozyuncu O, Beksac MS, Nemutlu E, et al. Maternal blood and amniotic fluid levels of moxifloxacin, levofloxacin and cefixime. J Obstet Gynaecol Res. 2010;36:484–7.
9. Kim JK, Cho JH. Change of external auditory canal pH in acute otitis externa. Ann Otol Rhinol Laryngol. 2009;118:769–72.
10. van Balen FAM, Smit WM, Zuithoff NPA, Verheij TJM. Clinical efficacy of three common treatments in acute otitis externa in primary care: randomised controlled trial. BMJ (Clin Res Ed). 2003;327:1201–5.

11. van Hasselt P, Gudde H. Randomized controlled trial on the treatment of otitis externa with one per cent silver nitrate gel. J Laryngol Otol. 2004;118:93–6.

12. Neher A, Nagl M, Appenroth E, et al. Acute otitis externa: efficacy and tolerability of N-chlorotaurine, a novel endogenous antiseptic agent. Laryngoscope. 2004;114:850–4.

13. Head K, Chong L, Bhutta MF, et al. Topical antiseptics for chronic suppurative otitis media. Cochrane Database Syst Rev. 2020;1(1):CD013055.

14. Caparroz FA, Gregorio LL, Bongiovanni G, et al. Rhinitis and pregnancy: literature review. Braz J Otorhinolaryngol. 2016;82:105–11.

15. Incaudo GA. Diagnosis and treatment of allergic rhinitis and sinusitis during pregnancy and lactation. CRIAI. 2004;27:159–78.

16. Brunworth J, Holmes J, Sindwani R. Inferior turbinate hypertrophy: review and graduated approach to surgical management. Am J Rhinol Allergy. 2013;27:411–5.

17. Bachert C, Hörmann K, Mösges R, et al. An update on the diagnosis and treatment of sinusitis and nasal polyposis. Allergy. 2003;58:176–91.

18. van Cauwenberge P, Bachert C, Passalacqua G, et al. Consensus statement on the treatment of allergic rhinitis. Eur Acad Allergol Clin Immunol Allergy. 2000;55:116–34.

19. Alhussien AH, Alhedaithy RA, Alsaleh SA. Safety of intranasal corticosteroid sprays during pregnancy: an updated review. Eur Arch Otorhinolaryngol. 2018;275:325–33.

20. Corren J. Intranasal corticosteroids for allergic rhinitis: how do different agents compare? J Allergy Clin Immunol. 1999;104:s144–9.

21. Sastre J, Mosges R. Local and systemic safety of intranasal corticosteroids. J Invest Allergol Clin Immunol. 2012;22(1):1–12.

22. Norjavaara E, de Verdier MG. Normal pregnancy outcomes in a population-based study including 2968 pregnant women exposed to budesonide. J Allergy Clin Immunol. 2003;111:736–42.

23. Bérard A, Sheehy O, Kurzinger ML, et al. Intranasal triamcinolone use during pregnancy and the risk of adverse pregnancy outcomes. J Allergy Clin Immunol. 2016;138(1):97–104.e7.

24. Dawes M, Chowienczyk PJ. Pharmacokinetics in pregnancy. Best Pract Res Clin Obstet Gynaecol. 2001;15:819–26.

25. Yau W-P, Mitchell AA, Lin KJ, et al. Use of decongestants during pregnancy and the risk of birth defects. Am J Epidemiol. 2013;178:198–208.

26. Kaliner MA, Berger WE, Ratner PH, Siegel CJ. The efficacy of intranasal antihistamines in the treatment of allergic rhinitis. Ann Allergy Asthma Immunol. 2011;106(2 Suppl):S6–S11.

27. Gonzalez-Estrada A. Allergy medications during pregnancy. Am J Med Sci. 2016;352(3):326–31.

28. Kanjanawasee D, Seresirikachorn K, Chitsuthipakorn W, Snidvongs K. Hypertonic saline versus isotonic saline nasal irrigation: systematic review and meta-analysis. Am J Rhinol Allergy. 2018;32(4):269–79.

29. Gilbert C, Mazzotta P, Loebstein R, Koren G. Fetal safety of drugs used in the treatment of allergic rhinitis: a critical review. Drug Saf. 2005;28:707–19.

30. Garavello W, Somigliana E, Acaia B, et al. Nasal lavage in pregnant women with seasonal allergic rhinitis: a randomized study. Int Arch Allergy Immunol. 2010;151:137–41.

31. Jiang H, Xiong X, Su Y, et al. Use of antiseptic mouthrinse during pregnancy and pregnancy outcomes: a randomised controlled clinical trial in rural China. BJOG. 2016;123:39–47.

32. Alabdulrazzaq F, Koren G. Topical corticosteroid use during pregnancy. Can Fam Physician. 2012;58(6):643–4.

33. Chi C-C, Wang S-H, Wojnarowska F, et al. Safety of topical corticosteroids in pregnancy. Cochrane Database Syst Rev. 2015;2015(10):CD007346.

Locoregional Anaesthesia During Pregnancy and the Post-partum Period

13

Hande Gurbuz, Hulya Topcu, K. Tolga Saracoglu, and Volker Wenzel

13.1 Introduction

Regional anaesthesia minimises the exposure of the foetus to potentially teratogenic drugs by preventing polypharmacy. It also helps to avoid the risk of potentially failed intubation and provides excellent postoperative analgesia. Therefore, regional anaesthesia should be preferred for surgical interventions in pregnant women [1]. However, local anaesthetics should be used in the minimum concentration and volume because of the increased sensitivity to local anaesthetic drugs in pregnant women and drug passage to the foetus. If it is not necessary, vasoconstrictors should not be added.

H. Gurbuz (✉)
Faculty of Medicine, Bursa Yuksek Ihtisas Research and Training Hospital, Department of Anaesthesiology and Reanimation, Health Sciences University, Bursa, Turkey

Faculty of Medicine, Department of Anatomy, Kocaeli University, İzmit, Turkey
e-mail: handegrbz@gmail.com

H. Topcu
Faculty of Medicine, Erol Olçok Research and Training Hospital, Department of Anaesthesiology and Reanimation, Hitit University, Çorum, Turkey
e-mail: drtopcuh@gmail.com

K. T. Saracoglu
Faculty of Medicine, Lütfi Kırdar Kartal Research and Training Hospital, Department of Anaesthesiology and Reanimation, Health Sciences University, İstanbul, Turkey
e-mail: saracoglukt@gmail.com

V. Wenzel
Department of Anaesthesiology, Intensive Care Medicine, Emergency Medicine and Pain Therapy, Bodensee Campus Medicine, Klinikum Friedrichshafen, Friedrichshafen, Germany
e-mail: V.Wenzel@klinikum-fn.de

13.2 The Anatomy and Techniques for Nerve Blocks of the Head and Neck

Regional anaesthesia techniques are frequently performed for postoperative pain management in ear, nose and throat surgery. However, head and neck interventions can also be carried out under regional anaesthesia in some circumstances. In head and neck surgery, field blocks (local infiltration) and nerve blocks can be used to anaesthetise the relevant area.

The trigeminal nerve and superficial cervical plexus derived from C2 to C4 cervical spinal nerve roots provide the skin of the face and neck a sensory innervation. These nerves are juxtaposed with several vital structures; therefore, the safety and efficacy of face and neck blocks depend on precise and thorough anatomical knowledge.

13.2.1 Trigeminal Nerve

The trigeminal nerve is the fifth and the thickest nerve among the cranial pairs. It is a hybrid nerve with both sensory and motor functions. It senses the whole face and part of the scalp and leaves the brainstem in two parts: radix sensoria and radix motoria. Trigeminal nerve fibres originate from four nuclei (three sensorial and one motor) found in the brainstem and spinal cord. Nucleus principalis (pontis) nervi trigemini receives primary sensory (both touch and pressure) input of the face through the trigeminal nerve and projects to the thalamic ventral posteromedial nucleus. Nucleus spinalis nervi trigemini receives the sensory fibres that descend along its lateral boundary as the spinal tract of the trigeminal nerve. Nucleus mesencephalici nervi trigemini is the proprioceptive nucleus of the masticatory muscles. Lastly, nucleus motorius nervi trigemini is the motor nucleus of the trigeminal nerve innervating through the skeletal muscles such as mylohyoideus, digastricus venter anterior, tensor veli palatini, tensor tympani and mastication muscles.

The trigeminal nerve intracranially passes through Meckel's cave, and in this fossa, it forms the sensorial Gasserian (semilunar) ganglion. As the trigeminal nerve fibres leave the Gasserian ganglion, the postganglionic fibres divide into three parts, each innervating a specific territory of the face. The three parts of the trigeminal nerve are ophthalmic division, maxillary division and mandibular division (Fig. 13.1). The maxillary and ophthalmic nerves enter the cavernous sinus and travel along its lateral border. The ophthalmic nerve exits the skull through the superior orbital fissure, whereas the maxillary nerve leaves the skull via the foramen rotundum, and the mandibular nerve exits the skull through the foramen ovale [2].

13.2.1.1 Trigeminal Nerve Blocks

Blockades of the Gasserian ganglion and the trigeminal nerve's superficial branches are primarily used in treating chronic pain conditions such as migraine, trigeminal neuralgia and herpes zoster. Besides, trigeminal nerve blocks are also used for

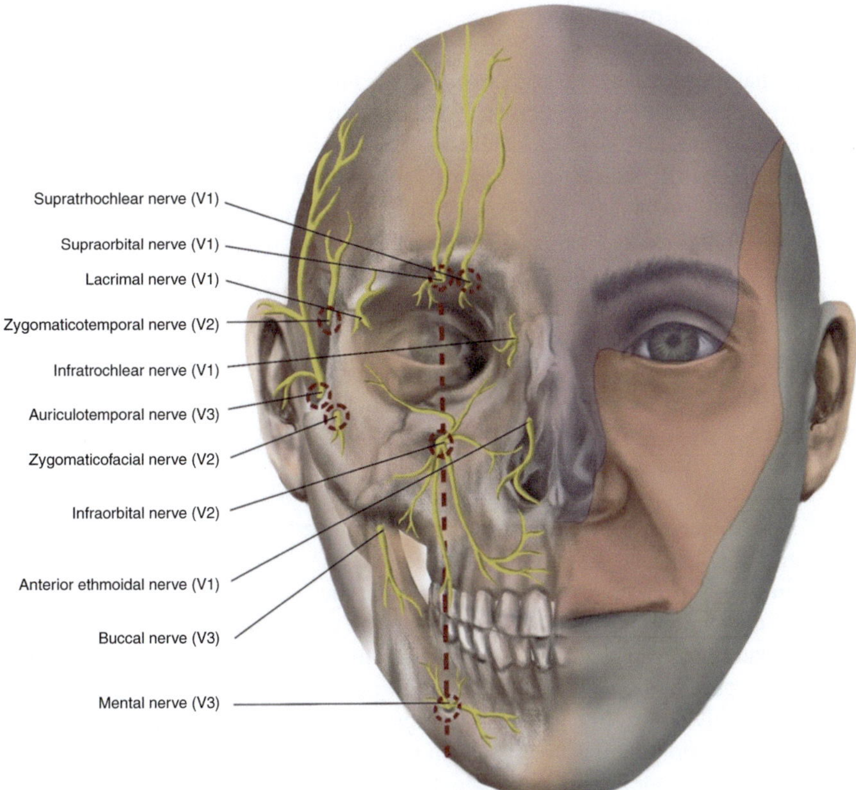

Fig. 13.1 Nerves of the face, the three parts of the trigeminal nerve are ophthalmic division, maxillary division and mandibular division

surgical procedures of their respective cutaneous areas, as anaesthesia techniques or adjunct to general anaesthesia to contribute analgesia.

13.2.1.2 The Trigeminal Cardiac Reflex

The trigeminal cardiac reflex is the sudden onset of asystole, bradycardia, hypotension, nausea, vomiting, gastrointestinal hypermotility or apnoea due to parasympathetic activity during manipulation of the sensory branches and nerve endings of the trigeminal nerve. The peripheral sensory neurons form the afferent pathway of the reflex arc via Gasserian ganglion to the sensorial nuclei of the trigeminal nerve—mainly the nucleus principalis nervi trigemini and the nucleus tractus spinalis nervi trigemini. Cardioinhibitory efferent nerve fibres that provoke negative chronotropic and inotropic responses arise from the vagal motor nucleus and end up on the myocardium [3].

The oculocardiac reflex is a type of the trigeminal cardiac reflex in which ophthalmic division constitutes the afferent pathway. It is triggered by mechanical stimulation of the ocular structures. The trigeminal cardiac reflex can occur while manipulating the trigeminal nerve divisions during head and neck surgeries [3].

13.2.2 Ophthalmic Nerve

The ophthalmic nerve derives of sensory fibres, and it takes the innervation of orbit, conjunctiva, lacrimal glands, cornea, paranasal sinuses, nasal mucosa, the skin of the nose and forehead, superior eyelids and the frontal part of the scalp. The ophthalmic nerve is the afferent pathway of the cornea reflex arc. Before leaving the cranium, it gives meningeal branches, and after exiting the superior orbital fissure is subdivided into three parts: frontal, nasociliary and lacrimal nerve [4].

13.2.3 Supraorbital and Supratrochlear Nerves

Supratrochlear and supraorbital nerve blocks are usually performed for the upper eyelid and lower forehead surgeries. These blocks can be used for the management of migraine headaches.

13.2.3.1 Supraorbital and Supratrochlear Nerve Blocks

The supratrochlear and supraorbital nerves can be anaesthetised together with a single injection of 1–3 mL of local anaesthetic. The supraorbital nerve can be palpated in the supraorbital notch by following the orbital rim and is located about 2–3 cm laterally from the midline. When a hypothetical sagittal line is drawn through the pupillary line, the supraorbital, infraorbital and mental nerves are positioned vertically on this line's trace. The supratrochlear nerve resides in about 1 cm medial to the supraorbital nerve. Thus, an injection to the supratrochlear nerve can be done after the supraorbital nerve blockade without removing the needle, by targeting the midline [5].

13.2.4 Nasociliary Nerve

Accompanied by nasociliary nerve, infraorbital nerve and pterygopalatine ganglion blocks, sufficient anaesthesia of the nose can be acquired.

13.2.4.1 Nasociliary Nerve Block

The needle is placed 1 cm above the medial canthus and advanced about 1.5 cm in a posterolateral direction. After entering the anterior ethmoidal foramen, 2 mL of the local anaesthetic is injected. Further advancement of the needle for 1 cm enables us to enter the posterior ethmoidal foramen and block the posterior ethmoidal nerve. The infratrochlear nerve block can be performed by infiltrating along the superior and medial boundaries of the orbit. An injection over the intersection of the nasal cartilage and bone is made to block the external nasal branch of the anterior ethmoidal nerve [5].

One should always keep in mind that when performing a nasociliary nerve block, the local anaesthetic should not contain epinephrine as it may cause retinal artery spasm.

13.2.5 Maxillary Nerve

The maxillary nerve is a thorough sensorial nerve, carrying impulses from the midface, inferior eyelids, superior lip, maxillary sinus, superior dental arch, gingiva, tonsilla palatina and soft and hard palates. The maxillary nerve is the afferent pathway of the sneeze reflex arc. It gives meningeal branches before leaving the cranial fossa through the foramen rotundum. After exiting the cranial cavity, it enters the pterygopalatine fossa, where it is situated above the pterygopalatine (sphenopalatine) ganglion (primarily facial nerve ganglion). The maxillary nerve subdivides into pterygopalatine branches, while zygomatic and posterior superior alveolar nerves arise from the maxillary nerve within the pterygopalatine fossa. The zygomatic nerve then divides into two sections: zygomaticofacial nerve and zygomaticotemporal nerve [6].

After leaving the pterygopalatine fossa, the maxillary nerve then reaches the infraorbital fissure, proceeds through the infraorbital canal and arises on the face via the infraorbital foramen, renaming as the infraorbital nerve. The infraorbital nerve divides into the external nasal, inferior palpebral, superior labial, middle and anterior superior alveolar nerves [4].

13.2.5.1 Maxillary Nerve Block

The truncal maxillary nerve block is practical to anaesthetise terminal branches of the nerves by a single injection. Maxillary nerve blocks can be used for dental procedures requiring injections for anaesthesia of multiple teeth, complementing general anaesthesia for maxillary surgeries, including maxillary trauma, osteotomy and cleft palate repair. Besides the pain management for surgical procedures, the maxillary nerve block is frequently used for trigeminal neuralgia. It should be recalled that a pterygopalatine ganglion blocked together with the maxillary nerve is expected after truncal maxillary nerve blocks within the pterygopalatine fossa.

The maxillary nerve can be blocked in the pterygopalatine fossa using a landmark technique or imaging guidance. Several techniques have been described for the maxillary nerve block:

Suprazygomatic Approach

Suprazygomatic approach is anticipated to reduce the risk of complications of the infrazygomatic approach such as maxillary artery puncture, orbital puncture and intracranial injection. In the suprazygomatic method, the needle insertion site is at the angle formed by the posterior orbital rim and the zygomatic arch. The needle is advanced perpendicular to the skin and advanced about 1.5–2 cm to touch the greater wing of the sphenoid bone. Then, the needle tip is redirected to the posterior and inferior and advanced about 3.5–4 cm. Following the loss of resistance, the pterygopalatine fossa is reached, and 5–8 mL of local anaesthetic is injected [7].

Greater Palatine Canal Approach

Blocking of the maxillary nerve in the pterygopalatine fossa through the greater palatine canal is an old technique, and not regularly preferred as a first option due to the risk of complications and the discomfort of the procedure. The greater palatine nerve and the descending palatine artery travel through the greater palatine canal from the pterygopalatine fossa to the oral cavity. The orifice of the canal is the greater palatine foramen, located on the palate 1 cm medial to the second molar teeth. This technique is contraindicated if the foramen cannot be located. The depression of the foramen can be identified by applying pressure on the palate with a cotton swab. The needle is inserted in the greater palatine foramen. It is then advanced approximately 3 cm in the canal at an angle of 45° to the long axis of the hard palate. After negative aspiration of blood, roughly 2 mL of the local anaesthetic is injected [8].

Coronoid Approach

Pain therapists usually use the coronoid approach in the pterygopalatine ganglion blockade, often conducted under fluoroscopy. Following a similar technique, blockage of the maxillary nerve located adjacent to the pterygopalatine ganglion in the pterygopalatine fossa is also feasible.

The needle is introduced perpendicularly at the centre of the coronoid notch below the zygomatic arch, anteroinferior to the tragus, and then advanced about 4–5 cm until it meets the nasal wall. At this level, the needle should be withdrawn slightly and redirected to the anterior and superior towards the maxillary nerve. Here, there may be paraesthesia in the region of the maxillary nerve. After negative aspiration of blood, 5–10 mL of local anaesthetic is administered [9].

13.2.6 Infraorbital Nerve

Infraorbital nerve block provides anaesthesia for the area between the lower eyelid, the lateral edge of the nose and the upper lip. The infraorbital nerve can be blocked after exiting the infraorbital foramen by using the infraorbital foramen as a landmark with intraoral or extraoral approaches. The infraorbital foramen can be easily spotted at the junction of the two imaginary drawn lines, one passing sagittally through the centre of the pupil and the other passing through the ala nasi horizontally, below the orbital rim. Regardless of the chosen block technique, the infraorbital foramen should not be penetrated to avoid eyeball damage and lower eyelid swelling.

13.2.6.1 Infraorbital Nerve Block

Intraoral Approach

While keeping the finger palpating the foramen, the needle is introduced into the buccal mucosa at the extent of the first premolar or the canine, and then directed upwards until palpated near the infraorbital foramen. 2–3 mL local anaesthetic is adequate for the blockage of the nerve [6].

Extraoral Approach

After locating the infraorbital foramen, a needle is introduced through the skin in a superomedial direction until touching the bone. A lateral-to-medial technique is recommended for preventing penetration into the foramen. Also, the facial artery and vein are very close to the needle in this technique; hence, utmost attention must be taken not to inject the drug intravascularly [6].

13.2.7 Zygomaticotemporal Nerve

Zygomaticotemporal nerve block provides anaesthesia in the region between the lateral orbital rim, the superior edge of the zygomatic arch and the temporal fusion line. It is usually used for cosmetic interventions of the face and as a component of the scalp blocks.

13.2.7.1 Zygomaticotemporal Nerve Block

The needle insertion site is behind the lateral orbital rim, posterior to the frontozygomatic suture at the lateral canthus level. The needle is directed downwards until reached a bony touch of the concave portion of the lateral orbital rim; then, 1–2 mL of local anaesthetic is injected [10].

13.2.8 Zygomaticofacial Nerve

Zygomaticofacial nerve block provides anaesthesia on the skin of a triangular area between the malar region along the zygomatic arch and the lateral canthus.

13.2.8.1 Zygomaticofacial Nerve Block

The zygomaticofacial nerve can be blocked on the inferolateral portion of the orbital rim by injecting 1–2 mL of local anaesthetic [10].

13.2.9 Mandibular Nerve

The mandibular nerve is a hybrid nerve consisting of both the motor and sensory fibres, passing through the foramen ovale, and reaches the infratemporal fossa. Here, it subdivides into the posterior and anterior trunks. Before the division, it gives two branches: the medial pterygoid nerve (motor) and the meningeal branch (sensory).

The masseteric nerve (motor), deep temporal nerves (motor), lateral pterygoid nerve (motor) and buccal nerve (sensory) arise from the anterior trunk. The masseteric nerve, lateral pterygoid nerve and deep temporal nerves innervate the same masticatory muscles. The buccal nerve carries sensory stimulus from the buccal mucosa.

There are three main branches that arise from the posterior trunk: auriculotemporal nerve (sensory), inferior alveolar nerve (sensory) and lingual nerve (sensory). The auriculotemporal nerve has two roots, encircling the middle meningeal artery. It emerges onto the face passing between the mandible neck and sphenomandibular ligament. The auriculotemporal nerve merges with the lesser petrosal nerve carrying postganglionic fibres (parasympathetic) from the ganglion oticum. It ascends and continues its course posteriorly to the superficial temporal artery after giving branches to the parotid gland. Then, it receives the cutaneous innervation of the temporal area of the scalp, the external acoustic meatus, auricle and external side of the tympanic membrane. The lingual nerve carries sensory impulses from the two-thirds anterior part of the tongue. The inferior alveolar nerve passes into the mandibular canal via mandibular foramen, in conjunction with the inferior alveolar artery and vein. Before entering into the mandibular canal, it gives the mylohyoid branch (supplying motor impulses to mylohyoid muscle and the anterior belly of the digastric muscle) that runs through the mylohyoid sulcus on the inner side of the mandible. The inferior alveolar nerve gives its terminal branches (incisive and mental nerves) at the first and second premolar teeth level. The mental nerve exits the mental foramen, at the level of the inferior second premolar tooth, to provide cutaneous innervation to the lower lip and chin [11].

13.2.9.1 Mandibular Nerve Block

The block of the main trunk of the mandibular nerve is useful for the pain management of surgeries involving the mandible and the nerve's respective innervation area. However, the blockage of the mandibular nerve's terminal branches is commonly preferred over the main trunk. Dentists frequently use mandibular nerve block when the inferior alveolar nerve block fails due to accessory innervation.

The mandibular nerve trunk block is performed before the nerve divides into its three main terminal branches. Different approaches have been described to perform the mandibular nerve block.

Gow-Gates Technique

While the mouth is open as large as possible, the second maxillary molar tooth is identified. The needle is introduced at the mesiopalatal cusp level, aligning the needle tip in the orientation of a hypothetical line on the inferior point of the tragus of the ear. The target point is the neck of the mandible condyle. Injection of 1–2 mL of local anaesthetic provides adequate anaesthesia of the mandibular nerve (auriculotemporal, mylohyoid, inferior alveolar, lingual and buccal nerves) [12].

Vazirani-Akinosi Closed-Mouth Technique

This technique is useful in patients unable to open their mouths. The needle is inserted in a lateral to medial direction, lateral to the maxillary tuberosity and medial to the coronoid process, aiming to enter the pterygomandibular space between the mandibular ramus and the medial pterygoid muscle while avoiding bony tissue contact [12].

Coronoid Approach

The mandibular nerve can be blocked with this technique at the skull base level on its exit from the foramen ovale. The needle is placed perpendicularly in the middle of the coronoid notch and advanced towards the skull base about a depth of 2–4 cm until it reaches the lateral pterygoid plate. Afterwards, the needle is withdrawn slightly and redirected towards inferoposterior. At this point, the needle tip placement can be confirmed with a nerve stimulator to obtain the mandible elevation twitch. A 5 mL of local anaesthetic injection would be adequate for the mandibular nerve block [6]. The potential complications of the method are the puncture of the middle meningeal and internal maxillary arteries. A transient facial nerve block can be observed with the deposition of large volumes of local anaesthetic.

13.2.10 Mental Nerve

The mental nerve block is advisable for the surgeries of the lower lip, chin and teeth.

13.2.10.1 Mental Nerve Block

The mental foramen resides in the mental process, on the hypothetical vertical line through the pupil in longitudinal alignment with supraorbital and infraorbital nerves. Like the infraorbital nerve block technique, the needle is positioned on the mental foramen in a lateral to medial direction, with the guidance of the palpating finger while not penetrating the foramen, and 1–3 mL of local anaesthetic is injected [6].

13.2.11 Auriculotemporal Nerve

Auriculotemporal nerve block provides anaesthesia to the helix and tragus of the ear and a part of the scalp as well.

13.2.11.1 Auriculotemporal Nerve Block

The auriculotemporal nerve is located behind the superficial temporal artery at the ear level; thus, the artery can be used as a landmark. While palpating the arterial pulsation, the needle is placed behind the artery at a point of anterior and superior to the tragus, and 3–4 mL of local anaesthetic is deposited [6].

13.2.12 Sphenopalatine Ganglion

The sphenopalatine ganglion is juxtaposed in front of the foramen rotundum and pterygoid canal, next to the sphenopalatine foramen. Within the pterygopalatine fossa, it remains below the maxillary nerve. It is one of the largest parasympathetic ganglia and associated topographically with the maxillary nerve and functionally with the facial nerve. The sphenopalatine ganglion has palatine, nasal, pharyngeal and orbital efferent branches. The parasympathetic fibres go to the lacrimal, nasal and palatal glands within the maxillary nerve branches and are responsible for secretion and vasodilation in these regions. The carotid plexus form the sympathetic part of the ganglion through the deep petrosal nerve. After separating from the genicular ganglion (parasympathetic), the great superficial petrosal nerve (facial nerve's first branch) joins with the deep petrosal nerve (sympathetic) arising from the carotid plexus; then together they form the nerve of the pterygoid canal (Vidian nerve). Lastly, the Vidian nerve enters the pterygopalatine fossa through the pterygoid canal and merges with the pterygopalatine ganglion [2].

13.2.12.1   Pterygopalatine Ganglion Block

Pterygopalatine ganglion block is commonly used in treating headaches and facial neuralgias. After a successful diagnostic block with a local anaesthetic, radiofrequency ablation or neurostimulation can be applied for managing chronic pain conditions.

There are several approaches in blocking the pterygopalatine ganglion in the pterygopalatine fossa. Due to the anatomic vicinity of the maxillary nerve and pterygopalatine ganglion, the block techniques are very similar to the maxillary nerve block (see Sect. 13.2.5). Because the pterygopalatine ganglion is located in caudomedial of the maxillary nerve, paraesthesia in the upper teeth indicates the maxillary nerve stimulation; hence, the needle ought to be redirected accordingly.

Topical Application Approach

Due to the proximity of ganglion to the posterior mucosal wall of the nose, the topical application approach can be employed as a non-invasive technique. The head is extended; then, 3 mL of 4% lidocaine-absorbed cotton-tipped pledget is inserted through the nostril perpendicularly to the face. The pledget is pushed forwards to the upper boundary of the middle turbinate until the tip touches the mucosal membrane, and left for 30 min, followed by their removal [13].

13.2.13   Cervical Plexus

The cervical plexus is a network of nerve fibres originating from the ventral rami of cervical spinal nerves from C1 to C5, providing both motor and sensorial supplies to the head and neck structures. Motor branches travel through anteromedial direction, while cutaneous branches out posteriorly. The cervical plexus also receives a contribution from the cervical sympathetic ganglions via rami communicantes grisea.

Motor branches of the cervical plexus comprise the ansa cervicalis innervating infrahyoid muscles and geniohyoid muscle via the hypoglossal nerve. The cervical spinal nerves emerging from C3 to C5 constitute the phrenic nerve, supplying the diaphragm, mediastinal pleura and pericardium. Muscular branches contribute to motor innervation of prevertebral muscles, muscles in the nuchal region, sternocleidomastoid, trapezius and levator scapulae muscles.

Sensory branches of the cervical plexus emerge along the posterior aspect of the sternocleidomastoid muscle, which corresponds to the junction point of the superior and middle thirds of the sternocleidomastoid muscle, called as the nerve point of the neck or punctum nervosum (a.k.a. Erb's point). Sensory branches of the cervical plexus innervate the scalp, ear, neck and upper thorax [2, 4] (Fig. 13.2).

The greater auricular nerve is comprised of C2 and C3 spinal nerves, innervating the skin covering the parotid gland, the posterior aspect of the external ear and the area between the mandibular angle and the mastoid process.

The lesser occipital nerve arises from C2 (and sometimes with a contribution from C3) and provides cutaneous innervation to the posterosuperior portion of the scalp and neck.

The transverse cervical nerve is stemmed from C2 and C3 spinal nerves and innervates the skin of the neck's anterior triangle.

The supraclavicular nerves arise from C3 and C4 spinal nerves and provide cutaneous sensation to the upper chest and shoulders.

The greater occipital nerve consisted of the medial branch of the posterior rami of C2 and C3 spinal nerves, innervating the skin of the upper neck, occiput and scalp up to the vertex.

13.2.13.1 Cervical Plexus Block

Cervical plexus blocks are indicated for carotid endarterectomy and superficial neck surgery. The cervical plexus can be successfully blocked using either the anatomic

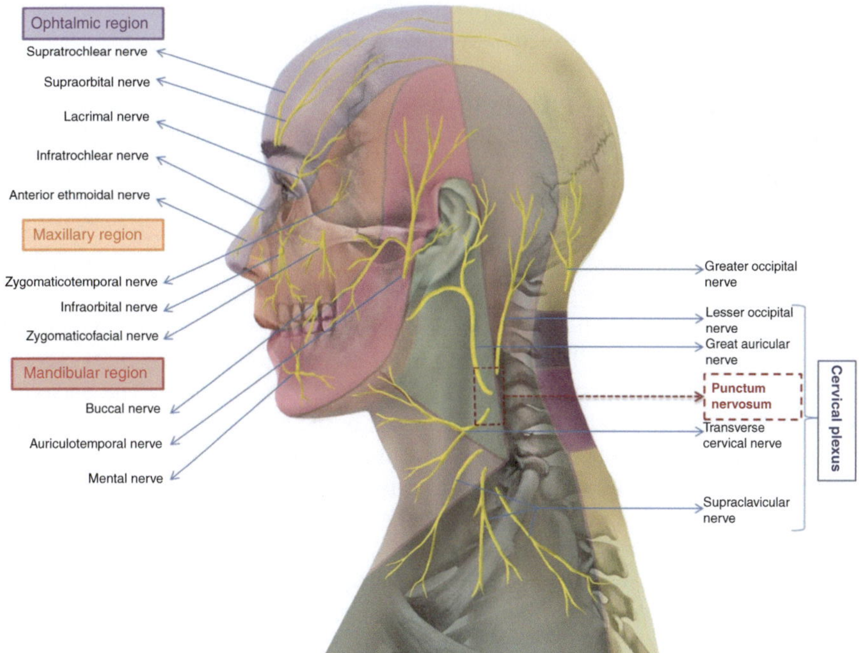

Fig. 13.2 Sensory branches of the cervical plexus innervate the scalp, ear, neck and upper thorax [2, 4]

landmark technique or ultrasound-guided technique. The procedure can be performed by injecting local anaesthetic under the deep cervical (prevertebral) facia (deep cervical block) or superficial to the investing layer of the prevertebral facia (superficial cervical block). The deep cervical plexus block is associated with severe complications, including inadvertent intravascular injection (vertebral artery) and intrathecal injection. The superficial cervical plexus block is simple and safer than the deep cervical plexus block. Also, the superficial cervical plexus block provides reliable anaesthesia as a deep technique for most circumstances.

The aim is to deposit local anaesthetic between the fascia cervicalis and the posterior sheath of the sternocleidomastoid muscle. For the landmark technique, the sternocleidomastoid muscle is identified, and the target is to infiltrate the lateral edge of the middle third of the sternocleidomastoid muscle (punctum nervosum or Erb's point) (Fig. 13.2). A 5–15 mL of local anaesthetic is sufficient for the block [14].

13.2.13.2 Greater Auricular Nerve Block

The greater auricular nerve block is used for anaesthesia of the auricle or as a part of the scalp blocks. Additionally, this block is also favoured for the management of headaches.

A single injection can be made at the tragus level, 1.5 cm behind the auricle, to block the postauricular branches. The ultrasound-guided technique has been successfully used to perform the block. A high-frequency linear probe is placed on the middle third of the sternocleidomastoid muscle in the short axis and then tracked upwards through the earlobe along the muscle's posterior edge. The nerve can be identified as a hypo-echoic structure approximately 4–5 cm inferior to the ear [15].

13.2.13.3 Greater Occipital and Lesser Occipital Nerve Blocks

Greater and lesser occipital nerve blocks are usually used to treat headaches (i.e. migraines, cervicogenic headaches and post-dural puncture headache). They are also beneficial for surgical pain (i.e. as a part of scalp blocks) and anaesthesia for the related surgical area. With the injection of a large enough local anaesthetic volume, it is possible to simultaneously block the greater and lesser occipital nerves by availing their proximity.

Granted a hypothetical line from mastoid process to the external occipital protuberance divided by three, the greater occipital nerve is found at the most medial third, whereas the lesser occipital nerve resides in the middle third. The occipital artery is palpated to identify the injection point of the greater occipital nerve. The injection place is medial to the artery. Occasionally, due to anatomic variations, the greater occipital nerve may be located laterally to the artery. Although single-shot blocks can be done, due to the proximity to the other occipital nerves, the block can be performed in a fan-like distribution with 3–5 mL of local anaesthetic, to block more than one nerve with a single injection [16]. Ultrasound-guided blocks help provide safety by avoiding the puncture of the occipital artery and improving the blocks' success rate.

13.3   The Anatomy and Techniques for Regional Blocks of the Head and Neck

13.3.1 Regional Anaesthesia of the Ear

Regional anaesthesia can be used in several auricular procedures: tympanoplasty, myringoplasty, auricular surgery, tympanostomy tube insertion, mastoidectomy and stapes surgery. Although general anaesthesia provides comfort to both surgeon and the patient, regional anaesthesia offers a bloodless surgical area, less operation time and a painless postoperative period.

The cutaneous innervation of the auricle is supplied by four nerves originating from cranial pairs and cervical plexus: (1) greater auricular nerve (cervical plexus), (2) lesser occipital nerve (cervical plexus), (3) auriculotemporal nerve (trigeminal nerve) and (4) auricular branch of the vagus nerve (Arnold's nerve). The auriculotemporal nerve supplies the innervation of the anterior and superior walls of the external acoustic canal, while Arnold's nerve provides sensation to the inferior and posterior walls [2, 11].

The auriculotemporal nerve and cervical plexus blocks can be done (see cervical plexus section) for anaesthesia of the auricle. Injecting a local anaesthetic around the auricle provides a field block, forming a ring (ring block). None of these techniques provides anaesthesia to the Ramsay Hunt area; thus, Arnold's nerve has to be blocked by inserting a needle into the tragus and injecting approximately 0.2 mL of local anaesthetic [6, 17].

The tympanic membrane is innervated by the auriculotemporal nerve, Arnold's nerve and tympanic branch of the glossopharyngeal nerve (Jacobson's nerve). Additional infiltration with a local anaesthetic is usually needed during tympanic procedures to block Jacobson's nerve [17].

13.3.1.1   Block Technique
The external ear block includes both field block and individual nerve blocks (described in detail in the relevant sections).

13.3.2 Regional Anaesthesia of the Nose

Nasal infiltration is usually used by the surgeons mostly as a routine part of the surgery to decrease bleeding using vasoconstrictors. Nerve blocks can also be used in most septoplasty cases, rhinoplasty, intranasal surgery and the repair of the skin laceration for anaesthesia and analgesia [18].

The sensory innervation of the nasal skin and cavity includes the trigeminal nerve (ophthalmic and maxillary branches) and pterygopalatine ganglion. Ethmoidal branches of the nasociliary nerve (ophthalmic branch) supply sensation to the sphenoidal, ethmoidal and frontal sinuses, as well as anterior and superior sections of the nasal cavity. Nasal branches of the anterior ethmoidal nerve (ophthalmic branch) provide a sensorial supply to the nasal cavity's lateral wall, the nasal bone, the anterior part of the septum and the skin to the tip of the nose. The sensorial output of the root of the nose is provided by the supratrochlear nerve (ophthalmic branch). The infraorbital nerve (maxillary branch) supplies cutaneous sensation to the wings of the nose. Nasal and palatal branches of the maxillary nerve and the pterygopalatine ganglion innervate the nasal cavity and posterior portion of the septum [4].

13.3.2.1 Block Technique

The nasal block includes the joint blocking of the trigeminal branches that innervate the nose and the sphenopalatine ganglion [6]. Blocking these nerves was explained in detail in the previous sections.

13.3.3 Regional Anaesthesia of the Scalp

Scalp blocks are indicated for many head and neck and neurosurgical procedures. They can be used as an anaesthesia method in superficial surgical procedures of the head and neck. Scalp blocks suppress the haemodynamic response to skull pin head holder insertion and skin incision in neurosurgery. Furthermore, scalp blocks are predominantly used in the diagnostic and therapeutic management of headache syndromes.

13.3.3.1 Block Technique

Scalp blocks are comprised of the blockage of seven nerves: (1) supraorbital nerve (ophthalmic branch), (2) supratrochlear nerve (ophthalmic branch), (3) zygomaticotemporal nerve (maxillary branch), (4) auriculotemporal nerve (mandibular branch), (5) greater occipital nerve (cervical plexus), (6) lesser occipital nerve (cervical plexus) and (7) great auricular nerve (cervical plexus).

The block method of these nerves was explained in detail in the previous sections.

13.3.4 Regional Anaesthesia of the Upper Airway

Surgical procedures in patients with known or anticipated difficult airway should be carried out under locoregional anaesthesia, if possible. In the later stages of pregnancy, pregnant women are prone to difficult airway changes. In cases requiring general anaesthesia and endotracheal intubation, awake intubation is an option that should be applied for difficult airway management. However, it is crucial to suppress airway reflexes (such as gag reflex, glottis closure reflex and coughing) for awake intubation and provide local and regional anaesthesia. Simultaneously, airway anaesthesia can provide anaesthesia and analgesia in some other head and neck procedures.

Airway anaesthesia can be provided with topical and nerve blocks by administering local anaesthetics via an atomiser device, nebuliser or spray [19]. The risk of nerve block complications is high because more than one individual nerve has to be blocked together. Blockade of three fundamental nerves or their branches is required for airway anaesthesia: (1) Trigeminal nerve, (2) glossopharyngeal nerve and (3) vagal nerve.

The upper airway consists of nasal and oral cavities, pharynx and larynx. According to the neuronal innervation, the upper airway can be examined in three regions: the trigeminal part, the glossopharyngeal part and the vagal part.

Trigeminal part: The trigeminal nerve provides sensory innervation to the nasal cavity, turbinates, oral cavity and the anterior two-thirds of the tongue.

Glossopharyngeal part: The oropharynx, nasopharynx, soft palate and posterior one-third of the tongue, the vallecula and the anterior part of the epiglottis.

Vagal part: The sensory innervation of the posterior part of the larynx, the posterior surface of the epiglottis and more distal airway structures. The sensation of the laryngeal mucosa above the plica vocalis level is supplemented by the internal branch of the superior laryngeal nerve, and the recurrent laryngeal nerve supports the sensory innervation of the larynx mucosa under the level of plica vocalis.

13.3.4.1 Trigeminal Nerve
(Explained in detail in the relevant sections)

13.3.4.2 Glossopharyngeal Nerve
The glossopharyngeal nerve leaves the cranium from the jugular foramen along with the vagal nerve and the hypoglossal nerve. It descends from the jugular foramen in a posteromedial direction to the styloid process along the posterior side of the stylopharyngeal muscle. In the upper airway, the glossopharyngeal nerve innervates the nasal cavity, turbinates, oral cavity and the posterior one-third of the tongue, vallecula, tonsils, pharyngeal wall and the anterior surface of the epiglottis. The glossopharyngeal nerve takes the somatic sensation of the middle ear cavity and tuba auditiva. It provides both tonsils and middle ear innervation; hence, referred pain can be felt in tonsillitis in the ear.

The glossopharyngeal nerve has two main branches:

The tympanic nerve joins the tympanic plexus in the middle ear cavity. The lesser petrosal nerve arising from this plexus unites with ganglion oticum. The parasympathetic fibres, emerging from this union, stretch out to the parotid gland.

The carotid sinus branch carries senses from baro-/chemoreceptors located in the aortic arch and the bifurcation of common carotid arteries.

The glossopharyngeal nerve forms the afferent pathway of the carotid sinus reflex (baroreceptor and barosympathetic reflexes), gag reflex and uvular reflex arches, while the vagal nerve constitutes the efferent pathway of these reflexes [2].

Glossopharyngeal Nerve Block
The glossopharyngeal nerve block is useful for glossopharyngeal neuralgia, abolishing gag reflex for surgery (transoral vocal cord surgery, endodontics, gastrointestinal endoscopy) and managing postoperative pain after tonsillectomy. The glossopharyngeal nerve can be blocked either extraorally or intraorally.

Extraoral-peristyloid approach: This technique is used for the management of the glossopharyngeal neuralgia. Although the peristyloid approach is beneficial in patients who cannot open their mouths, it is a relatively complicated technique despite fluoroscopy; thus, it is not recommended for the anaesthesia of the oropharynx. Unintended vagal block or internal carotid artery puncture can be observed because of the proximity. Landmarks should be identified clearly before performing the peristyloid glossopharyngeal nerve block. The needle is introduced perpendicularly to touch the styloid process (3.5–4.5 cm in depth) in the midpoint of the hypothetical line drawn from the mastoid process to the mandible angle. The injection place is just posterior to the styloid process. A volume of 5–7 mL of local anaesthetic provides anaesthesia for the glossopharyngeal nerve area [20].

Intraoral approach: Performing the intraoral glossopharyngeal block is more straightforward than the peristyloid technique. Thus, it can be used for temporary anaesthesia or analgesia in oropharyngeal interventions (i.e. tonsillectomy, laryngoscopy, gastrointestinal endoscopy). A study demonstrated that swishing and gargling with 2% lidocaine for 2 min, followed by 10% lidocaine spray administration, provided a superior route of anaesthesia according to glossopharyngeal nerve injections for awake direct laryngoscopy [21]. Glossopharyngeal nerve blocks provide better conditions for upper gastrointestinal endoscopic interventions in comparison with topical methods [22].

The intraoral glossopharyngeal nerve injections can be performed by both the anterior and posterior tonsillar pillar approaches. Anterior tonsillar pillar approach has been preferred predominantly for the ease of application and better patient tolerance [23]. Topical anaesthesia to the oropharynx is required before performing the intraoral glossopharyngeal blocks. Gargle or local anaesthetics can be sprayed for topical anaesthesia.

The anterior tonsillar pillar approach is performed by placing 5 mL of a local anaesthetic in the base of the anterior tonsillar pillar (palatoglossal arch) at a depth of 0.25–0.5 cm [24, 25].

The posterior tonsillar pillar approach is performed by injecting a local anaesthetic to the posterior tonsillar pillar base [26].

13.3.4.3 Vagal Nerve

The vagal nerve is a mixed nerve and leaves the cranium together with the glossopharyngeal and hypoglossal nerves. Major branches of the vagal nerve in relevance with airway innervation are the auricular and pharyngeal branches and superior and recurrent laryngeal nerves.

The auricular branch takes the somatic sensation of the external part of the tympanic membrane and the skin of the external acoustic meatus.

The pharyngeal branch is the main motor nerve of the pharynx. It forms the pharyngeal plexus over the constrictor pharynges muscle in conjunction with the pharyngeal branches of the glossopharyngeal nerve, the fibres arising from the external branch of the superior laryngeal nerve and sympathetic nerves. The pharyngeal plexus supplies innervation to all soft palate muscles except for tensor veli palatini and stylopharyngeus muscles.

The superior laryngeal nerve is divided into two branches below to the hyoid bone's greater horn. The internal branch is the sensorial nerve, innervating the laryngeal mucosa above the vocal folds. It pierces the thyrohyoid membrane in conjunction with the superior laryngeal artery and vein but then disperses under the mucosa in the pyriform recess. The external branch is the motor nerve and supplies motor innervation to the cricothyroid muscle. It travels on the lateral aspect of the larynx without piercing the thyrohyoid membrane.

The recurrent laryngeal nerve curves under the subclavian artery on the right and the arcus aorta on the left, then traverses upwards with the inferior thyroid artery and ends up as the inferior laryngeal nerve. It provides motor supply to all laryngeal muscles, except cricothyroid muscle (the external branch of the superior laryngeal nerve). It gives sensory innervation to the laryngeal mucosa below the vocal folds' level [2, 4].

The blockade of vagal nerve branches is performed for the anaesthesia of the related sensory area of the vagal nerve in the upper airways. The vagal nerve branches, which need to be blocked for airway anaesthesia, are the recurrent and superior laryngeal nerves. Performing these interventions with ultrasound guidance facilitates the applications and increases the block success in patients whose anatomic landmarks are difficult to identify.

Superior Laryngeal Nerve Block

Blocking the superior laryngeal nerve, particularly the internal branch, accompanying other nerve blocks is required for awake intubation or cricothyrotomies.

External approach: The superior laryngeal nerve can be blocked by direct infiltration into the place adjacent to the hyoid bone's greater cornu, from where the nerve penetrates the thyrohyoid membrane. The extension of the head eases the hyoid bone identification. The needle is inserted and advanced by targeting the greater cornu. When the needle tip is shifted towards the inferior part of the bone after the bony touch is detected, both the internal and external branches are blocked in this position. If the needle is moved further and the thyrohyoid membrane is pierced, the local anaesthetic is injected into this location, blocking only the internal branch.

In patients whose hyoid bones cannot be identified, thyroid cartilage is palpated. The needle is introduced and pushed forwards, targeting the superior cornu of the thyroid cartilage; then, a similar procedure can be performed in the cephalad direction. 2 mL of local anaesthetic is adequate for the block [27].

Internal approach: The blockage of the internal branch is targeted with the internal approach. The block takes place in the internal branch progressing towards the pyriform recess after piercing the thyrohyoid membrane. Local anaesthetic-soaked cotton pledgets are placed bilaterally in the pyriform fossa using forceps and left there for 5–10 min [28].

Recurrent Laryngeal Nerve Block

The recurrent laryngeal nerve has both sensory and motor fibres running cooperatively. Direct blockage of the nerve is contraindicated that it results in airway obstruction due to bilateral vocal fold paralysis because of the blockade of the motor fibres. Thus, the anaesthesia of the sensory fibres can be achieved by spraying the local anaesthetic solution on the mucosa at the level below the vocal folds by blocking only the mucosal branches.

The cricoid cartilage is palpated in the midline, and the cricothyroid membrane, juxtaposed superior to the cricoid cartilage, is identified. Then, the needle is inserted perpendicularly to the skin on the midline. When air is aspirated, quickly 4–5 mL of local anaesthetic is given, and then the needle is retracted. This manoeuvre causes coughing that helps disperse the local anaesthetic along the airway mucosa [27].

13.4 Local Anaesthetics

Local anaesthetics egress the placenta by passive diffusion, affected by several factors. Among these, liposolubility, degree of ionisation and protein binding rate play a prominent role. Drugs with low ionisation degrees, meaning non-ionised moiety is high, have high liposolubility, and hence, highly liposoluble drugs penetrate biologic membranes straightforwardly.

The active form of local anaesthetics in nerve blockage is the ionised form. Protein binding rate determines the toxicity of local anaesthetics: the more free-drug residue in the plasma without protein binding, the greater the risk of toxicity. Local anaesthetics are weak bases, with a low degree of ionisation, substantial lipid solubility and variable protein binding ratio. At steady state, maternal and foetal plasma non-ionised forms are found in equilibrium. However, in acidic environments, local anaesthetics tend to switch to the ionised form. Therefore, in foetal acidosis cases, foetal concentrations are expected to be higher than maternal plasma (i.e. ion trapping) [29].

Local anaesthetics bind primarily to α1-acid glycoprotein and secondarily to albumin. During pregnancy, maternal levels of both α1-acid glycoprotein and albumin decrease; therefore, the free form of protein-binding drugs increases [30]. The transfer of highly protein-bound local anaesthetics such as bupivacaine through the placenta is relatively slower [29]. Repeated injections and relatively high blood concentrations of drugs lead to an increased free-drug concentration and cause foetal accumulation. Also, neuronal sensitivity to local anaesthetics increases due to higher progesterone levels during pregnancy. Thus, the volume and concentration of local anaesthetics should be reduced in regional anaesthesia in pregnant women.

Serum concentrations of local anaesthetics vary depending on the injection site, injection technique and additives. Therefore, the utmost attention should be paid to ensure that the injection is not intravascular. The addition of a vasoconstrictor agent while injecting into a highly vascular area prolongs the elimination time of local anaesthetics by participating in the systemic circulation. Thus, vasoconstrictors reduce the risk of systemic toxicity and extend the duration of action by decreasing the plasma concentration of local anaesthetics. However, one should bear in mind that epinephrine injection may impair uteroplacental circulation in these pregnant women. Instead, bicarbonate buffering may be considered to increase the success and density of regional anaesthesia and to extend the duration of action.

While liver enzymes metabolise amide-type local anaesthetics such as bupivacaine, lidocaine and mepivacaine, ester drugs undergo rapid hydrolysis by nonspecific esterases in blood. In theory, the toxicity risk of ester local anaesthetics increases in cholinesterase deficiency (cholinesterase levels decrease in pregnant women), but there is no clinical report confirming such cases. As they are metabolised to para-aminobenzoic acid and cause anaphylaxis, procaine and benzocaine should not be used in pregnant women [31].

Prilocaine is an amide-type local anaesthetic with a high risk of methaemoglobinaemia. Lidocaine is less potent than bupivacaine with a protein binding rate of up to 70%. It is the most common local anaesthetic used in dental interventions, especially in pregnant women [32]. Until recently, there is no clinical report showing any adverse effects on the mother or baby. However, lidocaine has been measured at significantly higher levels in the umbilical cord when used in parturients [33]. Since bupivacaine is highly protein-bound (>90%), its transfer through the placenta is low. It is the most preferred drug for obstetric anaesthesia and analgesia in pregnant women. In repeated injections, the free amount in the maternal plasma increases and accumulates in the foetus. Bupivacaine is a racemic mixture, and levobupivacaine is the levo-isomer of bupivacaine, while ropivacaine is the propyl homolog of bupivacaine. Both levobupivacaine and ropivacaine are S (−) enantiomers. The S (−) isomers have a lower affinity for cardiac sodium channels than the R (+) bupivacaine isomer. Therefore, they are sorted as bupivacaine, levobupivacaine and ropivacaine in descending order as in cardiotoxicity risk [29]. However, cardiotoxicity doses of local anaesthetics have been tested only in the laboratory environment, and it has been observed that they do not cause cardiotoxicity until the blood concentration exceeds three times as much required to produce seizures. Since the biodynamics of the human body is highly variable, doses should be adjusted accordingly.

More neurobehavioral changes have been observed in newborns with general anaesthesia compared to regional anaesthesia [34]. Local anaesthetics are considered as safer when used in pregnant patients at appropriate doses with proper technique while considering the foetal condition.

13.5 LAST Treatment

The local anaesthetic systemic toxicity (LAST) treatment is dissimilar to other cardiac arrest events that it consists of seizure management, immediate administration of a lipid emulsion 20% and advanced cardiovascular life support. Benzodiazepines may be used to control seizure activity in haemodynamically stable patients, and large doses of propofol should be avoided. Arrhythmias, particularly those caused by bupivacaine toxicity, are generally refractory to the treatment, so emergency cardiopulmonary bypass can be life-saving until the drug leaves the heart tissue. During CPR, vasopressin works better in acidosis compared with catecholamine. Administration of any local anaesthetics should be terminated. Lipid emulsion 20%

treatment should be started immediately. An initial bolus of 1.5 mL/kg lipid emulsion 20% is given immediately over 2–3 min, and an infusion of 0.25 mL/kg/min—calculated for ideal body weight—is initiated. If there is no response, bolus injections with the same dose may be repeated one more time or twice, with the infusion rate doubled. Care must be taken not to exceed the maximum dosage of 12 mL/kg of lipid emulsion 20% [35].

References

1. Güngör I, Tezer T, Polat GG, et al. Popliteal sciatic nerve block in a pregnant patient in the last trimester. Turk J Anaesthesiol Reanim. 2015;43:279–81.
2. Ozan H, editor. Anatomi. 3rd ed. Klinisyen: Ankara; 2013.
3. Meuwly C, Golanov E, Chowdhury T, et al. Trigeminal cardiac reflex: new thinking model about the definition based on a literature review. Medicine (Baltimore). 2015;94:484. https://doi.org/10.1097/MD.0000000000000484.
4. Standring S, editor. Gray's anatomy: the anatomical basis of clinical practice. 41st ed. Elsevier: London; 2016.
5. Sola C, Dadure C, Choquet O, et al. Nerve blocks of the face; 2017. https://www.nysora.com/techniques/head-and-neck-blocks/nerve-blocks-face/. Accessed 29 Oct 2020.
6. von Arx T, Abdelkarim AZ, Lozanoff S. The face—a neurosensory perspective. Swiss Dent J. 2017;127:1066–75.
7. Mesnil M, Dadure C, Captier G, et al. A new approach for peri-operative analgesia of cleft palate repair in infants: the bilateral suprazygomatic maxillary nerve block. Paediatr Anaesth. 2010;20:343–9.
8. Aoun G, Zaarour I, Sokhn S, et al. Maxillary nerve block via the greater palatine canal: an old technique revisited. J Int Soc Prev Commun Dent. 2015;5:359–64.
9. McClenahan MF, Hillegass MG. Trigeminal nerve block. In: Yong RJ, Nguyen M, Nelson E, Urman RD, editors. Pain medicine: an essential review. Cham: Springer International Publishing; 2017.
10. Davies T, Karanovic S, Shergill B. Essential regional nerve blocks for the dermatologist: part 1. Clin Exp Dermatol. 2014;39:777–84.
11. Paulsen F, Böckers TM, Waschke J, editors. Sobotta anatomy textbook: English edition with Latin nomenclature. 1st ed. Munich: Elsevier; 2018.
12. Haas DA. Alternative mandibular nerve block techniques: a review of the Gow-Gates and Akinosi-Vazirani closed-mouth mandibular nerve block techniques. J Am Dent Assoc. 2011;142:8–12.
13. Piagkou M, Demesticha T, Troupis T, et al. The pterygopalatine ganglion and its role in various pain syndromes: from anatomy to clinical practice. Pain Pract. 2012;12:399–412.
14. Bendtsen TF, Abbas S, Chan V. Ultrasound-guided cervical plexus block. In: Hadzic A, editor. Hadzic's textbook of regional anesthesia and acute pain management. 2nd ed. Beijing: McGraw-Hill Education; 2017.
15. Ökmen K, Ökmen BM. Ultrasound guided superficial cervical plexus block versus greater auricular nerve block for postoperative tympanomastoid surgery pain: a prospective, randomised, single blind study. Agri. 2018;30:171–8.
16. Loukas M, El-Sedfy A, Tubbs RS, et al. Identification of greater occipital nerve landmarks for the treatment of occipital neuralgia. Folia Morphol (Warsz). 2006;65:337–42.
17. El-Begermy MA, El-Begermy MM, Rabie AN, et al. Use of local anesthesia in ear surgery: technique, modifications, advantages, and limitations over 30 years' experience. Egypt J Otolaryngol. 2016;32:161–9.
18. Molliex S, Navez M, Baylot D, et al. Regional anaesthesia for outpatient nasal surgery. Br J Anaesth. 1996;76:151–3.

19. Pani N, Rath SK. Regional and topical anaesthesia of upper airways. Indian J Anaesth. 2009;53:641–8.
20. Singh PM, Dehran M, Mohan V, et al. Analgesic efficacy and safety of medical therapy alone vs combined medical therapy and extraoral glossopharyngeal nerve block in glossopharyngeal neuralgia. Pain Med. 2013;14:93–102.
21. Sitzman BT, Rich GF, Rockwell JJ, et al. Local anesthetic administration for direct laryngoscopy. Are glossopharyngeal blocks superior? Anesthesiology. 1997;86:34–40.
22. Ramírez MO, Segovia BL, Cuevas MAG, et al. Glossopharyngeal nerve block versus lidocaine spray to improve tolerance in upper gastrointestinal endoscopy. Gastroenterol Res Pract. 2013;2013:264509. https://doi.org/10.1155/2013/264509.
23. Henthorn RW, Amayem A, Ganta R. Which method for intraoral glossopharyngeal nerve block is better? Anesth Analg. 1995;81:1113–4.
24. Benumof JL. Management of the difficult adult airway. Anesthesiology. 1991;75:1094–6.
25. Garg R, Singhal A, Agrawal K, et al. Managing endodontic patients with severe gag reflex by glossopharyngeal nerve block technique. J Endod. 2014;40:1498–500.
26. Barton S, Williams JD. Glossopharyngeal nerve block. Arch Otolaryngol. 1971;93:186–7.
27. Ahmad I. Regional and topical anesthesia for awake endotracheal intubation. In: Hadzic A, editor. Hadzic's textbook of regional anesthesia and acute pain management. 2nd ed. Beijing: McGraw-Hill Education; 2017.
28. Curran J, Hamilton C, Taylor T. Topical analgesia before tracheal intubation. Anaesthesia. 1975;30:765–8.
29. Butterworth J. Clinical pharmacology of local anesthetics. In: Hadzic A, editor. Hadzic's textbook of regional anesthesia and acute pain management. 2nd ed. Beijing: McGraw-Hill Education; 2017.
30. Anell-Olofsson M, Ahmadi S, Lönnqvist PA, et al. Plasma concentrations of alpha-1-acid glycoprotein in preterm and term newborns: influence of mode of delivery and implications for plasma protein binding of local anaesthetics. Br J Anaesth. 2018;121:427–31.
31. Carson BL. Final review of toxicological literature: local anesthetics that metabolize to 2,6-xylidine or o-toluidine. In: National Toxicology Program; 2000. https://ntp.niehs.nih.gov/ntp/htdocs/chem_background/exsumpdf/anesthetics_508.pdf. Accessed 29 Oct 2020.
32. Lee JM, Shin TJ. Use of local anesthetics for dental treatment during pregnancy; safety for parturient. J Dent Anesth Pain Med. 2017;17:81–90.
33. Kuhnert BR, Philipson EH, Pimental R, et al. Lidocaine disposition in mother, fetus, and neonate after spinal anesthesia. Anesth Analg. 1986;65:139–44.
34. Choi J, Germond L, Santos AC. Obstetric regional anesthesia. In: Hadzic A, editor. Hadzic's textbook of regional anesthesia and acute pain management. 2nd ed. Beijing: McGraw-Hill Education; 2017.
35. Weinberg GL. Treatment of local anesthetic systemic toxicity (LAST). Reg Anesth Pain Med. 2010;35:188–93.

General Anesthesia During Pregnancy and the Postpartum Period

Hande Gurbuz, Hulya Topcu, K. Tolga Saracoglu, and Volker Wenzel

14.1 Introduction

14.1.1 Anesthetic Considerations for Nonobstetric Surgery During Pregnancy

Hundreds of thousands of pregnant women undergo surgery for nonobstetric reasons each year. Surgery is performed on 0.75–2% of pregnant women with an indication at any gestational period for nonobstetric reasons [1]. Surgical indications for nonobstetric reasons during pregnancy include acute abdominal

H. Gurbuz (✉)
Faculty of Medicine, Department of Anaesthesiology and Reanimation, Bursa Yuksek Ihtisas Research and Training Hospital, Health Sciences University, Bursa, Turkey

Faculty of Medicine, Department of Anatomy, Kocaeli University, İzmit, Turkey
e-mail: handegrbz@gmail.com

H. Topcu
Faculty of Medicine, Department of Anaesthesiology and Reanimation, Erol Olçok Research and Training Hospital, Hitit University, Çorum, Turkey
e-mail: drtopcuh@gmail.com

K. T. Saracoglu
Faculty of Medicine, Department of Anaesthesiology and Reanimation, Lütfi Kırdar Kartal Research and Training Hospital, Health Sciences University, İstanbul, Turkey
e-mail: saracoglukt@gmail.com

V. Wenzel
Department of Anaesthesiology, Intensive Care Medicine, Emergency Medicine and Pain Therapy, Bodensee Campus Medicine, Klinikum Friedrichshafen, Friedrichshafen, Germany
e-mail: V.Wenzel@klinikum-fn.de

C. Cingi et al. (eds.), *ENT Diseases: Diagnosis and Treatment during Pregnancy and Lactation*, https://doi.org/10.1007/978-3-031-05303-0_14

163

diseases—appendicitis and cholecystitis—malignancies, trauma, and cardiac diseases [2–5]. Ear–nose–throat (ENT) emergencies such as epistaxis, head and neck trauma, tracheal stenosis, and cancer require surgery during pregnancy [6–12].

Surgery and anesthesia during pregnancy are critical since an intervention to the mother may also affect the baby. Anatomical, physiological, and pharmacodynamics/pharmacokinetic changes in pregnancy, limited time for preoperative anesthetic preparation due to the urgency of the intervention, and dealing with two patients at the same time are challenging even for a senior anesthesiologist. Potential risks and benefits of surgical and anesthetic interventions for a gravid patient should be taken into consideration for both mother and fetus. Thus, anesthesiologists should remodify the standard anesthetic protocols to achieve two principal goals: (1) maternal safety by having comprehensive knowledge in maternal physiology and (2) fetal safety by avoiding teratogenic agents, maintaining uteroplacental blood flow, and preventing abortion or preterm labor [13]. A multidisciplinary team of surgeons, obstetricians, anesthesiologists, and perinatologists must determine nonobstetric surgeries performed on pregnant women.

14.1.2 Timing of Surgery

The risk of abortion and preterm delivery have been predominant following nonobstetric surgeries performed during pregnancy [14]. The second trimester is considered safer for nonobstetric surgeries; however, epidemiological studies have demonstrated that the selection of the first trimester is widespread for interventions, followed by second and third trimesters [3, 4, 15]. However, when maternal hypotension and hypoxia are in control, it is suggested that the procedure performed in any period of pregnancy does not pose a higher risk to the mother and fetus than the sickness of the mother [16, 17].

Fetal mortality cannot be associated with a specific anesthetic agent or technique, but it has been suggested that the reason for surgery plays a critical role, particularly for pelvic surgeries and procedures performed for obstetric indication. In general, teratogenic effects of anesthetic agents have not been proven, but other factors such as maternal hypoxia, hypotension, vasopressor application, hypo/hypercarbia, and electrolyte disturbances remain as the major factors in teratogenicity than anesthetic agents [2]. The risk of preterm birth increases in surgeries performed in the last trimester. The timing and indications for surgery are crucial for both maternal and fetal outcomes. Thus, elective surgeries should be postponed until the postnatal period and breastfeeding. If surgery is inevitable, i.e., urgent surgeries, optimal timing is the second trimester. Only emergency surgeries should be considered during the first or the third trimester [18].

14.2   Maternal and Fetal Safety

14.2.1 Maternal Safety

14.2.1.1   Maternal Physiology and Anesthetic Implications

During pregnancy, adaptational changes affect all organ systems for the mother to tolerate pregnancy and delivery and provide maternal homeostasis as well as trigger the mother for lactation. Although hormonal fluctuations are the most responsible for changes in the first trimester, mechanical changes dominate in the second half of the pregnancy due to uterus enlargement.

Changes in the Cardiovascular System

Oxygen consumption of the cardiovascular system surges to fulfill metabolic needs of both the mother and fetus. With the mechanical pressure of the enlarged uterus in the later stages of pregnancy, the heart is shifted toward left and anteriorly. The heart expands as a consequence of blood volume increase. In echocardiographic studies, left ventricle hypertrophy occurs at the fourth gestational weeks, and the left ventricle may expand up to 50% at term [19, 20]. Dilatation occurs in the mitral, tricuspid, and pulmonary valves, but these changes are not observed in the aortic valve [21].

As of the week four of pregnancy, heart rate, stroke volume, and cardiac output increases by 20–30%, 20–50%, and 30–50%, respectively [22–24]. This elevation in cardiac output is the utmost in the first two trimesters but does not further increase in the third trimester. In the supine position, cardiac output measurements may be lower due to compression from vena cava. Escalated heart rate becomes evident in the first trimester and remains steady until the end of the pregnancy [20]. Therefore, stroke volume enlargement depends predominantly on the cardiac output increase. Ejection fraction is also heightened due to ventricular hypertrophy and dilatation [22–24], while colloid osmotic pressure decreases. In pregnant women close to term, the systemic vascular resistance and pulmonary vascular resistance reduce by 20–30%. Pulmonary artery pressure decreases slightly, but central venous pressure and pulmonary capillary wedge pressure remain unchanged [22, 23]. Postpartum measurements of these parameters return to pre-pregnancy values only in 24 weeks or longer. The perfusion of the uterus, kidneys, and extremities elevates along with an increase in the cardiac output.

Supine Hypotensive Syndrome

Gravid uterus imposes pressure on the abdominal aorta and vena cava inferior depending on the position and gestational age. The pressure on the filling of the vena cava inferior can be avoided by lifting the left lateral of the uterus by 30°. Studies have shown that vena cava inferior filling does not increase with 15° of lateral tilt position [25].

Venous return to the heart reduces drastically due to caval compression in the supine position, particularly after the 24th gestational weight. The initial response to compensate for this decrease in preload is tachycardia. If the cardiovascular system is unable to recompense in preload, bradycardia and hypotension emerge, known as the supine hypotensive syndrome. Up to 8–15% parturients experience supine hypotensive syndrome, while others are thought to maintain right atrial preload by collateral venous return [26]. The prevalent objective diagnostic criteria practiced are the reduction in the systolic blood pressure and the mean blood pressure by 15 mmHg and above, and 15–30 mmHg, respectively, concomitantly with an increase in heart rate of 20 beats/min and more.

Changes in the Respiratory System

Mucosal fragility increases due to vascular enlargement and extracellular fluid infiltration into the nasal, laryngeal, and oropharyngeal mucosa, thereby causing nasal congestion, rhinitis, or epistaxis. Airway edema can be more severe, particularly in preeclamptic pregnant women under tocolytic therapy. Besides, the difficult airway should be expected with the expansion of fat pads in the head and neck [27], thus increasing the risk of bleeding during airway manipulation. Breasts enlarge in preparation for breastfeeding but may cause difficulty in airway manipulation during intubation. Therefore, short-handled blades should be in consideration. An anesthesiologist should always be ready for potentially difficult airway in pregnant women.

In the later stages of pregnancy, due to the compression of the enlarged uterus, the vertical diameter of the chest cavity decreases by 4 cm, while the sagittal and transverse diameters expand only by 2 cm [28]. Tidal volume and alveolar ventilation also increase, accompanied by a slight rise in the breathing frequency. The net result of these changes sums up in an increase in the minute ventilation of up to 50%. Expiratory reserve volume, residual volume, and functional residual capacity diminish due to the enlarged uterus compressing the lung. However, vital capacity and total lung capacity remain consistent as a result of increased inspiratory reserve volume [29].

The closing capacity does not change in pregnant women, but a decrease in the functional residual capacity to closing capacity ratio causes smaller airways to clog faster [29]. Healthy pregnant women can tolerate this condition effortlessly, albeit it may cause hypoxemia in pregnant women with a secondary condition affecting closing capacities such as smoking, obesity, lung disease, and scoliosis.

Increased ventilation causes mild respiratory alkalosis. Arterial blood gas measurements demonstrate a decrease of $PaCO_2$ up to 30 mmHg, while PaO_2 increases to 105 mmHg [30, 31]. The acidity (pH) is stabilized by using bicarbonate buffer systems. Therefore, the $PaCO_2$ levels that are considered typical in a nonpregnant person may indicate hypercapnia for pregnant women. Adequate oxygenation for the fetus can be achieved by adjusting $PaO_2 \geq 65$ mmHg and $SpO_2 \geq 95\%$ in maternal blood. While physiological respiratory alkalosis during pregnancy shifts the oxyhemoglobin dissociation curve to the left, the maternal 2,3-diphosphoglycerate level also increases and facilitates oxygen passage to the fetus by skewing toward the left. Therefore, hyperventilation should be avoided during general anesthesia [2].

As a result of all these alterations in the lung capacity and respiratory dynamics, oxygen reserves of pregnant women diminish as well. Alveolar ventilation expansion and functional residual capacity decrease, thus accelerating intake and elimination of inhalation anesthetics. Hence, the minimal alveolar concentration (MAC) value decreases for all inhalation anesthetics in pregnant women [32]. Hypoxia develops swiftly during periods of apnea and hypoventilation, resulting in a decrease in the functional residual capacity and increased metabolic rate. By considering all these changes during pregnancy, inhalation anesthetics should be kept at lower MAC values [33]. Pre-oxygenation with 100% oxygen for 5 min is essential before general anesthesia induction.

Studies have shown that the maternal death rate due to anesthesia complications is higher with general anesthesia than with regional anesthesia for cesarean section [34]. The majority of anesthesia-related deaths occur due to airway-related problems such as aspiration, intubation difficulties, and insufficient ventilation during general anesthesia [34]. Therefore, these alarming deaths can be minimized by identifying changes in the maternal respiratory system, predicting potential complications, and taking essential precautions.

Changes in the Gastrointestinal System

Progesterone increase in pregnant women was previously associated with decreased gastrointestinal motility [35–37], but of late, it has been shown that gastric emptying time does not shorten at any period of pregnancy [38]. By contrast, gastric secretions are acidified during pregnancy, and intragastric pressure increases with the shift in the typical position of the stomach caused by the mechanical stress by the uterus. Lower esophageal sphincter tone is remarkably reduced, particularly in pregnant women with retrosternal burning. As a consequence, all pregnant women are prone to passive regurgitation, active vomiting, and pulmonary aspiration under general anesthesia. Therefore, endotracheal intubation should be performed in pregnant women undergoing general anesthesia, presuming the subject with a full stomach, and precautions should be taken into account for potential complications. Preferably, intubation should be performed with a video-assisted laryngoscope.

Other Changes

Perfusion in the skin, muscle tissue, uterus, kidney, and brain increase by cause of cardiac output and the reduction in the systemic vascular resistance during pregnancy. The half-life of neuromuscular blockers shortens in pregnant women due to increased muscle tissue perfusion. Skin temperature increase, palmar erythema, spider angioma, varicose dilatation, and hemorrhoids can also be observed as a result of vascular dilatation, angioproliferation, and congestion emerging with a direct effect of estrogen. Vasomotor instability identified by facial flushing, pallor, and Raynaud's phenomenon may be observed due to vasodilatation or vasospasm secondary to increased estrogen levels during pregnancy. Widespread nonpitting edema can be observed in the entire body, particularly in the extremities, due to the reduction in plasma oncotic pressure and capillary permeability and increased cardiac output and vena cava pressure in the later periods of pregnancy [39].

Mineralocorticoid levels increase in the plasma and total blood volume due to sodium and water retention. Physiological anemia transpires in conjunction with an increase in red blood cell volume [2]. Susceptibility to hypercoagulability and thromboembolism occurs due to increases in almost all procoagulant coagulation factors (I, VII, VIII, IX, X and XII) and fibrinogen levels [40].

Serum cholinesterase activity decreases by 20% in the term period [41], but a slight decrease in succinylcholine or ester local anesthetic (such as 2-chloroprocaine) metabolisms remains negligible. Pregnancy increases free-serum concentrations of drugs that bind to plasma proteins while hindering the albumin to globulin ratio [42]. As neural sensitivity to local anesthetics increases based upon progesterone, local anesthetic dose and concentration should be lowered in regional blocks [43, 44].

14.2.2 Fetal Safety

14.2.2.1 Fetal Effects of Anesthesia

Although in vitro and in vivo studies on fetal brain development have reported histological changes and neurodevelopmental adverse effects in the brain after exposure to most anesthetics during rapid brain development periods, there is no evidence that any specific anesthetic agent is hazardous in humans with limited exposures less than 3 h [18, 45, 46]. In 2016, the US Food and Drug Administration (FDA) issued a drug safety warning regarding the potential adverse effects of anesthetic and sedative drugs on neuronal development, especially in the third trimester of pregnancy and children under 3 years old [47]. Although human clinical studies involving young children have reported conflicting results, extensive studies indicate that a single and short anesthetic exposure does not show detrimental effects on neuronal development [48–50]. Both the FDA and the American College of Obstetrics and Gynecologists recommend not postponing inevitable surgeries during pregnancy. It is also worth noting that the cumulative dose plays a crucial role in developing congenital malformations for teratogenicity.

14.2.2.2 Fetal Effects of Maternal Factors

Healthy development of the fetus depends on sufficient oxygen intake from the placenta. Therefore, the well-being of the fetus is a function of the uteroplacental blood flow. It is obligatory to avoid hemodynamic and metabolic instabilities that cause vasoconstriction to maintain uteroplacental blood flow. In preventing hypotension, except for extreme conditions such as maternal renal failure and heart failure, a liberal fluid regimen is recommended in the perioperative period [13]. Ephedrine and phenylephrine, two vasopressor agents, can be safely used in pregnant women. The 20:1 mixture of caffeine/theodrenaline is another potent vasoactive drug that increases blood pressure by increasing cardiac output and stroke volume, without increasing the heart rate and maintaining the peripheral resistance unchanged [51]. It has a longer duration of action than ephedrine and phenylephrine, requiring less bolus administrations. There was also no significant difference in neonatal acidosis and APGAR scores in comparison with ephedrine and phenylephrine [52].

Similar to hypotension, hypertension causes uterine artery spasms and disrupts the fetoplacental circulation. The first options in the intravenous treatment of hypertension are labetalol and hydralazine. If signs of pulmonary edema develop, nitroglycerin may be administered [53]. Maternal hypoxia and hypo/hypercapnia may also cause vasoconstriction in the uterine artery and disrupt fetal circulation [54].

14.2.2.3 Placental Transfer of Drugs

Drugs penetrate the placenta by passive diffusion. Therefore, the placental transfer is proportional to the concentration gradient on both sides of the placenta (maternal–fetal). As only free-drug fractions can pass through the placenta, the placental transfer of highly bound drugs to maternal plasma proteins is also inadequate. Most anesthetic drugs such as local anesthetics and sedatives are weak bases and have a relatively low ionization degree [44]. Neuromuscular blockers with a high degree of ionization cannot be transferred from the placenta in substantial concentrations. Nonionized drugs are more lipophilic than ionized drugs, where lipophilic drugs can penetrate tissue barriers and are more prone to traverse the placenta. Acidosis causes an increase in the ionized form of the drug. In the case of fetal acidosis, ionized drugs cannot diffuse back across the placenta, causing accumulation of the drug in the fetal plasma, known as **ion trapping** [55].

14.2.2.4 Teratogenicity

A teratogen is an agent that can disturb the intrauterine development of the embryo or fetus, producing congenital malformations. It is of consensus that teratogenesis occurs after fertilization caused by several mechanisms. Theoretically, any drug can be teratogenic if administered at a sufficiently high dose for long periods, and precisely, at the right time of the development [56, 57]. The first 2 weeks of pregnancy are an **all-or-nothing** period, meaning that exposure to teratogenic agents before organogenesis causes either the loss or intact preservation of the fetus. Moreover, exposure during the organogenesis may lead to structural abnormalities, and hence, functional problems can occur in the post-embryonic organogenesis period [58].

Although many drugs used in anesthesia have been associated with teratogenic effects in vivo, such findings are intricate to extrapolate to humans due to cross-species variation and the high dose of agents used in animal studies [45, 46]. When evaluating the likelihood of teratogenicity in maternal drug applications, the following points should be considered: (1) human teratogenicity studies cannot be performed due to ethical issues, (2) studies on experimental animals are not sufficient, and (3) use of findings to predict outcome in humans is misappropriate. Moreover, since polypharmacy is often involved during anesthesia, it is unattainable to ascribe any fetal adverse effects to only a single drug.

In many comprehensive retrospective studies, the relationship between anesthetic drugs and congenital malformations in humans has remained unknown [18]. Instead, many studies have highlighted that surgery or anesthesia is associated with preterm labor or intrauterine death, especially when administered in the first trimester [56, 59–61]. It is thought that anesthesia complications are responsible for these adverse effects rather than the direct effects of the anesthetic drugs on the fetus [62, 63]. For instance, hypoxemia and hypotension can be teratogenic factors alone, causing physiological impairment.

In anesthesia during pregnancy, the management of risk factors in the mother as a result of physiological adaptation is crucial for the maintenance of the fetoplacental unit. Factors to consider for the fetal well-being are the needs of the growing fetus, the optimization of fetal oxygenation and uteroplacental perfusion, and both the direct and indirect impacts of the drugs. Accordingly, the anesthetic approach in nonobstetric surgery during pregnancy should be as follows:

1. Surgery should not be performed before the 16th gestational week, if possible, or at least, postponed to the second trimester.
2. The patient should be consulted with an obstetrician preoperatively.
3. Preoperative antacid administration should be considered for aspiration prophylaxis.
4. Perioperative normoxia, normocapnia, normotension, and normoglycemia should be provided.
5. Regional anesthesia should be preferred whenever possible, but nitrous oxide should be avoided if general anesthesia is preferred.
6. The fetal heart rate should be monitored before and after surgery [2].

Additionally, the use of tocolytic drugs should be discussed, and the uterus should be deviated to the left in the perioperative period, following the 16th gestational week [13, 64].

14.2.2.5 Risk Categorization of Drugs

The FDA has created a five-letter safety category for drug use in pregnancy with a system in 1979 that reviews the safety of commonly used drugs and grades the teratogenic effects of drugs (A, B, C, D, X). However, FDA implemented the Pregnancy and Lactation Labelling Final Rule, suggesting replacing the pregnancy letter categories with narrative subsections including pregnancy (labor and delivery), lactation (nursing mothers), and females and males with reproductive potential in 2015 [65, 66].

14.2.2.6 Fetal Heart Rate Monitoring

Fetal monitoring aims to detect the fetal heart rate changes that may result from maternal factors. It is recommended to document fetal heart rate before and after surgery regardless of gestational age [67, 68]. However, intraoperative fetal heart rate monitoring is challenging to interpret as there is an anticipated reduction in beat-to-beat variability under general anesthesia, and not all nonobstetric operations can be paused to allow emergency cesarean delivery. Thus, the absolute benefit to the fetus is unknown. The decision to use intermittent or continuous intraoperative fetal monitoring should be personalized based on gestational age, type of surgery, and available resources [18]. If continual fetal heart rate monitoring is selected, an obstetrician experienced in cesarean delivery should be present to monitor and interpret the fetal heart rate throughout the surgery.

Intraoperative fetal heart rate can be monitored by an electronic fetal heart rate monitor or Doppler ultrasound. Transabdominal monitoring may be technically challenging or impractical during abdominal surgeries. In such circumstances, the use of transvaginal Doppler ultrasonography may be considered. Drugs used for general and regional anesthesia can lead to changes in the fetal heart rate. All mainstream anesthetic drugs penetrate the placenta and may result in minimal fetal heart rate variability, simultaneously with a decrease in the fetal heart rate baseline of 10–25 bpm [2]. If instantaneous unexplained fluctuations occur in fetal heart rate, it is mandatory to evaluate the maternal condition to unravel the factors causing interruption of the uteroplacental blood flow. The objective of the optimization of the maternal condition is to improve the impaired uteroplacental blood flow. Parameters to consider for optimization are to increase left uterine displacement, to correct oxygenation and acid-base status, to treat hypotension, to ensure appropriate end-tidal CO_2 and hemoglobin levels, to check the surgical site to rule out any external compression impairing the uteroplacental perfusion, and to consider the administration of drugs to improve uterine relaxation (i.e., volatile agents, nitroglycerin) [2].

14.2.2.7 Avoidance and Treatment of Preterm Delivery

The incidence of spontaneous abortion, premature birth, and preterm delivery after nonobstetric surgery during pregnancy has increased due to surgery itself, manipulation of the uterus during surgery, and maternal systemic disease (i.e., infection) [69]. The risk of miscarriage during pregnancy is higher in the first and third trimesters. Routine prophylactic tocolytic application is controversial. However, in acute preterm labor, intravenous hydration, calcium channel blocking agents, cyclooxygenase inhibitors (NSAID), beta-mimetics, and magnesium sulfate can be given in agreement with an obstetrician's decision [54]. Antenatal corticosteroid administration should be considered for fetal lung maturation.

14.3 Anesthetic Drugs

14.3.1 Frequently Used Drugs for Anesthesia and Analgesia

14.3.1.1 Benzodiazepines

Benzodiazepines are often used during pregnancy to manage severe anxiety or agitation, or drugs with the shortest half-lives such as lorazepam and midazolam are of consideration. Some studies suggest that long-term use of benzodiazepines in early pregnancy is associated with cleft palate and congenital inguinal hernia [70, 71]. A single exposure to benzodiazepines in pregnant women for perioperative or operative purposes does not cause congenital malformations. It is further stated that benzodiazepines can be beneficial for the fetus by controlling the catecholamine level arising from preoperative surgical stress [72]. In postpartum use, benzodiazepines are transmitted to milk because of their lipophilic nature. Therefore, the utmost caution should be exercised in chronic use during the lactation period, and the administration doses should be adjusted accordingly.

14.3.1.2 Opioids

Opioids are commonly used in anesthesia to reduce the response to laryngoscopy and for analgesia. Opioids—highly lipophilic and low-molecular-weight drugs—easily egress the placenta. While the known maternal side effects of systemic opioids are sedation, respiratory depression, postural hypotension, constipation, delayed gastric emptying, bradycardia, and cardiac arrest, opioids in the placenta infiltrating into the fetus may cause respiratory depression and changes in the fetal heart rate [18]. Opioid elimination in newborns and fetuses is more prolonged than in adults. Although opioids used in general anesthesia are more likely to cause respiratory depression in the newborn, a meta-analysis of the use of opioids (alfentanil, remifentanil, and fentanyl) for the induction of cesarean delivery did not show a significant difference in the first- and fifth-minute APGAR scores post-opioid administration [73]. Opioids used in regional anesthesia have less maternal and fetal-neonatal side effects than their systemic use [74]. The long-term use of opioids during pregnancy for either medical reasons or drug addiction can cause neonatal opioid withdrawal syndrome that could be life-threatening [75, 76]. Several studies have shown that opioids may be associated with congenital disabilities, including neural tube defects, congenital heart defects, gastroschisis, or weak fetal growth, stillbirth, and premature birth due to chronic maternal use [77].

Morphine is a potent opioid with high μ-opioid receptor affinity with a longer half-life. UGT2B7 metabolizes morphine to morphine-3-glucuronide (70%) and morphine-6-glucuronide (M6G; 30%) in the liver [78]. M6G is an active metabolite and 13 times more potent than morphine. By rapidly egressing the placenta, drug levels in fetal blood in the fifth minute escalate to a value closer to the maternal serum levels [79]. Since the liver is immature in newborns, the half-life of M6G is longer in infants than in adults. Morphine causes respiratory depression predominantly in newborns due to the high brain permeability. Due to the altered pharmacodynamics and pharmacokinetics during pregnancy, the plasma clearance of morphine increases, and the half-life is shortened compared to nonpregnant women. Theoretically, these changes are expected to reduce fetal exposure. Morphine and its metabolites egress into breast milk in trace amounts. Detrimental effects are not expected in a single application, but the newborn should be monitored closely for a latent respiratory depression in repetitive usage.

Meperidine (pethidine) is a synthetic opioid that agonistically affects through μ- and κ-opioid receptors. It has a potency of 10% of morphine with a half-life of 2.5–3 h. Meperidine is metabolized to normeperidine in the liver, causing convulsions with a prolonged activity period (14–21 h) [79]. It reaches the balance in maternal and fetal blood by passing through the placenta due to its high liposolubility. It can be used as a single dose in the perinatal period and lactation. However, it is not recommended during lactation since it causes accumulation of normeperidine in infants with repeated use [80].

Fentanyl is a highly liposoluble and protein-bound synthetic opioid that binds to μ-opioid receptors. It is metabolized in the liver to inactive metabolites via CYP3A. It has a fast release and short duration of action, thus causing less neonatal respiratory depression than meperidine. Its single use is considered safe during breastfeeding, but there is insufficient data on its continual use [79, 81].

Alfentanil and sufentanil are potent synthetic mu-opioid receptor agonist analgesic drugs. Alfentanil is an analog of fentanyl that is only 10% potent but has a shorter duration of action and quicker onset. Available data on pregnant women are insufficient to relate the drug with birth defects and miscarriage. Sufentanil is ten times as potent as fentanyl. It has a half-life shorter than fentanyl but longer than alfentanil.

Remifentanil is a selective μ-opioid receptor agonist with a rapid onset of action and a very short half-life, as low as 3–10 min. The placental transfer is very low due to its rapid hydrolysis by nonspecific tissue and plasma cholinesterases. It is considered to be appropriate for use in anesthesia for surgical interventions during pregnancy and the peripartum period. However, one should not underestimate that it may impair uteroplacental circulation due to hypotension. Mothers administered with remifentanil should be closely monitored for respiratory depression [82].

Tramadol is a weak μ-opioid receptor agonist metabolized in the liver by demethylation and glucuronidation through CYP2D6 (codeine is also metabolized by CYP2D6) to its active metabolite *O*-desmethyl tramadol. Tramadol hinders the central neuronal reuptake of serotonin and norepinephrine. Analgesic potency of tramadol is comparable to meperidine, and 10–20% of morphine, causing less respiratory depression than morphine in analgesic doses equal to morphine [79]. Both tramadol and its metabolite *O*-desmethyl tramadol are excreted into breastmilk [83]. Similar to codeine, there are clinically critical consequences of tramadol metabolism via the cytochrome P450 isoenzyme CYP2D6. CYP2D6 has a considerable genetic polymorphism whose function is deficient in poor metabolizers, while relatively higher in ultra-rapid metabolizers [84]. The clinical reflection of this diversity is that the efficacy and side effects of the drug are low in poor metabolizers but are higher in ultra-rapid metabolizers. In ultra-rapid metabolizers, the drug passes into breast milk in substantial amounts. Prediction of both maternal and neonatal effects of tramadol and codeine is impractical since the type of CYP2D6 genotype is unknown in patients. Case reports of severe neonatal respiratory depression and even deaths due to tramadol use have been reported in the literature [81, 84]. Thus, the use of tramadol is not recommended during breastfeeding [85]. In some countries, the use of tramadol in children under 12 is prohibited.

14.3.1.3 Hypnotics

Propofol enables rapid and smooth induction of anesthesia with a short duration of action and fast recovery time. It effectively controls the cardiovascular response to laryngoscopy. Propofol also has an anti-emetic activity but not an analgesic effect. It is popular in a wide range of uses in general anesthesia and sedation. However, propofol may interfere with uteroplacental blood flow that ultimately causes cardiovascular depression and hypotension in a dose-dependent manner. Also, propofol is a nonionized and highly liposoluble anesthetic agent that can penetrate through the placenta [72]. It can be detected in breast milk in trace amounts since it is rapidly cleansed from the plasma.

Thiopentone is a barbiturate with neuroprotective and anticonvulsant effects and is favored in rapid serial induction for its rapid-onset characteristic. It has a longer context-sensitive half-life in comparison with propofol. Barbiturates have no analgesic effect but are associated with postoperative barbiturate-hyperalgesia. Thiopentone decreases cardiac output and causes hemodynamic instability and respiratory depression in a dose-dependent fashion; altogether, it may adversely affect uteroplacental blood flow.

It has high lipid solubility with affinity to plasma proteins and rapidly passes from the placenta to the fetus. It reaches the maximum dose approximately within a minute in the umbilical cord vein. It passes through the placenta immediately after anesthesia induction, but its effect is observed in the fetus within 45 s. After 2–3 min, thiopental concentrations in the maternal and fetal blood balance, and the drug concentration moderately decreases in both. The drug infiltrates into the fetal brain tissue, but the dose of thiopental lesser than 4 mg/kg in induction does not cause fetal depression, thus considered safe in obstetric patients [72].

Ketamine is an NMDA blocker used for anesthesia induction and sedation. Unlike propofol and thiopentone, ketamine has analgesic properties. It may be selected in asthmatic patients due to its bronchodilator effect but is not suitable for use in hypertensive patients due to its sympathomimetic activity. Relative hemodynamic stability makes ketamine a preferred agent for many emergency cases [86]. Ketamine is more liposoluble and less protein-bound than thiopental, so it rapidly passes through the placenta and saturates in the fetus 1–2 min after maternal administration. It increases uterine tone at doses above 1 mg/kg; hence, the dosage should be kept below 1 mg/kg when it is administered in pregnant women [72]. Ketamine is associated with awareness during anesthesia. Also, it can cause the emergence of delirium and hallucinations. These adverse effects can be prevented by administering benzodiazepines or barbiturates simultaneously.

Etomidate, a GABA-A agonist, is usually preferred for its safe hemodynamic profile. However, it can lead to nausea and vomiting, hiccups, myoclonus, and pain at the injection site. Moreover, it causes adrenal suppression in long-term use and lowers the seizure threshold. It can also cause adrenal suppression in the neonate and decrease the cortisol levels after maternal anesthesia induction. Therefore, etomidate use in obstetric patients is not recommended [87].

14.3.1.4　Volatile Anesthetics

MAC values of the inhalation agents used in anesthesia decrease due to the physiological changes during pregnancy. Therefore, providing adequate anesthesia with low-dose inhalation anesthesia reduces the depressive effects in infants.

Sevoflurane, desflurane, and isoflurane are commonly used in volatile anesthetics nowadays. No teratogenicity effect has been reported with the use of volatile anesthetics during pregnancy [57]. A critical disadvantage of volatile anesthetics is that they increase postpartum blood loss by decreasing uterine muscle tone in a dose-dependent manner. These effects can be reduced by using low concentrations with administrating oxytocin concomitantly.

Nitrous oxide is a low-molecular-weight and nonlipophilic molecule. It diffuses through the placenta depending on the exposure time but does not affect uterine contractions and fetal heart rate. Nitrous oxide causes the oxidation of vitamin B12 and prevents the activation of methionine synthase. Methionine synthase is an essential enzyme for DNA synthesis. Therefore, it should be avoided in the first trimester of pregnancy. Its use is not recommended because there are opioid alternatives to substitute its usage as an analgesic in early pregnancy. No adverse event has been reported due to its use in the later periods of pregnancy. Nitrous oxide is also widely used as an inhalational agent in labor analgesia [88].

14.3.1.5 Neuromuscular Blockers

Muscle relaxants are used to facilitate endotracheal intubation and to increase surgical comfort. Neuromuscular blocking agents have a polar molecular structure and cannot pass through the placenta; thus, no fetal adverse effects have been reported. Their metabolism may be affected depending on the physiological changes during pregnancy. No adverse effects in the infant have been reported as the transition of the drug into milk during the postpartum period is negligible.

Succinylcholine is a hydro-soluble depolarizing muscle relaxant. For this reason, the amount of the drug passed into the fetus is negligible and does not cause neonatal respiratory depression. Suitable conditions for intubation occur within 45 s after intravenous administration, and the drug is eliminated from the body by plasma cholinesterases. Plasma cholinesterase levels decrease by about 25% from the beginning of pregnancy until the postpartum 7 days [89].

Rocuronium has substituted succinylcholine due to its rapid onset of action. After introducing sugammadex, the relaxant binding agent selective for rocuronium and vecuronium, rocuronium becomes a non-depolarizing muscle relaxant in difficult airway management of choice. A regular dose of rocuronium is 0.6 mg/kg, and while it provides the suitable conditions for intubation in about 98 s, intubation can be achieved within 60 s by increasing the induction dose up to 1–1.2 mg/kg. The placental transfer of rocuronium is negligible. Having the least placental transfer among the neuromuscular blocking agents, rocuronium has become widespread for obstetric anesthesia [90].

Vecuronium is another non-depolarizing muscle relaxant that is not preferred in pregnant women due to its long onset time and prolonged duration of action [90].

Atracurium and cis-atracurium are neuromuscular blocking agents that undergo organ-independent elimination (Hoffman degradation). They may cause histamine discharge and hypotension in high doses for rapid onset. These muscle relaxants are not recommended in pregnant women as hypotension may cause fetal adverse effects with decreased uteroplacental blood flow. However, organ-independent elimination is a suitable option for repeated doses of muscle relaxants in pregnant women with liver or renal dysfunction [90].

14.3.1.6 Neuromuscular Block Reversal Agents

Neostigmine is a cholinesterase inhibitor used for the reversal of non-depolarizing muscle relaxants. Neostigmine is administered simultaneously with sympathomimetics such as atropine or glycopyrrolate to oppose its parasympathomimetic effects. It passes through the placenta in trace amounts. When combined with glycopyrrolate, fetal bradycardia may occur since the dosage of glycopyrrolate passing out the placenta is lower than neostigmine. Thus, neostigmine is recommended for use in conjunction with atropine [91].

Sugammadex is a gamma-cyclodextrin that inactivates steroid neuromuscular blocking agents by encapsulation. The dose of sugammadex depends on the level of neuromuscular blockade with the highest affinity for rocuronium, followed by vecuronium, pancuronium, and pipecuronium, respectively [92].

Sugammadex has several clinical advantages over neostigmine. However, sugammadex also diminishes free progesterone levels by binding progesterone with encapsulation. This effect may be significant, as progesterone is required for endometrial decidualization and uterine growth in the early pregnancy and is crucial for the maintenance of pregnancy. It is known that administration of anti-progesterone drugs such as onapristone or mifepristone results in miscarriage or preterm labor [93]. Therefore, the use of sugammadex in pregnant women, except for the cesarean section in the third trimester, has raised serious concerns due to progesterone interaction. Although in vivo studies have shown that sugammadex administration during the first trimester of pregnancy does not result in any fetal risk, there are no case reports or studies in humans [94]. Besides, sugammadex interacts with progesterone containing oral contraceptives, reducing the efficacy of the drug. Hence, a nonhormonal contraception method should be reconsidered for the following 7 days after sugammadex administration [95].

14.3.1.7 Anticholinergic Drugs

Atropine is an anticholinergic agent commonly used perioperatively for its anti-sialagogue and anti-asthmatic properties, constituting the first-line treatment in suppressing parasympathetic activation and treatment of life-threatening bradycardic rhythms and poisonings (i.e., organophosphate pesticides). Atropine passes the placenta, causing fetal tachycardia [91]. Although the use of atropine during pregnancy has not been shown to cause any teratogenicity, its safety has been uncorroborated. Therefore, it should only be used in cases when there is no other alternative. Atropine is excreted into milk and may cause anticholinergic effects in infants. Also, having been shown to inhibit lactation, its usage should be avoided for breastfeeding women unless indispensable [96].

Glycopyrrolate is a synthetic anticholinergic drug used perioperatively for the same indications with atropine. Because glycopyrrolate cannot cross the blood–brain barrier, it is less likely to cause altered mental status than atropine. Glycopyrrolate does not cross the placenta, and it does not excrete into breast-milk [97].

14.3.1.8 Nonopioid Analgesics

Nonopioid analgesics are used to avoid the unforeseen adverse effects of opioid analgesics.

Paracetamol is an analgesic used widespread during pregnancy. It can be used safely in the treatment of mild to moderate pain at any stage of pregnancy. However, in some studies, it has been argued that the maternal use of paracetamol in recurrent doses may be associated with neonatal asthma and neurobehavioral problems [98–100]. Paracetamol is considered to be safe to use during the lactation period. Although it passes into breastmilk at varying amounts, the dose of paracetamol uptaken by the baby with milk is lower than the therapeutic range [81].

Nonsteroidal anti-inflammatory drugs are associated with premature closure of fetal ductus arteriosus and oligohydramnios; thus, their use during pregnancy is generally contraindicated unless inevitable. For example, in some specific cases such as preeclampsia, antenatal low-dose aspirin use is recommended [101]. It has also been stated that ibuprofen, diclofenac, naproxen, celecoxib, ketorolac, and low-dose aspirin (not in analgesic doses) are compatible with breastfeeding during the lactation period [81].

14.4 Anesthesia Management

14.4.1 General Anesthesia

Although both regional and general anesthesia can be safely applied for operations performed for nonobstetric reasons during pregnancy, it is recommended to prefer regional techniques whenever possible [58, 72]. The type of anesthesia should be chosen according to the maternal and fetal conditions, indications, location, and the duration of surgery.

14.4.1.1 Preanesthetic Evaluation

The pregnancy status of the patients at childbearing age is not routinely checked before surgery. The ASA Practice Advisory for Preanesthesia Evaluation recommended that pregnancy testing may be offered to the patients, especially before the procedures that are expected to expose the fetus to potential teratogens [102–104].

Standard preoperative assessment should be held with meticulous attention to the airway. The mother should be informed about potential teratogenicity and difficult airway. The patient should be consulted preoperatively with an obstetrician and perinatologist. Also, a pediatrician should be involved in the team if preterm delivery is anticipated.

Verbal reassurance is preferred over pharmacologic premedication. Gastric emptying in pregnant women is comparable to nonpregnant patients [105]. However, antacid prophylaxis is required after 14 weeks of gestation [106]. A combination of nonparticulate antacids and H2-receptor blockers is sufficient to increase the gastric pH. Ultrasound assessment of gastric content can be used to individualize the risk of tracheal aspiration [107]. Besides, the prophylaxis of venous thromboembolism should be considered.

14.4.1.2 Rapid Sequence Induction and Intubation

Rapid sequence induction and intubation (RSII) for anesthesia is a technique designed to minimize the possibility of pulmonary aspiration in patients at risk by placing an endotracheal tube as quickly as possible after induction. The RSII is generally used in emergency services and procedures. Indications for RSII include patients with a full stomach, gastrointestinal physiological changes, increased abdominal pressure, and pregnancy after 20 weeks of gestation with increased aspiration risk with anesthesia induction.

Before RSII, a thorough airway evaluation is required. Not in all but the most urgent cases, a rapid airway assessment and questioning of previous airway problems should be conducted. If difficult airway management is anticipated, a modified RSII with awake intubation may alternatively be chosen.

The preparation of equipment for RSII should be similar to routine induction. Standard and alternative airway devices should be readily available, including small, medium, and large face masks, various sizes and types of laryngoscopes, oral and nasal airways, several sizes of supraglottic airways, and a bougie, which should be of reach. Alternative laryngoscopy devices, including video laryngoscopes and flexible bronchoscopes, and other emergency airway and aspiration apparatus should be available and quickly accessible.

Anxiolytics may be administered if the patient is hemodynamically stable. Generally, prokinetics and antacids can be administered before the procedure. Due to physiological changes in pregnant women, all patients should be pre-oxygenated with 10 L/min 100% oxygen before general anesthesia to increase oxygen reserve and provide additional time to secure the airway. Pre-oxygenation is particularly crucial before RSII, as the mask ventilation with this technique is usually not carried out between induction and intubation periods [108]. Immediately post-induction, cricoid pressure is recommended until the patient is intubated [109, 110]. However, the use of cricoid pressure is controversial as it may lead the airway more difficult when misapplied, and its efficacy in preventing pulmonary aspiration may be insufficient [111]. The patient is given an appropriate hypnotic agent, often thiopental and most often propofol, and a neuromuscular blocker, especially in pregnant women. The first choice is to inject succinylcholine (or high-dose rocuronium) intravenously and to make it suitable for intubation within approximately 45–60 s. The endotracheal cuff is inflated immediately following intubation.

Possible complications of RSII include the inability to intubate, hypoxemia, hypotension, and pulmonary aspiration, all of which have adverse effects on pregnant women and fetuses. Therefore, it may be worthwhile to determine the cricothyroid membrane position by palpating the cricothyroid membrane during pre-oxygenation since front-of-neck access is required in a possible failed intubation. Also, the use of ultrasound may help monitor the cricothyroid membrane [112, 113].

Airway complications and pulmonary aspiration can occur while emerging from anesthesia. In most cases, an orogastric or nasogastric tube should be put in during anesthesia to drain the gastric content by aspirating.

Patients should be kept intubated with the endotracheal tube cuff inflated until the airway reflexes are fully restored. It would be helpful to extubate obstetric patients in the left lateral or head-up position [110]. Patients should be transferred to the post-anesthesia care unit in a head-up position to reduce the possibility of regurgitation [114].

14.4.1.3 Difficult Airway Management

Difficult airway should always be expected due to physiological changes in pregnant women. If general anesthesia is required in patients with difficult airway anticipation, the procedure should be started with all the equipment and an experienced team for difficult airway management.

An experienced anesthesiologist should perform intubation due to the risk of pulmonary aspiration, difficult airway, and inadequate ventilation depending on physiological changes of pregnant women. Before the induction, the pregnant patient should be pre-oxygenated with 10 L/min 100% oxygen [109]. Short handled blades can be preferred to ease the manipulation of laryngoscopes because of the enlarged breasts. Multiple intubation attempts pose a risk for complications; therefore, successful intubation at the first attempt should be the priority [115]. No more than two attempts should be made with direct laryngoscopy because of airway difficulty increases due to the risk of bleeding and edema after each attempt [110]. Although video laryngoscopy provides excellent advantages, it should be discontinued after two unsuccessful attempts, but instead, supraglottic airway devices such as laryngeal masks should be considered [109, 116]. In the case of two failed attempts in the placement of supraglottic airway devices, the necessary procedures for invasive airway access (front-of neck access or surgical cricothyrotomy) should be applied immediately [109, 110].

Cannot Intubate–Cannot Ventilate

If the patient cannot be ventilated with a face mask or supraglottic airway devices, front-of neck access or surgical cricothyrotomy should be performed immediately. If the maternal condition deteriorates and cardiac arrest develops, maternal advanced life support should be started immediately, and perimortem cesarean delivery should be considered in pregnant women over 20 gestational weeks [110].

14.5 Anesthesia and Postoperative Analgesia in Lactation

During lactation, the breastfeeding mother may need anesthesia or analgesic medication. However, there are some concerns about using anesthetic or analgesic drugs during lactation due to potential harm to the infants by drug-tainted milk. The effect of drugs on the infant may vary depending on various factors such as the type of drugs, the amount of maternal exposure, the breastfeeding period, and the amount of milk. However, studies on this subject are limited.

Drugs contaminate breast milk through intracellular junctions between lactocytes. Intracellular junctions of lactocytes start narrowing 24–48 h after birth and are fully sealed on postpartum 7–10 days [81]. Since the amount of colostrum in the first 24–48 h in the postpartum period is meager, the transmission of maternally administered drugs to the newborn in the early postpartum period is deficient [117]. However, when the amount of milk increases in later periods, the transition of drugs to the infant would also increase. Hence, the exposure of the newborn to maternally administered drugs culminates between the postpartum third and tenth days [81].

As a thumb rule for systemic drug applications during the lactation period, it is recommended to use anesthetic and analgesic drugs at minimal doses as the drugs may pass into breast milk in incalculable amounts [118]. Multimodal analgesia methods are strongly recommended for reducing drug doses in treating maternal pain. In postoperative analgesia, nonsteroidal anti-inflammatory drugs, opioids, and nerve blocks can be used alone or in combination. Locoregional anesthesia and analgesia techniques should be considered part of the multimodal regimen in postoperative pain control during lactation and pregnancy. In some cases, for instance, ENT surgeries, regional anesthesia would provide adequate pain control without the need for additional systemic medication. The first-line systemic analgesic should be nonopioid analgesics in treating maternal pain. In the case of opioids usage, their use should be limited to a minimal effective dose momentarily [117].

Anesthetic drugs having extremely short half-life are rapidly redistributed in the body. For short-term interventions, it is suggested that the mother can start breastfeeding immediately after surgery, but not to pump and dump the milk [81]. It is also essential to monitor the alertness of both the mother and the baby attentively. When the mother receives high doses of medication, discarding the breastmilk for 24–48 h prevents the exposure of the infant to drugs. However, given that the drugs are excreted in breast milk in relatively lower amounts from the systemic circulation, and milk goes into the stomach, not intravenous, breastfeeding can still be continued if the benefits outweigh the risks [117].

14.6 Cardiopulmonary Resuscitation in Pregnancy

Cardiac arrest during pregnancy is infrequent and limited in merely case reports/series. Nonetheless, according to the data available, maternal survival is lower than in other reported epidemiological studies [119, 120]. Cardiopulmonary resuscitation (CPR) in pregnancy is complicated because the mother and fetus are affected concomitantly. Therefore, precautions should be taken for both maternal cardiac arrest and neonatal resuscitation. Besides, when perimortem cesarean delivery is required, the management of these patients requires multidisciplinary team collaboration. While applying basic and advanced cardiac life support algorithms in pregnant women, these protocols should be remodified depending on physiological and anatomical changes during the pregnancy. The resuscitation team should be aware of physiological changes in the pregnancy that may affect resuscitation techniques.

14.6.1 Differences in Basic Life Support and Advanced Cardiovascular Life Support in Pregnant Women

14.6.1.1 Basic Life Support

Pregnant women are more disadvantageous in respiration and hemodynamics than nonpregnant adults depending on the physiology of pregnancy. Also, they are more vulnerable to develop hypoxemia rapidly with apnea due to limited oxygen reserves with increased metabolism. When the uterus is at or above the umbilicus level, pregnant women tend to instigate hypotension due to aortocaval compression when lying in the supine position. In such cases, basic life support (BLS) should be applied immediately. While evaluating the responsiveness of the patient, the location of the uterus should also be spotted promptly with reference to the umbilicus level. Simultaneous Uterine displacement should also be added to the Circulation-Airway-Breathing assessment (i.e., C-A-B-U) [121–123]. All these tasks must be executed concurrently, not sequentially. The BLS requires a minimum of four responders to be present [123].

14.6.1.2 Circulation

As in all adult CPRs, high-quality chest compressions should be performed at a rate of at least 100 per minute at a depth of at least 5 cm allowing full recoil, and at a compression ventilation ratio of 30:2 with minimal interruptions. Manual uterine displacement should be performed by another rescuer to prevent aortocaval compression. For effective and high-quality chest compressions, the patient should be in the supine position, not left lateral tilt [124, 125]. Previous guidelines have suggested positioning the hands slightly above the sternum for chest compressions in CPR in pregnancy, but the evidence is not convincing. Thus, hands should be positioned in the middle of the chest and lower half of the sternum in pregnant women with chest compressions as in nonpregnant adults. Defibrillation protocol is identical to that of nonpregnant adults since the transthoracic impedance does not change [123]. Fetal monitoring is not recommended during CPR to avoid interruption of cardiac compressions. However, if delivery is still not achieved after a successful CPR, fetal heart rate can be monitored for fetal evaluation.

14.6.1.3 Airway

Airway management should always be considered problematic in pregnant women due to airway edema and obesity. Pregnant women are at risk of the rapid development of hypoxemia as a result of decreased functional residual capacity and increased oxygen consumption and increased intrapulmonary shunt. Early two-handed (not a single-handed technique) bag-mask ventilation with a 100% oxygen of 15 L/min while avoiding hyperventilation is crucial to prevent desaturation in a pregnant woman. Because of the risk of a difficult airway, intubation should be performed by an experienced laryngoscopist [126]. Alternative airway interventions such as supraglottic airway devices or cricothyrotomy should be considered after two unsuccessful laryngoscopy attempts [108, 127–130]. The cricoid pressure—Sellick maneuver—to prevent vomiting during intubation has not been effective [111, 131]. It also renders intubation attempts more difficult, thus not recommended during CPR [132]. If the fundus of the uterus is at or above the umbilicus level, a lower tidal volume should be applied compared to levels in nonpregnant women.

14.6.1.4 Perimortem Cesarean Delivery

If there is no response to CPR within 4 min, emergency perimortem cesarean delivery should be planned in pregnant women with a uterus extending to or above the umbilicus level regardless of the gestational age and fetal viability [133]. An emergency hysterotomy is not essential in all pregnant women but life-saving for the mother whose cardiac arrest is thought to be due to aortocaval compression [134, 135].

14.6.1.5 Drugs Used During Advanced Cardiovascular Life Support

All of the drugs used during CPR in nonpregnant adults are also recommended in the same dose for CPR in pregnant women. The lower extremity should not be preferred for intravenous access because the blood return to the heart is impaired due to caval pressure. In cases where intravenous access is not possible, the intraosseous route should be considered.

If hypovolemia or bleeding is considered a possible cause of cardiac arrest during pregnancy, fluid resuscitation and blood product replacement should be performed immediately.

If the patient is being infused with magnesium in the prearrest period and magnesium intoxication is considered a cause of cardiac arrest, magnesium infusion should be discontinued, and then calcium chloride (10 mL) or calcium gluconate (30 mL) should be given intravenously [136].

Regional anesthesia is the primary recommended method of anesthesia for patients during pregnancy. If local anesthetic systemic toxicity (LAST) is considered the cause of cardiac arrest, the LAST protocol should be conducted immediately (see: Chap. 13: Locoregional Anaesthesia During Pregnancy and the Post-partum Period).

References

1. Reitman E, Flood P. Anaesthetic considerations for non-obstetric surgery during pregnancy. Br J Anaesth. 2011;107:72–8.
2. Bauchat JR, van de Velde M. Nonobstetric surgery during pregnancy. In: Chestnut DH, editor. Chestnut's obstetric anesthesia: principles and practice. 6th ed. Philadelphia: Elsevier; 2019.
3. Devroe S, Bleeser T, van de Velde M, et al. Anesthesia for non-obstetric surgery during pregnancy in a tertiary referral center: a 16-year retrospective, matched case-control, cohort study. Int J Obstet Anesth. 2019;39:74–81.
4. Vujic J, Marsoner K, Lipp-Pump AH, et al. Non-obstetric surgery during pregnancy—an eleven-year retrospective analysis. BMC Pregnancy Childbirth. 2019;19:382. https://doi.org/10.1186/s12884-019-2554-6.
5. Arkenbosch JHC, van Ruler O, de Vries AC. Non-obstetric surgery in pregnancy (including bowel surgery and gallbladder surgery). Best Pract Res Clin Gastroenterol. 2020;44–45:101669. https://doi.org/10.1016/j.bpg.2020.101669.

6. Kastrinidis N, Kleinjung T. Blocked nose, nosebleeds, ringing in the ear: ENT diseases during pregnancy. Praxis (Bern 1994). 2019;108:329–34.
7. Lippincott LH, Amedee RG. ENT issues in pregnancy. J La State Med Soc. 1999;151:350–4.
8. Vlastarakos PV, Manolopoulos L, Ferekidis E, et al. Treating common problems of the nose and throat in pregnancy: what is safe? Eur Arch Otorhinolaryngol. 2008;265:499–508.
9. Kumar R, Hayhurst KL, Robson AK. Ear, nose, and throat manifestations during pregnancy. Otolaryngol Head Neck Surg. 2011;145:188–98.
10. Cornthwaite K, Varadharajan K, Oyarzabal M, et al. Management of prolonged epistaxis in pregnancy: case report. J Laryngol Otol. 2013;127:811–3.
11. Kiciński K, Skorek A, Stankiewicz C. Managment of head and neck cancers during pregnancy. Otolaryngol Pol. 2011;65:326–32.
12. Scholz A, Srinivas K, Stacey MRW, et al. Subglottic stenosis in pregnancy. Br J Anaesth. 2008;100:385–8.
13. Upadya M, Saneesh PJ. Anaesthesia for non-obstetric surgery during pregnancy. Indian J Anaesth. 2016;60:234–41.
14. Mazze RI, Källén B. Appendectomy during pregnancy: a Swedish registry study of 778 cases. Obstet Gynecol. 1991;77:835–40.
15. Mazze RI, Källén B. Reproductive outcome after anesthesia and operation during pregnancy: a registry study of 5405 cases. Am J Obstet Gynecol. 1989;161:1178–85.
16. Tolcher MC, Fisher WE, Clark SL. Nonobstetric surgery during pregnancy. Obstet Gynecol. 2018;132:395–403.
17. Balinskaite V, Bottle A, Sodhi V, et al. The risk of adverse pregnancy outcomes following nonobstetric surgery during pregnancy: estimates from a retrospective cohort study of 6.5 million pregnancies. Ann Surg. 2017;266:260–6.
18. American College of Obstetricians and Gynecologists and American Society of Anesthesiologists. ACOG Committee Opinion No. 775: nonobstetric surgery during pregnancy (interim update). Obstet Gynecol. 2019;133:285–6.
19. Schannwell CM, Zimmermann T, Schneppenheim M, et al. Left ventricular hypertrophy and diastolic dysfunction in healthy pregnant women. Cardiology. 2002;97:73–8.
20. Robson SC, Hunter S, Boys RJ, et al. Serial study of factors influencing changes in cardiac output during human pregnancy. Am J Phys. 1989;256:1060–5.
21. Campos O, Andrade JL, Bocanegra J, et al. Physiologic multivalvular regurgitation during pregnancy: a longitudinal doppler echocardiographic study. Int J Cardiol. 1993;40:265–72.
22. Abbas AE, Lester SJ, Connolly H. Pregnancy and the cardiovascular system. Int J Cardiol. 2005;98:179–89.
23. Fujitani S, Baldisseri MR. Hemodynamic assessment in a pregnant and peripartum patient. Crit Care Med. 2005;33:354–61.
24. Desai DK, Moodley J, Naidoo DP. Echocardiographic assessment of cardiovascular hemodynamics in normal pregnancy. Obstet Gynecol. 2004;104:20–9.
25. Higuchi H, Takagi S, Zhang K, et al. Effect of lateral tilt angle on the volume of the abdominal aorta and inferior vena cava in pregnant and nonpregnant women determined by magnetic resonance imaging. Anesthesiology. 2015;122:286–93.
26. Lanni SM, Tillinghast J, Silver HM. Hemodynamic changes and baroreflex gain in the supine hypotensive syndrome. Am J Obstet Gynecol. 2002;187:1636–41.
27. Pilkington S, Carli F, Dakin MJ, et al. Increase in Mallampati score during pregnancy. Br J Anaesth. 1995;74:638–42.
28. Crapo RO. Cardiopulmonary physiology during pregnancy. Clin Obstet Gynecol. 1996;39:3–16.
29. Kolarzyk E, Szot WM, Lyszczarz J. Lung function and breathing regulation parameters during pregnancy. Arch Gynecol Obstet. 2005;272:53–8.
30. Shankar KB, Moseley H, Vemula V, et al. Arterial to end-tidal carbon dioxide tension difference during anaesthesia in early pregnancy. Can J Anaesth. 1989;36:124–7.
31. Templeton A, Kelman GR. Maternal blood-gases, (PAO2-PaO2), physiological shunt and vd/vt in normal pregnancy. Br J Anaesth. 1976;48:1001–4.

32. Goodman S. Anesthesia for nonobstetric surgery in the pregnant patient. Semin Perinatol. 2002;26:136–45.
33. Fanzago E. Anaesthesia for non obstetric surgery in pregnant patients. Minerva Anestesiol. 2003;69:416–27.
34. Hawkins JL, Koonin LM, Palmer SK, et al. Anesthesia related deaths during obstetric delivery in the United States, 1979-1990. Anesthesiology. 1997;86:277–84.
35. Levy DM, Williams OA, Magides AD, et al. Gastric emptying is delayed at 8-12 weeks' gestation. Br J Anaesth. 1994;73:237–8.
36. Lawson M, Kern F Jr, Everson GT. Gastrointestinal transit time in human pregnancy: prolongation in the second and third trimesters followed by postpartum normalization. Gastroenterology. 1985;89:996–9.
37. Chiloiro M, Darconza G, Piccioli E, et al. Gastric emptying and orocecal transit time in pregnancy. J Gastroenterol. 2001;36:538–43.
38. Wong CA, McCarthy RJ, Fitzgerald PC, et al. Gastric emptying of water in obese pregnant women at term. Anesth Analg. 2007;105:751–5.
39. Panicker VV, Riyaz N, Balachandran PK. A clinical study of cutaneous changes in pregnancy. J Epidemiol Glob Health. 2017;7:63–70.
40. Thornton P, Douglas J. Coagulation in pregnancy. Best Pract Res Clin Obstet Gynaecol. 2010;24:339–52.
41. Wildsmith JA. Serum pseudocholinesterase, pregnancy and suxamethonium. Anaesthesia. 1972;27:90–1.
42. Evans RT, Wroe JM. Plasma cholinesterase changes during pregnancy. Their interpretation as a cause of suxamethonium-induced apnoea. Anaesthesia. 1980;35:651–4.
43. Datta S, Lambert DH, Gregus J, et al. Differential sensitivities of mammalian nerve fibers during pregnancy. Anesth Analg. 1983;62:1070–2.
44. Choi J, Germond L, Santos AC. Obstetric regional anesthesia. In: Hadzic A, editor. Hadzic's textbook of regional anesthesia and acute pain management. 2nd ed. Beijing: McGraw-Hill Education; 2017.
45. Bosnjak ZJ, Logan S, Liu Y, et al. Recent insights into molecular mechanisms of propofol-induced developmental neurotoxicity: implications for the protective strategies. Anesth Analg. 2016;123:1286–96.
46. Wu J, Bie B, Naguib M. Epigenetic manipulation of brain-derived neurotrophic factor improves memory deficiency induced by neonatal anesthesia in rats. Anesthesiology. 2016;124:624–40.
47. U.S. Food and Drug Administration. FDA drug safety communication: FDA review results in new warnings about using general anesthetics and sedation drugs in young children and pregnant women; 2016. https://www.fda.gov/media/101937/download. Accessed 29 Oct 2020.
48. Sun LS, Li G, Miller TL, et al. Association between a single general anesthesia exposure before age 36 months and neurocognitive outcomes in later childhood. JAMA. 2016;315:2312–20.
49. Sun LS. Introduction to "anesthesia and neurodevelopment in children": a supplement from the sixth pediatric anesthesia neurodevelopmental assessment (PANDA) symposium. J Neurosurg Anesthesiol. 2019;31:101–2.
50. Aytuluk HG. Evaluation of advanced behavior guidance techniques used in dentistry: sedation and general anesthesia. Osmangazi J Med. 2020;42:466–73.
51. Heller AR, Heger J, Gama de Abreu M, et al. Cafedrine/theodrenaline in anaesthesia: influencing factors in restoring arterial blood pressure. Anaesthesist. 2015;64:190–6.
52. Chappell D, Helf A, Gayer J, et al. Antihypotensive drugs in cesarean sections: treatment of arterial hypotension with ephedrine, phenylephrine and Akrinor (cafedrine/theodrenaline) during cesarean sections with spinal anesthesia. Anaesthesist. 2019;68:228–38.
53. Regitz-Zagrosek V, Roos-Hesselink JW, Bauersachs J, et al.; ESC Scientific Document Group (2018) 2018 ESC guidelines for the management of cardiovascular diseases during pregnancy. Eur Heart J. 39:3165–3241.
54. Maltepe F, Arkan A. Effects on the fetus of anesthesia and non-obstetric surgery for obstetric patient. Turkiye Klinikleri J Surg Med Sci. 2006;2:23–31.

55. Brown WU, Bell GC, Alper MH. Acidosis, local anesthetics and the newborn. Obstet Gynecol. 1976;48:27–30.
56. Okeagu CN, Anandi P, Gennuso S, et al. Clinical management of the pregnant patient undergoing non-obstetric surgery: review of guidelines. Best Pract Res Clin Anaesthesiol. 2020;34:269–81.
57. Kuczkowski KM. Nonobstetric surgery during pregnancy: what are the risks of anesthesia? Obsest Gynecol Surv. 2004;59:52–6.
58. van de Velde M, de Buck F. Anesthesia for non-obstetric surgery in the pregnant patient. Minerva Anestesiol. 2007;73:235–40.
59. Visser BC, Glasgow RE, Mulvihill KK, et al. Safety and timing of nonobstetric abdominal surgery in pregnancy. Dig Surg. 2001;18:409–17.
60. Fisher SC, Siag K, Howley MM, et al. Maternal surgery and anesthesia during pregnancy and risk of birth defects in the National Birth Defects Prevention Study, 1997-2011. Birth Defects Res. 2020;112:162–74.
61. Cohen-Kerem R, Railton C, Oren D, et al. Pregnancy outcome following non-obstetric surgical intervention. Am J Surg. 2005;190:467–73.
62. Brodsky JB, Cohen EN, Brown BW Jr, et al. Surgery during pregnancy and fetal outcome. Am J Obstet Gynecol. 1980;138:1165–7.
63. Duncan PG, Pope WD, Cohen MM, et al. Fetal risk of anesthesia and surgery during pregnancy. Anesthesiology. 1986;64:790–4.
64. Ravindra GL, Madamangalam AS, Seetharamaiah S. Anaesthesia for non-obstetric surgery in obstetric patients. Indian J Anaesth. 2018;62:710–6.
65. U.S. Department of Health and Human Services Food and Drug Administration, Center for Drug Evaluation and Research, Center for Biologics Evaluation and Research. Pregnancy, lactation, and reproductive potential: labeling for human prescription drug and biological products—content and format guidance for industry; 2020. https://www.fda.gov/media/90160/download. Accessed 29 Oct 2020.
66. Department of Health and Human Services Food and Drug Administration. In: Clinical pharmacology section of labeling for human prescription drug and biological products. Guidance for industry. Federal Register. 2016;81(233):87563–87565. Available online via the Government Publishing Office (www.gpo.gov). https://www.govinfo.gov/content/pkg/FR-2014-12-04/pdf/2014-28241.pdf. Accessed 29 Oct 2020.
67. Po' G, Olivieri C, Rose CH, et al. Intraoperative fetal heart monitoring for non-obstetric surgery: a systematic review. Eur J Obstet Gynecol Reprod Biol. 2019;238:12–9.
68. Kilpatrick CC, Puig C, Chohan L, et al. Intraoperative fetal heart rate monitoring during nonobstetric surgery in pregnancy: a practice survey. South Med J. 2010;103:212–5.
69. Yamashita M, Hayashi S, Endo M, et al. Incidence and risk factors for recurrent spontaneous preterm birth: a retrospective cohort study in Japan. J Obstet Gynaecol Res. 2015;41:1708–14.
70. Wikner BN, Stiller CO, Bergman U, et al. Use of benzodiazepines and benzodiazepine receptor agonists during pregnancy: neonatal outcome and congenital malformations. Pharmacoepidemiol Drug Saf. 2007;16:1203–10.
71. Dolovich LR, Addis A, Vaillancourt JM, et al. Benzodiazepine use in pregnancy and major malformations or oral cleft: meta-analysis of cohort and case-control studies. BMJ. 1998;317:839–43.
72. Kuczkowski KM. The safety of anaesthetics in pregnant women. Expert Opin Drug Saf. 2006;5:251–64.
73. White LD, Hodsdon A, An GH, et al. Induction opioids for caesarean section under general anaesthesia: a systematic review and meta-analysis of randomised controlled trials. Int J Obstet Anesth. 2019;40:4–13.
74. Guignard B, Bossard AE, Coste C, et al. Acute opioid tolerance: intraoperative remifentanil increases postoperative pain and morphine requirement. Anesthesiology. 2000;93:409–17.
75. Devroe S, van de Velde M, Rex S. General anesthesia for caesarean section. Curr Opin Anaesthesiol. 2015;28:240–6.

76. Patrick SW, Barfield WD, Poindexter BB, Committee on Fetus and Newborn, Committee on Substance Use and Prevention. Neonatal opioid withdrawal syndrome. Pediatrics. 2020;146(5):e2020029074. https://doi.org/10.1542/peds.2020-029074.

77. Lind JN, Interrante JD, Ailes EC, et al. Maternal use of opioids during pregnancy and congenital malformations: a systematic review. Pediatrics. 2017;139:e20164131. https://doi.org/10.1542/peds.2016-4131.

78. Peck T, Williams M (2008) Core drugs in anaesthetic practice. In: Peck T, Hill S (Authors) Pharmacology for anaesthesia and intensive care, 3rd edn. Cambridge: Cambridge University Press.

79. Gin T. Pharmacology during pregnancy and lactation. In: Chestnut DH, editor. Chestnut's obstetric anesthesia: principles and practice. 6th ed. Philadelphia: Elsevier; 2019.

80. Sachs HC, Committee on Drugs. The transfer of drugs and therapeutics into human breast milk: an update on selected topics. Pediatrics. 2013;132:796–809.

81. Mitchell J, Jones W, Winkley E, et al. Guideline on anaesthesia and sedation in breast-feeding women 2020: guideline from the Association of Anaesthetists. Anaesthesia. 2020;75:1482–93.

82. Kan RE, Hughes SC, Rosen MA, et al. Intravenous remifentanil: placental transfer maternal and neonatal effects. Anesthesiology. 1998;88:1467–74.

83. Ito S. Opioids in breast milk: pharmacokinetic principles and clinical implications. J Clin Pharmacol. 2018;58:151–63.

84. Minami K, Uezono Y, Ueta Y. Pharmacological aspects of the effects of tramadol on G-protein coupled receptors. J Pharmacol Sci. 2007;103:253–60.

85. U.S. Food and Drug Administration. Codeine and tramadol medicines: drug safety communication—restricting use in children, recommending against use in breast-feeding women; 2017. https://www.fda.gov/Safety/MedWatch/SafetyInformation/SafetyAlertsforHumanMedicalProducts/ucm554029.htm. Accessed 29 Oct 2020.

86. Wenzel V, Lindner KH. Best pharmacological practice in prehospital intubation. Lancet. 2009;374:267–826.

87. Downing JW, Buley RJ, Brock-Utne JG, et al. Etomidate for induction of anaesthesia at caesarean section: comparison with thiopentone. Br J Anaesth. 1979;51:135–40.

88. Rosen MA. Nitrous oxide for relief of labor procedure systemic review. Am J Obstet Gynecol. 2002;186:110–25.

89. Leighton BL, Cheek TG, Gross JB, et al. Succinylcholine pharmacodynamics in peripartum patients. Anesthesiology. 1986;64:202–5.

90. Magorian T, Flannery KB, Miller RD. Comparison of rocuronium, succinylcholine, and vecuronium for rapid-sequence induction of anesthesia in adult patients. Anesthesiology. 1993;79:913–8.

91. Clark RB, Brown MA, Lattin DL. Neostigmine, atropine, and glycopyrrolate: does neostigmine cross the placenta? Anesthesiology. 1996;84:450–2.

92. Amorim P, Lagarto F, Gomes B, et al. Neostigmine vs. sugammadex: observational cohort study comparing the quality of recovery using the postoperative quality recovery scale. Acta Anaesthesiol Scand. 2014;58:1101–10.

93. Yellon SM, Dobyns AE, Beck HL, et al. Loss of progesterone receptor-mediated actions induce preterm cellular and structural remodeling of the cervix and premature birth. PLoS One. 2013;8:e81340. https://doi.org/10.1371/journal.pone.0081340.

94. Et T, Topal A, Erol A, Tavlan A, et al. The effects of sugammadex on progesterone levels in pregnant rats. Balkan Med J. 2015;32:203–7.

95. Richardson MG, Raymond BL. Sugammadex administration in pregnant women and in women of reproductive potential: a narrative review. Anesth Analg. 2020;130:1628–37.

96. Howie WO, McMullen PC. Breastfeeding problems following anesthetic administration. J Perinat Educ. 2006;15:50–7.

97. Hale TW. Anesthetic medications in breastfeeding mothers. J Hum Lact. 1999;15:185–94.

98. Liew Z, Ritz B, Rebordosa C, et al. Acetaminophen use during pregnancy, behavioral problems, and hyperkinetic disorders. JAMA Pediatr. 2014;168:313–20.

99. Magnus MC, Karlstad O, Haberg SE, et al. Prenatal and infant paracetamol exposure and development of asthma: the Norwegian Mother and Child Cohort Study. Int J Epidemiol. 2016;45:512–22.
100. Migliore E, Zugna D, Galassi C, et al. Prenatal paracetamol exposure and wheezing in childhood: causation or confounding? PLoS One. 2015;10:e0135775. https://doi.org/10.1371/journal.pone.0135775.
101. Hauspurg A, Sutton E, Catov J, et al. Applying the new ACC/AHA aspirin effect on adverse pregnancy outcomes associated with stage 1 hypertension in a high-risk cohort. Hypertension. 2018;72:202–7.
102. Lamont T, Coates T, Mathew D, et al. Checking for pregnancy before surgery: summary of a safety report from the National Patient Safety Agency. BMJ. 2010;341:3402. https://doi.org/10.1136/bmj.c3402.
103. Apfelbaum JL, Connis RT, Nickinovich DG, et al. Practice advisory for preanesthesia evaluation. An updated report by the American Society of Anesthesiologists task force on preanesthesia evaluation. Anesthesiology. 2012;116:522–38.
104. American Society of Anesthesiologists. Pregnancy testing prior to anesthesia and surgery; 2016. https://www.asahq.org/standards-and-guidelines/pregnancy-testing-prior-to-anesthesia-and-surgery. Accessed 29 Oct 2020.
105. O'Sullivan G. Gastric emptying during pregnancy and the puerperium. Int J Obstet Anesth. 1993;2:216–24.
106. Nedjlova M, Johnson T. Anaesthesia for non-obstetric procedures during pregnancy. Continuing Educ Anaesthesia Crit Care Pain. 2012;12:203–6.
107. van de Putte P, Perlas A. Ultrasound assessment of gastric content and volume. Br J Anaesth. 2014;113:12–22.
108. Balki M, Cooke ME, Dunington S, et al. Unanticipated difficult airway in obstetric patients: development of a new algorithm for formative assessment in high-fidelity simulation. Anesthesiology. 2012;117:883–97.
109. Mushambi MC, Kinsella SM, Popat M, et al. Obstetric Anaesthetists' association and difficult airway society guidelines for the management of difficult and failed tracheal intubation in obstetrics. Anaesthesia. 2015;70:1286–306.
110. Bordoni L, Parsons K, Rucklidge MWM. Obstetric airway management. Update in Anaesthesia. 2019;34:7–13.
111. Ovassapian A, Salem MR. Sellick's maneuver: to do or not do. Anesth Analg. 2009;109:1360–2.
112. Zheng BX, Zheng H, Lin XM. Ultrasound for predicting difficult airway in obstetric anesthesia: protocol and methods for a prospective observational clinical study. Medicine (Baltimore). 2019;98:17846. https://doi.org/10.1097/MD.0000000000017846.
113. Kristensen MS, Teoh WH, Rudolph SS. Ultrasonographic identification of the cricothyroid membrane: best evidence, techniques, and clinical impact. Br J Anaesth. 2016;117:39–46.
114. Paranjothy S, Griffiths JD, Broughton HK, et al. Interventions at caesarean section for reducing the risk of aspiration pneumonitis. Cochrane Database Syst Rev. 2014;2:CD004943. https://doi.org/10.1002/14651858.CD004943.pub4.
115. Bernhard M, Becker TK, Gries A, et al. The first shot is often the best shot: first-pass intubation success in emergency airway management. Anesth Analg. 2015;121:1389–93.
116. Scott-Brown S, Russell R. Video laryngoscopes and the obstetric airway. Int J Obstet Anesth. 2015;24:137–46.
117. Martin E, Vickers B, Landau R, et al. ABM clinical protocol #28, peripartum analgesia and anesthesia for the breastfeeding mother. Breastfeed Med. 2018;13:164–71.
118. Tobolic TJ. Primum non nocere breastfeeding. Breastfeed Med. 2019;14:77–8.
119. Zelop CM, Grimes EP. Cardiopulmonary resuscitation in pregnancy. In: Field JM, Kudenchuk PJ, O'Connor RE, editors. The textbook of emergency cardiovascular care and CPR. Philadelphia: Wolters Kluwer; 2009.
120. Zelop CM, Einav S, Mhyre JM, et al.; American Heart Association's Get With the Guidelines-Resuscitation Investigators. Characteristics and outcomes of maternal cardiac arrest: a descriptive analysis of get with the guidelines data. Resuscitation. 2018;132:17–20.

121. Vanden Hoek TL, Morrison LJ, Shuster M, et al. Part 12: cardiac arrest in special situations: 2010 American Heart Association guidelines for cardiopulmonary resuscitation and emergency cardiovascular care. Circulation. 2011;122:829–61.
122. Kikuchi J, Deering S. Cardiac arrest in pregnancy. Semin Perinatol. 2018;42:33–8.
123. Jeejeebhoy FM, Zelop CM, Lipman S, et al.; American Heart Association Emergency Cardiovascular Care Committee, Council on Cardiopulmonary, Critical Care, Perioperative and Resuscitation, Council on Cardiovascular Diseases in the Young, and Council on Clinical Cardiology. Cardiac arrest in pregnancy: a scientific statement from the American Heart Association. Circulation. 2015;132:1747–1773.
124. Yun JG, Lee BK. Spatial relationship of the left ventricle in the supine position and the left lateral tilt position (implication for cardiopulmonary resuscitation in pregnant patients). Fire Sci Eng. 2013;27:75–9.
125. Archer TL, Suresh P, Shapiro AE. Cardiac output measurement, by means of electrical velocimetry, may be able to determine optimum maternal position during gestation, labour and caesarean delivery, by preventing vena caval compression and maximising cardiac output and placental perfusion pressure. Anaesth Intensive Care. 2011;39:308–11.
126. Apfelbaum JL, Hagberg CA, Caplan RA, et al., American Society of Anesthesiologists Task Force on Management of the Difficult Airway. Practice guidelines for management of the difficult airway: an updated report by the American Society of Anesthesiologists task force on management of the difficult airway. Anesthesiology. 2013;118:251–270.
127. Mhyre JM, Healy D. The unanticipated difficult intubation in obstetrics. Anesth Analg. 2011;112:648–52.
128. Panchal AR, Berg KM, Hirsch KG, et al. 2019 American Heart Association focused update on advanced cardiovascular life support: use of advanced airways, vasopressors, and extracorporeal cardiopulmonary resuscitation during cardiac arrest: an update to the American Heart Association guidelines for cardiopulmonary resuscitation and emergency cardiovascular care. Circulation. 2019;140:881–94.
129. Soar J, Maconochie I, Wyckoff MH, et al. 2019 international consensus on cardiopulmonary resuscitation and emergency cardiovascular care science with treatment recommendations: summary from the basic life support; advanced life support; pediatric life support; neonatal life support; education, implementation, and teams; and first aid task forces. Circulation. 2019;140:826–80.
130. Soar J, Nicholson TC, Parr MJ, et al.; International Liaison Committee on Resuscitation (ILCOR) Advanced Life Support Task Force. Advanced airway management during adult cardiac arrest: consensus on science with treatment recommendations; 2019. https://costr. ilcor.org/document/advanced-airway-management-during-adult-cardiac-arrest. Accessed 29 Oct 2020.
131. Boet S, Duttchen K, Chan J, et al. Cricoid pressure provides incomplete esophageal occlusion associated with lateral deviation: a magnetic resonance imaging study. J Emerg Med. 2012;42:606–11.
132. Neumar RW, Otto CW, Link MS, et al. Part 8: adult advanced cardiovascular life support: 2010 American Heart Association guidelines for cardiopulmonary resuscitation and emergency cardiovascular care. Circulation. 2010;122:729–67.
133. Svinos H. Towards evidence based emergency medicine: best BETs from the Manchester Royal Infirmary, BET 1: emergency caesarean section in cardiac arrest before the third trimester. Emerg Med J. 2008;25:764–5.
134. Finegold H, Darwich A, Romeo R, et al. Successful resuscitation after maternal cardiac arrest by immediate cesarean section in the labor room. Anesthesiology. 2002;96:1278.
135. Cardosi RJ, Porter KB. Cesarean delivery of twins during maternal cardiopulmonary arrest. Obstet Gynecol. 1998;92:695–7.
136. Cobb B, Lipman S. Cardiac arrest: obstetric CPR/ACLS. Clin Obstet Gynecol. 2017;60:425–30.

Pain Management in Pregnancy and Lactation

15

Vildan Kılıç Yılmaz, Alp Gurbet, and Desiderio Passali

15.1 Introduction

Pain is one of the most common symptoms that can be seen in all age groups and brings the person to the physician. Since pain may be the first sign of severe diseases, it should be investigated and treated effectively to avoid physiological and psychological dysfunctions in patients. According to the definition revised in 2020 by the International Association for the Study of Pain (IASP), pain is an unpleasant sensory and emotional experience associated with, or resembling that associated with, actual or potential tissue damage in any part of the body. The presence of emotional factors as well as objective stimuli causes differences in definition, perception, and behavioral responses to pain. Pain is a personal experience affected by biological, psychological, and social factors to varying degrees [1].

There are many physiological, anatomical, psychological, and biochemical changes during pregnancy in order to meet the needs of the developing fetus, as well as the adaptation of the mother to pregnancy [2]. Understanding these physiological

V. Kılıç Yılmaz (✉)
Faculty of Medicine, Department of Anesthesiology and Reanimation (Algology), Health Sciences University, Derince Research and Training Hospital, Kocaeli, Turkey
e-mail: vildancik@yahoo.com

A. Gurbet
Faculty of Medicine, Department of Anesthesiology and Reanimation, Uludağ University, Bursa, Turkey
e-mail: dragurbet@yahoo.com

D. Passali
Department of Medical, Surgical and Neuroscience Sciences, and Department of Otorhinolaryngology, Univerity of Siena, Siena, Italy
e-mail: d.passali@virgilio.it

C. Cingi et al. (eds.), *ENT Diseases: Diagnosis and Treatment during Pregnancy and Lactation*, https://doi.org/10.1007/978-3-031-05303-0_15

changes enables us to know the effects and side effects of analgesic, anesthetic, and adjuvant agents to be used in the treatment of pain during pregnancy by helping us to conduct an appropriate, complete, and effective pain treatment.

15.2 Physiological Changes in Pregnancy

15.2.1 Hormonal Changes

With fertilization, the corpus luteum secretes progesterone, estrogen, and relaxin in the ovary. The placenta, by undertaking the hormone production function, produces human chorionic somatomammotropin (hCS; previously known as human placental lactogen and chorionic growth hormone-prolactin) starting from 6–8 weeks of gestation [3]. Human chorionic gonadotrophin (hCG) released from syncyticotrophoblast cells is detected in blood 6 days after conception and in urine 2 or 3 weeks later. It reaches a maximum level in the first between 10 and 12 weeks of pregnancy and then falls and tends to plateau at a lower level throughout pregnancy [4, 5].

Progesterone production increases during pregnancy and reaches a value of 100–300 ng/mL at term [6]. Progesterone is the cause of dilatation within the renal tract, smooth muscle relaxation, generalized vasodilatation, bronchodilatation, slow gastrointestinal tract motility, constipation, and early nausea and vomiting [7–10]. It reduces the need for anesthetic agents in neuraxial anesthesia and the need for inhalation anesthetics in general anesthesia by decreasing the MAC (minimal alveolar concentration) value [11, 12]. Progesterone is a neurotransmitter and increases the pain threshold level together with endogenous endorphins in pregnancy [13–15]. It is also thermogenic and has a natriuretic effect unlike estrogen [16].

Estradiol concentrations reach 25,000 pg/mL at term [6]. It causes fluid retention by increasing Na+ and water retention coupled with increased aldosterone during pregnancy and increases the tendency to hypertension [17–20]. It makes the symphysis pubis elastic with relaxation, especially in the pelvic ligaments and sacroiliac joint. Although this situation facilitates labor, it becomes the main cause of musculoskeletal pain during pregnancy [21–23].

During pregnancy, thyroid-binding globulin (TBG), TT4 (total tyroxine), TT3 (total triiodothyronine) also increase. Free T3 and free T4 are normal or slightly lower. An increase is observed in the levels of 1,25-dihydroxyvitamin D, calcitonin, serum parathyroid hormone (PTH), insulin ACTH, renin–angiotensin, and aldosterone [24].

15.2.2 Cardiovascular and Hemodynamic Changes

Peripheral vasodilatation occurs in the endothelium by synthesis of estradiol, vasodilator prostaglandins (PGI2), and nitric oxide. Peripheral vasodilation causes a 25–30% decrease in systemic vascular resistance (SVR). In order to tolerate a decrease in SVR, cardiac output (CO) increases by 40–50%. Blood volume increases by 40–50% at term. While uterine blood flow is 50 mL/min in the tenth week of gestation, it reaches 850 mL/min at term [25, 26]. The heart rate also increases by an average of 10 beats per minute. Cardiac compliance and myocardial contractility increase. Ejection fraction (EF) does not decrease. Stroke volume increases by 20–30% above baseline [27]. The electrocardiogram in pregnancy may show sinus tachycardia, ectopic beats, shortening of the PR and uncorrected QT intervals, a Q wave and T wave inversion in the lateral leads or lead III, or left axis deviation [28].

15.2.3 Respiratory Changes

Tidal volume increases by 40–50%. Inspiratory capacity and oxygen intake increase. Progesterone increases the carbon dioxide sensitivity of the respiratory center, and the minute ventilation increases by 45–50%. Functional residual capacity (FRC) is decreased by 20%, and residual volume is decreased by 20%. Respiratory alkalosis is usually observed during pregnancy, but this situation can be compensated by renal bicarbonate excretion [8, 29, 30]. The incidence of obstructive sleep apnea (OSA) increases as a result of narrowing in the oropharyngeal area due to mucosal hyperemia, edema, fluid shifts, and increased maternal blood volume [31, 32].

15.2.4 Hematological Changes

While total blood volume increases by 30–50%, red cell mass increase by 20–30%, and this causes "physiological anemia." During pregnancy, the hemoglobin concentration drops to 10–20 g/L and returns to normal in 4–6 weeks after delivery. White blood cell account is at the level of $10–15 \times 10^9/L$, and an increase of $30 \times 10^9/L$ can be observed during delivery. It returns to a normal level in 6–7 days after pregnancy. Clotting factors (I, VII, VIII, X, XII, prekallikrein, von Willebrand factor, thrombin, activated partial thromboplastin time, prothrombin time, renal erythropoietin/reticulocyte count, and fibrinogen levels) increase by 50–79%. Platelets and antithrombin III decrease. The risk of hypercoagulability is higher in pregnancy [33, 34].

15.2.5 Renal Changes

In the 14th week of pregnancy, both the renal blood flow and the glomerular filtration rate (GFR) increase by 25% and 50%, respectively. Therefore, significant amounts of water and sodium are retained [35]. Creatinine level drops to 0.4–0.8 mg/ dL. The renin–angiotensin–aldosterone system is activated during normal pregnancy. Estrogen directly triggers angiotensinogen production. Protein excretion with urine increases up to 300 mg/per day. Increased frequency of urination, nocturia, and incontinence are also common [36, 37].

15.2.6 Gastrointestinal Changes

The increase in progesterone level during pregnancy reduces motility and leads to an increase in gastric acid secretion. Therefore, the incidence of gastroesophageal reflux (GER) increases. A slight decrease in transaminase and bilirubin levels, hypersalivation, decrease in lower esophagus, lower sphincter pressure, decrease in gastric motility, prolonged gastric emptying time, decrease in small intestine motility, constipation, cholestasis, and decrease in gallbladder motility are among the most common gastrointestinal symptoms seen during pregnancy [38].

15.2.7 Musculoskeletal Changes

The pregnant woman has elevated ligamentous laxity, secondary to increased relaxin release, which may cause increased joint mobility and instability (Table 15.1).

Table 15.1 Pathophysiological changes that may have an impact on the pharmacokinetics of certain drugs in pregnancy [38]

Changes	Potential effect on pharmacokinetics
Vomiting and nausea	↓ Absorption (↓ peak conc. and ↓ oral bioavailability)
Delayed motility	Delayed absorption (↑ time to peak conc.)
Decreased gastric acid secretion	↓ For anionic drugs, oral bioavailability
Body weight gain	↑ Apparent volume of distribution
Body fat gain	↑ For lipophilic drugs, apparent volume of distribution
Increased plasma volume	↑ Apparent volume of distribution
Changes in hepatic drug- metabolizing enzymes	Altered hepatic clearance for high extraction drugs given orally or low extraction ratio drugs applied intravenously
Increased hepatic blood flow	↑ Hepatic clearance for high extraction ratio drugs
Increased renal blood flow	↑ Renal clearance for unchanged drug
Increased glomerular filtration	↑ Renal clearance for unchanged drug
Chronic disease or pregnancy complications	Changes in ADMET/PD
Maternal poly-pharmacy	PK/PD drug interactions
Placenta	Placental transporters and drug metabolism in placenta
Fetus	Hepatic CYP3A7 has no effect on clearance. However, it can alter the concentration of the drug and its metabolites in the fetus as well as ↑ apparent volume of distribution
Amniotic fluid	↑ Apparent volume of distribution and drug accumulation

PD pharmacodynamics, *PK* pharmacokinetics, ↑ increase, ↓ decrease, *ADME drug* absorption, distribution, metabolism, and excretion, *CYP* cytochrome P450

15.3 Pharmacokinetic Mechanisms in Pregnancy

Pharmacokinetics examines the absorption, distribution, metabolism, and excretion processes, respectively, following the administration of the drug to the body, and evaluates the concentration of the drug in the target tissue in the body [39, 40]. Thus, it determines in which route, in what dosage, how, how long, and when the drug should be used [41]. In addition to the changes in the expectant mother, the pharmacokinetic route of drugs in the placenta and fetus leads to various concerns in terms of efficacy and teratogenicity in the treatment.

Bioavailability is a measure that shows how much the body benefits from the drug given for systemic purposes. Due to the decrease in drug absorption and increase in drug elimination during pregnancy, the drug concentration decreases and fluctuations can be seen in free drug concentration. For drugs taken orally, the decrease in intestinal motility due to the increase in progesterone and the increase in gastric pH because of the decrease in gastric secretion, as well as increased frequency of nausea and vomiting, affect drug absorption. In intramuscular applications, increased tissue blood flow may increase absorption. In addition, absorption may decrease in the presence of diffuse edema. An increase is observed in absorption of inhalation agents due to increased cardiac output and tidal volume [42–44].

The distribution of the drug that enters the systemic circulation in the body varies according to whether it is lipophilic or nonionized. Lipophilic drugs are much easier to cross the placenta and reach fetal circulation. Increasing total body fluid provides a larger area in which hydrophilic drugs can disperse (i.e., volume of distribution increases). As a result of this significant dilution, the maximum concentration of many hydrophilic drugs decreases, but this clinical effect is compensated by changes in plasma protein concentrations to some extent. Body fat rate also increases. As a result of this, a wider distribution volume is formed for lipophilic drugs [45, 46].

Drug elimination takes place in the liver, mucosa, and lumen of the gastrointestinal tract, kidneys, lungs, brain, and tissues by the process of enzymatic metabolism or direct excretion. Hepatic elimination kinetics, protein binding, metabolic enzyme activity, and portal blood flow can change during pregnancy due to many factors. Cytochrome P450 (CYP450) enzymes are induced by estrogen/progesterone, which increases the metabolic rate of drugs. The decrease in the activity of the CYP1A2 enzyme increases the duration of drug elimination [47].

Since an increase in renal blood flow and glomerular filtration rates by 25% and 50%, respectively, increases the excretion of drugs excreted through the kidneys during pregnancy, an effective dose adjustment should be considered [48, 49].

15.4 Placental Transfer of Drugs

It is important that the drugs given to the mother during pregnancy affect the fetus as well as the transition of the drugs given to the mother from the maternal circulation to the fetal circulation. It is important that the drugs given to the mother during pregnancy affect the fetus as well as the transition of the drugs given to the mother from the maternal circulation to the fetal circulation. The most important factor that affects the placental passage of drugs is the placental blood flow [50]. Drugs usually pass through the placenta by passive diffusion. Drugs with lipophilic structures enter the fetal circulation more easily than hydrophilic drugs [51]. Another important factor is their molecular weight. Drugs with a molecular weight less than 500 Da (Dalton) (many drugs, especially those entering the central nervous system are in this group) can easily cross the placenta, while those between 500 and 1000 Da can partially pass. Substances between 1000 and 5000 Da can hardly cross. Those above 5000 Da (such as insulin and heparin) cannot pass [52]. Although some molecules such as immunoglobulin G antibodies (160,000 Da) are large, they can easily reach the fetal circulation by a different mechanism called pinocytotic mechanism [53]. Glucose, one of the most important substrates for fetal development, cross the placental barrier with its own active transport system, although it has a small molecular weight. These findings show that the majority of drugs can cross the placenta [53, 54].

In the 8 weeks after post-conception, immature metabolization is performed in the fetal liver, but the insufficient enzymatic activity and the direct entrance of almost 50% of the fetal circulation coming from the umbilical vein to the fetal cardiovascular and cerebral circulation without coming to the fetal liver cause drug accumulation in the fetus. In addition, the plasma pH of the fetus is slightly more acidic than that of the maternal plasma. For this reason, basic drugs found in maternal plasma, which are more basic, pass easily through the placental barrier since they are nonionized (lipophilic). In the acidic fetal blood, these drugs become ionized and accumulate here. This situation is called "ion trapping."

15.5 Nonobstetric Pain Situations in Pregnancy

Especially in severe acute pain during pregnancy, obstetric emergencies that may require surgical intervention should be eliminated first. In addition, chronic pain treatments that existed before pregnancy may need to be continued during pregnancy and the postpartum period.

The most common nonobstetric pains during pregnancy are described in the following sections.

1. Back pain
   Hormonal changes and increased mechanical pressure during pregnancy cause weight gain, fluid retention, postural changes, and increased joint and ligament laxity. These changes cause low back pain, upper back pain, sacroiliac joint pain, sciatica/radiculopathy, spondylolisthesis, lumbar discopathy, and coccidinia pains in pregnancy.
2. Pregnancy-related pelvic pain
3. Hip pain (Osteonecrosis, transient osteoporosis of the hip)
4. Neuropathic pain (Meralgia paresthetica, Carpal Tunnel Syndrome, diabetic polynoropathy, intercostal neuralgia)

5. Headache is the most common complaint during pregnancy. Although it is a migraine-type headache, migraine that starts during pregnancy is rare. Generally, migraine improves during pregnancy, especially in the first trimester. The recovery rate is more pronounced in cases of migraine associated with menstruation. Treatment should be primarily nonpharmacological methods such as acupuncture relaxation exercises, biofeedback, behavioral cognitive therapy, and local ice applications. When these treatments fail, first-line drug therapy is paracetamol. Triptans should be avoided in the third trimester due to the slight increase in the risk of uterine atony and peripartum bleeding. Low-dose ergot derivatives pose a high teratogenic risk and should not be used in pregnancy as high doses can cause uterine contractions and miscarriage. Beta blockers can cause low fetal birth weight as a result of a moderate reduction of placental blood flow due to decreased maternal cardiac output. When used in the peripartum period, attention should be paid to the newborn due to the risk of bradycardia, hypotension, hypothermia, hypoglycemia, apnea, and respiratory distress.

With the increase of progesterone, estrogen, aldosterone, and cortisol, the cardiac output and total blood volume also increase. Edema is observed in mucosal membranes and extremities due to increased extravascular volume, especially in the third trimester of pregnancy. Mucosal edema, which occurs completely as a result of physiological changes, may cause ear, nose, and throat diseases, which existed before pregnancy, to be more severe. It may also lead to new complaints related to pregnancy. However, most of these complaints return to normal after pregnancy [55].

Diseases with increased frequency during pregnancy are hearing loss due to Eustachian tube dysfunction [56], osteosclerosis caused by the effect of estrogen, sudden sensorineural hearing loss [57–62], Meniere's disease caused by fluid retention, Bell's palsy as a result of peri-neural edema, rhinitis due to the anticholinesterase effect of estrogen, the incidence of allergic rhinitis as a result of the increase in corticosteroids, epistaxis due to vascular congestion, obstructive sleep apnea, gastroesophageal reflux, granuloma gravidarum (pregnancy tumor), ptyalism gravidarum, and tinnitus.

15.6 Pharmacological Pain Treatment in Pregnancy and Lactation

15.6.1 Medication in Pregnancy

For the drug to be used by the mother during pregnancy, two organisms, maternal and fetal, are considered. When pregnant and breastfeeding women are prescribed drugs, these drugs might have a teratogenic effect on the fetus and breastfed babies. Teratogens are substances that may cause an irreversible damage to the growth, structure, or function of the developing embryo or fetus [63].

For a substance to be teratogenic, it must have the following:

1. Exposure proven at critical times during development
2. Consistent dysmorphic data identified in well-conducted epidemiological studies
3. Certain syndromes or defects consistently related to specific teratogens
4. Uncommon anatomical defects due to environmental exposure (e.g., facial dysmorphology and carbamazepine nail hypoplasia) [64]

From the teratogenesis perspective, human pregnancy is divided into three periods.

1. Preimplantation (from fertilization to implantation): The preimplantation period is a gestation period traditionally characterized by the "all-or-nothing" phenomenon, and exposure to teratogenic substances during this period results in serious cell damage and embryonic loss.
2. Embryonic (2nd–9th week): Compared to other periods, more malformations are encountered in this period. The extent to which fetal organ systems will be affected by teratogen at what stage varies according to the order of formation (e.g., if the teratogen acts between 6.5 and 8 weeks of gestation, the heart is the most affected organ). Moreover, disorders resulting from changes in the structure and function of organs that are normally developed during embryogenesis can be seen [65].
3. Fetal (from the ninth week to term): Although it is known that most of the teratogens act at certain developmental stages of pregnancy, the same agent may present with different clinical outcomes at different stages. Nonsteroidal anti-inflammatory drugs (NSAIDs) (e.g., ibuprofen and indomethacin) are associated with gastroschisis and other fetal sequelae if the embryo is exposed to these drugs during early pregnancy. If the fetus is exposed to NSAIDs after 30 weeks, irreversible closure of the ductus (pulmonary hypertension) and kidney failure (oligohydramnios) may occur [66].

15.7 Medications in the Breastfeeding Mother

The use of drugs during breastfeeding is based on the principles of effective treatment of the mother as well as protecting the infant from possible side effects. A drug that is considered to be necessary for maternal health may be harmful to the embryo and fetus. However, the lack of a drug due to some health concerns may also cause problems for maternal health. For potential teratogenic and embryotoxic effects of drugs, the United States Food and Drug Administration (FDA) developed a five-category labeling system (A, B, C, D, and X) using scientific and evidence-based data for all drugs approved in the United States (Tables 15.2 and 15.3).

Table 15.2 Chart of the FDA pregnancy risk categories [67, 68]

Category A	Category B	Category C	Category D	Category E
Controlled human studies do not demonstrate fetal risk	In vivo studies demonstrate fetal risk not verified by human studies **or** animal studies do not demonstrate fetal risk and controlled human studies are not available	Controlled human studies are absent and animal studies are not available or demonstrate adverse effects on the fetus	Human studies or investigational or post-marketing data demonstrate fetal risk; advantages may be acceptable in spite of possible risks	Both animal and human studies or investigational or post-marketing data demonstrate fetal risk, which obviously outweighs possible benefits

In 2009, the FDA's Pregnancy Risk Categories classification was changed with a new system called Pregnancy and Lactation Labeling Rule (PLLR), and PLLR started to be used actively in 2015 [67–69]

Table 15.3 New pregnancy-risk categories [67, 68]

Pregnancy (including labor and delivery)	Lactation	Females and males of reproductive potential
Pregnancy exposure registry Risk summary Clinical considerations	Risk summary Clinical considerations	Pregnancy testing Contraception Infertility

The factors that reduce the placental transfer of drugs are ionized state (polar molecules), high molecular weight (larger molecules), increased protein binding, low lipophilicity and hydrophobicity, increased maternal metabolism, and early gestational age [70].

15.7.1 Drug Delivery Route

The bioavailability of orally administered drugs is different from parenteral drugs. In mothers using parenteral drugs, although these drugs are excreted in breast milk, the amount absorbed by the infant remains very low due to insufficient oral absorption (insulin, morphine, aminoglycosides) [70].

15.7.2 Pharmacokinetic Properties of the Drug

The serum concentration of the drug depends on its distribution, metabolism, and excretion. When drugs with a long half-life are taken, drug exposure in the fetus may gradually increase [71].

15.8 Infant-Related Features

Gestational and postnatal age affect drug metabolism. Since liver and kidney functions are lower in preterm infants compared to term infants, drug interactions may be different. Because the drug's half-life is longer in term infants, it should be considered that drug accumulation may be higher with repeated doses [71].

15.9 Factors Determining the Effect of Drugs on Infants

(a) Milk–plasma ratio (M/P): This ratio determines the amount of drug that passes into breast milk. The ratio of drug concentration in plasma to drug concentration in milk is calculated [72].
(b) Infant dose: Dose (infant) = Drug concentration in milk × Volume of milk received [73].
(c) Relative infant dose (RID): Relative infant dose = infant dose (mg/kg/day)/ maternal dose (mg/kg/day) × 100. It is one of the most useful methods in determining drug exposure. It should not exceed 10% of the relative infant dose value [74] (Table 15.4).

Table 15.4 Hale's lactation risk category [75]

L1	Compatible	Drugs have been administered by numerous breastfeeding women without increased adverse effects on the infant. Controlled studies fail to indicate risk to the infant in breastfeeding women, and the possible damage to the infant is remote, or the drug is not orally bioavailable in an infant
L2	Probably compatible	Drugs have been tested in a limited number of breastfeeding women without any increase in adverse effects on the infant. And/or findings of an exhibited risk likely to follow the use of the product in a breastfeeding woman is remote
L3	Possibly compatible	Drugs without any controlled studies in breastfeeding women, but the risk of untoward effects to an infant is likely, or controlled studies demonstrate only minimal nonthreatening adverse effects. As long as the potential benefits outweigh the potential risks to the infant, drugs should be administered
L4	Possibly hazardous	Positive findings of risk to breast milk production or to a breastfed infant; however, the advantages of use in breastfeeding mothers may be confirmed in spite of the possible risk to the infant (e.g., if the drug is necessary for a critical situation or for a severe disease for which safer drugs are not available)
L5	Hazardous	Major and confirmed risk to the infant. Drug should not be given because the risk justifies any possible benefit

15.10 Frequently Used Drugs for Pain Management

15.10.1 Acetaminophen

Mechanism: Like other NSAIDs, cyclooxygenase (COX) is known to act by inhibiting the COX enzyme, prostaglandin, and thromboxane pathways in the central nervous system. Cyclooxygenase is thought to provide this inhibition by binding on COX3 and not COX 1 and COX 2. However, this pathway has not been demonstrated in humans [76, 77]. Another mechanism is thought to have a stimulating effect on the descending serotonergic pathways in the central nervous system (CNS). Some studies have indicated that acetaminophen or one of its metabolites has an analgesic effect by activating the cannabinoid system [78].

Metabolism: Acetaminophen is metabolized in the liver.

Risk during pregnancy: It is accepted as Category B in FDA pregnancy risk classification.

Risk during breastfeeding: It is considered safe during pregnancy and lactation. Although it is the best option during pregnancy, intermittent use is still recommended because it causes asthma and wheeze in infants [78]. Although it is recommended to avoid regular use during 8–14 weeks of pregnancy due to the risk of cryptorchidism, further studies are needed on this subject [72, 79]. In the literature, there are two cohort studies revealing a relationship between acetaminophen use during pregnancy and increased attention deficit hyperactivity disorder (ADHD) [80]. Disruption of the maternal endocrine system, regulating fetal brain development, by paracetamol used during pregnancy is considered to be the possible cause of ADHA [81]. Paracetamol remains the drug option for the pregnant requiring a simple analgesic when nondrug measures are not effective. The daily dose should not exceed the recommended 4 g/day, and the duration of use should not be extended.

15.10.2 Nonsteroid Anti-inflammatory Drugs (NSAIDs)

Mechanism: Cyclooxygenase (COX 1 and 2) acts as an analgesic anti-inflammatory antipyretic by inhibiting the synthesis of prostaglandins and thromboxanes through enzyme inhibition.

Metabolism: They are hepatically metabolized through CYP450.

Risk during pregnancy: They are accepted as Category C until the third trimester and become Category D in the third trimester.

Risk during breastfeeding: Low-dose aspirin (up to 81 mg/day), ibuprofen, indomethacin, and naproxen are regarded to be safe in lactation [82–84].

All NSAIDs easily cross the placenta. Their safety during pregnancy depends on the timing, dose, and duration of exposure. When used in the first trimester, they may cause birth defects (miscarriage, neural tube defects, pulmonary valve stenosis, limb reduction defects, amniotic bands, and diaphragmatic hernia) [67]. In a controlled study, naproxen used in the first trimester was identified as the cause of oral clefts. Similarly, an increased risk of ventricular septal defects was observed in the first trimester (aspirin, ibuprofen, and naproxen) [85]. The second trimester is relatively safer for NSAIDs, but evidence at the final 2b level identified an association with infant cryptorchism. In the third trimester, the usage of these drugs should be avoided due to the risk of premature closure of ductus arteriosus resulting in the potential of persistent primary hypertension, oligohydramnios caused by decreased fetal renal flow, necrotizing enterocolitis, bleeding disorders during delivery, and intracranial hemorrhage in the mother and newborn [67, 85]. Ibuprofen ranks second after paracetamol as an analgesic and first as an anti-inflammatory until the 28th week of pregnancy. Diclofenac can be considered the second anti-inflammatory agent after ibuprofen. If possible, no NSAI agents should be used after the gestational week. Acetylsalicylic acid should never be the first option, but low-dose aspirin (50–150 mg) can be used throughout the entire pregnancy for necessary (antiphospholipid syndrome, preeclampsia) indications. Long-term use of high doses (500 mg) in the first trimester may result in miscarriage and congenital defects. There are studies demonstrating that its use at the time of conception resulted in miscarriage [86]. An increased risk of gastroschisis has been shown in exposures during the first trimester of pregnancy [87]. Acetylsalicylic acid is also used in assisted reproductive technology (ART)/intracytoplasmic sperm injection (ICSI) from early pregnancy to late pregnancy [88–90]. Acetylsalicylic acid should be avoided during breastfeeding because of the risk of Reye's syndrome.

Cyclooxygenase-2-selective (COX2) NSAIDs are related to impaired fertilization and implantation as well as congenital malformations. Therefore, it is not recommended for use when pregnancy is planned and during pregnancy [85]. COX-2 inhibitors such as rofecoxib, sulindac, ketorolac, and nimesulide are also known to have tocolytic effects [91] (Table 15.5).

15.10.3 Opioid Analgesia

Mechanism: Opioids are found especially in the central nervous system and spinal cord, as well as in organ systems including the gastrointestinal system, cardiovascular system, lung, and bladder. They perform their effects through endogenous opioid receptors (mu, kappa, delta, sigma, epsilon, opioid-like receptor OPL1). Tramadol and methadone are double-acting drugs with both opioid and nonopioid mechanisms. Tramadol serotonin does noradrenaline presynaptic reuptake inhibition (SNRI). Methadone N-methyl-D-aspartate (NMDA) has a receptor antagonist effect.

Risk during pregnancy: Opioids (Category C) are powerful analgesics that can be used for moderate and severe pain in pregnancy. The pregnant mostly use opioids as combined drugs together with analgesics such as acetaminophen or cough medicines [92]. Opioids can rapidly cross the placenta and blood–brain barrier because of their low molecular weight and high lipophilicity and pose a risk to the fetus [93].

Table 15.5 Nonsteroid anti-inflammatory drugs (NSAIDs)

Drugs	Hale's lactation risk category	Briggs breastfeeding recommendation categories	FDA pregnancy risk categories		RID%
Acetaminophen	L1	Compatible	B		10–25% [74]
Aspirin	L3	Potential toxicity	D		9–21% [91]
Diclofenac	L2	Probably compatible	C D	a	1% [75]
Ibuprofen	L1	Compatible	C D	a	0.6% [75]
Indomethacin	L3	Probably compatible	C D	a	0.4% [75]
Ketorolac	L2	Probably compatible	C D	a	0.2–0.4% [91]
Naproxen	L3 or L4	Probably compatible	C D	a	1–3% [91]

Briggs breastfeeding recommendation categories [67]
Hale's lactation risk category [78]
RID relative infant dose [85]
[a] They are accepted as Category C until the third trimester and become Category D in the third trimester

Opioid use, 1 month before pregnancy and in the first trimester, may cause congenital anomalies that affect the CNS [94], congenital heart disease (CHD) [95], premature rupture of membranes, preeclampsia, placental abruption, and fetal death. When opioids are taken in the late stages of pregnancy, depending on the week of gestation in the infant, preterm birth, decreased head circumference, small for gestational age infants, sudden infant death syndrome, congenital heart disease, and abdominal wall defect (gastroschisis) may be encountered. Another important problem is neonatal abstinence syndrome (NAS). NAS is mostly a self-limiting syndrome, which has effects, including gastrointestinal (vomiting, diarrhea, and poor feeding,), autonomic (tachypnea, diaphoresis, and temperature dysregulation), and central nervous system (irritability, tremors, crying, and seizures). It may occur in the first 72 h and last for weeks. Consequently, potential benefits and harms should be compared before opioid analgesic treatment is started [96].

Another opioid-related disease that can be encountered in pregnancy is opioid use disorder (OUD). OUD increases the risk of intrauterine growth restriction, obstetric preterm labor, stillbirth, and maternal death. Moreover, it causes neonatal and long-term childhood problems [97]. Methadone has been the standard medicine for the treatment of opioid addiction in pregnant women [98]. Higher doses, especially in the third trimester, are generally required because of the increased methadone metabolism in pregnancy [99].

Risk during breastfeeding: Although all opioids pass into breast milk in low quantities, opioids in breast milk rarely have toxic effects due to poor oral

Table 15.6 Opioid analgesia

Drugs	Hale's lactation risk category	Briggs breastfeeding recommendationcategory	FDA pregnancy risk categories	RID%
Morphine	L3	Probably compatible	B	2.5–7.5% [96, 101]
Codeine	L3	Potential toxicity	C	0.3–1.2% [96, 101]
Oxycodone	L3	Probably compatible	B	2.6–7.6% [96, 101]
Tramadol	L3		C	2.3% [96, 101]
Fentanyl	L3	Probably compatible	C	1.2% [96, 101]
Hydromorphone	L3	Probably compatible	C	0.7% [96, 101]
Hydrocodone	L3	Potential toxicity	C	1.6–3.7% [96, 101]
Methadone	L3	Compatible	C	1.2–7% [96, 101]
Buprenorphine	L2	Compatible	C	0.4% [96, 101]
Meperidin	L2–L3	Compatible	C	1.4–13.9% [96, 101]

Briggs breastfeeding recommendation categories [68]
RID relative infant dose [85]

absorption in newborns. Morphine should be preferred if opioids are required during breastfeeding. The metabolism of drugs containing codeine may vary due to differences in enzyme levels in individuals. While codeine may be ineffective in enzyme deficiencies, it may also be over-metabolized and affect the infant. For this reason, codeine should not be preferred during breastfeeding [100] (Tables 15.6 and 15.7).

Opioids are not the first-line therapy for mild to moderate pain in the pregnant or general population [102]. With increased clearance, decreased half-life, and rapid transition through the placenta, the pharmacokinetics of morphine are especially affected by pregnancy [103]. Meperidine should not be given in repeated doses as it may cause myoclonus and generalized seizures due to normeperidine, a metabolite with a long half-life (18 h) that accumulates after several doses. Opioids including butorphanol, codeine/acetaminophen, and tramadol/acetaminophen are not more effective than NSAIDs in migraine headaches during pregnancy [104]. Fentanyl patch can be used in the treatment of long-term chronic pain during breastfeeding, provided that the baby is closely monitored for side effects [105].

Low-affinity opioid agonists, including tramadol and tapentadol, are frequently prescribed for pain, partly due to the notion that their potential for abuse and addiction is lower than full opioid agonists [106]. Tramadol is used in

Table 15.7 Equianalgesic doses of different routes of administrations of opioids [92]

Drug	Dose (mg)	Conversion factor
Morphine, oral	30	1
Morphine, i.v., i.m., s.c.	10	0.3
Morphine, epidural	3	0.1
Morphine, intrathecal	0.3	0.01
Oxycodone, oral	20	1.5
Hydromorphone, oral	8	3.75
Methadone, oral	10	0.3
Tramadol, oral	150	0.2
Tramadol, i.v.	100	0.1
Meperidine, i.v.	75	0.13
Fentanyl, i.v.	0.1	100
Sufentanil, i.v.	0.01	1000
Buprenorphine, s.l.	0.3	100

somatic and visceral pain and is likely effective in neuropathic pain. Tramadol, along with its active metabolites, easily crosses the placenta; however, studies evaluating its safety and efficacy in pregnancy are limited. The use of tramadol should be avoided in women with preeclampsia or eclampsia and a high risk of seizures or in women taking other drugs that increase central nervous system serotonin levels.

Tapentadol is a centrally acting analgesic that acts by opioid receptor agonism (MOR) and noradrenaline reuptake inhibition (NRI) [107]. Tapentadol effectively reduces pain, eliminates functional losses, improves the quality of life of the patient, and has a good safety profile, and gastrointestinal tolerability has strengthened its use in chronic pain [108]. There is a lack of sufficient studies evaluating the use of tapentadol in pregnancy. However, this situation will be changed due to the increasing use of tapentadol in the treatment of acute and chronic pain. Although it is not sufficient in terms of safety in pregnant women, no birth defects were observed among women exposed to tapentadol in clinical and safety data-based case studies [109].

15.11 Local Anesthetics

Mechanism: They act by preventing nerve membrane depolarization with sodium channel blockage.

Metabolism: They are almost completely metabolized through the liver (CYP450), about 3% absorbed systemically.

Risk during pregnancy: Lidocaine, 5% lidocaine patches (Category B), prilocaine (Category C), bupivacaine (Category C; fetal bradycardia), mepivacaine (Category C; fetal bradycardia), ropivacaine (Category B).

Low fetal pH compared to maternal pH ion entrapment leads to easy placental transition. Moreover, the high rate of fetal-free drug (low binding protein) theoretically suggests that local anesthetic toxicity is more common in the newborn. However, the mother is more likely to experience toxic side effects before the fetus is affected. It has been shown that fetuses are more resistant to local anesthetic toxicity than adults. The data of multiple studies did not indicate a significant difference in the rate of birth defects for pregnant women exposed to local anesthetics compared to women not exposed [110].

Risk during breastfeeding: Lidocaine is excreted in breast milk; caution needs to be exercised in breastfeeding women.

Lidocaine passes into breast milk in small quantities with a RID of 0.5–3.1% and is rated L2. Bupivacaine has a RID of 0.78–0.9% and is also rated L2 [110]. Local anesthetics are used in pregnant women, central blocks, headache treatment (occipital nerve blocks, trigeminal nerve end bundle blocks, sphenopalatine block), and peripheral nerve blocks in other painful conditions. Lidocaine, bupivacaine, and ropivacaine are safe during pregnancy and breastfeeding. In terms of its overall safety profile, lidocaine ropivacaine is safer than bupivacaine [111], whereas ropivacaine is safer than bupivacaine [112].

15.11.1 Glucocorticoids

They can be used together with local anesthetics in neuraxial block and peripheral nerve block treatment for antirheumatic pain, headache, and other pain during pregnancy. Glucocorticoids are metabolized in the placenta by nonfluorinated glucocorticoids (such as prednisone, prednisolone, hydrocortisone, methylprednisone, and methylprednisolone) and 11-β-hydroxysteroid dehydrogenase enzyme and are compatible with pregnancy since less than 10% reaches the fetus [113].

Prednisolone is compatible with each trimester of pregnancy, breastfeeding, and paternal exposure. Similar to prednisolone, methylprednisolone has rates of placental transfer with equivalent anti-inflammatory effects at 79% of the prednisolone dose. Therefore, it should be compatible with pregnancy, breastfeeding, and paternal exposure [114].

Fluorinated steroids (betamethasone and dexamethasone) are metabolized at a much lower rate, and fluticasone has accelerating effects on fetal lung development as it passes through the placental barrier without being metabolized. It should not be used to treat pain during pregnancy [115]. Steroids are safe for short-term use; if used continuously or in the first trimester, the risk of cleft lip or cleft palate and low birth weight increases. The risk of hypoadrenalism in babies born to mothers using steroids should be considered [116] (Table 15.8).

Table 15.8 American Academy of Pediatrics (AAP)

Agent	FDA pregnancy category	Lactation category	Advice of AAP
Lidocaine	B	L2	Compatible
Prilocaine	B	Unknown	Unknown
Bupivacaine	C	L2	Unknown
Prednisolon	B	L2	Compatible
Methylprednisolone	B	L2 (except for long-term high dosage)	Compatible
Triamcinolone	C	L3 (not reported via milk)	Unknown
Dexamethasone	C	L3 (avoid high doses)	Unknown
Betamethasone	C	L3 (none reported)	Unknown
Botulinum toxin	C	Unknown	Unknown

15.12 Anticonvulsants

15.12.1 Pregabaline–Gabapentine

Mechanism: It is a structural analog of GABA; it acts by binding to the voltage-gated calcium channel alpha2-delta subunit by reducing presynaptic depolarization and excitatory neurotransmitters (glutamate, noradrenaline, and substance P).

Metabolism: Renal excretion without being metabolized.

Risk during pregnancy: Category C.

Although there are not enough studies, the fact that pregabalin increases major birth defect suggests that it should be used carefully in women of childbearing age. Gabapentin is related to craniofacial abnormalities, neural tube defects, and mental disability. When used in mandatory indications, the fetus should be followed-up closely [117].

Risk during breastfeeding: It is not known whether it is excreted in breast milk. It is advised to discontinue receiving the medication or bottle-feed. The infant should be followed up for adverse effects if the mother continues to take the medication while breastfeeding [118]. Low levels of the drug were found in the serum of babies of mothers who used gabapentin up to 2.1 g/day. A single oral dose of 300 or 600 mg given to the mother prior to cesarean section had no effect on breastfeeding initiation [119].

15.12.2 Topiramat

Mechanism: GABA (A) receptor augmentation and sodium channel blocker.

Metabolism: Renally excreted.

Risk during pregnancy: Category C.

Risk during breastfeeding: Highly recommended to discontinue medication before breastfeeding or bottle-feed.

15.12.3 Carbamazepine

Mechanism: It reacts with sodium channels inhibiting the release of glutamate.

Risk during pregnancy: Category D studies on mice have demonstrated a large number of fetuses with congenital defects of the CNS or urogenital system. Usage during pregnancy may lead to neural tube defects.

Risk during breastfeeding: Carbamazepine has relatively high levels in breast milk, and breastfed infants have measurable serum levels, but they are mostly below the antiepileptic therapeutic range. The medication or bottle-feed should be stopped. The infant should be monitored for adverse effects if the mother continues to take the medication while breastfeeding [119].

15.12.4 Antidepressants

Mechanism: Tricyclic antidepressants (TCAs) (amitriptylin, nortriyptilin, imipramine) act on serotonin-noradrenaline presynaptic reuptake inhibition, N-methyl-D-aspartate (NMDA) receptor inhibition, and an increasing mechanism of postsynaptic 5HT1A serotonin receptor sensitivity.

SSRI (selective serotonin reuptake inhibitor): Paroxetine, fluoxetine, and escitalopram.

SNRI (serotonin-noradrenaline presynaptic reuptake inhibitor): Venlafaxine and duloxetine.

Tricyclic antidepressants (TCAs) make sodium (Na+) channel blockade by modulating inhibitory descending pathways with serotonin-noradrenaline presynaptic reuptake inhibition. This causes suppression of peripheral sensitization and reduction in pain.

Metabolism: Hepatic metabolism via CYP 1A2 and CYP 2D6 isoenzymes.

Risk during pregnancy: Antidepressants are often used as adjuvant agents in the analgesic treatment of chronic pain or as primary treatment for concomitant depression. Although there are few studies examining the safety and efficacy of antidepressants for pregnant women with chronic pain, the studies contain reassuring information regarding use in pregnancy [120]. Antidepressant agents are important in terms of continuing the treatment used for neuropathic pain before pregnancy or adding to the treatment of neuropathic pain that occurs during pregnancy. For women who regularly take antidepressants, abrupt discontinuation can accelerate discontinuation syndrome and increase pain perception through stress and anxiety [121].

Developmental delay and limb abnormalities were reported when amitriptyline was taken in early pregnancy. When taken in the third trimester, it can lead to cardiac problems, irritability, respiratory distress, muscle spasms, urinary retention, seizures, and withdrawal symptoms. Some studies have demonstrated a small increase in the risk of cardiovascular malformations in women who were treated with certain SSRIs such as sertraline, paroxetine, and fluoxetine in early pregnancy although this has not been demonstrated in subsequent systematic reviews and meta-analyzes [122–124]. Approximately 20% of newborns have a risk of postnatal adaptation syndrome (PNAS), involving cyanosis, respiratory distress, apnea, feeding difficulties, temperature instability, vomiting, hypoglycemia, hypotonia or hypertonia, jitteriness, persistent crying, and hyper-reflexia. However, the symptoms of postnatal adaptation syndrome (PNAS) are usually mild and disappear spontaneously in most newborns [125]. While the prenatal exposure of venlafaxine, the SNRI, may be regarded as relatively safe for neonates, data on duloxetine are too little to draw a conclusion [126]. Neonatal withdrawal syndrome and serotoninergic syndrome were observed in the babies of mothers who used duloxetine, but studies are not sufficient for reliability in pregnant women [127].

Risk during breastfeeding: Amitriptyline passes very little into breast milk and is found in the plasma and urine of breastfed children. No side effects have been reported. Therefore, it can be considered safe in breastfeeding [128]. Paroxetine levels in breast milk are low and have not been detected in the serum of most breastfed babies. It is one of the antidepressant options during breastfeeding [129]. Levels of escitalopram in breast milk are low or largely undetectable and well tolerated by breastfed infants. Transfer of sertraline to a breastfed infant is minimal, and no significant adverse effects have been reported. Sertraline is considered one of the antidepressant options during breastfeeding (Hale's L2). Breastfed babies of mothers receiving venlafaxine should be monitored for excessive sedation and adequate weight gain, especially if they are newborns or preterm. Newborn babies of mothers taking the drug during pregnancy may experience neonatal withdrawal syndrome [130]. An infant who is breastfed by a mother taking duloxetine requires monitoring for behavioral changes, sleep disturbance, feeding changes, growth, and neurodevelopment [131].

15.12.5 Triptanes and Ergot Alkaloids

Triptans bind to serotonin receptors as serotonin (5-hydroxytryptamine) (5-HT) agonists in acute treatments of migraine-type headaches and act as neural inhibitors and vasoconstrictors [132]. Dihydroergotamine (DHE) is a semi-synthetic and hydrogenated ergot alkaloid, and, like triptans, they act through the 5HT1D, 5HT1B, and 5HT1F receptors. Ergots (FDA Category X) should be avoided during pregnancy due to their effects on the uterus. On the contrary, triptans are considerably safer during pregnancy. An observational study established no link between sumatriptan used in the first trimester (528 pregnancies) and teratogenicity or negative pregnancy outcomes [133]. For triptans, the relationship between sumatriptan and the risks of low birth weight, preterm delivery, and minor fetal anomalies expected during pregnancy could not be proven, while this risk is higher for eletriptan and frovatriptan. This information suggests that sumatriptan can be used more safely during pregnancy [134]. Despite the controversy, sumatriptan may be considered during pregnancy, especially for patients with migraines accompanied by severe nausea and vomiting that are functionally prohibitive or cause maternal dehydration [103, 134]. Since the level exposing the baby of the mother using sumatriptan is relatively low in infant dose and oral bioavailability, this drug is considered to be safe during breastfeeding [135].

15.12.6 Neuroleptics (Dopamine Antagonists)

Other drugs used in the acute treatment of migraine headaches in nonpregnant women phenothiazines (prochlorperazine, chlorpromazine, promethazine), butyrophenones (droperidol, haloperidol), and metoclopramide. Metoclopramide can be prescribed for pregnant women with acute migraine headaches in addition to NSAIDs or triptans to prevent nausea and vomiting. Metoclopramide is compatible with breastfeeding and also increases prolactin levels. Therefore, it is sometimes used as a galactagogue to stimulate milk production [136]. Although the risk of fetal malformation related to promethazine has not been demonstrated, platelet aggregation inhibition, irritability, or extrapyramidal effects have been shown in infants up to 2 weeks before birth. Although no fetal malformation has been demonstrated in prochlorperazine use, there is a risk of jaundice, reflex changes, extrapyramidal symptoms, and potentially severe withdrawal effects when received in the third trimester. Diphenhydramine, which is frequently used with phenothiazines to reduce extrapyramidal side effects, has not been shown to have a risk of fetal malformation, but it may cause neonatal withdrawal in the third-trimester use. Since promethazine and diphenhydramine reduce milk production, prochlorperazine is not recommended for breastfeeding due to the risk of sedation and apnea in the baby [136, 137] (Table 15.9).

15.12.7 Muscle Relaxants

Baclofen GABA (B) agonist. It prevents mono- and polysynaptic spinal reflexes. When taken orally, it is also associated with fetal malformations such as omphalocele. When administered intrathecally, it appears to have a low concentration in breast milk and to have no side effects on the fetus [142].

Cyclobenzaprine is considered safe during pregnancy. This drug is used in pregnant women. Despite a report of early closure of ductus arteriosus, approximately 50% of the drug passes into breast milk during breastfeeding [143].

Thiocolchicoside is a commonly used muscle relaxant in the treatment of acute painful muscle spasms. This drug is contraindicated in children less than 16 years of age during pregnancy and breastfeeding [144] (Table 15.10).

15.12.8 Interventional Analgesics in Pregnancy and Lactation

The presence of the fetus in the treatment of acute or chronic pain during pregnancy causes concerns due to the risk of teratogenicity. Therefore, nonpharmacological treatments are considered first, and medical treatments are planned in the

Table 15.9 Anticonvulsants drugs

Drugs	Hale's lactation risk category	Briggs breastfeeding recommendation category	FDA pregnancy risk categories	RID%
Anticonvulsants				
Gabapentin	**L2**	Probably compatible	C	1.3–6.6 [138]
Pregabalin	**L3**	Potential toxicity	C	7 [139]
Topiramate	**L3**	Potential toxicity	C	**24.5** [110, 138]
Carbamazepine	**L2**	Probably compatible	D	**3.8–5.9** [74]
Antidepressants				
Amitriptyline	**L2**	Potential toxicity	C	1.9–2.8 [110]
Fluoxetine	**L2**	Potential toxicity	C	0.8–16.3 [140]
Paroxetine	**L2**	Potential toxicity	C	1.2–2.8 [75]
Escitalopram	**L2**	Potential toxicity	C	5.2–7.9 [75]
Sertraline	**L2**	Potential toxicity	C	0.4–2.2 [75]
Venlafaxine	**L3**	Potential toxicity	C	3.5–9.2 [140]
Duloxetine	**L3**	Potential toxicity	C	**0.1** [140]
Neuroleptics				
Metoclopramide	**L2**	Potential toxicity	B	4.7–14.3 [110]
Promethazine	**L2**	Probably compatible	C	
Prochlorperazine	**L2**	Potential toxicity	C	
Ergots (dihydroergotamine, ergotamine)	**L3**	Potentially hazardous	X	
Triptans	L3		C	
Eletriptan	L2	Compatible	C	0.02 [110, 141]
Sumatriptan	L3	Probably compatible	C	3.5–15.3 [75, 141]
Frovatriptan	L3	Probably compatible	C	**NR** [141]
Zolmitriptan	L3	Probably compatible	C	**NR** [141]
Vitamin B12	**L1**	Compatible	C	
Magnesium	**L1**	Compatible	B	**0.17**
Diphenhydramin	**L2**	Probably compatible		0.7–1.4 [74]

NR not reported

Table 15.10 Muscle relaxants drugs

Drugs	FDA pregnacy classification	Risk during breastfeeding
Cyclobenzaprine	Category B	Not known if it is excreted in breast milk
Baklofen	Category C	Oral baclofen is excreted in breast milk and should not be used
Tizanidine	Category C	Not known if it is excreted in breast milk
Methocarbamol	Category C	Excreted in breast milk
Metaxalone	Category B	Not known if it is excreted in breast milk
Carisoprodol	Category C	Drug is excreted in breast milk and can cause sedation
Chlorzoxazone	Category C	Not known if excreted in breast milk; safety advised

second line in pain that is common during pregnancy. However, with its rapid onset and long duration of action, interventional analgesia is desired to be used in pregnant women, but the lack of sufficient scientific data causes abstention in cases.

In cases of PLBP (pregnancy-related low back pain), PGP (pregnancy-related pelvic girdle pain), symphysis pubis dysfunction, lumbar radiculopathy, musculoskeletal pain, and neuropathic pain, which are common during pregnancy, interventional treatments can be planned in order not to use drugs or to reduce the doses of drugs when no response is obtained despite all conservative and medical treatments. Although fluoroscopy is used in interventional treatments except in pregnancy, it is contraindicated in pregnant women. Blind injections via anatomical points, magnetic resonance imaging (MRI)-guided injections, and ultrasound are safer. Since blind injections have the risk of complications and magnetic resonance imaging (MRI) is not cost effective, ultrasound blocks are considered the most ideal method in terms of safety and cost [145].

Using ultrasound, interlaminar epidural steroid injection (ILESI), ganglion impar and sacrococcygeal ligament injection, diagnostic or therapeutic sacroiliac joint injection, caudal epidural steroid injection, symphysis pubis injection, therapeutic intra-articular zygapophysial joint injection, and lumbar diagnostic medial branch injection can be performed. Although there are case reports showing injections such as intercostal block, lateral femoral cutaneous nerve block [145], carpal tunnel block [146], ultrasound-guided erector spinae plane block [147], intra-articular injections, and trigger point injections, more data are needed [148–153].

Spinal cord stimulation (SCS), another invasive procedure, is a neuromodulation method used in chronic pain syndromes. Although cases have been presented showing that SCS is a suitable option for chronic pain management during pregnancy for women with CRPS (complex regional pain syndrome), information on this issue is not yet sufficient [154, 155].

15.13 Physical Therapy

Postural techniques and physical therapy, manual therapy, water therapy, transcutaneous nerve stimulation, stabilization belts, yoga, osteopathic manipulative treatment (OMT), cognitive behavioral therapy, biofeedback, and chiropractic care can be performed [156].

15.14 Acupuncture

Acupuncture is considered to be beneficial in muscle skeletal pain in pregnancy, avoiding uterine and cervical reference points in order not to trigger labor. Acupuncture also seems to be effective in the management of tension headache [157, 158].

15.15 Botulinum Toxin

Data on botulinum toxin during pregnancy are mostly related to women who received it without being aware of the pregnancy. Despite limited data, no congenital anomaly has been reported in the first trimester use [159, 160].

References

1. Raja SN, Carr DB, Cohen M, Finnerup NB, Flor H, Gibson S, et al. The revised International Association for the Study of Pain definition of pain: concepts, challenges, and compromises. Pain. 2020;161(9):1976–82.
2. Hall JE, Hall ME. Guyton and Hall textbook of medical physiology e-book. Elsevier Health Sciences; 2020.
3. Monteiro R, Salman M, Yentis S, Malhotra S. Analgesia, anaesthesia and pregnancy: a practical guide. Cambridge: Cambridge University Press; 2019.
4. Phung J, Paul J, Smith R. Maintenance of pregnancy and parturition. In: Maternal-fetal and neonatal endocrinology. Cambridge: Academic; 2020. p. 169–87.
5. Feghali M, Venkataramanan R, Caritis S. Pharmacokinetics of drugs in pregnancy. Semin Perinatol. 2015;39:512–9.
6. Tal R, Taylor HS, Burney RO, Mooney SB, Giudice LC. Endocrinology of pregnancy. In: Endotext [Internet]. MDText.com; 2015
7. Di Renzo GC, Giardina I, Clerici G, Brillo E, Gerli S. Progesterone in normal and pathological pregnancy. Horm Mol Biol Clin Invest. 2016;27(1):35–48.
8. Talbot L, Maclennan K. Physiology of pregnancy. Anaesth Intensive Care Med. 2016;17(7):341–5.
9. Dekkers GW, Broeren MA, Truijens SE, Kop WJ, Pop VJ. Hormonal and psychological factors in nausea and vomiting during pregnancy. Psychol Med. 2020;50(2):229–36.
10. Mohamadi S, Garkaz O, Abolhassani M, Bolbol Haghighi N. The relationship of nausea and vomiting during pregnancy with pregnancy complications. J Midwifery Reprod Health. 2020;8(3):1–7.

11. Manji Z, Figueroa AD. Pregnancy. In: Oral board review for oral and maxillofacial surgery. Cham: Springer. p. 459–63.
12. Erden V, Yangn Z, Erkalp K, Delatioglu H, Bahçeci F, Seyhan A. Increased progesterone production during the luteal phase of menstruation may decrease anesthetic requirement. Anesth Analg. 2005;101(4):1007–11.
13. Carvalho B, Angst MS, Fuller AJ, Lin E, Mathusamy AD, Riley ET. Experimental heat pain for detecting pregnancy-induced analgesia in humans. Anesth Analg. 2006;103(5):1283–7.
14. Draisci G, Catarci S, Vollono C, Zanfini BA, Pazzaglia C, Cadeddu C, et al. Pregnancy-induced analgesia: a combined psychophysical and neurophysiological study. Eur J Pain. 2012;16(10):1389–97.
15. Kashanian M, Dadkhah F, Zarei S, Sheikhansari N, Javanmanesh F. Evaluation the relationship between serum progesterone level and pain perception after cesarean delivery. J Matern Fetal Neonatal Med. 2019;32(21):3548–51.
16. Grant LK, Gooley JJ, St Hilaire MA, Rajaratnam SM, Brainard GC, Czeisler CA, et al. Menstrual phase-dependent differences in neurobehavioral performance: the role of temperature and the progesterone/estradiol ratio. Sleep. 2020;43(2):zsz227.
17. Chesnutt AN. Physiology of normal pregnancy. Crit Care Clin. 2004;20(4):609–15.
18. Tan EK, Tan EL. Alterations in physiology and anatomy during pregnancy. Best Pract Res Clin Obstet Gynaecol. 2013;27(6):791–802.
19. Wiegel RE, Jan Danser AH, Steegers-Theunissen RP, Laven JS, Willemsen SP, Baker VL, et al. Determinants of maternal renin-angiotensin-aldosterone-system activation in early pregnancy: insights from 2 cohorts. J Clin Endocrinol Metabol. 2020;105(11):3505–17.
20. Lumbers ER. The physiological roles of the renin-angiotensin aldosterone system and vasopressin in human pregnancy. In: Maternal-fetal and neonatal endocrinology. Cambridge: Academic; 2020. p. 129–45.
21. Ren S, Gao Y, Yang Z, Li J, Xuan R, Liu J, et al. The effect of pelvic floor muscle training on pelvic floor dysfunction in pregnant and postpartum women. Phys Act Health. 2020;4(1):130–41.
22. Bai J, Qi QR, Li Y, Day R, Makhoul J, Magness RR, Chen DB. Estrogen receptors and estrogen-induced uterine vasodilation in pregnancy. Int J Mol Sci. 2020;21(12):4349.
23. Casagrande D, Gugala Z, Clark SM, Lindsey RW. Low back pain and pelvic girdle pain in pregnancy. J Am Acad Orthop Surg. 2015;23(9):539–49.
24. Sel G. Physiological changes during pregnancy. In: Practical guide to oral exams in obstetrics and gynecology. Cham: Springer; 2020. p. 29–37.
25. Spiegelman J, Meng ML, Haythe J, Goffman D. Cardiovascular physiology of pregnancy and clinical implications. In: Cardio-obstetrics: a practical guide to care for pregnant cardiac patients; 2020.
26. Soma-Pillay P, Nelson-Piercy C, Tolppanen H, Mebazaa A. Physiological changes in pregnancy. Cardiovasc J Afr. 2016;27(2):89–94.
27. Liu S, Jassal DS, Zelop CM. Cardiovascular changes in pregnancy. In: Principles and practice of maternal critical care, 2020. pp. 101–108.
28. Cordina R, McGuire MA. Maternal cardiac arrhythmias during pregnancy and lactation. Obstet Med. 2010;3(1):8–16.
29. Kepley JM, Bates K, Mohiuddin SS. Physiology, maternal changes. StatPearls [Internet]; 2020.
30. LoMauro A, Aliverti A. Respiratory physiology of pregnancy: physiology masterclass. Breathe (Sheff). 2015;11(4):297–301.
31. Roca GQ, Anyaso J, Redline S, Bello NA. Associations between sleep disorders and hypertensive disorders of pregnancy and materno-fetal consequences. Curr Hypertens Rep. 2020;22(8):1–9.
32. Garbazza C, Hackethal S, Riccardi S, Cajochen C, Cicolin A, D'Agostino A, et al. Polysomnographic features of pregnancy: a systematic review. Sleep Med Rev. 2020;50:101249.
33. Rodger M, Sheppard D, Gándara E, Tinmouth A. Haematological problems in obstetrics. Best Pract Res Clin Obstet Gynaecol. 2015;29(5):671–84.

34. Barrett JF, Whittaker PG, Williams JG, Lind T. Absorption of non-haem iron from food during normal pregnancy. BMJ. 1994;309(6947):79–82.
35. Ramarao K, Guptha CSJ, Mohammed AM, Mohammed SUR, Ahmed SM, Nayak SS. Evaluation of physiological changes and pharmacokinetic variations in pregnancy condition. OSP J Health Care Med. 2020;1(3):1–5.
36. Lumbers ER, Pringle KG. Roles of the circulating renin-angiotensin-aldosterone system in human pregnancy. Am J Phys Regul Integr Comp Phys. 2014;306(2):R91–R101.
37. Odutayo A, Hladunewich M. Obstetric nephrology: renal hemodynamic and metabolic physiology in normal pregnancy. Clin J Am Soc Nephrol. 2012;7(12):2073–80.
38. Zielinski R, Searing K, Deibel M. Gastrointestinal distress in pregnancy. J Perinat Neonatal Nurs. 2015;29(1):23–31.
39. Costantine M. Physiologic and pharmacokinetic changes in pregnancy. Front Pharmacol. 2014;5:65.
40. Anderson GD. Pregnancy-induced changes in pharmacokinetics. Clin Pharmacokinet. 2005;44(10):989–1008.
41. Yadava SM. Normal physiology of pregnancy. Ob/Gyn Secrets E-Book. 2016. 149.
42. Frederiksen MC. Physiologic changes in pregnancy and their effect on drug disposition. In: Seminars in perinatology, vol. 25, no. 3. Philadelphia: WB Saunders; 2001. pp. 120–123.
43. Kazma JM, van den Anker J, Allegaert K, Dallmann A, Ahmadzia HK. Anatomical and physiological alterations of pregnancy. J Pharmacokinet Pharmacodyn. 2020;47(4):271–85.
44. Stika SC, Frederiksen MC. Drug therapy in pregnant and nursing women. In: Atkinson AJ, Abernethy DR, Daniels CE, Dedrick RL, Markey SP, editors. Principles of clinical pharmacology. 2007.
45. Katzung BG. Basic and clinical pharmacology. New York: McGraw Hill; 2012.
46. Dawes M, Chowienczyk PJ. Pharmacokinetics in pregnancy. Best Pract Res Clin Obstet Gynaecol. 2001;15(6):819–26.
47. Zhao Y, Hebert MF, Venkataramanan R. Basic obstetric pharmacology. In: Seminars in perinatology, vol. 38, no. 8. Philadelphia: WB Saunders; 2014. pp. 475–486.
48. Avram MJ. Pharmacokinetic studies in pregnancy. In: Seminars in perinatology, vol. 44, no. 3. Philadelphia: WB Saunders; 2020. p. 151227.
49. Anger GJ, Piquette-Miller M. Pharmacokinetic studies in pregnant women. Clin Pharmacol Therap. 2008;83(1):184–7.
50. Syme MR, Paxton JW, Keelan JA. Drug transfer and metabolism by the human placenta. Clin Pharmacokinet. 2004;43(8):487–514.
51. Wunsch MJ, Stanard V, Schnoll SH. Treatment of pain in pregnancy. Clin J Pain. 2003;19(3):148–55.
52. Della-Giustina K, Chow G. Medications in pregnancy and lactation. Emerg Med Clin North Am. 2003;21(3):585.
53. Gude NM, Roberts CT, Kalionis B, King RG. Growth and function of the normal human placenta. Thromb Res. 2004;114(5–6):397–407.
54. Anderson PO, Sauberan JB. Modeling drug passage into human milk. Clin Pharmacol Therap. 2016;100(1):42–52.
55. Sherlie VS, Varghese A. ENT changes of pregnancy and its management. Indian J Otolaryngol Head Neck Surg. 2014;66(1):6–9.
56. Bhagat DR, Chowdhary A, Verma S. Physiological changes in ENT during pregnancy. Indian J Otolaryngol Head Neck Surg. 2006;57(3):268–70.
57. Sharma K, Sharma S, Chander D. Evaluation of audio-rhinological changes during pregnancy. Indian J Otolaryngol Head Neck Surg. 2011;63(1):74–8.
58. Goh AY, Hussain SSM. Sudden hearing loss and pregnancy: a review. J Laryngol Otol. 2012;126(4):337.
59. Xie S, Wu X. Clinical management and progress in sudden sensorineural hearing loss during pregnancy. J Int Med Res. 2020;48(2):0300060519870718.
60. Wang YP, Young YH. Experience in the treatment of sudden deafness during pregnancy. Acta Otolaryngol. 2006;126(3):271–6.

61. Yin T, Huang F, Ren J, Liu W, Chen X, Li L, et al. Bilateral sudden hearing loss following habitual abortion: a case report and review of literature. Int J Clin Exp Med. 2013;6(8):720.
62. Zeng XL, He JC, Li P. Sudden sensorineural hearing loss during pregnancy: a 21 cases report. Chin J Otol Chinese. 2014;12:207–10.
63. Wiles NM, Hunt BJ, Callanan V, Chevretton EB. Sudden sensorineural hearing loss and antiphospholipid syndrome. Haematologica. 2006;91(12 Suppl):ECR46.
64. John T, Spong Catherine Y. Management of high-risk pregnancy: an evidence-based approach. Hoboken: Blackwell Publishing; 2007.
65. Shepard TH, Lemire RJ. Catalog of teratogenic agents. Baltimore: JHU Press; 2004.
66. Cabrera RM, Hill DS, Etheredge AJ, Finnell RH. Investigations into the etiology of neural tube defects. Birth Defects Res C Embryo Today. 2004;72(4):330–44.
67. Antonucci R, Zaffanello M, Puxeddu E, Porcella A, Cuzzolin L, Dolores Pilloni M, Fanos V. Use of non-steroidal anti-inflammatory drugs in pregnancy: impact on the fetus and newborn. Curr Drug Metab. 2012;13(4):474–90.
68. Leek JC, Arif H. Pregnancy medications; 2019.
69. Pernia S, DeMaagd G. The new pregnancy and lactation labeling rule. Pharm Therap. 2016;41(11):713.
70. Fantasia HC, Harris AL. Changes to pregnancy and lactation risk labeling for prescription drugs. Nurs Womens Health. 2015;19(3):266–70.
71. Hale TW. Maternal medications during breastfeeding. Clin Obstet Gynecol. 2004;47(3):696–711.
72. Ostrea EM, Mantaring JB, Silvestre MA. Drugs that affect the fetus and newborn infant via the placenta or breast milk. Pediatr Clin. 2004;51(3):539–79.
73. Verstegen RH, Anderson PO, Ito S. Infant drug exposure via breast milk. Br J Clin Pharmacol. 2020;
74. Newton ER, Hale TW. Drugs in breast milk. Clin Obstet Gynecol. 2015;58(4):868–84.
75. Chandrasekharan NV, Dai H, Roos KLT, Evanson NK, Tomsik J, Elton TS, Simmons DL. COX-3, a cyclooxygenase-1 variant inhibited by acetaminophen and other analgesic/antipyretic drugs: cloning, structure, and expression. Proc Natl Acad Sci U S A. 2002;99(21):13926–31.
76. Ilett KF, Kristensen JH. Drug use and breastfeeding. Expert Opin Drug Saf. 2005;4(4):745–68.
77. Hutchinson S, Marmura MJ, Calhoun A, Lucas S, Silberstein S, Peterlin BL. Use of common migraine treatments in breast-feeding women: a summary of recommendations. Headache. 2013;53(4):614–27.
78. Gerriets V, Anderson J, Nappe TM. Acetaminophen. StatPearls [Internet]; 2020.
79. Magnus MC, Karlstad Ø, Håberg SE, Nafstad P, Davey Smith G, Nystad W. Prenatal and infant paracetamol exposure and development of asthma: the Norwegian mother and child cohort study. Int J Epidemiol. 2016;45(2):512–22.
80. Souza AMD, Menezes SL. Safe use of analgesics in pregnancy. In: Nitte Gulabi Shetty Memorial Institute of Pharmaceutical Sciences, 4.
81. Liew Z, Ritz B, Virk J, Olsen J. Maternal use of acetaminophen during pregnancy and risk of autism spectrum disorders in childhood: AD Anish National Birth Cohort Study. Autism Res. 2016;9(9):951–8.
82. Pangtey GS, Agarwal N. Nonsteroidal anti-inflammatory drug use during pregnancy and lactation: effects on mother and child. In: Women's health in autoimmune diseases. Singapore: Springer; 2020. p. 215–9.
83. Dharmanand BG. Fibromiyalji. Gelen *Kadın Sağlığı Otoimmun Hastalıklar*. Singapur, Springer; 2020. s. 269–278.
84. Adams K, Bombardier C, van der Heijde DM. Safety of pain therapy during pregnancy and lactation in patients with inflammatory arthritis: a systematic literature review. J Rheumatol Suppl. 2012;90:59–61.
85. Ericson A, Källén BA. Nonsteroidal anti-inflammatory drugs in early pregnancy. Reprod Toxicol. 2001;15(4):371–5.

86. Li DK, Ferber JR, Odouli R, Quesenberry C. Use of nonsteroidal antiinflammatory drugs during pregnancy and the risk of miscarriage. Am J Obstet Gynecol. 2018;219(3):275.e1–8.

87. Kozer E, Nikfar S, Costei A, Boskovic R, Nulman I, Koren G. Aspirin consumption during the first trimester of pregnancy and congenital anomalies: a meta-analysis. Am J Obstet Gynecol. 2002;187(6):1623–30.

88. Berliana A. Aspirin Dosis Rendah untuk Mencegah Preeklamsia pada Kehamilan. Jurnal Ilmiah Kesehatan Sandi Husada. 2020;12(2):1029–36.

89. Massimo R, Irene C, Elena R, Grazietta FS, Alice B, Elisa M, et al. Treatment of antiphospholipid syndrome. Clin Immunol. 2020;221:108597.

90. Wang L, Huang X, Li X, Lv F, He X, Pan Y, et al. Efficacy evaluation of low-dose aspirin in IVF/ICSI patients evidence from 13 RCTs: a systematic review and meta-analysis. Medicine. 2017;96(37):e7720.

91. Bloor M, Paech M. Nonsteroidal anti-inflammatory drugs during pregnancy and the initiation of lactation. Anesth Analg. 2013;116(5):1063–75.

92. Tobon AL, Habecker E, Forray A. Opioid use in pregnancy. Curr Psychiatry Rep. 2019;21(12):118.

93. Chan F, Koren G. Is periconceptional opioid use safe? Can Fam Physician. 2015;61(5):431–3.

94. Tosounidou S, Gordon C. Medications in pregnancy and breastfeeding. Best Pract Res Clin Obstet Gynaecol. 2020;64:68–76.

95. Broussard CS, Rasmussen SA, Reefhuis J, Friedman JM, Jann MW, Riehle-Colarusso T, et al. Maternal treatment with opioid analgesics and risk for birth defects. Am J Obstet Gynecol. 2011;204(4):314.e1–314.e11.

96. Zipursky J, Juurlink DN. Opioid use in pregnancy: an emerging health crisis. Obstet Med. 2021;14(4):211–9.

97. Maeda A, Bateman BT, Clancy CR, Creanga AA, Leffert LR. Opioid abuse and dependence during pregnancy temporal trends and obstetrical outcomes. J Am Soc Anesthesiol. 2014;121(6):1158–65.

98. Jumah NA, Graves L, Kahan M. The management of opioid dependence during pregnancy in rural and remote settings. CMAJ. 2015;187(1):E41–6.

99. Fullerton CA, Kim M, Thomas CP, Lyman DR, Montejano LB, Dougherty RH, et al. Medication-assisted treatment with methadone: assessing the evidence. Psychiatr Serv. 2014;65(2):146–57.

100. Hendrickson RG, McKeown NJ. Is maternal opioid use hazardous to breast-fed infants? 2012.

101. Zipursky J, Juurlink DN. The implausibility of neonatal opioid toxicity from breastfeeding. Clin Pharm Therap. 2020;108(5):964–70.

102. Flood P, Raja SN. Balance in opioid prescription during pregnancy. Anesthesiology. 2014;120(5):1063–4.

103. Pritham UA, McKay L. Safe management of chronic pain in pregnancy in an era of opioid misuse and abuse. J Obstet Gynecol Neonatal Nurs. 2014;43(5):554–67.

104. Ong JJY, De Felice M. Migraine treatment: current acute medications and their potential mechanisms of action. Neurotherapeutics. 2018;15(2):274–90.

105. Cohen RS. Fentanyl transdermal analgesia during pregnancy and lactation. J Hum Lact. 2009;25(3):359–61.

106. Nagpal G, Rathmell JP. Chapter 35. Practical management of pain. Philadelphia: Mosby; 2014. pp. 474–491.

107. Tzschentke TM, Christoph T, Kögel BY. The mu-opioid receptor agonist/noradrenaline reuptake inhibition (MOR–NRI) concept in analgesia: the case of tapentadol. CNS Drugs. 2014;28(4):319–29.

108. Baron R, Eberhart L, Kern KU, Regner S, Rolke R, Simanski C, Tölle T. Tapentadol prolonged release for chronic pain: a review of clinical trials and 5 years of routine clinical practice data. Pain Pract. 2017;17(5):678–700.

109. Stollenwerk A, Sohns M, Heisig F, Elling C, von Zabern D. Review of post-marketing safety data on tapentadol, a centrally acting analgesic. Adv Ther. 2018;35(1):12–30.

110. Wells RE, Turner DP, Lee M, Bishop L, Strauss L. Managing migraine during pregnancy and lactation. Curr Neurol Neurosci Rep. 2016;16(4):40.
111. Lee JM, Shin TJ. Use of local anesthetics for dental treatment during pregnancy; safety for parturient. J Dental Anesth Pain Med. 2017;17(2):81–90.
112. Hansen TG. Ropivacaine: a pharmacological review. Expert Rev Neurother. 2004;4(5):781–91.
113. Skorpen CG, Hoeltzenbein M, Tincani A, Fischer-Betz R, Elefant E, Chambers C, et al. The EULAR points to consider for use of antirheumatic drugs before pregnancy, and during pregnancy and lactation. Ann Rheum Dis. 2016;75(5):795–810.
114. Heilskov S, Deleuran MS, Vestergaard C. Immunosuppressive and immunomodulating therapy for atopic dermatitis in pregnancy: an appraisal of the literature. Dermatol Ther. 2020;10(6):1215–28.
115. Blumenfeld A, Ashkenazi A, Grosberg B, Napchan U, Narouze S, Nett B, et al. Patterns of use of peripheral nerve blocks and trigger point injections among headache practitioners in the USA: results of the American Headache Society Interventional Procedure Survey (AHS-IPS). Headache. 2010;50(6):937–94.
116. Temprano KK, Bandlamudi R, Moore TL. Antirheumatic drugs in pregnancy and lactation. In: Seminars in arthritis and rheumatism, vol. 35. 2005.
117. Winterfeld U, Merlob P, Baud D, Rousson V, Panchaud A, Rothuizen LE, et al. Pregnancy outcome following maternal exposure to pregabalin may call for concern. Neurology. 2016;86(24):2251–7.
118. Cross AL, Viswanath O. Pregabalin. StatPearls [Internet]; 2020.
119. Anderson PO. Antiepileptic drugs during breastfeeding. Breastfeed Med. 2020;15(1):2–4.
120. Källén B, Reis M. Ongoing pharmacological management of chronic pain in pregnancy. Drugs. 2016;76(9):915–24.
121. Pariante CM, Seneviratne G, Howard L. Should we stop using tricyclic antidepressants in pregnancy? Psychol Med. 2011;41(1):15–7.
122. Malm H, Artama M, Gissler M, Ritvanen A. Selective serotonin reuptake inhibitors and risk for major congenital anomalies. Obstet Gynecol. 2011;118(1):111–20.
123. Gentile S, Galbally M. Prenatal exposure to antidepressant medications and neurodevelopmental outcomes: a systematic review. J Affect Disord. 2011;128(1–2):1–9.
124. Huybrechts KF, Sanghani RS, Avorn J, Urato AC. Preterm birth and antidepressant medication use during pregnancy: a systematic review and meta-analysis. PLoS One. 2014;9(3):e92778.
125. Grigoriadis S, VonderPorten EH, Mamisashvili L, Eady A, Tomlinson G, Dennis CL, et al. The effect of prenatal antidepressant exposure on neonatal adaptation: a systematic review and meta-analysis. J Clin Psychiatry. 2013;74(4):309–20.
126. Bellantuono C, Vargas M, Mandarelli G, Nardi B, Martini MG. The safety of serotonin–noradrenaline reuptake inhibitors (SNRIs) in pregnancy and breastfeeding: a comprehensive review. Hum Psychopharmacol Clin Exp. 2015;30(3):143–51.
127. Einarson A. Antidepressants and pregnancy: complexities of producing evidence-based information. CMAJ. 2010;182(10):1017–8.
128. Hale's LT. Medications and mother's milk . Amarillo; 2008.
129. Berle JO, Spigset O. Antidepressant use during breastfeeding. Curr Womens Health Rev. 2011;7(1):28–34.
130. Davanzo R, Copertino M, De Cunto A, Minen F, Amaddeo A. Antidepressant drugs and breastfeeding: a review of the literature. Breastfeed Med. 2011;6(2):89–98.
131. Dhaliwal JS, Spurling BC, Molla M. Duloxetine. StatPearls [Internet]. 2020. Accessed 5 May 2021.
132. Soldin OP, Dahlin J, O'Mara DM. Triptans in pregnancy. Ther Drug Monit. 2008;30(1):5.
133. Ephross SA, Sinclair SM. 16 Yıllık S umatriptan, N aratriptan ve T reximet P regnancy R egistry'den Nihai Sonuçlar. Baş Ağrısı: Baş ve Yüz Ağrısı Dergisi. 2014;54(7):1158–1172.

134. Spielmann K, Kayser A, Beck E, Meister R, Schaefer C. Pregnancy outcome after anti-migraine triptan use: a prospective observational cohort study. Cephalalgia. 2018;38(6):1081–92.
135. Parikh SK. Unique populations with episodic migraine: pregnant and lactating women. Curr Pain Headache Rep. 2018;22(12):80.
136. Burch R. Epidemiology and treatment of menstrual migraine and migraine during pregnancy and lactation: a narrative review. Headache. 2020;60(1):200–16.
137. Hale TW. Hale's medications & mothers' milk™ 2019. Springer Publishing Company; 2018.
138. Davanzo R, Dal Bo S, Bua J, Copertino M, Zanelli E, Matarazzo L. Antiepileptic drugs and breastfeeding. Ital J Pediatr. 2013;39(1):1–11.
139. Crettenand M, Rossetti AO, Buclin T, Winterfeld U. Use of antiepileptic drugs during breastfeeding: what do we tell the mother? Nervenarzt. 2018;89(8):913–21.
140. Fortinguerra F, Clavenna A, Bonati M. Psychotropic drug use during breastfeeding: a review of the evidence. Pediatrics. 2009;124(4):e547–56.
141. Davanzo R, Bua J, Paloni G, Facchina G. Breastfeeding and migraine drugs. Eur J Clin Pharmacol. 2014;70(11):1313–24.
142. Hara T, Nakajima M, Sugano H, Karagiozov K, Hirose E, Goto K, Arai H. Pregnancy and breastfeeding during intrathecal baclofen therapy—a case study and review. NMC Case Rep J. 2018;5(3):65.
143. Moreira A, Barbin C, Martinez H, Aly A, Fonseca R. Maternal use of cyclobenzaprine (Flexeril) may induce ductal closure and persistent pulmonary hypertension in neonates. J Matern Fetal Neonatal Med. 2014;27(11):1177–9.
144. Kamath A. Thiocolchicoside: a review. DHR Int J Med Sci. 2013;4(2):39–45.
145. Mabie WC. Peripheral neuropathies during pregnancy. Clin Obstet Gynecol. 2005;48(1):57–66.
146. Petrover D, Richette P. Treatment of carpal tunnel syndrome: from ultrasonography to ultrasound guided carpal tunnel release. Joint Bone Spine. 2018;85(5):545–52.
147. Samerchua A. Ultrasound-guided erector spinae plane catheter provides analgesia for a pregnant and a pediatric patient. Thai J Anesthesiol. 2020;46(2):114–8.
148. Comlek S. Ultrasound-guided interventions during pregnancy for lumbosacral pain unresponsive to conservative treatment: a retrospective review. J Clin Ultrasound. 2021;49(1):20–7.
149. Connolly TM, Nadav D, Gungor S. Ultrasound-guided caudal epidural steroid injection for successful treatment of radiculopathy during pregnancy. Pain Manag. 2020;10(2):67–71.
150. Pyke MR, Shutt LE. The management of nonobstetric pains in pregnancy. Reg Anesth Pain Med. 2003;28(1):54–7.
151. Mcgoldrick NP, Green C, Burke N, Quinlan C, Mccormack D. Pregnancy and the orthopaedic patient. Orthop Trauma. 2012;26(3):212–9.
152. Ahn SG, Lee J, Park HJ, Kim YH. Ultrasound-guided pararadicular block using a paramedian sagittal oblique approach for managing low back pain in a pregnant woman: a case report. Anesth Pain Med. 2016;11(3):291–4.
153. Scalercio L, Vitter J, Elliott CE. Placement of a continuous stellate ganglion block for treatment of refractory ventricular fibrillation in the setting of known prinzmetal angina during pregnancy: a case report. A&A Pract. 2019;12(4):106–8.
154. Ito S, Sugiura T, Azami T, Sasano H, Sobue K. Spinal cord stimulation for a woman with complex regional pain syndrome who wished to get pregnant. J Anesth. 2013;27(1):124–7.
155. Ahmed S, Lindsay JM, Snyder DI. Spinal cord stimulation for complex regional pain syndrome: a case study of a pregnant female. Pain Physician. 2016;19(3):E487–93.
156. Shah S, Banh ET, Koury K, Bhatia G, Nandi R, Gulur P. Pain management in pregnancy: multimodal approaches. Pain Res Treat. 2015;2015:987483.
157. Ternov NK, Grennert L, Åberg A, Algotsson L, Åkeson J. Acupuncture for lower back and pelvic pain in late pregnancy: a retrospective report on 167 consecutive cases. Pain Med. 2001;2(3):204–7.

158. Endres HG, Böwing G, Diener HC, Lange S, Maier C, Molsberger A, et al. Acupuncture for tension-type headache: a multicentre, sham-controlled, patient-and observer-blinded, randomised trial. J Headache Pain. 2007;8(5):306.
159. de Oliveira Monteiro E. Botulinum toxin and pregnancy. SKINmed. 2006;5(6):308.
160. Qerama E, Fuglsang-Frederiksen A, Jensen TS. The role of botulinum toxin in management of pain: an evidence-based review. Curr Opin Anesthesiol. 2010;23(5):602–6. multi-modal intervention that included.

Oral Mucosal Lesions During Pregnancy and in the Postpartum Period

16

Işıl Taylan Cebi, Abdullah Karataş, and Chae-Seo Rhee

16.1 Introduction

Pregnancy is a distinctive period during which intricate physiological and hormonal changes occur regarding the development of the fetus. The oral mucosal disorders experienced during pregnancy are mostly related to hormonal and immunological changes [1]. These changes occur due to the increased production of progesterone, estrogen, and chorionic gonadotropins. Due to the elevated levels of sexual hormones, vascular permeability and proliferation also increase. These changes lead to a pro-inflammatory state [2]. In addition, the impaired immunological function creates a predisposition for several oral infections [3].

The most prevalent oral mucosal lesions during pregnancy are oral candidiasis, gingival hyperplasia, pyogenic granuloma, cheek biting, benign migratory glossitis, and aphthous ulcers. In this chapter, these disorders are going to be evaluated and summarized in order to help otorhinolaryngologists and dental professionals in the diagnosis and management of these disorders.

Knowledge of the oral mucosal lesions that occur during pregnancy will contribute to early detection and management, as well as facilitate the provision of appropriate instructions to patients.

I. T. Cebi (✉) · A. Karataş
Faculty of Medicine, Department of Otorhinolaryngology, Health Sciences University, İstanbul Haseki Research and Training Hospital, İstanbul, Turkey
e-mail: drisiltaylan@hotmail.com; akrts2000@yahoo.ca

C.-S. Rhee
Department of Otorhinolaryngology, Head and Neck Surgery, Seoul National University, College of Medicine, Seoul, South Korea
e-mail: csrhee@snu.ac.kr

C. Cingi et al. (eds.), *ENT Diseases: Diagnosis and Treatment during Pregnancy and Lactation*, https://doi.org/10.1007/978-3-031-05303-0_16

## 16.2	Anatomy of the Oral Cavity

The oral cavity consists of the upper and lower lips, buccal mucosa, upper and lower alveolar ridges, hard palate, retromolar trigones, oral tongue anterior to the circumvallate papillae, and the floor of the mouth. The boundaries of the oral cavity are the vermilion border anteriorly, the junction of the hard and soft palate superiorly, the circumvallate papillae posteriorly, and the buccal mucosa laterally. The oral cavity is separated into two parts by the teeth and the alveolar ridge. The external part is the oral vestibule, and the internal part is the true oral cavity.

The major arterial supply is from the external carotid artery. The tongue is supplied by the lingual artery, the submental artery supplies the floor of the mouth, the fascial and buccal arteries supply the buccal mucosa, and the ascending and descending pharyngeal arteries supply the palate.

Venous drainage in the oral cavity is carried out by the veins corresponding to their namesake arteries. The chief drainage is by way of the fascial and retromandibular veins into the internal jugular vein and also posteriorly by way of the pterygoid plexus into the cavernous sinus.

## 16.3	Structure and Function of the Oral Mucosa

The oral cavity is completely lined by a mucous membrane called oral mucosa. The epithelium of the tongue is derived from the endoderm, while the epithelium of the lips, oral vestibule, buccal mucosa, gingiva, palate, and floor of the mouth is derived from the ectoderm. The oral mucosa consists of two layers: the stratified squamous epithelium (keratinized or not keratinized) and the underlying connective tissue layer called lamina propria. Beneath the lamina propria lies the submucosa consisting of vessels, adipose tissues, and salivary glands. The surface is kept moist by the major and minor salivary glands that produce mucus.

The major functions of the oral mucosa are as follows: (1) mechanical protection against compressive and shearing forces; (2) barrier function to microorganisms, toxins, and antigens; (3) protection by humoral and cell-mediated immunity; (4) lubrication and buffering provided by the salivary glands; and (5) the sensory function providing input for touch, taste, pain, and temperature.

## 16.4	Oral Mucosal Lesions During Pregnancy

### 16.4.1	Oral Candidiasis

Approximately 30–60% of healthy individuals carry *Candida* species within their oral cavity. These microorganisms usually exist as commensal colonies. The pathologic colonization of *Candida* species is related to various factors such as malnutrition, metabolic diseases, concurrent infections, salivary gland hypofunction, antibiotherapy, immunocompromising conditions, transplant patients, and long-term steroid therapy [4]. During the gestational period, the decrease in salivary bicarbonate buffer, gastroesophageal reflux, and frequent vomiting leads to a decrease in salivary pH levels. This results in the shift of oral microbiota and proliferation of yeasts [5–7].

The classic presentation of candidiasis is in a pseudomembranous form commonly known as thrush. Salivary gland hypofunction and xerostomia may be the causes of this acute presentation. Creamy white plaques occur on the tongue, buccal mucosa, gingiva, palate, and oropharynx. Most of the cases are asymptomatic, but a burning oral sensation, soreness that causes difficulty in eating or swallowing, loss of taste, and minor bleeding at the affected sites may be observed. White plaques can be wiped off easily, and an erythematous mucosa can be observed underneath. This is a classical marker for oral candidiasis [4, 8].

The medical history of the patient and the examination of oral cavity are required for diagnosis. Periodic acid-Schiff (PAS) stain applied to the smear sample can confirm the diagnosis. Ten percent potassium hydroxide (KOH), Gram stain, or methylene blue may also be used for the presentation of pseudohyphal elements and budding yeast [8].

The treatment of choice is 10 mg of oral clotrimazole troches. A 14-day course of five troches a day should be prescribed. The patients should be instructed not to put anything in their mouth for 30 min after use. In addition, meticulous oral hygiene is essential for treating oral candidiasis. Frequent water consumption is also recommended for xerostomia [4].

16.4.2 Pregnancy Gingivitis

Pregnancy gingivitis or gingival hyperplasia is the hyperplastic growth of the gingiva through the gestational period. It affects 30–75% of all pregnant women [9]. The gingival changes range from asymptomatic gingivitis to a serious condition with bleeding and pain. These changes usually begin at the second month of gestation and increase through the eighth month [10–12]. Pregnancy gingivitis usually occurs due to the massive sex hormone production during pregnancy, namely, up to 40-fold estrogen and up to ten-fold progesterone levels from normal concentrations [5]. The elevated estrogen and progesterone levels in circulation increase the permeability of capillaries and decrease immune defense, therefore increasing the predisposition to gingival inflammation. Estrogen plays a role in the reduction of periodontal tissue keratinization and decreases the efficiency of the epithelial barrier. Progesterone, which is partly metabolized in inflamed gingiva, generates a greater amount of active progesterone, thereby favoring the proliferation of endothelial cells [13]. Pregnancy gingivitis appears due to pre-existing gingivitis caused by dental plaque and bacterial deposits on oral surfaces. Therefore, pregnancy is not the reason but an exacerbating factor [7, 10, 14]. The inflammation subsides at the end of pregnancy due to the reduction of sexual steroid secretion. Proper hygiene of the mouth and proper dental care with plaque control are recommended. The safest period for providing routine dental care is the second trimester [10, 11].

16.4.3 Pyogenic Granuloma

Pyogenic granuloma, also known as lobular capillary hemangioma, is a benign reactive inflammatory lesion due to the hyperplasia of fibroblasts and capillaries. It can arise in skin and mucous membranes. When mucosal surfaces are considered, the female to male ratio is 2:1 [15]. The most frequent sites involved in the oral cavity are the anterior maxillary gingiva, lower lip, tongue, buccal mucosa, and upper lip (Fig. 16.1). The prevalence in pregnant women is approximately 2% [5, 10, 14]. A prevalence of 0.22–14.2% has been reported in several studies [5]. Due to its increased frequency during pregnancy, pyogenic granuloma is also called granuloma gravidarum. It may arise in any trimester. The lesion is a sessile or pedinculated, raspberry-like nodule that may become overgrown and cover the neighboring teeth. Depending on the vascularity, the color varies from red, reddish purple to pink. It is usually painless and asymptomatic, but bleeding may occur easily.

The exact etiopathology is not fully understood, but the combination of factors such as increased female sex hormone levels during pregnancy, local irritants (e.g., foreign material within the gingival crevice), repeated trauma during brushing, dental plaque, and periodontal inflammation may be responsible [16–18]. The high levels of sex hormones induce the vascularity of gums stricken by periodontitis and gingivitis. Due to the inflammation, the metabolism of progesterone slows down and the level of active progesterone within the gingiva rises. This leads to the dilation of the gingival capillaries, stasis, and increased sensitivity to local irritants, trauma, dental plaque, and bacterial deposits [14, 19].

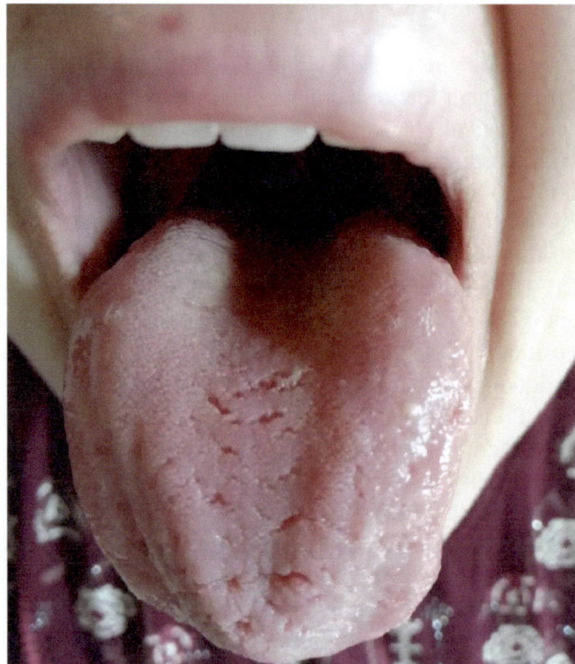

Fig. 16.1 Pedinculated pyogenic granuloma on the lower lip

The differential diagnosis consists of peripheral giant cell granuloma, peripheral ossifying fibroma, hemangioma, and foreign body reaction [16, 17, 20]. The peripheral giant cell granuloma seems similar to pyogenic granuloma but bluer in color. Peripheral ossifying fibroma consists of cellular fibroblastic connective tissue with randomly dispersed foci of dystrophic calcification and appears as a nodule on gingiva. Hemangioma is a benign tumor of endothelial cells consisting of an increased number of blood vessels [16].

After delivery, with the reduction of hormone levels, apoptosis and regression of the tumor take place. The usual course postpartum is spontaneous regression. Therefore, intervention should be avoided. Regular follow-ups with a dental surgeon and maintenance of good oral hygiene are recommended. Rarely, severe or recurrent bleeding may occur, and excision may be necessary. In such a case, the patient should be informed that recurrence is common [10, 11, 16].

16.4.4 Morsicatio Buccarum

Biting the buccal mucosa for a long period of time leads to traumatic erosive ulcers at the level of the occlusal planes. These ulcerative lesions are associated with white and thickened areas in the buccal mucosa, which are called morsicatio buccarum [5, 17]. Increased buccal fat tissue and weight gain, joined with anxiety and stress, may lead to this disorder. It may be confused clinically with other mucosal lesions such as lichen planus, pemphigus, gestational pemphigoid, and oral candidiasis [5, 6, 21].

16.4.5 Benign Migratory Glossitis

Benign migratory glossitis or geographical tongue was first described as a migratory rash of the tongue in 1831 [22]. It is a common condition characterized by an asymptomatic presentation of multiple, well-demarcated, erythematous areas of variable size surrounded by yellow-white borders (Fig. 16.2). The lesions usually occur on the anterior two-thirds of the dorsal tongue, heal frequently, and subsequently develop in other areas. The etiology remains unclear. The commonly proposed risk factors are genetic factors, hormonal changes and oral contraceptive pills, diabetes mellitus, and pregnancy. In some studies, benign migratory glossitis showed a higher prevalence in pregnant women (2.97–3.23%). However, further studies are needed to explore the increased prevalence during pregnancy [6, 14, 21, 23].

16.4.6 Aphthous Ulcers

Aphthous ulcers are recurrent, painful, self-limiting lesions that are generally restricted to non-keratinized oral mucosa. They are more prevalent in the second and third decades of life. Simple aphthous ulcers are self-limiting lesions and heal

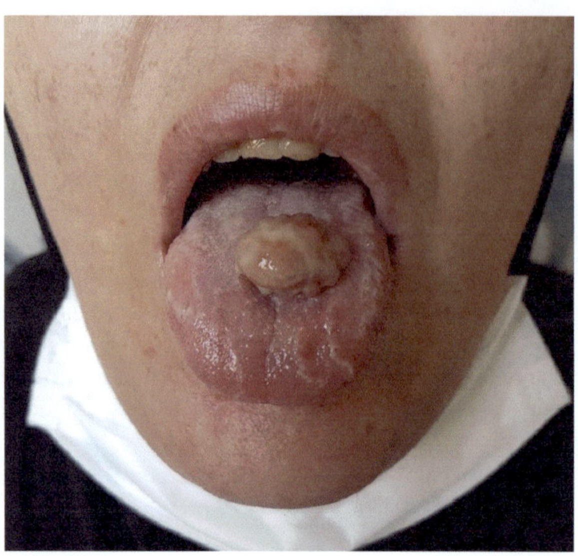

Fig. 16.2 Benign migratory glossitis

within a short period of time without scarring. Complex aphthosis involves lesions healing with scar and persisting beyond 10–14 days [24]. Their exact etiology is unknown, and they are supposed to be multifactorial with immune-mediated damage to epithelial cells [25]. The triggering factors are trauma, infection, poor oral hygiene, malnutrition, and hormonal changes. However, several studies indicate that aphthous ulcers flare premenstrually and then clear during pregnancy [26], but this is not supported by large studies.

Aphthous ulcers during pregnancy may be managed by observation. They can be ascribed to hematinic deficiencies, so serum iron, B12, folate, and zinc levels should be checked. Topical corticosteroid gel application 4–6 times a day may be used for the treatment of complex aphthosis. In rare cases, short-term oral corticosteroid therapy may be appropriate. Colchicine and dapsone, which are prescribed for serious, complex aphthae, fall under pregnancy class-C; thalidomide, although very efficient, falls under pregnancy class-X [10].

16.4.7 Behcet's Disease

It is a rare inflammatory condition that affects multiple organ systems chronically. It is characterized by mucocutaneous lesions, as well as ocular, vascular, and central nervous system manifestations. Oral involvement presents with aphthous ulcerations, which are usually the initial symptoms. The aphthous lesions usually heal without scarring within 7–12 days, but the pain due to multiple aphthous ulcerations may debilitate the patient and impair oral intake. The peak incidence is in the second and third decades. The etiology is unknown, but a genetic predisposition with most patients having the HLA-B51 allele is apparent in some populations. Vasculitis leads to an inflammatory response and damage, resulting in multisystem involvement. The natural course involves remissions and relapses [10, 11].

The course of Behcet's disease during gestation varies. A recent study showed that 27.3% of pregnant women experienced relapse, 52.3% had remission, and 20.4% had no change in their disease [27]. For those who experienced relapse, the most frequent symptom was multiple severe aphthous ulcerations. The course of Behcet's disease during gestation is variable. Therefore, it is suggested that gestation is insignificant regarding the course of the disease. In addition, no maternal or fetal adverse outcome due to Behcet's disease is expected during pregnancy [28]. The treatment of oral lesions is similar to that employed for aphthous ulcers discussed previously.

16.4.8 Pemphigus Vulgaris

Pemphigus vulgaris is an immunobullous intraepithelial disease affecting both skin and mucosae. Although rare during pregnancy, it has great clinical importance due to the fetal morbidity and mortality risk. Oral involvement is much more frequent than cutaneous lesions. Furthermore, no location other than the oral cavity may be involved. The oral lesions can be defined as erosive bullae, which heal with no scar tissue [29, 30].

The disease is induced by autoantibodies against desmogleins. Desmogleins are transmembranous desmosomal units and also elements of cell adhesion proteins. The IgG and C3 deposition in the epidermis is revealed through direct immunofluorescence studies [31]. Indirect immunofluorescence studies are also positive, with an apparent correlation between the disease activity and antibody titers. Neonatal involvement takes place due to the transplacental transfer of IgG autoantibodies [32, 33]. There is no correlation between the disease severity and antibody titers in neonates. Moreover, neonatal pemphigus vulgaris is not likely to advance into adulthood [11, 29, 34].

The disease may occur or progress during the gestational period. During the first and second trimesters, changes in disease activity are more prevalent. The production of endogenous steroids by the placenta in the third trimester may lead to a relative improvement or stabilization of the disease [30]. No direct correlation between the severity of maternal disease and the extent of neonatal involvement has been detected. Patients in remission may give birth to neonates with severe disease [35, 36]. Patients with active pemphigus may also deliver healthy neonates [30, 37]. Pemphigus patients often deliver healthy neonates with localized skin lesions, which resolve in 2–4 weeks [11, 35]. The fetal outcome is unpredictable due to the lack of related cases in the literature. Similarly, the recurrence rates in subsequent pregnancies are unknown. The first line of treatment for active pemphigus during pregnancy is topical and oral corticosteroids. Plasmapheresis may also be useful in some cases [38].

16.4.9 Gestational Pemphigoid

Gestational pemphigoid, also known as herpes gestationis, is a rare autoimmune blistering disease during pregnancy. It causes blistering on the mucosal membranes and the skin. Mucosal involvement is detected in 20% of the cases [39]. It mostly occurs during the second and last trimesters and tends to resolve after the gestational period. The mean duration of the disease is 6 months postpartum. Relapses may happen due to the use of combined oral contraceptives after delivery and during menstruation. The prevalence is approximately 0.002–0.005% [39–41].

Gestational pemphigoid is induced by IgG autoantibodies against the structural components of the dermo-epidermal junction. The BP180 is a transmembrane glycoprotein and a significant autoantigen that is highly immunodominant in gestational pemphigoid. Autoantibodies targeting BP180 play a key role in blister formation. The transmission of autoantibodies to the fetus may result in preterm delivery, bullous or papular rash, and low birth weight in neonates [42, 43].

Topical corticosteroids can be used in mild and moderate disease. Oral corticosteroids are often used for severe and debilitating disease [40, 41]. The risks of exposure to systemic corticosteroids should be considered when treating gestational pemphigoid.

Immunoglobulins or cyclosporin treatment may be considered in persistent and severe cases, but the potential risks to the fetus should always be considered [44–46].

References

1. de Araujo S, Figueiredo C, Goncalves Carvalho Rosalem C, et al. Systemic alterations and their oral manifestations in pregnant women. J Obstet Gynaecol Res. 2017;43(1):16–22.
2. Zachariasen RD. Ovarian hormones and oral health: pregnancy gingivitis. Compendium. 1989;10(9):508–12.
3. Xiao J, Fogarty C, Wu TT, et al. Oral health and Candida carriage in socioeconomically disadvantaged US pregnant women. BMC Pregnancy Childbirth. 2019;19:480. https://doi.org/10.1186/s12884-019-2618-7.
4. Hellstein JW, Marek CL. Candidiasis: red and white manifestations in the oral cavity. Head Neck Pathol. 2019;13(1):25–32.
5. Bett JVS, Batistella EA, Melo G, et al. Prevalence of oral mucosal disorders during pregnancy: a systematic review and meta-analysis. J Oral Pathol Med. 2019;48:270–7. https://doi.org/10.1111/jop.12831.
6. Sarifakioglu E, Gunduz C, Gorpelioglu C. Oral mucosa manifestations in 100 pregnant versus non-pregnant patients: an epidemiological observational study. Eur J Dermatol. 2006;16(6):674–6.
7. Jain K, Kaur H. Prevalence of oral lesions and measurement of salivary pH in the different trimesters of pregnancy. Singap Med J. 2015;56(1):53–7. https://doi.org/10.11622/smedj.2015010.
8. Millsop JW, Fazel N. Oral candidiosis. Clin Dermatol. 2016;34(4):487–94. https://doi.org/10.1016/j.clindermatol.2016.02.02.
9. Barak S, Oettinger-Barak O, Oettinger M, et al. Common oral manifestations during pregnancy: a review. Obstet Gynecol Surv. 2003;58:624–8.
10. Torgerson RR, Marnach ML, Bruce AJ, et al. Oral and vulvar changes in pregnancy. Clin Dermatol. 2006;24:122–32. https://doi.org/10.1016/j.clindermatol.2005.10.004.

11. Ramos-E-Silva M, Martins NR. Oral and genital changes in pregnancy. Clin Dermatol. 2016;34(3):353–8. https://doi.org/10.1016/j.clindermatol.2016.02.007.
12. Henry F, Quatresooz P, Valverde-Lopez JC, et al. Blood vessel changes during pregnancy: a review. Am J Clin Dermatol. 2006;7:65–9.
13. Amar S, Chung KM. Influence of hormonal variation on the periodontium in women. Periodontol 2000. 1994;6:79–87. https://doi.org/10.1111/j.1600-0757.1994.tb00028.x.
14. Diaz-Guzman LM, Castellanos-Suarez JL. Lesions of the oral mucosa and periodontal disease behaviour in pregnant patients. Med Oral Patol Oral Cir Bucal. 2004;9:430–7.
15. Harris MN, Desai R, Chuang TY, et al. Lobular capillary hemangiomas: an epidemiologic report, with emphasis on cutaneous lesions. J Am Acad Dermatol. 2000;42:1012–6.
16. Purwar P, Dixit J, Sheel V, et al. 'Granuloma gravidarum': persistence in puerperal period an unusual presentation. BMJ Case Rep. 2015;2015:bcr2014206878. https://doi.org/10.1136/bcr-2014-206878.
17. Neville BW, Damm DD, Chi AC, et al. Oral and maxillofacial pathology. Amsterdam: Elsevier Health Sciences; 2015.
18. Regezi JA, Sciubba JJ, Jordan RC. Oral pathology: clinical pathologic considerations. 4th ed. Philadelphia: WB Saunders; 2000.
19. Ojanotko-Harri AO, Harri MP, Hurttia HM, et al. Altered tissue metabolism of progesterone in pregnancy gingivitis and granuloma. J Clin Periodontol. 1991;18:262–6.
20. Dutra KL, Longo L, Grando LJ, et al. Incidence of reactive hyperplastic lesions in the oral cavity: a 10 year retrospective study in Santa Catarina, Brazil. Braz J Otorhinolaryngol. 2019;85(4):399–407. https://doi.org/10.1016/j.bjorl.2018.03.006.
21. Rezazadeh F, Falsafi N, Sarraf Z. Mucosal disorders in pregnant versus non-pregnant women. Dent J. 2014;2(4):134–41. https://doi.org/10.3390/dj.2040134.
22. Shulman JD, Carpenter WM. Prevalence and risk factors associated with geographic tongue among US adults. Oral Dis. 2006;12:381–6. https://doi.org/10.1111/j.1601-0825.2005.01208.x.
23. Assimakopoulos D, Patrikakos G, Fotika C, et al. Benign migratory glossitis or geographic tongue: an enigmatic oral lesion. Am J Med. 2002;113(9):751–5.
24. Rogers RS III. Complex aphthosis. Adv Exp Med Biol. 2003;528:311–6.
25. Rogers RS III. Recurrent aphthous stomatitis: clinical characteristics and associated systemic disorders. Semin Cutan Med Surg. 1997;16:278–83.
26. McCartan BE, Sullivan A. The association of menstrual cycle, pregnancy, and menopause with recurrent oral aphthous stomatitis: a review and critique. Obstet Gynecol. 1992;80:455–8.
27. Uzun S, Alpsoy E, Durdu M, et al. The clinical course of Behcet's disease in pregnancy: a retrospective analysis and review of the literature. J Dermatol. 2003;30:499–502.
28. Marsal S, Falga C, Simeon CP, et al. Behcet's disease and pregnancy relationship study. Br J Rheumatol. 1997;36:234–8.
29. Ruach M, Ohel G, Rahav D, et al. Pemphigus vulgaris and pregnancy. Obstet Gynecol Surv. 1995;50:755–60.
30. Muhammad JK, Lewis MA, Crean SJ. Oral pemphigus vulgaris occurring during pregnancy. J Oral Pathol Med. 2002;31:121–4.
31. Anhalt GJ. Making sense of antigens and antibodies in pemphigus. J Am Acad Dermatol. 1999;40:763–6.
32. Green D, Maize JC. Maternal pemphigus vulgaris with in vivo bound antibodies in the stillborn fetus. J Am Acad Dermatol. 1982;7:388–92.
33. Moncada B, Kettelsen S, Hernandez-Moctezuma JL, et al. Neonatal pemphigus vulgaris: role of passively transferred pemphigus antibodies. Br J Dermatol. 1982;106:465–7.
34. Chowdhury MM, Natarajan S. Neonatal pemphigus vulgaris associated with mild oral pemphigus vulgaris in the mother during pregnancy. Br J Dermatol. 1998;139:500–3.
35. Egea L, Le Borgne H, Samson M, et al. Oral infections and pregnancy: knowledge of health professionals. Gynecol Obstet Fertil. 2013;41:635–40.
36. Tope WD, Kamino H, Briggaman RA, et al. Neonatal pemphigus vulgaris in a child born to a woman in remission. J Am Acad Dermatol. 1993;29:480–5.

37. Hern S, Vaughan Jones SA, Setterfield J, et al. Pemphigus vulgaris in pregnancy with favourable foetal prognosis. Clin Exp Dermatol. 1998;23:260–3.
38. Shieh S, Fang YV, Becker JL, et al. Pemphigus, pregnancy, and plasmapheresis. Cutis. 2004;73:327–9.
39. Kneisel A, Hertl M. Autoimmune bullous skin diseases. Part 1: clinical manifestations. JDDG. 2011;9(10):844–57. https://doi.org/10.1111/j.1610-0387.2011.07793.x.
40. Amber KT, Murrell DF, Schmidt E, et al. Autoimmune subepidermal bullous diseases of the skin and mucosae: clinical features, diagnosis, and management. Clin Rev Allergy Immunol. 2017;54(1):26–51. https://doi.org/10.1007/s12016-017-8633-4.
41. Lobato-Berezo A, Fernández Figueras MT, Moreno Romero JA, et al. Pemphigoid gestationis mimicking erythema multiforme with mucosal involvement. Actas Dermosifiliogr. 2019;110:696–7.
42. Lipozencic J, Ljubojevic S, Bukvic-Mokos Z. Pemphigoid gestationis. Clin Dermatol. 2012;30:51–5. https://doi.org/10.1016/j.clindermatol.2011.03.009.
43. Jenkins RE, Hern S, Black MM. Clinical features and management of 87 patients with pemphigoid gestationis. Clin Exp Dermatol. 1999;24:255–9.
44. Doiron P, Pratt M. Antepartum intravenous immunoglobulin therapy in refractory pemphigoid gestationis: case report and literature review. J Cutan Med Surg. 2010;14:189–92.
45. Ozdemir O, Atalay CR, Asgarova V, et al. A resistant case of pemphigus gestationis successfully treated with cyclosporine. Interv Med Appl Sci. 2016;8:20–2. https://doi.org/10.1556/1646.8.2016.1.3.
46. Hapa A, Gurpinar A, Akan T, et al. A resistant case of pemphigus gestationis successfully treated with intravenous immunoglobulin plus cyclosporine. Int J Dermatol. 2014;53:269–71. https://doi.org/10.1111/ijd.12236.

Snoring and Sleep Apnea During Pregnancy and Postpartum Period

17

Duygu Erdem, Sultan Şevik Eliçora, and Giulio Cesare Passali

17.1 Introduction

Sleep-disordered breathing (SDB) is a group of disorders that includes a spectrum ranging from simple snoring to obstructive sleep apnea (OSA). Sleep disorders impair the quality of life in pregnant women and cause many symptoms such as daytime sleepiness, fatigue, and lack of concentration, and it also has very severe obstetric (hypertension, preeclampsia, diabetes, and depression) and fetal (small for gestational age, preterm birth, intrauterine growth retardation, low APGAR, etc.) consequences. The diagnosis and management of SDB in pregnancy are challenging due to most symptoms being indistinguishable from the general symptoms and signs of pregnancy. Although the gold standard method for diagnosis is all-night polysomnography, it is not always applicable during pregnancy. Management of SDB in pregnancy is also a subject of debate. Prescribing drugs in pregnant patients is not recommended. It is important to prevent weight gain and obesity during pregnancy. Continuous positive airway pressure (CPAP) remains the most effective treatment modality in SDB during pregnancy.

D. Erdem (✉) · S. Şevik Eliçora
Medical School, Department of Otorhinolaryngology, Zonguldak Bülent Ecevit University, Zonguldak, Turkey
e-mail: duygualtuntas@gmail.com; drsultan@mynet.com

G. C. Passali
Department of Otorhinolaryngology, Catholic University of Sacred Heart, Rome, Italy
e-mail: GiulioCesare.Passali@unicatt.it

C. Cingi et al. (eds.), *ENT Diseases: Diagnosis and Treatment during Pregnancy and Lactation*, https://doi.org/10.1007/978-3-031-05303-0_17

17.2   Sleep Disorders and Pregnancy

Sleep disorders are typically classified as disturbed sleep quality, poor sleep continuity, short or long sleep duration, restless legs syndrome, and sleep-disordered breathing (SDB). Approximately 75% of women experience different types of sleep disruptions during pregnancy [1]. Hormonal, anatomical, and physiological changes during pregnancy contribute to this situation. The term SDB includes a wide spectrum of disorders characterized by ventilation abnormalities during sleep. This spectrum ranges from habitual snoring to obstructive sleep apnea (OSA).

Snoring is the most common form of SDBs and has been the subject of many studies since it can be diagnosed using scales (Pittsburgh Sleep Quality Index—PSQI, Modified Berlin Questionnaire—MBQ, Epworth Sleepiness Scale—ESS, etc.) [2, 3]. OSA, on the other hand, is a more serious form of SDB and requires polysomnography (PSG) for diagnosis. However, difficulties may be encountered in the application and standardization of PSG in pregnant women. Both snoring and OSA impair the quality of life in pregnant women and cause many symptoms such as daytime sleepiness, fatigue, and lack of concentration, as well as very severe obstetric (hypertension, preeclampsia, diabetes, and depression) and fetal (small for gestational age-SGA, preterm birth, intrauterine growth retardation, low APGAR, etc.) consequences.

17.3   Physiological Changes in Pregnancy

Although SDB is rare in women of reproductive age, it is very common in pregnant women. There are various mechanisms that both facilitate and prevent SDB during pregnancy. The balance of these mechanisms contributes to the oxygenation of the fetus.

17.3.1 Factors that Prevent SDB During Pregnancy

1. The increase in the progesterone level causes an increase in ventilation response to hypoxia and hypercapnia [4, 5], which increases the tidal volume.
2. Progesterone causes relaxation and dilatation in upper airway muscles and protects upper airway blockage [6].
3. Decreased rapid eye movement phase and reduced sleep in the supine position affect the quality of sleep and its related outcomes [7].

17.3.2 Factors that Facilitate SDB During Pregnancy

1. Upper airway edema occurs due to hormonal changes, the pharyngeal diameter becomes narrow, and there is resistance in the upper airway [8].
2. Estrogen-dependent nasal congestion and rhinitis occur [7].

3. Physiological hypervolemia is seen [9].
4. The diaphragm rises due to the enlargement of the uterus. Functional residual capacity in the lung decreases due to diaphragm elevation [10].
5. The upper airway narrows due to the decrease in tracheal traction [10].
6. Weight gain occurs in pregnancy [10].
7. The Mallampati score also increases during pregnancy [8, 11].
8. Arousal threshold decreases due to frequent awakenings caused by pregnancy-related discomfort.

As a result of all these changes, pregnancy is associated with shorter sleep times and superficial sleep status. When these are accompanied by problems such as urinary fullness, frequent urination at night, back pain, fetal movements, and restless legs syndrome, poor sleep quality is inevitable during the pregnancy period. However, the apnea–hypopnea index, arterial oxyhemoglobin desaturation, and flow limitation do not differ between pregnant and nonpregnant women of similar age [12, 13].

17.4 Snoring in Pregnancy

Snoring, which is a sign of increased upper airway resistance, usually occurs as a result of the vibration of the pharyngeal walls due to compromised upper airways during sleep [14]. Habitual snoring is defined as snoring that occurs at least three to four times a week [15, 16]. While previous studies have shown that 14–41.3% of pregnant women have habitual snoring, this rate is reported to be 4% in nonpregnant women [17–19]. While the frequency of snoring is 7.9% in the first trimester, it increases to 21.2% in the third trimester. It has also been reported that the pre-pregnancy weight of women plays a role in snoring experienced during early pregnancy [20–22].

17.4.1 Epidemiology and Risk Factors

Age [23], obesity [24], overweight during pregnancy [25], smoking [24], alcohol or drug use [26], snoring history before pregnancy [25], wide neck diameter [25, 27], passive smoking [28], and poverty [29] increase the risk of SDB during pregnancy. Another factor that plays a role in snoring is whether the pregnant woman has asthma. In a study conducted by Williams et al., it was shown that snoring was seen 1.79 times more common in pregnant women with asthma, and this increased to 5.39 times when excess weight was also considered [30].

The most important of these risk factors is weight before the pregnancy. Guinhouya et al. assumed that pre-pregnancy weight and weight gained during pregnancy were critical in sleep disorders [31].

17.4.2 Maternal Morbidity

17.4.2.1 Hypertension and Preeclampsia

Studies have shown that snoring is an independent risk factor for gestational hypertension [3, 17, 19, 32–34]. In relation to this, various theories have been proposed:

1. Patients with SDB have chronic hypoxemia, which leads to preeclampsia [35].
2. Intermittent hypoxemia attacks cause epithelial dysfunction and result in preeclampsia [36].
3. Increased oxidative stress markers initiate placental changes and lead to preeclampsia [37].
4. Snoring has been shown to increase erythropoiesis, defined as increasing red blood cells in the umbilical cord. This leads to restriction in uterine growth and maternal hypertension [38, 39].
5. In snoring, inflammation and fluid increase, which is a risk factor for gestational hypertension and preeclampsia [40]. Studies have shown that if SDB is treated, patients' blood pressure values improve [41, 42].

17.4.2.2 Diabetes

There are conflicting results concerning the relationship between diabetes and SDB. Some studies suggest that poor sleep quality increases insulin resistance and causes hyperglycemia in pregnant women, and increased oxidative stress, inflammation, sympathetic activity, and cortisol levels contribute to this situation [43]. Qui et al. reported that snoring increased the risk of gestational diabetes by 1.86 times. The authors also showed that when overweight women were included in the evaluation, this risk further increased up to 6.9 times [22, 44].

17.4.2.3 Depression

Maternal snoring is also a risk factor for depression [34, 45].

17.4.2.4 Obstetrical Outcomes

Qiou et al. and Ayrım et al. did not find a connection between snoring and obstetric outcomes [14, 22]. In contrast, O'Brien et al., who evaluated 1673 women, reported habitual snoring in a total of 35% (26% with pregnancy-onset snoring and 9% with chronic snoring). Chronic snoring was found to be associated with SGA and elective cesarean delivery, while snoring that started during pregnancy was determined to be associated with emergency cesarean delivery [46]. In a study of 1000 patients, unplanned cesarean delivery was found to be related to snoring [27].

17.5 Fetal/Infantile Morbidity

17.5.1 Infant Birth Weight

In most studies, no significant relationship was found between the mean birth weight and snoring [14, 18, 35, 47]. In contrast, Micheli et al. reported a significant relationship between snoring and low birth weight [48].

17.5.2 SGA/Intrauterine Growth Retardation

Franklin et al. found that SGA was seen approximately three times more in mothers that snored [17]. O'Brien et al. and Micheli et al. found that SGA was associated with chronic snoring [46, 48]. Micheli et al. also observed a relationship between severe snoring and SGA [48]. However, Tauman et al. did not find a relationship between these two conditions [49].

17.5.3 Preterm Delivery

Dunietz et al. showed that loud and frequent snoring was associated with preterm birth [34, 50–52].

17.5.4 Cesarian Section

Yang et al. showed that snoring increases the probability of cesarean delivery [34].

17.5.5 APGAR

While there are many publications stating that snoring does not affect the APGAR score [14, 18, 47], some suggest that it does have an effect, but they are limited in number [17].

17.5.6 Genetic Disorder

It has been shown that the telomere length of infants is shortened in patients with SDB. This is considered to be due to SDB accelerating chromosomal aging in pregnant women [53].

17.5.7 Treatment

For the treatment of SDB during pregnancy, first, conservative methods, including controlling pregnancy weight gain, head elevation, avoiding supine position, and reducing alcohol and sedatives can be tried. The treatment of pregnancy-related rhinitis using medical agents or sodium hyaluronate [54] can also contribute to the reduction of snoring. However, the most effective way to prevent snoring and its complications is continuous positive airway pressure (CPAP). In a study by Guilleminault et al., a significant improvement was noted in daytime sleepiness, snoring, and fatigue scores in pregnant women who underwent CPAP [33]. Poyares et al. showed that early CPAP application was successful in controlling hypertension and pregnancy outcomes in pregnant women with hypertension and chronic snoring [42].

17.6 Sleep Apnea in Pregnancy

OSA is the most severe form of SDB and includes multiple apnea and hypopnea episodes during sleep due to decreased airflow through the upper airway despite the respiratory effort. OSA can lead to interruption of sleep, hype-carbia, and cycles of hypoxemia and re-oxygenation [55]. In the obstetric literature, the terms OSA and SDB are sometimes used interchangeably. Pregnancy complications and adverse pregnancy outcomes are more common in women with OSA [55, 56].

During pregnancy, OSA can occur in two main clinical forms: chronic OSA, which develops before pregnancy and continues during pregnancy, and gestational OSA, which develops during pregnancy without a previous history. In women with gestational OSA, an increase in OSA severity can be expected due to physiological and hormonal changes related to pregnancy. Again, depending on the same mechanisms, it can be assumed that gestational OSA will improve after pregnancy. However, the term gestational OSA has not yet been fully defined [55, 56].

17.6.1 Epidemiology and Risk Factors

The prevalence of OSA is approximately 3% among women of reproductive age. However, among pregnant women, the prevalence ranges from 8 to 20% [57]. According to some authors, obesity and weight gain during pregnancy are the main risk factors for pregnancy-related OSA. However, some studies suggest that independent of obesity, pregnant women with OSA are at increased risk of adverse maternal and neonatal outcomes. Pregnancy itself has been recognized as an independent risk factor for OSA, with a prevalence of 11% in the first trimester increasing throughout gestation to 27% in the third trimester [58].

OSA is also associated with some comorbidities such as gestational diabetes, gestational hypertension, preeclampsia, cardiac arrhythmias, and cardiovascular diseases. Women who have cardiovascular risk factors may be at increased risk of OSA during pregnancy [55].

Recurrent placental hypoxemia episodes, vascular changes, damage of oxygen radicals, endothelial dysfunction, and sympathetic hyperactivity are among the possible pathophysiological mechanisms of the effect of OSA on maternal or fetal outcomes [59]. The pathophysiologic pathways of OSA and preeclampsia are similar [55, 60]. They both seem to be pro-inflammatory states, triggered by sympathetic nervous system activation. There is an increase in antiangiogenic proteins that cause endothelial dysfunction by a similar mechanism in both OSA and preeclampsia. This endothelial dysfunction leads to tension abnormalities, vascular tone changes, and proteinuria and cardiovascular disturbances in preeclampsia [55].

17.6.2 Symptoms

Many symptoms detected in patients with OSA are already common during pregnancy due to many hormonal changes, such as over-fatigue, frequent awaking at night, and increased daytime sleepiness. Pregnant women may think that these symptoms are due to the natural course of pregnancy and thus may not report them as a complaint [57].

17.6.3 Screening and Diagnosis

There is no evidence that various questionnaires routinely used to diagnose OSA, such as the Epworth Sleepiness Scale, Berlin questionnaire, and STOP-BANG questionnaire, are useful in the obstetric population [58]. The gold standard technique for the diagnosis of OSA remains to be PSG [59, 61]; however, PSG is not available in many medical centers, and long waiting times make it impossible to use it during pregnancy [55, 59].

17.6.4 Maternal Morbidity

Retrospective data have shown that OSA is associated with increased maternal mortality and morbidity during the course of pregnancy [56]. Pregnant women with a diagnosis of OSA are more likely to have gestational hypertension, preeclampsia, gestational diabetes, cardiomyopathy, and preterm or cesarean delivery [55, 59–63]. OSA can lead to adverse maternal outcomes in pregnancy and should be questioned in pregnant women, especially those with chronic diseases. Pregnant women with OSA should be routinely checked for diabetes and hypertension before and after delivery. These adverse outcomes are also reported to be exacerbated in the presence of obesity [60].

There are many studies focusing on the association between OSA and gestational hypertension or preeclampsia. These two entities are found to be associated with significant maternal and neonatal morbidity and mortality [59]. In addition, OSA is also associated with a threefold increased risk of cardiomyopathy, congestive heart failure, and hysterectomy [61].

Maternal obesity is the main risk factor for the development of gestational diabetes mellitus (GDM), a condition associated with many adverse maternal, fetal, and neonatal outcomes. The association of simple snoring with GDM has not been demonstrated, but OSA has been associated with an increased risk [59, 61]. SDB disrupts glucose metabolism regardless of body weight, especially in the third trimester [61].

OSA is also associated with the prenatal symptoms of depression. In a study by Redhead et al., OSA severity was found to be associated with depression symptoms [64].

It should be kept in mind that all of these disorders are multifactorial, and SDB is not the only reason for the adverse maternal outcomes of pregnancy [61].

17.6.5 Neonatal Morbidity

Intermittent hypoxia and placental ischemia are the main mechanisms responsible for adverse fetal outcomes [59]. Maternal OSA has been found to be associated with preterm delivery, SGA, low birth weight, increase in assisted vaginal delivery, and cesarean section (elective or emergent). Low Apgar scores and stillbirth have also been shown to be increased in pregnant women with OSA [59]. OSA diagnosis is associated with a longer hospital stay and increased risk of intensive care requirement after delivery [59]. However, there is no evidence of an increased risk of fetal death or miscarriage associated with OSA [62].

17.6.6 Treatment

There are no accepted guidelines for the management of OSA during pregnancy. Treatment strategies are similar to those provided by guidelines for the management of OSA in general population [59]. There is no evidence that treatment during pregnancy improves maternal or neonatal outcomes, and strategies for treating OSA in the general population are usually modified for pregnancy. The aim of pregnancy-specific treatments is to minimize maternal and fetal complications and improve birth outcomes [55].

OSA management during pregnancy should be carried out in a multidisciplinary manner and continued during the postpartum period [55].

The effectiveness of nonpharmacological strategies, such as controlling weight gain, left lateral or elevated head in bed when sleeping, restricting smoking, alcohol, and caffeine intake, treating nasal congestion, exercising regularly, and following good sleep hygiene measures in pregnancy is still controversial.

Dietary management, weight loss, and positional therapy used during mild OSA in the general population may not be applicable during pregnancy; thus, they may have negative effects on the developing fetus [61]. In addition, it may not be possible to keep the lateral position throughout sleep, which is frequently recommended in mild OSA [61].

There is no proven medication to prevent or treat OSA. Positive airway pressure (PAP) therapy is the main option in the treatment of OSA in pregnancy as in the general population [61]. PAP is generally safe and well tolerated during pregnancy. The patient adherence rates to PAP in pregnancy are similar to the general population at approximately 50–60%. No significant side effects have been reported due to PAP treatment in pregnant women compared with the general population [61].

While oral appliances are a treatment option in patients with OSA in the general population, there are no proven data on their use in pregnancy. They are not practical during pregnancy, and multiple fitting sessions make their use uncomfortable during a short period of time.

Surgery is another treatment option for the management of OSA in the general population. However, due to the risks involved, surgical operations should be avoided during pregnancy. Tracheostomy is another treatment option in pregnant women with OSA, but it should not be performed unless it is absolutely necessary [59].

17.7 Postpartum Period

There are limited studies on the continuity of gestational OSA in the postpartum period. In a study by Street et al. evaluating 65 women with valid data at two different times, 24 women were determined to be positive for OSA during the third trimester of pregnancy (37%), and this proportion did not meaningfully decline at the first postpartum visit (23 subjects, 35%) [58]. Of the eight participants whose OSA resolved after delivery, all except one had mild OSA, and of the seven participants that developed OSA in the postpartum period, all had mild OSA. The data from the many studies suggest that gestational OSA differs from these diseases in that it may resolve considerably more slowly after delivery, but is potentially similar in that it may serve as a marker or predisposition to chronic OSA. These data demonstrate that OSA pathologies can continue for 2–3 months after delivery, with approximately 20% of cases suffering from this condition until 6–8 months after delivery.

The increased likelihood of OSA during pregnancy has been speculated to reflect weight gain, upper airway edema primarily due to increased estrogen effects, increased airflow caused by the progesterone-induced increase in tidal volume, and altered sleeping position due to the enlarging uterus. All of these conditions should rapidly resolve following delivery and are unlikely to explain the unchanged prevalence of OSA at 7.4 weeks after delivery. It is conceivable that lactation effects, sleep deprivation, and sleep fragmentation because of neonatal care may explain the changes in overall prevalence and the new-onset, mild OSA, during this period, but they are less likely to explain the persistence of OSA for 6–8 months after delivery. Postpartum weight retention is minimal and does not differ between groups, making it unlikely to solely account for such a high rate of persistent OSA [58].

In conclusion, gestational OSA is common, occurring in more than one of three women in the third trimester. It is not resolved in most of these women within the first 2–3 months after delivery, and the reduction in the OSA prevalence, if any, is slow for 6–8 months after delivery. Women diagnosed with OSA during pregnancy should be reevaluated for the persistence of this condition in the postpartum period.

References

1. Pien GW, Schwab RJ. Sleep disorders during pregnancy. Sleep. 2004;27:1405–17.
2. Buysse DJ, Reynolds CF, Monk TH, et al. The Pittsburgh Sleep Quality Index (PSQI): a new instrument for psychiatric research and practice. Psychiatry Res. 1989;28:193–213.
3. Sharma SK, Nehra A, Sinha S, et al. Sleep disorders in pregnancy and their association with pregnancy outcomes: a prospective observational study. Sleep Breath. 2016;20(1):87–93.
4. Moore LG, McCullough RE, Weil JV. Increased HVR in pregnancy: relationship to hormonal and metabolic changes. J Appl Physiol. 1985;62(1):158–63.
5. Jensen D, Wolfe LA, Slatkovska L, et al. Effects of human pregnancy on the ventilatory chemoreflex response to carbon dioxide. Am J Physiol Regul Integr Comp Physiol. 2005;288(5):R1369–75.
6. Popovic RM, White DP. Upper airway muscle activity in normal women: influence of hormonal status. J Appl Physiol. 1998;84(3):1055–62.
7. Ursavaş A, Karadağ M. Sleep breathing disorders in pregnancy. Tuberk Toraks. 2009;57:237–43.
8. Izci B, Vennelle M, Liston WA, et al. Sleep-disordered breathing and upper airway size in pregnancy and post-partum. Eur Respir J. 2006;27(2):321–7.
9. Venkata C, Venkateshiah SB. Sleep-disordered breathing during pregnancy. J Am Board Fam Med. 2009;22(2):158–68.
10. Maasilta P, Bachour A, Teramo K, et al. Sleep-related disordered breathing during pregnancy in obese women. Chest. 2001;120(5):1448–54.
11. Pilkington S, Carli F, Dakin MJ, et al. Increase in Mallampati score during pregnancy. Br J Anaesth. 1995;74(6):638–42.
12. Young T, Palta M, Dempsey J, et al. The occurrence of sleep-disordered breathing among middle-aged adults. N Engl J Med. 1993;328:1230–5.
13. Rimpilä V, Jernman R, Lassila K, et al. Upper-airway flow limitation and transcutaneous carbon dioxide during sleep in normal pregnancy. Sleep Med. 2017;36:67–74.
14. Ayrım A, Keskin EA, Ozol D, et al. Influence of self-reported snoring and witnessed sleep apnea on gestational hypertension and fetal outcome in pregnancy. Arch Gynecol Obstet. 2011;283:195–9.
15. Kump K, Whalen C, Tishler PV, et al. Assessment of the validity and utility of a sleep symptom questionnaire. Am J Respir Crit Care Med. 1994;150:735–41.
16. Young T, Shahar E, Nieto FJ, et al. Predictors of sleep-disordered breathing in community-dwelling adults: the Sleep Heart Health Study. Arch Intern Med. 2002;162:893–900.
17. Franklin KA, Holmgren PA, Jonsson F, et al. Snoring, pregnancy-induced hypertension, and growth retardation of the fetus. Chest. 2000;117:137–41.
18. Loube DI, Poceta JS, Morales MC, et al. Self-reported snoring in pregnancy: association with fetal outcome. Chest. 1996;109:885–9.
19. Tsai SY, Lee PL, Lee CN. Snoring and blood pressure in third-trimester normotensive pregnant women. J Nurs Scholarsh. 2018;50(5):522–9.
20. Pien GW, Fife D, Pack AI, et al. Changes in symptoms of sleep-disordered breathing during pregnancy. Sleep. 2005;28:1299–305.
21. O'Brien LM, Bullough AS, Owusu JT, et al. Pregnancy-onset habitual snoring, gestational hypertension, and preeclampsia: prospective cohort study. Am J Obstet Gynecol. 2012;207(6):487.
22. Qiu C, Enquobahrie D, Frederick IO, et al. Glucose intolerance and gestational diabetes risk in relation to sleep duration and snoring during pregnancy: a pilot study. BMC Womens Health. 2010;10:17.
23. Louis JM, Koch MA, Reddy UM, et al. Predictors of sleep-disordered breathing in pregnancy. Am J Obstet Gynecol. 2018;218(5):521.e1–521.e12.
24. Champagne KA, Kimoff RJ, Barriga PC, et al. Sleep disordered breathing in women of childbearing age & during pregnancy. Indian J Med Res. 2010;131:285–301.
25. Izci-Balserak B, Pien GW. Sleep-disordered breathing and pregnancy: potential mechanisms and evidence for maternal and fetal morbidity. Curr Opin Pulm Med. 2010;16:574–82.

26. Epstein LJ, Kristo D, Strollo PJ Jr, et al. Clinical guideline for the evaluation, management and long-term care of obstructive sleep apnea in adults. J Clin Sleep Med. 2009;5:263–76.
27. Bourjeily G, Raker CA, Chalhoub M, et al. Pregnancy and fetal outcomes of symptoms of sleep-disordered breathing. Eur Respir J. 2010;36(4):849–55.
28. Ohida T, Kaneita Y, Osaki Y, et al. Is passive smoking associated with sleep disturbance among pregnant women? Sleep. 2007;30(9):1155–61.
29. Kalmbach DA, Cheng P, Sangha R, et al. Insomnia, short sleep, and snoring in mid-to-late pregnancy: disparities related to poverty, race, and obesity. Nat Sci Sleep. 2019;11:301–15.
30. Williams MA, Gelaye B, Qiu C, et al. Habitual snoring and asthma comorbidity among pregnant women. J Asthma. 2011;48(1):91–7.
31. Guinhouya BC, Bisson M, Dubois L, et al. Body weight status and sleep disturbances during pregnancy: does adherence to gestational weight gain guidelines matter? J Womens Health. 2019;28(4):535–43.
32. Pérez-Chada D, Videla AJ, O'Flaherty M, et al. Snoring, witnessed sleep apneas and pregnancy-induced hypertension. Acta Obstet Gynecol Scand. 2007;86(7):788–92.
33. Guilleminault C, Kreutzer M, Chang JL. Pregnancy, sleep disordered breathing and treatment with nasal continuous positive airway pressure. Sleep Med. 2004;5(1):43–51.
34. Yang Z, Zhu Z, Wang C, et al. Association between adverse perinatal outcomes and sleep disturbances during pregnancy: a systematic review and meta-analysis. J Matern Fetal Neonatal Med. 2022;35(1):166–74.
35. Köken G, Sahin FK, Cosar E, et al. Oxidative stress markers in pregnant women who snore and fetal outcome: a case control study. Acta Obstet Gynecol Scand. 2007;86:1317–21.
36. Connolly G, Razak AR, Hayanga A, et al. Inspiratory flow limitation during sleep in pre-eclampsia: comparison with normal pregnant and non-pregnant women. Eur Respir J. 2001;18:672–6.
37. Fung AM, Wilson DL, Barnes M, et al. Obstructive sleep apnea and pregnancy: the effect on perinatal outcomes. J Perinatol. 2012;32:399–406.
38. Tauman R, Many A, Deutsch V, et al. Maternal snoring during pregnancy is associated with enhanced fetal erythropoiesis—a preliminary study. Sleep Med. 2011;12:518–22.
39. Hermansen MC. Nucleated red blood cells in the fetus and newborn. Arch Dis Child Fetal Neonatal Ed. 2001;84:F211–5.
40. Su MC, Chiu KL, Ruttanaumpawan P, et al. Difference in upper airway collapsibility during wakefulness between men and women in response to lower-body positive pressure. Clin Sci. 2009;116:713–20.
41. Edwards N, Blyton DM, Kirjavainen T, et al. Nasal continuous positive airway pressure reduces sleep-induced blood pressure increments in preeclampsia. Am J Respir Crit Care Med. 2000;162:252–7.
42. Poyares D, Guilleminault C, Hachul H, et al. Pre-eclampsia and nasal CPAP, part 2: hypertension during pregnancy, chronic snoring, and early nasal CPAP intervention. Sleep Med. 2007;9:15–21.
43. Gooley JJ, Mohapatra L, Twan DCK. The role of sleep duration and sleep disordered breathing in gestational diabetes mellitus. Neurobiol Sleep Circadian Rhythms. 2017;4:34–43.
44. Reutrakul S, Zaidi N, Wroblewski K, et al. Sleep disturbances and their relationship to glucose tolerance in pregnancy. Diabetes Care. 2011;34(11):2454–7.
45. O'Brien LM, Owusu JT, Swanson LM. Habitual snoring and depressive symptoms during pregnancy. BMC Pregnancy Childbirth. 2013;13:113.
46. O'Brien LM, Bullough AS, Owusu JT, et al. Snoring during pregnancy and delivery outcomes: a cohort study. Sleep. 2013;36(11):1625–32.
47. Sahin FK, Köken G, Cosar E, et al. Obstructive sleep apnea in pregnancy and fetal outcome. Int J Gynaecol Obstet. 2008;100:141–6.
48. Micheli K, Komninos I, Bagkeris E, et al. Sleep patterns in late pregnancy and risk of preterm birth and fetal growth restriction. Epidemiology. 2011;22(5):738–44.
49. Tauman R, Sivan Y, Katsav S. Maternal snoring during pregnancy is not associated with fetal growth restriction. J Matern Fetal Neonatal Med. 2012;25(8):1283–6.

50. Dunietz GL, Shedden K, Schisterman EF, et al. Associations of snoring frequency and intensity in pregnancy with time-to-delivery. Paediatr Perinat Epidemiol. 2018;32(6):504–11.
51. Cai XH, Li ML, Xu XF, et al. Zhonghua Jie He He Hu Xi Za Zhi. 2010;33(5):331–5.
52. August EM, Salihu HM, Biroscak BJ, et al. Systematic review on sleep disorders and obstetric outcomes: scope of current knowledge. Am J Perinatol. 2013;30(4):323–34.
53. Salihu HM, King L, Patel P, et al. Association between maternal symptoms of sleep disordered breathing and fetal telomere length. Sleep. 2015;38(4):559–66.
54. Favilli A, Laurenti E, Stagni GM, et al. Effects of sodium hyaluronate on symptoms and quality of life in women affected by pregnancy rhinitis: a pilot study. Gynecol Obstet Invest. 2019;84(2):159–65.
55. Dominiguez JE, Street L, Louis J. Management of obstructive sleep apnea in pregnancy. Obstet Gynecol Clin North Am. 2018;45(2):233–47.
56. Dominiguez JE, Krystal AD, Habib AS. Obstructive sleep apnea in pregnant women: a review of pregnancy outcomes and an approach to management. Anesth Analg. 2018;127(5):1167–77.
57. Balserak Bİ, Zhu B, Grandner MA, et al. Obstructive sleep apnea in pregnancy: performance of a rapid screening tool. Sleep Breath. 2019;23:425–32.
58. Street LM, Aschenbrenner CA, Houle TT, et al. Gestational obstructive sleep apnea: biomarker screening models and lack of postpartum resolution. J Clin Sleep Med. 2018;14(4):549–55.
59. Ayyar L, Shaib F, Guntupalli K. Sleep-disordered breathing in pregnancy. Sleep Med Clin. 2018;13(3):349–57.
60. Karaduman M, Sarı O, Aydoğan Ü, et al. Evaluation of obstructive sleep apnea symptoms in pregnant women with chronic disease. J Matern Fetal Neonatal Med. 2016;29(20):3379–85.
61. Gupta R, Rawat VS. Sleep and sleep disorders in pregnancy. In: Steegers EAP, Cipolla MJ, Miller EC, editors. Handbook of clinical neurology, vol. 172. Elsevier; p. 169–186.
62. Pearson F, Batterham AM, Cope S. The STOP-Bang questionnaire as a screening tool for obstructive sleep apnea in pregnancy. J Clin Sleep Med. 2019;15(5):705–10.
63. Bin YS, Cistulli PA, Ford JB. Population-based study of sleep apnea in pregnancy and maternal and infant outcomes. J Clin Sleep Med. 2016;12(6):871–7.
64. Redhead K, Walsh J, Galbally M, et al. Obstructive sleep apnea is associated with depressive symptoms in pregnancy. Sleep. 2020;43(5):zsz270.

Dysphagia During Pregnancy and the Postpartum Period

18

Hüseyin Köseoğlu, Mesut Sezikli, and Gordon Soo

18.1 Introduction

Dysphagia is commonly defined as difficulty with swallowing. This term was derived from the Greek words "dys" and "fagein," which mean "bad" and "to eat," respectively [1–3]. Other swallowing-related complaints, which are commonly confused, are odynophagia and globus sensation. Odynophagia refers to painful swallowing, and globus sensation refers to the sensation of a lump in the throat.

18.2 Initial Approach to a Patient with Dysphagia

It is important to distinguish oropharyngeal dysphagia from esophageal dysphagia [4]. Oropharyngeal dysphagia is defined as difficulty in transporting bolus from the mouth to the esophagus, whereas esophageal dysphagia is delayed transit of the food throughout the esophagus. Patients with oropharyngeal dysphagia report difficulty initiating swallowing and may have regurgitation, aspiration, and the feel of residual food in the pharynx. These patients often change their position during swallowing to help the transfer of food to the esophagus, like extending their arms and neck or using their finger to push the food. Patients with esophageal dysphagia feel difficulty in swallowing several seconds after initiating the swallowing process. The main causes of dysphagia according to this classification are summarized in

H. Köseoğlu (✉) · M. Sezikli
Faculty of Medicine, Department of Gastroenterology, Hitit University, Çorum, Turkey
e-mail: huseyinko@yahoo.com; drsezikli@hotmail.com

G. Soo
Department of Otorhinolaryngology, Head and Neck Surgery, Hong Kong, The Chinese University of Hong Kong, Hong Kong Special Administrative Region, China
e-mail: gordonsoo@gmail.com

C. Cingi et al. (eds.), *ENT Diseases: Diagnosis and Treatment during Pregnancy and Lactation*, https://doi.org/10.1007/978-3-031-05303-0_18

Table 18.1 The main causes of dysphagia

Oropharyngeal dysphagia		Esophageal dysphagia	
Mechanic obstruction	Cervical osteophyte	**Extraesophageal obstruction**	Aberrant subclavian artery
	Cricopharyngeal bar		Thoracic aorta aneurysm
	Zenker's diverticulum		Mediastinal mass
	Goiter	**Intraesophageal obstruction**	Benign tumors
	Neoplasms of the larynx, pharynx, and tongue		Esophageal carcinoma
Motility disorders	Cerebrovascular event		Caustic esophagitis
	Parkinson's disease		Eosinophilic esophagitis
	Amyotrophic lateral sclerosis		Radiation injury
	Multiple sclerosis		Peptic stricture
	Myasthenia gravis	**Motility disorders**	Achalasia
	Myotonic dystrophy		Distal esophageal spasm
Miscellaneous	Decreased saliva secretion		Hypercontractile esophagus
			Hypertensive LES

LES lower esophageal sphincter

Table 18.1. Because the etiology differs between the two types of dysphagia, all patients should be evaluated according to this classification.

Subsequently, all patients should be evaluated according to types of food-producing symptoms, the time course, and the severity of the symptoms and associated symptoms. Taking a careful history focusing on these questions helps the clinician for making an appropriate differential diagnosis and planning diagnostic testing. For example, acute onset of inability to swallow foods suggests impaction of a foreign body. Oropharyngeal dysphagia in an older patient, especially with weight loss, pain, and a history of smoking, may be due to malignancies of the base of the tongue, larynx, and pharynx. Oropharyngeal dysphagia with speech changes suggests neuromuscular disorders. A combination of hoarseness, nasal speech, and dysphonia with oropharyngeal dysphagia may indicate muscular dystrophy. Oropharyngeal dysphagia, which progresses during the meal, may be due to myasthenia gravis. Progressive esophageal dysphagia is commonly due to esophageal carcinoma, peptic stricture, or achalasia, whereas intermittent esophageal dysphagia may be seen in esophageal strictures. Dysphagia for solids alone usually develops in patients with anatomic obstruction, whereas dysphagia for both solids and liquids is often associated with motility disorders. Chronic heartburn in a patient with esophageal dysphagia may be due to complications of gastroesophageal reflux disease, such as peptic stricture, erosive esophagitis, and even esophageal adenocarcinoma. Associated weight loss may be an indicator of obstructing esophageal malignancies. The physical examination should include a careful examination of the oral cavity, head, and neck and also include neurologic examination [3, 4].

After taking adequate history and doing a proper physical examination, clinicians should plan diagnostic testing according to the symptoms. Central nervous system imaging and nasoendoscopy may be indicated in patients with oropharyngeal dysphagia. Further testing for oropharyngeal dysphagia includes videofluoroscopic swallowing studies and manometry, according to the initial diagnosis. Commonly used tests for esophageal dysphagia are barium contrast esophagogram, upper gastrointestinal endoscopy, and esophageal manometry. Upper endoscopy should be performed in patients with esophageal dysphagia, with the aim of determining the underlying cause, excluding malignancy, and performing therapy if indicated. Barium contrast esophagogram is commonly performed before endoscopy when proximal esophageal lesions (such as laryngeal cancer, Zenker's diverticulum) are suspected and after endoscopy when a negative upper gastrointestinal endoscopy is present in patients in whom mechanical obstruction is still the suspected diagnosis. In patients whose upper endoscopy suspects esophageal motility disorders or could not detect any reason for dysphagia, esophageal manometry should be performed [5–7].

18.3 General Considerations About Dysphagia in Pregnancy and Postpartum Period

Due to the rarity of dysphagia causing illnesses, no specific guidelines are present about dysphagia or dysphagia causing diseases in pregnancy. But if a pregnant patient presents with dysphagia, the same initial questions should be asked to her and a possible diagnosis for dysphagia should be made. The diagnostic tests should be performed carefully in pregnant patients. Although diagnostic imaging studies with ionizing radiation expose the fetus less than the level with evidence of a risk for fetal anomalies, barium esophagogram should be used with caution. Fetal risk with radiation decreases with gestation age, but there is no evidence that esophagogram is contraindicated in pregnant patients. Central nervous system imaging may be performed if indicated, but magnetic resonance imaging should be preferred over computed tomography. Ionizing radiation has no unfavorable effect on babies of breastfeeding mothers [8].

Upper gastrointestinal endoscopy is an important diagnostic test in patients with dysphagia, especially esophageal dysphagia. The safety of gastrointestinal endoscopy in pregnancy is not widely studied. Although upper endoscopy is safe and effective in pregnancy in case series and case–control studies, it is accepted to be risky for the fetus because the fetus is sensitive to maternal hypoxia and hypotension. Sedation may cause hypotension or hypoventilation. Another mechanism for fetal hypoxia is decreased uterine blood flow due to inferior vena cava compression with maternal positioning. Endoscopy in pregnancy should be performed only if the indication is strong and it should be deferred until to the second trimester if it is possible [9]. The American Society for Gastrointestinal Endoscopy (ASGE) defined dysphagia and odynophagia as indications for endoscopy in pregnant patients [9]. Cautious administration of sedation should be performed because of the increased risk of aspiration and difficult airway. When used in standard concentrations, none of the currently used anesthetic agents have been shown to have teratogenic effects in humans [10]. Commonly used drugs such as meperidine, midazolam, propofol, ketamine, and fentanyl have a FDA category of safety in pregnancy of grade B but should be used with the lowest effective dose and close monitoring. Consultation with an obstetrician should be made before endoscopy and fetal heart rate should be monitored if indicated. Upper endoscopy may be performed in lactating women, but caution should be exercised in using medication for sedation because they may be excreted in breast milk. Esophageal manometry is not contraindicated in pregnant and breastfeeding patients.

18.4 Considerations About some Specific Causes of Dysphagia in Pregnancy and Postpartum Period

18.4.1 Achalasia

Achalasia is an esophageal motility disorder, which is characterized by incomplete lower esophageal sphincter relaxation with increased sphincter tone and non-peristaltic contractions of the esophagus. It is a rare disease with an incidence of 0.5–1/100000 population per year. The disease affects most commonly patients between 25 and 60 years and therefore may appear in pregnancy. Dysphagia, regurgitation, vomiting, chest pain, coughing, and weight loss are main symptoms of achalasia. In pregnancy, achalasia was found to be associated with maternal malnutrition and death, preterm delivery, fetal growth restriction, and even fetal demise. Upper gastrointestinal endoscopy may help differentiate from mechanical obstruction, and it may suggest the diagnosis of achalasia. But manometry is critical in the diagnosis of achalasia. The diagnosis should be made with upper endoscopy and esophageal motility in pregnant patients, with caution as mentioned above. The treatment options of achalasia are pharmacological therapy with smooth muscle relaxants, endoscopic botulinum toxin injection, endoscopic pneumatic dilatation, peroral endoscopic myotomy, and Heller myotomy. The most commonly used medications for achalasia are isosorbide dinitrate and nifedipine, which both have a FDA category of safety in pregnancy of grade C. Botulinum toxin (FDA category C medication) injection has the risk of miscarriage but may be used with caution as a bridging therapy until delivery. Case reports are present in the literature performing successful pneumatic balloon dilatation and surgical myotomy in pregnant patients. Esophageal rupture at pneumatic dilatation and general anesthesia risks at myotomy should be kept in mind. In our literature search, no pregnant case receiving peroral endoscopic myotomy was present. Because none of the therapy alternatives are without risk, conservative therapy with enteral or parenteral nutrition support until delivery may be an alternative method in pregnant patients with achalasia [11–15].

18.4.2 Other Motility Disorders

Distal esophageal spasm (formerly known as diffuse esophageal spasm) is the impaired inhibitory innervation, which leads to premature and propagated contractions seen in the distal part of the esophagus. Hypercontractile (jackhammer) esophagus is named when vigorous esophageal contractions exist in a patient with dysphagia. The real incidences of these diseases are unknown, but both diseases are seen very rarely. The patients commonly present with dysphagia for solids and liquids and noncardiac chest pain, and the precise diagnosis is made by manometry studies. Nitrates, calcium channel blockers, hydralazine, tricyclic antidepressants, and anxiolytics may be used for these diseases, but a widely accepted treatment algorithm does not exist. Endoscopic botulinum toxin injection and surgery are further treatment options. Most of the patients may also have symptoms of gastroesophageal reflux disease (GERD), and acid suppression with PPIs may be needed. No data is available about these motility disorders in pregnancy because of the rarity of these conditions. In our opinion, the treatment of such patients may be delayed until delivery. But the aforementioned treatment options may be considered in patients with severe symptoms and nutritional deficiencies [15].

18.4.3 Esophageal Tumors

Esophageal benign and malignant tumors are other causes of dysphagia. The most common esophageal cancers are malign epithelial tumors, and the two most common types of epithelial tumors are squamous cell cancer and adenocarcinoma. The most common symptoms are progressive dysphagia and weight loss. Chronic gastrointestinal blood loss may occur and result in iron deficiency anemia. Esophageal cancers are more commonly seen in males compared to females. Additionally, the median age at diagnosis for esophageal cancer is 69 years, and only about 3% of patients with esophageal cancers are under 45 years. Due to this epidemiologic data, esophageal cancers are very rare during pregnancy. But esophageal tumors should always kept in mind as an etiological reason in patients presenting with dysphagia and upper gastrointestinal endoscopy should be performed if indicated. Only several case reports about esophageal cancer in pregnancy are present in the literature, and there is no consensus about the management and treatment of esophageal cancer during pregnancy. Magnetic resonance imaging or endoscopic ultrasonography may be performed safely for the staging of esophageal carcinoma in pregnancy. The treatment should be individualized according to the tumor size, gestational age, and fetus maturation. Successful resection of esophageal tumors in pregnancy is present in the literature [16, 17].

18.4.4 Gastroesophageal Reflux Disease, Peptic Stricture, and Schatzki's Ring

Dysphagia may be seen over 30% of patients with GERD. It develops mostly when GERD causes peptic stricture, but severe esophageal inflammation alone may also present with dysphagia [18, 19]. GERD is frequently seen in pregnancy, and its incidence increases with gestational age. Commonly, no testing is required in pregnant patients with reflux symptoms, and the diagnosis of GERD should be based on symptoms and treatment response [20]. Alginic acid and calcium- and magnesium-based antacids are safe treatment options in the treatment of GERD in pregnancy. Ranitidine has been used for years, which has a FDA pregnancy category of B. PPIs may be used if the aforementioned drugs are not sufficient for symptom relief. Omeprazole is categorized as category C by FDA, whereas the other PPIs are categorized as group B. A recently published meta-analysis showed that PPI use was associated with an increased risk of congenital malformations [21]. Other probable problems of the use of PPIs in pregnancy are childhood asthma in offspring and increased risk of cholestasis. Because of safety concerns, PPIs should only be used if the benefit outweighs the risk to the fetus. Peptic strictures develop in 7–23% of patients with reflux esophagitis without treatment and are the most common cause of benign esophageal strictures. Schatzki's ring is widely considered the form of an early peptic stricture, which is most commonly seen in older men. The diagnosis of peptic strictures is made by upper endoscopy, with the advantage of performing endoscopic therapy at the same session. The treatment of peptic stricture includes acid-suppressive therapy with PPIs and endoscopic dilatation with bougie or balloon. Based on studies, healing the coexistent esophagitis with acid suppression is essential for the longer clinical benefit of endoscopic dilatation. Because of the risk of perforation and other complications, endoscopic dilatation should be preferably delayed until delivery. But endoscopic dilatation may be performed cautiously in pregnant patients with severe symptoms, who cannot maintain adequate nutritional status [22].

18.4.5 Other Benign Strictures

The most common etiologic reason for benign esophageal strictures is gastroesophageal reflux, whereas around 25% of patients have other reasons for stricture development. Examples are radiation injury, history of esophageal sclerotherapy, surgical anastomosis, and caustic ingestion. The diagnosis of these conditions is made with the help of endoscopy. The therapy should focus on relieving dysphagia with endoscopic dilatation and prevent stricture recurrence. Mechanical dilators and balloon dilators may be used for dilatation in symptomatic patients. The complication of endoscopic dilatation includes perforation, chest pain, bacteremia, and hemorrhage, which may all be life threatening [22]. No consensus about endoscopic dilatation in pregnancy exists, but if these complications develop in a pregnant patient, the results may be more catastrophic for the patients and even for the clinician. Because of these complications, it is thought to be logical to defer such interventions until the postpartum period. Nutritional support with oral nutritional products may be given to such patients.

18.4.6 Eosinophilic Esophagitis

Eosinophilic esophagitis is a chronic immune-mediated esophageal disease, which is characterized by esophageal dysfunction symptoms and by eosinophil-dominant inflammation on histologic analysis [23]. Its incidence has increased in recent years. EoE commonly presents with dysphagia, food impaction, or chest pain. It often affects young patients and may be commonly detected at reproductive age. Little is known about the association between EoE and pregnancy. Recently, it was published that most patients with EoE reported that symptoms improved with pregnancy [24]. EoE has probably no unfavorable effect on pregnancy outcomes. The first-line treatment of EoE is dietary therapy. Avoidance of known food allergens should be suggested to these patients. The diet therapy can be continued throughout the pregnancy, but attention should be paid to the risk of nutritional deprivation. Acid suppression therapy with PPIs and topical glucocorticoids are pharmacologic therapies used in patients with EoE. PPIs should be used with caution because of safety reasons mentioned above. Corticosteroids are classified as category C in pregnancy, with a risk of adrenal insufficiency, but corticosteroids are widely used for various diseases and a large cohort study showed no statistically significant risk of congenital malformations [25]. Local corticosteroids are used in EoE, and it is expected to be safer than systemic corticosteroids. Because symptoms tend to worsen during pregnancy, the medical therapy should be continued throughout pregnancy. Corticosteroids are also safe in breastfeeding patients and may be used [26]. EoE may lead to esophageal strictures, which may worsen dysphagia. The first therapy for these strictures should be medical, but endoscopic dilatation may be performed in patients with strictures who have not responded to medical therapy. Dilatation should be performed carefully because of the increased risk of perforation [27]. Pregnancy is not a contraindication for endoscopic dilatation and can be performed in indicated patients with maximum attention, preferably in the second trimester.

18.4.7 Functional Dysphagia

Globus sensation, functional dysphagia, functional chest pain, functional heartburn, and reflux hypersensitivity are diseases that are called functional swallowing disorders [28]. Symptoms in functional swallowing disorders are not due to gastroesophageal reflux, dysmotility, or mechanical obstruction. The diagnosis of functional dysphagia needs exclusion of oropharyngeal reasons of dysphagia, structural lesions of the esophagus, GERD, EoE, and motility disorders. Hypersensitivity and hypervigilance are important components of the pathogenesis of these diseases.

The treatment of functional dysphagia includes cognitive behavioral therapy, esophageal-directed hypnotherapy, and medical therapy with antidepressants and PPIs [29]. Gastrointestinal symptoms including nausea, vomiting, and heartburn are commonly seen in pregnancy. Theoretically functional dysphagia should not be affected by pregnancy, but because hypersensitivity and hypervigilance are major pathogenetic factors in functional dysphagia, symptoms other than dysphagia occurring through pregnancy may exacerbate dysphagia. Pregnancy may be a challenging period for some patients and cause stress. Functional dysphagia is a stress-sensitive disorder, and the increased level of stress may exacerbate functional dysphagia in pregnancy. Behavioral therapy and PPIs may be continued through pregnancy. PPI use in pregnancy has some safety risks and should only be used if other therapies fail. The use of antidepressants should be withheld if possible due to probable risks of antidepressant use during pregnancy, but low-dose antidepressants may be continued in indicated patients with caution. Another important problem with functional dysphagia in pregnancy is receiving adequate nutrition for the fetus and mother. The pain or discomfort associated with swallowing may lead to avoidance of food intake, and this may cause malnutrition. The patients should be warned about this issue, and adequate dietary intake should be encouraged.

18.4.8 Neurological Disorders

Virtually any neuromuscular disease may cause dysphagia, especially oropharyngeal dysphagia. Some examples include stroke, poliomyelitis, amyotrophic lateral sclerosis, Parkinson's disease, oculopharyngeal dystrophy, myotonic dystrophy, myasthenia gravis, multiple sclerosis, medullary and vagal tumors, and surgical manipulation of the medullary and vagal region. Most of these diseases are seen in elderly patients and are rarely seen in pregnant patients. The management of these kinds of dysphagia includes the treatment of underlying disorder and additional interventions such as swallow rehabilitation, therapeutic endoscopy, and surgery. Multiple sclerosis is commonly seen in young women, and therefore its effect on pregnancy is important. Although the effect of pregnancy on dysphagia due to multiple sclerosis is not widely investigated, pregnancy has beneficial effects on multiple sclerosis symptoms and relapse rates. Pregnant patients with multiple sclerosis should be evaluated for medications risk/benefit ratio and be treated if the benefit outweighs the risks for treatment [30]. Myasthenia gravis is more commonly seen in women and mostly develops in the third decade. Therefore, an overlap of myasthenia gravis with pregnancy is expected. About 15% of patients with myasthenia gravis have bulbar symptoms including dysphagia. A large case series showed that most patients experienced worsening of the symptoms of myasthenia gravis in pregnancy, but 29% of the patients had relief of symptoms. The effect of pregnancy on dysphagia in patients with myasthenia gravis has not been studied to date. When the symptoms are mild, no treatment is needed during pregnancy. Pyridostigmine and corticosteroids may be used with caution, and intravenous immunoglobulin and plasma exchange may also be used for severe forms [31]. Oculopharyngeal muscular dystrophy is a rare hereditary disease causing ptosis, dysarthria, and dysphagia due to ocular and pharyngeal muscle involvement. Regardless of the neurological disease-causing dysphagia, the most important issue is to provide necessary nutrition for the mother and fetus. Nutritional assessment should be performed, and support should be given to patients with inadequate nutrition.

References

1. Smout AJ. Approach to the patient with dysphagia, odynophagia, or noncardiac chest pain. In: Podolsky DK, Camilleri M, Fitz JG, Kalloo AN, Shanahan F, Wang TC, editors. Yamada's textbook of gastroenterology. 6th ed. Hoboken: Wiley; 2016.
2. Francis DL. Dysphagia. In: DeVault KR, Wallace MB, Aqel BA, Lindor KD, editors. Practical gastroenterology and hepatology board review toolkit. 2nd ed. Hoboken: Wiley; 2016.
3. Trate DM, Parkman HP, Fisher RS. Dysphagia. Evaluation, diagnosis, and treatment. Prim Care. 1996;23:417–32.
4. Rothstein RD. A systematic approach to the patient with dysphagia. Hosp Pract. 1997;32:169–75.
5. Barloon TJ, Bergus GR, Lu CC. Diagnostic imaging in the evaluation of dysphagia. Am Fam Physician. 1996;53:535–46.
6. Varadarajulu S, Eloubeidi MA, Patel RS, et al. The yield and the predictors of esophageal pathology when upper endoscopy is used for the initial evaluation of dysphagia. Gastrointest Endosc. 2005;61:804–8.
7. Ott DJ. Radiographic techniques and efficacy in evaluating esophageal dysphagia. Dysphagia. 1990;5:192–203.
8. Committee on Obstetric Practice. Committee opinion no. 723: guidelines for diagnostic imaging during pregnancy and lactation. Obstet Gynecol. 2017;130:e210–6. https://doi.org/10.1097/AOG.0000000000002355.
9. ASGE Standard of Practice Committee, Shergill AK, Ben-Menachem T, et al. Guidelines for endoscopy in pregnant and lactating women. Gastrointest Endosc. 2012;76:18–24. https://doi.org/10.1016/j.gie.2012.02.029.
10. Committee on Obstetric Practice. ACOG Committee opinion no. 775: nonobstetric surgery during pregnancy. Obstet Gynecol. 2019;133:e285–6. https://doi.org/10.1097/AOG.0000000000003174.
11. Spiliopoulos D, Spiliopoulos M, Awala A. Esophageal achalasia: an uncommon complication during pregnancy treated conservatively. Case Rep Obstet Gynecol. 2013;2013:639698. https://doi.org/10.1155/2013/639698.
12. Khudyak V, Lysy J, Mankuta D. Achalasia in pregnancy. Obstet Gynecol Surv. 2006;61:207–11. https://doi.org/10.1097/01.ogx.0000201893.92103.94.
13. Palanivelu C, Rangarajan M, Maheshkumaar GS, Parthasarathi R. Laparoscopic Heller's cardiomyotomy for achalasia of the cardia in a pregnant patient. Ann Acad Med Singap. 2008;37:442–3.
14. Neubert ZS, Stickle ET. Bridging therapy for achalasia in a second trimester pregnant patient. J Fam Med Prim Care. 2019;8:289–97. https://doi.org/10.4103/jfmpc.jfmpc_389_18.
15. Pandolfino JE, Kahrilas PJ. Esophageal neuromuscular function and motility disorders. In: Feldman M, Friedman LS, Brandt LJ, editors. Sleisenger and Fordtran's gastrointestinal and liver disease. 10th ed. Philadelphia: Elsevier Inc; 2016.
16. Patel NC, Ramirez FC. Esophageal tumors. In: Feldman M, Friedman LS, Brandt LJ, editors. Sleisenger and Fordtran's gastrointestinal and liver disease. 10th ed. Philadelphia: Elsevier Inc; 2016.
17. Şahin M, Kocaman G, Özkan M, et al. Resection of esophageal carcinoma during pregnancy. Ann Thorac Surg. 2015;99:333–5. https://doi.org/10.1016/j.athoracsur.2014.01.080.

18. Richter JE, Friedenberg FK. Gastroesophageal reflux disease. In: Feldman M, Friedman LS, Brandt LJ, editors. Sleisenger and Fordtran's gastrointestinal and liver disease. 10th ed. Philadelphia: Elsevier Inc; 2016.

19. Pregun I, Hritz I, Tulassay Z, Herszényi L. Peptic esophageal stricture: medical treatment. Dig Dis. 2009;27:31–7. https://doi.org/10.1159/000210101.

20. Katz PO, Gerson LB, Vela MF. Guidelines for the diagnosis and management of gastro-esophageal reflux disease. Am J Gastroenterol. 2013;108(3):308–29. https://doi.org/10.1038/ajg.2012.444.

21. Li CM, Zhernakova A, Engstrand L, et al. Systematic review with meta-analysis: the risks of proton pump inhibitors during pregnancy. Aliment Pharmacol Ther. 2020;51:410–20. https://doi.org/10.1111/apt.15610.

22. Standards of Practice Committee, Egan JV, Baron TH, et al. Esophageal dilation. Gastrointest Endosc. 2006;2006(63):755–60.

23. Liacouras CA, Furuta GT, Hirano I, et al. Eosinophilic esophagitis: updated consensus recommendations for children and adults. J Allergy Clin Immunol. 2011;128:3–20.

24. Schreiner P, Meissgeier S, Safroneeva E, et al. Disease progression and outcomes of pregnancies in women with eosinophilic esophagitis. Clin Gastroenterol Hepatol. 2019;S1542-3565(19):31397–7. https://doi.org/10.1016/j.cgh.2019.11.057.

25. Hviid A, Molgaard-Nielsen D. Corticosteroid use during pregnancy and risk of orofacial clefts. CMAJ. 2011;183:796–804.

26. Burk CM, Long MD, Dellon ES. Management of eosinophilic esophagitis during pregnancy. Dig Dis Sci. 2016;61:1819–25. https://doi.org/10.1007/s10620-016-4077-6.

27. Dougherty M, Runge TM, Eluri S, et al. Esophageal dilation with either bougie or balloon technique as a treatment for eosinophilic esophagitis: a systematic review and meta-analysis. Gastrointest Endosc. 2017;86:581–91.

28. Aziz Q, Fass R, Gyawali CP, et al. Functional esophageal disorders. Gastroenterology. 2016;S0016-5085(16):00178–5. https://doi.org/10.1053/j.gastro.2016.02.012.

29. Guadagnoli LA, Pandolfino JE, Yadlapati R. Functional swallowing disorders. In: Beniwal-Patel P, Shaker R, editors. Gastrointestinal and liver disorders in women's health. Cham: Springer; 2019.

30. Voskuhl R, Momtazee C. Pregnancy: effect on multiple sclerosis, treatment considerations, and breastfeeding. Neurotherapeutics. 2017;14(4):974–84. https://doi.org/10.1007/s13311-017-0562-7.

31. Waters J. Management of myasthenia gravis in pregnancy. Neurol Clin. 2019;37(1):113–20. https://doi.org/10.1016/j.ncl.2018.09.003.

Temporomandibular Joint Disorders During Pregnancy and the Postpartum Period

19

Mehmet Birol Özel and Berna Özel

19.1 Introduction

Temporomandibular joint (TMJ) is a unique structure in the body, forming a twin joint between the mandibular bone and the skull, exhibiting complex biomechanical properties. With the lower joint space allowing rotation and the upper joint space allowing sliding movement, it is considered a "ginglymoarthroidal joint" [1]. The muscles of mastication, suprahyoid, and infrahyoid muscles produce jaw movements [2]. It is continuously functional in chewing, speaking, and swallowing. It also aids in important functions such as taste and breathing. The maximum opening movement is 40–60 mm, lateral movement is 10–12 mm, and maximum protrusive movement is approximately 8–11 mm depending on the age and size of the individual, and the interocclusal space measured at the incisors is 1–10 mm with the mandible in the rest position and head in the upright position [3].

19.2 Signs and Symptoms of Temporomandibular Disorders

Costen was a pioneer in describing signs and symptoms that may be referred to as temporomandibular disorders (TMDs) today [4]. A meta-analysis and a systematic review that reported a high prevalence of otologic signs and symptoms such as ear fullness, otalgia, tinnitus, vertigo, and hearing loss among adult patients with TMD might be a confirmation of his early observations [5]. Although TMD is an umbrella

M. B. Özel
Faculty of Dentistry, Department of Orthodontics, Kocaeli University, Kocaeli, Turkey
e-mail: birolozel@hotmail.com

B. Özel (✉)
Private Dental Center, Trabzon, Turkey
e-mail: berna0980@yahoo.com

251

C. Cingi et al. (eds.), *ENT Diseases: Diagnosis and Treatment during Pregnancy and Lactation*, https://doi.org/10.1007/978-3-031-05303-0_19

term for symptoms of pain and dysfunction at the masticatory muscles, temporomandibular joint (TMJ) and the head and neck region with restricted jaw movements, TMJ sounds, headaches, and ear pain as common findings, it is advised to make a clear distinction between muscle and joint problems [6]. Due to the complex structure and functionality of the craniofacial region and the diversity of signs and symptoms of TMD, diagnosis and treatment of temporomandibular disorders require a multidisciplinary approach and collaboration among medical specialties. Specialties in various branches of dentistry and ear, nose, and throat, physical therapy and rehabilitation, plastic surgery, neurology, and psychiatry are often involved in the diagnosis and treatment of TMD.

Due to the sampling, selection criteria, and data collection methods, reported prevalence values vary [7]. The prevalence of TMD was reported to be between 5 and 12% by the National Institute of Dental and Craniofacial Research [8]. According to a recent systematic review and meta-analysis conducted by Valesan et al., the overall prevalence of TMD was found to be 31% in adults/elderly and 11% in children/adolescents. The most prevalent TMD was disk displacement, with a reduction of 26% in adults/elderly and 7.5% in children/adolescents [9].

Although there are studies reporting that there is no difference in the prevalence of TMD between genders [10], in many studies it has been stated that TMD is more common in women [11–14].

## 19.3	Etiology

Despite the fact that the exact etiology of TMD may not be resolved accurately in many cases, trauma, clenching, third molar removal, somatization, and female gender were reported as risk factors [15, 16]. According to neuromuscular theory, occlusal interferences creating an imbalance in the neuromuscular mechanism through proprioceptive feedback may also produce pain and spasm in the masticatory system [17], but the effect of the occlusion on the development of TMD has not been clearly demonstrated [18, 19]. Even though a direct cause–effect relationship has not been established, oral parafunctions such as thumb sucking, nail biting, and bruxism may be predisposing factors and should be eliminated [20, 21]. TMD has also been attributed to psychosocial factors [22–24], and myofascial pain dysfunction syndrome patients have been shown to demonstrate higher salivary cortisol and anxiety levels than controls [25]. In a schizophrenia population, which is a serious mental disorder, the prevalence of TMD signs and tooth wear was found to be higher than in controls, which could be attributed to the disease itself, psychotropic medications, and altered lifestyle and oral health [26]. Also, axis II of the Diagnostic Criteria for TMD (DC/TMD), which is utilized as a tool for the assessment of TMDs, includes an assessment of psychosocial status and pain-related disability [27]. Higher levels of somatization and psychoticism were also found to hinder efforts for treatment [28]. Sarlani et al. emphasized the role of the central nervous system and reported greater temporal summation of pain and aftersensations from digital stimulation exhibited by TMD patients than controls suggesting a generalized hyperexcitability of the central nociceptive system that could contribute to the development and/or maintenance of chronic TMD pain. They also found greater temporal summation of pain and aftersensations in healthy females than males, which could be a possible reason for the predominance of TMD among women [29]. Higher levels of IL-8 and IgG found in female TMD patients may also suggest that chronic inflammation and autoimmunity may also be involved in TMD [30]. Although conclusive results could not have been drawn to date, genetic polymorphisms, rs6269 and rs9332377, in COMT were shown to be significantly associated with TMD [31].

19.4 Diagnosis

Diagnosis of TMDs is made by a careful anamnesis, clinical examination, and medical imaging. Information about the main complaint, onset, duration, intensity of pain, trauma related to the jaw, dental interventions, previous treatments, parafunctional activities (pencil biting, bruxism, clenching, lip biting, tongue thrusting), extraoral habits (holding a phone between the shoulder and chin, playing violin, holding the mandible in the palm while resting), head and ear pain, and cervical diseases are gathered within a detailed history. Clinical examination basically consists of inspection, palpation, and auscultation. The aim of visual examination is to observe the presence of deviations/deflections during opening and closing movements of the jaw. Also, the range of mouth opening, lateral and protrusive movements, are measured and recorded. Body posture, level of the shoulders, asymmetry of the face, and any visible swelling in the joint region should be included in inspection. External palpation of the joint and palpating the posterior aspect of the condyle by placing little fingers inside the external auditory canal during mouth opening and closing is performed in order to evaluate the balance between the right and left condyles and feel TMJ sounds. In many instances, a stethoscope may be used for auscultation of TMJ sounds that could not be felt on palpation. Palpation of muscles of mastication and neck for soreness and trigger points should also be performed.

The clinical examination is usually supported by medical imaging methods for TMJ diagnosis. Panoramic radiographs, transcranial radiographs, computerized tomography, digital fluoroscopy, ultrasonography, scintigraphy, and magnetic resonance imaging are utilized for imaging of the TMJ. Posteroanterior cephalograms, panoramic radiographs, transcranial radiographs, and computerized tomography are used for imaging the osseous structures of TMJ for developmental anomalies, trauma, and arthritis-related bony changes. Dynamic display of the joint movement may be obtained by digital fluoroscopy [32]. Despite its limitations in imaging the hard tissues and operator dependency for accuracy, ultrasonography is a noninvasive, relatively simple, and low-cost imaging technique used for evaluating disk position and effusion in TMJ and studying painful joints [33]. Nuclear imaging (scintigraphy) provides supplemental physiological information in the evaluation of skeletal growth, condylar hyperplasia, synovitis, and appraisal of rheumatoid arthritis or osteoarthritis [34]. Magnetic resonance imaging is used for the evaluation of the position and morphology of the disc and is regarded as the gold standard for soft tissue imaging of the TMJ [34]. Although arthroscopic and arthrographic imaging are also available methods, they have limited utility due to the special skills needed for performing the procedures and their invasive nature [35].

Research diagnostic criteria for temporomandibular disorders (RDC/TMD) [36] and diagnostic criteria for temporomandibular disorders (DC/TMD) [27] are internationally accepted classification tools for TMD diagnosis. RDC/TMD consists of two parts. The first part is for the diagnosis of malfunctions of masticatory muscles and TMJ. The severity of pain experienced in chronic painful conditions and TMD and the extent of the pathological change in tissues may not necessarily overlap. Therefore, there are questions to evaluate pain and psychosocial status in the second part [36]. International Classification of Orofacial Pain (ICOP) is a recent attempt to increase the standardization and reproducibility [37]. The development of diagnostic systems for TMDs is a dynamic process and depends on the reduction of heterogeneity and the ability to reduce a complex disease to a phenotype that can be detected by simple clinical evaluations [38].

For clinical purposes, Laskin proposed a simplified TMD classification consisting of problems related to the articular origin and muscular origin. Muscle problems are summarized as myalgia, myofascial pain, myositis, myospasm, hyperkinesia, hypokinesia, hypertrophy, and contracture, whereas joint problems are summarized as congenital anomalies, developmental anomalies, traumatic injuries, ankylosis, arthritis, neoplasia, internal derangements, subluxation, and/or dislocation [6]. Musculoskeletal conditions were found to be the most common cause of TMDs, which constituted almost 50% of cases, where disc displacement, in which the condyle-disc relationship is impaired, was diagnosed in 41.1% and inflammatory degenerative disorders were diagnosed in 30.1% of the patients [39, 40].

Myofascial TMDs show spontaneous facial pain or pain in mandibular movements and sensitivity to palpation in musculature, especially the masticatory muscles and the presence of trigger points [41]. Myofascial TMD may overlap with tension-type headache [42] and fibromyalgia and a differential diagnosis may not be available [43, 44]. Manfredini et al. used two self-report questionnaires to compare psychopathological symptoms in groups of patients with myofascial pain, disc displacement, joint disorders, and no TMD in terms of mood and panic-agoraphobic spectrum. They found that depressive symptoms for mood spectrum and stress sensitivity, panic, separation anxiety, hypochondriac, and agoraphobic symptoms for panic-agoraphobic spectrum were significantly higher in myofascial pain patients, indicating that psychological factors may have an important impact in this group of patients [45]. Catastrophization can be defined as a pessimistic expectation about the future that is not based on facts, while in terms of pain, it is the actual or expected level of pain experience showing an exaggerated negativity bias and has been shown to affect both the symptom severity and treatment outcome in TMD patients [46].

19.5   TMD in Relation to Pregnancy/Lactation

It was previously mentioned that most of the epidemiological studies show a consensus that the prevalence of TMD symptoms is higher in women. The incidence of TMD in women in patient populations was reported to be higher than that in the general population [47]. This has been largely attributed to sex hormones, especially estrogen. The effects of serum estrogen, exogenous estrogen, and locally synthesized estrogen were emphasized [48]. During the pregnancy period, which comprises the development of the fetus, the woman body undergoes important physiological changes that create a serious burden on the female body. During pregnancy, both estrogen and progesterone levels rise. Estrogens are thought to play a role in the development of TMD by increasing joint laxity during pregnancy and inducing a series of specific inflammatory responses in the TMJ [49]. Solak et al. compared the prevalence of TMD and systemic joint hypermobility in pregnant women with a matched nonpregnant women sample and found no correlation between systemic joint hypermobility and TMD [50]. Also, improvement of musculoskeletal symptoms of TMD or protective effects of pregnancy have also been reported [51, 52]. Almubarak et al. reported lower estrogen levels in patients with TMD in a cross-sectional study conducted in a female population in the Aseer region [53]. The percentage of TMD and non-TMD patients was investigated by Muñoz Lora et al. and has been found to be similar in postmenopausal women who were receiving hormone replacement therapy and not receiving hormone replacement therapy, suggesting that usage of exogenous hormones was not associated with TMD [54]. Patil et al. measured serum levels of estrogen and progesterone by the enzyme immunoassay competition method in the luteal phase of the menstrual cycle and reported increased serum levels of estrogen and progesterone with increasing severity of TMD [55]. The role of sex hormones in the development of TMD was also investigated on the basis of polycystic ovary syndrome, and the frequency and severity of TMD were found to be higher in polycystic ovary syndrome patients than in matched controls [56]. Another study confirmed these results reporting a seven times higher incidence of TMD in polycystic ovary syndrome patients, and also matrix metalloproteinase (MMP) 1–8, tumor necrosis factor (TNF)-alpha, and progesterone levels were found to be significantly higher than in healthy controls. Moreover, only the progesterone levels differed between the polycystic ovary syndrome patients with and without TMD, suggesting that lower levels of progesterone may be associated with TMD [57]. The relief of TMD symptoms during pregnancy was attributed to the increasing level of progesterone. Progesterone was shown to downregulate Sodium channel 1.7 (Nav1.7), which is important for pain perception, and progesterone receptor antagonist RU-486 partially reversed the effect of progesterone. These findings may even bring up the use of progesterone as a potential drug for TMD pain [58]. Although joint laxity increased in peripheral joints during pregnancy and postpartum, it was not found to be correlated with serum relaxin levels [59].

Although uncommon, temporomandibular joint dislocation has been reported as a complication of hyperemesis gravidarum in pregnancy [60].

19.6 Treatment

It is well known that successful treatment depends on correct diagnosis and appropriate treatment. Although some TMDs have identifiable objective findings and good response to treatment and even spontaneous improvement, in many instances the underlying physical factor may not be fully identified and cannot be fully resolved despite all treatment modalities [61].

It is necessary to understand the natural course of the disease in treatment planning. Most TMJ symptoms improve over a period of approximately 1 year or more. Main aims of the treatment are elimination of pain, improvement of dysfunction, and slowing the progression of the disease.

Although there is a lack of knowledge and there is no consensus among clinicians on the modality of treatment and a standardized evidence-based approach toward TMD treatment, available options may include patient education, psychological and behavioral interventions (relaxation techniques and stress management), therapeutic exercises, manual treatment methods, physical therapy agents, nonsteroidal anti-inflammatory drugs (NSAIDs), muscle relaxants, antidepressants, antipsychotics, anxiolytics, antiepileptics, narcotic analgesics, acupuncture, occlusal splint therapy, various intra-articular injection applications, and surgical treatment methods to be applied individually or in combination. Although the role of malocclusion in the etiology of TMD has not been clearly established [62], orthodontic treatment of a severe and obvious malocclusion may be a beneficial approach to eliminating one of the possible factors [63].

Prioritizing reversible approaches in treatment interventions may provide satisfactory relief in most cases [64]. Application of more sophisticated treatment modalities necessitates the involvement of appropriate medical specialties [41]. In terms of pregnancy and lactation, it is also important to note that pharmacotherapy is limited in order to ensure maternal and fetal safety during these periods.

19.7 Conclusion

TMD is a multifactorial condition in which the role of psychosocial factors should not be overlooked. The prevalence of TMD shows a tendency toward female gender, but the effect of sex hormones on pathogenesis has been found to be controversial to date. There is no consensus on the effect of pregnancy on TMD. Various medical specialties are involved in the evaluation and treatment of TMD, and treatment modalities may depend on the specialty involved.

References

1. Okeson J. Etiology of functional disturbances in the masticatory system. In: Management of temporomandibular disorders and occlusion. 6th ed. St. Louis: Mosby Year Book Publication; 2008. p. 130–63.

2. Atkinson M. The temporomandibular joints, muscles of mastication, and the infratemporal and pterygopalatine fossa. In: Anatomy for dental students. 4th ed. Oxford: Oxford University Press; 2013. p. 241–56.
3. Nelson SJ, Ash MM. The temporomandibular joints, teeth, and muscles, and their functions. In: Wheeler's dental anatomy, physiology, and occlusion. 9th ed. St. Louis: Elsevier; 2010. p. 259–74.
4. Costen JB. A syndrome of ear and sinus symptoms dependent upon disturbed function of the temporomandibular joint. 1934. Ann Otol Rhinol Laryngol. 1997;43(1):1–15.
5. Porto De Toledo I, Stefani FM, Porporatti AL, Mezzomo LA, Peres MA, Flores-Mir C, De Luca CG. Prevalence of otologic signs and symptoms in adult patients with temporomandibular disorders: a systematic review and meta-analysis. Clin Oral Investig. 2017;21(2):597–605.
6. Laskin DM. Temporomandibular disorders: a term whose time has passed! J Oral Maxillofac Surg. 2020;78(4):496–7.
7. Lim PF, Smith S, Bhalang K, Slade GD, Maixner W. Development of temporomandibular disorders is associated with greater bodily pain experience. Clin J Pain. 2010;26(2):116–20.
8. National Institute of Dental and Craniofacial Research. Prevalence of TMJD and its signs and symptoms; 2018. https://www.nidcr.nih.gov/research/data-statistics/facial-pain/prevalence. Accessed 1 May 2021.
9. Valesan LF, Da-Cas CD, Réus JC, Denardin ACS, Garanhani RR, Bonotto D, Januzzi E, de Souza BDM. Prevalence of temporomandibular joint disorders: a systematic review and meta-analysis. Clin Oral Investig. 2021;25(2):441–53.
10. Alpaslan C, Yaman D. Clinical evaluation and classification of patients with temporomandibular disorders using 'diagnostic criteria for temporomandibular disorders'. Acta Odontol Turcica. 2020;37:1–6.
11. Fichera G, Polizzi A, Scapellato S, Palazzo G, Indelicato F. Craniomandibular disorders in pregnant women: an epidemiological survey. J Funct Morphol Kinesiol. 2020;5(2):36.
12. Wang J, Chao Y, Wan Q, Zhu Z. The possible role of estrogen in the incidence of temporomandibular disorders. Med Hypotheses. 2008;71(4):564–7.
13. Locker D, Slade G. Prevalence of symptoms associated with temporomandibular disorders in a Canadian population. Community Dent Oral Epidemiol. 1988;16(5):310–3.
14. Magnusson T, Egermark I, Carlsson GE. A longitudinal epidemiologic study of signs and symptoms of temporomandibular disorders from 15 to 35 years of age. J Orofac Pain. 2000;14(4):310–9.
15. Huang GJ, LeResche L, Critchlow CW, Martin MD, Drangsholt MT. Risk factors for diagnostic subgroups of painful temporomandibular disorders (TMD). J Dent Res. 2002;81(4):284–8.
16. Silveira EB, Rocabado M, Russo AK, Cogo JC, Osorio RA. Incidence of systemic joint hypermobility and temporomandibular joint hypermobility in pregnancy. Cranio. 2005;23(2):138–43.
17. Suvinen TI, Reade PC, Kemppainen P, Könönen M, Dworkin SF. Review of aetiological concepts of temporomandibular pain disorders: towards a biopsychosocial model for integration of physical disorder factors with psychological and psychosocial illness impact factors. Eur J Pain. 2005;9(6):613–33.
18. Türp JC, Schindler H. The dental occlusion as a suspected cause for TMDs: epidemiological and etiological considerations. J Oral Rehabil. 2012;39(7):502–12.
19. Celić R, Jerolimov V, Pandurić J. A study of the influence of occlusal factors and parafunctional habits on the prevalence of signs and symptoms of TMD. Int J Prosthodont. 2002;15(1):43–8.
20. Sari S, Sonmez H. Investigation of the relationship between oral parafunctions and temporomandibular joint dysfunction in Turkish children with mixed and permanent dentition. J Oral Rehabil. 2002;29(1):108–12.
21. Lobbezoo F, Lavigne GJ. Do bruxism and temporomandibular disorders have a cause-and-effect relationship? J Orofac Pain. 1997;11(1):15–23.
22. Rollman GB, Gillespie JM. The role of psychosocial factors in temporomandibular disorders. Curr Rev Pain. 2000;4(1):71–81.
23. Auerbach SM, Laskin DM, Frantsve LM, Orr T. Depression, pain, exposure to stressful life events, and long-term outcomes in temporomandibular disorder patients. J Oral Maxillofac Surg. 2001;59(6):628–33.

24. Nifosì F, Violato E, Pavan C, Sifari L, Novello G, Guarda Nardini L, Manfredini D, Semenzin M, Pavan L, Marini M. Psychopathology and clinical features in an Italian sample of patients with myofascial and temporomandibular joint pain: preliminary data. Int J Psychiatry Med. 2007;37(3):283–300.
25. Nadendla LK, Meduri V, Paramkusam G, Pachava KR. Evaluation of salivary cortisol and anxiety levels in myofascial pain dysfunction syndrome. Korean J Pain. 2014;27(1):30–4.
26. Gurbuz O, Alatas G, Kurt E. Prevalence of temporomandibular disorder signs in patients with schizophrenia. J Oral Rehabil. 2009;36(12):864–71.
27. Schiffman E, Ohrbach R, Truelove E, Look J, Anderson G, Goulet JP, List T, Svensson P, Gonzalez Y, Lobbezoo F, Michelotti A, Brooks SL, Ceusters W, Drangsholt M, Ettlin D, Gaul C, Goldberg LJ, Haythornthwaite JA, Hollender L, Jensen R, John MT, De Laat A, de Leeuw R, Maixner W, van der Meulen M, Murray GM, Nixdorf DR, Palla S, Petersson A, Pionchon P, Smith B, Visscher CM, Zakrzewska J, Dworkin SF, International RDC/TMD Consortium Network, International association for Dental Research; Orofacial Pain Special Interest Group, International Association for the Study of Pain. Diagnostic criteria for temporomandibular disorders (DC/TMD) for clinical and research applications: recommendations of the International RDC/TMD Consortium Network and Orofacial Pain Special Interest Group. J Oral Facial Pain Headache. 2014;28(1):6–27.
28. Jung W, Lee KE, Suh BJ. Influence of psychological factors on the prognosis of temporomandibular disorders pain. J Dent Sci. 2021;16(1):349–55.
29. Sarlani E, Greenspan JD. Why look in the brain for answers to temporomandibular disorder pain? Cells Tissues Organs. 2005;180(1):69–75.
30. Son C, Park YK, Park JW. Long-term evaluation of temporomandibular disorders in association with cytokine and autoantibody status in young women. Cytokine. 2021;144:155551. https://doi.org/10.1016/j.cyto.2021.155551. Epub 2021 May 1.
31. Brancher JA, Bertoli FMP, Michels B, Lopes-Faturri A, Pizzatto E, Losso EM, Orsi JS, Feltrin de Souza J, Küchler EC, Wambier LM. Is catechol-O-methyltransferase gene associated with temporomandibular disorders? A systematic review and meta-analysis. Int J Paediatr Dent. 2021;31(1):152–63.
32. Bandai N, Sanada S, Ueki K, Funabasama S, Tsuduki S, Matsui T. [Morphological analysis for kinetic X-ray images of the temporomandibular joint]. Nihon Hoshasen Gijutsu Gakkai Zasshi. 2003;59(8):951–957.
33. Tognini F, Manfredini D, Melchiorre D, Bosco M. Comparison of ultrasonography and magnetic resonance imaging in the evaluation of temporomandibular joint disc displacement. J Oral Rehabil. 2005;32(4):248–53.
34. Lewis EL, Dolwick MF, Abramowicz S, Reeder SL. Contemporary imaging of the temporomandibular joint. Dent Clin North Am. 2008;52(4):875–90.
35. Westesson PL. Reliability and validity of imaging diagnosis of temporomandibular joint disorder. Adv Dent Res. 1993;7(2):137–51.
36. Dworkin SF, LeResche L. Research diagnostic criteria for temporomandibular disorders: review, criteria, examinations and specifications, critique. J Craniomandib Disord. 1992;6(4):301–55.
37. International Classification of Orofacial Pain, 1st ed. (ICOP). Cephalalgia. 2020;40(2):129–221.
38. Ohrbach R, Dworkin SF. The evolution of TMD diagnosis: past, present, future. J Dent Res. 2016;95(10):1093–101.
39. Manfredini D, Guarda-Nardini L, Winocur E, Piccotti F, Ahlberg J, Lobbezoo F. Research diagnostic criteria for temporomandibular disorders: a systematic review of axis I epidemiologic findings. Oral Surg Oral Med Oral Pathol Oral Radiol Endod. 2011;112(4):453–62.
40. Okeson J. Differential diagnosis and management of TMDs. In: Orofacial pain guidelines for assessment, diagnosis, and management, the American Academy of Orofacial Pain, 6th ed. Hanover Park: Quintessence Publishing; 2018.
41. Fernández-de-las-Penas C, Svensson P. Myofascial temporomandibular disorder. Curr Rheumatol Rev. 2016;12(1):40–54.

42. Svensson P. Muscle pain in the head: overlap between temporomandibular disorders and tension-type headaches. Curr Opin Neurol. 2007;20(3):320–5.
43. Fraga BP, Santos EB, Farias Neto JP, Macieira JC, Quintans LJ Jr, Onofre AS, De Santana JM, Martins-Filho PR, Bonjardim LR. Signs and symptoms of temporomandibular dysfunction in fibromyalgic patients. J Craniofac Surg. 2012;23(2):615–8.
44. Pimentel MJ, Gui MS, Martins de Aquino LM, Rizzatti-Barbosa CM. Features of temporomandibular disorders in fibromyalgia syndrome. Cranio. 2013;31(1):40–5.
45. Manfredini D, Bandettini di Poggio A, Cantini E, Dell'Osso L, Bosco M. Mood and anxiety psychopathology and temporomandibular disorder: a spectrum approach. J Oral Rehabil. 2004;31(10):933–40.
46. Häggman-Henrikson B, Bechara C, Pishdari B, Visscher CM, Ekberg E. Impact of catastrophizing in patients with temporomandibular disorders—a systematic review. J Oral Facial Pain Headache. 2020;34(4):379–97. Rammelsberg et al reported a 31% persistence, 33% remittence and 36% recurrence in myofascial pain patients according to RDC/TMD criteria at 5 years follow up. (Rammelsberg P, LeResche L, Dworkin S, Mancl L. Longitudinal outcome of temporomandibular disorders: a 5-year epidemiologic study of muscle disorders defined by research diagnostic criteria for temporomandibular disorders. J Orofac Pain. 2003 Winter;17(1):9–20.
47. Kapila S. Does the relaxin, estrogen and matrix metalloproteinase axis contribute to degradation of TMJ fibrocartilage? J Musculoskelet Neuronal Interact. 2003;3(4):401–5.
48. Yu S, Xing X, Liang S, Ma Z, Li F, Wang M, Li Y. Locally synthesized estrogen plays an important role in the development of TMD. Med Hypotheses. 2009;72(6):720–2.
49. Bayramova A. TMD and pregnancy? Clin J Obstet Gynecol. 2018;1:1–6.
50. Solak Ö, Turhan-Haktanır N, Köken G, Toktas H, Güler Ö, Kavuncu V, et al. Prevalence of temporomandibular disorders in pregnancy. Eur J Gen Med. 2009;6(4):223–8.
51. LeResche L, Sherman JJ, Huggins K, Saunders K, Mancl LA, Lentz G, Dworkin SF. Musculoskeletal orofacial pain and other signs and symptoms of temporomandibular disorders during pregnancy: a prospective study. J Orofac Pain. 2005;19(3):193–201.
52. Mayoral VA, Espinosa IA, Montiel AJ. Association between signs and symptoms of temporomandibular disorders and pregnancy (case control study). Acta Odontol Latinoam. 2013;26(1):3–7.
53. Almubarak H, Alzahrani FA, Kaleem SM, Zakirulla M. Prevalence of temporomandibular disorders (TMDs) in relation to estrogen levels among females in Aseer region, Saudi Arabia. Ann Trop Med Public Health. 2020;23(16):SP231624.
54. Lora VR, Canales Gde L, Gonçalves LM, Meloto CB, Barbosa CM. Prevalence of temporomandibular disorders in postmenopausal women and relationship with pain and HRT. Braz Oral Res. 2016;30(1):e100.
55. Patil SR, Yadav N, Mousa MA, Alzwiri A, Kassab M, Sahu R, Chuggani S. Role of female reproductive hormones estrogen and progesterone in temporomandibular disorder in female patients. J Oral Res Rev. 2015;7(2):41.
56. Soydan SS, Deniz K, Uckan S, Unal AD, Tutuncu NB. Is the incidence of temporomandibular disorder increased in polycystic ovary syndrome? Br J Oral Maxillofac Surg. 2014;52(9):822–6.
57. Yazici H, Taskin MI, Guney G, Hismiogullari AA, Arslan E, Tulaci KG. The novel relationship between polycystic ovary syndrome and temporomandibular joint disorders. J Stomatol Oral Maxillofac Surg. 2020;S2468-7855(20):30263–9.
58. Bi RY, Zhang XY, Zhang P, Ding Y, Gan YH. Progesterone attenuates allodynia of inflamed temporomandibular joint through modulating voltage-gated sodium channel 1.7 in trigeminal ganglion. Pain Res Manag. 2020;2020:6582586.
59. Schauberger CW, Rooney BL, Goldsmith L, Shenton D, Silva PD, Schaper A. Peripheral joint laxity increases in pregnancy but does not correlate with serum relaxin levels. Am J Obstet Gynecol. 1996;174(2):667–71.
60. Khatıb G, Büyükkurt S, Küçükgöz Güleç Ü, Tuncay Özgünen F, Evrüke C, Demir C. Hiperemezis Gravidaruma Bağlı Alışılmadık Bir Komplikasyon; Akut Bilateral Temporomandibuler Eklem Dislokasyonu. J Clin Obstet Gynecol. 2013;23(4):266–8.

61. Li DTS, Leung YY. Temporomandibular disorders: current concepts and controversies in diagnosis and management. Diagnostics (Basel). 2021;11(3):459.
62. Motro PFK, Motro M, Oral K. Orthodontics and temporomandibular disorders. Are they related? Turk J Orthod. 2015;28:71–6.
63. Martin D, Rozencweig S, Maté A, Valenzuela J. Importance de la position du condyle dans le diagnostic, le traitement et la prévention des DAM [The importance of condyle position in the diagnosis, treatment and prevention of TMD]. Orthod Fr. 2015;86(2):125–149.
64. Fernandes G, Gonçalves DAG, Conti P. Musculoskeletal disorders. Dent Clin North Am. 2018;62(4):553–64.

Odontogenic Diseases During Pregnancy and Postpartum Period

20

E. Alper Sinanoglu, Umut Seki, and Marcel Noujeim

20.1 Introduction

Odontogenic diseases occurring during pregnancy and the postpartum period are discussed in this chapter. Due to hormonal changes, essential for the development of the fetus, oral cavity may also be subject to reversible and irreversible changes during pregnancy. Accumulation of hormones in oral mucosa tissues, increase of certain salivary cariogenic microorganisms, and decrease in salivary pH may result in gingivitis, epulis gravidarum, dental erosion, caries, and odontogenic inflammatory lesions. Pregnancy alone does not cause those lesions, but it may aggravate preexisting diseases or conditions. On the other hand, odontogenic and stomatologic diseases during pregnancy may cause complications such as preeclampsia, preterm birth, and low birth weight. In the postpartum period, there is a regression in predisposing conditions of diseases and resolution for most of them.

20.2 Stomatologic Changes Due to Alterations of Pregnancy

Pregnancy is a complex condition where the female body undergoes physiological, hormonal, immunological, and metabolic changes to ensure the growth and developmental needs of fetus. All systems undergo important physiological alterations

E. A. Sinanoglu (✉) · U. Seki
Department of Oral and Maxillofacial Radiology, Faculty of Dentistry, Kocaeli University, Kocaeli, Turkey
e-mail: alpersinanoglu@yahoo.com; dtumut@outlook.com

M. Noujeim
American Board of Oral and Maxillofacial Radiology, Advanced Imaging Diagnostics, San Antonio, TX, USA
e-mail: marcelnoujeim@gmail.com

© The Author(s), under exclusive license to Springer Nature Switzerland AG 2022
C. Cingi et al. (eds.), *ENT Diseases: Diagnosis and Treatment during Pregnancy and Lactation*, https://doi.org/10.1007/978-3-031-05303-0_20

and adaptations with metabolic demands. Increased secretion of various hormones such as estrogen and progesterone may cause local or systemic conditions. Oral mucosa, microbiota, and saliva are affected by those processes, which may result in stomatologic and odontologic manifestations.

20.2.1 Changes in Oral Mucosa

The oral mucosa is a mucous membrane that consists of epithelium and underlying connective tissue. It has a dynamic nature and provides a physical barrier to infection. The epithelial cells respond actively to bacteria by various mechanisms such as increased proliferation, the alteration of cell-signaling events, changes in differentiation, and cell death [1]. The oral mucosa is continuous with the skin of the lips and the mucosa of the soft palate and pharynx. It consists of three zones. The masticatory mucosa has a keratinized epithelium and includes the gingiva and the hard palate, the specialized mucosa that covers the dorsum of the tongue with the papillae and associated taste buds, and the remaining part called the lining mucosa; it has a nonkeratinized epithelium and covers striated muscle, bone, and glands [1–3].

Gingiva covers the alveolar process and surrounds the cervical portion of the teeth. As a part of masticatory mucosa, it consists of an epithelial layer and underlying connective tissue layer called lamina propria. Together with gingiva, the alveolar bone proper, periodontal ligament, and root cementum constitute the periodontium. The main function of the periodontium is to attach the tooth to the bone and to maintain the integrity of the surface of the masticatory mucosa [2].

Increased levels of two main hormones lead to both transient and irreversible changes in oral mucosa. Considering its stimulatory effect on both metabolism of collagen and angiogenesis, estrogen is one of them. It also decreases keratinization of the gingival epithelium during pregnancy. However, in terms of its effect on the levels of proinflammatory mediators and on the gingival vasculature, progesterone has the major effect in the gingival tissues. It is responsible for the highly vascular edematous inflammatory response via increasing vascularity and permeability of the gingival tissues [2]. Additionally, estrogen and progesterone may also alter the cell-mediated immune function in oral mucosa, resulting in a delayed immune response to infection [4]. Reduction of antimicrobial activity of peripheral neutrophils and depression of the maternal T-lymphocyte response are also associated with the altered tissue response observed during pregnancy [1, 5].

20.2.2 Changes in Oral Microbiota

Pregnancy-related changes of oral mucosa result in the accumulation of hormones in gingival tissues and alterations in the composition of saliva. Estrogens stimulate the proliferation and desquamation of epithelial cells, which provides a better nutritional environment for bacteria [6]. Numerous anaerobic and aerobic bacterial species such as *Fusobacterium nucleatum, Bacteroides melaninogenicus, Prevotella intermedia*, and *Porphyromonas gingivalis* are known to be stimulated by the sex hormones [5, 7]. Estradiol, the sex hormone involved in the main endocrine events at the beginning of pregnancy, has been found to be metabolized by *Streptococcus mutans* and *Streptococcus sanguis* [8]. In saliva, increasing numbers of *Streptococcus mutans*, yeast, and lactobacilli were also reported for the last trimester and lactation period [6]. During pregnancy, these conditions have the potential to promote bacterial growth and lead to increased oral microbial load.

20.2.3 Changes in Saliva

Protective functions of saliva depend on a large group of innate and acquired factors such as immunoglobulins, lysozyme, lactoferrin, peroxidase systems, and agglutinins, together with buffering effect and mechanical cleansing [9]. During pregnancy, alterations in the saliva may decrease those functions and may promote odontogenic and mucosal lesions.

Although a decreased flow rate during pregnancy was reported in some studies [9], significant alterations were not reported according to the results of longitudinal studies [8, 10, 11]. The main changes are associated with the composition of the saliva, such as the decreased pH, which is found to be lower in pregnancy [11]. Calcium and phosphate concentrations are also reported to be slightly lower in the saliva of pregnant women as well [8]. Changes in dietary habits such as regular consumption of sugary drinks and citrus foods and snacks favor an increase in the levels of acidophilic microorganisms [5].

An important function of the saliva is its buffering effect, which works by counteracting the decrease in pH and is determined primarily by the concentration of bicarbonate ion. Toward the third trimester period, this capacity of saliva shows a significant decrease and immediately recovers to normal after birth [8].

20.3 Odontogenic and Stomatologic Diseases of Pregnancy

20.3.1 Gingivitis Gravidarum

Gingivitis is the inflammatory disease of gingival tissues caused by bacterial plaque. It is characterized by edema, hyperplasia, erythema of the gingival, and increased bleeding [12]. As with other systemic conditions, the hormonal changes accentuate the gingival response. The pregnancy is not the cause of gingivitis but may be a predisposing factor for aggravation of a preexisting condition (Fig. 20.1) [8]. In other words, no notable changes occur for individuals with an optimum oral hygiene [13].

Gingivitis gravidarum is an acute inflammation of the gingival tissues during the second and third trimester of pregnancy [13, 14]. Regarding oral hygiene maintenance, gingivitis gravidarum is common and occurs in 30–100% of all pregnant

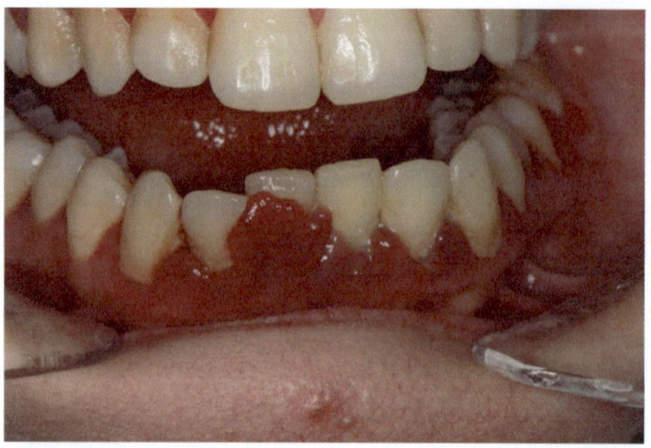

Fig. 20.1 Gingivitis gravidarum. Please note the presence of dental calculus, which leads to plaque accumulation indicating the poor oral hygiene

women [15]. This is often the case during pregnancy when toothbrushing may be less frequent because it may induce nausea [16].

The gingiva is inflamed and varies in color from bright red to bluish red. The gingivae may be edematous and pliable, pit on pressure, appear smooth and shiny, and sometimes may present a raspberry-like appearance [13]. The extreme redness results from marked vascularity, and there is an increased tendency to bleed [13]. The tissue is tender to palpation, and the severity is related to plaque accumulation and poor oral hygiene [16]. Accompanied with an acute infection, gingivitis gravidarum may become painful [13].

The generally accepted mechanisms are related to the increased levels of progesterone, which lead to increased permeability and dilatation of gingival capillary vessels, resulting in increased vascular flow and exudation. These effects are partly mediated by an increased synthesis of prostaglandin [14]. During pregnancy, there are two peaks in the course of the disease, first one is during the first trimester, due to overproduction of gonadotropins, and the second one is during the third trimester, presenting the highest estrogen and progesterone levels [13]. The increased sex hormones cause the destruction of gingival mast cells and the resultant release of histamine and proteolytic enzymes, which may also contribute to the exaggerated inflammatory response to local factors [13]. This disease is usually transitory and responds to meticulous home care, oral prophylaxis, and standard oral hygiene measures. Severe gingivitis may require periodontal treatment in order to stop progression [17].

20.3.2 Epulis Gravidarum (Pregnancy Tumor)

The hyperplastic response of the gingiva may exacerbate epulis gravidarum, which is a pyogenic granuloma and is also known as the pregnancy tumor [16]. This lesion progresses with preexisting gingivitis and poor oral hygiene. Epulis gravidarum usually appears in the first trimester of pregnancy with a rate of 0.2%–9.6% [13].

This proliferation presents as a rapidly growing gingival mass that may be sessile or pedunculated. Vascularity of the lesion and degree of venous stasis change the color of the lesion from purplish red to deep blue. Pyogenic granulomas usually do not cause alveolar bone loss [13]. Most frequently, they arise from the interdental papilla of the gingiva and can enlarge to several centimeters in size [16]. Epulis gravidarum may bleed profusely when touched and gradually become hyperplastic and nodular [18]. Based on histological features, the lesion consists of mainly hyperplastic granulation tissue with notable capillary content [19]. Pathogenesis of the lesion has been associated with increased local synthesis of angiogenic factors such as vascular endothelial growth factor and angiopoietin-2, which are stimulated by the sex hormones [18].

In many cases, the lesions undergo partial or complete resolution at the postpartum period, especially if local irritants are removed. During pregnancy, if it becomes large and symptomatic, treatment may include surgical removal. However, the lesion displays a tendency for post-surgical recurrence when excised before birth. Therefore, maintaining good oral hygiene to reduce plaque retention is important in the postoperative period [12, 18]. The differential diagnosis group is also relatively large for epulis gravidarum. As a red gingival mass, its clinical appearance may be similar to peripheral giant cell granuloma. A peripheral odontogenic or ossifying fibroma may also be considered. Less commonly, other conditions include Kaposi's sarcoma, bacillary angiomatosis, non-Hodgkin's lymphoma, and, rarely, metastatic cancer [19].

20.3.3 Dental Erosion

Dental erosion is the loss of tooth structure surface. The outermost part of the tooth, the enamel is the first affected layer, followed by the underlying dentin. Erosion is a chemical process causing demineralization due to a low pH. A pH of 5.5 is critical for dissolving dental enamel [20]. The defective areas of teeth seem yellowish or brown due to exposed dentin. Endogenous acidic agents such as gastric fluids cause generalized erosion on the lingual, incisal, and occlusal surfaces of the teeth [21]. The pH value of gastric acid is 1–1.5 and thus far below the critical level for dissolving enamel [20].

Pregnancy-related exposure of teeth to gastric acid causes erosions due to several reasons. The first possible reason is the morning sickness, the hyperemesis gravidarum, which causes frequent vomiting over a period of several weeks. On the other hand, it should be kept in mind that vomiting is a common occurrence during pregnancy. In pregnancies, detectable dental erosions are rare because the period of pregnancy is limited. If hyperemesis gravidarum presents an increased frequency of vomiting in the first trimester, then dental erosions become apparent [20]. In the later stages, the acid reflux is the second reason. The smooth muscle–relaxing effects of progesterone and estrogen are likely responsible for the decreased tone of upper esophageal and gastroesophageal sphincters, which lead to increased reflux of stomach contents into oral cavity. The upward pressure from the gravid uterus may also result in exaggerated acid reflux. When reflux is excessive, it becomes gastroesophageal reflux disease and may cause severe forms of erosions on the enamel [22]. Toothbrushing may be a contributing factor just after being exposed by a low pH agent, which may result in easy abrasion of the softened dental surface [21].

Management of the erosion involves dietary and lifestyle changes and aims to reduce acid exposure [17]. The patients should rinse with fluoride mouthwash or a solution that contains sodium bicarbonate thoroughly after vomiting. Application of casein phosphopeptide amorphous calcium phosphate on the teeth can also be suggested. Considering the risk of the progression, the expectant mother should be warned not to brush her teeth immediately after vomiting and to use a soft toothbrush to avoid further damage [23].

20.3.4 Odontogenic Inflammatory Lesions

The jaws are unique in the sense that teeth create a direct pathway for agents and pathogenic microorganisms to enter bone [24]. Inflammatory lesions are commonly encountered in oral cavity and mostly related to microbial infections that reach the bone through nonvital teeth, periodontal lesions, and traumatic injuries. The primary reason for pulpitis is the presence of dental caries, and numerous sequelae may follow untreated pulp necrosis. The inflammatory process extends into the periapical area of the root and may exacerbate as a cyst or a granuloma or an abscess [19]. Pregnancy alone does not appear to cause those lesions but may aggravate a preexisting condition and has the potential to create an environment favoring such lesions.

20.3.5 Caries in Pregnancy

Dental caries is a multifactorial and infectious oral disease caused primarily by the complex interaction of oral flora with fermentable dietary carbohydrates. This interaction results in demineralization and loss of tooth structure [21]. After the destruction of the enamel, the underlying dentin is exposed to the oral environment and bacterial proteolytic enzymes [25]. Primary and recurrent caries constitute the most common reasons for pulpal inflammation and necrosis [26].

During pregnancy, the susceptibility to odontogenic problems increases, and there is a common belief that teeth will be damaged. It has been reported that the chemical analysis presented similar results in terms of the total mineral composition for the extracted teeth of the pregnant and nonpregnant women [27]. Considering the slow progress of an initial caries lesion, it is hard to evaluate the effect of pregnancy on dental health. But due to predisposing changes in saliva, increased demineralization (due to lowered buffering effect and pH) and decreased remineralization potential (due to lowered calcium and phosphate concentrations) together with increased levels of cariogenic bacteria, all can increase the risk of dental caries. As mentioned before, it is a multifactorial process, and other factors may also contribute to the process. For example, dietary change toward sugary snacks and citrus foods may lead to a drop in salivary pH. Gingival bleeding has a negative effect for the maintenance of oral hygiene and may result in less attention toward oral health [8].

20.3.6 Dental Abscesses in Pregnancy

Dental caries are not self-limiting. If they are left untreated, bacteria and their toxic products will reach the dental pulp. Thus, as an inflammatory response, pulpitis occurs. Subsequently, toxic substances from the pulp space diffuse through the apical foramen of the dental root into the adjacent periapical part of the periodontal ligament and surrounding bone tissue [25]. Due to inflammation of periradicular tissues, discomfort may occur when the teeth come into contact. Swelling may often accompany pain and may be localized to the mucogingival and also to fascial planes or spaces [28].

The submandibular space is the most frequently involved location of odontogenic abscesses. During pregnancy, severe odontogenic and orofacial infections have the potential to cause serious complications for the mother and fetus. The risk of morbidity with progressing infection and the potential risks related to dental or surgical management must be evaluated together. Definitive treatment of abscesses is surgical exploration and drainage. The second trimester is the optimal period for nonemergent dental treatment procedures. On the other hand, emergency procedures can and should be provided at any time in pregnancy. Furthermore, a progressing infection is more harmful for the fetus than the stress of dental treatment. It is also stated that early and aggressive surgical management is likely to be less harmful than prolonged use of i.v. antibiotics [29].

20.3.7 Odontogenic Inflammatory Cysts in Pregnancy

Caries progress to pulpitis, and pulp necrosis progress to apical granuloma. Triggered by bacteria or their toxic products, apical granuloma has the potential to transform into an inflammatory cyst. Radicular cysts are by far the most commonly seen inflammatory cysts and constitute approximately one half to three-fourths of all types of cysts in the jaws (Table 20.1) [19, 30]. Proliferation of small odontogenic epithelial residues, the rests of Malassez in the vicinity of the periapical area of the root, may show reactive proliferation leading to the formation of a radicular cyst [25]. Usually, they do not cause any symptoms and are often identified as an incidental finding [19].

Considering the formerly mentioned potential of pregnancy to aggravate a preexisting condition, an untreated asymptomatic radicular cyst has a chance of being symptomatic by getting secondarily infected. When complicated by secondary infection, radicular cysts may be characterized by pain and swelling [25]. But in the

Table 20.1 World Health Organization classification of odontogenic cysts[a]

A—Odontogenic cysts of inflammatory origin
Radicular cyst
Inflammatory collateral cysts
B—Odontogenic and nonodontogenic developmental cysts
Dentigerous cyst
Odontogenic keratocyst
Lateral periodontal and botryoid odontogenic cyst
Gingival cyst
Glandular odontogenic cyst
Calcifying odontogenic cyst
Orthokeratinised odontogenic cyst
Nasopalatine duct cyst

[a]Adapted from World Health Organization Classification of Tumours of the Head and Neck [30]

diagnostic process, evaluation of clinical symptoms must be accompanied by radiological findings, which is a concerning issue for both expectant mothers and clinicians. The American Dental Association (ADA) states that routine radiographs should be avoided during pregnancy, but pregnancy is not a reason to delay clinically indicated dental radiographs [31]. The American College of Obstetricians and Gynecologists also published that "Women should be counseled that X-ray exposure from a single diagnostic procedure does not result in harmful fetal effects" [32]. In the case of a full-mouth dental radiographic examination, total exposure is 0.25 mGy with the use of radiation protection equipment such as aprons and thyroid collars [24]. Specifically, exposure to less than 50 mGy has not been associated with an increase in fetal anomalies or pregnancy loss [32].

In radiologic examination, a radicular cyst is seen as a round or oval radiolucency with well-defined cortical boundaries. Generally, the epicenter of a radicular cyst is located approximately at the apex of a nonvital tooth. Treatment of a tooth with a radicular cyst may include extraction, endodontic therapy, or apical surgery. In pregnancy, for large radicular cysts, marsupialization is the recommended treatment instead of surgical removal [24]. Dental treatment can be provided safely at any period of gestation. However, many health care professionals regard the second trimester as the optimal time to perform nonemergent procedures [33].

20.4 Alterations in Preexisting Diseases with Oral Manifestations During Pregnancy

20.4.1 Odontogenic Tumors

Pregnancy hormones help provide the requirements for the development, growth, and birth of an infant. Regarding their effects, it is speculated that these hormones may induce several alterations in cell metabolism, which may affect the benign or malignant growth of a lesion. On the other hand, there is no direct evidence, and steps of this mechanism are not confirmed yet [34].

Table 20.2 World Health Organization classification of odontogenic tumors[a]

A—Malignant odontogenic tumors
Odontogenic carcinomas
Ameloblastic carcinoma
Primary intraosseous carcinoma
Sclerosing odontogenic carcinoma
Clear cell odontogenic carcinoma
Ghost cell odontogenic carcinoma
Odontogenic carcinosarcoma
Odontogenic sarcomas
B—Benign epithelial odontogenic tumors
Ameloblastoma
Squamous odontogenic tumor
Calcifying epithelial odontogenic tumor
Adenomatoid odontogenic tumor
C—Benign mixed epithelial and mesenchymal odontogenic tumors
Ameloblastic fibroma
Primordial odontogenic tumor
Odontoma
Dentinogenic ghost cell tumor
D—Benign mesenchymal odontogenic tumors
Odontogenic fibroma
Odontogenic myxoma/myxofibroma
Cementoblastoma
Cemento-ossifying fibroma

[a]Adapted from World Health Organization Classification of Tumours of the Head and Neck [30]

Odontogenic tumors originate from epithelial and mesenchymal remnants of the tooth germs, which are located exclusively in tooth-bearing areas of the maxilla and the mandible [19]. According to the World Health Organization, these neoplasms can be classified regarding their possession of odontogenic epithelium and ectomesenchyme tissue (Table 20.2) [24, 30]. Clinically, odontogenic tumors are typically asymptomatic, although they have the potential to cause expansion, bone loss, displacement, and root resorption of adjacent teeth [19].

20.4.1.1 Ameloblastoma

Regarding the local and multi-systemic alterations of pregnancy hormones, it was suggested that pregnancy hormones could induce hyperplasia, modulate the lesion, and promote rapid growth of the ameloblastoma [34]. However, there are a few studies reporting the development of this benign odontogenic tumor in the pregnancy period [34–36].

Ameloblastoma is the most common benign odontogenic tumor that has aggressive characteristic features with high recurrence rates [24, 34]. Remnants of the dental lamina and the enamel organ are the source of odontogenic epithelium from which ameloblastoma arises [24]. Although these remnants of the odontogenic epithelium may be located in any tooth-bearing areas in the jaws, most ameloblastomas (80%) develop in the molar/ramus region of the mandible, and it is seen rarely in the premolar and anterior regions [24, 34]. The tumor is asymptomatic and slow-growing in nature. Ameloblastoma may present significant expansion and perforation of the cortical bone, which may result in infiltration of the tumor to adjacent soft tissues [34]. The oral mucosa over the lesion is intact, and patients rarely report pain or paresthesia. Most patients refer to the clinic with swelling and facial asymmetry [24]. But the swelling of jaws is a common symptom and may easily be misdiagnosed without radiological examination.

The radiographic appearance of ameloblastoma is not pathognomonic [35]. It may be present as a unilocular or multilocular radiolucency, with or without cortical outlines in the radiography [34, 35]. Unilocular lesions may resemble odontogenic keratocysts, or dentigerous, radicular cysts, whereas multilocular lesions have a wide range of differentials such as the central giant cell granuloma, odontogenic myxoma, and odontogenic keratocysts [35].

20.4.1.2 Adenomatoid Odontogenic Tumor

Due to the 2:1 female predilection for adenomatoid odontogenic tumor (AOT), it can be suggested that estrogen or progesterone may play some role in the development and growth of the lesion. Similar to ameloblastoma, developing AOTs in pregnancy are rarely reported [37–39]. Estrogen receptor expression in AOTs is also investigated, and no immunoreactivity was observed [38].

AOT is an uncommon, nonaggressive, mixed odontogenic tumor. It contains connective tissue elements and also calcifications that may be dentin- or enamel-like material. It is slow-growing and enlarges gradually with painless swelling manifesting asymmetry. AOTs usually occur in the anterior maxilla and mandible, especially the canine region. AOT may be present with an impacted tooth, mostly canine [24].

20.4.2 Temporomandibular Disorders

Temporomandibular disorder (TMD) is a collective term for the group of disturbances that affect the masticatory system, the temporomandibular joints (TMJ), and associated structures [40]. Functional disorders of masticatory muscles are the most common complaint, and others are characterized by pain in the preauricular area and TMJ, limitation or deviation in the mandibular range of motion, and TMJ sounds (clicking, popping, and crepitus) during mandibular function [41].

Orthopedic instability, sources of deep pain, and muscle hyperactivity are significantly implicated etiologic factors of TMD, and they may be induced by pregnancy-specific sleep disruption, morning sickness. For the expectant mother, emotional stress is another important provoking factor in this period as well. In addition to above-mentioned factors, the relationship between circulating estrogen levels and TMD has also been investigated. Estrogen receptors are localized in the TMJ tissues, such as chondroid tissue of condyle and retrodiscal tissues. Depending on the pain signaling type and estrogen is speculated to be in relation to TMD for regulating the pain mechanisms [42]. It is also described as a promoter for the degenerative changes in the TMJ via increasing the synthesis of specific cytokines and profoundly influencing several cell activities that may be associated with remodeling or degenerative processes [43].

Throughout pregnancy, the ligaments of the pubic symphysis and sacroiliac joints loosen, possibly because of the hormones relaxin and estrogen [41]. It is also speculated that female reproductive hormones represent a risk factor for the development of TMD [44]. In addition to the increase of estrogen, relaxin also increases two to threefold during pregnancy. Elevated levels of relaxin were related to the tenderness of joint tissues, including the TMJ [45, 46], presenting an increased systemic joint laxity [41]. As the hypermobile TMJ may be more prone to dysfunction, the laxity of the TMJ is affected by elevated estrogen and relaxin levels, which may be a contributing factor in the development of TMDs [47].

20.5 Effects of Odontogenic and Stomatologic Diseases on Systemic Conditions

Regarding the etiology of pregnancy complications such as preeclampsia, preterm birth, and low birth weight, it has been suggested that bacterial infections may be correlated and may even induce these conditions [48, 49]. As a destructive inflammation, periodontitis affects approximately 30% of women of child-bearing age [17]. It is characterized by the destruction of the periodontal ligament, bone, and soft tissue as a result of a local host immune response to microbial plaques on the tooth surface [49]. As a potential reservoir for inflammatory mediators, periodontal infections may pose a threat to the placenta and fetus [50]. Progressing inflammation may also cause alveolar bone resorption and, eventually, tooth loss [49]. Additionally, any pulpal disease extending into the periradicular tissues may cause inflammation. Together with periodontal disease, both diseases have the potential to induce bacteremia, which can affect pregnancy.

In these processes, the release of PGE2 may restrict placental blood flow and may result in intrauterine growth restriction and low birth weight [17]. A number of studies have linked an increased risk of preeclampsia with elevated serum levels of C-reactive protein, which contributes to periodontal infections [18]. The management of periodontal disease is based on early diagnosis, and the treatment decreases the levels of a variety of cytokines, chemokines, and prostaglandins in the affected sites [49]. The risk reduction of preterm birth was demonstrated to be related to deep root scaling treatment as well. Considering those relations, all women who are pregnant or planning to become pregnant are recommended to undergo a periodontal examination and any necessary treatment [17].

20.6 The Postpartum Period

Considering the potential of pregnancy on preexisting conditions of odontogenic and stomatologic diseases, the postpartum may be considered the resolution period for most of those lesions. Regression of gingivitis occurs by 2 months after birth due

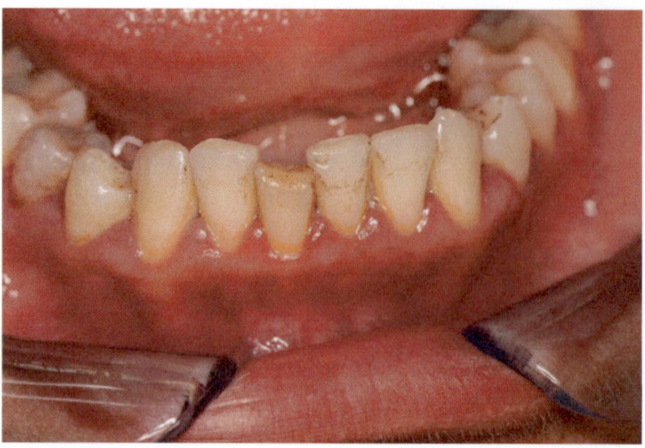

Fig. 20.2 Recession of bleeding of a preexisting gingivitis gravidarum in the postpartum period. Please note the dental calculus deposition, which is an etiological factor

to decreasing hormone levels. Furthermore, symptoms such as tooth mobility, pocket depth, and gingival bleeding start to decrease in the postpartum period (Fig. 20.2). When comparing periodontal changes in pregnancy and postpartum, no significant loss of attachment is observed [13]. Epulis gravidarum also regresses 1–2 months postpartum [22]. However, in some cases, surgical excision may be required for complete resolution [12]. Regarding the regression of the changes in saliva and microbiota, the conditions favoring the tendency of dental caries formation also return to the individuals' potential before pregnancy. After 1 year, the conditions of the mother's gingiva become the same circumstances as nonpregnant women [13].

References

1. Fiorellini JP, Stathopoulou PG. Anatomy of the periodontium. In: Newman MG, Takei H, Klokkevold PR, Carranza FA, editors. Carranza's clinical periodontology. St. Louis, MO: Elsevier Saunders; 2015.
2. Lindhe J, Karring T, Araújo M. Anatomy of periodontal tissues. In: Lang NP, Lindhe J, editors. Clinical periodontology and implant dentistry, 2 volume set. John Wiley & Sons, Blackwell; 2015.
3. Ross MH, Pawlina W. Histology. Lippincott Williams & Wilkins; 2006.
4. Boutigny H, de Moegen ML, Egea L, et al. Oral infections and pregnancy: knowledge of gynecologists/obstetricians, midwives and dentists. Oral Health Prev Dent. 2016;14(1):41–7.
5. Silva de Araujo Figueiredo C, Gonçalves Carvalho Rosalem C, Costa Cantanhede AL, et al. Systemic alterations and their oral manifestations in pregnant women. J Obstet Gynaecol Res. 2017;43(1):16–22.
6. Laine M, Tenovuo J, Lehtonen OP. Pregnancy-related increase in salivary Streptococcus mutans, lactobacilli and IgA. In: Cimasoni G, Lehner T, editors. Borderland between caries and periodontal disease. 3rd ed. Geneve: Médecine et Hygiene; 1986.
7. Hassan MN, Belibasakis GN, Gumus P, et al. Annexin-1 as a salivary biomarker for gingivitis during pregnancy. J Periodontol. 2018;89(7):875–82.
8. Laine MA. Effect of pregnancy on periodontal and dental health. Acta Odontol Scand. 2002;60(5):257–64.

9. Laine M, Tenovuo J, Lehtonen OP, et al. Pregnancy-related changes in human whole saliva. Arch Oral Biol. 1988;33(12):913–7.

10. Laine M, Tenovuo J, Lehtonen OP, et al. Pregnancy-related changes in human whole saliva. Arch Oral Biol. 1988;12:913–7.

11. Laine M, Pienihäkkinen K. Salivary buffer effect in relation to late pregnancy and postpartum. Acta Odontol Scand. 2000;58:8–10.

12. Steinberg BJ, Hilton IV, Iida H, et al. Oral health and dental care during pregnancy. Dental Clin. 2013;57(2):195–210.

13. Klokkevold PR, Mealey BL. Influence of systemic conditions. In: Newman MG, Takei H, Klokkevold PR, Carranza FA, editors. Carranza's clinical periodontology. St. Louis, MO: Elsevier Saunders; 2015.

14. Mariotti A. Plaque-induced gingival diseases. In: Lang NP, Lindhe J, editors. Clinical periodontology and implant dentistry, 2 volume set. John Wiley & Sons, Blackwell; 2015.

15. Wu M, Chen SW, Jiang SY. Relationship between gingival inflammation and pregnancy. Mediat Inflamm. 2015; https://doi.org/10.1155/2015/623427.

16. Langlais RP, Miller CS, Gehrig JS. Color atlas of common oral diseases. Philadelphia: Wolters Kluwer, Lippincott Williams & Wilkins; 2009.

17. Silk H, Douglass AB, Douglass JM, et al. Oral health during pregnancy. Am Fam Physician. 2008;77(8):1139–44.

18. Armitage GC. Bi-directional relationship between pregnancy and periodontal disease. Periodontol. 2013;61(1):160–76.

19. Regezi JA, Sciubba J, Jordan RC. Oral pathology: clinical pathologic correlations. St. Louis, MO: Elsevier Saunders; 2016.

20. Scheutzel P. Etiology of dental erosion–intrinsic factors. Eur J Oral Sci. 1996;104(2):178–90.

21. Scott Eidson R, Shugars DA. Patient assessment, Examiantion and diagnosis, and treatment planning. In: Heymann HO, Swift EJ, Ritter AV, editors. Sturdevant's art and science of operative dentistry. 6th ed. St. Louis: Elsevier Mosby; 2013.

22. Funk E, Gelbard A. ENT complaints in pregnancy second of two parts: the ear and the throat. OBG Management. 2010;22(9):28.

23. Kandan PM, Menaga V, Kumar RRR. Oral health in pregnancy (guidelines to gynaecologists, general physicians & oral health care providers). JPMA J Pak Med Assoc. 2011;61(10):1009–14.

24. White SC, Pharoah MJ, editors. Oral radiology: principles and interpretation. St. Louis, MO: Elsevier Health Sciences.

25. Slootweg PJ. Dental pathology. Berlin, Heidelberg: Springer; 2013.

26. Boynton TT, Ferneini EM, Goldberg MH. Odontogenic infections of the facial spaces. In: Hupp JR, Ferneini EM, editors. Head, neck, and orofacial infections: an interdisciplinary approach. St. Louis, MO: Elsevier Health Sciences; 2015.

27. Dragiff DA, Karshan M. Effect of pregnancy on the chemical composition of human dentin. J Dent Res. 1943;22:261–5.

28. Patel B. Endodontic diagnosis, pathology and treatment planning. Classification of pulp and perio-apical disease. Cham: Springer International Publishing; 2015.

29. Tocaciu S, Robinson BW, Sambrook PJ. Severe odontogenic infection in pregnancy: a timely reminder. Aust Dent J. 2017;62(1):98–101.

30. El-Naggar AK, Chan JKC, Grandis JR, Takata T, Slootweg PJ. WHO classification of Tumours of the head and neck, chapter 8. 4th ed. Lyon: IARC Press; 2017.

31. American Dental Association Council on Access, Prevention, and Interprofessional Relations. Women's oral health issues. Chicago: American Dental Association; 2006. p. 3–8.

32. American College of Obstetricians and Gynecologists Committee Opinion. Guidelines for diagnostic imaging during pregnancy. Obstet Gynecol. 2004;104(3):647–51.

33. Kloetzel MK, Huebner CE, Milgrom P. Referrals for dental care during pregnancy. J Midwifery Women's Health. 2011;56(2):110–7.

34. da Silva HEC, Costa EDSR, Medeiros ACQ, et al. Ameloblastoma during pregnancy: a case report. J Med Case Rep. 2016;10(1):1–7.

35. Gordy FM, Holder R, Carroll MKO, et al. Growth of an ameloblastoma during pregnancy: opportunity lost? Spec Care Dentist. 1996;16(5):199–203.
36. Herberts BG, Sandström J. Ameloblastoma occurring and recurring during pregnancies. Acta Otolaryngol. 1957;48(4):327–32.
37. Bhandari N, Kothari M. Adenomatoid odontogenic tumour mimicking a periapical cyst in pregnant woman. Singap Dent J. 2010;31(1):26–9.
38. Shinozaki Y, Jinbu Y, Kusama M, et al. A case report of adenomatoid odontogenic tumor arising in a pregnant woman. Oral Med Pathol. 2004;9(1):31–4.
39. Sekiya R, Yamazaki H, Izawa K, et al. Case of adenomatid odontogenic tumor during pregnancy. Tokai J Exp Clin Med. 2011;36(4):124–7.
40. Okeson JP. Management of temporomandibular disorders and occlusion-E-book. St. Louis, MO: Elsevier Health Sciences; 2013.
41. Solak Ö, Turhan-Haktanir N, Köken G, et al. Prevalence of temporomandibular disorders in pregnancy. Eur J Gen Med. 2009;6(4):223–8.
42. Fichera G, Polizzi A, Scapellato S, et al. Craniomandibular disorders in pregnant women: an epidemiological survey. J Funct Morphol Kinesiol. 2020;5(2):36.
43. Haskin CL, Milam SB, Cameron IL. Pathogenesis of degenerative joint disease in the human temporomandibular joint. Crit Rev Oral Biol Med. 1995;6(3):248–77.
44. LeResche L, Saunders K, Von Korff MR, et al. Use of exogenous hormones and risk of temporomandibular disorder pain. Pain. 1997;69:153–60.
45. Matarese G, Isola G, Anastasi GP, et al. Transforming growth factor Beta 1 and vascular endothelial growth factor levels in the pathogenesis of periodontal disease. Eur J Inflamm. 2013;11:479–88.
46. Trenti A, Tedesco S, Boscaro C, et al. Estrogen, angiogenesis, immunity and cell metabolism: solving the puzzle. Int J Mol Sci. 2018;19:859.
47. Westling L. Temporomandibular joint dysfunction and systemic joint laxity. Swed Dent J Suppl. 1992;81:1–79.
48. Nuriel-Ohayon M, Neuman H, Koren O. Microbial changes during pregnancy, birth, and infancy. Front Microbiol. 2016;7:1031.
49. Penova-Veselinovic B, Keelan JA, Wang CA, et al. Changes in inflammatory mediators in gingival crevicular fluid following periodontal disease treatment in pregnancy: relationship to adverse pregnancy outcome. J Reprod Immunol. 2015;112:1–10.
50. Gaffield ML, Gilbert BJC, Malvitz DM, et al. Oral health during pregnancy: an analysis of information collected by the pregnancy risk assessment monitoring system. J Am Dent Assoc. 2001;132(7):1009–16.

Tonsillopharyngitis During Pregnancy and the Postpartum Period

Bahar Alagöz, Nuray Bayar Muluk, and Jeffrey C. Bedrosian

21.1 Introduction

Infections during pregnancy may occur at any time from the first implantation of the blastocyst to the point at which the mother gives birth and the period surrounding birth. These infections may also harm the fetus or neonate. Since bacterial infections during pregnancy often produce no symptoms, doctors need to remain alert to the possibility of infection and carry out sufficiently careful infective screening [1].

The most frequently occurring bacterial infection that poses a risk to the life of the neonate and potentially the mother is the Group B *Streptococcus* (GBS), i.e., *Streptococcus agalactiae*. Infections with *S. agalactiae* have the following features [1]:

- *S. agalactiae* may be a commensal bacterium within the vagina, rectum, or oral cavity.
- Intrapartum transmission involves either spread from the vagina higher up into the genital tract or as delivery occurs.

B. Alagöz (✉)
ENT Department, Ordu State Hospital, Ordu, Turkey
e-mail: raufoguzhankum@gmail.com

N. Bayar Muluk
Department of Otorhinolaryngology, Faculty of Medicine, Kırıkkale University, Kırıkkale, Turkey
e-mail: btahsin@hotmail.com

J. C. Bedrosian
St. Luke's Medical Center, Rhinology and Skull Base Surgery, Specialty Physician Associates, Bethlehem, PA, USA
e-mail: jbedrosi16@gmail.com

C. Cingi et al. (eds.), *ENT Diseases: Diagnosis and Treatment during Pregnancy and Lactation*, https://doi.org/10.1007/978-3-031-05303-0_21

- During pregnancy, GBS is responsible for infections of the urinary bladder, amnion, and endometrium and may cause stillbirth. Somewhat rarely, hematogenous spread leads to endocarditis or meningitis.
- During the postpartum period, GBS may be responsible for urinary tract infections and may produce an abscess in the pelvis of the mother.
- Early-onset infection with *S. agalactiae* takes place before the neonate reaches the age of 1 week and usually presents as sepsis without an identifiable focus, pneumonia, or meningitis. The mean age at which it presents is 12 h.
- Late-onset GBS infection in newborns is between the ages of 7 and 89 days, with the average onset being at 36 days of age. The most frequently noted signs are bacteremia without a definite focus of infection and meningitis.
- Neonates who recover from the infection are prone to long-term neurological complications, including auditory loss, visual impairment, and learning disability.

The US Centers for Disease Control recommend the following actions [1]:

- All mothers-to-be should have swabs taken from the vagina and rectum when the pregnancy reaches the 35–37-week stage [2].
- The site where vaginal swabs have the highest specificity is the introitus, slightly inside the ring of the hymen. For rectal swabs, the highest specificity is far beyond the anal sphincter. Swabs taken from the cervix, around the anus or rectum, or the perineum are unsuitable. When collecting the swab, a speculum must not be employed [3].
- A positive result on culture should lead to a decision to treat the mother when she goes into labor.

21.2 Tonsillopharyngitis

The principal pathogenic bacteria responsible for tonsillopharyngitis at all ages and in every country are Group A Streptococci (GAS), especially *S. pyogenes*. Although the majority of cases of tonsillopharyngitis or pharyngitis do not merit antibiotic therapy, infections with GAS do call for antibiotics [4].

GAS are capable of both colonizing the oropharynx and causing symptoms of infection.

- The term "active infection" describes an infection by GAS that results in symptoms.
- The term "persistent infection" describes an infection by GAS that results in symptoms that persist even following correct antibiotic therapy. Thus, a persistent infection means one where pharmacotherapy has failed.
- The term "recurrent infection" denotes an infective episode with GAS, producing symptoms, following appropriate antimicrobial pharmacotherapy. The pathogen responsible for the recurrent episode may be an identical or a different serotype from the original infection. This type of infection is most common

when several people pass the infection among each other, such as people living in the same house or attending the same school or daycare facility [5].

- When GAS are present long-term as a colonizer in the oropharynx, but this produces no immune reaction by the host nor any symptoms, the term "chronic carriage" is used. Exactly how frequently chronic carriage occurs remains to be established, although reports in the literature suggest a frequency of between 4 and 5% in healthy adults [6], while the frequency in children ranges from 2 to 20% [6–13]. This state may continue for a period lasting a few months or even a few years [12, 14].

It has been proven [15, 16] that antibiotics can alleviate the symptoms of pharyngitis secondary to streptococcal infection and speed recovery. Nonetheless, it is usual for symptomatic resolution to occur within the space of 3–5 days in the majority of cases [17], and thus the main rationale for the use of antibiotics is to prevent the case from becoming complicated.

21.3 Etiology

Tonsillitis (both complicated and uncomplicated) is caused by infection by a virus or bacterium, as well as immune system factors. Overcrowding and a poor nutritional status render patients more susceptible to tonsillitis. The majority of cases of acute pharyngitis or tonsillitis are viral in origin. The following are the usual causative viral pathogens [18]:

- Herpes simplex virus
- Epstein–Barr virus (EBV)
- Cytomegalovirus
- Herpesviridae of other types
- Adenovirus
- Measles virus

Between 15 and 30% of instances of pharyngotonsillitis are bacterial in origin, with anaerobes being particularly significant in this respect. Bacterial tonsillitis is most frequently the result of infection with Group A β-hemolytic *Streptococcus pyogenes* (GABHS). GABHS is able to attach itself to the epithelial cells of the tonsil via adhesin receptors expressed by the epithelium. It is likely that a key component in the development of bacterial tonsillitis is the attachment of antibodies over the surface of the bacterium [18].

Recurrent tonsillitis: When swabs taken from the core of tonsils in patients with repeated episodes of tonsillitis are cultured, multiple microbes are isolated. Both aerobes and anaerobes are found. In pediatric cases of recurrent GABHS tonsillitis, the flora differs from pediatric cases where recurrence is not a feature. In recurrent cases, GABHS overgrow at the expense of other bacteria, and thus other bacteria do not keep the infection in check. For recurrent cases, the usual pathogens detected are *Streptococcus pneumoniae*, *Staphylococcus aureus*, and *Haemophilus influenzae*. The anaerobe most likely to be isolated is *Bacteroides fragilis* [18].

Pediatric and adult cases of recurrent tonsillitis differ microbiologically. It is more common to isolate bacterial pathogens in adults, and organisms from the genera *Prevotella* and *Porphyromonas*, as well as *B. fragilis*, are more common in adults. GABHS are more commonly isolated in pediatric cases. A further difference is the higher prevalence of beta-lactamase expressing bacteria in adults [18].

21.4 Signs and Symptoms

The presenting features in patients suffering from acute tonsillitis are as follows [18]:

- Pyrexia
- Painful throat
- Offensive-smelling breath
- Patients finding it hard to swallow
- Pain when swallowing
- Tender cervical lymphadenopathy

21.5 Antibiotics in Pregnancy

In pregnant patients, the decision to treat with antibiotic medications needs to involve careful consideration of the risks to both mother and fetus. All antimicrobial agents have the ability to enter the fetal circulation, and this means that the mother cannot take any antibiotic without at least potential harm to the fetus. Prescribed medications are, in fact, implicated in no more than 1 in 100 congenital anomalies, but antibiotics are among the most commonly prescribed pharmacological agents, and thus their teratogenic potential is a matter of great significance [1].

21.5.1 Classification

There is a severe lack of evidence about how teratogenic the majority of antibiotics may be in humans. The US FDA (Food and Drug Administration) has a classification scheme for medications that categorizes their teratogenic potential. Drugs may be classified in the following way [1]:

- Category A agents have been studied in pregnant women, and no risk to the mother or fetus has been identified.
- Category B agents have not been shown to present a teratogenic risk in animal studies. Evidence in humans may be limited, or animal studies may indicate a risk that does not seem present in humans.

- Category C agents are toxic in animals, but there is insufficient evidence to decide on toxicity in human beings.
- For Category D agents, there are data indicating teratogenic risk in humans.
- In Category X, reports linking particular fetal abnormalities to the agent exist.

Regardless of the categorization of any particular antibiotic, the decision to treat during pregnancy is only justified where the benefit is greater than the potential risk.

21.5.2 Antibiotics in Frequent Use

The following agents are often used [1]

- Penicillins all fall under category B. Among these agents, those prescribed with the highest frequency to pregnant patients are penicillin itself, amoxicillin, and ampicillin, thanks to a generous safety margin and the absence of known teratogenicity. A collaborative study of perinatal women established that there were no harms observed in a sample of 3546 women administered penicillin within the initial trimester. Pregnancy does, however, lead to a higher circulating volume in the woman and an increased rate of filtration by the glomeruli; therefore, an upward dose adjustment may be required to reach an appropriate concentration within the circulation.
- Cephalosporins are also category B agents. Since there is an absence of research evidence concerning the use of cephalosporins in the initial trimester of pregnancy, they cannot be considered suitable as first-choice agents. However, in general, they may be thought safe.
- Metronidazole is under category B. Research has identified mutagenic potential in vitro. Nonetheless, the risk of mutations does not appear raised in actual data from use in pregnancy. Thus, metronidazole may be a controversial choice. It is advisable not to use metronidazole within the initial trimester, unless absolutely necessary.
- Macrolides, including azithromycin, do not have any demonstrable association with congenital anomalies and are thought safe for employment in pregnant women. Macrolides are within category B.
- Clindamycin has no data indicating teratogenicity and is in category B.

21.6 Antibiotic Use During Breastfeeding

There may be many reasons why a breastfeeding mother may need to be prescribed medication. Breastfeeding is known to be highly beneficial for the infant; hence, it should only be halted if the mother is using an agent with the potential to harm the baby and excreted in significant quantities into breast milk. Most medications do not appear from the data to result in harm to breastfeeding infants, and stopping breastfeeding even temporarily may make the resumption of the activity hard to achieve. Accordingly, where a decision is needed on breastfeeding in the context of medication use, this decision needs to be supported by accurate and up-to-date information [19].

There are two mechanisms by which a substance may be incorporated into breast milk, namely by diffusing passively or by being actively transported. The degree to which the drug enters breast milk is determined by the physical and chemical nature of the drug molecule, of which the key parameters to consider are the degree of protein binding, ionization potential, hydrophobicity, and molecular mass [20, 21].

21.6.1 Milk-to-Plasma Ratio

The milk-to-plasma (M/P) ratio is the ratio of $[\text{drug}]_{\text{milk}}/[\text{drug}]_{\text{plasma}}$. It can be derived experimentally. The ratio exhibits time-variability and depends on both the dose given and how long after dosing the concentration in milk is measured. The curve showing concentration in milk over time reflects that of plasma concentration over time, but with a delay. The M/P ratio offers an indication of the amount of agent the infant is exposed to while feeding, although this also depends on the bioavailability of the drug and the renal clearance in the child [19].

21.6.2 Excretion of Antibiotics in Breast Milk

21.6.2.1 Penicillins

The American Academy of Pediatrics has given approval to amoxicillin and ampicillin, both of which are aminopenicillins, for prescription to lactating mothers [22], although there is no discussion of the other agents in this group. Penicillins are present in breast milk, albeit at relatively low levels. Following administration of benzylpenicillin 100,000 IU by intramuscular injection, the M/P has been calculated to lie between 0.03 and 0.13. There is plentiful evidence to confirm that penicillins may be safely employed in breastfeeding patients [23, 24]. When cloxacillin and dicloxacillin, two agents that resist degradation by beta-lactamase, are given by mouth, the concentration in breast milk was found to be very low [23, 25].

The antibiotics nafcillin and methicillin may only be administered by a parenteral route. Nafcillin is very poorly absorbed through the gut, and methicillin breaks apart in the acidic environment of the stomach. While there are no specific accounts in the literature detailing the M/P ratio for these agents, it is reasonable to conclude it will be low, by analogy with other penicillins. One further factor is that the infant's absorption of these agents from the gut would also be very low due to the same issues affecting their bioavailability in adults [19].

Among penicillins that are active against *Pseudomonas*, the sole agent with approval from the American Academy of Pediatrics for use during lactation is ticarcillin [22]. Ticarcillin also suffers from minimal bioavailability when taken via the gut and is thus administered by a parenteral route [23]. There is no published evidence for the M/P ratio in mezlocillin. As is the case with other penicillins administered parenterally, the M/P ratio is thought to be very low and the bioavailability following ingestion in breast milk is likely to be negligible [23, 25].

Thus, in conclusion, lactation is not a contraindication for prescription of any antibiotic of penicillin-type.

21.6.2.2   Clavulanic Acid

Clavulanic acid is typically combined with amoxicillin (i.e., co-amoxiclav) since clavulanic acid inhibits the action of bacterial beta-lactamases. Clavulanic acid is suitable for oral administration and is secreted into breast milk [23]. There are no reports of harm to breastfeeding infants of mothers prescribed clavulanic acid, and thus it may be considered acceptable for use during lactation [19].

21.6.2.3   Cephalosporins

Cephalosporins, like penicillins, have a very low M/P ratio [26]. Multiple cephalosporins have been investigated pharmacodynamically, with evidence indicating that they are suitable for use during lactation [26–33].

21.6.2.4   First-Generation Cephalosporins

Cephalosporins of the first generation, whether given by mouth or a parenteral route, have a low M/P ratio. The plasma concentrations in infants breastfed by mothers taking cefazolin and cefalotin were beneath the level of detection [26, 27, 32]. The American Academy of Pediatrics approves first-generation cephalosporins for prescription to lactating women [22].

21.6.2.5   Second-Generation Cephalosporins

Despite the widespread prescription of cefuroxime and cefaclor, there are no data published showing the M/P ratio in humans. Nonetheless, there are no reports to date showing adverse effects in the children of mothers to whom these agents were administered while breastfeeding [25, 32]. Second-generation cephalosporins are generally accepted as suitable agents for use in lactating mothers [19].

21.6.2.6   Third-Generation Cephalosporins

When ceftazidime at a dose of between 1 and 2 g was administered parenterally, the peak level in breast milk occurred 5 h post-administration, and around 4.4% of the agent entered the milk [30]. The AAP has given its approval to the third-generation agents cefotaxime, ceftazidime, and ceftriaxone for prescription to lactating mothers [22].

21.6.2.7   Metronidazole

The AAP recommendation is to halt breastfeeding for between 12 and 24 h in lactating mothers given a single dose of metronidazole [22]. However, Bar-Oz et al. [19] state their recommendation that administration of metronidazole for brief periods or at low doses should not be the basis for a decision to halt breastfeeding.

21.6.2.8 Fluoroquinolones

There are reports indicating that fluoroquinolones may result in arthropathy in juvenile animals [34, 35]. The FDA, taking these data into consideration, does not grant approval to use these agents in either infants or children generally [19].

21.6.2.9 Macrolides

Erythromycin was the first agent of the macrolide antibiotics discovered. Its peak concentration in breast milk reaches between 0.4 and 1.6 mg L^{-1}, following administration of 400 mg t.d.s, while a dosage regime consisting of 2 g daily produced a peak of 1.6–3.2 mg L^{-1} [36]. There is a single case report linking infantile pyloric stenosis to exposure to erythromycin in breast milk [37]. However, despite this report, the AAP still approves erythromycin for use in lactating mothers [22].

Clarithromycin acts as a weak base, in common with other macrolide antibiotics, and thus may potentially be subject to ion trapping in breast milk. A study investigating the excretion of clarithromycin into breast milk found a peak M/P ratio of 0.25, whereas the highest recorded M/P ratio for the metabolite of clarithromycin was 0.75 [38].

References

1. Smith DS. Bacterial infections and pregnancy. In: Smith CV, editor. Medscape. Updated: Sep 11, 2018. https://emedicine.medscape.com/article/235054-overview. Accessed 31 March 2021.
2. Schrag S, Gorwitz R, Fultz-Butts K, Schuchat A. Prevention of perinatal group B streptococcal disease. Revised guidelines from CDC. MMWR Recomm Rep. 2002;51:1–22.
3. Centers for Disease Control and Prevention. Procedures for collecting clinical specimens for culture of group B Streptococcus (GBS) at 35–37 weeks' gestation. CDC; November 2010. http://www.cdc.gov/groupbstrep/guidelines/downloads/procedure-collecting.pdf. Accessed 24 Aug 2016.
4. Pichichero ME. Treatment and prevention of streptococcal pharyngitis in adults and children. In: Sexton DJ, Edwards MS, Bond S, Kunins L, editors. UpToDate. Last updated: Jan 16, 2020.
5. Efstratiou A, Lamagni T. Epidemiology of streptococcus pyogenes. In: Ferretti JJ, Stevens DL, Fischetti VA, editors. Streptococcus pyogenes: basic biology to clinical manifestations. Oklahoma City: University of Oklahoma Health Sciences Center; 2016.
6. Gunnarsson RK, Holm SE, Söderström M. The prevalence of beta-haemolytic streptococci in throat specimens from healthy children and adults. Implications for the clinical value of throat cultures. Scand J Prim Health Care. 1997;15(149)
7. Schwartz RH, Wientzen RL Jr, Pedreira F, et al. Penicillin V for group A streptococcal pharyngotonsillitis. A randomized trial of seven vs ten days' therapy. JAMA. 1981;246(1790)
8. Pontin IP, Sanchez DC, Di Francesco R. Asymptomatic group A streptococcus carriage in children with recurrent tonsillitis and tonsillar hypertrophy. Int J Pediatr Otorhinolaryngol. 2016;86:57.
9. Abdissa A, Asrat D, Kronvall G, et al. Throat carriage rate and antimicrobial susceptibility pattern of group A Streptococci (GAS) in healthy Ethiopian school children. Ethiop Med J. 2011;49:125.
10. Nayiga I, Okello E, Lwabi P, Ndeezi G. Prevalence of group a streptococcus pharyngeal carriage and clinical manifestations in school children aged 5–15 yrs in Wakiso District, Uganda. BMC Infect Dis. 2017;17:248.

11. Marshall HS, Richmond P, Nissen M, et al. Group A streptococcal carriage and Seroepidemiology in children up to 10 years of age in Australia. Pediatr Infect Dis J. 2015;34:831.
12. Martin JM, Green M, Barbadora KA, Wald ER. Group A streptococci among school-aged children: clinical characteristics and the carrier state. Pediatrics. 2004;114:1212.
13. Shaikh N, Leonard E, Martin JM. Prevalence of streptococcal pharyngitis and streptococcal carriage in children: a meta-analysis. Pediatrics. 2010;126:e557.
14. Kaplan EL. The group A streptococcal upper respiratory tract carrier state: an enigma. J Pediatr. 1980;97:337.
15. Spinks A, Glasziou PP, Del Mar CB. Antibiotics for sore throat. Cochrane Database Syst Rev. 2013:CD000023.
16. Little P, Hobbs FD, Moore M, et al. Clinical score and rapid antigen detection test to guide antibiotic use for sore throats: randomised controlled trial of PRISM (primary care streptococcal management). BMJ. 2013;347:f5806.
17. Brink WR, Rammelkamp CH Jr, Denny FW, Wannamaker LW. Effect in penicillin and aureomycin on the natural course of streptococcal tonsillitis and pharyngitis. Am J Med. 1951;10:300.
18. Shah UK. Tonsillitis and peritonsillar abscess. In: Meyers AD (Ed). Medscape. Updated: Apr 06, 2020. https://emedicine.medscape.com/article/871977-overview. Accessed online at March 31, 2021.
19. Bar-Oz B, Bulkowstein M, Benyamini L, Greenberg R, Soriano I, Zimmerman D, Bortnik O, Berkovitch M. Use of antibiotic and analgesic drugs during lactation. Drug Saf. 2003;26(13):925–35. https://doi.org/10.2165/00002018-200326130-00002.
20. Tadio A, Ito S. Drugs and breast-feeding. In: Koren G, editor. Maternal-fetal toxicology. 3rd ed. New York, NY: Marcel Dekker; 2001. p. 177–232.
21. Chung AM, Reed MD, Blumer JL. Antibiotics and breastfeeding. Pediatr Drugs. 2002;4(12):817–37.
22. American Academy of Pediatrics. The transfer of drugs and other chemicals into human milk. Pediatrics. 2001;108:776–89.
23. Matsuda S. Transfer of antibiotics into maternal milk. Biol Res Pregnancy Perinatol. 1984;5:57–60.
24. Nau H. Clinical pharmacokinetics in pregnancy and perinatology: II. Penicillins. Dev Pharmacol Ther. 1987;10:174–98.
25. Hale T. Medications and mothers' milk. 9th ed. Amarillo, TX: Pharmasoft Medical Publishing; 2000.
26. Kafetzis DA, Siafas CA, Georgakopoulous PA, et al. Passage of cephalosporins and amoxicillin into breast milk. Acta Paediatr Scand. 1981;70:285–6.
27. Yoshioka H, Cho K, Takimoto M, et al. Transfer of cefazolin into human milk. J Pediatr. 1979;94:151–2.
28. Dresse A, Lambotte R, Dubois M, et al. Transmammary passage of cefoxitin: additional results. J Clin Pharmacol. 1983;23:438–40.
29. Shyu WC, Shah VR, Campbell DA, et al. Excretion of cefprozil into human breast milk. Antimicrob Agents Chemother. 1992;36:938–41.
30. Blanco JD, Jorgensen JH, Castaneda YS, et al. Ceftazidime levels in human breast milk. Antimicrob Agents Chemother. 1983;23:479–80.
31. Bourget P, Quinquis-Desmaris V, Fernandez H. Ceftriaxone distribution and protein binding between maternal blood and milk postpartum. Ann Pharmacother. 1993;27:294–7.
32. Gilbert DN, Moellering RC Jr, Sande MA, editors. The Sanford guide to antimicrobial therapy. 29th ed. Antimicrobial Therapy Inc.; 1999. p. 58.
33. Kafetzis DA, Brater DC, Fanourgakis JE, et al. Ceftriaxone distribution between maternal blood and fetal blood and tissues at parturition and between blood and milk postpartum. Antimicrob Agents Chemother. 1983;23:870–3.
34. Product information, Noroxin (norfloxacin): Merck & Co Inc.; 2001.
35. Burkhardt JE, Hill MA, Carton WW. Morphologic and biochemical changes in articular cartilages of immature beagle dogs dosed with difloxacin. Toxicol Pathol. 1992;20:246–52.

36. Briggs GG, Freeman RK, Yaffe SJ. Drugs in pregnancy and lactation. 5th ed. Baltimore, MD: Williams & Wilkins; 1998.
37. Stang H. Pyloric stenosis associated with erythromycin ingested through breast milk. Minn Med. 1986;69:669–70.
38. Sedlmayr T, Peters F, Raasch W, et al. Clarithromycin, a new macrolide antibiotic: effectiveness in puerperal infections and pharmacokinetics in breast milk. Geburtshilfe Frauenheilkd. 1993;53(7):488–91.

Facial and Deep Cervical Infections During Pregnancy and the Postpartum Period

22

Derya Cebeci, Fatih Alper Akcan, and Sergei Karpischenko

22.1 Introduction

Facial and deep cervical infections comprise a portion of the infective conditions to affect the head and neck region. They may result in serious complications and may even pose a risk to life. This type of infection may occur during pregnancy or in the puerperium when the associated physiological changes may render the woman more susceptible to infection and prone to a more severe clinical course. In such patients, special care is needed to protect the fetus and mother, to ensure the pregnancy proceeds as normal, and to allow for breastfeeding. Following the discovery of antibiotics, deep neck infections have become relatively rare due to the widespread use of antibiotics, especially penicillin, worldwide [1]. For this reason, many clinicians may not be familiar with these types of infections. The purpose of this chapter is to raise awareness among ENT specialists and other clinicians and thus facilitate proper diagnosis and treatment and the prevention of complications.

D. Cebeci (✉)
Department of Otorhinolaryngology, Şanlıurfa Viranşehir State Hospital, Şanlıurfa, Turkey
e-mail: drderyacebeci@gmail.com

F. A. Akcan
Department of Otorhinolaryngology, Düzce University, Faculty of Medicine, Düzce, Turkey
e-mail: f.akcan@yahoo.com

S. Karpischenko
Department of Otorhinolaryngology, The First Pavlov State Medical University of Saint Petersburg, Saint Petersburg, Russia
e-mail: karpischenkos@mail.ru

C. Cingi et al. (eds.), *ENT Diseases: Diagnosis and Treatment during Pregnancy and Lactation*, https://doi.org/10.1007/978-3-031-05303-0_22

22.2 Etiology

Deep cervical bacterial infections originate in the upper aerodigestive tract and affect the deep cervical tissues. Odontogenic infections are the most common type, followed by oropharyngeal infections, such as tonsillitis or pharyngitis [2, 3]. The periodontal tissues increase in sensitivity and susceptibility to irritation as a result of the hormonal alterations that accompany pregnancy and the postpartum period. Furthermore, many women consume extra snacks while they are pregnant. This results in the accumulation and hardening of dental plaque. These plaques may infect the gingiva and lead to bleeding when the woman brushes her teeth. Plaque formation also produces new dental caries or accelerates pre-existing decay [4, 5]. Odontogenic infections are more of a risk in patients with poor dental hygiene or who are of low socioeconomic status [6]. Endoscopic manipulation and oral surgery may result in iatrogenic trauma to the lumen of the upper aerodigestive tract. Foreign bodies lodged in the upper aerodigestive canal may become a focus of infection, which then spreads to the deep cavities of the cervical region. Cutaneous cellulitis starts as a superficial infection but may track into the deeper cervical structures along the planes of the face. Sialadenitis, acquired or congenital masses (such as thyroglossal duct cysts, laryngoceles, or branchial cleft cysts), may become infected and result in deep cervical infections. Acute mastoiditis can extend to the upper part of the neck and develop into a Bezold's abscess. Lymph nodes affected by malignancy may undergo necrosis and form an abscess in patients over the age of 40 years [7]. Penetrating trauma to the face or neck or intravenous (IV) drug misuse may also be responsible. In pregnant and postpartum women, those who are immunosuppressed, have diabetes mellitus, or are HIV positive, infections may be more virulent and may involve atypical organisms [6].

22.3 Microbiology

Deep cervical infections are typically bacterial in type and may consist of the same organisms as are found in the normal bacterial flora of the adjacent mucosal surfaces [8]. A similar situation is observed in pregnant and breastfeeding women. Normal oral flora can contain aerobic and anaerobic bacterial species, various fungal species, viruses, and even protozoans. Following advances in molecular identification techniques, more than 700 types of bacteria have now been identified in the oral cavity [9]. Most of these normal flora bacteria can cause odontogenic infections. The most common microorganisms isolated are *Streptococcus viridans*, *Staphylococcus epidermidis*, *S. aureus*, *Streptococcus pyogenes* (Group A β-hemolytic streptococci), *Fusobacterium*, *Bacteroides*, and *Peptostreptococcus* species [10]. Less frequently encountered bacteria include *Pseudomonas*, *Haemophilus*, *Neisseria*, and *Escherichia* species. The organisms isolated from deep cervical infections arising from causes other than odontogenic are somewhat different. For example, the typical organisms in deep cervical infections originating from acute bacterial rhinosinusitis are *Streptococcus pneumoniae*, *Moraxella catarrhalis*, *H. influenzae*, and *S. aureus* [11]. Anaerobes are seen in head and deep neck infections secondary to chronic rhinosinusitis [12]. Facultative Gram-negative bacilli such as *P. aeruginosa* and *S. aureus* may also be involved, where there is an extension from chronic otitis media or mastoiditis [13, 14]. Patients with co-morbid disorders (such as diabetes mellitus), or who are immunocompromised, may harbor pathogens such as *P. aeruginosa* and other drug-resistant pathogens, e.g., *Klebsiella pneumoniae* and extended-spectrum beta-lactamase (ESBL)-producing Enterobacteriaceae [15, 16]. An infection of the cervical vertebral column (e.g., vertebral osteomyelitis or discitis) developing after esophageal or tracheal instrumentation may cause a prevertebral infection and hematogenous spread. Intravenous drug misuse, alcoholism, immunosuppression, and diabetes mellitus are specific known risk factors for infections of the prevertebral space. Gram-positive bacteria, specifically *S. aureus* and methicillin-resistant *S. aureus* (MRSA), often predominate.

Gram-negative bacilli (*P. aeruginosa*), fungi, and mycobacteria may also be isolated [17–19]. Atypical organisms, such as *Actinomyces* and *Bartonella henselae*, are among the causes of deep cervical infections. Actinomyces infection provokes granuloma formation. There are so-called sulfur granules within a central abscess. *Bartonella henselae* is the organism responsible for cat scratch disease. Nontuberculous and tuberculous infections of the head and neck may appear as cervical lymphadenopathy. Surgical treatment is generally best avoided in atypical deep neck infections to prevent chronic scarring and fistula formation.

22.4   Anatomy

Knowledge of the complex anatomy of the facial and neck cavities is key to appreciating the pathogenesis, spread, and clinical course of infections.

There are two cervical fasciae within the neck, namely the deep and the superficial fascia. The superficial cervical fascia (SCF) is located between the dermis and the deep cervical fascia. Fat and loose connective tissues surround the superficial lymph nodes, platysma, and muscles of facial expression. The deep cervical fascia is subdivided into superficial, middle, and deep layers (Table 22.1). The superficial layer of the deep cervical fascia (SLDCF) is located between the SCF and the neck muscles. The SLDCF wraps around two muscles (the trapezius and sternocleidomastoid), as well as two glands (the parotid and submandibular). The middle layer of the deep cervical fascia (MLDCF) attaches to the base of the skull and extends into the mediastinum. The muscular lamina envelops the strap muscles, while the visceral lamina envelops the pharynx, larynx, trachea, esophagus, and thyroid. The deepest layer of the cervical deep fascia is divided into two components: the prevertebral and the alar fascia. The prevertebral layer surrounds the paraspinal muscles, scalene muscles, and the levator scapulae muscle [20]. The alar layer surrounds the posterior and lateral walls of the retropharyngeal space. All the layers of the deep cervical fascia unite to form the carotid sheath. The carotid sheath contains the carotid artery, tenth cranial nerve, and jugular vein. It extends from the base of the

Table 22.1 Deep neck and facial spaces' content and possible sources of infections

	Contents	Possible source of infection[a]
1. Facial region		
(a) Buccal space	Adipose tissue, the facial artery and vein, Stensen's duct, branches of CN VII and IX	Three maxillary molars infections
(b) Canine space		Apical infections of maxillary canine tooth
(c) Masticator space		
• Masseter space • Pterygoid space • Temporal space	Mandibular nerve (V3), the internal maxillary artery, temporalis muscle, ramus of mandible	Infections of molar teeth
(d) Parotid space	The parotid gland with lymph nodes, the facial nerve (CN VII), the external carotid, internal maxillary and retromandibular vein	Acute parotitis, intraparotid lymphadenitis
2. Suprahyoid region		
(a) Sublingual space	Deep portion of submandibular gland, sublingual gland, glossopharyngeal (CN IX) and hypoglossal (CN XII) nerves, lingual artery, vein and nerve	Dental sepsis, sialolithiasis, an infected ranula
(b) Submental space	Lymph nodes, fat tissue, and the anterior jugular vein	Lymphadenitis, odontogenic origin, infected ranula, extension of infections of submandibular space
(c) Submandibular space		Odontogenic origin, sialoadenitis, lymphadenitis, trauma
(d) Ludwig's angina (IIa + IIb + IIc)	Cellulitis of the submental, sublingual, and submandibular spaces	Odontogenic origin
(e) Parapharyngeal space		
• Prestyloid compartment • Poststyloid compartment	Parotid gland, fat tissue, internal maxillary artery, lingual nerve, inferior alveolar, and auriculotemporal nerve The internal carotid artery, internal jugular vein, CN IX–XII, sympathetic trunk	A central contact zone for all other deep neck spaces
(f) PERITONSILLAR SPACE	Loose connective tissue	Acute tonsillitis
3. Infrahyoid region		
(a) Pretracheal space (anterior visceral zone)	Trachea, thyroid gland, anterior wall of the esophagus	Traumatic perforation of esophagus, thyroiditis

Table 22.1 (continued)

	Contents	Possible source of infection[a]
4. Entire neck		
(a) Retropharyngeal space	Fatty areolar tissue, lymph nodes (from skull base to T2 thoracic vertebral level)	Nasopharynx, oropharynx, sinonasal region
(b) Danger space	A small amount of loose connective tissue (from pharynx to mediastinum)	A potential path for spread of infections
(c) Carotid space	The internal carotid artery, internal jugular vein, CN IX-XII, sympathetic trunk	
(d) Prevertebral space	Prevertebral muscles, vertebral artery and vein	Infective spondylodiscitis, penetrating injuries

[a] Most frequently sources

skull to the upper mediastinum and is a key route (a "Lincoln's Highway") from the chest up through the neck. This anatomical conformation is important when anticipating the spread of infection in this area.

The deep fascia forms important cavities deep within the neck, some of which are interconnected. The buccal space in the facial region is bordered by the buccinator muscle and buccopharyngeal fascia medially, the skin laterally, the lip muscles anteriorly, and the pterygomandibular line posteriorly. The superior border of this space is the zygomatic arch, while the mandible forms the inferior border. The canine space is also referred to as the infraorbital space. It is located between the levator anguli oris muscle superiorly, and the levator labii superioris muscle inferiorly. The masticator cavity consists of closely related sub-spaces. The masseter space lies between the masseter muscle and the ramus of the mandible, the pterygoid space lies between the pterygoid muscles and the mandible, and the temporal space lies between the temporal fascia and the temporalis muscle. The masticator space is adjacent to the buccal space anteriorly, the parotid space posteriorly, the skull base superiorly, and the parapharyngeal space medially. The parotid space is formed by the superficial layer of the deep cervical fascia as it envelops the parotid gland. The sublingual space, located in the suprahyoid region, is bordered by the mucosa of the oral cavity floor superiorly, the mylohyoid muscle inferiorly, and the mandible anterolaterally. The submandibular space is located between the mylohyoid muscle and the hyoid bone and is in direct communication with the contralateral submandibular space. Laterally, there is the anterior belly of the digastric muscle and anteriorly the submental space, surrounded by the lower border of the mandible. Ludwig's angina, with involvement of the bilateral submandibular, submental, and sublingual spaces, generally develops from an odontogenic infection. In the cases of Ludwig's angina, the airway patency should be secured urgently and drainage and antibiotic treatment rapidly initiated. The parapharyngeal space is also termed the pharyngomaxillary or lateral pharyngeal space. This space, which has the shape of an inverted pyramid, extends from the skull base superiorly to the hyoid bone inferiorly and is in close proximity to the other spaces. The region consists of two subunits: the prestyloid and poststyloid. The peritonsillar space is between the palatine tonsils and the superior constrictor muscle. In the infrahyoid region, anterior to the trachea, lies the pretracheal space (anterior visceral space), which extends from the level of the thyroid cartilage to the superior mediastinum. There are four spaces that run along the entire neck. The retropharyngeal space extends from the skull base to the level of the T1-2 thoracic vertebrae. It is located between the alar and buccopharyngeal fascia. The danger space (alar space) is between the alar fascia anteriorly and the prevertebral fascia posteriorly. This space extends from the skull base to the diaphragm and may permit infections to spread rapidly into the mediastinum. The prevertebral space is located between the prevertebral fascia and the vertebral column. The potential space within the carotid sheath is called the carotid space. All these spaces contain vital structures (Table 22.1).

22.5 Clinical Assessment

22.5.1 History

As with every disease, the diagnosis of facial and deep neck infections begins by obtaining an accurate history. Fever, pain, redness, and swelling are commonly seen in patients. Other symptoms that may develop, depending on the location of the infection, are a sore throat, odynophagia, dysphagia, hoarseness, "hot potato" speech, trismus, ear pain, and shortness of breath. It should be noted that these symptoms may be masked by antibiotic treatment, as often occurs due to their widespread use. First of all, the patient should be asked about the onset and duration of symptoms. Enquiry should be made about past medical history, including chronic conditions such as diabetes mellitus, hematological malignancy, hepatitis, and human immunodeficiency virus (HIV). Note whether the patient smokes and consumes alcohol. Ask about steroid use, previous chemotherapy, and any immunodeficiency and record any (drug) allergies. If the patient is pregnant, obtain the history of the pregnancy (which trimester currently, the course of the pregnancy, any history of preeclampsia or gestational diabetes) and enquire about breastfeeding status in postpartum women. It should be recorded whether the patient has a recent history of intubation or upper airway surgery, oral/dental intervention, pharyngitis, sinusitis, otitis, IV medication, hospitalization, blunt or penetrating soft tissue trauma, recent neck surgery, or radiation exposure. If the origin of the infection can be identified, the probable pathogenic microorganisms (including both typical and atypical bacteria) involved and the pattern of spread can be predicted. To take a particular example, a prolonged hospital admission to an intensive care unit where jugular vein catheters were inserted may develop suppurative thrombophlebitis of the internal jugular vein (Lemierre's syndrome). Or, to take another example, diffuse cellulitis and lymphoedema may disguise otherwise prominent clinical features in patients who have undergone neck surgery or have received neck radiotherapy for cancer.

22.5.2 Physical Examination

Any patient with a possible deep neck infection should have the head and neck examined. On inspection, patients may appear toxic and listless. In the majority of cases, pyrexia is noted. Erythema, swelling, asymmetry, and regional lymphadenitis can be observed in the neck. During palpation, localized areas of fluctuation or tenderness and crepitation may be identified. The cause of crepitation may be gas-producing bacteria or airway trauma. Abscesses in this area may not be fluctuant due to being deeply located and overlaid by tense muscles and fascia. Diagnostic imaging will be required to localize the lesion. Examination of the oral cavity and oropharynx should be carefully performed. Use of a headlamp facilitates bimanual examination. In the presence of decayed or broken teeth, an odontogenic source of infection should be suspected. To ensure the safety of the airway, evaluate carefully any swelling in the floor of the mouth and edema of the tongue base and check how mobile the tongue is. Trismus occurs due to local pressure on the trigeminal nerve or masticatory muscles. The salivary gland ducts (Wharton and Stensen ducts) should be monitored for any purulent discharge and palpated for sialolithiasis. Medial displacement of the lateral pharyngeal wall strongly suggests a parapharyngeal space infection, while lateral displacement of the uvula suggests a peritonsillar abscess. In the absence of inflammatory symptoms, unilateral pharyngeal wall swelling should make the clinician consider the possibility of a parapharyngeal tumor. Patients with dysphagia but no shortness of breath, hoarseness, stridor and/or odynophagia or oropharyngeal cause should, where possible, have the upper airway evaluated in the awake state using a flexible fiberoptic endoscope. Since the mucosa of pregnant and puerperal women is very friable, the examination should be performed very gently. If an obstructed airway is suspected, patency of the airway should be secured by tracheal intubation or tracheotomy prior to undertaking any examination or other intervention. A complete cranial nerve examination is recommended (especially cranial nerves IX to XII). Horner syndrome may occur due to the involvement of the cervical sympathetic plexus within the carotid sheath.

22.6 Laboratory Evaluation

22.6.1 Blood Tests

Many physiological hematological changes occur during pregnancy [21]. These changes revert to normal after the puerperium [22]. There are increases in the number of circulating leukocytes and erythrocytes. Despite this, a relatively larger increase in the plasma volume can result in physiological anemia [23]. Hypercoagulability is a further hematological alteration and is due to an increase in various pro-coagulation factors and a decrease in other anti-coagulation factors during pregnancy [24]. Gestational diabetes is also common. In face and deep neck infections, there is generally leukocytosis apparent when a complete blood count (CBC) is performed. Measuring the white blood cell (WBC) count on a daily basis can help monitor the patient's response to treatment. Routine biochemical analyses, such as glucose level, erythrocyte sedimentation rate (ESR), C-reactive protein (CRP), liver enzymes (aspartate transaminase and alanine transaminase), and renal function tests (blood urea nitrogen, creatinine, albumin, total protein, serum potassium, and sodium electrolytes) should be evaluated initially and then every 2 or 3 days throughout the hospital stay. Fluid and nutritional requirements go up during pregnancy or breastfeeding, and these factors should be considered when treating the patient. The coagulation profile is particularly important to consider if patients require surgical drainage. If an aspiration sample is obtainable from the infected area, it should be sent to the laboratory for culture. If the patient has sepsis, blood culture should also be undertaken.

22.6.2 Imaging Studies

In the presence of signs or symptoms suggestive of deep neck/facial infection, imaging studies should be rapidly ordered to confirm the diagnosis and localize the lesion, as well as evaluate possible spread, complications, and airway compression.

Ultrasonography, which does not entail exposure to radiation and is easily accessible and noninvasive, is the initial investigation of choice. Ultrasound is a safe option during pregnancy and the postpartum period. It is the gold standard to differentiate between cellulitis and an abscess. Drainage and aspiration can be performed under ultrasonic guidance. However, the inability of ultrasonography to furnish detailed anatomical views reduces its value.

Plain radiography is an inexpensive, noninvasive, and fast imaging method; however, it is of limited value in the evaluation of facial and deep neck infections. Lateral neck films are helpful in evaluating the upper aerodigestive tract, especially in detecting supraglottis or retropharyngeal abscess. Increased thickness of the prevertebral soft tissues and air or air–fluid levels are signs of an infection of the retropharyngeal space. Chest radiography may be indicated if mediastinitis or aspiration is suspected. Suspicion of an odontogenic cause should prompt a request for an oral panoramic or plain X-ray.

Computed tomography (CT) is usually the preferred imaging method to determine and evaluate the location and spread of deep neck cavity infections [25]. The use of intravenous contrast for CT scanning provides excellent visualization of most soft tissue and bone structures of the head and neck. CT requires the use of iodine-containing contrast agents. There have been no reports of teratogenicity arising from the use of iodinated contrast agents, but the inorganic iodine dose used for imaging is around 0.1% of the dose that can be used to intervene in thyroid metabolism disorders. Nonionic contrast agents have been shown to cross the placenta and inhibit type II and type III deiodinases. Subsequently, the decreased triiodothyroxine level in the cell directly affects the transcription of multiple genes that are critical for fetal development [26]. Intravenous iodinated contrast media falls into Class B of the Food and Drug Administration's (FDA) drug classification scheme. Intravenous contrast media, as with all drugs in pregnancy, should only be administered when essential and only after informed consent has been obtained. CT scanning in the postpartum period is safer and IV contrast can be used, provided the patient has no allergy to contrast agents or renal impairment. Current guidelines do not support cessation of breastfeeding following administration of contrast agents. However, if the mother remains concerned about possible effects, a conservative approach (waiting for 12–24 h, expressing and discharging milk during this time) may be suggested [27, 28]. Radiation exposure during imaging in pregnant women remains the subject of controversy. Recent studies have shown that doses below 5–10 centigray (cGy) have no association with intrauterine growth retardation or the development of congenital defects [29]. The radiation exposure from a CT scan is lower than the normal safe radiation level (i.e., 5–10 cGy) [30]. All radiation doses are, however, potentially cumulative. Therefore, it is best to avoid CT scans in pregnant patients and use CT scans only in those patients who do not respond to surgical treatment [31]. Measures, such as the use of an abdominal lead shield, can be taken to minimize fetal exposure. When a pregnant woman requires radiological investigation to make a diagnosis, the risks from the imaging procedure and the benefits to be obtained in diagnosis and treatment need to be balanced.

Magnetic resonance imaging (MRI) is not usually undertaken for suspected deep neck infections, but MRI may be an alternative when fetal exposure is a concern. MRI does not involve ionizing radiation. Furthermore, MRI scans can provide greater detail than CT on the spread of infection to the intracranial, prevertebral, and parotid spaces. The potential effects of strong magnetic fields on the fetus are not fully known.

22.7 Treatment

In treating pregnant patients, clinicians should plan how to provide maximum benefit to the mother while minimizing risk to the fetus. Planning also needs to consider both mother and child in the postpartum period. A multidisciplinary approach is key to the diagnosis–treatment process in pregnant or puerperal women. The team should be composed of specialists in ENT, anesthesia, and gynecology.

22.7.1 Airway Management

The first step in treatment is to secure the airway since the most common causes of mortality in deep neck infections are hypoxia or asphyxia [32]. Damage to the normal airway anatomy, tissue edema, immobilization, and restricted mouth opening render intubation or tracheotomy especially difficult [33]. In addition, many of the physiological and anatomical changes occurring during pregnancy can cause airway difficulty. Congestion of the respiratory tract mucosal capillaries may produce edema within the oropharynx, nasopharynx, larynx, and trachea [34, 35]. Pregnancy-related changes, i.e., an increased circulatory volume and high estrogen levels, may contribute to increased mucosal edema [36]. These changes in the mucosa can be significantly aggravated by preeclampsia or an upper respiratory tract infection [37–39]. To preempt possible airway complications, it is important to evaluate the upper airway first by fiberoptic endoscopy. The patient should not be taken to the radiology department for imaging studies until the airway has been secured. If a pregnant or puerperal woman shows moderate airway symptoms and mild edema is detected when evaluating the airway, medical treatments such as humidified oxygen mask fitting, nebulized adrenaline, or intravenous steroids can be administered. With the exception of budesonide (category B), all inhaled corticosteroids fall within pregnancy risk category C [40]. If systemic corticosteroids are used, the lowest effective dose should be used. Patients should be closely monitored for the potential side effects of corticosteroids. No adverse effects in babies whose mothers used corticosteroids during breastfeeding have been noted. High doses may occasionally cause transient reductions in milk production [41]. The decision to prescribe such agents should be undertaken only after canvassing the opinion of specialists in the multidisciplinary team and evaluating benefits against risk. In cases like this, it may be difficult to use a rigid laryngoscope for tracheal intubation due to deformation in the airway anatomy, limited mouth opening, and tissue stiffness. On occasion, attempted intubation actually exacerbates an already threatened airway. It should be kept in mind that there may be an urgent need for tracheotomy [42]. For a difficult airway, awake fiberoptic intubation is recommended [43]. However, this procedure calls for substantial experience and knowledge of the airway and equipment. A 5–6-mm flexible bronchoscope may be suitable. Nasal intubation during pregnancy can cause epistaxis. Generally, oral fiberoptic intubation is preferable. It is important to sit the patient upright and to clear the secretions from the airway to allow for good visibility. Topical anesthesia is used to prevent the gag reflex and swallowing [44]. The most important problem to be aware of is sudden airway loss caused by airway irritation and bronchospasm provoked by an inexperienced operator attempting fiberoptic bronchoscopy [45, 46]. The recently introduced video-laryngoscopes have the advantage of being easier to use [47]. The tracheostomy set should be held in readiness. If tracheal intubation is predicted to be difficult when the patient is initially evaluated, tracheotomy under local anesthesia may be the first option to consider.

22.7.2 Medical Treatment

22.7.2.1 Metabolic Support and Liquid Replacement

Normally, fluid requirements increase in pregnant and breastfeeding women. The European Food Safety Authority (EFSA) recommends pregnant women drink 2.3 L per day and breastfeeding women, 2.7 L [48]. In deep neck infections, any fluid deficit increases alongside low oral intake due to dysphagia, odynophagia, and trismus and increased losses through high fever. Maternal shock, in which uteroplacental blood flow falls, resulting in fetal hypoxia, is the main cause of fetal death [49]. Sufficient fluids should be administered orally or intravenously. Normal saline, 5% dextrose, or Hartmann's solution (Ringer's lactate solution (RL)) are all suitable for this purpose. The rate of intravenous infusion may be set at 75–125 mL/h over a 24-h period [50]. Care should be exercised to prevent central pontine myelinolysis, which may develop as a complication of too rapid infusion [51].

If the patient has no oral intake, parenteral nutritional support should be provided, following consultation with appropriate specialists.

22.7.2.2   Antibiotic Treatment

The mainstay of treatment for deep neck infections is antibiotic therapy and surgical drainage to gain a specimen for microbiological culture. Empirical antibiotic therapy should be initiated even before culture results are obtained to prevent the progression of the infection [52]. In the selection of empirical antibiotics, it is important that the antibiotic selected have a broad spectrum of efficacy against streptococci and anaerobes since these pathogens are among the most frequently isolated organisms.

Antibiotic intolerance or allergy should be noted. If the patient has recently used antibiotics, the possibility of resistant strains should be kept in mind and antibiotic selection should be made accordingly. Since an abscess cavity is avascular, antibiotics may not penetrate the site of infection.

Any medicine given to women during pregnancy or lactation has the potential to cause adverse effects on the fetus or newborn. In 1979, the FDA (Food and Drug Administration) categorized drugs into five groups (A, B, C, D, or X), which indicates their potential to cause birth defects when used in pregnancy. Thus, drugs in category A are safe to use during pregnancy, while the teratogenicity of agents in class X is definitely established.

Penicillin and cephalosporin are safe in pregnant women. Clindamycin may be used where the patient has a penicillin allergy. Tetracycline and aminoglycosides are generally contraindicated during pregnancy because of their effects: tooth discoloration, impaired bone development, and ototoxicity [53]. The fluoroquinolones (moxifloxacin, ciprofloxacin, levofloxacin) should not be used in pregnant women due to their toxic effects on cartilaginous development.

In cases where the general condition of the patient is good, empirical IV antibiotic treatment for 2–3 days may be sufficient, provided the area of the neck involved is limited and any abscess does not exceed 2.5 cm in size [54]. Patients not taking oral fluids should be hospitalized to permit close follow-up and facilitate the provision of fluid replacement. Obstetric follow-up of pregnant women should also be arranged. If the patient's clinical condition worsens or there is no response to treatment, further imaging studies and surgical intervention may be required. If clinical improvement is seen following administration of IV antibiotics, treatment should be continued for 24 h after symptoms resolve. Following completion of a course of antibiotics intravenously, treatment, given orally, should go on for a further fortnight in pregnant or puerperal women.

22.7.2.3 Analgesia

Paracetamol (acetaminophen) is usually the first choice of analgesic in pregnant and breastfeeding women [55]. Since the use of NSAIDs after the 30th week of pregnancy may cause neonatal pulmonary hypertension and early closure of the ductus arteriosus, it is recommended their use be avoided [56]. Information on the use of NSAIDs during breastfeeding is very limited.

Opioids are potentially dangerous as they may cause respiratory depression, especially in the last few hours before giving birth.

22.7.3 Surgical Treatment

Surgical procedures for the management of deep neck infections in pregnant and postpartum patients resemble the approach taken in nonpregnant patients. Surgical drainage is required if the abscess is large in size, complications have developed, or there is a poor response to medication (i.e., following 2–3 days of empirical IV antibiotic therapy). The purpose of surgical drainage is to evacuate and irrigate the infected area, to place a drain in order to prevent recycling, and to obtain samples for culture. Local anesthesia is preferable to general anesthesia, wherever feasible, since it avoids the potential complications of a general anesthetic in the mother and fetus. Lidocaine (Anelok) is the generally preferred category B local anesthetic agent. Since lidocaine can cross the placenta, as can all local anesthetics, the lowest effective dose should be used. Lidocaine has been classified by the American Academy of Pediatrics as a suitable agent to use in breastfeeding women [57].

Other than in emergency cases where an urgent airway needs to be established, all women should undergo a gynecological and obstetric evaluation to determine their condition and that of the fetus before surgery is undertaken.

After 18–20 weeks of gestation, the position in which the woman lies during surgery is key. With the patient supine, the inferior vena cava is compressed due to an increase in abdominopelvic mass, resulting in supine hypotension syndrome. To prevent or reduce supine hypotension, a pillow should be placed under the patient's right gluteal region and the right hip should be raised 10–12 cm so that the pregnant woman ends up positioned between 5 and 15 degrees toward the left [58]. This position ensures there will be adequate uteroplacental and renal perfusion.

Imaging-guided needle aspiration is an effective alternative to surgery for deep neck area infections that do not compress the airway and have clearly defined borders.

Different surgical approaches have been defined according to the site of infection and which structures are adjacent [59], such as the transoral, transcervical, transoral, transcervical combined, and endoscopic approaches.

In peritonsillar area infections, a transoral approach utilizing a topical anesthetic spray (lidocaine) is preferred where the patient is co-operative and there is no trismus. It is not recommended that local anesthetic containing added adrenaline be used for pregnant women. Aspiration is performed with a needle and 10-mL syringe, inserting the needle at the point of greatest fluctuance. If aspiration fails, an approximately 1-cm long incision can be made following the course of the anterior tonsillar plica. Repeated drainage may sometimes be required. Acute tonsillectomy (quinsy tonsillectomy) may be a preferred option in the treatment of peritonsillar abscess, but this procedure entails considerable risks for the mother and fetus. To avoid surgical procedures that require a pregnant or postpartum woman to be under general anesthesia, tonsillectomy is usually deferred until later.

Odontogenic infections can cause fatal conditions such as Ludwig's angina and mediastinitis if intervention is delayed. It is best to have dental treatment of an elective type in the second trimester of pregnancy, but if there is a situation that requires urgent treatment, the necessary intervention may be undertaken in any trimester [60]. If a deep neck lesion is caused by a dental root infection, the tooth should be extracted as soon as possible. In the cases of Ludwig's angina, drainage can be performed transcervically and transorally on both sides.

In buccal space infections, transoral drainage can be achieved by an intraoral incision just below the orifice of the parotid duct.

For infections within the masticator space, intraoral access is possible by making a vertical incision along the pterygomandibular raphe. The wound may be left open to heal by secondary intention or be sutured with an absorbable suture. Drains are generally not used where a transoral approach is used.

Retropharyngeal infections with small abscesses may be aspirated transorally with a needle in a patient able to tolerate the procedure. Larger abscesses require incision and drainage via a transcervical and/or transoral approach.

In transcervical approaches, the location of the incision can be planned to occur both where the best view of the anatomy is obtainable and to be most cosmetically acceptable, depending on which area is infected.

A preauricular parotid incision is beneficial in parotid space and temporal space infections.

Horizontal neck incisions allow access to the parapharyngeal, masticator, pterygoid, prevertebral, submandibular, retropharyngeal, lateral neck, and carotid spaces.

A horizontal submental incision can be made to access the floor of the mouth and the bilateral submandibular spaces.

All pus and fluid draining from infections of the face and deep neck area should be sent to microbiology for culture. In multilocular abscesses, in particular, the whole cavity should be opened by blunt finger dissection to clear out any purulent material [61]. The cavity should be washed repeatedly with isothermal normal saline. A Penrose drain is placed and attached to the skin of the neck. The incision is loosely closed with a 4-0 nylon suture.

Endoscopic methods enjoy several key advantages over external approaches, notably a shorter operation time, absence of cervical scarring, and minimal occurrence of complications. There are case histories in the literature where transnasal endoscopic drainage has been used for a retropharyngeal abscess, and transoral endoscopic drainage has been employed in a case of parapharyngeal abscess [62, 63].

22.8 Complications

All infections that are inadequately treated, diagnosed, or treated late, and thus able to spread to other cavities, entail the risk of complications. The complications that may arise in facial and deep cervical infections produce morbidity and risk mortality, whether during pregnancy and the postpartum period in a woman or at other times in both sexes. However, for pregnant women, early diagnosis and aggressive treatment of complications are crucial to protect the health of both mother and fetus. A multidisciplinary approach should be adopted. Potentially life-threatening and frequently occurring complications include the following [64, 65]:

- Respiratory distress linked to tracheal compression
- Airway obstruction
- Aspiration
- Sepsis, septic shock, and septic embolism
- Necrotizing fasciitis
- Vascular complications: jugular vein thrombosis, Lemierre's syndrome (LS), cavernous sinus thrombosis, and carotid artery pseudoaneurysm or rupture
- Mandibular or cervical osteomyelitis
- Mediastinitis (descending necrotizing mediastinitis)
- Brain abscess
- Cranial nerve paralysis
- Disseminated intravascular coagulation (DIC)
- Spontaneous abortion and intrauterine death

In deep neck infections, complications must be rapidly identified and diagnosed, and emergency treatments, including airway management, rapid surgical drainage, and administration of broad-spectrum antibiotics, are initiated without delay. If anticoagulant agents are required, low-molecular-weight heparin (LMWH) is the agent of choice for pregnant and puerperal patients. LMWH does not cross the placenta, nor does it carry a risk of fetal bleeding or teratogenicity [66].

References

1. Weed HG, Forest LA. Deep neck infection. In: Cummings CW, Flint PW, Harker LA, et al., editors. Otolaryngology: head and neck surgery. 4th ed. Philadelphia, PA: Mosby Elsevier; 2005. p. 2515–24.

2. Olvier ER, Gillespie MB. Deep neck infections. In: Flint PW, Haughey BH, et al., editors. Cummings otolaryngology head and neck surgery. Philadelphia, PA: Mosby Elsevier; 2010. p. 201–9.

3. Huang TT, Liu TC, Chen PR. Deep neck infection: analyssis of 185 cases. Head Neck. 2004;26:853–60.

4. López NJ, Smith PC, Gutierrez J. Periodontal therapy may reduce the risk of preterm low birth weight in women with periodontal disease: a randomized controlled trial. J Periodontol. 2002;73:911–24.

5. Jarjoura K, Devine PC, Perez-Delboy A, Herrera-Abreu M, D'Alton M, Papapanou PN. Markers of periodontal infection and preterm birth. Am J Obstet Gynecol. 2005;192:513–9.

6. Vieira F, Allen SM, Stocks RMS, Thompson JW. Deep neck infection. Otolaryngol Clin N Am. 2008;41:459–83.

7. Lin YY, Hsu CH, Lee JC, et al. Head and neck cancers manifested as deep neck infection. Eur Arch Otorhinolaryngol. 2012;269:585–90.

8. Todd JK. Bacteriology and clinical relevance of nasopharyngeal and oropharyngeal cultures. Pediatr Infect Dis. 1984;3:159.

9. Marsh PD, Martin MV. Oral microbiology. 5th ed. Edinburgh, UK: Churchill Livingston; 2009.

10. Boscolo-Rizzo P, Stellin M, Muzzi E, et al. Deep neck infections: a study of 365 cases highlighting recommendations for management and treatment. Eur Arch Otorhinolaryngol. 2012;269:1241–9.

11. Brook I. Current management of upper respiratory tract and head and neck infections. Eur Arch Otorhinolaryngol. 2009;266:315.

12. Stephenson MF, Mfuna L, Dowd SE, et al. Molecular characterization of the polymicrobial flora in chronic rhinosinusitis. J Otolaryngol Head Neck Surg. 2010;39:182.

13. Hull MW, Chow AW. An approach to Oral infections and their management. Curr Infect Dis Rep. 2005;7:17.

14. Laulajainen Hongisto A, Aarnisalo AA, Lempinen L, et al. Otogenic intracranial abscesses, our experience over the last four decades. J Int Adv Otol. 2017;13:40.

15. Huang TT, Tseng FY, Yeh TH, et al. Factors affecting the bacteriology of deep neck infection: a retrospective study of 128 patients. Acta Otolaryngol. 2006;126:396.

16. Lin HT, Tsai CS, Chen YL, Liang JG. Influence of diabetes mellitus on deep neck infection. J Laryngol Otol. 2006;120:650.

17. Jackson KA, Bohm MK, Brooks JT, et al. Invasive methicillin resistant Staphylococcus aureus infections among persons who inject drugs—six sites, 2005–2016. MMWR Morb Mortal Wkly Rep. 2018;67:625.

18. Gordon RJ, Lowy FD. Bacterial infections in drug users. N Engl J Med. 2005;353:1945.

19. Issa K, Diebo BG, Faloon M, et al. The epidemiology of vertebral osteomyelitis in the United States from 1998 to 2013. Clin Spine Surg. 2018;31:E102.

20. Sutcliffe P, Lasrado S. Anatomy, head and neck, deep cervical neck fascia. StatPearls Publishing; 2020.

21. Chandra S, Tripathi A, Mishra S, Amzarul M. Physiological changes in hematological parameters during pregnancy. Indian J Hematol Blood Transfus. 2012;28(3):144–6.

22. Dennen F, Ocaña J, Karasik S, Egan L, Paredes N, Flisser A, et al. Comparison of hemodynamic, biochemical and hematological parameters of healthy pregnant women in the third trimester of pregnancy and the active labor phase. BMC Pregnancy Childbirth. 2011;11:33.

23. Turner M, Aziz SR. Management of the pregnant oral and maxillofacial patient. J Oral Maxillofac Surg. 2002;60:1479–88.

24. Valera MC, Parant O, Vayssiere C, Arnal JF, Payrastre B. Physiological and pathologic changes of platelets in pregnancy. Platelets. 2010;21(8):587–95.

25. Hurley MC, Heran MK. Imaging studies for head and neck infections. Infect Dis Clin N Am. 2007;21:305.

26. Agrawal NK. Maternal-fetal thyroid interactions. In: Thyroid hormone. Chapter 5. London: InTech Open Access Publisher; 2012. p. 125–56.

27. Tremblay E, Thérasse E, Thomassin-Naggara I, et al. Quality initiatives: guidelines for use of medical imaging during pregnancy and lactation. Radiographics. 2012;32(3):897–911. https://doi.org/10.1148/rg.323115120.
28. Wang PI, Chong ST, Kielar AZ, et al. Imaging of pregnant and lactating patients: part 1, evidence-based review and recommendations. AJR Am J Roentgenol. 2012;198(4):778–84. https://doi.org/10.2214/AJR.11.7405.
29. Giglio JA, Lanni SM, Laskin DM, Giglio NW. Oral health care for the pregnant patient. J Can Dent Assoc. 2009;75:43–8.
30. Nickoloff E, Alderson P. Radiation exposure to patients from CT: reality, public perception, and policy. AJR Am J Roentgenol. 2001;177:285–7.
31. Czeizel AE, Pataki T, Rockenbauer M. Reproductive outcome after exposure to surgery under anesthesia during pregnancy. Arch Gynecol Obstet. 1998;261:193–9.
32. Jenkins A, Wong DT, Correa R. Management choices for the difficult airway by anaesthesiologists in Canada. Can J Anesth. 2002;49:850–6.
33. Karkos PD, Leong SC, Beer H, et al. Challenging airways in deep neck space infections. Am J Otolaryngol. 2007;28:415–8.
34. Jouppila R, Jouppila P, Hollmen A. Laryngeal oedema as an obstetric anaesthesia complication: case reports. Acta Anaesthesiol Scand. 1980;24:97–8.
35. Kuczkowski KM, Reisner LS, Benumof JL. Airway problems and new solutions for the obstetric patient. J Clin Anesth. 2013;15:552–63.
36. Norwitz ER, Robinson JN, Malone FD. Pregnancy-induced physiologic alterations. In: Dildy GA, Belfort MA, Saade GR, et al., editors. Critical care obstetrics. 4th ed. Malden, MA: Blackwell Science; 2004. p. 19–42.
37. Seager SJ, Macdonald R. Laryngeal oedema and pre-eclampsia. Anaesthesia. 1980;35:360–2.
38. Brimacombe J. Acute pharyngolaryngeal oedema and pre-eclamptic toxaemia. Anaesth Intensive Care. 1992;20:97–8.
39. Brock-Utne JG, Downing JW, Seedat F. Laryngeal oedema associated with pre-eclamptic toxaemia. Anaesthesia. 1977;32:556–8.
40. Kallen B, Rydhstraem H, Aberg A. Congenital malformations after the use of inhaled budesonide in early pregnancy. Obstet Gynecol. 1999;93:392–5.
41. McGuire E. Sudden loss of milk supply following high-dose triamcinolone (Kenacort) injection. Breastfeed Rev. 2012;20:32–4.
42. Osborn TM, Assael LA, Bell RB. Deep space neck infection: principles of surgical management. Oral Maxillofacial Surg Clin N Am. 2008;20:353–65.
43. Cho SY, Woo JH, Kim YJ, Chun EH, Han JI, Kim DY, Baik HJ, Chung RK. Airway management in patients with deep neck infections a retrospective analysis. Medicine (Baltimore). 2016;95(27):e4125.
44. Munnur U, Boisblanc B, Suresh M. Airway problems in pregnancy. Crit Care Med. 2005;33(10)
45. McGuire G, El-Beheiry H. Complete upper airway obstruction during awake fibreoptic intubation in patients with unstable cervical spine fractures. Can J Anaesth. 1999;46:176–8.
46. Shaw IC, Welchew EA, Harrison BJ, et al. Complete airway obstruction during awake fibreoptic intubation. Anaesthesia. 1997;52:582–5.
47. Niforopoulou P, Pantazopoulos I, Demestiha T, et al. Video-laryngoscopes in the adult airway management: a topical review of the literature. Acta Anaesthesiol Scand. 2010;54:1050–61.
48. Authority EFS. Scientific opinion on dietary reference values for water. EFSA J. 2010;8(3)
49. Turner M, Aziz SR. Management of the pregnant oral and maxillofacial surgery patient. J Oral Maxillofac Surg. 2002;60:1479–88.
50. Tan PC, Norazilah MJ, Omar SZ. Dextrose saline compared with normal saline rehydration of hyperemesis gravidarum: a randomized controlled trial. Obstet Gynecol. 2013;121(2 Pt 1):291–8.
51. Nelson-Piercy C. Treatment of nausea and vomiting in pregnancy: when should it be treated and what can be safely taken? Drug Saf. 1998;19:155–64.
52. Huang TT, Tseng FY, Yeh TH, Hsu CJ, Chen YS. Factors affecting the bacteriology of deep neck infections: a retrospective study of 128 patients. Acta Otolaryngol. 2006;126:396–401.

53. Naseem M, Khurshid Z, Khan HA, Niazi F, Zohaib S, Zofar MS. Oral health challenges in pregnant women: recommendations for dental care professionals. Saudi J Dental Res. 2016;7:138–46.
54. Wong DK, Brown C, Mills N, et al. To drain or not to drain—management of pediatric deep neck abscesses: a case-control study. Int J Pediatr Otorhinolaryngol. 2012;76:1810–3.
55. UK Medicines Information. Can opioids be used for pain relief during pregnancy? UKMi; 2018. Accessed 2018 Oct 17.
56. Antonucci R, Zaffanello M, Puxeddu E, Porcella A, Cuzzolin L, Pilloni MD, et al. Use of non-steroidal anti-inflammatory drugs in pregnancy: impact on the fetus and newborn. Curr Drug Metab. 2012;13:474–90.
57. Butler DC, Heller MM, Murase JE. Safety of dermatologic medications in pregnancy and lactation. J Am Acad Dermatol. 2014;70:417.e1–417.e10.
58. Duvekot JJ, Peeters LL. Maternal cardiovascular hemodynamic adaptation to pregnancy. Obstet Gynecol Surv. 1994;49(Suppl):S1–14.
59. Toshima M. Deep neck infection. Antibiot Chemother. 2000;16:1715–20.
60. Moore HB, Juarez-Colunga E, Bronsert M, et al. Effect of pregnancy on adverse outcomes after general surgery. JAMA Surg. 2015;150:637–43.
61. Sethi DS, Stanley RE. Parapharyngeal abscesses. J Laryngol Otol. 1991;105:1025–30.
62. Nagy M, Pizzuto M, Backstrom J, Brodsky L. Deep neck infections in children: a new approach to diagnosis and treatment. Laryngoscope. 1997;107:1627–34.
63. Nicolai P, Lombardi D, Berlucchi M, Farina D, Zanetti D. Drainage of retro-parapharyngeal abscess: an additional indication for endoscopic sinus surgery. Eur Arch Otorhinolaryngol. 2005;262:722–30.
64. Vieira F, Allen SM, Stocks RSM, Thompson JW. Deep neck infections. Otolaryngol Clin N Am. 2008;12:459–83.
65. Wills PI, Vernon RP. Complications of space infections of the head and neck. Laryngoscope. 1981;91:1129–36.
66. Bates SM. Treatment and prophylaxis of venous thromboembolism during pregnancy. Thromb Res. 2003;108:97–106.

Influenza Occurring in Pregnant Women

23

Dilara Tütüncü Yavuz, İbrahim Çukurova,
and Codrut Sarafoleanu

23.1 Influenza Virus

Influenza is a respiratory infection caused by influenza viruses. The influenza is quite widespread infection for the human race from the old times. The word "influenza" was originated from the Italian language, meaning "influence." Since the disease caused by influenza virus infection occurs more often in winter seasons, it was thought in the ancient world to be caused by the influence of astrological movements [1]. Influenza virus continues to cause yearly seasonal epidemics worldwide and periodically pandemics.

Influenza virus is well documented with its structural parts. Influenza is a single-stranded RNA virus in the Orthomyxoviridae family. Three types—A, B, and C—have been identified, but only types A and B cause widespread outbreaks [2]. Among the three types, influenza A viruses are clinically the most important pathogens and have been responsible for severe epidemics in humans. Influenza A viruses are further classified into subtypes based on antigenic differences between the hemagglutinin and neuraminidase surface glycoproteins [3]. The virus usually causes a respiratory disease in humans. The hemagglutinin glycoprotein on the surface of the

D. T. Yavuz (✉)
Department of Otorhinolaryngology, Istanbul Sisli Hamidiye Etfal Training and Research Hospital, Istanbul, Turkey
e-mail: dilarattnc@yahoo.com.tr

İ. Çukurova
Section of Otorhinolaryngology, Tepecik Training and Research Hospital, İzmir Faculty of Medicine, University of Health Sciences, İzmir, Turkey
e-mail: Cukurova57@gmail.com

C. Sarafoleanu
ENT&HNS Department, University of Medicine and Pharmacy "Carol Davila", Sfanta Maria Clinical Hospital, Bucharest, Romania
e-mail: csarafoleanu@gmail.com

C. Cingi et al. (eds.), *ENT Diseases: Diagnosis and Treatment during Pregnancy and Lactation*, https://doi.org/10.1007/978-3-031-05303-0_23

virus facilitates attachment to respiratory epithelial cells by binding to sialic acid receptors. The neuraminidase glycoprotein facilitates the release of progeny virions by catalyzing the cleavage of glycosidic linkages to sialic acid (neuraminic acid). Subsequently, the virus particle is taken up via endocytosis [4].

The disease is transmitted through an air-borne route from respiratory droplets. Contaminated hands are most responsible for the transmission. The virus can survive for 8–48 h on surfaces, depending on environmental factors. Virus invades the respiratory epithelium, initially in the tracheobronchial tree but later throughout the whole respiratory tract. The infection in humans is normally limited to the respiratory tract. Viral shedding begins after around 1 day and peaks before the onset of symptoms. Adults can transmit the virus to healthy individuals for 5 days and transmission period for pediatric population can last for 10 days. Typical symptoms include fever, myalgia, headache, and fatigue, peaking 2–3 days after infection and resolving within 1–2 weeks. Coughing and overall weakness can persist for up to 2 weeks. If the virus spreads from the bronchiolar tract to the alveoli, viral pneumonia and interstitial pneumonitis with mononuclear and hemorrhage infiltration and finally lysis of the interalveolar space are all possible [5]. The replication of the virus leads to the lysis of the epithelial cells and enhanced mucus production, causing runny nose and cough. Also, inflammation and edema at the replication site due to cytokines released contribute to the disease. This can lead to fever and related symptoms. Innate immunity as well as the adaptive immune system will normally restrict virus propagation. Serious illness occurs in a minority of cases, often due to secondary bacterial infections or exacerbation of cardiovascular and respiratory illness. Although most people recover within a week without requiring medical attention, influenza can lead to severe illness, hospitalization, and death, especially in elder adults, infants, pregnant women, overweight individuals, and individuals with chronic medical conditions (Fig. 23.1).

23.2 Influenza in Pregnancy

Pregnant women are considered vulnerable to serious influenza disease and related complications, on the basis of evidence documenting excess influenza-related mortality in pregnant women during historical and recent pandemics [6]. The impact of pandemic influenza on pregnant women and their unborn children was first examined systematically during the 1889 and more substantially during the 1918 pandemics. The 1918 "Spanish flu" killed 675,000 persons in the United States, with an overall case fatality rate of 1–2%. Numerous studies indicated that pregnant women were at greatly elevated risk of severe disease and death, with overall fatality rates calculated to be as high as 27%, and as high as 50% or higher in pregnant women who developed secondary bacterial pneumonia. The 1957 and 1968 influenza pandemics caused significantly lower overall mortality, with 70,000 and 30,000 US deaths in the first year, respectively, but pregnant women again accounted for significant and disproportionate numbers of deaths [7].

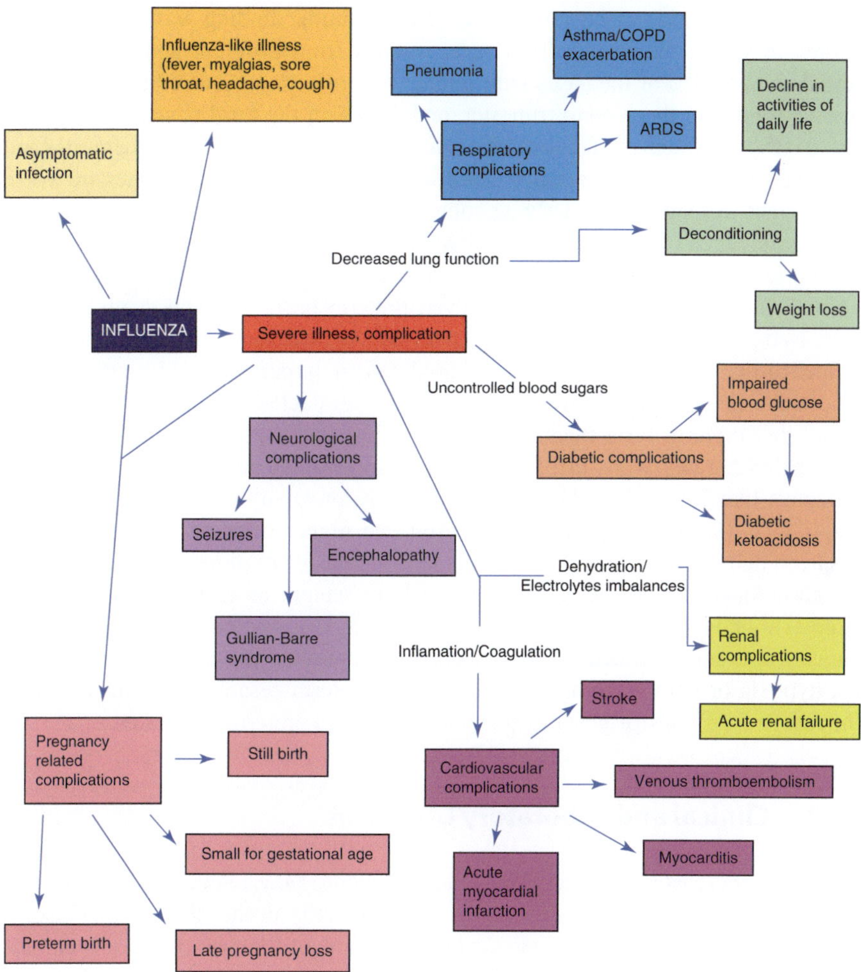

Fig. 23.1 The course of influenza infection and pregnancy-related complications

Both seasonal and pandemic influenza have a significant impact on the fetus as well as the mother. In recent years of seasonal influenza virus circulation, infection during pregnancy has been associated with an approximately fivefold increase in perinatal mortality, including miscarriages, stillbirths, and early neonatal diseases and death [8, 9]. Pregnant women appear to be at an increased risk of influenza virus infection or influenza-like illness, especially during the third trimester of pregnancy [10]. Studies found that pregnant women with influenza have a higher risk of hospitalization than nonpregnant same-aged patients with influenza [11]. Severity of clinical course in influenza differs between trimesters. Pregnant women with influenza infection present with severe disease later in pregnancy, women presenting in the second trimester have a 1.2-fold increase, and women in the third trimester have

2.3-fold higher odds of hospitalization [12]. A similar finding was observed in a review in which the results from seven studies from different geographic areas revealed that 9.1% of the cases with influenza A infection occurred in the first trimester, 29.8% in the second trimester, and 47.0% in the third trimester [13]. The risk of severe influenza infection and pneumonia is highest in the third trimester and during the early postpartum period (2 weeks postdelivery) [14]. Outcomes are worse in pregnant women with underlying comorbidities, including asthma [15, 16].

The influence of influenza virus infection on pregnancy outcome appears to be related to the severity of maternal infection. In outpatients, pregnancy outcome is normal. In hospitalized patients, however, preterm birth and fetal death rates are increased. These effects are in line with previous reports on the influence of influenza-like illness. In a population-based and an outpatient study, no differences in pregnancy outcome between infected and uninfected pregnant women were found, but preterm birth rates, the number of small-for-gestational age neonates, and stillbirth rates were increased in pregnant women hospitalized because of influenza-like illness [17]. Also, in another study, pregnant women hospitalized for respiratory illness during influenza season had higher odds of preterm delivery, cesarean delivery, and fetal distress, and their infants were more likely to be small-for-gestational age and have lower mean birth weight as compared to pregnant women not hospitalized for respiratory illness [18, 19]. Another study found that in patients with severe infection, preterm cesarean sections were carried out for maternal hypoxia or hemodynamic instability [20]. Preterm cesarean sections could be the reason for small-for-gestational age neonates and preterm birth rates.

23.3 Clinical and Laboratory Diagnosis

The influenza season runs every year from October to May, but the exact timing and duration can vary. Transmission occurs predominantly during the winter seasons. However, pandemic influenza can occur at any time of the year. If there is an outbreak of influenza that is announced by the health authority and the patient's anamnesis includes a contact history with an infected patient, the diagnosis can be decided upon the anamnesis easily. Even if the patient has got an influenza vaccine for the season, this does not rule out the influenza virus infection.

The diagnosis of influenza infection can be based on clinical symptoms (influenza-like illness) or confirmed infection. Clinical manifestations of influenza infection during pregnancy are similar to those in the nonpregnant patient and include generalized fever, myalgias, sore throat, headache, and cough [21] (Table 23.1).

Typically, symptoms peak 2–3 days after infection and resolve within 1–2 weeks. Coughing and overall weakness can persist for up to 2 weeks.

On physical examination, the pharynx may be erythematous and inflamed and auscultation of the lungs may demonstrate rales and rhonchi, especially in the setting of superimposed pneumonia [22]. The standardized definition of influenza-like illness of the Centers for Disease Control and Prevention (CDC) is widely used for

Table 23.1 Influenza signs and symptoms in confirmed influenza

Sign	Frequency of symptoms (%)
Fever	97
Cough	94
Headache	47
Sore throat	35
Myalgias	35

the clinical diagnosis of influenza: the presence of fever (>37.8 °C) and sore throat or dry cough occurring during the flu season in the absence of other explanatory causes such as pyelonephritis or other infections [23].

Mostly, the diagnosis of influenza infection can be made clinically. The diagnostic tests are usually unnecessary. But if it is necessary, the diagnosis can also be confirmed by identification of the virus from respiratory secretions through a nasopharyngeal or oropharyngeal swab. Although the sensitivity of influenza virus detection confirmed via culture and real-time reverse transcription-polymerase chain reaction assay is reported to be as high as 99% by the CDC, the clinical utility of these tests is limited due to the time (up to 1 week) required to obtain results. Serology-based rapid influenza diagnostic tests are available for immediate clinical use (results available within 1 h or less); however, the overall sensitivity is much lower (40–69% for detection of 2009 novel A H1N1 virus and 60–80% for seasonal A H1N1) [24]. If the diagnosis is possible influenza based on the anamnesis and clinical examination, even there is a negative diagnostic test result, the test result is not significant for the final decision. Therefore, initiation of antiviral therapy should not be withheld based on a negative rapid test for influenza as this does not rule out influenza infection and can delay needed treatment in susceptible groups.

Other ancillary testing methods such as complete blood count and chest X-ray are usually normal except in the setting of complications such as bacterial superinfection, when leukocytosis and radiological signs of pneumonia may be present [21, 25].

23.4 Complications

Influenza infection is usually self-limiting upper respiratory tract infection, but sometimes very aggressive clinical course can be observed. Different systemic complications can be observed in influenza infection. The disease can decrease lung function and cause pneumonia, asthma\COPD attack, and acute respiratory distress syndrome (ARDS). Because of respiratory complications, the patient can experience fatigue, lose weight, and become tired of daily life activities. The influenza infection can cause dehydration and electrolyte imbalances and so it can progress with renal complications such as acute renal failure. The virus can stimulate the inflammation\coagulation system, and infection can complicate with cardiovascular problems such as stroke, venous thromboembolism, and acute myocardial infarction. The virus itself or the immune system can affect the cardiac muscle directly and can cause myocarditis complication. It can also cause neurological complications like seizures, Guillain–Barré syndrome, or encephalopathy. If the patient already has uncontrolled blood sugar, diabetic complications can be observed (Fig. 23.1).

The most common complication of influenza infection is lower respiratory tract infection (pneumonia), either from primary infection with influenza or due to bacterial superinfection. Other complications include the development of acute respiratory distress syndrome, respiratory failure, ICU admission, and death [26].

In the last century, increased influenza risk for pregnant women has been reported in multiple clinical and epidemiological studies undertaken during pandemic years as well as during seasonal influenza epidemics. The 2009 pandemic served as a strong reminder that influenza-induced disease can have a great impact on certain at-risk populations, and those pregnant women are one such important population. The increased risk of fatal and severe disease in these women was appreciated more than 500 years ago, and during the last century, pregnant women and their newborns have continued to be greatly affected by both seasonal and pandemic influenza [7]. Pregnant women can have all systemic complications explained above; also, these complications can progress with pregnancy-related complications. A pregnant patient can have pregnancy-related influenza complications even though she does not have any other systemic complications.

Pregnancy-related complications of influenza are preterm birth, small-for-gestational age, late pregnancy loss, and stillbirth.

23.5 Pregnancy-Related Complications

The antenatal influenza can affect both birth and perinatal outcomes. It has been hypothesized to result in inflammatory responses or immune dysregulation that might increase the risk for spontaneous abortion, stillbirth, and preterm birth and alter the placental transfer of nutrients and cytokines to the developing fetus, which might affect fetal growth [27]. According to some studies, influenza infection during pregnancy has been associated with an approximately fivefold increase in perinatal mortality, including miscarriages, stillbirths, and early neonatal diseases and death [9].

Although sequelae from infection with some viral pathogens in pregnancy are well understood (e.g., congenital cytomegalovirus, rubella, varicella), potential pathogenic effects of influenza viruses on the fetus are not. As the influenza virus is rarely transmitted across the placenta, influenza virus infection is more likely to be associated with adverse birth outcomes through other mechanisms such as maternal fever and inflammation. Immunological responses, such as elevated proinflammatory cytokine levels, can also influence placental function and are recognized as an important pathway to preterm birth [6, 28, 29]. Part of this risk seems to have resulted from a nearly doubling of Cesarean section deliveries in influenza-infected mothers, in many cases being performed on an emergent basis due to worsening maternal status. Such premature births due to spontaneous delivery or Cesarean section were presumably associated with maternal infection and not infection of the fetus [30].

Birth defects have not yet been sufficiently studied. However, in a meta-analysis, it is demonstrated a medium to strong association between first-trimester influenza exposure and congenital abnormalities such as neural tube defects, anencephaly, encephalocele, spina bifida, and hydrocephaly [31].

23.6 Preterm Birth

In a review of influenza in pregnancy, among women with influenza disease, the range of preterm birth risks extended from 4.0 to 25.8% [6]. Two studies that analyzed severe 2009 pH1N1 influenza disease reported a preterm birth risk of 24% among women with influenza [9, 32]. Three other 2009 pH1N1 studies based on a wider range of illness severity reported no significantly elevated risk of preterm birth [33–35]. In the two highest-quality studies from seasonal epidemic years, no association was observed between influenza and preterm birth, whether based on hospitalization for influenza disease or broader ascertainment criteria [19, 35]. About preterm birth and maternal influenza infection, firm conclusions are difficult to draw, although several studies suggest that severe maternal disease due to 2009 pH1N1 influenza is associated with preterm birth. But there is no evidence for an association with mild-to-moderate 2009 pH1N1 influenza, or with seasonal influenza of any severity. According to a study, women hospitalized with 2009 pH1N1 influenza illness have a significantly increased risk of preterm delivery if they develop secondary pneumonia compared with those who do not develop pneumonia (71 versus 27%) [9].

23.7 Small-for-Gestational Age

Small-for-gestational age (SGA) birth is sex-specific birthweight lower than <tenth percentile [33]. Baseline risks of SGA birth range from 3.9 to 14.1% in women with no influenza disease during pregnancy and from 2.8 to 15.3% among women who had influenza disease [19, 36, 37]. Some studies found relationships with influenza infection and SGA [19]. But some others did not identify any significant increase in the risk of SGA for either influenza or non-influenza hospitalizations diagnosed in any trimester of pregnancy [38]. Studying the relationship between maternal influenza and perinatal outcomes is challenging. Even though there are contrary results for SGA, SGA should always be considered as a possible complication of influenza.

23.8 Stillbirth

Stillbirth is defined as fetal death after 20 weeks' gestation among all births, and perinatal mortality includes stillbirths and neonatal deaths before 7 days of age [39]. There are many studies about the relationship of stillbirth with antenatal influenza in the literature. Findings from individual-level epidemiologic studies are inconsistent, and many studies are limited by an inadequate number of events (particularly for fetal death) and methodological weaknesses. Considering the multifactorial etiology of fetal death, an association may not be detectable in a time-series analysis at the population level.

A study found that influenza A virus infection is associated with nearly 2.4 times more stillbirths than the control [40]. Secondary pneumonia was also identified as a contributing factor to excess fetal deaths during the influenza pandemic of 1918–1919 [41].

Drawing any overall conclusions on the risk of fetal death following maternal influenza is challenging due to insufficient mortality events in most studies and inconsistent study definitions of fetal death. Two highest-quality studies reported significantly increased risks of fetal death following maternal 2009 pH1N1 influenza illness, but high-quality evidence from seasonal influenza time periods is lacking. Although a small subgroup of higher-quality studies found that severe pH1N1 influenza disease during pregnancy increased the risk of fetal death, there was little evidence that mild 2009 pH1N1 influenza, seasonal influenza disease of any severity, or subclinical infection in pregnant women was associated with the outcomes [6].

23.9 Pathophysiologic Mechanisms Underlying Increased Influenza Risk to Pregnant Women

Influenza virus infection is a common and usually self-limiting infection. In specific populations like pregnant women, however, complications of the disease appear to be more prevalent. Significant anatomic and physiologic changes during normal pregnancy include changes that increase the risk of respiratory failure and complicate the treatment of respiratory illness. These changes include nasal mucosal edema, elevation of the diaphragm to accommodate the uterus, increased respiratory rate, increased intra-abdominal pressure, decreased chest compliance, and as a consequence, increased risk of aspiration. Decreased functional residual capacity due to a greater expiratory volume can lead to alveolar collapse. Because increased tidal volume is necessary to meet increased oxygenation needs, minute ventilation is increased, leading to falling arterial CO_2 partial pressure and compensated metabolic acidosis. These cardiopulmonary changes and the increased respiratory rate needed to compensate for the metabolic acidosis make pregnant women more susceptible to respiratory compromise, predispose to the development of pulmonary edema, and make such complications more difficult to treat [42].

Pregnancy has been considered an immunomodulating and even an immunosuppressive state. The effect of immunomodulatory changes of pregnancy upon influenza infection is unclear, but some studies suggest effects on disease progression [43]. During pregnancy, changes in maternal immunity are required to prevent the fetus from being rejected by the mother's immune system [44]. The placenta produces progesterone, prostaglandin E2, and interleukins (IL) 4 and 10, which inhibit the T helper (Th) 1 response of maternal immune defense. In addition, both CD4+ and CD8+ T cells in the peripheral blood downregulate Th1 cytokines (e.g., IFN-gamma and IL-2) and upregulate Th2 cytokines (e.g., IL-4). Thus, the maternal immune system shifts toward Th2-type immunity [45].

Immune changes of pregnancy might exacerbate influenza disease but may not fully explain the increased risk of death in influenza-infected pregnant women. Cellular immune responses following influenza virus infection lead to increased pulmonary inflammation, potentially accounting for the increased morbidity and mortality in this patient population. Because physiologic and anatomic risk factors for severe influenza in pregnancy are poorly understood, this is still an important research topic. Despite vulnerability to influenza, pregnancy confers no greater risk than the risk associated with conditions such as cardiorespiratory disease, obesity, or advanced age [46].

23.10 Prevention and Treatment of Influenza in Pregnancy

Prevention strategies for influenza infection in pregnant women begin with limiting the exposure of the virus. This includes hand washing, respiratory hygiene, cough etiquette, and social distancing. Importance of influenza infection in pregnancy and droplet precautions should be introduced to all pregnant women during the first obstetric visit.

23.10.1 Vaccination

Influenza vaccination is the most effective way to prevent influenza virus infection and hence severe outcomes. Although the influenza vaccine is classified as a category C agent in pregnancy, the positive safety profile has led to recommendations of the CDC, American College of Obstetrics and Gynecology (ACOG), and WHO that all pregnant women should be vaccinated with seasonal inactivated influenza vaccine—trivalent influenza vaccine (TIV). The live attenuated influenza vaccine is not recommended for use in pregnant women but can be used postpartum. Data from the Vaccine Adverse Event Reporting System (VAERS) on over two million vaccinated pregnant women detected few or no adverse effects on fetuses or infants whose mothers received influenza vaccine during pregnancy, the finding supported by evidence from numerous case–control studies [47–50].

For neonates, effects of maternal influenza vaccination during pregnancy are evident. It prevents neonatal morbidity and hospitalization from influenza virus infection in the first 6 months of life [51–53]. This is probably due to the transplacental passage of protective maternal antibodies against the influenza virus. Neonatal/cord blood levels of these antibodies are at approximately the same level as in maternal blood [51, 54, 55]. Also, vaccination results in the presence of influenza-specific immunoglobulin A levels in breast milk [56].

Despite evidence of the significantly increased morbidity and mortality from influenza infection during pregnancy and good safety and efficacy data of influenza vaccination, vaccine uptake in this at-risk population remains universally poor, including in the late gestational period [57]. During the 2014/2015 influenza season, vaccine uptake in pregnant women was 44.1–56.1% in the UK (England, Scotland, Wales, and Northern Ireland) and 50.3% in the USA [58, 59]. An Australian study revealed that one-third of general practitioners did not believe influenza virus infection to be a significant risk to mother or baby, and more than half had significant concerns about the safety of influenza vaccination during pregnancy [60]. Thus, worldwide influenza vaccination during pregnancy is still at low rates.

Contrary to beliefs, according to some research, vaccination is safe during all stages of pregnancy, including the first trimester [61, 62]. No significant long-term adverse effects (teratogenic, carcinogenic, or neurologic) have been shown in pregnant women receiving the influenza vaccine during the first trimester and would not be expected from an inactivated vaccine. In addition, there have been no observed associations between inactivated influenza vaccination and gestational diabetes, gestational hypertension, preeclampsia/eclampsia, or chorioamnionitis in vaccinated women [63, 64].

23.10.2 Nonspecific Treatment

Both nonpharmaceutical and pharmaceutical interventions can be used for nonspecific treatment in pregnancy. The management of influenza infection in pregnancy is similar to that in the nonpregnant general population. Mostly, increasing fluid intake is enough, and acetaminophen can be used to control fever. The disease usually resolves itself in 10 days.

Respiratory support may be necessary in the presence of inadequate oxygenation, and prompt evaluation for superimposed pneumonia should be undertaken with hospitalization and initiation of broad-spectrum antibiotic coverage against common bacteria, including *Staphylococcus aureus*, *Streptococcus pneumonia*, and *Haemophilus influenza*.

23.10.3 Antiviral Treatment

No randomized controlled trials on the benefits and/or risks of treatment of pregnant women with antiviral medication are found in the literature. Neuraminidase inhibitors (oseltamivir and zanamivir) have become the current antivirals of choice for influenza. These influenza antiviral agents are classified as category C drugs in pregnancy, meaning that no clinical studies have been performed in pregnant women and that animal studies either have not been carried out or have shown an adverse fetal effect in at least one species [65].

Table 23.2 Dosage of oseltamivir

Oseltamivir	Dosage	Duration
Treatment	75 mg, twice daily	5 days
Chemoprophylaxis	75 mg, daily	10 days

Only limited data exist on the pharmacokinetics of oseltamivir in pregnant women. Retrospective studies generally have found a minimal risk to mother and fetus, although low levels of oseltamivir drug metabolites are transferred transplacentally [66, 67]. Safety reports on the outcome of pregnancy after oseltamivir use during pregnancy are reassuring. Pregnancy outcomes were reported for approximately 2500 pregnant women who used oseltamivir during pregnancy. There was no increased risk of congenital malformations or other adverse pregnancy outcomes for both the mother and neonate [17]. These data suggest that current antivirals are likely to be safe in pregnancy, but further study is needed.

Using neuraminidase inhibitors for prophylaxis in pregnancy is also uncertain. Despite incomplete data, recommendations for post-exposure prophylaxis and early initiation of treatment of pregnant women suspected of influenza infection are important to reduce morbidity and mortality for pregnant women that have additional comorbidities. According to studies, it is recommended that, in women who are pregnant or 2 weeks postpartum highly suspected to have influenza virus infection, antiviral therapy should be commenced as soon as possible after the onset of symptoms and should not be delayed until test results are available [68].

The dose of antiviral therapy for the treatment of influenza during pregnancy consists of oseltamivir 75 mg twice daily for 5 days. Dosing for chemoprophylaxis consists of oseltamivir 75 mg once daily for 10 days [26] (Table 23.2).

Early initiation of treatment is associated with reduced illness duration, severity, mortality, need for antibiotics, and hospitalization [14, 16]. Available data suggest that early initiation of antiviral treatment (within 2 days of symptom onset) was associated with an 84% reduction in the odds of admission to an intensive care unit during the 2009 pandemic. Similarly, another study revealed that significantly fewer pregnant women who received oseltamivir treatment within 2 days of symptom onset had severe illness compared with women who initiated treatment 3–4 days or 5 days or more after symptom onset, respectively [21, 69–71].

By taking into consideration influenza morbidity and mortality, antiviral treatment seems relatively safe during pregnancy.

23.11 Conclusion

Influenza in pregnancy is an important public health problem, and it is underappreciated both by the public and healthcare staff. Its potential morbidity and mortality can be decreased by educating women and their physicians about available preventative and therapeutic modalities such as vaccination. Maternal vaccination is safe and effective in preventing influenza infection in both mothers and their infants, and it should be prioritized. It is important that physicians educate their patients regarding the increased severity of influenza infection in pregnancy and describe precautions for prevention of the infection. Influenza vaccination should be offered to every pregnant woman and every woman considering becoming pregnant.

- Studies suggest that pregnant women with influenza have a higher risk of hospitalization than nonpregnant patients with influenza.
- Significant anatomic and physiologic changes during normal pregnancy include changes that increase the risk of respiratory failure and complicate the treatment of respiratory illness.
- The risk of severe influenza infection and pneumonia is highest in the third trimester and during the early postpartum period (2 weeks postdelivery).
- Preterm birth rates, the number of small-for-gestational age neonates, and stillbirth rates are increased in pregnant women hospitalized because of influenza-like illness.
- Early initiation of antiviral therapy is associated with reduced illness duration, severity, mortality, need for antibiotics, and hospitalization.
- Unless contraindicated, all pregnant women irrespective of gestational age should be vaccinated against influenza to prevent influenza virus infection.

References

1. Luo M. Influenza virus entry. Adv Exp Med Biol. 2012;726:201–21. https://doi.org/10.1007/978-1-4614-0980-9_9.
2. Olshaker JS. Influenza. Emerg med Clin north. America. 2003;21:353–61.
3. Nicholson KG, Wood JM, Zambon M. Influenza. Lancet. 2003;362:1733–45.
4. Pleschka S. Overview of Influenza viruses. Curr Top Microbiol Immunol. 2012;1–20 https://doi.org/10.1007/82_2012_272.
5. Wilschut J, McElhaney JE. Influenza. Mosby Elsevier Limited; 2005.
6. Fell DB, Savitz DA, Kramer MS, et al. Maternal influenza and birth outcomes: systematic review of comparative studies. BJOG. 2017;124:48–59.
7. Memoli M, Harvey H, Morens D, et al. Influenza in pregnancy. Influenza Other Respir Viruses. 2013;7(6):1033–9.
8. Michaan N, Amzallag S, Laskov I, et al. Maternal and neonatal out- come of pregnant women infected with H1N1 influenza virus (swine flu). J Matern Fetal Neonatal Med. 2012;25:130–2.
9. Pierce M, Kurinczuk JJ, Spark P, et al. Perinatal outcomes after maternal 2009/H1N1 infection: national cohort study. BMJ. 2011;342:d3214.
10. Dodds L, McNeil SA, Fell DB, et al. Impact of influenza exposure on rates of hospital admissions and physician visits because of respiratory illness among pregnant women. CMAJ. 2007;176:463–8.
11. Mertz D, Geraci J, Winkup J, et al. Pregnancy as a risk factor for severe outcomes from influenza virus infection: a systematic review and meta-analysis of observational studies. Vaccine. 2017;35(4):521–8. https://doi.org/10.1016/j.vaccine.2016.12.012.
12. Lim ML. 2009/H1N1 infection in pregnancy association with adverse perinatal outcomes. Evid Based Nurs. 2012;15(1):11–2.
13. Liu SL, Wang J, Yang XH, et al. Pandemic influenza a (H1N1) 2009 virus in pregnancy. Rev Med Virol. 2013;23(1):3–14.

14. Siston AM, Rasmussen SA, Honein MA, et al. Pandemic 2009 influenza a(H1N1) virus illness among pregnant women in the United States. JAMA. 2010;303(15):1517–25.
15. Hartert TV, Neuzil KM, Shintani AK, et al. Maternal morbidity and perinatal outcomes among pregnant women with respiratory hospitalizations during influenza season. Am J Obstet Gynecol. 2003;189(6):1705–12.
16. Somerville LK, Basile K, Dwyer DE, et al. The impact of influenza virus infection in pregnancy. Future Microbiol. 2018;13:263–74. https://doi.org/10.2217/fmb-2017-0096.
17. Meijer WJ, van Noortwijk AGA, Bruinse HW, et al. Influenza virus infection in pregnancy: a review. Acta Obstet Gynecol Scand. 2015;94:797–819.
18. Martin A, Cox S, Jamieson DJ, et al. Respiratory illness hospitalizations among pregnant women during influenza season, 1998–2008. Matern Child Health J. 2013;17(7):1325–31.
19. McNeil SA, Dodds LA, Fell DB, et al. Effect of respiratory hospitalization during pregnancy on infant outcomes. Am J Obstet Gynecol. 2011;204(6):S54–7.
20. ANZIC Influenza Investigators and Australasian Maternity Outcomes Surveillance System. Critical illness due to 2009 A/H1N1 influenza in pregnant and postpartum women: population based cohort study. BMJ. 2010;340:–c1279.
21. Tita A, Cantu J. Management of Influenza in pregnancy. Am J Perinatol. 2012;30(02):099–104. https://doi.org/10.1055/s-0032-1331033.
22. Rasmussen SA, Jamieson DJ, Bresee JS. Pandemic influenza and pregnant women. Emerg Infect Dis. 2008;14:95–100.
23. Centers for Disease Control and Prevention (CDC). Overview of influenza surveillance in the United States; 2011. http://www.cdc.gov/flu/weekly/overview.htm. Accessed 7 Oct 2011.
24. Centers for Disease Control and Prevention (CDC). Interim guidance for the detection of novel influenza A virus using rapid influenza diagnostic tests; 2009. http://www.cdc.gov/h1n1flu/guidance/rapid_testing.htm. Accessed 10 Aug 2009.
25. Duff P, Sweet R, Edwards R. Maternal and fetal infections. In: Creasy and Resnik's maternal-fetal medicine. 6th ed. Philadelphia, PA: Saunders Elsevier; 2009.
26. Centers for Disease Control and Prevention (CDC). 2011–2012 Influenza antiviral medications: summary for clinicians; 2011. http://www.cdc.gov/flu/professionals/antivirals/summary-clinicians.htm. Accessed 31 Aug 2011.
27. Raj RS, Bonney EA, Phillippe M. Influenza, immune system, and pregnancy. Reprod Sci. 2014;21:1434–51.
28. Steinhoff MC, MacDonald NE. Influenza pandemics—pregnancy, pathogenesis, and perinatal outcomes. JAMA. 2012;308:184–5.
29. Steinhoff MC, Omer SB. A review of fetal and infant protection associated with antenatal influenza immunization. Am J Obstet Gynecol. 2012;207:S21–7.
30. Mosby LG, Rasmussen SA, Jamieson DJ. 2009 pandemic influenza A (H1N1) in pregnancy: a systematic review of the literature. Am J Obstet Gynecol. 2011;205:10–8.
31. Luteijn JM, Brown MJ, Dolk H. Influenza and congenital anomalies: a systematic review and meta-analysis. Hum Reprod. 2014;29(4):809–23. https://doi.org/10.1093/humrep/det455.
32. Doyle TJ, Goodin K, Hamilton JJ. Maternal and neonatal outcomes among pregnant women with 2009 pandemic influenza A(H1N1) illness in Florida, 2009–2010: a population-based cohort study. PLoS One. 2013;8:e79040.
33. Naresh A, Fisher BM, Hoppe KK, et al. A multicenter cohort study of pregnancy outcomes among women with laboratory-confirmed H1N1 influenza. J Perinatol. 2013;33:939–43.
34. Haberg SE, Trogstad L, Gunnes N, et al. Risk of fetal death after pandemic influenza virus infection or vaccination. N Engl J Med. 2013;368:333–40.
35. Hansen C, Desai S, Bredfeldt C, et al. A large, population-based study of 2009 pandemic Influenza A virus subtype H1N1 infection diagnosis during pregnancy and outcomes for mothers and neonates. J Infect Dis. 2012;206:1260–8.
36. Nieto-Pascual L, Arjona-Berral JE, Marin-Martin EM, et al. Early prophylactic treatment in pregnant women during the 2009-2010 H1N1 pandemic: obstetric and neonatal outcomes. J Obstet Gynaecol. 2013;33:128–4.

37. Irving WL, James DK, Stephenson T, et al. Influenza virus infection in the second and third trimesters of pregnancy: a clinical and seroepidemiological study. BJOG. 2000;107:1282–9.
38. Regan AK, Feldman B, Azziz-Baumgartner E, et al. An international cohort study of birth outcomes associated with hospitalized acute respiratory infection during pregnancy. J Infect. 2020;81(1):48–56. https://doi.org/10.1016/j.jinf.2020.03.057.
39. Fell DB, Buckeridge DL, Platt RW, et al. Circulating influenza virus and adverse pregnancy outcomes: a time-series study. Am J Epidemiol. 2016;184(3):163–75. https://doi.org/10.1093/aje/kww044.
40. He J, Liu ZW, Lu YP, et al. Systematic review and meta-analysis of influenza A virus infection during pregnancy associated with an increased risk for stillbirth and low birth weight. Kidney Blood Press Res. 2017;42(2):232–43. https://doi.org/10.1159/000477221.
41. Harris J. Influenza occurring in pregnant women. J Am Med Assoc. 1919;72:978–80.
42. Mighty HE. Acute respiratory failure in pregnancy. Clin Obstet Gynecol. 2010;53:360–8.
43. Elenkov IJ, Wilder RL, Bakalov VK, et al. IL-12, TNF-alpha, and hormonal changes during late pregnancy and early postpartum: implications for autoimmune disease activity during these times. J Clin Endocrinol Metab. 2001;86:4933–8.
44. Figueiredo AS, Schumacher A. The T helper type 17/regulatory T cell paradigm in pregnancy. Immunology. 2016;148:13–21.
45. Reinhard G, Noll A, Schlebusch H, et al. Shifts in the TH1/TH2 balance during human pregnancy correlate with apoptotic changes. Biochem Biophys Res Commun. 1998;245:933–8.
46. Gonzalez-Candelas F, Astray J, Alonso J, et al. Sociodemographic factors and clinical conditions associated to hospitalization in influenza A (H1N1)2009 virus infected patients in Spain, 2009–2010. PLoS One. 2012;7:e33139. https://doi.org/10.1371/journal.pone.0033139.
47. Fiore AE, Uyeki TM, Broder K, et al. Prevention and control of influenza with vaccines: recommendations of the Advisory Committee on Immunization Practices (ACIP), 2010. MMWR Recomm Rep. 2010;59:1–62.
48. Moro PL, Broder K, Zheteyeva Y, et al. Adverse events following administration to pregnant women of influenza A (H1N1) 2009 monovalent vaccine reported to the Vaccine Adverse Event Reporting System. Am J Obstet Gynecol. 2011;205(473):e1–9.
49. American College of Obstetricians and Gynecologists Committee on Obstetric Practice. ACOG Committee Opinion No. 468: influenza vaccination during pregnancy. Obstet Gynecol. 2010;116(4):1006–7. https://doi.org/10.1097/AOG.0b013e3181fae845.
50. Grohskopf LA, Sokolow LZ, Olsen SJ, et al. Prevention and control of influenza with vaccines: recommendations of the advisory committee on immunization practices, United States, 2015–16 influenza season. MMWR Morb Mortal Wkly Rep. 2015;64(30):818–25.
51. Madhi SA, Cutland CL, Kuwanda L, et al. Influenza vaccination of pregnant women and protection of their infants. N Engl J Med. 2014;371:918–31.
52. Zaman K, Roy E, Arifeen SE, et al. Effectiveness of maternal influenza immunization in mothers and infants. N Engl J Med. 2008;359:1555–64.
53. Eick AA, Uyeki TM, Klimov A, et al. Maternal influenza vaccination and effect on influenza virus infection in young infants. Arch Pediatr Adolesc Med. 2011;165:104–11.
54. Zuccotti G, Pogliani L, Pariani E, et al. Transplacental antibody transfer following maternal immunization with a pandemic 2009 influenza A(H1N1) MF59-adjuvanted vaccine. JAMA. 2010;304:2360–1.
55. Steinhoff MC, Omer SB, Roy E, et al. Influenza immunization in pregnancy—antibody responses in mothers and infants. N Engl J Med. 2010;362:1644–6.
56. Schlaudecker EP, Steinhoff MC, Omer SB, et al. IgA and neutralizing antibodies to influenza A virus in human milk: a randomized trial of antenatal influenza immunization. PLoS One. 2013;8:e70867.
57. Hewagama S, Walker SP, Stuart RL, et al. 2009 H1N1 influenza A and pregnancy outcomes in Victoria. Aust Clin Infect Dis. 2010;50(5):686–90.
58. Ding H, Black CL, Ball S, et al. Influenza vaccination coverage among pregnant women—United States, 2014–15 influenza season. MMWR Morb Mortal Wkly Rep. 2015;64(36):1000–5.

59. Public Health England. Surveillance of influenza and other respiratory viruses in the United Kingdom: Winter 2014–2015; 2015. www.gov.uk/government/uploadsattachmentdata/file429617/Annualreport March2015ver4.pdf

60. Maher L, Dawson A, Wiley K, et al. Influenza vaccination during pregnancy: a qualitative study of the knowledge, attitudes, beliefs, and practices of general practitioners in central and South-Western Sydney. BMC Fam Pract. 2014;15(1):102.

61. Baum U, Leino T, Gissler M, et al. Perinatal survival and health after maternal influenza A(H1N1)pdm09 vaccination: a cohort study of pregnancies stratified by trimester of vaccination. Vaccine. 2015;33(38):4850–7.

62. McHugh L, Andrews RM, Lambert SB, et al. Birth outcomes for Australian mother–infant pairs who received an influenza vaccine during pregnancy, 2012–2014: the FluMum study. Vaccine. 2017;35(10):1403–9.

63. Mak TK, Mangtani P, Leese J, et al. Influenza vaccination in pregnancy: current evidence and selected national policies. Lancet Infect Dis. 2008;8(1):44–52.

64. Naleway AL, Irving SA, Henninger ML, et al. Safety of influenza vaccination during pregnancy: a review of subsequent maternal obstetric events and findings from two recent cohort studies. Vaccine. 2014;32(26):3122–7.

65. Pregnant Women and Novel Influenza A (H1N1) Virus: Considerations for Clinicians; 2010. http://www.cdc.gov/h1n1flu/clini-cian_pregnant.htm

66. Donner B, Niranjan V, Hoffmann G. Safety of oseltamivir in pregnancy: a review of preclinical and clinical data. Drug Saf. 2010;33:631–42.

67. Tomi M, Nishimura T, Nakashima E. Mother-to-fetus transfer of antiviral drugs and the involvement of transporters at the placental barrier. J Pharm Sci. 2011;100:3708–18.

68. Fiore AE, Fry A, Shay D, et al. Antiviral agents for the treatment and chemoprophylaxis of influenza—recommendations of the advisory committee on immunization practices (ACIP). MMWR Recomm Rep. 2011;60(1):1–24.

69. Creanga AA, Johnson TF, Graitcer SB, et al. Severity of 2009 pandemic influenza A (H1N1) virus infection in pregnant women. Obstet Gynecol. 2010;115:717–26.

70. Yates L, Pierce M, Stephens S, et al. Influenza A/H1N1v in pregnancy: an investigation of the characteristics and management of affected women and the relationship to pregnancy outcomes for mother and infant. Health Technol Assess. 2010;14:109–82.

71. Varner MW, Rice MM, Anderson B, et al. Eunice Kennedy Shriver National Institute of Child Health and Human Development (NICHD) maternal-fetal medicine units network (MFMU). Influenza-like illness in hospitalized pregnant and postpartum women during the 2009–2010 H1N1 pandemic. Obstet Gynecol. 2011;118:593–600.

Management of COVID-19 During Pregnancy and the Postpartum Period

24

Selcan Arslan Özel and Tuğba Sarı

24.1 Introduction

Severe acute respiratory syndrome coronavirus 2 (SARS-CoV-2) causes coronavirus disease 2019 (COVID-19). The course of COVID-19 in pregnant women, which continues to spread rapidly worldwide, on which many studies and researches are ongoing and has many unknowns, is also controversial.

In this section, epidemiology, transmission routes, clinic, complications, diagnosis, treatment, prevention measures, and follow-up of COVID-19 in pregnant women are discussed.

24.2 COVID-19 in Pregnant Women

24.2.1 COVID-19 Epidemiology in Pregnant Women

Until now, the data in the literature were that pregnancy and birth did not increase the risk of SARS-CoV-2 transmission and that COVID-19 showed a similar course in pregnant women compared to non-pregnant women. During the disease in pregnant women, more than 90% heals before birth. Although pregnancy is not reported as a risk factor for COVID-19, it should be kept in mind that symptoms may

S. A. Özel (✉)
Infectious Diseases and Clinical Microbiology Department, Health Sciences University, Derince Training and Research Hospital, Derince, Kocaeli, Turkey
e-mail: selcandr@yahoo.com

T. Sarı
Medical Faculty, Infectious Diseases and Clinical Microbiology Department, Pamukkale University, Denizli, Turkey
e-mail: drtugba82@gmail.com

C. Cingi et al. (eds.), *ENT Diseases: Diagnosis and Treatment during Pregnancy and Lactation*, https://doi.org/10.1007/978-3-031-05303-0_24

progress more seriously due to physiological changes during the natural course of pregnancy [1–15].

On the contrary, in the report, where more than 90,000 COVID-19 cases are examined in the United States; it has been reported that the rates of hospitalization in the intensive care unit (1.5% versus 0.9%) and intubation (0.5% versus 0.3%) are higher than non-pregnant women [16]. Symptomatic disease and mortality rates do not increase in pregnant women. It has been reported that the rate of being affected by SARS-CoV-2 infection in black and Hispanic pregnant women is much higher than in other pregnant women. This study, which was inconsistent with previous data, showed that pregnant women with COVID-19 should be followed closely [17].

In one of the studies conducted in New York, where the prevalence of COVID-19 is high, 215 pregnant women were screened for COVID-19, and 33 (15%) pregnant women, four of whom were symptomatic, were found to be SARS-CoV-2 positive [2]. In the other study, 10 (71%) of 14 SARS-CoV-2 positive pregnant women who were asymptomatic at presentation became symptomatic during delivery or in the postpartum period [1]. It may be wrong to generalize these study findings to regions with lower COVID-19 prevalence [17]. SARS-CoV-2 favorable rates, most of which are asymptomatic, have been reported in the range of 2.6–3.9% in pregnancy screenings performed in different regions of the United States, where the prevalence is lower [18–20].

## 24.3	SARS-CoV-2 Virus Transmission Routes During Pregnancy

24.3.1 Mother-to-Baby Transmission

Limited information is available on peripartum COVID-19. A few possible causes of in utero infection have been reported. Although vertical transmission has not been confirmed, this possibility exists [21–25]. For the risk of transmission by breastfeeding, viruses have been detected in several breast milk samples. It can be transmitted to the newborn through droplets due to close contact during breastfeeding [21, 26, 27].

## 24.4	Diagnosis of SARS-CoV-2 During Pregnancy

Diagnostic criteria for SARS-CoV-2 infection during pregnancy are the same as those who are not pregnant. The possibility of COVID-19 should be considered in patients with new-onset of fever/chills and/or respiratory symptoms (e.g., cough, shortness of breath), nausea/vomiting, diarrhea, headache, loss of smell/taste, sore throat, myalgia, and weakness.

It should also be considered in patients with severe lower respiratory tract disease of unexplained etiology. Residing or traveling in a community contaminated area of SARS-CoV-2 in the past 14 days or close contact with a confirmed or suspected COVID-19 case should raise suspicion.

Patients meeting the test criteria should also be tested for other respiratory pathogens. Detection of another viral or bacterial pathogen does not exclude SARS-CoV-2. In areas where the infection is common, prenatal (or one day before if elective) SARS-CoV-2 testing is recommended for all patients if testing is available [17].

RT-PCR (reverse transcriptase-polymerase chain reaction) test, which is the primary method used in diagnosis, is used to confirm the diagnosis of COVID-19, but false positivity may also be seen [28]. On the other hand, false negativity can be seen in tests taken on the 4 days before symptoms and on the first day of symptoms [29, 30]. The test's sensitivity depends on several factors, such as the quality of the sample and the duration of the disease. Nasopharyngeal specimens have higher sensitivity than oropharyngeal or nasal specimens [28]. If the first test is negative in patients with COVID-19 clinic and persistent suspicion, the test should be repeated 24 hours to a few days. Infection control measures for COVID-19 should continue throughout this test. The second test's negativity usually excludes infection but should be decided according to the patient's clinic [31]. If clinical suspicion of COVID-19 infection persists and for treatment decisions, the test may be repeated in higher sensitivity lower respiratory tract samples (e.g., sputum, bronchoalveolar lavage) [32]. The reliability of tests that detect Ig G and Ig M, such as ELISA and rapid antibody tests, is still controversial.

In addition to laboratory tests, imaging methods are also susceptible in diagnosis. There are concerns that methods such as chest radiography and thoracic computed tomography (CT) may cause fetal teratogenicity due to the X-rays and radiation they contain. Chest radiography is sufficient for the initial evaluation of patients with COVID-19 diagnosis. A single radiograph carries a shallow radiation dose of 0.05–0.1 rad. The fetal radiation dose for thorax CT is 1.5 rad, and it is pretty low. The safe radiation dose limit during pregnancy is 5 rad. Studies have shown that CT imaging does not increase the risk of fetal anomalies or pregnancy loss. Therefore, CT can be used if necessary in the evaluation of pregnant women. In some studies, it has been reported that thorax ultrasonography can be performed in the evaluation of pregnant women diagnosed with COVID-19 because it is fast and reliable. Bilateral subpleural ground-glass areas can be detected as hyperechogenic lung foci on ultrasonography [33, 34].

24.5 Clinical Findings in Pregnancy

All pregnant women, especially if they have been in close contact with confirmed or suspected cases, should be monitored to develop symptoms and signs of COVID-19 (similar to those in non-pregnant individuals). (>8200) reported a similar rate of symptomatic cases compared to non-pregnant women (>83,000), while one-third of pregnant women and 10% of non-pregnant women reported symptomatic status unknown [16].

Symptoms such as weakness, shortness of breath, nasal congestion, nausea/vomiting during a normal pregnancy's physiological course can be confused with the clinical signs of COVID-19 with a fever course [17].

When pregnant women are compared in terms of symptoms of COVID-19 compared to non-pregnant women, cough (52% vs. 54%) and shortness of breath (30%) symptoms were similar in proportion to headache (41% vs. 52%), muscle aches (38% vs. 47%), and fever (up to 34%). It has been reported that symptoms such as tremor (29% versus 36%) and diarrhea (14% versus 23%) were observed at a lower rate in pregnant women. Less common symptoms include sore throat, runny nose/stuffy nose, nausea/vomiting, and loss of smell and/or taste.

The most common laboratory findings during COVID-19 infection in pregnant women are; It has been reported as 47% lymphopenia and 17% as mild increases in liver enzymes [35].

Classification of disease severity: In the United States, the National Institutes of Health classified disease severity in non-pregnant individuals as follows [36]:

- *Asymptomatic or presymptomatic infection:* SARS-CoV-2 test positive but no symptoms.
- *Mild disease:* Those who do not have shortness of breath or have standard lung imaging but have clinical symptoms such as fever, cough, sore throat, weakness, headache, and muscle pain.
- *Moderate disease:* Those with pneumonia detected by clinical evaluation or imaging and oxygen saturation (SaO2)> 93 percent in room air.

Severe disease: Those with tachypnea (respiratory rate >30/min), $SaO_2 \leq 93\%$ in room air, the ratio of arterial partial pressure of oxygen to inhaled oxygen fraction (PaO_2/FiO_2) <300 or >50% involvement in the lung parenchyma.

- *Critical illness:* Respiratory failure, septic shock, and/or multiple organ dysfunction.

The course of SARS CoV-2 infection in pregnant women is generally similar to that of non-pregnant persons, except in severe and critical conditions [37]. According to the results of the study conducted on the clinical course in pregnant women:

In a prospective cohort study of 241 pregnant women with SARS-CoV-2 infection in New York, 61% of pregnant women were asymptomatic at presentation, while 30% of them became symptomatic before delivery [38].

It has been reported that 27% of the pregnant women who were found to have COVID-19 during hospitalization were mild, 26% severe, and 5% critical. It has been reported that severe disease is more common in pregnant women with comorbidities in advanced weeks of gestation compared to early pregnancy [39]. In a review in which 538 pregnant women were examined, it was reported that 15% (32/209) had severe disease and 1.4% (3/209) had the acute disease, and 3% (8/263) required maternal ICU hospitalization [35].

Similar laboratory abnormalities (hemolysis, elevated liver enzyme levels, thrombocytopenia) can be detected in pregnant women in COVID-19 infection, pre-eclampsia, and HELLP syndrome (hemolysis, elevated liver enzymes, low platelets). These diagnoses should also be considered in the differential diagnosis [40–42].

It is known that some pregnant women with severe disease have laboratory findings compatible with an increased inflammatory response similar to cytokine release syndrome. It is unknown whether the regular immunological changes of pregnancy affect this picture's formation and course [17].

24.6 Pregnancy Complications

Complications of SARS-CoV-2 infection include acute respiratory distress syndrome and myocardial damage, but other organ systems may also be affected [17].

Serious sequelae of maternal COVID-19 infection include the need for long-term ventilation support and extracorporeal membrane oxygenation (ECMO) [43–45]. It is observed that pregnant women with COVID-19 pneumonia have an increased risk of preterm and cesarean delivery [17]. Besides, maternal deaths, sometimes due to multi-organ failure and cardiopulmonary complications, have been reported in pregnant women, most of whom were healthy before SARS-CoV-2 infections [45–50]. The risk of death in pregnancy does not appear to be increased than non-pregnant women of reproductive age [16].

Fever and hypoxemia secondary to COVID-19 may increase the risk of premature birth, premature rupture of membranes, and increased fetal heart rate, but premature births may also occur in patients without severe respiratory disease. Although there is a general tendency for elective cesarean delivery with the concern that maternal respiratory failure may increase during expected delivery, this hypothesis has not been proven.

A review of 538 pregnant COVID-19 patients reported that 20% delivered before 37 weeks and 85% by cesarean section [35]. In a prospective cohort study in which 427 pregnant women with a confirmed diagnosis of COVID-19 were examined in England, it was reported that 27% delivered preterm and 59% by cesarean section [45]. In New York, 241 pregnant women with confirmed COVID-19 infection had a preterm delivery rate of 15%, a cesarean section rate of 52% in those with a severe clinical course, and a cesarean rate of 92% in critically ill patients [38]. The rate of symptomatic pregnant women in these studies is high.

24.6.1 Fetal Complications

The incidence of spontaneous abortion secondary to COVID-19 infection does not appear to be increased, but data on infections in the first trimester of pregnancy are limited [14, 51, 52]. It has been reported that five pregnancies with a required clinical course resulted in fetal death, and maternal death occurred in four of them, and the mother was still in ECMO in one [43, 46].

While more than 95% of the newborns were in good condition at birth, neonatal complications have been associated mainly with preterm labor and adverse uterine conditions caused by acute maternal disease [46, 51, 53].

There are concerns regarding the effect of hyperthermia seen during COVID-19 on organogenesis. Although it is thought that febrile diseases in the first trimester affect organogenesis and may cause congenital anomalies such as neural tube defects and low birth weight, no increased incidence was observed regarding these results. In patients with high fever, it should also be evaluated in terms of intrapartum and postpartum infections (e.g., chorioamnionitis, endometritis), and a PCR test SARS-CoV-2 should also be requested. The use of acetaminophen during pregnancy, including the first trimester, is generally safe and can reduce pregnancy risks associated with fever exposure [17].

The possible horizontal transition has been reported in several cases of peripartum maternal infection during the third trimester, indicating that congenital infection is possible but uncommon (<3% of maternal infections) [54].

Babies of mothers with suspected or confirmed COVID-19 are considered suspected to have COVID-19 and should be tested for SARS-CoV-2 RNA by RT-PCR from a swab sample nasopharynx oropharynx, or nasal region [122]. If the first test is negative, the retest should be done approximately 48 hours later; however, for asymptomatic newborns expected to be discharged after <48 h, a single test performed between 24 and 48 h is sufficient. Serological testing is not recommended to diagnose acute infection in newborns.

In a review of babies born to 936 COVID-19-infected mothers, neonatal viral RNA testing in 27/936 (2.9%) nasopharyngeal samples taken immediately after or 48 hours after birth, 1/34 cord blood sample, and 2/26 placental samples were positive. Besides, 3/82 immunoglobulin M (IgM) positivity was found in SARS-CoV-2 serological examination [54].

There are no accepted criteria for evidence of congenital SARS-CoV-2 infection. The number of criteria has been determined by Shah et al. [55]. These criteria include maternal symptoms and contact status, maternal test results, the newborn's clinical status, and neonatal test results [55].

Intrauterine fetal death/stillbirth due to congenital SARS-CoV-2 infection can only be confirmed by PCR detection of the virus from fetal tissues or placental tissues or the detection of viral particles in the tissue virus fetal/placental tissue culture by electron microscopy. Virus detection by PCR from a fetal surface of the placenta or a fetal is classified as a possible infection. The likelihood of infection is low if the virus is detected by PCR only on the placenta's surface swab from the maternal side and if it is not detected or tested by PCR from the fetal or placental tissue. The virus is not detected in fetal tissues by PCR, or autopsy by electron microscopy indicates no infection [17]. Until now, no evidence of infection has been reported in the literature in studies examining placental specimens, except for a few cases [21, 24, 56–58].

In studies conducted with COVID-19 patients, the viremia level was very low at approximately 1%. This suggests that placental and horizontal transition will be rare [59].

The entry of SARS-CoV-2 into the cell is thought to be dependent on the angiotensin-converting enzyme 2 (ACE 2) receptor and serine protease, which are minimally expressed in the placenta [60, 61]. This may explain the rare occurrence of placental SARS-CoV-2 infection and fetal transmission.

Although it is not fully proven whether there is a horizontal transition, two cases with SARS-CoV-2 RNA positivity have been reported so far in samples taken from newborn and placental samples [21, 56]. In one of these case reports, mild hypothermia, hypoglycemia, and feeding difficulties compatible with premature were reported in the newborn, but it was reported that there was no respiratory distress. In the other case, it was reported that neonatal resuscitation was performed after birth but was extubated within 6 h, and then recovered after developing irritability, poor nutrition, axial hypertonia, and opisthotonus on the third day of life.

Congenital SARS-CoV-2 infection diagnosis in a baby born alive depends on the presence or absence of the newborn's clinical features and the mother's infection. In symptomatic cases, congenital infection is confirmed if PCR detects a virus in the cord blood taken within the first 12 h after birth or in the neonatal blood or amniotic fluid is taken before membrane rupture. In asymptomatic cases, neonatal infection is confirmed if PCR detects the virus in cord blood or neonatal blood was taken within 12 h of birth [17].

The newborn may be infected with intrapartum. In symptomatic newborns of infected mothers, intrapartum infection is confirmed at birth (after cleansing the baby). If SARS-CoV-2 PCR from nasopharyngeal swabs is positive, there is no alternative diagnosis for symptoms [17].

In asymptomatic newborns of infected mothers, intrapartum infection is confirmed if both SARS-CoV-2 PCR from nasopharyngeal swabs is positive at birth (after cleansing the baby) between 24 and 48 h [17].

Transmission to newborns is thought to be primarily through exposure to respiratory droplets from mothers with SARS-CoV-2 infection and other caregivers [35, 62].

Vaginal and amniotic fluid samples are negative to date, except for two cases in most women who test positive for SARS-CoV-2 in the nasopharynx [12, 21, 56, 63, 64].

24.7 Approach to Pregnant Women with Suspected or Diagnosed COVID-19

24.7.1 Monitoring at Home

Most pregnant women with suspected or definite COVID-19 diagnosis (at least 86%) can be followed up at home if hospitalization is not required for other reasons. However, it should be ensured that there are no obstetric problems (e.g., preterm labor), there is no possibility that the clinical situation may deteriorate rapidly. If it occurs, immediate hospital admission should be recommended [35]. Besides, fetal movement count should be performed in pregnant women in the third trimester, and it should be reported that fetal movement is reduced. Pregnant women diagnosed with COVID-19 should have symptoms (shortness of breath, tachypnea, persistent fever higher than 39 °C despite appropriate acetaminophen use, inability to take orally) for at least 2 weeks [31].

24.7.2 Follow-up of Pregnant Women Diagnosed with COVID-19 in the Hospital

Pregnant women with mild illness and comorbidities (e.g., hypertension, pregestational diabetes, chronic kidney disease, chronic cardiopulmonary disease, immunosuppressive conditions) or moderate to critical illness are hospitalized [65].

Follow-up should be done in a hospital with gynecologists, obstetricians, perinatology, infectious diseases, chest diseases, anesthesiology and reanimation, and neonatal specialists.

All pregnant women should have a confirmed case for signs and symptoms of COVID-19 (fever and/or new cough, shortness of breath, sore throat, muscle aches, rhinorrhea/nasal congestion, and smell and taste abnormalities) entering the hospital for hospitalization. It should be questioned whether there is close contact, and also temperature measurement should be done [66]. The CDC recommends screening for pregnant women with suspected COVID-19 or developing symptoms at admission [67].

Considering that asymptomatic patients and presymptomatic patients may pose a risk for healthcare personnel and newborns in the United States, the SARS-CoV-2 test is performed for all pregnant women prepared for delivery [1, 68, 69].

Being diagnosed with COVID-19 alone is not a reason for referral to a higher center. Pregnant women with severe disease, oxygen requirement, comorbidities, or critical illness should be followed up in a hospital with obstetric services and a level III or IV adult intensive care unit (ICU), in an isolated room with negative pressure, if possible, prepared in a way that does not pose a risk of contamination to other patients. Labor follow-up and delivery should be carried out with a limited number of personnel by respecting the isolation rules [29, 70]. The algorithm for pregnancy follow-up with a diagnosis of COVID-19 prepared by ACOG (American College of Obstetrics and Gynecology) and SMFM (Society for Maternal-Fetal Medicine) is presented as follows.

For assessment of disease severity if there are symptoms of fever ≥38 °C or cough, shortness of breath, nausea, vomiting/diarrhea; shortness of breath, effort dyspnea, hemoptysis (more than a teaspoon), chest pain when coughing, dysphagia, dehydration, orientation, and cooperation limitation are evaluated. If any is detected, the patient is evaluated as high-risk and referred to the upper center following the isolation rules. Suppose there are comorbidity, obstetric problems, socio-economic status disorder, insufficiency in self-care, and difficulty in follow-up, in that case, the patient is evaluated as medium risk, isolated for monitoring, and imaging is performed if necessary. If respiratory distress develops, the patient is evaluated in the high-risk category.

In addition to routine laboratory tests, blood cultures should be taken for accompanying bacterial infections. The fluid-electrolyte balance should be monitored. Since aggressive hydration may cause pulmonary edema and worsen maternal oxygenation, appropriate hydration of <75 ccs/h should be performed by following up the fluid taken out [111]. Conservative fluid therapy is recommended for pregnant women with severe COVID-19 clinic to avoid hypotension and organ hypoperfusion.

24.8 Treatment

24.8.1 Maternal Respiratory Support

Among critically ill COVID-19 patients, profound acute hypoxemic respiratory failure resulting from acute respiratory distress syndrome (ARDS) is expected. General supportive treatment in critically ill COVID-19 pneumonia is similar to that in ARDS patients due to other causes. Common complications of ARDS associated with COVID-19 include acute kidney injury, elevated liver enzymes, and heart damage (e.g., cardiomyopathy, pericarditis, pericardial effusion, arrhythmia, sudden cardiac death).

Maternal peripheral oxygen saturation (SpO_2) should be kept at 95% during pregnancy if SpO_2 drops below 95% and arterial blood gas should be obtained to measure the partial pressure of oxygen (PaO_2). To ensure a proper oxygen diffusion gradient from the maternal side to the fetal side, the maternal PaO_2 must be greater than 70 mmHg. The World Health Organization (WHO) recommends that maternal SpO_2 be maintained at $\geq$92–95 after the patient is stable [71].

In the Intensive Care Unit, severe patients with COVID-19 are usually followed up in a prone position. Sleeping in the prone position during sleep allows the pregnancy to increase oxygen saturation and escape intubation [72–74]. Permissive hypercapnia (PCO_2 <60 mmHg) and extracorporeal membrane oxygenation (ECMO) are not harmful to the fetus and can be applied if indicated for the treatment of ARDS, but data are limited [73, 74]. High positive end-expiratory pressure strategies (>10 mmHg) require close and continuous maternal and fetal monitoring as they reduce preload and cardiac output [72].

24.8.2 Use and Type of Venous Thromboembolism Prophylaxis

While direct data on thromboembolic risk with COVID-19 are limited, there is an increased risk. American Society of Hematology, Critical Care Medicine Association, and International Society of Thrombosis and Hemostasis; In patients hospitalized with COVID-19, prophylaxis is recommended for pregnant/

postpartum women COVID-19 unless there is a contraindication (e.g., bleeding, severe thrombocytopenia). For antepartum prophylaxis in pregnant women with no severe or critical illness and expected delivery within a few days, 5000 units of unfractionated heparin subcutaneously every 12 h is a recommended dose [75–77].

Since unfractionated heparin is more easily reversed than low molecular weight heparin, it is generally preferred in pregnant women near birth. Low molecular weight heparin (e.g., enoxaparin 40 mg daily) makes sense in those who are not expected to deliver within a few days and are postpartum [75–77].

24.8.3 Dexamethasone

The use of 6 mg/day dexamethasone for ten days or up to discharge in critically ill patients who receive oxygen supplements or ventilator support in COVID-19 infection is used to manage refractory shock.

The harm of glucocorticoid therapy for lung maturation has not been demonstrated, but a multidisciplinary decision should be made before administration. In pregnant women who meet the criteria for the use of glucocorticoids for maternal treatment of COVID-19 and are at high risk for preterm labor, dexamethasone (four doses of 6 mg 12 h apart) or betamethasone (two 12 mg doses) to induce fetal pulmonary maturation dose), followed by prednisolone (40 mg orally daily) or hydrocortisone (80 mg intravenously twice daily). This prevents the fetus from prolonged exposure to dexamethasone or betamethasone that crosses the placenta in a metabolically active form and can have side effects.

24.8.4 Antiviral Drug Therapy

Although it is not a definite option for COVID-19, studies of some drugs used in other indications are ongoing. Among these studies, SOLIDARITY and RECOVERY are studied, including pregnant women [78, 79]. In some centers, remdesivir is used in pregnant women with severe forms of COVID-19. Remdesivir is a novel with activity against SARS-CoV-2 [80] and similar coronaviruses (including severe acute respiratory syndrome [SARS] and coronavirus associated with the Middle East respiratory syndrome [MERS-CoV]), both in vitro and in vivo. It is a nucleotide analog [80, 81]. It has been reported to be used in pregnant women with Ebola and Marburg virus disease without fetal toxicity [82]. However, in all randomized studies performed with remdesivir, pregnant women and breastfeeders were excluded from the study.

Data from randomized studies generally show that hydroxychloroquine or chloroquine preparations have no benefit. Also, adverse maternal effects may cause abnormal heart rhythms (QT interval prolongation and ventricular tachycardia), particularly in patients taking other drugs that cause QTc prolongation. Hydroxychloroquine crosses the placenta. In animal studies, an accumulation in fetal ocular tissue has been observed, but no increased risk of fetal ocular abnormalities has been observed in humans. This is safe considering that the drug is used by pregnant women to treat systemic lupus erythematosus or for the prevention of malaria disease. However, the available data are limited, and the fetus's risk should be considered as they are used at different doses in COVID-19 infection [83].

Another drug used in pregnant women with COVID-19 is lopinavir-ritonavir which is also used to treat HIV infection. It crosses the placenta and may increase the risk of premature birth but has no teratogenic effect in humans. Ribavirin and baricitinib are teratogenic, among other drugs used for COVID-19.

24.8.5 Convalescent Plasma

Convalescent plasma therapy is a method used as supportive therapy in the treatment of COVID-19. Successful use of convalescent plasma has been reported in a few pregnant cases, sometimes with drug therapy (e.g., steroids, remdesivir, lopinavir/ritonavir, azithromycin) [84–86].

24.8.6 Low-dose Aspirin and Nonsteroidal Anti-inflammatory Drugs (NSAIDs)

For pregnant women without COVID-19, ACOG noted that low-dose aspirin as medically indicated should continue to be recommended (e.g., prevention of pre-eclampsia) [70].

Concerns about NSAIDs' possible adverse effects have developed due to a case of serious illness taking NSAIDs (ibuprofen) in the early stages of the pandemic [87]. In South Korea, patients hospitalized for COVID-19 were associated with a worse clinical condition when compared with those who used NSAIDs and those who did not use them within the seven days before hospitalization. However, this study found that those with poor clinical conditions were older and had a higher underlying comorbidity rate [88]. In a retrospective study from Israel; when NSAID use was compared with acetaminophen use or antipyretic use [89]. Given the uncertainty in the relationship between NSAID use and poor prognosis, acetaminophen may be recommended as an analgesic, if possible. However, the American College of Obstetrics and Gynecologists, WHO, and the European Medicines Agency recommend not avoiding NSAIDs in COVID-19 patients when clinically indicated [70, 71, 90].

24.8.7 Tokolysis

In women with known or suspected COVID-19, the preferred tocolytic is nifedipine. Indomethacin is a suitable alternative among beta sympathomimetics that can further increase the maternal heart rate. Magnesium sulfate should be used with caution in terms of respiratory depression.

24.9 Fetal Monitoring

Usually, the fetus has viability around 25 weeks. Fetal monitoring should be performed with fetal heart rate, contraction follow-up, amount of amniotic fluid, and doppler USG. For hospitalized patients, fetal heart rate monitoring can be provided with an external Bluetooth-enabled fetal monitor. Continuous monitoring can be performed in unstable hospitalized patients who will undergo emergency cesarean delivery with fetal heart rate monitoring. The fetal stress test can be performed once or twice a day in patients with stable oxygen saturation (SaO_2).

Limited data are available on fetal growth in pregnant women infected with COVİD-19. Acute and chronic intervillous inflammation due to COVID-19 may be focal avascular villus and chorionic plate and placental insufficiency due to thrombus and uteroplacental vascular malperfusion in fetal vascular structures in the trunk villi and suboptimal fetal growth related to this. These lesions may also be caused by coagulopathy associated with COVID-19, placental hypoxia during acute maternal illness, placental viral infection, or a combination of these factors [21, 56, 91–93].

24.10 Follow-up of Women Recovering from COVID-19

Fetal growth retardation, identified with other SARS infections, is a theoretical problem [94, 95]. It is recommended that pregnant women with a definite diagnosis be controlled by ultrasonography in fetal growth and amniotic fluid volume starting 14 days after symptoms resolve [21, 56, 91–93]. For those infected in the first or second trimester, 18–23 A detailed fetal screening is recommended during the weeks of gestation.

The following isolation removal criteria have been established for mothers with suspected or confirmed COVID-19 [96]:

- At least ten days have passed after the first appearance of symptoms (this period can be extended to 20 days if there is a critical and severe clinical situation).
- Twenty-four hours have passed since the last height of fever.
- Other symptoms have improved.

These criteria must be followed to prevent contamination. However, the continuation of the SARS-CoV-2 RT-PCR result for weeks does not always mean that the contamination continues despite the presence of viral RNA [28].

24.11 Planning Delivery in COVID-19 Pregnant Women

- There is no emergency delivery indication for pregnant women diagnosed with COVID-19 with mild symptoms if there is no medical/obstetric indication for an emergency delivery. Delivery after a positive mother has a negative test result or after isolation is removed will minimize the risk of postnatal transmission to the newborn [70]. Vital signs should be followed up after birth. Follow-up should be done every 4 h for 24 h after vaginal delivery and 48 h after cesarean delivery. For pregnant women with a diagnosis of preterm COVID-19 and medical/obstetric complications (e.g., premature rupture of membranes, preeclampsia), the timing of delivery is determined by protocols for medical/obstetric disorder.

- For patients with moderate illness, continuous pulse oximetry monitoring is recommended for the first 24 h until symptoms resolve. Laboratory tests and imaging are determined according to the course of the disease.
- For patients with severe or critical illness, very close maternal monitoring and care in the maternity and maternity unit or intensive care unit is indicated. Deciding on the timing of delivery for women with severe disease should be made by considering many factors on a patient basis [31, 97].

Whether the mother's respiratory symptoms will improve with birth and the risk of transmission during the mother's birth with acute illness should be considered. It should also be kept in mind that maternal antibody production and, therefore, the newborn's passive immunity may not have time to develop. On the other hand, increased oxygen consumption and decreased functional residual capacity during pregnancy may cause clinical deterioration in pregnant women with pneumonia [98].

In multiple pregnancies, excessive uterine distension or severe polyhydramnios in the third trimester may further compromise lung function.

Some authors recommend delivery between 32 and 34 weeks for pregnant women with COVID-19 infected with pneumonia but not intubated. Maternal hypoxia, which may develop when lung involvement increases, may put the fetus at risk. Some authors also do not advocate for delivery. However, the mother's condition may worsen in the second week, given the known morbidity and mortality of babies that will occur before 32 weeks of gestation.

It is challenging to plan the delivery timing of a critically ill hospitalized pregnant woman who was intubated due to COVID-19. One group advocates delivery if the patient is stable after 32–34 weeks, while others advocate delivery only for patients with refractory hypoxemic respiratory failure or who are critically ill [72].

Maternal support should continue with fetal monitoring as much as possible in <32 weeks of gestation. In some cases, maternal ECMO may be required [74]. With intense breathing from the infected patient, especially during active delivery, the spread of respiratory droplets and virus is facilitated, and the effectiveness of the mask may be reduced [99, 100]. The risk of transmission with feces-containing viruses with defecation during pushing during labor should also be considered [57, 101]. Pregnant women with suspected or confirmed COVID-19 are instructed to wear surgical masks during labor and delivery [100, 102].

According to many opinions, COVID-19 infection alone is not an indication for cesarean section. In a study evaluating 37 cesarean sections and 41 standard vaginal deliveries, maternal clinical deterioration after cesarean was 22%, while this rate was reported as 5% in standard vaginal delivery [103]. However, the small number of patients in this study and the delivery method's bias may affect the findings. In asymptomatic women, labor and cesarean deliveries should not be delayed or rescheduled with appropriate medical indications [17].

24.11.1 Analgesia and Anesthesia

In patients known or suspected to have COVID-19, the neuraxial anesthetic is not contraindicated and has several advantages in giving birth: it provides good analgesia and thus reduces cardiopulmonary stress caused by pain and anxiety and thus virus shedding. It also eliminates the need for general anesthesia in case of emergency cesarean delivery. The Society of Obstetric Anesthesia and Perinatology recommends suspending the use of nitrous oxide for birth analgesia in these patients due to insufficient data on cleaning, filtering, and potential aerosolization of nitrous oxide systems [104].

General anesthesia (intubation and extubation) causes aerosol scattering, so all healthcare professionals must wear complete personal protective equipment (N-95 masks, etc.) during cesarean delivery.

Most COVID-19 patients with postpartum hemorrhage are managed according to standard protocols. However, some authors recommend avoiding tranexamic acid in COVID-19 patients because its antifibrinolytic properties may increase thrombosis risk in those with severe or critically ill health [105].

24.11.2 Psychological Support

All postpartum patients should be screened for postpartum depression four to eight weeks after birth. The most widely used scale is the 10-item Edinburgh Postpartum Depression Scale, but alternatives are also available. The psychological impact of COVID-19 should also be acknowledged, and support should be provided for moderate to severe anxiety [106].

24.12 Protective Measures

Pregnant women should follow the same recommendations as non-pregnant persons to avoid exposure to the virus (e.g., social distancing, hand hygiene, wearing a mask). Pregnant women with a history of close contact without a mask with a confirmed, probable, or suspected COVID-19 person should be isolated for up to 14 days and monitored for symptoms [17]. It is recommended for pregnant women not to hinder pregnancy follow-up. However, hygiene and social isolation measures should be followed at every examination, and unnecessary visits should not be made. However, taking such measures may be difficult for the homeless, those staying in the shelter, those living in migrant camps, and refugee pregnant women.

There are many ways to reduce the time patients spend in healthcare facilities, including pregnant women with high-risk pregnancies. In order to prevent transmission to pregnant women, examinations via the internet such as telemedicine, telephone consultation, reduction of the number of face-to-face examinations, collective requests for follow-up tests on examination days (e.g., aneuploidy, diabetes, infection screening), restriction of attendants during examinations and tests, and obstetric ultrasound are recommended to reduce the frequency of examinations (e.g., gestational age, fetal abnormality, fetal growth, placental attachment) and to respect social distance [107].

Generally, it is recommended that pregnant women come for control (ultrasound and/or laboratory tests) only at about 12, 20, 28, and 36 weeks of gestation. Even some practices should be done with telemedicine, and a single visit at the 32nd week is recommended. Baseline evaluation should be made at each examination. Complete urine analysis and blood pressure measurement should be done. In the first 3 months, control with ultrasonography and detailed USG evaluation between 18 and 22 weeks is recommended. Supportive treatments such as folic acid and vitamin D recommended during pregnancy should be continued [31].

It is recommended that these examinations be performed by patients and healthcare professionals wearing their masks, and video communication is encouraged. Besides, the psychological impact of COVID-19 should be considered, and psychological support should be provided as depression and anxiety, which can be severe in pregnant women, are also common [108–110].

Considering the possibility of transmission of SARS-CoV-2 from asymptomatic individuals (or individuals who show no symptoms in the incubation period), since COVID-19 in children can often be mild and asymptomatic, pregnant women with children should be more careful [111–117]. The CDC recommends that children limit the time when playing with other children and play outdoors and wear masks [118].

There is no standard vocational guidance for pregnant healthcare workers, specifying which jobs should be restricted [70, 119]. Pregnant workers in non-healthcare professions may continue to work until they give birth. However, risk-reducing measures (less risky positions or self-isolation) may be considered to reduce the individual's risk of peripartum infection [70].

24.13 Follow-up of a Newborn Born from a Mother Diagnosed with COVID-19

The newborn's risk of receiving SARS-CoV-2 from its mother is low, and the data show that there is no difference in the risk of neonatal SARS-CoV-2 infection, whether the newborn is cared for in a separate room or the mother's room. Mothers should wear a mask and apply hand hygiene during contact with their babies, and maintain physical distance between mother and newborn at other times.

The risk of SARS-CoV-2 transmission through breast milk is not yet clear, although several case series reported that all breast milk samples from mothers with COVID-19 were negative [51, 120]. In later studies, it was reported by some investigators that viruses were detected in breast milk samples [21, 26, 27].

In a WHO study, breast milk samples from 43 mothers were found to be SARS-CoV-2 negative by RT-PCR, and three mothers' samples were found positive. However, no additional tests for viability and infectivity of the virus were performed [121]. Eighty-two babies of mothers who tested positive for SARS-CoV-2 and continued to breastfeed were tested, and no babies were found positive for SARS-CoV-2 after birth [122].

In conclusion, it is recommended to continue breastfeeding, considering the benefits of breast milk and antibodies contained in breast milk can provide passive antibody protection for the baby. However, one should pay attention to hand hygiene before and after breastfeeding and wear a mask during breastfeeding.

In mothers with confirmed COVID-19 or symptomatic mothers with suspected COVID-19, ideally, to minimize direct contact, the baby can be pumped if it is preferred to give breastmilk expressed by another caregiver mother has recovered or the other healthy caregiver. In such cases, the mother should wear a mask and clean her hands and breasts thoroughly before pumping; pump parts and bottles must be cleaned. During caregiver-provided procedures (e.g., changing diapers, bathing, feeding), they should wear appropriate personal protective equipment (gowns, gloves, face mask, and eye protection) [17].

References

1. Breslin N, Baptiste C, Gyamfi-Bannerman C, Miller R, Martinez R, Bernstein K, Ring L, Landau R, Purisch S, Friedman AM, Fuchs K, Sutton D, Andrikopoulou M, Rupley D, Sheen J-J, Aubey J, Zork N, Moroz L, Mourad M, Wapner R, Simpson LL, D'Alton ME, Goffman D. COVID-19 infection among asymptomatic and symptomatic pregnant women: Two weeks of confirmed presentations to an affiliated pair of New York City hospitals. Am J Obstet Gynecol MFM. 2020:100118. https://doi.org/10.1016/j.ajogmf.2020.100118.
2. Sutton D, Fuchs K, D'Alton M, Goffman D. Universal screening for SARS-CoV-2 in women admitted for delivery. N Engl J Med. 2020;382:2163–4. https://doi.org/10.1056/NEJMc2009316.
3. Wu Z, McGoogan JM. Characteristics of and important lessons from the coronavirus disease 2019 (COVID-19) outbreak in China: summary of a report of 72 314 cases from the Chinese Center for Disease Control and Prevention. JAMA. 2020; https://doi.org/10.1001/jama.2020.2648.
4. Hospitalization Rates and Characteristics of Patients Hospitalized with laboratory-confirmed Coronavirus Disease 2019—COVID-NET, 14 States, March 1–30, 2020—PubMed. https://pubmed.ncbi.nlm.nih.gov/32298251/. Accessed 15 Aug 2020
5. Report of the WHO-China Joint Mission on Coronavirus Disease 2019 (COVID-19); 16–24 Feb 2020. https://www.who.int/docs/default-source/coronaviruse/who-china-joint-mission-on-covid-19-final-report.pdf. Accessed 14 April 2020.
6. Di Mascio D, Khalil A, Saccone G, Rizzo G, Buca D, Liberati M, Vecchiet J, Nappi L, Scambia G, Berghella V, D'Antonio F (2020) Outcome of Coronavirus spectrum infections (SARS, MERS, COVID 1-19) during pregnancy: a systematic review and meta-analysis. Am J Obstet Gynecol MFM 100107. doi: https://doi.org/10.1016/j.ajogmf.2020.100107
7. Schwartz DA. An analysis of 38 pregnant women with COVID-19, their newborn infants, and maternal-fetal transmission of SARS-CoV-2: maternal coronavirus infections and pregnancy outcomes. Arch Pathol Lab Med. 2020; https://doi.org/10.5858/arpa.2020-0901-SA.

8. Khan S, Jun L, Null N, Siddique R, Li Y, Han G, Xue M, Nabi G, Liu J. Association of COVID-19 with pregnancy outcomes in healthcare workers and general women. Clin Microbiol Infect Off Publ Eur Soc Clin Microbiol Infect Dis. 2020;26:788–90. https://doi.org/10.1016/j.cmi.2020.03.034.

9. Yang H, Sun G, Tang F, Peng M, Gao Y, Peng J, Xie H, Zhao Y, Jin Z. Clinical features and outcomes of pregnant women suspected of coronavirus disease 2019. J Infect. 2020;81:e40–4. https://doi.org/10.1016/j.jinf.2020.04.003.

10. Della Gatta AN, Rizzo R, Pilu G, Simonazzi G. Coronavirus disease 2019 during pregnancy: a systematic review of reported cases. Am J Obstet Gynecol. 2020;223:36–41. https://doi.org/10.1016/j.ajog.2020.04.013.

11. Qiancheng X, Jian S, Lingling P, Lei H, Xiaogan J, Weihua L, Gang Y, Shirong L, Zhen W, GuoPing X, Lei Z, Sixth batch of Anhui medical team aiding Wuhan for COVID-19. Coronavirus disease 2019 in pregnancy. Int J Infect Dis IJID Off Publ Int Soc Infect Dis. 2020;95:376–83. https://doi.org/10.1016/j.ijid.2020.04.065.

12. Yang Z, Wang M, Zhu Z, Liu Y. Coronavirus disease 2019 (COVID-19) and pregnancy: a systematic review. J Matern-Fetal Neonatal Med Off J Eur Assoc Perinat Med Fed Asia Ocean Perinat Soc Int Soc Perinat Obstet. 2020:1–4. https://doi.org/10.1080/14767058.2020.1759541.

13. Li N, Han L, Peng M, Lv Y, Ouyang Y, Liu K, Yue L, Li Q, Sun G, Chen L, Yang L. Maternal and neonatal outcomes of pregnant women with COVID-19 pneumonia: a case-control study. Clin Infect Dis Off Publ Infect Dis Soc Am. 2020; https://doi.org/10.1093/cid/ciaa352.

14. Juan J, Gil MM, Rong Z, Zhang Y, Yang H, Poon LC. Effect of coronavirus disease 2019 (COVID-19) on maternal, perinatal and neonatal outcome: systematic review. Ultrasound Obstet Gynecol Off J Int Soc Ultrasound Obstet Gynecol. 2020;56:15–27. https://doi.org/10.1002/uog.22088.

15. Kasraeian M, Zare M, Vafaei H, Asadi N, Faraji A, Bazrafshan K, Roozmeh S. COVID-19 pneumonia and pregnancy; a systematic review and meta-analysis. J Matern-Fetal Neonatal Med Off J Eur Assoc Perinat Med Fed Asia Ocean Perinat Soc Int Soc Perinat Obstet. 2020:1–8. https://doi.org/10.1080/14767058.2020.1763952.

16. Ellington S, Strid P, Tong VT, Woodworth K, Galang RR, Zambrano LD, Nahabedian J, Anderson K, Gilboa SM. Characteristics of Women of Reproductive Age with laboratory-confirmed SARS-CoV-2 Infection by Pregnancy Status - United States, January 22-June 7, 2020. MMWR Morb Mortal Wkly Rep. 2020;69:769–75. https://doi.org/10.15585/mmwr.mm6925a1.

17. Coronavirus disease 2019 (COVID-19): Pregnancy issues—UpToDate. https://www.uptodate.com/contents/coronavirus-disease-2019-covid-19-pregnancy-issues?search=covid%20pregnancy&source=search_result&selectedTitle=1~150&usage_type=default&display_rank=1. Accessed 6 Aug 2020

18. Campbell KH, Tornatore JM, Lawrence KE, Illuzzi JL, Sussman LS, Lipkind HS, Pettker CM. Prevalence of SARS-CoV-2 among patients admitted for childbirth in southern Connecticut. JAMA. 2020; https://doi.org/10.1001/jama.2020.8904.

19. LaCourse SM, Kachikis A, Blain M, Simmons LE, Mays JA, Pattison AD, Salerno CC, McCartney SA, Kretzer NM, Resnick R, Shay RL, Savitsky LM, Curtin AC, Huebner EM, Ma KK, Delaney S, Delgado C, Schippers A, Munson J, Pottinger PS, Cohen S, Name S, Bourassa L, Bryan A, Greninger A, Jerome KR, Roxby AC, Lokken E, Cheng E, Adams Waldorf KM, Hitti J. Low prevalence of SARS-CoV-2 among pregnant and postpartum patients with universal screening in Seattle, Washington. Clin Infect Dis Off Publ Infect Dis Soc Am. 2020; https://doi.org/10.1093/cid/ciaa675.

20. Goldfarb IT, Diouf K, Barth WH, Robinson JN, Katz D, Gregory KE, Ciaranello A, Yawetz S, Shenoy ES, Klompas M. Universal SARS-CoV-2 testing on admission to the labor and delivery unit: low prevalence among asymptomatic obstetric patients. Infect Control Hosp Epidemiol. 2020:1–2. https://doi.org/10.1017/ice.2020.255.

21. Kirtsman M, Diambomba Y, Poutanen SM, Malinowski AK, Vlachodimitropoulou E, Parks WT, Erdman L, Morris SK, Shah PS. Probable congenital SARS-CoV-2 infection in a neonate born to a woman with active SARS-CoV-2 infection. CMAJ Can Med Assoc J J Assoc Medicale Can. 2020;192:E647–50. https://doi.org/10.1503/cmaj.200821.
22. Dong L, Tian J, He S, Zhu C, Wang J, Liu C, Yang J. Possible vertical transmission of SARS-CoV-2 from an infected mother to her newborn. JAMA. 2020; https://doi.org/10.1001/jama.2020.4621.
23. Zeng L, Xia S, Yuan W, Yan K, Xiao F, Shao J, Zhou W. Neonatal early-onset infection with SARS-CoV-2 in 33 neonates born to mothers with COVID-19 in Wuhan, China. JAMA Pediatr. 2020; https://doi.org/10.1001/jamapediatrics.2020.0878.
24. Baud D, Greub G, Favre G, Gengler C, Jaton K, Dubruc E, Pomar L. Second-trimester miscarriage in a pregnant woman with SARS-CoV-2 infection. JAMA. 2020; https://doi.org/10.1001/jama.2020.7233.
25. Zeng H, Xu C, Fan J, Tang Y, Deng Q, Zhang W, Long X. Antibodies in infants born to mothers with COVID-19 pneumonia. JAMA. 2020;323:1848–9. https://doi.org/10.1001/jama.2020.4861.
26. Wu Y, Liu C, Dong L, Zhang C, Chen Y, Liu J, Zhang C, Duan C, Zhang H, Mol BW, Dennis C-L, Yin T, Yang J, Huang H. Coronavirus disease 2019 among pregnant Chinese women: case series data on the safety of vaginal birth and breastfeeding. BJOG Int J Obstet Gynaecol. 2020; https://doi.org/10.1111/1471-0528.16276.
27. Groß R, Conzelmann C, Müller JA, Stenger S, Steinhart K, Kirchhoff F, Münch J. Detection of SARS-CoV-2 in human breastmilk. Lancet Lond Engl. 2020;395:1757–8. https://doi.org/10.1016/S0140-6736(20)31181-8.
28. Interpreting Diagnostic Tests for SARS-CoV-2. https://pubmed.ncbi.nlm.nih.gov/32374370/. Accessed 17 Aug 2020
29. Kucirka LM, Lauer SA, Laeyendecker O, Boon D, Lessler J. Variation in false-negative rate of reverse transcriptase polymerase chain reaction-based SARS-CoV-2 tests by time since exposure. Ann Intern Med. 2020; https://doi.org/10.7326/M20-1495.
30. Kelly JC, Dombrowksi M, O'neil-Callahan M, Kernberg AS, Frolova AI, Stout MJ. False-negative COVID-19 testing: considerations in obstetrical care. Am J Obstet Gynecol MFM. 2020:100130. https://doi.org/10.1016/j.ajogmf.2020.100130.
31. Donders F, Lonnée-Hoffmann R, Tsiakalos A, Mendling W, Martinez de Oliveira J, Judlin P, Xue F, Donders GGG, Isidog Covid-Guideline Workgroup Null. ISIDOG recommendations concerning COVID-19 and pregnancy. Diagn Basel Switz. 2020;10 https://doi.org/10.3390/diagnostics10040243.
32. World Health Organization. Coronavirus disease (COVID-19) technical guidance: Surveillance and case definitions. https://www.who.int/emergencies/diseases/novel-coronavirus-2019/technical-guidance/surveillance-and-case-definitions. Accessed 28 Feb 2020.
33. How to perform lung ultrasound in pregnant women with suspected COVID-19. https://pubmed.ncbi.nlm.nih.gov/32207208/. Accessed 17 Aug 2020
34. Buonsenso D, Raffaelli F, Tamburrini E, Biasucci DG, Salvi S, Smargiassi A, Inchingolo R, Scambia G, Lanzone A, Testa AC, Moro F. Clinical role of lung ultrasound for diagnosis and monitoring of COVID-19 pneumonia in pregnant women. Ultrasound Obstet Gynecol Off J Int Soc Ultrasound Obstet Gynecol. 2020;56:106–9. https://doi.org/10.1002/uog.22055.
35. Huntley BJF, Huntley ES, Di Mascio D, Chen T, Berghella V, Chauhan SP. Rates of maternal and perinatal mortality and vertical transmission in pregnancies complicated by severe acute respiratory syndrome coronavirus 2 (SARS-Co-V-2) infection: a systematic review. Obstet Gynecol. 2020;136:303–12. https://doi.org/10.1097/AOG.0000000000004010.
36. NIH COVID-19 Treatment Guidelines. https://covid19treatmentguidelines.nih.gov/overview/management-of-covid-19/. Accessed 22 April 2020.
37. Pierce-Williams RAM, Burd J, Felder L, Khoury R, Bernstein PS, Avila K, Penfield CA, Roman AS, DeBolt CA, Stone JL, Bianco A, Kern-Goldberger AR, Hirshberg A, Srinivas SK, Jayakumaran JS, Brandt JS, Anastasio H, Birsner M, O'Brien DS, Sedev HM,

Dolin CD, Schnettler WT, Suhag A, Ahluwalia S, Navathe RS, Khalifeh A, Anderson K, Berghella V. Clinical course of severe and critical COVID-19 in hospitalized pregnancies: a US cohort study. Am J Obstet Gynecol MFM. 2020:100134. https://doi.org/10.1016/j.ajogmf.2020.100134.

38. Characteristics and outcomes of 241 births to women with severe acute respiratory syndrome coronavirus 2 (SARS-CoV-2) infection at five New York City medical centers. https://pubmed.ncbi.nlm.nih.gov/32555034/. Accessed 15 Aug 2020.

39. Crovetto F, Crispi F, Llurba E, Figueras F, Gómez-Roig MD, Gratacós E. Seroprevalence and presentation of SARS-CoV-2 in pregnancy. Lancet Lond Engl. 2020; https://doi.org/10.1016/S0140-6736(20)31714-1.

40. COVID-19 and HELLP: overlapping clinical pictures in two gravid patients. https://pubmed.ncbi.nlm.nih.gov/32566368/. Accessed 18 Aug 2020

41. Mendoza M, Garcia-Ruiz I, Maiz N, Rodo C, Garcia-Manau P, Serrano B, Lopez-Martinez RM, Balcells J, Fernandez-Hidalgo N, Carreras E, Suy A. Pre-eclampsia-like syndrome induced by severe COVID-19: a prospective observational study. BJOG Int J Obstet Gynaecol. 2020; https://doi.org/10.1111/1471-0528.16339.

42. Zitiello A, Grant GE, Ben Ali N, Feki A. Thrombocytopaenia in pregnancy: the importance of differential diagnosis during the COVID-19 pandemic. J Matern-Fetal Neonatal Med Off J Eur Assoc Perinat Med Fed Asia Ocean Perinat Soc Int Soc Perinat Obstet. 2020:1–3. https://doi.org/10.1080/14767058.2020.1786527.

43. Mullins E, Evans D, Viner RM, O'Brien P, Morris E. Coronavirus in pregnancy and delivery: rapid review. Ultrasound Obstet Gynecol Off J Int Soc Ultrasound Obstet Gynecol. 2020;55:586–92. https://doi.org/10.1002/uog.22014.

44. Clinical findings and disease severity in hospitalized pregnant women with coronavirus disease 2019 (COVID-19). https://pubmed.ncbi.nlm.nih.gov/32433453/. Accessed 15 Aug 2020

45. Knight M, Bunch K, Vousden N, Morris E, Simpson N, Gale C, O'Brien P, Quigley M, Brocklehurst P, Kurinczuk JJ, UK Obstetric Surveillance System SARS-CoV-2 Infection in Pregnancy Collaborative Group. Characteristics and outcomes of pregnant women admitted to hospital with confirmed SARS-CoV-2 infection in UK: national population-based cohort study. BMJ. 2020;369:m2107. https://doi.org/10.1136/bmj.m2107.

46. Hantoushzadeh S, Shamshirsaz AA, Aleyasin A, Seferovic MD, Aski SK, Arian SE, Pooransari P, Ghotbizadeh F, Aalipour S, Soleimani Z, Naemi M, Molaei B, Ahangari R, Salehi M, Oskoei AD, Pirozan P, Darkhaneh RF, Laki MG, Farani AK, Atrak S, Miri MM, Kouchek M, Shojaei S, Hadavand F, Keikha F, Hosseini MS, Borna S, Ariana S, Shariat M, Fatemi A, Nouri B, Nekooghadam SM, Aagaard K. Maternal death due to COVID-19. Am J Obstet Gynecol. 2020;223:109.e1–109.e16. https://doi.org/10.1016/j.ajog.2020.04.030.

47. Ahmed I, Azhar A, Eltaweel N, Tan BK. First COVID-19 maternal mortality in the UK associated with thrombotic complications. Br J Haematol. 2020;190:e37–8. https://doi.org/10.1111/bjh.16849.

48. Blitz MJ, Rochelson B, Minkoff H, Meirowitz N, Prasannan L, London V, Rafael TJ, Chakravarthy S, Bracero LA, Wasden SW, Pachtman Shetty SL, Santandreu O, Chervenak FA, Schwartz BM, Nimaroff M. Maternal mortality among women with coronavirus disease 2019 admitted to the intensive care unit. Am J Obstet Gynecol. 2020; https://doi.org/10.1016/j.ajog.2020.06.020.

49. Takemoto MLS, Menezes M d O, Andreucci CB, Nakamura-Pereira M, Amorim MMR, Katz L, Knobel R. The tragedy of COVID-19 in Brazil: 124 maternal deaths and counting. Int J Gynaecol Obstet Off Organ Int Fed Gynaecol Obstet. 2020; https://doi.org/10.1002/ijgo.13300.

50. Weekly COVID-19 Pregnancy Data www.cdc.gov. Accessed 11 Aug 2020.

51. Elshafeey F, Magdi R, Hindi N, Elshebiny M, Farrag N, Mahdy S, Sabbour M, Gebril S, Nasser M, Kamel M, Amir A, Maher Emara M, Nabhan A. A systematic scoping review of COVID-19 during pregnancy and childbirth. Int J Gynaecol Obstet Off Organ Int Fed Gynaecol Obstet. 2020;150:47–52. https://doi.org/10.1002/ijgo.13182.

52. Coronavirus disease 2019 in pregnant women: a report based on 116 cases. https://pubmed. ncbi.nlm.nih.gov/32335053/. Accessed 15 Aug 2020

53. Li J, Wang Y, Zeng Y, Song T, Pan X, Jia M, He F, Hou L, Li B, He S, Chen D. Critically ill pregnant patient with COVID-19 and neonatal death within two hours of birth. Int J Gynaecol Obstet Off Organ Int Fed Gynaecol Obstet. 2020;150:126–8. https://doi.org/10.1002/ ijgo.13189.

54. Kotlyar A, Grechukhina O, Chen A, Popkhadze S, Grimshaw A, Tal O, Taylor HS, Tal R. Vertical transmission of COVID-19: a systematic review and meta-analysis. Am J Obstet Gynecol. 2020; https://doi.org/10.1016/j.ajog.2020.07.049.

55. Shah PS, Diambomba Y, Acharya G, Morris SK, Bitnun A. Classification system and case definition for SARS-CoV-2 infection in pregnant women, fetuses, and neonates. Acta Obstet Gynecol Scand. 2020;99:565–8. https://doi.org/10.1111/aogs.13870.

56. Vivanti AJ, Vauloup-Fellous C, Prevot S, Zupan V, Suffee C, Do Cao J, Benachi A, De Luca D. Transplacental transmission of SARS-CoV-2 infection. Nat Commun. 2020;11:3572. https://doi.org/10.1038/s41467-020-17436-6.

57. Detection of SARS-COV-2 in placental and fetal membrane samples. https://pubmed.ncbi. nlm.nih.gov/32391518/. Accessed 15 Aug 2020.

58. Patanè L, Morotti D, Giunta MR, Sigismondi C, Piccoli MG, Frigerio L, Mangili G, Arosio M, Cornolti G. Vertical transmission of COVID-19: SARS-CoV-2 RNA on the fetal side of the placenta in pregnancies with COVID-19 positive mothers and neonates at birth. Am J Obstet Gynecol MFM. 2020:100145. https://doi.org/10.1016/j.ajogmf.2020.100145.

59. Wang W, Xu Y, Gao R, Lu R, Han K, Wu G, Tan W. Detection of SARS-CoV-2 in different types of clinical specimens. JAMA. 2020; https://doi.org/10.1001/jama.2020.3786.

60. Pique-Regi R, Romero R, Tarca AL, Luca F, Xu Y, Alazizi A, Leng Y, Hsu C-D, Gomez-Lopez N. Does the human placenta express the canonical cell entry mediators for SARS-CoV-2? eLife. 2020;9 https://doi.org/10.7554/eLife.58716.

61. Hecht JL, Quade B, Deshpande V, Mino-Kenudson M, Ting DT, Desai N, Dygulska B, Heyman T, Salafia C, Shen D, Bates SV, Roberts DJ. SARS-CoV-2 can infect the placenta and is not associated with specific placental histopathology: a series of 19 placentas from COVID-19-positive mothers. Mod Pathol Off J U S Can Acad Pathol Inc. 2020; https://doi. org/10.1038/s41379-020-0639-4.

62. Walker KF, O'Donoghue K, Grace N, Dorling J, Comeau JL, Li W, Thornton JG. Maternal transmission of SARS-COV-2 to the neonate, and possible routes for such transmission: a systematic review and critical analysis. BJOG Int J Obstet Gynaecol. 2020; https://doi. org/10.1111/1471-0528.16362.

63. Qiu L, Liu X, Xiao M, Xie J, Cao W, Liu Z, Morse A, Xie Y, Li T, Zhu L. SARS-CoV-2 is not detectable in the vaginal fluid of women with severe COVID-19 infection. Clin Infect Dis Off Publ Infect Dis Soc Am. 2020;71:813–7. https://doi.org/10.1093/cid/ciaa375.

64. Chen H, Guo J, Wang C, Luo F, Yu X, Zhang W, Li J, Zhao D, Xu D, Gong Q, Liao J, Yang H, Hou W, Zhang Y. Clinical characteristics and intrauterine vertical transmission potential of COVID-19 infection in nine pregnant women: a retrospective review of medical records. Lancet Lond Engl. 2020;395:809–15. https://doi.org/10.1016/S0140-6736(20)30360-3.

65. https://smfm.org

66. Centers for disease control and prevention. interim infection prevention and control recommendations for healthcare personnel during the coronavirus disease 2019 (COVID-19) pandemic. https://www.cdc.gov/coronavirus/2019-ncov/hcp/infection-control-recommendations.html. Accessed 14 July 2020.

67. Interim considerations for infection prevention and control of coronavirus disease 2019 (COVID-19) in inpatient obstetric healthcare settings. https://www.cdc.gov/coronavirus/2019-ncov/hcp/inpatient-obstetric-healthcare-guidance.html. Accessed 09 April 2020.

68. Breslin N, Baptiste C, Miller R, Fuchs K, Goffman D, Gyamfi-Bannerman C, D'Alton M. Coronavirus disease 2019 in pregnancy: early lessons. Am J Obstet Gynecol MFM. 2020;2:100111. https://doi.org/10.1016/j.ajogmf.2020.100111.

69. Berghella V. Coronavirus guidance—from AJOG MFM. NOW!: Protection for obstetrical providers and patients . https://els-jbs-prod-cdn.jbs.elsevierhealth.com/pb/assets/raw/Health%20Advance/journals/ymob/Proetection_Ob_Prov_Pts-1584979215463.pdf. Accessed 31 March 2020.
70. www.ACOG.org. Accessed 02 July 2020.
71. World Health Organization (WHO). Clinical management of severe acute respiratory infection (SARI) when COVID-19 disease is suspected interim guidance 27 May 2020.
72. Tolcher MC, McKinney JR, Eppes CS, Muigai D, Shamshirsaz A, Guntupalli KK, Nates JL. Prone positioning for pregnant women with hypoxemia due to coronavirus disease 2019 (COVID-19). Obstet Gynecol. 2020;136:259–61. https://doi.org/10.1097/AOG.0000000000004012.
73. Pacheco LD, Saad A. Ventilator management in critical illness. In: Phelan JP, Pacheco LD, Foley MR, et al., editors. Critical care obstetrics. 6th ed. Wiley-Blackwell; 2018.
74. Webster CM, Smith KA, Manuck TA. Extracorporeal membrane oxygenation in pregnant and postpartum women: a ten-year case series. Am J Obstet Gynecol MFM:20202100108.
75. Thachil J, Tang N, Gando S, Falanga A, Cattaneo M, Levi M, Clark C, Iba T. ISTH interim guidance on recognition and management of coagulopathy in COVID-19. J Thromb Haemost JTH. 2020;18:1023–6. https://doi.org/10.1111/jth.14810.
76. American Society of Hematology. COVID-19 and VTE/anticoagulation: frequently asked questions. https://www.hematology.org/covid-19/covid-19-and-vte-anticoagulation. Accessed 24 April 2020.
77. Society of Critical Care Medicine. COVID-19 guidelines. https://www.sccm.org/SurvivingSepsisCampaign/Guidelines/COVID-19. Accessed 24 April 2020.
78. Public health emergency SOLIDARITY trial of treatments for COVID-19 infection in hospitalized patients. http://www.isrctn.com/ISRCTN83971151. Accessed 20 July 2020.
79. RECOVERY. Randomised evaluation of COVID-19 therapy. https://www.recoverytrial.net/. Accessed 20 July 2020.
80. Wang M, Cao R, Zhang L, Yang X, Liu J, Xu M, Shi Z, Hu Z, Zhong W, Xiao G. Remdesivir and chloroquine effectively inhibit the recently emerged novel coronavirus (2019-nCoV) in vitro. Cell Res. 2020;30:269–71. https://doi.org/10.1038/s41422-020-0282-0.
81. Sheahan TP, Sims AC, Graham RL, Menachery VD, Gralinski LE, Case JB, Leist SR, Pyrc K, Feng JY, Trantcheva I, Bannister R, Park Y, Babusis D, Clarke MO, Mackman RL, Spahn JE, Palmiotti CA, Siegel D, Ray AS, Cihlar T, Jordan R, Denison MR, Baric RS. Broad-spectrum antiviral GS-5734 inhibits both epidemic and zoonotic coronaviruses. Sci Transl Med. 2017;9 https://doi.org/10.1126/scitranslmed.aal3653.
82. Mulangu S, Dodd LE, Davey RT, Tshiani Mbaya O, Proschan M, Mukai D, Lusakibanza Manzo M, Nzolo D, Tshomba Oloma A, Ibanda A, Ali R, Coulibaly S, Levine AC, Grais R, Diaz J, Lane HC, Muyembe-Tamfum J-J, PALM Writing Group, Sivahera B, Camara M, Kojan R, Walker R, Dighero-Kemp B, Cao H, Mukumbayi P, Mbala-Kingebeni P, Ahuka S, Albert S, Bonnett T, Crozier I, Duvenhage M, Proffitt C, Teitelbaum M, Moench T, Aboulhab J, Barrett K, Cahill K, Cone K, Eckes R, Hensley L, Herpin B, Higgs E, Ledgerwood J, Pierson J, Smolski's M, Sow Y, Tierney J, Sivapalasingam S, Holman W, Gettinger N, Vallée D, Nordwall J, PALM Consortium Study Team. A randomized, controlled trial of ebola virus disease therapeutics. N Engl J Med. 2019;381:2293–303. https://doi.org/10.1056/NEJMoa1910993.
83. Lacroix I, Bénévent J, Damase-Michel C. Chloroquine and hydroxychloroquine during pregnancy: what do we know? Therapie. 2020; https://doi.org/10.1016/j.therap.2020.05.004.
84. Grisolia G, Franchini M, Glingani C, et al. Convalescent plasma for COVID-19 in pregnancy: a case report and review. Am J Obstet Gynecol MFM. 2020;
85. Zhang B, Liu S, Tan T, Huang W, Dong Y, Chen L, Chen Q, Zhang L, Zhong Q, Zhang X, Zou Y, Zhang S. Treatment with convalescent plasma for critically ill patients with severe acute respiratory syndrome coronavirus 2 infection. Chest. 2020;158:e9–e13. https://doi.org/10.1016/j.chest.2020.03.039.

86. Anderson J, Schauer J, Bryant S, Graves CR. The use of convalescent plasma therapy and remdesivir in the successful management of a critically ill obstetric patient with novel coronavirus 2019 infection: a case report. Case Rep. Womens Health. 2020:e00221. https://doi.org/10.1016/j.crwh.2020.e00221.

87. Day M. Covid-19: ibuprofen should not be used for managing symptoms, say doctors and scientists. BMJ. 2020;368:m1086. https://doi.org/10.1136/bmj.m1086.

88. Jeong HE, Lee H, Shin HJ, Choe YJ, Filion KB, Shin J-Y. Association between NSAIDs use and adverse clinical outcomes among adults hospitalized with COVID-19 in South Korea: A nationwide study. Clin Infect Dis Off Publ Infect Dis Soc Am. 2020; https://doi.org/10.1093/cid/ciaa1056.

89. Rinott E, Kozer E, Shapira Y, Bar-Haim A, Youngster I. Ibuprofen use and clinical outcomes in COVID-19 patients. Clin Microbiol Infect Off Publ Eur Soc Clin Microbiol Infect Dis. 2020; https://doi.org/10.1016/j.cmi.2020.06.003.

90. European Medicines Agency. EMA gives advice on the use of nonsteroidal anti-inflammatories for COVID-19. https://www.ema.europa.eu/en/news/ema-gives-advice-use-non-steroidal-anti-inflammatories-covid-19. Accessed 19 March 2020.

91. Shanes ED, Mithal LB, Otero S, Azad HA, Miller ES, Goldstein JA. Placental pathology in COVID-19. Am J Clin Pathol. 2020;154:23–32. https://doi.org/10.1093/ajcp/aqaa089.

92. Prabhu M, Cagino K, Matthews KC, Friedlander RL, Glynn SM, Kubiak JM, Yang YJ, Zhao Z, Baergen RN, DiPace JI, Razavi AS, Skupski DW, Snyder JR, Singh HK, Kalish RB, Oxford CM, Riley LE. Pregnancy and postpartum outcomes in a universally tested population for SARS-CoV-2 in New York City: a prospective cohort study. BJOG Int J Obstet Gynaecol. 2020; https://doi.org/10.1111/1471-0528.16403.

93. Smithgall MC, Liu-Jarin X, Hamele-Bena D, Cimic A, Mourad M, Debelenko L, Chen X. Third trimester placentas of SARS-CoV-2-positive women: histomorphology, including viral immunohistochemistry and in situ hybridization. Histopathology. 2020; https://doi.org/10.1111/his.14215.

94. Wong SF, Chow KM, Leung TN, Ng WF, Ng TK, Shek CC, Ng PC, Lam PWY, Ho LC, To WWK, Lai ST, Yan WW, Tan PYH. Pregnancy and perinatal outcomes of women with severe acute respiratory syndrome. Am J Obstet Gynecol. 2004;191:292–7. https://doi.org/10.1016/j.ajog.2003.11.019.

95. Ng WF, Wong SF, Lam A, Mak YF, Yao H, Lee KC, Chow KM, Yu WC, Ho LC. The placentas of patients with severe acute respiratory syndrome: a pathophysiological evaluation. Pathology (Phila). 2006;38:210–8. https://doi.org/10.1080/00313020600696280.

96. CDC. Care for newborns. https://www.cdc.gov/coronavirus/2019-ncov/hcp/caring-for-newborns.html Accessed 04 August 2020.

97. Chen D, Yang H, Cao Y, Cheng W, Duan T, Fan C, Fan S, Feng L, Gao Y, He F, He J, Hu Y, Jiang Y, Li Y, Li J, Li X, Li X, Lin K, Liu C, Liu J, Liu X, Pan X, Pang Q, Pu M, Qi H, Shi C, Sun Y, Sun J, Wang X, Wang Y, Wang Z, Wang Z, Wang C, Wu S, Xin H, Yan J, Zhao Y, Zheng J, Zhou Y, Zou L, Zeng Y, Zhang Y, Guan X. Expert consensus for managing pregnant women and neonates born to mothers with suspected or confirmed novel coronavirus (COVID-19) infection. Int J Gynaecol Obstet Off Organ Int Fed Gynaecol Obstet. 2020;149:130–6. https://doi.org/10.1002/ijgo.13146.

98. Stephens AJ, Barton JR, Bentum N-AA, Blackwell SC, Sibai BM. General guidelines in the management of an obstetrical patient on the labor and delivery unit during the COVID-19 pandemic. Am J Perinatol. 2020;37:829–36. https://doi.org/10.1055/s-0040-1710308.

99. Jamieson DJ, Steinberg JP, Martinello RA, Perl TM, Rasmussen SA. Obstetricians on the coronavirus disease 2019 (COVID-19) front lines and the confusing world of personal protective equipment. Obstet Gynecol. 2020;135:1257–63. https://doi.org/10.1097/AOG.0000000000003919.

100. Boelig RC, Manuck T, Oliver EA, Di Mascio D, Saccone G, Bellussi F, Berghella V. Labor and delivery guidance for COVID-19. Am J Obstet Gynecol MFM. 2020;2:100110. https://doi.org/10.1016/j.ajogmf.2020.100110.

101. Zhang W, Du R-H, Li B, Zheng X-S, Yang X-L, Hu B, Wang Y-Y, Xiao G-F, Yan B, Shi Z-L, Zhou P. Molecular and serological investigation of 2019-nCoV infected patients: implication of multiple shedding routes. Emerg Microbes Infect. 2020;9:386–9. https://doi.org/10.108 0/22221751.2020.1729071.

102. Berghella V. NOW!: protection for obstetrical providers and patients. Am J Obstet Gynecol MFM. 2020:100109. https://doi.org/10.1016/j.ajogmf.2020.100109.

103. Martínez-Perez O, Vouga M, Cruz Melguizo S, Forcen Acebal L, Panchaud A, Muñoz-Chápuli M, Baud D. Association between mode of delivery among pregnant women with COVID-19 and maternal and neonatal outcomes in Spain. JAMA. 2020; https://doi.org/10.1001/jama.2020.10125.

104. Considerations for obstetric anesthesia care related to COVID-19. https://soap.org/education/provider-education/expert-summaries/interim-considerations-for-obstetric-anesthesia-care-related-to-covid19/. Accessed 30 March 2020.

105. Ogawa H, Asakura H. Consideration of tranexamic acid administration to COVID-19 patients. Physiol Rev. 2020;100:1595–6. https://doi.org/10.1152/physrev.00023.2020.

106. Cox JL, Holden JM, Sagovsky R. Detection of postnatal depression. Development of the 10-item Edinburgh postnatal depression scale. Br J Psychiatry J Ment Sci. 1987;150:782–6. https://doi.org/10.1192/bjp.150.6.782.

107. Boelig RC, Saccone G, Bellussi F, Berghella V. MFM guidance for COVID-19. Am J Obstet Gynecol MFM. 2020:100106. https://doi.org/10.1016/j.ajogmf.2020.100106.

108. Immediate psychological responses and associated factors during the initial stage of the 2019 coronavirus disease (COVID-19) epidemic among the general population in China. https://pubmed.ncbi.nlm.nih.gov/32155789/. Accessed 18 Aug 2020.

109. Berthelot N, Lemieux R, Garon-Bissonnette J, Drouin-Maziade C, Martel É, Maziade M. Uptrend in distress and psychiatric symptomatology in pregnant women during the coronavirus disease 2019 pandemic. Acta Obstet Gynecol Scand. 2020;99:848–55. https://doi.org/10.1111/aogs.13925.

110. Wu Y, Zhang C, Liu H, Duan C, Li C, Fan J, Li H, Chen L, Xu H, Li X, Guo Y, Wang Y, Li X, Li J, Zhang T, You Y, Li H, Yang S, Tao X, Xu Y, Lao H, Wen M, Zhou Y, Wang J, Chen Y, Meng D, Zhai J, Ye Y, Zhong Q, Yang X, Zhang D, Zhang J, Wu X, Chen W, Dennis C-L, Huang H-F. Perinatal depressive and anxiety symptoms of pregnant women during the coronavirus disease 2019 outbreak in China. Am J Obstet Gynecol. 2020;223:240.e1–9. https://doi.org/10.1016/j.ajog.2020.05.009.

111. Rothe C, Schunk M, Sothmann P, Bretzel G, Froeschl G, Wallrauch C, Zimmer T, Thiel V, Janke C, Guggemos W, Seilmaier M, Drosten C, Vollmar P, Zwirglmaier K, Zange S, Wölfel R, Hoelscher M. Transmission of 2019-nCoV infection from an asymptomatic contact in Germany. N Engl J Med. 2020;382:970–1. https://doi.org/10.1056/NEJMc2001468.

112. Kupferschmidt K. Study claiming new coronavirus can be transmitted by people without symptoms was flawed. In: Sci. AAAS; 2020. https://www.sciencemag.org/news/2020/02/paper-non-symptomatic-patient-transmitting-coronavirus-wrong. Accessed 6 Aug 2020

113. Yu P, Zhu J, Zhang Z, Han Y. A familial cluster of infection associated with the 2019 novel coronavirus indicating possible person-to-person transmission during the incubation period. J Infect Dis. 2020;221:1757–61. https://doi.org/10.1093/infdis/jiaa077.

114. Bai Y, Yao L, Wei T, Tian F, Jin D-Y, Chen L, Wang M. Presumed asymptomatic carrier transmission of COVID-19. JAMA. 2020; https://doi.org/10.1001/jama.2020.2565.

115. Hu Z, Song C, Xu C, Jin G, Chen Y, Xu X, Ma H, Chen W, Lin Y, Zheng Y, Wang J, Hu Z, Yi Y, Shen H. Clinical characteristics of 24 asymptomatic infections with COVID-19 screened among close contacts in Nanjing, China. Sci China Life Sci. 2020;63:706–11. https://doi.org/10.1007/s11427-020-1661-4.

116. Qian G, Yang N, Ma AHY, Wang L, Li G, Chen X, Chen X. COVID-19 transmission within a family cluster by presymptomatic carriers in China. Clin Infect Dis Off Publ Infect Dis Soc Am. 2020;71:861–2. https://doi.org/10.1093/cid/ciaa316.

117. He X, Lau EHY, Wu P, Deng X, Wang J, Hao X, Lau YC, Wong JY, Guan Y, Tan X, Mo X, Chen Y, Liao B, Chen W, Hu F, Zhang Q, Zhong M, Wu Y, Zhao L, Zhang F, Cowling BJ, Li

F, Leung GM. Temporal dynamics in viral shedding and transmissibility of COVID-19. Nat Med. 2020;26:672–5. https://doi.org/10.1038/s41591-020-0869-5.
118. United States Centers for Disease Control and Prevention. Coronavirus disease 2019 (COVID-19). Help stop the spread of COVID-19 in children. Tips to protect children during a COVID-19 outbreak. https://www.cdc.gov/coronavirus/2019-ncov/daily-life-coping/children/protect-children.html. Accessed 29 July 2020.
119. RCOG. COVID-19 virus infection and pregnancy. Occupational health advice for employers and pregnant women during the COVID-19 pandemic. https://www.rcog.org.uk/en/guidelines-research-services/guidelines/coronavirus-pregnancy/covid-19-virus-infection-and-pregnancy.
120. Liu W, Wang J, Li W, Zhou Z, Liu S, Rong Z. Clinical characteristics of 19 neonates born to mothers with COVID-19. Front Med. 2020;14:193–8. https://doi.org/10.1007/s11684-020-0772-y.
121. WHO. Breastfeeding and COVID-19. Scientific brief. 23 June 2020. https://www.who.int/publications/i/item/10665332639. Accessed 25 June 2020.
122. Salvatore CM, Han J-Y, Acker KP, Tiwari P, Jin J, Brandler M, Cangemi C, Gordon L, Parow A, DiPace J, DeLaMora P. Neonatal management and outcomes during the COVID-19 pandemic: an observation cohort study. Lancet Child Adolesc Health. 2020; https://doi.org/10.1016/S2352-4642(20)30235-2.

Head and Neck Trauma During Pregnancy and the Postpartum Period

25

Hacer Baran, Ömer Hızlı, and Gabriela Kopacheva-Barsova

25.1 Introduction

Trauma is the most common cause of non-obstetric deaths during pregnancy, and it affects 8% of all pregnant women. The post-traumatic mortality rate of pregnant women is twice as that of non-pregnant women [1, 2]. The most common trauma type is blunt trauma (69%), while penetrating traumas are least common (1.5%) in pregnant women [3]. Motor vehicle accidents are the most common cause of trauma-related deaths in pregnant women, with falling, domestic violence, burns, assault and stabbing being the other causes [4, 5].

Regardless of the aetiology of trauma, certain pearl points need to be considered in the management of trauma during pregnancy to eliminate or minimise the morbidity and mortality of both the baby and the mother. The physicians dealing this condition should be aware of the fact they are responsible for the lives of two people and that the best treatment approach for the foetus is to treat the mother. However, trauma management in pregnancy and in the early postpartum period is often challenging and depends on anatomical and physiological changes. Care should be

H. Baran (✉)
Department of Otolaryngology—Head and Neck Surgery, Health Sciences University, Faculty of Medicine, İstanbul Dr. Lütfi Kırdar Research and Training Hospital, İstanbul, Turkey
e-mail: baranhacer@hotmail.com

Ö. Hızlı
Department of Otolaryngology—Head and Neck Surgery, Giresun Research and Training Hospital, Giresun, Turkey
e-mail: hizliomer@gmail.com

G. Kopacheva-Barsova
Cyril and Methodius University of Skopje, Faculty of Medicine, Skopje, Republic of Macedonia

C. Cingi et al. (eds.), *ENT Diseases: Diagnosis and Treatment during Pregnancy and Lactation*, https://doi.org/10.1007/978-3-031-05303-0_25

taken during the postpartum period as the administration of contrast agents and drugs as part of post-traumatic interventions may affect the child through breast milk [6, 7].

## 25.2	Pregnancy-Related Changes to be Monitored

During pregnancy, an increase in the total blood volume and cardiac output and a decrease in the systemic vascular resistance are observed in the cardiovascular system. A 40%–50% increase in the total blood volume is seen, which is accompanied by a hike of only around 30% in the red blood cells (RBCs), resulting in dilutional anaemia [8, 9]. A tolerance to haemorrhagic shock may develop as a result of the increased blood volume and RBCs, and symptoms such as tachycardia and hypotension that occur before the shock can only be observed after a 35% loss in the total blood volume. If the pregnant woman's blood pressure is <80/40 mmHg, her heart rate is >140 or <50 beats per minute, her respiratory rate is >24 or <10 breaths per minute, or the foetal heart rate is >160 or <110 beats per minute, adequate care should be taken as there is a high risk of maternal or foetal morbidity and mortality. With regard to the circulatory system, a decrease in the venous return as a result of the compression of the inferior vena cava by the uterus in the supine position during the second and third trimesters is often seen in pregnant women. Consequently, hypotension may develop, which is accompanied by dizziness, sweating and nausea (supine hypotension syndrome). To prevent this syndrome, the woman should be placed in the left lateral decubitus position by manually relocating the uterus to the left side. By doing so, increased cardiac output is achieved and hypotension is prevented. The physicians should ensure that the cervical spine remains immobile in the trauma patients during this manoeuvre [10–12].

During and after pregnancy, various physiological changes related to the respiratory system are observed. The upper respiratory tract mucosa, tongue and soft palate become more oedematous and fragile. As the pregnancy progresses, the incidence of Mallampati Class III airway increases. The occurrence of nasal congestion and epistaxis increases. Furthermore, a 10%–15% hike in oxygen consumption occurs. There are possibilities for hyperventilation and respiratory alkalosis. In addition, with the enlargement of the uterus, the diaphragm shifts upwards and the functional residual capacity decreases by 20% while the tidal volume increases by 40%. While the pregnant women become more susceptible to hypoxia, they cannot compensate for acidosis. To prevent hypoxia in pregnant patients, oxygenation with 100% oxygen should be performed for 3–5 min before intubation. In case of a respiratory distress, early intubation should not be avoided. Mask ventilation should be avoided because of the risk of aspiration [13–15].

During pregnancy, leucocyte count, erythrocyte sedimentation rate and most of the coagulation factors are elevated. Dilutional anaemia is observed during pregnancy as mentioned above. The increase in the level of all coagulation factors except

XI and XIII is responsible for the hyper-coagulopathy seen during pregnancy and the resulting thromboembolic events [9, 15, 16]. In pregnant women, low molecular weight heparin is the preferred prophylactic agent before surgery because it does not cross the placenta and is unlikely to cause spontaneous bleeding [15, 17]. Supine position should be avoided because of the heightened venous stasis and clot formation caused by vena cava pressure [15].

The surge in progesterone level during pregnancy lowers the oesophageal tone as well as stomach and intestinal motility. During the last two trimesters, particularly from the 36th week, the risk of reflux oesophagitis becomes apparent owing to the decrease in the oesophageal tone. Simultaneously, the intensified intra-gastric pressure exerted by the expanding foetus increases the development of reflux with a slow gastric ejaculation period. During general anaesthesia, a nasogastric tube should be inserted to prevent stomach aspiration [15].

25.3 Assessment of Trauma

Head and neck trauma in pregnant women should be managed by a multidisciplinary team comprising an otolaryngologist, a maxillofacial surgeon, a neurosurgeon, an obstetrician, a paediatrician, an anaesthesiologist, and a radiologist. During the evaluation of a pregnant or postpartum trauma patient, the lateral decubitus position should initially be provided; subsequently, a rapid primary assessment should be performed to identify and manage the life-threatening conditions of the mother. After the evaluation of the foetal situation, other essential evaluations pertaining to the secondary trauma should be performed and a treatment plan should be chalked-out [18, 19].

25.3.1 Primary Evaluation

A rapid evaluation is required to identify and effectively manage the life-threatening conditions. Owing to the changes in plasma volume observed in pregnancy, symptoms such as tachycardia or hypotension may not be noted until the blood loss is >35%. Since these conditions affect placental perfusion, vasopressor drugs (such as norepinephrine and phenylephrine) should be administered in case of a response to the appropriate volume loading with crystalloid. Nevertheless, if necessary, resuscitation drugs could be administered in the same doses as recommended for a non-pregnant patient, in line with the life-supporting guidelines. Pregnant women are prone to hypoxia because of the respiratory changes occurring in pregnancy; therefore, oxygen support should be provided. Since the risk of aspiration is enhanced due to gastrointestinal tract changes, a nasogastric tube should be introduced for decompression [10–18].

25.3.2 Evaluation of Foetal Condition

Once the initial evaluation is completed and the maternal haemodynamics are stabilised, foetal monitoring should be immediately initiated. Information about obstetric history, including gestational age, foetal maturity, date of birth and the presence of other complications during pregnancy should be obtained. The condition of the foetus can be effectively monitored using the ultrasound (USG), Doppler or Pinard horn. Foetal arrhythmia is often the first sign of impairment of maternal haemodynamics. In the event of a cardiac arrest occurring in the pregnant woman, a Caesarean section can be performed by resuscitation if the foetus is older than 24 gestational weeks. Perimortem Caesarean delivery of living foetuses may also be successful if performed within 4 minutes of the maternal cardiac arrest [1, 18, 20, 21].

25.3.3 Secondary Evaluation

After the evaluation of the pregnant woman and the foetus, examinations regarding the secondary trauma should be performed and a treatment plan should be created. The effect of imaging during pregnancy on foetal development is controversial. However, if these tests are clinically required, the indications are the same as for non-pregnant trauma patients and should not be delayed. Computed tomography scans can identify maternal and foetal injuries, but the evaluation must be performed only after the haemodynamic stabilisation of the patient. In trauma patients, the optimal treatment algorithm should be designed after physical examination, imaging and radiological evaluation [18].

25.3.4 Radiological Evaluation

Evaluation of trauma by imaging is the first step in fracture management. Nonetheless, selecting the appropriate radiological evaluation method is crucial. In this regard, since the head and neck area is relatively farther away from the foetus, performing radiological examinations of this region by protecting the abdominal area is possible [15, 22].

The physicians should pay attention to several issues such as radiation exposure, contrast agent use and magnetic field exposure while choosing the imaging method. The effects of radiation on the foetus vary depending on the radiation dose and the stage of pregnancy. While the foetal radiation dose is lower in case of head, neck and extremity injuries, it is higher in abdominal and pelvic injuries [22]. If the radiation exposure is <50 mGy, the risks of foetal anomaly and foetal loss are low. Considering the very low absorption rate, breastfeeding is allowed after contrast administration [22].

Since no definite data on teratogenic effects and acoustic trauma related to magnetic resonance imaging (MRI) are available for pregnant patients, MRI during pregnancy and lactation has not been contraindicated. However, as the procedure increases the tissue temperature, an MRI under 1.5 Tesla should be preferred [23]. Considering the uncertainty of the effects of gadolinium-based contrast agents on the foetus, they are recommended only if the benefits clearly outweigh the risks [22, 24].

The teratogenic effects of USG during pregnancy have not been established; hence, this technique may be the first choice [22].

25.4 Choosing the Anaesthetic Method

25.4.1 General Anaesthesia (GA)

GA is generally not recommended in the first and third trimesters because of the potential foetal damage caused by anaesthetic anoxia [25]. In addition, intubation may be difficult depending on the fragile and oedematous upper respiratory tract mucosa. Supine position should be avoided, and lateral decubitus position should be preferred [18]. Thiopental and propofol are safe induction agents. Besides, halothane, isoflurane, enflurane and desflurane are safe in pregnancy when used at appropriate doses. However, surgery under GA during pregnancy and the postpartum period should be performed only when absolutely warranted. An indication of surgical intervention should be evaluated based on the trimester. In the first trimester, the operation should be planned only if the mother is under a high risk of mortality or morbidity. However, if the risk is minimal or absent, the procedure can be postponed to a later period of the pregnancy. Elective surgeries should be postponed to the postpartum period, if possible. Emergency surgeries should be performed immediately in due consideration of the mother's life being at stake; a multidisciplinary approach, along with an adequate foetal follow-up, is required [1, 3, 18].

25.4.2 Local Anaesthesia (LA)

Since LA is safer than the volatile anaesthetic agents that can be teratogenic, it is preferred for any surgical intervention during the first and third trimesters. According to Donaldson et al., even though the LA agents cross the placental barrier, foetal toxicity has not been demonstrated in humans even at doses above the maximum recommended dose [25, 26]. The safety of LA in a pregnant patient depends on the type and dosage of the agent. Those considered safe in pregnancy belong to pregnancy risk category B [27].

Lidocaine is safe in all three trimesters of pregnancy. Bupivacaine belongs to category C, which poses a risk to the foetus [18]. During pregnancy, physiological changes such as increased vascular permeability and volume lead to a predisposition of LA overdose. Previous studies have reported that pregnancy is associated with an increase in unbound LA molecules, which predisposes the foetus to toxicity [28]. Hence, decreasing the dose of the LA agent is considered a safe measure. The maximum lidocaine dose with 1:100,000 epinephrine is 7.7 mg/kg in a non-pregnant woman but 4.4 mg/kg in a pregnant woman [18].

25.5 Choice of Treatment

Since some medications are known to cause miscarriage, teratogenicity and low birth weight in the foetus, any medication should be carefully prescribed to a pregnant woman [15, 29].

25.5.1 Analgesics

Acetaminophen is the most common analgesic agent used in pregnancy because it is safe and effective. It is known as not being associated with an increased risk of congenital anomalies [30]. Non-steroidal anti-inflammatory drugs (NSAIDs) should be avoided since they inhibit the synthesis of prostaglandins essential for endometrial integrity. The use of NSAIDs in the last trimester may cause early closure of the ductus arteriosus and delayed delivery [15, 31].

25.5.2 Antibiotics

Penicillin and cephalosporins are the most common antibiotics prescribed in head and neck infections, and these drugs have been found to be safe in pregnancy. Macrolides, such as erythromycin and clindamycin, may be prescribed for patients with penicillin allergy [15]. In >17.000 foetuses exposed to metronidazole in the first trimester, no increase in the rate of congenital abnormalities was observed. Metronidazole can be used in case of maxillofacial infections [32].

25.5.3 Corticosteroids

Corticosteroids are used to alleviate inflammation in the head and neck region [15]. Prednisone and prednisolone were reported as not causing serious adverse effects on the foetus when used in pregnant women. Triamcinolone and beclomethasone are associated with foetal defects. These drugs are locally safe; however, their systemic use can damage the foetus and should therefore be avoided in pregnancy. Pregnancy-specific complications such as early membrane rupture, hypertension and gestational diabetes mellitus are associated with steroid use. American College of Obstetricians and Gynecologists Committee of Obstetricians and Gynecologists stated that a single dose of corticosteroids can be given to all women between 24 and 34 weeks of pregnancy. There exists a risk of preterm birth within 7 days of administration of the drug [15, 33].

25.6 Conclusion

During pregnancy and lactation, the trauma patients should be evaluated by a multidisciplinary team owing to the physiological changes, and necessary interventions should be carried out. Since the condition of the mother affects the foetus too, extra caution should be exercised. Nonetheless, it should not be forgotten that the priority is to save the life of the mother. The necessary surgical interventions, especially in case of maxillofacial traumas, can be postponed and electively performed as long as the patient's condition allows it. The preferred diagnostic and treatment methods and the surgical interventions to be applied should be decided by taking into account the pregnancy or lactation status of the patient.

Although there is no generally accepted directive regarding the approach to head and neck trauma in pregnancy and in the postpartum period, the inference from case-based evaluations is that pregnancy status should be ignored in case of emergency surgical interventions, and saving the mother's life should be prioritised. Elective surgeries should be postponed until after delivery, if possible. Surgical interventions that cannot be postponed, on the other hand, should be performed with the least harm to the foetus after appropriate evaluations.

References

1. Huls CK, Detlefs C. Trauma in pregnancy. Semin Perinatol. 2018;42(1):13–20. https://doi.org/10.1053/j.semperi.2017.11.004.
2. Deshpande NA, Kucirka LM, Smith RN, Oxford CM. Pregnant trauma victims experience nearly 2-fold higher mortality compared to their nonpregnant counterparts. Am J Obstet Gynecol. 2017;217(5):590.e1–9. https://doi.org/10.1016/j.ajog.2017.08.004.
3. Petrone P, Jiménez-Morillas P, Axelrad A, Marini CP. Traumatic injuries to the pregnant patient: a critical literature review. Eur J Trauma Emerg Surg. 2019;45(3):383–92. https://doi.org/10.1007/s00068-017-0839-x.
4. Fischer PE, Zarzaur BL, Fabian TC, Magnotti LJ, Croce MA. Minor trauma is an unrecognized contributor to poor fetal outcomes: a population-based study of 78,552 pregnancies. J Trauma. 2011;71(1):90–3. https://doi.org/10.1097/TA.0b013e31821cb600.
5. Weiss HB, Songer TJ, Fabio A. Fetal deaths related to maternal injury. JAMA. 2001;286(15):1863–8. https://doi.org/10.1001/jama.286.15.1863.
6. Mathur S, Pillenahalli Maheshwarappa R, Fouladirad S, et al. Emergency Imaging in Pregnancy and Lactation [Formula: see text]. Can Assoc Radiol J. 2020;71(3):396–402. https://doi.org/10.1177/0846537120906482.
7. Sakamoto J, Michels C, Eisfelder B, Joshi N. Trauma in Pregnancy. Emerg Med Clin North Am. 2019;37(2):317–38. https://doi.org/10.1016/j.emc.2019.01.009.
8. Duvekot JJ, Peeters LL. Renal hemodynamics and volume homeostasis in pregnancy. Obstet Gynecol Surv. 1994;49(12):830–9. https://doi.org/10.1097/00006254-199412000-00007.
9. Suresh L, Radfar L. Pregnancy and lactation. Oral Surg Oral Med Oral Pathol Oral Radiol Endod. 2004;97(6):672–82. https://doi.org/10.1016/j.tripleo.2004.02.002.
10. Petrone P, Marini CP. Trauma in pregnant patients. Curr Probl Surg. 2015;52(8):330–51. https://doi.org/10.1067/j.cpsurg.2015.07.001.
11. Mendez-Figueroa H, Dahlke JD, Vrees RA, Rouse DJ. Trauma in pregnancy: an updated systematic review. Am J Obstet Gynecol. 2013;209(1):1–10. https://doi.org/10.1016/j.ajog.2013.01.021.

12. Petrone P, Asensio JA. Trauma in pregnancy: assessment and treatment. Scand J Surg. 2006;95(1):4–10. https://doi.org/10.1177/145749690609500102.
13. Gordon MC. Maternal physiology in pregnancy. In: Gabbe SG, Niebyl JR, Simpson J, editors. Obstetrics: normal and problem pregnancies. 4th ed. New York: Churchill Livingstone; 2002.
14. Thornburg KL, Jacobson SL, Giraud GD, Morton MJ. Hemodynamic changes in pregnancy. Semin Perinatol. 2000;24(1):11–4. https://doi.org/10.1016/s0146-0005(00)80047-6.
15. Shetty L, Shete A, Gupta AA, Kheur S. Pregnant oral and maxillofacial patient—catch 22 situation. Dentistry. 2015;5:329. https://doi.org/10.4172/2161-1122.1000329.
16. Hamaoui E, Hamaoui M. Nutritional assessment and support during pregnancy. Gastroenterol Clin North Am. 2003;32(1):59–121., v. https://doi.org/10.1016/s0889-8553(02)00132-2.
17. Turner M, Aziz SR. Management of the pregnant oral and maxillofacial surgery patient. J Oral Maxillofac Surg. 2002;60(12):1479–88. https://doi.org/10.1053/joms.2002.36132.
18. Sridharan G, Panneerselvam E, Ponvel K, Tarun S, Krishna Kumar Raja VB. Maxillofacial trauma in a pregnant patient: contemporary management principles with a case report & review of literature. Chin J Traumatol. 2020;23(2):78–83. https://doi.org/10.1016/j.cjtee.2020.02.003.
19. Zhang M, Alexander AL, Most SP, Li G, Harris OA. Intracranial dislocation of the mandibular condyle: a case report and literature review. World Neurosurg. 2016;86:514.e1–11. https://doi.org/10.1016/j.wneu.2015.09.007.
20. Rose CH, Faksh A, Traynor KD, Cabrera D, Arendt KW, Brost BC. Challenging the 4- to 5-minute rule: from perimortem cesarean to resuscitative hysterotomy. Am J Obstet Gynecol. 2015;213(5):653–6, 653.e1. https://doi.org/10.1016/j.ajog.2015.07.019.
21. Katz VL. Perimortem cesarean delivery: its role in maternal mortality. Semin Perinatol. 2012;36(1):68–72. https://doi.org/10.1053/j.semperi.2011.09.013.
22. Raptis CA, Mellnick VM, Raptis DA, Kitchin D, Fowler KJ, Lubner M, Bhalla S, Menias CO. Imaging of trauma in the pregnant patient. Radiographics. 2014;34(3):748–63. https://doi.org/10.1148/rg.343135090.
23. Committee opinion No. 723: guidelines for diagnostic imaging during pregnancy and lactation. Obstet Gynecol. 2017;130(4):e210–6. https://doi.org/10.1097/AOG.0000000000002355. Erratum in: Obstet Gynecol. 2018 Sep;132(3):786.
24. Pearce C, Martin SR. Trauma and considerations unique to pregnancy. Obstet Gynecol Clin North Am. 2016;43(4):791–808. https://doi.org/10.1016/j.ogc.2016.07.008.
25. Howe GL, editor. Minor oral surgery. 3rd ed. Oxford: John Wright; 1985. p. 29e31.
26. Donaldson M, Goodchild JH. Pregnancy, breast-feeding and drugs used in dentistry. J Am Dent Assoc. 2012;143(8):858–71. https://doi.org/10.14219/jada.archive.2012.0290.
27. Ninan D, editor. Dentistry and the pregnant patient. Batavia, IL: Quintessence Publishing Co Inc; 2018.
28. Rosenberg PH, Veering BT, Urmey WF. Maximum recommended doses of local anesthetics: a multifactorial concept. Reg Anesth Pain Med. 2004;29(6):564–75; discussion 524. https://doi.org/10.1016/j.rapm.2004.08.003.
29. Broe A, Pottegård A, Lamont RF, Jørgensen JS, Damkier P. Increasing use of antibiotics in pregnancy during the period 2000-2010: prevalence, timing, category, and demographics. BJOG. 2014;121(8):988–96. https://doi.org/10.1111/1471-0528.12806.
30. Di Sessa TG, Moretti ML, Khoury A, Pulliam DA, Arheart KL, Sibai BM. Cardiac function in fetuses and newborns exposed to low-dose aspirin during pregnancy. Am J Obstet Gynecol. 1994;171(4):892–900. https://doi.org/10.1016/s0002-9378(94)70056-7.
31. Burtin P, Taddio A, Ariburnu O, Einarson TR, Koren G. Safety of metronidazole in pregnancy: a meta-analysis. Am J Obstet Gynecol. 1995;172(2 Pt 1):525–9. https://doi.org/10.1016/0002-9378(95)90567-7.
32. Committee on Obstetric Practice. ACOG committee opinion: antenatal corticosteroid therapy for fetal maturation. Obstet Gynecol. 2002;99(5 Pt 1):871–3. https://doi.org/10.1016/s0029-7844(02)02023-9.
33. Aramanadka C, Gadicherla S, Shukla A, Kudva A. Facial fracture in pregnancy: case report and review. J Int Oral Health. 2018;10:99–102. https://doi.org/10.4103/jioh.jioh_263_17.

Head and Neck Trauma During Pregnancy and the Postpartum Period: General Overview

Mustafa Salış, Bartu Badak, and Necdet Fatih Yaşar

26.1 Introduction

Trauma is a condition that endangers the lives of both the mother and the fetus. It is one of the leading causes of non-obstetric maternal deaths. It occurs in 6–7% of all pregnancies. Moderate and severe traumas may result in a maternal mortality rate of 46% and a fetal mortality rate of 40%. The most common causes of traumas are: 49% were motor vehicle accidents, 25% falls, 22% assault and gunshot injuries, and 1% burns [1–4].

No matter how traumas occur during pregnancy, some points should not be forgotten in management. The aim is to reduce the morbidity and mortality of the baby together with the mother. The best treatment for the fetus is to treat the mother. However, anatomical and physiological changes during pregnancy can make diagnosis and treatment difficult.

If physiological changes occurring during pregnancy are known, the approach to the patient will be more optimal, and maternal-fetal mortality and morbidity will decrease. In maternal hypoxia, uterine artery perfusion will deteriorate due to contraction in uterine arteries due to catecholamines, and maternal heart rate and blood pressure will become insufficient for fetal nutrition. If we consider the physiological changes that occur during pregnancy:

- The heartbeat is higher than usual, as early decompensation.
- Ventilation and oxygen consumption per minute are high, which are more susceptible to hypoxia.

M. Salış (✉) · B. Badak · N. F. Yaşar
Department of General Surgery, Eskisehir Osmangazi University, Eskisehir, Turkey
e-mail: salismustafa@gmail.com

C. Cingi et al. (eds.), *ENT Diseases: Diagnosis and Treatment during Pregnancy and Lactation*, https://doi.org/10.1007/978-3-031-05303-0_26

True anemia should not be confused with physiological dilutional anemia.

With the enlargement of uterus, the diaphragm rises and the intercostal space required for thoracostomy shifts upward. Because of the compression of the inferior vena cavae by the uterus, the patient should be placed in the left lateral position if there is no contraindication. Thereby the symptoms of hypotension, sweating, and nausea are not confused with other reasons [5]. While the intestines are protected against traumas by the enlarged uterus, the fetus and the bladder are more prone to damage.

- With the increase of uterine blood flow (having a blood flow of 600 mL per minute), the risk of bleeding and retroperitoneal bleeding increases in traumas [5].
- With decreased lung compliance, cardiopulmonary resuscitation will be difficult. Some studies indicate that resuscitation may not be fully effective in the later weeks of pregnancy due to aortocaval compression. Perimortem cesarean performed after unsuccessful resuscitation will decrease fetal mortality in the first 4–5 min [6].
- BUN and creatine values require closer monitoring due to renal increased blood flow.
- Attention should be paid to hydronephrosis, especially on the right, which may develop due to hypomobility in the urinary system. Leukocytosis during pregnancy (6000–16,000 cells/mm^3) is not specific to trauma.

While increasing levels of factor 2,7,8,9,10 create susceptibility to thrombosis during pregnancy, it requires attention after trauma. Fibrinogen levels during pregnancy are >200 mg/dL. The reduction of fibrinogen supports thrombocytopenia DIC. As the cause of gastrointestinal hypomobility and increased intra-abdominal pressure, the risk of aspiration increases during pregnancy.

In the ECG, changes such as temporary ST-T wave changes, the appearance of the Q waveform, and inverted T waves in V1, V2, and V3 can be observed. With all these changes in mind, pregnant patients should be monitored more closely and carefully when exposed to trauma.

26.2 Fetal and Maternal Injury Mechanisms

Head injuries and hemorrhagic shock (splenic rupture and pelvic fracture due to blunt trauma) are the most frequent causes of death in pregnant women presenting with trauma. Minor traumas may result in fetal losses, stillbirths, and neonatal deaths despite no maternal injury. Since the uterus is in the pelvis in the first trimester and amniotic fluid acts as a buffer against traumas for the fetus, indirect fetal injuries and deaths are more common in these weeks. Impaired uteroplacental flow may cause embryo losses weeks and months after the accident. Direct fetal injuries can develop due to penetrating traumas in the lower abdomen and perineum and pelvic fractures. The uterus and fetus are prone to injury in the later weeks of pregnancy. Fetal death risk increases to 70%. However, there is a decrease in maternal deaths, particularly as a result of penetrating injuries. The muscular structure of the uterus and amniotic fluid prevent other organ injuries by absorbing the damage [7, 8].

26.3   Blunt Abdominal Trauma

Of the blunt traumas, we encounter in pregnant women occur 40% after motor vehicle accidents, 30% after falls, and 20% after attacks. Fetal deaths occur in a wide range of 3.4–38%, and the most common cause is maternal death [9]. In cases where the mother is kept alive, the reason of fetal death is the premature separation of the placenta [10]. The most common injuries are head and neck injuries, intra-abdominal bleeding, pelvic fractures, and large vessel injuries. Splenic, hepatic, and uterine injuries are frequent in the abdominal trauma. Intestines are rarely injured [11]. Fetal losses in the first trimester occur due to uterine hypoperfusion and maternal hypotension since the bony pelvis protects the uterus. Direct fetal injuries are less than 1% in these weeks. Another cause of fetal death is uterine rupture, which occurs at a rate of 0.6% [9]. It often manifests with acute abdomen and maternal hypotension. Increased pelvic vascularity makes pelvic injuries as mortal as splenic and hepatic injuries. Abruptio placenta, which is more common in the last two trimesters (rate of 40–50% in major traumas, 3% in minor traumas), causes 30–75% fetal death and 1% maternal death. Placental separation usually occurs within the first six days after trauma. Fetal death often occurs within 48 h [8]. Vaginal bleeding may present along with abdominal or back pain or cramps, uterine tenderness, uterine rigidity or tetany, fetal distress, fetal bradycardia, hemodynamic instability, and disseminated intravascular coagulation. Although direct fetal injuries are rarely seen, in the last weeks of pregnancy, when the fetal head is engaged to the pelvis, skull bone fractures, brain injuries, and intracranial hemorrhages can be seen [12].

26.3.1 Protection

Vehicle accidents are the most common cause of blunt trauma, and seat belts are life-saving for mother and fetus. While the belts prevent ejection from the seat, they may cause uterine rupture and fetal death with the compressive effect of sudden flexion when misused. For this reason, instead of wearing only a horizontal arch that allows flexion, diagonal and horizontal arches that provide protection from three points should be worn together. The horizontal belt should be under the uterine corpus while the cross belt should be between the breasts, and over-tightening should be avoided. Fetal and maternal injuries can be reduced by 50% with the use of seat belts alone [13].

26.4 Penetrating Traumas

Penetrating traumas during pregnancy usually occur in the form of gunshot wounds and stabbing. Maternal mortality occurs 1/3 less than in non-pregnant women. Anatomically, the upward displacement of the intestines and the buffer function of the uterus significantly reduce other organ injuries, while fetal death occurs at a rate of 60%. If injuries occur in the upper abdomen and multiple bowel injuries are suspected, the best management is surgical exploration. In penetrating injuries, antibiotherapy should be initiated early against gram positives and *Clostridium* sp. In case of bowel injury, antibiotherapy should be added against gram-negative and anaerobes. After a trauma in the lower abdomen, uterine injuries are more common, and bleeding may occur due to dilated uterine vessels. In penetrating traumas, observation, laparoscopy, or exploration can be planned for treatment, depending on the patient's condition. Explorative laparotomy is not a cesarean indication if the fetal condition is good. In cases where uteroplacental flow may be impaired, such as obstetric reasons and uterine artery injury, cesarean delivery can be performed [12, 13].

26.5 Evaluation, Diagnosis, and Treatment

26.5.1 Pre-Hospital Environment

Transfer to the health center with maternal and neonatal intensive care is required as soon as possible. The most critical point in transport is that if there is no suspicion of a spinal injury in the second and third trimesters, transferring in the left lateral decubitus position. If spine injury is suspected, the patient should be immobilized with 15 degrees left inclination. As in non-pregnant trauma patients, following a rapid assessment, first, the airway must be assessed for patency, oxygen support should be given, and PaO2 should be kept above 70 mmHg. A rapid fluid replacement should contribute to the plasma volume. If unconscious, a nasogastric tube should be inserted to prevent aspiration. Meanwhile, the injury mechanisms, vital signs, and the patient's condition should be noted, and the use of vasopressors should be avoided, which may reduce uterine blood flow. Recording of information such as the week of pregnancy and the time of the last meal contributes to the acceleration of the treatment management in the health institution reached [14].

26.5.2 First Evaluation

First of all, the patient should be assessed in terms of ABC (Airway, Breathing, Circulation). If the pregnancy is greater than 24 weeks, the patient is placed in the left lateral position. Fetal heart rate is evaluated, and fetal monitoring and obstetric evaluation are provided at the earliest period after maternal stabilization [9].

26.5.2.1 Airway

In the case of cervical spine injury, the risk of aspiration should be taken into account, and early intubation should be performed using fiberoptic laryngoscopy if necessary. Pressing the jack while ventilating with the Ambu reduces the risk of aspiration. The possibility of difficult intubation in pregnant women should be kept in mind, and the endotracheal tube should be used with a diameter 0.5–1 mm smaller than usual. It should not be forgotten that intracranial pressure may increase in patients who had brain trauma during rapid intubation [9, 13, 15, 16].

26.5.2.2 Breathing

Attention should be paid to deformities in chest wall inspection. Thoracic trauma may cause rib fractures, as well as pneumothorax, chylothorax, hemothorax, tension pneumothorax, and pulmonary collapse, which may present with respiratory problems [13]. Taking into account the displacement of the diaphragm during pregnancy, it may be advisable to insert a thoracostomy tube, when indicated, one to two intercostal spaces higher than usual [17].

26.5.2.3 Circulation

Bleeding areas such as abdomen, retroperitoneum, thorax, pelvis, thigh, and uterus, which can abruptly cause shock, should be evaluated promptly, and direct pressure should be applied on the peripheral bleeding site. If there are any, long bone fractures should be reduced to control bleeding. Other findings of shock, such as tachycardia, decreased pulse pressure, pallor, and prolonged capillary filling, should be evaluated [18]. A palpable radial pulse indicates a systolic blood pressure over 80 mmHg. When the need for defibrillation develops, the same voltages should be applied as for the non-pregnant. There is no up-to-date information that there is any harm to the fetus. CPR should not be interrupted, and if any medication has to be applied, the upper extremities should be preferred because the lower extremities are under pressure [19]. The femoral pulse under uterine compression is unreliable to check the maternal heartbeat. At least two short and wide (14/16 gauge) peripheral intravenous catheters should be placed to allow rapid fluid infusion. Arterial catheterization enables continuous blood pressure measurement, gas-bicarbonate, lactate levels, and response to resuscitation [20]. Crystalloid fluids should be used for fluid replacement, and if hypovolemia does not improve despite 2–3 L, blood transfusion should be considered. Urinary output and urinary tract injury are evaluated with urinary catheterization. When hypovolemia is resolved, lactate levels should be maintained below 1.5 mEq/L as a sign of well-oxygenated tissue [1, 9].

In a pregnant woman who does not respond to resuscitation, other pathologies such as neurogenic shock, hypothermia, cardiac tamponade, pressurized pneumothorax, electrolyte, and acid–base imbalance, placental detachment, insufficient volume replacement, amniotic fluid, and air embolism should be considered as well. In the 24–32 week pregnant woman who does not respond to external cardiac massage and the systemic circulation does not restore within 5 min, open cardiac massage may be performed. In case of failure, performing an immediate cesarean section may save the fetus. If the external cardiac massage is not successful in pregnant women older than 32 weeks, cesarean section is performed immediately and the external table is continued. If there is still no return, CPR is continued with internal massage [21, 22].

26.5.2.4 Disability

A quick neurological evaluation is done. Orientation and pupillary responses are checked. The patient's condition is determined according to the Glasgow scale [21].

26.5.2.5 Exposure

All clothing is removed and all extremities are evaluated [21].

26.5.3 Second Evaluation

After ABCDE evaluation and the patient is stabilized, further examinations, such as imaging, obstetric examination, rectal and vaginal examination, should be carried on. The obstetric examination evaluates any possible feto-maternal hemorrhage, preterm labor, detachment placenta, and membrane rupture. In speculum examination, cervical and vaginal lacerations, hematomas, amniorrhexis, bleeding, and prolapse of fetal appendages are investigated. The fetus in the limits of viability should be monitored closely and the best approach is determined [12, 21, 23].

26.5.3.1 Routine Laboratory Tests

Routinely blood type is determined and, complete blood count, coagulation panel, fibrinogen, and D-dimer levels are studied [24]. Arterial blood gas also provides information about maternal peripheric perfusion as well as fetal perfusion. Electrolyte and glucose levels also provide information about the metabolic state. During the evaluation, pregnancy values should be taken into account [23].

26.5.3.2 Radiography

The embryo is most sensitive to radiation in the first trimester. Since organogenesis occurs in 2–8 weeks, radiation exposure may cause growth retardation, teratogenic and postnatal carcinogenic effects. While the teratogenic effect decreases between the 8 and 40 weeks of pregnancy, postnatal neoplastic effects, growth retardation, and particularly functional abnormalities in the central nervous system may develop. Acceptable cumulative radiation dose to avoid these effects is 5–10 rad. The level of exposure of the fetus or embryo to radiation depends on the size of the area that is imaged, the position of the patient, and the number of films. However, when mandatory, radiography should never be avoided [12, 14]. It has been accepted that the total absorbed dose on plain radiographs is 0.02–0.07 mrad and these values do not harm the fetus regardless of the gestational age. Multiple plan imaging can also be completed safely during pregnancy by using uterine protectors. In unprotected radiography, it has been calculated that the fetus is exposed to only 30% of the dose absorbed by the mother.

26.5.4 Ultrasonography

Ultrasonography (USG) is the most reliable radiological examination during pregnancy. The presence of free fluid inside the abdomen can be detected [25]. USG provides information about fetal status, gestational age, amnion fluid, fetal movements, and fetal presentation. Fetal fractures and retroplacental hematomas may be detected. However, placental abruption can be overlooked at a rate of 50–80% [26, 27].

26.5.5 Magnetic Resonance Imaging

MRI is an imaging method widely used for central nervous system injuries and ligament injuries and does not use ionizing radiation. However, its use in emergency conditions is more limited due to the long duration of the shootings [21].

26.5.6 Computed Tomography Scan

CT scan is a non-invasive, rapid, and specific method for showing the status of trauma patients. It is used more commonly than MRI. The patient is exposed to more radiation than in the scans of the head and chest regions. Techniques that may expose the fetus to less radiation should be preferred unless necessary [21].

26.5.7 Diagnostic Peritoneal Lavage

If it is considered that pregnancy might be masking the findings, then peritoneal lavage may be performed to determine whether the surgery is necessary [28]. A catheter is placed through an incision in the midline above the fundus. If hemoperitoneum is not detected, the catheter is placed toward the pelvis, 1 L of saline is given and allowed to return by gravity [23]. When significant abdominal blood is detected, an exploratory laparotomy with a midline incision should be performed.

26.5.8 Fetomaternal Hemorrhage

After blunt trauma, feto-maternal hemorrhage occurs at a rate of 8.8–30%. 0.07 mL of fetal blood is sufficient for the mother to be sensitized. This may cause neonatal anemia and fetal death with maternal Rh sensitization. Therefore, a pregnant trauma patient with Rh (−) blood type should be screened with Kleihauer-Betke (KB) test in terms of fetomaternal hemorrhage. If the test is negative, AntiD Ig 300 μg IM is administered within 72 h [12]. The Kleihauer-Betke test was found to be 100% specific and 96% sensitive for uterine contractions, and it was suggested that it could be used as a precursor of abruptio placentae and premature delivery [29].

26.5.9 Fetal Monitoring

If there is fetal distress following the stabilization of the mother, early diagnosis may save the fetus [30]. Gestational age should be calculated with ultrasound measurements by monitoring with cardiotocography. If the gestational age is greater than 24 weeks, the fetus should be followed up with continuous monitoring for 4–6 h after trauma. Most of the obstetric complications that occur are expected during this period including ablatio placenta (80% of all posttraumatic ablatio placenta cases). Although 20% of them are reported to develop within 24 h, there are cases of placental ablation even 5 days after the trauma. Therefore, patients with obstetric signs and symptoms should be observed for a longer time and fetal monitoring should be performed. Pregnant women who are asymptomatic (absence of vaginal bleeding and uterine contractions, absence of abdominal and uterine tenderness) or exposed to minor insignificant trauma can be discharged after brief and reassuring maternal and fetal monitoring. In pregnancies at less than 24 weeks of gestation without a fetal heartbeat or in unstable fetal conditions, the approach is planned according to the status of the mother. In cases where there is a stable course for 24 h, the mother may be discharged with warnings. In the presence of instability of the fetus or the mother, the patient is followed up in the hospital. Pregnant women with preterm contractions are treated with antibiotherapy, antenatal corticosteroid (2 doses of betamethasone or 4 doses of dexamethasone in 24–34 weeks), and tocolytic agents. If tocolysis is to be performed with ß-mimetic agents, the possibility of masking tachycardia secondary to trauma should be considered. Prolonged immobilization and prophylaxis against deep vein thrombosis should be considered [21].

26.6   Specific Maternal Injuries

26.6.1 Thermal Burns

When more than 50% of the total body surface is burned, the prognosis is bad for the mother and fetus, and it generally results in preterm labor, maternal hypotension, sepsis, and lung failure. Even though there is no direct fetal injury, fetal losses can be seen as a result of maternal hypovolemia and vasoconstriction in the uterine arteries [23].

26.6.2 Electric Injuries

It can appear in the form of contractions or fractures in all muscles. Neurological defects can happen due to falls. However, the fetus in amniotic fluid suffers more damage than the mother in electrical injuries [23, 31].

26.7 Postpartum Period

In the postpartum period, all principles of approach to trauma are valid for trauma patients. It should be kept in mind that the uterine volume is still large, considering the patient's recent birth. Also; the operation area should be examined in detail.

References

1. Gezginç K, Göktepe H. Gebelikte travmaya yaklaşım Selçuk. Üniv Tıp Derg. 2011;27(4):250. 2011;54.
2. Kuo C, Jamieson DJ, McPheeters ML, Meikle SF, Posner SF. Injury hospitalizations of pregnant women in the United States, 2002. Am J Obstet Gynecol. 2007;196(2):161.e1–6.
3. Chames MC, Pearlman MD. Trauma during pregnancy: outcomes and clinical management. Clin Obstet Gynecol. 2008;51(2):398–408.
4. El Kady D, Gilbert WM, Anderson J, Danielsen B, Towner D, Smith LH. Trauma during pregnancy: an analysis of maternal and fetal outcomes in a large population. Am J Obstet Gynecol. 2004;190(6):1661–8.
5. Stone IK. Trauma in the obstetric patient. Obstet Gynecol Clin North Am. 1999;26(3):459–67.
6. Katz V, Balderston K, DeFreest M. Perimortem cesarean delivery: were our assumptions correct? Am J Obstet Gynecol. 2005;192(6):1916–20.
7. Taviloğlu K, Ertekin C, Güloğlu R. Travma ve resüsitasyon kursu. İstanbul: Logos Yayıncılık; 2006.
8. Srinarmwong C. Trauma during pregnancy: a review of 38 cases. Thai J Surg. 2007;28(4):138–42.
9. Reddy SV, Shaik NA, Gunakala K. Trauma during pregnancy. J Obstet Anaesthesia Critical Care. 2012;2(1):3.
10. Al B, Bastürk M, Tekbaş G, Evsen MS, Sariçiçek V, Yücel Y, et al. Trauma management in pregnancy. J Acad Emerg Med/Akademik Acil Tip Olgu Sunumlari Dergisi. 2010;9(2)
11. Agboola AD, Osuala PC, Afuwape OO, Omigbodun AO. Traumatic splenic rupture in pregnancy with favourable pregnancy outcome: case report. Trop J Obstet Gynaecol. 2020;37(1):204–6.
12. Mirza FG, Devine PC, Gaddipati S. Trauma in pregnancy: a systematic approach. Am J Perinatol. 2010;27(07):579–86.
13. Oxford CM, Ludmir J. Trauma in pregnancy. Clin Obstet Gynecol. 2009;52(4):611–29.
14. Doan-Wiggins L. Trauma in pregnancy. In: Benrubi GI (Ed). Obstetric and gynecologic emergencies. Philadelphia, PA: Lippincott; 1996. p. 57–76.
15. Kirkpatrick AW, Ball CG, D'Amours SK, Zygun D. Acute resuscitation of the unstable adult trauma patient: bedside diagnosis and therapy. Can J Surg. 2008;51(1):57.
16. Suresh MS, Wali A. Failed intubation in obstetrics: airway management strategies. Anesthesiol Clin North Am. 1998;16(2):477–98.
17. Tsuei BJ. Assessment of the pregnant trauma patient. Injury. 2006;37(5):367–73.
18. Surgeons A. ATLS, advanced trauma life support for doctors. Chicago, Illinois: Amer College of Surgeons; 2008.
19. Rees G, Willis B. Resuscitation in late pregnancy. Anaesthesia. 1988;43(5):347–9.
20. Sperry JL, Minei JP, Frankel HL, West MA, Harbrecht BG, Moore EE, et al. Early use of vasopressors after injury: caution before constriction. J Trauma Acute Care Surg. 2008;64(1):9–14.
21. Corrina M, Oxford LJ. Trauma in pregnancy. Clin Obstet Gynecol. 2009;4(52):611.
22. Prentice-Bjerkeseth R. Perioperative anesthetic management of trauma in pregnancy. Anesthesiol Clin North Am. 1999;17(1):277–94.
23. Doan-Wiggins L. Trauma in pregnancy. Obstetric and gynecologic emergencies. Philadelphia: Lippincott; 1994. p. 57–76.

24. Hellgren M, Blombäck M. Studies on blood coagulation and fibrinolysis in pregnancy, during delivery and in the puerperium. Gynecol Obstet Investig. 1981;12(3):141–54.
25. Goodwin H, Holmes JF, Wisner DH. Abdominal ultrasound examination in pregnant blunt trauma patients. J Trauma Acute Care Surg. 2001;50(4):689–94.
26. Pearlman MD, Tintinalli JE, Lorenz RP. A prospective controlled study of outcome after trauma during pregnancy. Am J Obstet Gynecol. 1990;162(6):1502–10.
27. Dahmus MA, Sibai BM. Blunt abdominal trauma: are there any predictive factors for abruptio placentae or maternal-fetal distress? Am J Obstet Gynecol. 1993;169(4):1054–9.
28. Meyer D, Thal ER, Weigelt JA, Redman HC. Evaluation of computed tomography and diagnostic peritoneal lavage in blunt abdominal trauma. J Trauma. 1989;29(8):1168–70; discussion 70.
29. Muench MV, Canterino JC. Trauma in pregnancy. Obstet Gynecol Clin North Am. 2007;34(3):555–83.
30. Shah KH, Simons RK, Holbrook T, Fortlage D, Winchell RJ, Hoyt DB. Trauma in pregnancy: maternal and fetal outcomes. J Trauma Acute Care Surg. 1998;45(1):83–6.
31. Jaffe R, Fejgin M, Aderet NB. Fetal death in early pregnancy due to electric current. Acta Obstet Gynecol Scand. 1986;65(3):283.

The Effects of Vitamin D Deficiency and Its Replacement in the Gestation and Lactation Periods

Onur Tunca and Alper Sarı

27.1 Introduction

Vitamin D deficiency is still accepted as a global public health problem. The levels of vitamin D of the individuals in the USA, Canada, and European countries which are recognized socioeconomically as developed countries are not even at the desired level. With the discovery of the receptors of vitamin D in numerous tissues and organs, notably the musculoskeletal system, it is no more accepted as the hormone having a part only in the calcium-phosphorus metabolisms. Vitamin D level <30 ng/mL is considered a deficiency by many authors. Thus far, many studies have instantiated that vitamin D deficiency may be related to many disorders such as cardiovascular, metabolic, autoimmune diseases and gestational diabetes mellitus, preeclampsia, low birth weight, especially osteomalacia and rickets. Though there is not a consensus for the optimal dose, it is suggested by most of the researchers to get vitamin D support of 2000 IU during the gestation and lactation periods considering the negative maternal and neonatal effects.

27.2 Background and Epidemiology

Vitamin D deficiency is accepted as a global public health problem and individuals cannot meet the vitamin D requirements in quite a few countries [1–6]. On a global scale, the incidence rate of vitamin D deficiency is 30% in children while it is 60% in adults [3, 7]. Its prevalence rates of 25 hydroxy (OH) D <12 ng/mL (30 nmol/L)

O. Tunca (✉) · A. Sarı
Department of Internal Medicine, Faculty of Medicine, Afyon University of Health Sciences, Afyon, Turkey
e-mail: dronurtunca@hotmail.com; alpersari_@hotmail.com

C. Cingi et al. (eds.), *ENT Diseases: Diagnosis and Treatment during Pregnancy and Lactation*, https://doi.org/10.1007/978-3-031-05303-0_27

are reported to be 5.9%, 13%, and 7.4% in the USA [8, 9], Europe [8, 10], and Canada [8, 11], respectively. The annual prevalence of 25(OH)D <50 nmol/L is detected to be 24%, 40.4%, and 36.8% in the USA, Europe, and Canada, respectively [9–12]. According to the results of the National Health and Nutrition Examination Survey (NHANES) belonging to the period between 2007 and 2010, which evaluated the ethnic groups, the prevalence of 25(OH)D <30 nmol/L is reported to be 2.3%, 6.4%, and 24% in white, Hispanic and non-Hispanic colored people, respectively [9, 12]. However, the situation is much more serious in low and middle-income countries since the prevalence is observed to be 25(OH)D <30 nmol/L (12 ng/mL) in over 20% of the populations of Mongolia, Afghanistan, India, and Pakistan [12–14]. In addition to these epidemiological data, the ethnicity and gender differences in cutaneous pigmentation may indicate that individuals undergo evolutionary processes to meet their vitamin D requirements. However, the evolutionary pressure on light skin might have happened so as to meet the physiological needs of the organism. Additionally, the fact that women have lighter skin compared to men may arise from the requirements improving during the gestation and lactation periods [15, 16].

When taking a glance at the first steps of vitamin D in history, the story began with the findings of Polish Dr. Jedrzej Sniadecki about the direct effects of the lack of solar exposure on rachitis in 1822 [17]. Afterward, Dr. Elmer McCollum et al. defined vitamin D empirically [17, 18]. At a later stage, vitamin D receptors (VDR) were discovered [17, 19]. The historical journey of vitamin D has continued with the discovery of many more features organizing more than 2000 genes and affecting quite a few tissues beyond the skeletal system [15, 16]. A great number of developments and defined features mentioned above have increased the importance given to vitamin D. Many countries have put various policies into practice so as to enrich the levels of vitamin D in foods, especially milk. Upon the detection of the high prevalence of lactose intolerance in its public, the USA regarded the initiative to enrich orange juice in vitamin D as a necessary approach in 2003 [16, 20, 21]. The main purpose of all these initiatives was to sanitate public health and raise awareness among society.

Vitamin D deficiency, which is quite common around the world, has some general features: it is a steroidal prohormone [22, 23]; its receptors appear in many bodily tissues, notably in the musculoskeletal system [22, 24]. Vitamin D has a pivotal role in the maintenance of bone mineral metabolism, calcium, and phosphorus balance [25]. Its deficiency has been found to be relevant to both maternal and fetal adverse outcomes such as osteomalacia, rickets, neonatal hypocalcemia, craniotabes [26, 27], gestational diabetes mellitus (GDM), preeclampsia, small for gestational age (SGA), low birth weight (LBW), and preterm labor [22, 28]. Moreover, it has been proved that vitamin D affects fetal and postnatal growth with the impacts on the insulin-like growth factor regulation beyond its role in calcium and phosphorus metabolism [29]. Additionally, researchers have mentioned the contingent relationships between low vitamin D levels and cardiovascular, autoimmune, metabolic diseases [6, 30, 31]. As for vitamin D deficiency, 25(OH)D is the optimal reagent to interpret the vitamin D level [8, 32, 33] and the values below 30 ng/mL (75 nmol/L) are regarded as vitamin D deficiency by most of the authors [8, 34]. However, the field of medicine still has uncertainties about the replacement quantity and duration; moreover, whether replacements endure or not remains controversial.

27.3   The Metabolism of Vitamin D

Vitamin D is a fat-soluble hormone that has a role in maintaining bone health in addition to playing an extra-skeletal role. Vitamin D to be taken with foods consists of D_3 (cholecalciferol) and D_2 (ergocalciferol) forms. The foods rich in the forms of D_2 and D_3 are high-fat fishes such as salmon, sardine, cod, and some species of mushroom [16]. Vitamin D_2 and D_3 taken at low levels with foods are absorbed through the proteins existing on the enterocyte apical surface of small intestines. These proteins are defined as SR-BI (Scavenger Receptor Class B type 1), CD36 (Cluster Determinant 36), and NPC1L1 (Niemann-Pick C1-Like 1). It has been suggested that the high-dose pharmacological vitamin D forms are subject to passive transition. The way of absorption of hydroxyl vitamin D forms is still an uncertain issue. The only known point is that the hydroxyl forms are absorbed better than the non-hydroxyl ones [35]. The chemical structures of the forms of dietary D_2, D_3, and 25(OH)D are shown in Fig. 27.1.

The main source of vitamin D is obtained by endogenous absorption of sunlight (UVB) from the skin and the transformation of vitamin D3 from 7-dehydrocholesterol [6, 22]. This stage does not contain chemically enzymatic transactions but involves a heat-sensitive process under the effect of UVB. The short-term UVB exposure through extremities and face on sunny days provide almost 200 IU D_3 synthesis [36]. In addition, the UVB wavelength required for conversion of D_3 on the skin is approximately at a level of 290–315 nm. The carnation on the body after a 24-h sunbath of the entire body is named minima erythema dose (MED) and vitamin D synthesized in this way is claimed to be equal to approximately 25,000 IU D_2 taken through oral route [16]. Many factors are affecting the utilization of the above-mentioned UVB impacts, which can be summarized as the current location on the

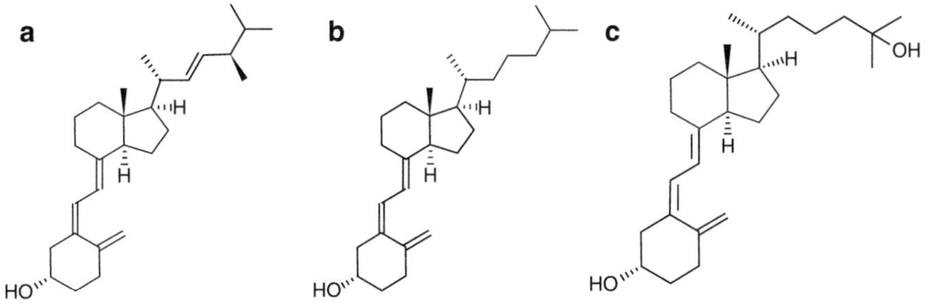

Fig. 27.1 Chemical structures of natural dietary forms of vitamin D: (**a**) ergocalciferol (vitamin D2), (**b**) cholecalciferol (vitamin D3), and (**c**) 25-hydroxycholecalciferol

world, the increased pigmentation on the skin, the features of the clothes on, aged above 65, seasonal loops, and sun protectors [16, 37].

Vitamin D forms synthesized by the skin, obtained from foods through the gastrointestinal system, are inactive. Moreover, vitamin D_2 differs from D_3 since it has a double bond between carbon 22 (C22) and carbon 24 (C24) and consists of C24 methyl groups. This feature of vitamin D_2 decreases its affinity to the vitamin D-binding protein (DBP) while it accelerates its elimination [38, 39]. The first spot of the inactive forms before active vitamin D form is the liver where they are subjected to complex and enzymatic processing. The enzymes playing active roles in vitamin D metabolism are members of the cytochrome P450 (CYP) enzyme superfamily and are included in the endoplasmic reticulum or mitochondrion [38, 40]. The prominent enzymes in the given condition are CYP2R1 (2 family, R subfamily, 1 polypeptide), CYP27A1, and CYP24A1. Both forms of vitamin D are metabolized in the liver to 25 (OH) vitamin D (calcidiol) form by CYP2R1 enzyme activity, and the resulting calcidiol forms the main circulating form. CYP27A1 is a mitochondrial enzyme and participates in the hydroxylation process of vitamin D_2. In addition, CYP27A1 is involved in other tissues of the body besides the liver. On the other hand, CYP24A1 catalyzes the metabolite formation of $24,25(OH)_2D_3$, which is an inactive form, from $25(OH)D_3$ in the liver while it catalyzes the formation of the active metabolites of $1,24,25(OH)_3D_3$ and lactone in the kidneys from $1,25(OH)_2D_3$. These reactions catalyzed by CYP24A1 are thought to inhibit the cumulation of 25(OH)D and $1,25(OH)_2$ D at a toxic level [38, 41, 42].

Vitamin D is ultimately transferred from the liver to the kidneys by DBP and metabolized into the 1,25-dihydroxyvitamin $(OH)_2$ D (calcitriol) by the activity of the enzyme 1-alpha (α) hydroxylase (CYP27B1). This process occurs in the renal tissues and proximal tubules and the megalin-cubilin protein pair plays a fairly crucial role in the cellular ingestion of the inactive vitamin D forms [43, 44]. The active form takes effect by binding to VDR which are located in the class II steroid hormone receptor family in the target cell [45]. CYP27B1 is not an enzyme active in the renal tissue; there have been researchers claiming it to involve in the cells of the lung, cutaneous, prostate gland, pancreas, and immune system. In conclusion, the aforementioned CYP27B1 is subjected to a strict modulation by three hormones, namely parathyroid hormone (PTH), active vitamin D itself, and fibroblast growth factor 23 (FGF23). FGF23 is a hormone the level of which increases with the progression of the stage within the chronic kidney diseases (CKD) and has a phosphaturic impact. Besides, the enzyme 1-alpha (α) hydroxylase has a downregulating feature; hence, the production of vitamin D decreases, and the absorption of calcium and phosphorus from intestines is interrupted [46]. PTH shows the effect of increasing the production of vitamin D while vitamin D has a negative impact on the PTH [38, 46]. Vitamin D metabolism is depicted in Fig. 27.2.

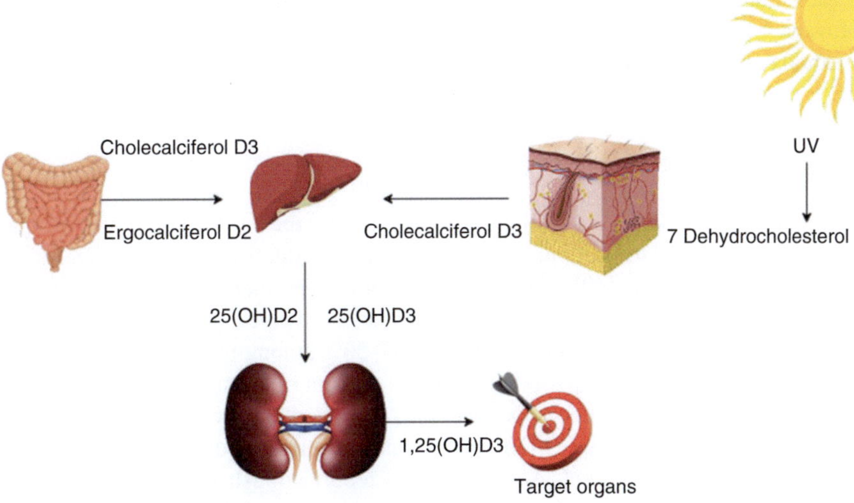

Fig. 27.2 Vitamin D has a crucial role both in calcium-phosphorus balance and bone metabolism. The most important impact is to increase the absorption of calcium and phosphorus from the intestines, to suppress parathyroid hormone (PTH) secretion, and to regulate the osteoblast-osteoclast functions in bone tissues. The other hormone to have a role in the aforementioned calcium-phosphorus balance is PTH and it increases the active vitamin D synthesis by influencing the enzyme 1-α hydroxylase in contrast to vitamin D

27.4   Measurement Methods of Vitamin D

There have been many laboratory methods used in the measurement of 25(OH) vitamin D from past to present. The initial method was developed pursuant to DBP in the early 1970s; the first radioimmunoassay (RIA) gained its place among the measurement methods in 1985 following the high-performance liquid chromatography (HPLC) in the late 1970s [47]. The following years witnessed new methods, namely liquid chromatography-tandem mass spectrometry (LC-MS/MS) and chemiluminescent immunoassay (CLIA) which have progressively increasing usage [48].

The measurement methods of vitamin D are classified under three main technical categories: manual immunoassay (RIA, enzyme immunoassay, etc.); automatic immunoassay (CLIA, etc.); and direct detection methods (HPLC, LC-MS/MS). While the first two of these methods involve a measurement based upon the immunological and chromatographic isolation, the last one depends on direct isolation. Thus, there are problems in terms of comparability due to the lack of a standard reference value among them. The levels of $25(OH)D_2$ and D_3 can be measured more precisely by the methods of HPLC and LC-MS/MS while they are more expensive compared to the RIA methods. Moreover, direct detection methods are disadvantageous in excessive need for specialists and their non-automated nature. However, the difficulties in procurement of radioactive substances within the RIA methods are highly challenging [47].

27.5   Vitamin D Deficiency

Vitamin D deficiency is a prevalent problem all over the world. The levels of vitamin D are measured low among all age groups in the countries such as India, Japan, the USA, and Australia [49]. The vitamin D requirement increases during the gestation period and the pregnant women become riskier in respect of deficiency. Vitamin D deficiency is estimated to be at the rate of 5–50% among pregnant women in the USA [50, 51]. A research involving the measurement of vitamin D in the pregnant and fetal blood in the Netherlands concludes that the rate of severe vitamin D deficiency is detected as 21% [52]. There have been different guideline suggestions for the optimal vitamin D level. According to a report published by the Institute of Medicine in the USA in 2010, the level of 25(OH)D below 20 ng/mL (50 nmol/L) is defined as vitamin D deficiency. The new view suggested by the association of endocrine determines the cut-off value of vitamin D as 30 ng/mL (75 nmol/L) [53]. Some experts define vitamin D deficiency as the level of 25(OH)D below 32 ng/mL (80 nmol/L) by the reagents of PTH, calcium absorption, and the activity of bone mineral [54]. The optimal level of vitamin D during the gestation period cannot be determined accurately and the studies are still underway [55]. The Endocrine Society 2011 guideline states that the level of 25(OH)D should be raised over 30 ng/ml during the gestation and lactation periods [34].

Although the optimal level of vitamin D is controversial, the level of vitamin D is accepted as follows: 25(OH)D <10 ng/mL (severe deficiency); 25(OH)D <20 ng/mL (deficiency); 25(OH)D between 20 and 30 ng/mL (insufficiency); 25(OH)D >30 ng/mL (sufficiency); and 25(OH)D >150 ng/mL (intoxication) [56].

27.6   The Maternal and Fetal Outcomes of Vitamin D Deficiency Seen During the Gestation Period

There have been many randomized controlled trials proving that the replacement of vitamin D during pregnancy prevents pregnancy complications. Some researches also show that vitamin D deficiency detected during pregnancy has no negative impacts on the mother and fetus. Thus, the effects of vitamin D deficiency on pregnancy are still controversial. Chen et al. in a cohort study conclude that many complications such as GDM, LBW, preterm birth, and cesarean section are significantly detected low in the group the level of vitamin D is measured high compared to the one with the low level of vitamin D [57].

27.7 The Maternal Outcomes Seen During Pregnancy Depending Upon Vitamin D Deficiency

Preeclampsia is a pregnancy-specific disorder that impairs 2–8% of the pregnancies going along with high blood pressure and proteinuria after the 20th gestational week [58, 59]. Eight meta-analyses including only pregnant women show that vitamin D deficiency increases the risk of preeclampsia significantly [60, 61]. Another case-control study also demonstrates that the pregnant women having severe preeclampsia before the 34th gestational week have lower vitamin D levels than the control group [62].

The pathophysiology of vitamin D on changing the risk of preeclampsia has not been proved yet. Preeclampsia has an endothelial dysfunction which means the breakdown of angiogenesis and the increase of adhesion molecules in maternal blood. The in vitro studies reveal that vitamin D recures angiogenesis and this recruitment occurs by inhibition of the expression of adhesion molecules in endothelial cells [63, 64]. However, some researches do not offer any clear relations between vitamin D level and preeclampsia [65]. It is required to have wider cohorts to clarify the studies in the field.

GDM is a glucose tolerance disorder that is initially diagnosed during pregnancy and is one of the common complications of pregnancy [66]. It also has maternal, fetal, and neonatal outcomes. Despite the relationship detected between vitamin D deficiency and GDM, the results of the studies are not clear. 31 meta-analyses including vitamin D insufficiency conclude that the risk of GDM may be related to vitamin D insufficiency [60]. Moreover, though there have been studies revealing that the relationship between the level of vitamin D and GDM is connected with ethnicity, there have been the ones that cannot prove that connection. A research, the majority of which is constituted by 16-week pregnant white women, proves that the patients with GDM have a low level of vitamin D; on the contrary, another research including 30-week pregnant Indian women does not reveal any relationship between GDM and vitamin D [67, 68].

Although the biological mechanism of the relationship between GDM and vitamin D has not been clarified yet, there have been publications on the fact that vitamin D can directly affect beta cells of the pancreas. The mechanism suggested by the researchers is stated to ease the transfer of glucose into the target tissues by regulating insulin resistance through the intracellular calcium levels of vitamin D [69]. It is obvious that more comprehensive studies are required in order to prove the relationship between vitamin D and GDM in a clearer way.

Births before the 37th week of pregnancy are called preterm births. It is seen in 10% of the pregnant [70]. A study carried out in the Netherlands reveals that there is a correlation between the level of vitamin D of the mother in the second trimester and preterm birth [71]. Another study carried out in South Korea shows that 79% of preterm infants have a deficient level of vitamin D at birth [72]. When the strong relationship between maternal and fetal vitamin D levels [13] is considered, the level of maternal vitamin D in pregnancy is proved to be important in terms of termination. This condition is associated with the causation of vitamin D into cytokine secretion and has immunomodulatory and anti-inflammatory impacts by regulating neutrophil functions [73].

There have been studies examining the relationship between vitamin D deficiency in pregnant and delivery methods and some of them reveal that vitamin D deficiency increases the rate of primary cesarian section [74]. The calcium loss depending on vitamin D deficiency may lead to decreased pelvic muscle power. This may cause prolonged labor, consequently leading to a cesarian section, which currently has no certainty. Another study including the pregnant women having maternal vitamin D deficiency between 11 and 13 gestational weeks does not offer a significant difference between cesarian and vaginal delivery [75].

Postpartum depression is an affective disorder that is seen together with biological, physical, and social changes during the lactation period following the labor. Its rate of incidence is 10–15% in developed countries while it is 15–20% in developing ones. Some researchers have provided evidence about the relation between vitamin D level and depression in the postpartum period. It has been revealed that the replacement of 2000 IU vitamin D is effective in decreasing postpartum depression [76]. However, it has been associated with the existence of VDR in cranial parts, particularly the hippocampus and cingulate gyrus, which have a place in depression pathology [77].

Vitamin D is known to regulate neutrophil functions and to have immunomodulatory and anti-inflammatory effects [73]. Moreover, it has also been revealed by some researches that vitamin D deficiency is related to bacterial vaginosis [78, 79].

27.8 The Effects of Vitamin D on Fetus

Maternal calcium and vitamin D occupy an important position in the development of the fetus. The calcium and 25(OH)D required by the fetus are provided through active transport from the blood. Thus, the maternal vitamin D deficiency redounds on fetus and neonates. The researches have detected a positive correlation between maternal vitamin D deficiency and femur volume, tibial sectional area, and bone mineral density [80]. Another meta-analysis including many researches reveals that the replacement of vitamin D during the gestational period is beneficial to birth weight and tall stature. The infants of pregnant women having vitamin D deficiency are seen to have low bone mass after birth [81]. Another study, on the other hand, provides no evidence of the relationship between vitamin D deficiency seen in pregnancy and neonatal bone mass [82].

The condition in which the neonatal birth weight is below the 10th percentile for the gestational age is defined as SGA (Small for Gestational Age) [83]. There have been many studies investigating the relationship between maternal vitamin D level and SGA. In a cohort study including more than 3000 pregnant women from multiple ethnic groups, it is found that vitamin D deficiency in the first trimester is connected with the risk of SGA and increased SGA [55]. Another study carried out in

China indicates that there is a positive correlation between maternal vitamin D level and neonatal birth weight [84]. A meta-analysis including more than 30 studies has detected a positive correlation between vitamin D concentrations and fetal growth, and birth weight [85].

There have been researches investigating the relationship between vitamin D deficiency and asthma. According to a study, the infants of the women who have maternal vitamin D deficiency or cannot take sufficient vitamin D have more tendency to have asthma, eczema, and wheezing [86]. In another study, the rate of incidence of eczema, and wheezing among the infants of the pregnant with high vitamin D level is 60% less than the ones with low vitamin D levels [87].

The other study investigating the relation between vitamin D levels and upper respiratory tract infections includes the measurement of vitamin D levels in umbilical cord blood. It reveals that the infants of the pregnant women in the group with low vitamin D levels have two times more tendency to have respiratory tract infections than the ones of the women with high vitamin D level [88].

Consequently, it wouldn't be wrong to claim that the maternal and fetal effects of vitamin D deficiency have not been clarified yet though there are many studies on this subject in the literature. Some of them can prove the relations between maternal, fetal complications, and vitamin D while this relation cannot be clarified in others. It is required in the field to carry out more comprehensive studies including long-term results of vitamin D so as to clarify the subject.

27.9 Vitamin D Treatment

The first and main factor to maintain the vitamin D balance is the sufficient dose of exposure of sunlight while the second one is to provide sufficient dietary vitamin D. Hence, pregnant women should be told that sunlight is the most crucial source of vitamin D and be necessarily suggested to take sufficient sunlight. It is accepted to be enough to have daily 15–20-min exposure for sufficient sunlight intake. However, this duration is affected by some parameters such as season, skin color, usage of skin-sparing cream, and the position of the sun.

World Health Organization (WHO) suggests a daily 200 IU vitamin D supplements together with a balanced diet for pregnant women with vitamin D deficiency [89]. Endocrine Society suggests 400 IU vitamin D intake on a daily basis in the pre-pregnancy period while it can be increased up to a daily dose of 1000 IU during the gestation period. Institute of Medicine (IOM) suggests 600 IU vitamin D supplements for all women during gestation and lactation periods in the guideline [90].

The General Directorate of Mother and Child Care and Family Planning affiliated with the Ministry of Health apply the 'Vitamin D Supplement Program for Pregnant Women' in Turkey since April 2011. All the pregnant women are given a daily single dose of 1200 IU vitamin D supplement starting from the 12th gestational week until the 6th month of the lactation period.

The treatment is suggested to start at the end of the first trimester. However, there is not a clear consensus upon treatment dose and its start time. It can be said that

6–8 weeks high dose (50,000 IU/week) vitamin D treatment recommended as loading dose in adult population is not included in the guideline reports prepared for pregnancy and lactation period.

There have been a great number of security surveys examining the maternal and fetal effects of the replacement of vitamin D started in the women in the gestation and lactation periods. Within a study, the replacement of 400, 2000, and 4000 IU vitamin D is applied on the 192 pregnant women having severe vitamin D deficiency in their 12–16th gestational weeks; afterward, the levels of vitamin D are measured during pregnancy and following the delivery. The group given 4000 IU dose is detected to have the highest vitamin D concentration and no adverse condition is reported to occur in the respective study. In addition, all the doses are found to be safe [91].

There are still a number of ongoing randomized controlled trials upon the optimum vitamin D level and replacement dose during gestation and lactation periods nowadays. The guideline suggestions are likely to have changes in the immediate future.

Vitamin D deficiency during gestation and lactation periods may hereby influence both maternal and fetal health negatively. Thus, the women in gestation and lactation periods should be informed about adequate nutrition for vitamin D and sufficient utilization of sunlight. Both pregnant and lactant women should have vitamin D replacement within the framework of vitamin D supplement programs, which should be followed by the examination of vitamin D levels and their scientific shares.

References

1. Cashman KD, Ritz C, Kiely M. Improved dietary guidelines for vitamin D: application of individual participant data (IPD)-level meta-regression analyses. Nutrients. 2017;9 https://doi.org/10.3390/nu9050469.
2. Consequences T. Recommendations abstracted from the american geriatrics society consensus statement on vitamin D for prevention of falls and their consequences. J Am Geriatr Soc. 2014;62:147–52. https://doi.org/10.1111/jgs.12631.
3. Holick MF. The vitamin D deficiency pandemic: approaches for diagnosis, treatment and prevention. Rev Endocr Metab Disord. 2017;18:153–65. https://doi.org/10.1007/s11154-017-9424-1.
4. Nesby-O'Dell S, Scanlon KS, Cogswell ME, et al. Hypovitaminosis D prevalence and determinants among African American and white women of reproductive age: Third National Health and Nutrition Examination Survey, 1988-1994. Am J Clin Nutr. 2002;76:187–92. https://doi.org/10.1093/ajcn/76.1.187.
5. Pilz S, März W, Cashman KD, et al. Rationale and plan for vitamin D food fortification: a review and guidance paper. Front Endocrinol (Lausanne). 2018a;9:1–16. https://doi.org/10.3389/fendo.2018.00373.
6. Pilz S, Zittermann A, Obeid R, et al. The role of vitamin D in fertility and during pregnancy and lactation: a review of clinical data. Int J Environ Res Public Health. 2018b;15 https://doi.org/10.3390/ijerph15102241.
7. Hossein-Nezhad A, Holick MF. Vitamin D for health: a global perspective. Mayo Clin Proc. 2013;88:720–55. https://doi.org/10.1016/j.mayocp.2013.05.011.

8. Amrein K, Scherkl M, Hoffmann M, et al. Vitamin D deficiency 2.0: an update on the current status worldwide. Eur J Clin Nutr. 2020;74:1498–513. https://doi.org/10.1038/s41430-020-0558-y.

9. Schleicher RL, Sternberg MR, Looker AC, et al. National estimates of serum total 25-hydroxyvitamin D and metabolite concentrations measured by liquid chromatography-tandem mass spectrometry in the US population during 2007-2010. J Nutr. 2016;146:1051–61. https://doi.org/10.3945/jn.115.227728.

10. Cashman KD, Dowling KG, Škrabáková Z, et al. Vitamin D deficiency in Europe: pandemic? Am J Clin Nutr. 2016;103:1033–44. https://doi.org/10.3945/ajcn.115.120873.

11. Sarafin K, Durazo-Arvizu R, Tian L, et al. Standardizing 25-hydroxyVitamin D values from the Canadian Health Measures Survey. Am J Clin Nutr. 2015;102:1044–50. https://doi.org/10.3945/ajcn.114.103689.

12. Cashman KD. Vitamin D deficiency: defining, prevalence, causes, and strategies of addressing. Calcif Tissue Int. 2020;106:14–29. https://doi.org/10.1007/s00223-019-00559-4.

13. Cashman KD, Sheehy T, O'Neill CM. Is vitamin D deficiency a public health concern for low middle income countries? A systematic literature review. Eur J Nutr. 2019;58:433–53. https://doi.org/10.1007/s00394-018-1607-3.

14. Roth DE, Abrams SA, Aloia J, et al. Global prevalence and disease burden of vitamin D deficiency: a roadmap for action in low- and middle-income countries. Ann N Y Acad Sci. 2018;1430:44–79. https://doi.org/10.1111/nyas.13968.

15. Jablonski NG, Chaplin G. The evolution of human skin coloration. J Hum Evol. 2000;39:57–106. https://doi.org/10.1006/jhev.2000.0403.

16. Wacker M, Holiack MF. Vitamin D-effects on skeletal and extraskeletal health and the need for supplementation. Nutrients. 2013;5:111–48. https://doi.org/10.3390/nu5010111.

17. Dzik KP, Kaczor JJ. Mechanisms of vitamin D on skeletal muscle function: oxidative stress, energy metabolism and anabolic state. Eur J Appl Physiol. 2019;119:825–39. https://doi.org/10.1007/s00421-019-04104-x.

18. McCollum EV, Simmonds N, Becker JE, Shipley PG. Studies on experimental rickets. J Biol Chem. 1922;53:293–312. https://doi.org/10.1016/s0021-9258(18)85783-0.

19. Haussler MR, Norman AW. Chromosomal receptor for a vitamin D metabolite. Nutr Rev. 2009;43:181–3. https://doi.org/10.1111/j.1753-4887.1985.tb02413.x.

20. Biancuzzo RM, Young A, Bibuld D, et al. Fortification of orange juice with vitamin D2 or vitamin D 3 is as effective as an oral supplement in maintaining vitamin D status in adults. Am J Clin Nutr. 2010;91:1621–6. https://doi.org/10.3945/ajcn.2009.27972.

21. Tangpricha V, Koutkia P, Rieke SM, et al. Fortification of orange juice with vitamin D: A novel approach for enhancing vitamin D nutritional health. Am J Clin Nutr. 2003;77:1478–83. https://doi.org/10.1093/ajcn/77.6.1478.

22. Agarwal S, Kovilam O, Agrawal DK. Vitamin D and its impact on maternal-fetal outcomes in pregnancy: a critical review. Crit Rev Food Sci Nutr. 2018;58:755–69. https://doi.org/10.1080/10408398.2016.1220915.

23. Weinert LS, Silveiro SP. Maternal–fetal impact of vitamin D deficiency: a critical review. Matern Child Health J. 2015;19:94–101. https://doi.org/10.1007/s10995-014-1499-7.

24. Joergensen JS, Lamont RF, Torloni MR. Vitamin D and gestational diabetes: an update. Curr Opin Clin Nutr Metab Care. 2014;17:360–7. https://doi.org/10.1097/MCO.0000000000000064.

25. Apaydin M, Can AG, Kizilgul M, et al. The effects of single high-dose or daily low-dosage oral colecalciferol treatment on vitamin D levels and muscle strength in postmenopausal women. BMC Endocr Disord. 2018;18:48. https://doi.org/10.1186/s12902-018-0277-8.

26. Curtis EM, Moon RJ, Harvey NC, Cooper C. Maternal Vitamin D supplementation during pregnancy. Br Med Bull. 2018;126:57–77. https://doi.org/10.1093/bmb/ldy010.

27. Soliman A, Salama H, Alomar S, et al. Clinical, biochemical, and radiological manifestations of vitamin D deficiency in newborns presented with hypocalcemia. Indian J Endocrinol Metab. 2013;17:697. https://doi.org/10.4103/2230-8210.113764.

28. Palaniswamy S, Williams D, Järvelin M-R, Sebert S. Vitamin D and the promotion of long-term metabolic health from a programming perspective. Nutr Metab Insights. 2015;8(1):NMI. S29526. https://doi.org/10.4137/nmi.s29526.
29. Ciresi A, Giordano C. Vitamin D across growth hormone (GH) disorders: From GH deficiency to GH excess. Growth Horm IGF Res. 2017;33:35–42. https://doi.org/10.1016/j.ghir.2017.02.002.
30. Gaksch M, Jorde R, Grimnes G, et al. Vitamin D and mortality: Individual participant data meta-analysis of standardized 25-hydroxyvitamin D in 26916 individuals from a European consortium. PLoS One. 2017;12:1–15. https://doi.org/10.1371/journal.pone.0170791.
31. Muscogiuri G, Altieri B, Annweiler C, et al. Vitamin D and chronic diseases: the current state of the art. Arch Toxicol. 2017;91:97–107. https://doi.org/10.1007/s00204-016-1804-x.
32. De Pascale G, Quraishi SA. Vitamin D status in critically ill patients: the evidence is now bioavailable! Crit Care. 2014;18:1–2. https://doi.org/10.1186/cc13975.
33. Martucci G, Tuzzolino F, Arcadipane A, et al. The effect of high-dose cholecalciferol on bioavailable vitamin D levels in critically ill patients: a post hoc analysis of the VITdAL-ICU trial. Intensive Care Med. 2017;43:1732–4. https://doi.org/10.1007/s00134-017-4846-5.
34. Holick MF, Binkley NC, Bischoff-Ferrari HA, et al. Evaluation, treatment, and prevention of vitamin D deficiency: an Endocrine Society clinical practice guideline. J Clin Endocrinol Metab. 2011;96:1911–30.
35. Borel P, Caillaud D, Cano NJ. Vitamin D bioavailability: state of the art. Crit Rev Food Sci Nutr. 2015;55:1193–205. https://doi.org/10.1080/10408398.2012.688897.
36. Haddad JG. Vitamin D-solar rays, the Milky Way, or both? N Engl J Med. 1992;326:1213–5. https://doi.org/10.1056/NEJM199204303261808.
37. Webb AR, DeCosta BRHM. Sunlight regulates the cutaneous production of vitamin D3 by causing its photodegradation. J Clin Endocrinol Metab. 1989;68:882–7. https://doi.org/10.1210/jcem-68-5-882.
38. Bikle DD. Vitamin D metabolism, mechanism of action, and clinical applications. Chem Biol. 2014;21:319–29. https://doi.org/10.1016/j.chembiol.2013.12.016.
39. Houghton LA, Vieth R. The case against ergocalciferol (vitamin D2) as a vitamin supplement. Am J Clin Nutr. 2006;84:694–7. https://doi.org/10.1093/ajcn/84.4.694.
40. Sugimoto H, Shiro Y. Diversity and substrate specificity in the structures of steroidogenic cytochrome P450 enzymes. Biol Pharm Bull. 2012;35:818–23. https://doi.org/10.1248/bpb.35.818.
41. White JH. Vitamin D metabolism and signaling in the immune system. Rev Endocr Metab Disord. 2012;13:21–9.
42. Zhu JG, Ochalek JT, Kaufmann M, et al. CYP2R1 is a major, but not exclusive, contributor to 25-hydroxyvitamin D production in vivo. Proc Natl Acad Sci U S A. 2013;110:15650–5. https://doi.org/10.1073/pnas.1315006110.
43. Nykjaer A, Dragun D, Walther D, et al. An endocytic pathway essential for renal uptake and activation of the steroid 25-(OH) vitamin D3. Cell. 1999;96:507–15. https://doi.org/10.1016/S0092-8674(00)80655-8.
44. Nykjaer A, Fyfe JC, Kozyraki R, et al. Cubilin dysfunction causes abnormal metabolism of the steroid hormone 25(OH) vitamin D3. Proc Natl Acad Sci U S A. 2001;98:13895–900. https://doi.org/10.1073/pnas.241516998.
45. DeLuca HF. Overview of general physiologic features and functions of vitamin D. Am J Clin Nutr. 2004;80:1689–96. https://doi.org/10.1093/ajcn/80.6.1689s.
46. Blau JE, Collins MT. The PTH-Vitamin D-FGF23 axis. Rev Endocr Metab Disord. 2015;16:165–74. https://doi.org/10.1007/s11154-015-9318-z.
47. Wallace AM, Gibson S, de la Hunty A, et al. Measurement of 25-hydroxyvitamin D in the clinical laboratory: current procedures, performance characteristics and limitations. Steroids. 2010;75:477–88. https://doi.org/10.1016/j.steroids.2010.02.012.
48. Atef SH. Vitamin D assays in clinical laboratory: past, present and future challenges. J Steroid Biochem Mol Biol. 2018;175:136–7. https://doi.org/10.1016/j.jsbmb.2017.02.011.
49. Dunlop AL, Taylor RN, Tangpricha V, et al. Maternal micronutrient status and preterm versus term birth for black and white US women. Reprod Sci. 2012;19:939–48.

50. Burris HH, Rifas-Shiman SL, Kleinman K, et al. Vitamin D deficiency in pregnancy and gestational diabetes mellitus. Am J Obstet Gynecol. 2012;207:182–e1.
51. Maghbooli Z, Hossein-nezhad A, Karimi F, et al. Correlation between vitamin D3 deficiency and insulin resistance in pregnancy. Diabetes Metab Res Rev. 2008;24:27–32.
52. von Websky K, Hasan AA, Reichetzeder C, et al. Impact of vitamin D on pregnancy-related disorders and on offspring outcome. J Steroid Biochem Mol Biol. 2018;180:51–64.
53. Holick MF, Binkley NC, Bischoff-Ferrari HA, et al. Guidelines for preventing and treating vitamin D deficiency and insufficiency revisited. J Clin Endocrinol Metab. 2012;97:1153–8.
54. Baker AM, Haeri S, Camargo CA Jr, et al. A nested case-control study of midgestation vitamin D deficiency and risk of severe preeclampsia. J Clin Endocrinol Metab. 2010;95:5105–9.
55. Leffelaar ER, Vrijkotte TGM, van Eijsden M. Maternal early pregnancy vitamin D status in relation to fetal and neonatal growth: results of the multi-ethnic Amsterdam Born Children and their Development cohort. Br J Nutr. 2010;104:108–17.
56. Wilson RL, Leviton AJ, Leemaqz SY, et al. Vitamin D levels in an Australian and New Zealand cohort and the association with pregnancy outcome. BMC Pregnancy Childbirth. 2018;18:1–10.
57. Chen G, Pang T, Li P, et al. Early pregnancy vitamin D and the risk of adverse maternal and infant outcomes: a retrospective cohort study. BMC Pregnancy Childbirth. 2020;20:1–8.
58. James JL, Whitley GS, Cartwright JE. Pre-eclampsia: fitting together the placental, immune and cardiovascular pieces. J Pathol. 2010;221:363–78.
59. Steegers EAP, Von Dadelszen P, Duvekot JJ, Pijnenborg R. Pre-eclampsia. Lancet. 2010;376:631–44.
60. Aghajafari F, Nagulesapillai T, Ronksley PE, et al. Association between maternal serum 25-hydroxyvitamin D level and pregnancy and neonatal outcomes: systematic review and meta-analysis of observational studies. Bmj. 2013;346
61. Tabesh M, Salehi-Abargouei A, Tabesh M, Esmaillzadeh A. Maternal vitamin D status and risk of pre-eclampsia: a systematic review and meta-analysis. J Clin Endocrinol Metab. 2013;98:3165–73.
62. Robinson CJ, Alanis MC, Wagner CL, et al. Plasma 25-hydroxyvitamin D levels in early-onset severe preeclampsia. Am J Obstet Gynecol. 2010;203:366–e1.
63. Cho GJ, Hong S-C, Oh M-J, Kim H-J. Vitamin D deficiency in gestational diabetes mellitus and the role of the placenta. Am J Obstet Gynecol. 2013;209:560–e1.
64. McManus R, Summers K, de Vrijer B, et al. Maternal, umbilical arterial and umbilical venous 25-hydroxyvitamin D and adipocytokine concentrations in pregnancies with and without gestational diabetes. Clin Endocrinol (Oxf). 2014;80:635–41.
65. Lee CL, Ng BK, Wu LL, et al. Vitamin D deficiency in pregnancy at term: risk factors and pregnancy outcomes. Horm Mol Biol Clin Investig. 2017;31
66. Association AD. Gestational diabetes mellitus. Diabetes Care. 2004;27:S88.
67. Farrant HJW, Krishnaveni GV, Hill JC, et al. Vitamin D insufficiency is common in Indian mothers but is not associated with gestational diabetes or variation in newborn size. Eur J Clin Nutr. 2009;63:646–52.
68. Panel IA of D and PSGC. International association of diabetes and pregnancy study groups recommendations on the diagnosis and classification of hyperglycemia in pregnancy. Diabetes Care. 2010;33:676–82.
69. Alvarez JA, Ashraf A. Role of vitamin D in insulin secretion and insulin sensitivity for glucose homeostasis. Int J Endocrinol. 2010;2010
70. Yadama AP, Mirzakhani H, McElrath TF, et al. Transcriptome analysis of early pregnancy vitamin D status and spontaneous preterm birth. PLoS One. 2020;15:e0227193.
71. Miliku K, Vinkhuyzen A, Blanken LME, et al. Maternal vitamin D concentrations during pregnancy, fetal growth patterns, and risks of adverse birth outcomes. Am J Clin Nutr. 2016;103:1514–22.
72. Kim I, Kim SS, Song JI, et al. Association between vitamin D level at birth and respiratory morbidities in very-low-birth-weight infants. Korean J Pediatr. 2019;62:166.

73. Karras SN, Wagner CL, Castracane VD. Understanding vitamin D metabolism in pregnancy: from physiology to pathophysiology and clinical outcomes. Metabolism. 2018;86:112–23.
74. Merewood A, Mehta SD, Chen TC, et al. Association between vitamin D deficiency and primary cesarean section. J Clin Endocrinol Metab. 2009;94:940–5.
75. Savvidou MD, Makgoba M, Castro PT, et al. First-trimester maternal serum vitamin D and mode of delivery. Br J Nutr. 2012;108:1972–5.
76. Wang J, Liu N, Sun W, et al. Association between vitamin D deficiency and antepartum and postpartum depression: a systematic review and meta-analysis of longitudinal studies. Arch Gynecol Obstet. 2018;298:1045–59.
77. Vaziri F, Nasiri S, Tavana Z, et al. A randomized controlled trial of vitamin D supplementation on perinatal depression: in Iranian pregnant mothers. BMC Pregnancy Childbirth. 2016;16:1–12.
78. Bodnar LM, Krohn MA, Simhan HN. Maternal vitamin D deficiency is associated with bacterial vaginosis in the first trimester of pregnancy. J Nutr. 2009;139:1157–61.
79. Hensel KJ, Randis TM, Gelber SE, Ratner AJ. Pregnancy-specific association of vitamin D deficiency and bacterial vaginosis. Am J Obstet Gynecol. 2011;204:41–e1.
80. Curtis EM, Moon RJ, Dennison EM, Harvey NC. Prenatal calcium and vitamin D intake, and bone mass in later life. Curr Osteoporos Rep. 2014;12:194–204.
81. Roth DE, Leung M, Mesfin E, et al. Vitamin D supplementation during pregnancy: state of the evidence from a systematic review of randomised trials. Bmj. 2017:359.
82. Basile LA, Taylor SN, Wagner CL, et al. Neonatal vitamin D status at birth at latitude 32 72′: evidence of deficiency. J Perinatol. 2007;27:568–71.
83. Battaglia FC, Lubchenco LO. A practical classification of newborn infants by weight and gestational age. J Pediatr. 1967;71:159–63.
84. Chen Y-H, Fu L, Hao J-H, et al. Maternal vitamin D deficiency during pregnancy elevates the risks of small for gestational age and low birth weight infants in Chinese population. J Clin Endocrinol Metab. 2015;100:1912–9.
85. Lo T-H, Wu T-Y, Li P-C, Ding D-C. Effect of Vitamin D supplementation during pregnancy on maternal and perinatal outcomes. Tzu-Chi Med J. 2019;31:201.
86. Barrett H, McElduff A. Vitamin D and pregnancy: an old problem revisited. Best Pract Res Clin Endocrinol Metab. 2010;24:527–39.
87. Miyake Y, Sasaki S, Tanaka K, Hirota Y. Dairy food, calcium and vitamin D intake in pregnancy, and wheeze and eczema in infants. Eur Respir J. 2010;35:1228–34.
88. Camargo CA, Ingham T, Wickens K, et al. Cord-blood 25-hydroxyvitamin D levels and risk of respiratory infection, wheezing, and asthma. Pediatrics. 2011;127:e180–7.
89. W.H.O. Guideline: vitamin D supplementation in pregnant women. Geneva: World Heal Organ; 2012.
90. Ross AC, Manson JE, Abrams SA, et al. The 2011 report on dietary reference intakes for calcium and vitamin D from the Institute of Medicine: what clinicians need to know. J Clin Endocrinol Metab. 2011;96:53–8.
91. Dawodu A, Saadi HF, Bekdache G, et al. Randomized controlled trial (RCT) of vitamin D supplementation in pregnancy in a population with endemic vitamin D deficiency. J Clin Endocrinol Metab. 2013;98:2337–46.

Reliability of Frequently Used Ear, Nose, and Throat Drugs During Pregnancy and the Postpartum Period

28

Elif Hilal Vural and Ismail Mert Vural

28.1 Introduction

Drug use during pregnancy is a process that may cause adverse effects on both pregnant women and fetuses, but the risk can be reduced by certain precautions. During pregnancy, women can use drugs for various acute or chronic reasons. Although the frequency of drug use during pregnancy may differ between countries, recent studies have shown that the rate of pregnant women using at least one drug during pregnancy is over 50% [1–4]. In a retrospective study (between the years 2008 and 2012), it has been shown that a considerable number of pregnant women used more than one drug, an average of 4,6 medications, in their pregnancy period, excluding vitamins and minerals. [1]. In a multinational study, the frequency of different drug types used in pregnancy has been investigated. While the frequency of drug use for the treatment of acute/short-term illnesses occurred is 68.4%, the frequency of drug use for the treatment of chronic/long-term illnesses occurred is 17%. Over-the-counter (OTC) drug use had a similar frequency with short-term drug use [2]. In another cohort study, it has been demonstrated that the prescription rate for drugs used for pregnancy-related symptoms increased, whereas the prescription rate for drugs used for chronic diseases and for short-time use declined during pregnancy [3]. Physiological variations during pregnancy alter the pharmacokinetics (absorption, distribution, metabolism, elimination) and

E. H. Vural (✉)
Department of Medical Pharmacology, Faculty of Medicine, Lokman Hekim University, Ankara, Turkey
e-mail: elif.vural@lokmanhekim.edu.tr

I. M. Vural
Department of Pharmacology, Gülhane Pharmacy Faculty, Health Sciences University, Ankara, Turkey
e-mail: ismailmert.vural@sbu.edu.tr

C. Cingi et al. (eds.), *ENT Diseases: Diagnosis and Treatment during Pregnancy and Lactation*, https://doi.org/10.1007/978-3-031-05303-0_28

pharmacodynamics of drugs [5]. Many pharmaceutical clinical experiments are performed on men or non-pregnant women due to ethical considerations and fetal risk. Prediction of the effect, side effect, and fetal risks of drug use in pregnancy is quite complicated due to both maternal pharmacokinetic/pharmacodynamic alterations and limited clinical data.

The changes that alter drug pharmacokinetics during the pregnancy include the decrease in intestinal motility and gastric acid secretion, nausea and vomiting in early pregnancy, increase in cardiovascular output and all body fluid compartment volumes, reduction in plasma binding protein concentration, increase in cytochrome P450 (CYP) family of enzymes and conjugation enzymes, increase in renal blood flow and the glomerular filtration rate. Although an increase in gastric pH and a decrease in intestinal motility alter the drug absorption, these changes have a minimal overall effect on the bioavailability and therapeutic effect of long-term medications. In oral administration variations in absorption ratio and rate as well as first-pass metabolism alter the bioavailability of the drugs. It is noteworthy that the variability in drug absorption is higher in oral administration than that in intramuscular and subcutaneous administration. An increase in cardiovascular output and plasma volume may increase absorption in intramuscular, subcutaneous, and inhaler administration. Another critical point is that an increase in drug clearance may worsen disease control during pregnancy in chronic diseases. In the postpartum period, drug doses, especially doses of drugs with a narrow therapeutic window, may need to be adjusted to avoid the toxic effects. The changes in CYP enzyme activity can alter activation and plasma concentrations of prodrugs which are the medications that are metabolized into a pharmacologically active drug after administration. Care should be taken in terms of toxic effects in pregnant patients using prodrug and dose adjustment should be made if necessary. When using renally excreted drugs, such as heparin, clearance also increases in pregnancy because of the alterations in renal functions described above [5–7]. The half-life, which is the time required for the plasma concentration of the drug to decrease up to 50% after the drug is discontinued, is an essential parameter in determining the dosage range [8]. Both variations of body fluid compartment volume and clearance alter the half-life of drugs in pregnancy. While the increase in clearance decreases the half-life, the increase in the volume of distribution increases the half-life. Half-life may increase, decrease, or does not alter during the pregnancy. Therefore, each drug must be assessed individually for the alternation in its half-life. In the absence of specific pharmacokinetic data, esp. half-life data, drugs should be dosed with the same frequency in both pregnant and nonpregnant women [5].

Hormonal alterations and placental physiology may affect drug pharmacodynamics. The placenta, which is the functional unit between fetal blood and maternal blood, is like a gate for the transplacental drug transition. According to the pharmacological properties such as molecular weight, electrical charge, and hydrophily of the drug, the transition can be facilitated or prevented by the placenta. Primary transplacental transition mechanisms are passive diffusion, carrier-mediated transport, and transcytosis. The human placenta expresses drug-metabolizing enzymes in various types and amounts depending on the stage of pregnancy [9]. Although various studies have demonstrated physiological and pharmacokinetic alterations during pregnancy, there are no examples of pregnancy-specific dose schedules [10].

Agents that can impair the development of the embryo or fetus are called teratogens. Teratogens cause congenital malformation, especially in the early stages of pregnancy, or can cause stillbirths. According to the World Health Organization (WHO) data, about 6% of babies worldwide are born with a congenital anomaly [11]. However, terminated pregnancies and stillbirths are not generally considered in most studies. The human embryo is susceptible to drugs during the first three months of pregnancy. Outside this period, chemical factors mostly cause retardation or dysfunction in the intrauterine development of the fetus without causing a significant malformation. The Food and Drug Administration (FDA) introduced pregnancy risk categories in 1979 to standardize how experimental animal and human studies were conducted on the effects of drugs on pregnancy. With this decision, manufacturers were obliged to include FDA pregnancy risk categories (A, B, C, D, and X) in the package insert for drugs that were not absorbed systemically or known to have no adverse effects on the fetus. On June 30, 2015, FDA changed the rule of pregnancy and lactation labeling as the letter categories could give rise to confusion about toxicity risk and often failed to provide meaningful clinical information. With this change, the FDA aims to give more information to health care providers, pregnant women, and nursing mothers. With the new rules, the prescription drug/biologic labeling is required to include the sections of "Pregnancy," "Lactation," and "Females and Males of Reproductive Potential." These sections contain detailed information about the risks and benefits of prescription drugs, or the use of biological products during pregnancy and lactation and by females and males of reproductive potential. Information obtained from clinical studies is insufficient in terms of teratogenicity risk [12]. It should be kept in mind that for many drugs, only the information obtained through experimental animal studies is available since the opportunity to conduct clinical studies in pregnant women is very limited due to ethical reasons. As they can cross the placenta to reach the fetus and cause harm to the fetus, drugs should be avoided during pregnancy unless absolutely necessary. Basic principles must be considered first, to ensure that the drug treatment is safe and rational. The critical point is that the period most susceptible to the teratogenic effect coincides with the period during which the woman is not likely to know that she is pregnant. Therefore, the physician when using new drugs and drugs that are likely to have teratogenic effects should be careful not only in pregnant women but also in all women who are likely to become pregnant.

Various studies have shown that the rate of compliance of pregnant women varies depending on the trimester or the duration of the drug use. It is thought that maternal fear for fetotoxicity may be influential on this rate. Antihistamines, antibiotics, antacids, non-steroid anti-inflammatory drugs, and gynecologic drugs are examples of short-term treatments used in pregnancy [13]. In a study, the prescriptions of all women patients in the Danish National Birth Cohort (DNBC) have been examined in one of the Danish regions. In that study, it has been shown that compliance was lower for short-term treatments, and the lowest compliance was seen for local treatments of cough and cold and the use of ophthalmologic and dermatologic preparations. The compliance ratio of corticosteroids, nasal preparations, and antihistamine drugs was 20%, 43%, and 59%, respectively. Conversely, it was observed that compliance with the drugs used in the treatment of chronic diseases and the prescribed analgesics was high [14]. It is important to stress that the compliance rate does not indicate that these drugs have a low risk of congenital anomaly. In a different study on women who had babies with a congenital anomaly, relatively low compliance has been demonstrated for corticosteroids, dermatological preparations, systemic antibacterial drugs, anti-emetics, ear, eye, nose, and throat preparations [15].

Breastfeeding is the optimal form of infant feeding for the first months of an infant's life. Drugs are usually passed through the milk in the mammary glands by passive diffusion in breastfeeding women. Alkaline drugs can accumulate in the milk since human milk is more acidic than plasma. Non-ionizing small molecule drugs, such as alcohol and ether, are found in milk and plasma in approximately equal concentrations. The exposure and potential for toxic effects are highest in premature neonates. The risk decreases in the first few months of life as the baby's clearance mechanisms mature. When maternal drug therapy is required, risk assessments should take into account the natural toxicity of the drug and the amount of drug distribution in milk. The infant should be regularly assessed for adverse effects and growth retardation during the treatment [8, 16].

Many physiological changes caused by estrogen and progesterone levels occur in pregnancy. Many of these changes cause exacerbation of Ear, Nose, and Throat (ENT) symptoms and some ENT diseases depending on the trimester of the pregnancy [17, 18]. For example, auditory or vestibular changes lead to hearing or balance symptoms. The most frequent symptoms are tinnitus, pressure in the ear, a decrease in hearing and otalgia, while less common symptoms include increase in the ear secretion, and better hearing. Auditory-related symptoms do not differ between trimesters. Dizziness is more common in the first and second trimesters. Vertigo, instability, imbalance, and gait balance are frequently observed in the first two trimesters of pregnancy [19]. Epistaxis can be observed due to increased vascularity and diffuse edema of respiratory mucosa. Also, some diseases seen in ENT pathologies during pregnancy, such as hypertension and pregnancy toxemia and hypercoagulable state, can lead to sudden loss of hearing [20]. On the other hand, some of the drugs used in ENT practice in the pregnant women are antipyretics and analgesics, nonsteroidal anti-inflammatory drugs (NSAIDs), nasal topicals and antihistamines, decongestants and expectorants, antacids and antidiarrheals, and dermatological topicals. Some of these drugs are OTC medications in some countries, therefore, access to these medications may be easier [21]. Medical treatments of ENT diseases are discussed below.

28.2 Drug Groups Which are Used in Ear, Nose, and Throat Practice

28.2.1 Medical Treatment of Infections in Ear, Nose, and Throat

Chemotherapy, which is a concept defined by Paul Ehrlich at the end of the nineteenth century, is the drug treatment of diseases caused by parasites, fungi, viruses, bacteria, and neoplasms that invade the human body. The main principle is to show an excellent toxic or lethal effect on the disease agent organism while showing little toxic effect on the host. The selective effect occurs due to structural and biochemical differences between the pathogenic microorganism cell and the human cell [8, 22].

The coexistence of infection is frequent with pregnancy, and many pregnant women are exposed to chemotherapeutic use. Although the most common infections during this period are the urinary tract infections, ENT infections are also seen in pregnant women. Generally, this group of drugs pass through the placenta at different rates in pregnant women and may potentially have some effects on the fetus. Besides, it may pass into milk during the lactation period and have effects in the neonatal period [8, 23–25].

28.2.1.1 Antibiotics

Antibiotics are chemotherapy agents that are used to treat or prevent bacterial infections. Antibiotics are divided into two groups according to their degree of effect on microorganisms at their concentrations in body fluids. While some antibiotics have a bacteriostatic effect by preventing the growth or reproduction of bacteria, some of them have a bactericidal effect by destroying bacteria directly. Antibiotic classes are divided into five groups according to their typical antibacterial action mechanism (Table 28.1). Antibiotics and their classes are listed in Table 28.1 [8, 22].

Antibiotics are one of the most commonly used drug groups in pregnancy. Physiologic changes in pregnancy lead to pharmacokinetic alterations in antibiotics. This may require dose adjustment or monitoring. It is particularly necessary to know the spectrum of antibiotics very well when used in pregnant women. If the causative agent of the infection is unknown or empirical treatment is to be started, then treatment with broad-spectrum antibiotics should be preferred. In cases where the causative agent of the infection is known, narrow-spectrum antibiotics should be chosen. If possible, single-agent therapy should be preferred over polypharmacy. Rational antibiotic choices provide the benefit-harm balance, minimize the duration of treatment and potential adverse effects. Whether the patient has comorbidity or not is another critical criterion. Failure of elimination organs affects the choice and dosage of antibiotics. Other medications used by pregnant women should be considered in terms of drug interaction [23, 26]. On the other hand, plasma concentrations of antibiotics vary due to their pharmacokinetic changes, such as increased volume

Table 28.1 Antibiotic classes according to their antibacterial action mechanism

Antibacterial action mechanism	Antibiotic classes [8, 22]
By inhibiting bacterial cell wall synthesis and activating lytic enzymes	• Beta-Lactams (Penicillins, Cephalosporins, Carbapenems, Monobactams, Beta-lactamase Inhibitors) • Glycopeptides
By increasing cytoplasm membrane permeability	• Polymyxins • Amphotericin B
By inhibiting protein synthesis in bacterial ribosomes	• Aminoglycosides • Macrolides • Tetracyclines • Chloramphenicol • Lincosamides • Streptogramins • Oxazolidinones
By inhibiting DNA or mRNA synthesis	• Fluoroquinolones • Rifamycin • 5-Nitroimidazole • Mitomycins
By inhibiting the metabolism	• Sulfonamides • Trimethoprim • Isoniazid

of distribution, increased renal clearance, and reduced protein binding in pregnancy. The increased volume of distribution and increased renal clearance prevent decreased protein binding from increasing the free plasma concentration of antibiotics. As a result, free plasma concentration and antimicrobial efficacy of antibiotics may reduce in pregnant women [5].

It has been reported for a long time in various literature that the use of antibiotics during pregnancy causes lower birth weight and different diseases such as childhood obesity, childhood asthma, atopic dermatitis, and epilepsy [23–25]. Many antibiotic exposures during pregnancy, especially beta-lactams, macrolides, clindamycin, and fosfomycin, are generally considered safe in the literature. On the other hand, quinolones, tetracyclines, sulfonamides, and metronidazole use during early pregnancy have been associated with an increased risk of spontaneous abortion. Aminoglycosides pass through the placenta, and their use in the first trimester of pregnancy may cause fetal toxicity [24]. It is stated that fluoroquinolone use in pregnancy may be associated with renal toxicity, cardiac defects, and central nervous system toxicity in the fetus [25, 27]. Tetracyclines, which cause permanent discoloration in bones and teeth by binding calcium in the fetus by passing through the placenta, especially in the second trimester, are contraindicated in pregnancy [24]. In Canada, 139,938 pregnancies, of which 15,469 included exposures to an antibiotic, between the years 1998 and 2008 have been included in a cohort study. It has been observed that in utero exposure to clindamycin, doxycycline, macrolide, quinolone, and phenoxymethylpenicillin increased the risk of major congenital malformations in infants [28].

28.2.1.2 Beta-Lactam Antibiotics and Pregnancy

Beta-lactam antibiotics act by blocking the transpeptidase activity of penicillin-binding proteins (PBP), which are responsible for cell wall synthesis in bacteria and inhibit peptidoglycan synthesis. The common characteristics of this class of antibiotics are the presence of a beta-lactam ring in their structure, the same mechanism of action, and resistance mechanism against them. Beta-lactam antibiotics show a bactericidal effect. Penicillins, cephalosporins, carbapenems, monobactams, and beta-lactamase inhibitors are the groups of beta-lactam antibiotics [29]. Beta-lactamases, which are activated by breaking the beta-lactam ring, are involved in bacterial resistance to beta-lactam antibiotics. Beta-lactamase inhibitors are co-administered with beta-lactam antibiotics to prevent this kind of resistance [29, 30].

Penicillins and cephalosporins are generally safe to use in pregnancy. Detailed information on the use of these antibiotics in pregnancy is given below.

28.2.1.3 Penicillin Antibiotics and Pregnancy

Penicillins are a class of antibiotics that has been in use since the 1940s. They are used as a first-line antibiotic in many cases. Different drugs that have different pharmacokinetic properties and spectrum have been created by making changes in the beta-lactam ring in this group of antibiotics (Table 28.2). Their effects are related to the development and reproduction phase of the bacteria. They are prescribed to treat various infections, including upper respiratory tract caused by group B Streptococci and ear infections [8, 29].

Penicillins are the most widely prescribed antibiotic class during pregnancy in various bacterial infections. They pass through the placenta and reach the fetus at different levels, mostly in high concentrations. Amoxicillin-clavulanate is recommended as empiric antimicrobial therapy for acute bacterial rhinosinusitis in pregnancy. In contrast anti-staphylococcal penicillins (except methicillin) produce lower fetal tissue concentrations due to their increased ratio of protein binding. Serum penicillin concentrations may decrease in pregnant women due to increased plasma volume and creatinine clearance. Penicillin concentration may need to be increased because of these physiological changes [5]. Caution should be exercised for possible allergic reactions also in pregnant women.

Although penicillins, like other medications, should be used during pregnancy only when the potential benefits outweigh the risks, their use in pregnancy is probably safe. In various studies, it has been demonstrated that no adverse effects in the fetus or newborn were attributable to penicillin. Natural (penicillin G and penicillin V) and aminopenicillins (ampicillin and amoxicillin) have the most robust safety data [23, 26]. Similarly, in a cohort study in Canada, it has been demonstrated that exposure to amoxicillin in pregnancy did not increase the incidence of major congenital malformations [28].

28.2.1.4 Cephalosporins Antibiotics and Pregnancy

Cephalosporin antibiotics are commonly used in various bacterial infections. They inhibit the last step of the synthesis of the murein layer of the bacterial cell wall and activate autolytic enzymes. They also disrupt the structural integrity of the gram (−)

Table 28.2 Penicillin classes and their spectrums

Classes	Drugs	Spectrum
Natural Penicillins	• Penicillin G • Penicillin V	Non-beta-lactamase producing gram-positive cocci, limited gram-negative cocci (*Neisseria meningitides*, non-penicillinase-producing *Neisseria gonorrhea*, *Pasteurella multocida*)
Antistaphylococcal Penicillins	• Methicillin • Nafcillin • Oxacillin • Cloxacillin • Dicloxacillin • Flucloxacillin	*Staphylococcus* sp. (including penicillinase-producing strains)
Aminopenicillins	• Ampicillin • Amoxicillin • Bacampicillin	Includes natural penicillins spectrum and gram-negative bacilli (*H. influenzae*, *E. coli*, *Proteus mirabilis*, *Salmonella* sp., *Shigella* sp.)
Carboxypenicillins	• Carbenicillin • Ticarcillin	Includes aminopenicillins spectrum and *Enterobacter*, *Providencia*, *Morganella*, indole-positive *Proteus*, and *Pseudomonas aeruginosa*
Ureidopenicillins	• Azlocillin • Mezlocillin • Piperacillin	Includes carboxypenicillins spectrum and *Klebsiella*, *Serratia*, *Enterococcus*, anaerobic bacteria. The activity against Streptococci is slightly less than others
Beta-lactamase inhibitor combinations	• Ampicillin-sulbactam • Amoxicillin-clavulanate • Ticarcillin-clavulanate • Piperacillin-tazobactam	Beta-lactamase inhibitors extend the antibiotic's spectrum and increase stability against β-lactamases

bacteria wall. There are five generations of cephalosporins with different characteristics and molecular structures (Table 28.3) [8, 29]. Unlike penicillins, they cause fewer allergic reactions and are resistant to inducible beta-lactamases. Although it has been noted in the past that there is a 10% cross-reactivity rate between penicillins and cephalosporins, recent studies suggest a lower rate of cross-reactivity. [31]. Cephalosporins can cross the placenta, and their use in pregnancy is probably safe. Since distribution volume and renal clearance of most cephalosporins increase in pregnancy, dose adjustment is required to keep plasma concentration above minimal inhibitory concentration (MIC) [5, 23]. In a cohort study in Canada, it has been shown that the incidence of major congenital malformations did not increase in 1005 newborns exposed to cephalosporins in utero [28].

Cefazolin, a member of the first generation cephalosporins, is the most used parenteral (iv and im) antibiotic in pregnancy. Since the distribution volume and renal excretion of cefazolin increase in pregnancy, dose adjustment should be made in pregnant women. Also, caution should be used in breastfeeding as a small amount of cefazolin enters the breast milk. Similarly, dose adjustment is required for

Table 28.3 Cephalosporin classes and their spectrums

Generations	Drugs	Spectrum
1st Generation	• Cephalexin[a] • Cefadroxil[a] • Cephradine[b] • Cefazolin • Cefalotin	Gram-positive cocci effective against *Proteus mirabilis*, some *Escherichia coli*, *Klebsiella pneumonia*
2nd Generation	• Cefaclor[a] • Cefuroxime[b] • Cefprozil[a] • Cefoxitin • Cefotetan • Loracarbef[a]	Less effective against gram-positive cocci compared to the 1st generation, but more effective against gram negatives
3rd Generation	• Cefixime[a] • Ceftibuten[a] • Cefpodoxime[a] • Cefoperazone • Ceftriaxone • Cefotaxime • Ceftazidime • Cefdinir[a] • Ceftizoxime • Cefsulodin	More effective against gram negatives than first and second generations, some of them have an anti-pseudomonal activity (cefoperazone, ceftazidime, cefsulodin), less effective against gram positives
4th Generation	• Cefepime • Cefpirome	Similar spectrum with 3rd generation and anti-pseudomonal activity
5th Generation	• Ceftaroline	Similar gram-negative activity with 3rd generation, effective against *Staphylococcus* sp., *Streptococcus pneumoniae*

[a] Oral administration
[b] Both oral and parenteral administration

cefepime, a fourth-generation cephalosporin, and cefoxitin, a second-generation cephalosporin, when used in pregnancy. On the other hand, one-third of a dose of ceftriaxone, a third-generation cephalosporin, is excreted unchanged in the urine and two-thirds by hepatic metabolism and the pharmacokinetics of ceftriaxone is not significantly altered during pregnancy [5]. Similarly, renal excretions of cefoperazone, a third-generation antipseudomonal cephalosporin, and moxalactam, a third-generation cephalosporin, are lower than other cephalosporin excretions [22]. Therefore, there is no need for dose adjustment for these antibiotics during pregnancy. However, ceftriaxone should not be given at term if not necessarily due to the risk of developing kernicterus [23].

28.2.1.5   Glycopeptides and Pregnancy

Glycopeptides inhibit the transglycosylation reaction and peptidoglycan formation for cell wall synthesis by binding to the terminal D-Ala-D-Ala sequence of peptides forming the cell wall of gram-positive bacteria. They have a bactericidal effect and are active against only gram-positive bacteria and anaerobes. There are two generations of glycopeptides. While vancomycin and teicoplanin are the members of the first generation, telavancin, dalbavancin, and oritavancin are the members of the second generation. The second generation of glycoproteins was introduced to the market in the 2010s. Glycopeptide is used for the treatment of serious infections such as endocarditis, enterocolitis, pneumonia, and skin caused by methicillin-resistant *Staphylococcus aureus* (MRSA), *Streptococcus*, or *Enterococcus* bacteria, which are resistant to other antibiotics [32].

The use of glycopeptides as a first-line therapy during pregnancy is not recommended. However, sometimes the benefits of treatment may outweigh the risks. At the end of the 1980s, it was demonstrated in a study that vancomycin uses during the second and third trimesters of pregnancy did not produce hearing loss or nephrotoxicity in the infant [33]. In various animal studies, while telavancin caused malformations and fetal weight loss, dalbavancin increased embryo lethality and offspring death at higher doses [23]. Therefore, second-generation glycopeptides are not recommended at pregnancy unless needed.

Due to excretion into human milk, the use of glycopeptides during breastfeeding is discouraged.

28.2.1.6 Fosfomycin and Pregnancy

Fosfomycin, which has a broad spectrum of activity against both gram-positive and gram-negative organisms, inhibits bacterial cell wall and biosynthesizes it irreversibly. Fosfomycin use in pregnancy is safe and effective. Oral fosfomycin is only indicated for the treatment of acute uncomplicated lower urinary tract infections in adults. However, iv fosfomycin can be used to treat infections at the central nervous system, soft tissues, bone, lungs, and abscesses caused by multidrug-resistant organisms [23, 34].

28.2.2 Agents That Increase the Permeability of the Outer Membrane

28.2.2.1 Polymyxin and Pregnancy

Polymyxin, which was first isolated in 1947, disorganizes the structures of the bacterial cell which are responsible for the maintenance of the osmotic equilibrium. The members of this group of antibiotics, polymyxin B and colistin, are bactericidal and narrow-spectrum antibiotics. They are only effective in gram-negative bacteria. Their absorption from the gastrointestinal tract is very weak, and they are not administered enterally. Due to their severe adverse effects, such as nephrotoxicity and neurotoxicity, their systemic use in treatment was very limited in the 1980s. However, in recent years, colistin has been used for the treatment of severe systemic infections caused by gram-negative bacteria with multiple drug resistance. On the other hand, polymyxin B is administered topically to the eyes, ears, and skin [35]. Local polymyxin B treatment is recommended in pregnant women with otitis externa provided there is no evidence of a tympanic membrane perforation [36]. Since the safety of polymyxin has not been shown in human pregnancy, it should be used only when the potential benefits outweigh the risks.

28.2.3 Protein Synthesis Inhibitors and Pregnancy

28.2.3.1   Macrolide Antibiotics and Pregnancy

Macrolide antibiotics act by inhibiting protein synthesis in bacterial ribosomes. Macrolides bind to the 50s subunit of the bacterial ribosome and prevent the t-RNA molecule from binding to the same. Although they have a bacteriostatic effect, they have a bactericidal effect against susceptible bacteria such as streptococci at high doses. Macrolides are widely used for respiratory system infections such as tonsil tonsillitis, sinusitis, otitis media, bronchitis, and pneumonia. Macrolides are an essential alternative in patients allergic to beta-lactam antibiotics also in pregnancy [37, 38].

Erythromycin is the first generation of macrolides, clarithromycin, azithromycin, and roxithromycin are the second generation of macrolides, and telithromycin is the third generation of macrolides. Half-life of the second-generation macrolides is longer, and their oral bioavailability is higher than the first-generation macrolides [37, 38]. Macrolides are effective against gram-positive bacteria (cocci/bacilli), mycoplasma, mycobacteria, some rickettsia species, and chlamydia. Their effectiveness against gram-negative bacteria is low and limited to *Neisseria gonorrhoea*, *Bordetella pertussis*, *Haemophilus influenzae*, and *Legionella pneumophila*. The effect of azithromycin against *H. influenzae* and *M. catarrhalis* is higher than the effect of erythromycin and clarithromycin, and less on the gram-positive bacteria [37].

Although it has been reported in various studies that macrolides exposure was not associated with an increased risk of major congenital malformations, some opposite findings have also been published. Erythromycin transplacental transmission is quite limited [39]. Azithromycin and roxithromycin also have limited transplacental transmission, similar to erythromycin. Although macrolides penetrate the cell easily, limited transplacental transfer of these macrolides provides an advantage for fetal exposure [40]. In a study that included 105.492 pregnant women between 1999 and 2009, results show that neither the first trimester nor the last trimester exposure to macrolides increased neonatal risk [41]. However, in another study, it has been observed that erythromycin exposure could lead to endocardial cushion defect and coarctation of the aorta [42]. Also, in a cohort study in Canada, digestive system malformations due to azithromycin exposure and urinary system malformations due to erythromycin exposure were observed [28]. While azithromycin use in pregnancy is probably safe, caution is recommended for erythromycin and clarithromycin. At higher doses, telithromycin has been shown to delay fetal maturation. Therefore, its use in pregnant women is not recommended [23].

Macrolides may cause cardiac arrhythmias such as torsade des pointes, ventricular tachycardia, ventricular fibrillation by prolonging the QT and QTc interval. While erythromycin has the highest tendency for prolonging the QT interval, azithromycin has the lowest tendency. The risk of arrhythmias is related to the plasma concentration of the drugs, and in the absence of additional risk factors, the risk is very low [43, 44]. Erythromycin, solithromycin, clarithromycin, telithromycin, and azithromycin can lead to liver injury at varying levels from moderate ALT increase to hepatic failure with different mechanisms such as mitochondrial dysfunction, oxidative stress, and bile acid transporter inhibition [45]. Due to the fact that macrolides inhibit hepatic cytochrome p450 enzymes, care should be taken in terms of drug interactions. Telithromycin has rare but severe side effects including hepatic failure, exacerbation of myasthenia gravis, syncope, and visual disturbances. Telithromycin license has been withdrawn from the markets of some countries due to these side effects [37, 46].

28.2.3.2 Clindamycin and Pregnancy

Clindamycin is a lincosamide antibiotic that binds to the 50s subunit of the bacterial ribosome and inhibits protein synthesis in bacterial ribosomes. Clindamycin has a bacteriostatic effect and is active against only gram-positive bacteria and anaerobes. However, it has bactericidal against some strains of staphylococci, streptococci, and Bacteroides fragilis at higher doses. Clindamycin is used to treat head and neck, dental, respiratory, bone and soft tissue, abdominal, and pelvic infections [47].

Clindamycin passes through the placenta and reaches the fetus at 50% of maternal plasma levels. Congenital malformations due to clindamycin have not been demonstrated in the literature, and animal studies have failed to demonstrate fetal risk with clindamycin therapy. However, in a cohort study in Canada, it has been demonstrated that clindamycin exposure in pregnancy increased the risk of musculoskeletal system malformation and ventricular/atrial septal defect [28]. In clinical use, it is an alternative therapy for pelvic infections and bacterial vaginosis in pregnancy [47]. In pregnancy, increased dosing for clindamycin may be required due to the degree of protein binding [23]. Clindamycin is also present in breast milk but safe to use in breastfeeding mothers [16].

28.2.3.3 Aminoglycosides and Pregnancy

Aminoglycosides inhibit protein synthesis by irreversibly binding to the ribosome 30S subunit of the bacterium. Members of this group of antibiotics are bactericidal and narrow-spectrum antibiotics. They are only effective on gram-negative bacteria, including pseudomonas and other resistant bacteria, and have low effects on anaerobic bacteria. Due to the fact that the aminoglycosides absorption from the gastrointestinal tract is very weak, they are not administered enterally. Since they cannot enter the central nervous system, they are administered intrathecally in meningitis and other central nervous system infections. Streptomycin was the first member of aminoglycosides introduced into clinical use in the 1940s. Since then, several other natural or semisynthetic members of the class were introduced into clinical use, including neomycin, kanamycin, gentamicin, netilmicin, tobramycin, sisomicin, and amikacin. Aminoglycosides are used as single agents and in combination with other antibiotics in therapy for a broad range of indications including intra-abdominal, genito-urinary, surgical, respiratory tract, central nervous system infections, sepsis, and surgical prophylaxis [48, 49]. Aminoglycoside antibiotics can be used in the treatment of otologic infections such as external otitis. Since aminoglycosides, neomycin, and gentamicin are effective on bacteria that cause acute external otitis, ear drop forms of these antibiotics are indicated in external otitis [50]. Local sensitivity, burning sensation, dermatitis, ototoxicity, vestibular disorder, and hearing loss are the side effects that can be seen in local administration. Nephrotoxicity, neurotoxicity, and ototoxicity, both cochlear and vestibular disorders, are the serious adverse effects of aminoglycoside antibiotics when administrating systemically. However, systemic absorption following topical administration does not appear to pose a risk of nephrotoxicity [48, 49].

Short-term use of aminoglycoside antibiotics, except streptomycin, is acceptable with monitoring, after careful assessment of the potential risks and benefits. Aminoglycosides pass through the placenta and may result in toxicities, especially in the first trimester of pregnancy [23]. It has been reported that streptomycin uses in the first trimester caused irreversible bilateral congenital deafness in the fetus [51]. Serum aminoglycoside concentration may decrease in pregnant women due to increased distribution volume and creatinine clearance. In the case of systemic use in pregnant women, it may be necessary to increase the frequency of dosing or the dose [5]. Local neomycin treatment is recommended in pregnant women with otitis externa if there is no evidence of a tympanic membrane perforation [36].

28.2.4 DNA or mRNA Synthesis Inhibitors

28.2.4.1 Quinolones and Pregnancy

Quinolones, which are broad-spectrum synthetic antibiotics, have a bactericidal effect. They inhibit the separation of bacterial chromosomes, replication, and transcription of DNA by inhibiting the enzymes DNA gyrase and Topoisomerase IV [8, 52]. There are four generations of quinolones (Table 28.4).

Quinolones are widely used for various infections such as urinary tract infections, prostatitis, gonorrhea, diarrheal disease, and ocular infections [52]. Quinolones are also used in the treatment of ENT infections by both local and systemic administration. It was reported that both acute otitis externa and acute otitis media could

Table 28.4 Quinolone classes and their spectrums

Generations	Drugs	Spectrum
1st Generation	Nalidixic acid Oxolinic acid	Active against gram-negative bacteria
2nd Generation	Ciprofloxacin Ofloxacin Norfloxacin Enoxacin Lomefloxacin Pefloxacin	Improved activity against gram-negative bacteria
3rd Generation	Levofloxacin	Active against both gram-negative and gram-positive bacteria
4th Generation	Moxifloxacin Gatifloxacin	Active against both gram-negative and gram-positive bacteria, also active against anaerobes and atypical bacteria.

be safely treated with combination therapy of ciprofloxacin and dexamethasone ear drops [53]. Similarly, in the Cochrane systematic review, it has been demonstrated that quinolone ear drops are more effective than other classes of antibiotics both in reducing ear discharge and in eradicating bacteria in chronic otitis media [36, 54].

Although teratogenicity of quinolone in animal and experimental studies has been discussed in the literature, the teratogenic effect in humans is controversial [23, 28, 55]. In a meta-analysis including 14 studies, it has been demonstrated that quinolones are not associated with unfavorable pregnancy outcomes, such as the increased risk for fetal malformation, preterm delivery, stillbirth, and miscarriage [55]. On the other side, in a cohort study in Canada, increased risk of urinary system malformations associated with quinolone exposure in pregnancy has been demonstrated. In addition, moxifloxacin exposure increases the risk of respiratory system malformations and ofloxacin use increases the risk of major congenital malformations according to the results of that study [28]. Ciprofloxacin and hydrocortisone are recommended in external otitis treatment by intra-otic administration if tympanic membrane perforation cannot be safely ruled out. Also, quinolones such as levofloxacin or moxifloxacin are recommended as an alternative agent to macrolides for empiric antimicrobial therapy for acute bacterial rhinosinusitis in pregnant women who are allergic to penicillin [36]. When all this information from clinical and animal studies is evaluated together, it is possible to conclude that quinolones should be used during pregnancy only when the potential benefits outweigh the risks and should not be used systemically as a first-line therapy during the first trimester.

28.2.5 Antiviral Treatments

Antiviral agents are chemotherapy agents that are used to treat or prevent viral infections. Viruses are obligate intracellular parasites whose replication needs host cells, and they survive by synthesizing their genetic material and new viral proteins into those cells. Viruses can be grouped according to their genetic material as DNA and RNA viruses. DNA viruses enter the cell nucleus. The mRNA required for new DNA synthesis is synthesized. Enzymes are synthesized in the cell via mRNAs in the early protein synthesis phase. On the other hand, RNA viruses directly affect the ribosomes in the host cell and synthesize the enzymes and structural proteins required for them. RNA retroviruses synthesize a DNA copy of viral RNA via viral reverse transcriptase, and this copy integrates into the host genome. Then cellular effect occurs through these DNA copies [8, 56, 57].

Antiviral agents show their effects by preventing the virus from entering or leaving the cell or activity within the host cell. Therefore, nonselective viral inhibitors can also cause host cell damage. With a better understanding of the viral replication stages, suitable targets for antivirals have been determined. Antiviral agents and their mechanisms of action are given in Table 28.5. All antiviral drugs are virostatic and can only affect replicating viruses [8, 58].

Table 28.5 Antiviral agents and their mechanism of action

Mechanism of action	Antiviral agents and the virus they affect
By blocking viral attachment and entry	• Enfuvirtide, Maravirok (HIV) • Docosanol (HSV) • Palivizumab (RSV)
By blocking penetration	• Interferon-alfa (HBV-HCV)
By blocking uncoating	• Amantadine, Rimantadine (influenza)
By blocking early protein synthesis	–
By blocking the nucleic acid synthesis	• Nucleoside Reverse Transcriptase Inhibitor/NRTI (HIV, HBV) • Non-Nucleoside Reverse Transcriptase Inhibitors/NNRTI (HIV) • Acyclovir, Valaciclovir (HSV, VZV) • Foscarnet (CMV) • Entecavir (HBV)
By blocking late protein synthesis and processing	• Protease inhibitors (HIV)
By blocking packaging and assembly	–
By blocking the viral release	• Neuraminidase inhibitors (influenza)

Pregnant women and postpartum women, especially in the first two weeks of postpartum, are at increased risk for severe illness from influenza compared to non-pregnant women. Early initiation of the antiviral treatment, within 48 h, is more likely to be beneficial. It was shown that the need for intensive care and the mortality rate reduced with the early antiviral treatment in pregnant women [59]. Antiviral treatments widely used for influenza include M2 inhibitors (amantadine and rimantadine) and neuraminidase inhibitors (oseltamivir, laninamivir, peramivir, and zanamivir).

28.2.5.1 Oseltamivir and Zanamivir

Recent meta-analyses have suggested that oseltamivir, when effectively used for the decrease of influenza symptoms, reduces the hospitalization rate, the risk of otitis media, and antibiotic usage. Nausea, vomiting, diarrhea, kidney damage, and mental reactions are common adverse reactions of oseltamivir [60]. It has been observed that oseltamivir is the most studied medicine for influenza virus treatment in pregnant women with randomized controlled trials, and the most preferred agent is oral oseltamivir in pregnant women. Limited data exist on the transplacental transfer of oseltamivir. There has been no indication of an association between congenital malformations and oseltamivir exposure during pregnancy [61, 62]. In Japan, 90 pregnant women who took oseltamivir during the first trimester were assessed, and the malformation ratio was %1, similar to the general population [61]. Zanamivir is administered by inhalation with a dry powder inhaler. Clinical experience with zanamivir is less in pregnant women compared to that with oseltamivir. Zanamivir and oseltamivir use during pregnancy have been associated with late transient hypoglycemia, but there is no association with congenital malformations, small gestational age, low birth weight, or birth-related death [63, 64]. It was demonstrated that the infant would have been exposed to much smaller concentration of oseltamivir via milk than the pediatric use of dosage [65].

28.2.5.2 Amantadine and Rimantadine

Amantadine and rimantadine affect the influenza virus via inhibition of M2 proton channels; thereby, it inhibits the replication of influenza A viruses. It has been reported that resistance is observed with neuraminidase inhibitors via the neuraminidase gene or hemagglutinin gene [66]. Amantadine and rimantadine have similar toxicity profiles, such as renal or hepatic failure. Teratogenic effects of amantadine and rimantadine have been shown with laboratory animals and are not recommended for human use [67]. Breastfeeding is not recommended during the use of these drugs due to the potential adverse effects on infants.

28.2.5.3 Acyclovir and Valacyclovir

Acyclovir, which is effective against HSV and VZV, acts as a competitive substrate of DNA polymerase and causes chain termination after combining with viral DNA. It can be administered topically, orally, and iv. Valacyclovir is a pro-drug which is metabolized to acyclovir in the liver. It is administered orally and has a longer duration of action than acyclovir [8, 56, 58]. Acyclovir is recommended for the treatment of varicella during the second and third trimesters. Also, they are treatment options in Bell's palsy, but their efficacy is controversial according to the literature [68, 69]. In a cohort study, congenital malformation and acyclovir or valacyclovir relation were investigated in all infants born alive in Denmark from 1996 to 2008. The study has demonstrated that the exposure to acyclovir or valacyclovir in the first trimester of pregnancy was not associated with an increased risk of major congenital malformations [70].

28.2.6 Antifungal Treatments

Otomycosis is a fungal infection that affects the ears. It mostly affects people with diabetes or other chronic illness, immunosuppressive patients, people who have instrumentation of the ear, or who swim frequently. There are several treatment options as local debridement, local, and systemic antifungal agents for otomycosis, but it can become chronic [71]. Systemic antifungals are used in the case of a malignant invasive otitis externa. Oral triazole antifungals such as voriconazole, and posaconazole which show adequate penetration of bone tissue and the central nervous system, are recommended in the treatment of patients with malignant fungal otitis externa complicated by mastoiditis and meningitis [72]. However, there are severe risks of fetal malformations associated with the exposure of various antifungals, including voriconazole. Amphotericin B is still one of the drug choices for the treatment of systemic fungal infections during pregnancy in spite of its serious adverse effects such as nephrotoxicity and neurotoxicity. On the other hand, the use of topical azoles for the treatment of superficial fungal infections is safe in pregnant women [73].

Fungal disease of the nose and paranasal sinuses can be encountered in immuno-suppressive patients or patients with uncontrolled diabetes mellitus. Topical and systemic antifungal agents can play a critical role in surgical intervention and in the management of patients with invasive fungal rhinosinusitis [74].

28.3 Rhinitis and Rhinosinusitis Treatment

Allergic rhinitis disease has a high prevalence all over the world. Symptoms of disease change the quality of life. There is a wide range of pharmacological treatment options. Clinical Practice Guideline recommends topical (intranasal) steroids, oral antihistamines, oral leukotriene antagonists combination therapy, or immunotherapy for rhinitis primary clinical manifestations [75]. Allergic rhinitis also occurs during pregnancy. However, the most common subtype of rhinitis in pregnancy is hormonal rhinitis. Pregnancy rhinitis has been reported in nearly one-quarter of all pregnancies, and it increases the risk of life-threatening conditions such as obstructive sleep apnea, gestational hypertension, and lower Apgar Scores in neonates. Pregnancy-induced vascular changes due to endogenous hormones can result in increased nasal congestion and secretions. Symptoms resolve with the end of pregnancy. Nasal lavage is an acceptable therapy for pregnancy-associated rhinitis. Pharmacological treatment options are targeted to restrain nasal obstruction improvement [76, 77]. Ideally, all drug therapy should be avoided during pregnancy, especially in the first trimester. Treatment options and side effects in pregnancy are discussed below.

28.3.1 Intranasal Corticosteroids

Intranasal corticosteroids show their effect by binding to glucocorticoid receptors. There are two generations of these drugs that have different pharmacokinetic and safety profiles: first and second generations. While triamcinolone acetonide, flunisolide, beclomethasone, and dexamethasone are defined as the first-generation, mometasone furoate, fluticasone propionate/furoate, and ciclesonide are the members of the second generation. Corticosteroids are lipophilic molecules, and they are exposed to the first-pass metabolism depending on the administration route. Lipophilicity and first past metabolism effects are decisive for the administration route, dose, effect, and side effect profile. Lipophilicity increases the absorption of the drug and its passage into the systemic circulation. Intranasal corticosteroids show their effects locally; some of them can be absorbed and directly enter the systemic circulation without first-pass metabolism [78]. Systemic bioavailability of the second generation including ciclesonide, mometasone furoate, fluticasone furoate/propionate is less than 1% (ciclesonide level below assay limit). The first-generation intranasal corticosteroids such as budesonide, beclomethasone dipropionate, triamcinolone acetonide, and flunisolide have more systemic bioavailability (greater than 34%). Epistaxis, throat irritation, and nasal dryness, burning, and stinging are the most common local side effects of intranasal corticosteroids. Nasal mucosal atrophy or ulceration and septal perforation are other rare local side effects [78, 79]. NHS guidelines recommend intranasal corticosteroids for the first-line therapy for moderate to severe allergic rhinitis persistent symptoms [80].

In various studies, it has been demonstrated that there is no statistically significant relation between major congenital malformation and intra-nasal use of budesonide, mometasone, fluticasone propionate/furoate, and beclomethasone. On the other hand, according to those studies, triamcinolone increases the congenital respiratory malformation risk significantly [81, 82]. Controversy remains about using intranasal corticosteroids during pregnancy. Except budesonide nasal spray, the use of which in pregnancy is acceptable, they are recommended during pregnancy only if other safer options do not provide enough relief. Intranasal beclomethasone is recommended as a first-line therapy for pregnant women with rhinitis [83, 84]. However, it is shown that exposure to budesonide nasal preparations in early pregnancy is associated with a significantly increased risk of cardiovascular defect, primarily ventricular septal defect and atrial septum defect [42]. The Drugs and Lactation Database states that the amounts of nasal corticosteroids absorbed into the maternal bloodstream and excreted into breastmilk are probably too small to affect an infant [85].

28.3.2 Antihistamines

Histamine plays a prominent role in rhinorrhea, especially itching and sneezing symptoms, except nasal obstruction. Although H_1 receptor antagonists are widely used in allergies and related symptoms, H_4 antagonists are also a prominent target in the treatment of allergies. There are two generations of antihistamines, H_1 receptor antagonists (Table 28.6). Levocetirizine and desloratadine are enantiomers of cetirizine and loratadine, respectively, and fexofenadine, which is the primary active metabolite of terfenadine. These later developed antihistamines are classified as the third generation of antihistamines by some authors, although they are mostly accepted as belonging to the second generation [86, 87].

The first-generation H1-antihistamines can penetrate the brain, and they lead to drowsiness and impairment of cognitive ability such as learning or driving ability. The second-generation antihistamines penetrate less than the first-generation antihistamines, and they show minimal sedative effects [88]. H1 receptor antagonists are effectively used for the first-trimester nausea and vomiting symptoms particularly on, mild-moderate cases. Drowsiness, dizziness, muscle twitches, dry-mouth, headache, rash, tachycardia are common adverse effects of cyclizine, which is indicated in motion sickness, nausea, and vomiting caused by various reasons, Menière's disease, and morning sickness [89]. It should be kept in mind that H1 antihistamines, especially short-term use of cyclizine, can cause ventricular tachyarrhythmia [90]. Promethazine, brompheniramine, and diphenhydramine may be associated with prolonged QTc and cardiac arrhythmias when taken in large doses or overdoses [88]. Increased or decreased teratogenicity risk of the first generation of

Table 28.6 Antihistamine agent classes

Generations	Subgroup	Drugs
1st Generations	*Alkylamines*	Brompheniramine Chlorpheniramine Dexclorpheniramine Triprolidine
	Ethanolamines	Carbinoxamine Clemastine Diphenhydramine Dimenhydrinate
	Ethylenediamine	Tripelennamine Pyrilamine maleate
	Piperazines	Hydroxyzine Cyclizine
	Piperidines	Azatidine Cyproheptadine
2nd Generations	*Alkylamines*	Acrivastine
	Piperazines	Cetirizine
	Piperidines	Loratadine Astemizole Terfenadine Bilastine

antihistamines is demonstrated in various animal studies. Some congenital malformations are detected with maternal exposure to the first-generation antihistamines, but "specific malformations" are not defined in humans [91]. In a meta-analysis to determine the relative risk for major malformations associated with the exposure to H1 receptor antagonist during the first period of pregnancy, a literature research has been conducted covering the period between 1960 and 1991. Twenty-four controlled studies have been examined as part of the study, and it has been concluded that the exposure to H1 receptor antagonist in pregnancy did not increase the teratogenic risk in humans [92]. On the basis of all these studies, it is assumed that antihistamine medications are safe during pregnancy despite the typical side effects. The first-generation antihistamines such as chlorpheniramine, dexchlorpheniramine, and hydroxyzine may be used during pregnancy. However, their anticholinergic adverse effect, such as drying of the mucous membrane, should not be forgotten [93]. Also, hydroxyzine should be used cautiously during first trimester due to animal data [94].

The second-generation antihistamines are the first-choice treatment during pregnancy with a minimal sedative side effect, although most of them have no or limited safety data in pregnancy [91]. Astemizole and terfenadine have been withdrawn from the market in some countries as they could lead to ventricular arrhythmias via elongation of the QT interval. In addition, their use in pregnancy is not preferred in other countries due to their cardiotoxic adverse effect, although they do not have teratogenicity risk [88]. The clinically antimuscarinic effect, such as dry mouth, and urinary retention, does not occur with desloratadine, fexofenadine, and levocetirizine. Levocetirizine leads to impairment of driving performance and cognitive functions or memory and psychomotor performance while fexofenadine and desloratadine do not. None of them affect cardiac potassium channels [95]. Human epidemiological studies with astemizole, cetirizine, and terfenadine have not shown any association between teratogenicity and maternal exposure. Although concerns have been raised that loratadine and desloratadine may cause hypospadias, this has not been proven [91]. According to a more recent safety study, exposure to cetirizine generally occurs in the first trimester; both prospective and retrospective findings showed that there is no increased risk of adverse pregnancy outcomes [96]. Human data on second-generation antihistamines are generally considered to be reassuring for congenital malformations [94]. Bilastine is a new-generation antihistamine drug that is a highly safe and effective medicine for chronic urticaria and allergic rhinitis without sedation, anticholinergic activity, or cardiac side effects. Although Bilastine has advantages for drug-food or disease interaction, there is minimal data for the use of Bilastine in pregnancy [97]. Fexofenadine is among the top 20 most prescribed medicines in the first trimester between 1997 and 2003 in the USA [4]. A cohort study with 1.287.668 pregnancies between 2001 and 2016 in Denmark showed that fexofenadine exposure during pregnancy was not associated with significant congenital malformations, spontaneous abortion, small gestational age, preterm, or stillbirth. In the same study, it has been demonstrated that there was no increased risk for fexofenadine exposure when compared to cetirizine and loratadine with a sensitivity analysis [98].

28.3.3 Intranasal Antihistamines

Levocabastine and azelastine are examples of intranasally administered antihistamines. Their effect occurs faster than oral H_1 antihistamines and well-tolerated medicines for allergic rhinitis [87]. Intranasal antihistamine exposure associated with an increased risk of congenital malformations has not been proven [94, 99]. However, it has been demonstrated that oral administration of azelastine can lead to developmental toxicities in animal studies. There are not any clinical studies in pregnancy for this group of antihistamines, but they are not specifically contraindicated during pregnancy [100].

28.3.4 Leukotriene Modifiers

Leukotriene modifier agents mainly consist of two categories, which are leukotriene receptor antagonist and 5-lipoxygenase pathway inhibitors. Zafirlukast and montelukast are potent and highly selective antagonists of leukotriene receptors. Oral absorption of leukotriene receptor antagonists is rapid, and peak plasma concentrations are generally achieved three hours after oral administration. Taking with food reduces the mean bioavailability by approximately 40%. They bind to plasma proteins at high levels, and their major elimination route is hepatic biotransformation and biliary excretion. Zafirlukast inhibits CYP3A and CYP2C9 enzymes. They are generally well-tolerated agents [87, 101]. Although leukotriene receptor antagonists are as effective as antihistamines, they are less effective than nasal corticosteroids in improving symptoms of allergic rhinitis [102]. Combination therapy of leukotriene receptor antagonists and intranasal glucocorticoids is recommended in the initial treatment of patients with moderate/severe seasonal allergic rhinitis. However, monotherapy of leukotriene receptor antagonists is not recommended for the first-line treatment of allergic rhinitis [103]. Leukotriene receptor antagonists are generally used as a member of multi-medication therapies for asthma control due to their effectiveness being less than inhaled corticosteroids [104].

It has been shown in a cohort study in Denmark that pregnant women's exposure to montelukast increased the risk of preterm delivery, preeclampsia, and gestational diabetes. It has been stated that this increase was associated with maternal asthma rather than montelukast exposure. Besides, montelukast exposure has not been found to be associated with an increased risk of significant congenital anomalies [105]. Zafirlukast has a similar safety profile with montelukast in terms of major congenital malformations [106]. Exposure to leukotriene receptor antagonists seems to be safe in pregnancy [94, 107].

Zileuton, which is a 5-lipoxygenase inhibitor and has oral administration, is indicated for the prophylaxis and chronic treatment of asthma. Animal studies with zileuton have not been conclusive, and there are no well-controlled studies in pregnant women. Zileuton generally has not recommended in pregnancy. It should be used during pregnancy only if the potential benefit justifies the potential risk to the fetus [94, 108].

28.3.5 Nasal Decongestants

Sympathomimetic amines such as adrenaline, ephedrine, phenylephrine, tuaminoheptane, and phenylpropanolamine and imidazoline derivatives such as naphazoline, oxymetazoline, tetryzoline, tramazoline, xylometazoline, and clonazoline are the two main groups of nasal decongestants. Their sympathomimetic efficacy occurs via stimulations of alfa-adrenergic receptors. Sympathomimetic amines act on alfa-1 receptors as a selective agonist on mostly capacitance vessels. They also can stimulate alpha-2 and beta receptors [109]. Imidazoline derivatives act on both capacitance and resistance vessels via alfa-2 receptor agonism. The latency time of sympathomimetic amines is 10–15 min (excluding adrenaline which has a latency time of 5–6 s), and their duration of action is 1.5–4 h. Although the latency time of imidazoline derivatives is as much as that of sympathomimetic amines, their duration of action is much longer. The action time of both xylometazoline and tramazoline is almost 11 h [110]. Nasal decongestants' well-known adverse effects are rebound congestion, hypertension, headache, nausea, insomnia, and dizziness. Generally, nasal decongestant use is limited with a maximum of 5 days. Rebound stimulation can occur "a few hours" after the administration of nasal decongestant. Rebound congestion may occur because of nasal decongestants' affinity to beta-adrenoreceptors. Firstly, the vasoconstriction effect occurs, then vasoconstriction disappears since the beta-receptor stimulation effect takes longer than the alfa-receptor effect, and the vasodilation becomes evident. If the patient is not informed, a nasal decongestant is used repeatedly to maintain the vasoconstriction effect. Repeated medicine use may result in tachyphylaxis [110].

The pregnant women may tend to use these medications over a more extended period or at higher doses than recommended because pregnancy rhinitis takes longer than common cold symptoms. Rhinitis medicamentosa occurs with overuse or prolonged use of nasal decongestants [77]. Chronic vasoconstriction, the fatigue of the constrictor mechanisms, vasomotor tone alterations, and rebound vasodilatation via beta receptors may be responsible for the development of rhinitis medicamentosa [109]. Nasal decongestants can be considered as a second-line therapy for the short-term when other safer options do not provide enough relief [83, 84]. Nasal decongestions have limited systemic absorption in the mother, and their risks for infants have not been shown in the literature. Nevertheless, it should not be used for the long term in lactating women.

28.3.6 Systemic Decongestants

Orally administered decongestant phenylephrine, phenylpropanolamine, and pseudoephedrine are recommended as a second-line therapy or, if necessary, for rhinitis during pregnancy [77, 84, 111]. In addition, recommendations are also existing that they should not be used during pregnancy due to the risk of causing congenital malformations mentioned below [94]. Pseudoephedrine is a sympathomimetic vasoconstrictor, and previous studies indicate that pseudoephedrine exposure in pregnancy is associated with gastroschisis [112, 113]. Similarly, results of later studies show that pseudoephedrine exposure is associated with an increased risk of gastroschisis (1.8-fold) and small intestine atresia (2-fold), but the statistical significance of this association is in borderline. On the other hand, using pseudoephedrine and acetaminophen together during pregnancy statistically increases the risk of gastroschisis significantly to 4.2-fold and small intestine atresia to 3-fold [114]. According to these data, it can be said that pseudoephedrine should not be used during pregnancy unless the benefit outweighs the risk to the fetus. Also, it was demonstrated that phenylephrine has been associated with clubfoot and eye/ear malformations. Except these congenital malformation risks, oxymetazoline may cause uteroplacental insufficiency at higher doses [94]. In a single-blind randomized study, the effect of pseudoephedrine has been compared to placebo in eight lactating women. While a single dose of pseudoephedrine significantly reduced milk production, the calculated infant dose delivered via milk was less than 10% of the maternal dose [115]. When pseudoephedrine is used by nursing mothers, especially by mothers who have difficulties in producing sufficient milk, caution is recommended.

28.3.7 Inhaled and Oral Preparations of Corticosteroids

Corticosteroids are administered in pregnancy to treat symptoms of autoimmune conditions due to their immunosuppressive and anti-inflammatory effects. They are, if indicated, considered safe in pregnancy during the second and especially the third trimester. Inhaled or oral preparations of corticosteroids are sometimes used for the treatment of chronic rhinosinusitis, asthma, and other ENT diseases such as Meniere's disease, sudden sensorineural hearing loss, and Bell's palsy [116, 117]. Prednisone, prednisolone, methylprednisolone, betamethasone, dexamethasone, and triamcinolone are examples of synthetic corticosteroids. There are several forms of corticosteroid therapies according to their administration route as oral, parenteral (intravenous, intramuscular), inhalation, and topical (intra-articular, ocular, intranasal, in-ear). Corticosteroids are considered safe for the treatment of various medical conditions during pregnancy.

Increased risk of cleft lip with or without cleft palate due to first-trimester corticosteroid exposure has been demonstrated in different studies [116–118]. However, it has been expressed in a mini-review that exposure to corticosteroids in early pregnancy was not associated with an increased risk of congenital malformations, including oral clefts [119]. In a cohort study in Denmark with 832.636 live births between 1996 and 2008, it has been demonstrated that corticosteroid exposure via different administration routes (oral, inhalant, nasal spray, or dermatologic and other topicals) during pregnancy was not associated with orofacial clefts [120]. There is limited evidence in the literature that the exposure of systemic corticosteroids during pregnancy causes an increase in the risks of preterm labor, low birth weight, or preeclampsia, and in some studies, these risks related to corticosteroid exposure were not seen [94, 116]. While there is no association between miscarriage and oral corticosteroid exposure in pregnancy, there is a slightly increased risk for inhaled corticosteroid exposure [119]. There is not sufficient data in the literature regarding whether corticosteroid exposure contributes to gestational diabetes mellitus [116]. If systemic steroids have to be used in the treatment, maternal blood glucose monitoring is recommended due to blood glucose irregularities [121].

28.3.8 Monoclonal Antibodies

Omalizumab is a recombinant monoclonal antibody for the free and membrane IgE. Omalizumab is used for asthma and chronic idiopathic urticaria subcutaneously. Omalizumab treatment dosage determines body weight (not more than 150 kg) and IgE level (30–700 IU/mL) [122]. In patients with inadequately controlled allergic rhinitis, it has been demonstrated that omalizumab significantly decreased the symptoms and rescue medication use and improved the quality of life [123]. Anaphylaxis is a rare but severe side effect during treatment [124]. No risk of omalizumab-related congenital malformation has been reported in recent studies, though with a small sample size [100, 125]. Due to limited data, omalizumab should only be used during pregnancy if necessary. There is no randomized design clinical data on its administration during breastfeeding. It has been demonstrated that omalizumab is excreted in breast milk with a limited level in cynomolgus monkeys [126]. As a result, the use of omalizumab may be considered during breast-feeding if clinically needed.

28.3.9 Anticholinergic Agents

Ipratropium bromide is an inhaled anticholinergic agent that has bronchodilator effect for asthma patients. The bronchodilatation effect of ipratropium is less than beta-2 adrenergic agonists, which are used in asthma and chronic obstructive pulmonary disease treatment [127]. Intranasal ipratropium is effective in decreasing rhinorrhea but does not affect nasal obstruction and sneezing in rhinitis [82]. Double-blind, placebo-controlled studies show that ipratropium bromide can reduce rhinorrhea in nonallergic rhinitides, such as gustatory and weather-induced rhinitis, but little information on its effect on allergic rhinitis is available [128]. It has been shown that ipratropium has no teratogenic effect on pregnant animals when administered by inhalation or gavage [129].

28.3.10   Theophylline

Theophylline, which is a methylxanthines derivate, is used for treating the symptoms of asthma. Allergic rhinitis is a common comorbidity of asthma. It is expressed that allergic rhinitis has been associated with both an increased risk of asthma development and asthma severity [130]. In a double-blind, randomized study, it has been demonstrated that low-dose theophylline had no significant effects on total nasal symptom scores and rhinosinusitis symptoms [131].

It has been reported that theophylline is associated with higher teratogenicity and embryotoxicity with zebrafish which is a pharmacological and toxicological studies model [132]. Earlier studies reported that theophylline exposure had a potential risk for heart defects, oral clefts, and urinary tract defects [133, 134]. In a case-control study in pregnant women with asthma, it has been reported that exposure to moderate doses of theophylline during the second and third trimester did not produce statistically significant differences between groups for complications and malformations [135]. Some literature considers that theophylline is generally used for severe or uncontrolled asthma patients and within multidrug therapy [136]. Theophylline levels must be monitored for toxicity, due to a decrease in theophylline clearance during pregnancy [94, 137, 138].

28.4 Meniere's Disease Treatment

Meniere's disease is an inner-ear condition that can cause vertigo, tinnitus, and sensorineural hearing loss. It is seen due to fluid retention, and estrogen and progesterone increase worsen the symptoms. Reduction of caffeine and salt consumption and, high water intake are recommended in the management of the Meniere's disease. While betahistine and diuretics are generally used as a first-line treatment, intratympanic dexamethasone application is considered as a second-line treatment [139]. However, the use of betahistine during pregnancy, also in nursing mothers, is not recommended as the potential risk for humans is unknown and studies in experimental animals are insufficient [117]. In a study, a limited number of pregnant women who were exposed to betahistine outcomes have been investigated in Turkey. Among 20 live births, 17 normal results, one major and two minor congenital malformations were shown. Two miscarriages were also seen [140]. It is recommended to avoid diuretics and histamines during pregnancy, as they may cause hypotension and hypovolemia and reduce cardiac output. During an acute attack, dimenhydrinate and meclizine may be administrated safely in pregnancy. In a randomized study, dimenhydrinate was effective in the treatment of nausea and vomiting in early pregnancy [141]. Metoclopramide can be used for persistent vomiting [142]. Detailed information about antiemetics is explained below.

28.4.1 Antiemetics

Nausea and vomiting are common clinical conditions during the first trimester. Usually, dietary or lifestyle changes provide adequate treatment for the control of these symptoms. If pharmacological treatment is required, pyridoxine and doxylamine or pyridoxine monotherapy is recommended in the first-line therapy and diphenhydramine or metoclopramide or ondansetron in the second-line therapy. Multiple antiemetic treatments can be used for antiemetic resistant nausea and vomiting or hyperemesis gravidarum [143, 144]. In a review that compares the efficacy of the commonly used antiemetics, it is demonstrated that neither of metoclopramide, ondansetron, and promethazine has superiority in symptomatic relief [143]. H_1 receptor antagonists such as promethazine and diphenhydramine have been widely used for nausea and vomiting treatment for a long while. Metoclopramide is an effective antiemetic via dopamine receptor antagonism, but its use is recommended as a second-line therapy due to extrapyramidal side effects such as dystonia and anticholinergic side effects such as drowsiness and dry mouth [143, 144]. Recent studies do not indicate an association between the metoclopramide use and major congenital malformations [145]. Ondansetron is a serotonin receptor antagonist prominently used for chemotherapy-induced nausea and vomiting. Ondansetron has been found useful in all range of nausea and vomiting severity during pregnancy [89]. Some epidemiological and animal studies report that ondansetron is associated with teratogenic side effects such as fetal rhythm disturbances and cleft palate [146]. Ten epidemiologic studies investigating the relation between congenital malformation risk and ondansetron exposure have been included in a systematic review. Among the studies in question, an association between prenatal exposure to ondansetron and cleft palate was identified in one case-control study and an increased risk of cardiovascular defects was demonstrated in one cohort study [147]. A retrospective cohort study of 1,816,414 pregnancies, of which 88,467 pregnancies were exposed to ondansetron, has been investigated in terms of the association between teratogenicity and ondansetron exposure. First-trimester exposure to ondansetron was associated with a small increase in the risk of oral clefts but not with cardiac malformations [148]. Systemic corticosteroids can be considered for refractory hyperemesis gravidarum treatment. When deciding to use systemic corticosteroids, particularly in the first trimester, harm-benefit balance should be evaluated due to the increased risk of oral cleft development [117, 144].

28.5　Bell's Palsy Treatment

Bell's palsy is usually seen during the third trimester or early postpartum. Perineural edema and mechanical compression due to viral inflammatory reactivation with subsequent demyelinization are thought to be etiology [117]. Bell's palsy is more common under the age of 40 or over the age of 60. It has been found that there is a relationship between Bell's palsy and pregnancy. Furthermore, pregnancy is thought to be responsible for the peak before the age of 40. Many cases of Bell's palsy appear during the third trimester, and medical treatment options such as diuretics, antivirals, pentoxifylline, and corticosteroids are recommended for treatment [69]. Corticosteroids are considered safe for the treatment of various medical conditions during pregnancy. However, the harm-benefit balance should be evaluated due to the increased risk of oral cleft development in the first trimester [117, 144]. According to the literature, the efficacy of acyclovir is a controversial issue, but corticosteroid treatment is recommended to start within the first 72 h of palsy [68, 69]. Inflammation of the facial nerve in Bell's palsy might be related to the herpes simplex virus, and antiviral agents are used in the treatment [149]. In a randomized, double-blind, placebo-controlled trial, prednisolone has been found to significantly shorten the total recovery time in patients with Bell's palsy. However, acyclovir given alone or in combination with prednisolone had no clinically significant effect [150]. It has been demonstrated that valacyclovir treatment does not affect the recovery time of facial paralysis [151].

28.6   Anticoagulant Medications, Epistaxis, and Treatment in Pregnancy

Anticoagulants and antiplatelets are the groups of drugs that are widely used, and their use is increasing year by year. For the peri-operative surgical planning and the acute management of complications such as bleeding and hematoma, clinical and pharmacokinetic knowledge of anticoagulant drugs is essential [152]. Brief information about the anticoagulants and antiplatelet drugs is given below.

28.6.1 Anticoagulants

Heparin, heparan sulfate, low molecular weight heparin (LMWH), and ultra-low molecular weight are the main classes of heparin. Heparin has a biological role in mainly the coagulation system, inflammation, angiogenesis, and growth factor signaling. It has been observed that thromboembolism risk increases during pregnancy. Heparin is widely used for venous thromboembolism. It is known that heparin has critical side effects, such as bleeding, osteoporosis, and heparin-induced thrombocytopenia [153]. Heparin is not suitable across the placenta barrier due to its high molecular weight [9]. Low molecular weight heparins (LMWH) are enoxaparin, dalteparin, tinzaparin, and nadroparin. These are used for venous thromboembolism treatment subcutaneously, and at the same doses for the non-pregnant women. LMWH does not cross the placenta barrier and breast milk. Osteopenia has not been shown with long-term use of LMWH during pregnancy. In deep vein thromboembolism or venous thromboembolism treatment switch from LMWH to UFH is recommended nearer the birth, due to the longer half-life of LMWH. UFH must be monitored and adjusted for achieving anticoagulation activity [154]. UFH is recommended in renal insufficiency conditions [155]. Heparin clearance increases in pregnancy as it is excreted from kidneys and dose adjustment may be needed in pregnancy [5]. If heparin therapy is to continue after delivery, the dose should be readjusted.

28.6.2 Oral Anticoagulants

Warfarin treatment is widely used for the prevention and treatment of thromboembolism in the general population. Studies have shown that the warfarin dose regimen is varied to achieve anticoagulant effectiveness because of the personal differences, particularly genetics of biotransformation enzymes. *CYP2C9*, *CYP4F2*, and *VKORC1* polymorphisms are highly studied genes to achieve optimal warfarin dosing and decrease adverse effects. Warfarin use contraindicated during pregnancy due to risks of the congenital malformations and fetal bleeding risk [154, 156].

Other anticoagulant drugs such as dabigatran, rivaroxaban, and apixaban are effective via Factor Xa inhibitions. These drugs do cross the placenta [155]. Although hemorrhagic complications are less common with dabigatran, rivaroxaban, and apixaban than with warfarin, pregnancy loss and fetal harm have been shown in animal studies for dabigatran and rivaroxaban. Edoxaban and apixaban showed no maternal or fetal harm in animal studies. The use of dabigatran, edoxaban, or apixaban should be decided upon by an evaluation of the harm-benefit balance. Rivaroxaban is not recommended during pregnancy [154, 156, 157].

28.6.3 Antiplatelet Drugs

Guidelines give less information about antiplatelet drugs because arterial thrombosis is less common than venous thrombosis during pregnancy. Antiplatelet drugs such as aspirin, ticlopidine, clopidogrel, and cilostazol inhibit platelet aggregation with different mechanisms on the platelet aggregation pathway. Most of them have side effects characterized by hemorrhage and related symptoms; in cases where these drugs are used, the risk and benefit should be well evaluated [156].

Due to increased vascularity of the nasal mucosa, the number of epistaxis incidences is higher in pregnancy. Although epistaxis is common during pregnancy, large volume epistaxis is rare and mostly seen in patients who have preexisting risk factors such as anticoagulant use or blood clotting disorders. IV tranexamic acid, an antifibrinolytic agent, administration, anterior packing, and bipolar cautery are recommended for the first-line therapy. If the first-line therapies fail, then vessel ligation or termination of pregnancy is recommended [158]. As pregnant patients are already hypercoagulable, antifibrinolytic treatment should carefully be managed.

28.7 Others

Vestibular migraine and sudden deafness can occur in the third trimester during pregnancy [159]. Sudden sensorineural hearing loss is relatively rare but it is an emergency medical condition in pregnancy. Although the exact etiology in pregnant women has not been identified, hormonal changes, autoimmune system disorders, hypercoagulability, and vascular occlusion are possible etiologies [160]. While the most common treatment is systemic corticosteroids, intratympanic corticosteroids are increasingly used [161].

Pharyngitis is often secondary to gastroesophageal reflux disease due to progesterone-induced decreased lower esophageal tone in pregnancy, and symptoms generally tend to dissipate postpartum. Lifestyle modifications, dietary changes, and antacids are applied as a first-line therapy. H_2 receptor antagonists are preferred as a second-line therapy. There is no association between H_2 receptor antagonists and neither congenital malformations nor intrauterine death risks. There are more efficacy and safety data available for ranitidine than other H_2 receptor antagonists. Patients with complicated reflux disease may be treated with proton-pump inhibitors [162]. Also, exposure to these drugs in pregnancy is not associated with a significantly increased risk of major congenital malformations [163].

During pregnancy pain is common. Acetaminophen and nonsteroidal anti-inflammatory drugs (NSAIDs) are used for mild to moderate pain. If needed, the lowest therapeutic dose and shortest possible duration are usually recommended [5, 164]. Exposure to NSAIDs is associated with a low increased risk of miscarriage and congenital malformations in early pregnancy. Also, premature closure of the fetal ductus arteriosus and oligohydramnios risk increase with NSAIDs exposure in late pregnancy [165, 166]. Therefore, NSAIDs should be used with caution in the first trimester and should be withdrawn at gestational week 32 except low-dose aspirin. Although NSAIDs are excreted into breast milk, evidence of harm has not been published yet [166]. Acetaminophen, which is an acceptable option all through pregnancy, is commonly used for analgesia and fever reduction in pregnancy [167]. Pharmacokinetics of oral acetaminophen does not change in pregnant women [5]. But long-term use in pregnancy is not recommended due to its association with a small risk of childhood asthma and prolonged paracetamol. Paracetamol is also a good choice for analgesia and fever reduction in breastfeeding mothers [166].

References

1. Ventura M, Maraschini A, D'Aloja P, et al. Drug prescribing during pregnancy in a central region of Italy, 2008-2012. BMC Public Health. 2018;18:623. https://doi.org/10.1186/s12889-018-5545-z.
2. Lupattelli A, Spigset O, Twigg MJ, et al. Medication use in pregnancy: a cross-sectional, multinational web-based study. BMJ Open. 2014;4(2):e004365. https://doi.org/10.1136/bmjopen-2013-004365.
3. Bakker MK, Jentink J, Vroom F. Drug prescription patterns before, during and after pregnancy for chronic, occasional and pregnancy-related drugs in the Netherlands. BJOG. 2006;113(5):559–68. https://doi.org/10.1111/j.1471-0528.2006.00927.x.
4. Mitchell AA, Gilboa SM, Werler MM. National birth defects prevention study. Medication use during pregnancy, with particular focus on prescription drugs: 1976–2008. Am J Obstet Gynecol. 2011;205(1):51.e1–8. https://doi.org/10.1016/j.ajog.2011.02.029.
5. Ansari J, Carvalho B, Shafer SL, et al. Pharmacokinetics and pharmacodynamics of drugs commonly used in pregnancy and parturition. Anesth. 2016;122(3):786–804. https://doi.org/10.1213/ANE.0000000000001143.
6. Feghali M, Venkataramanan R, Caritis S. Pharmacokinetics of drugs in pregnancy. Semin Perinatol. 2015;39(7):512–9.
7. Pavek P, Ceckova M, Staud F. Variation of drug kinetics in pregnancy. Curr Drug Metab. 2009;10(5):520–9. https://doi.org/10.2174/138920009788897993.
8. Katzung BG. Basic and clinical pharmacology. 14th ed. New York: The McGraw-Hill Companies; 2018.
9. Tetro N, Moushaev S, Rubinchik-Stern M, et al. The placental barrier: the gate and the fate in drug distribution. Pharm Res. 2018;35(4):71. https://doi.org/10.1007/s11095-017-2286-0.
10. Koren G, Pariente G. Pregnancy-associated changes in pharmacokinetics and their clinical implications. Pharm Res. 2018;35(3):61. https://doi.org/10.1007/s11095-018-2352-2.
11. WHO. Congenital anomalies; 2020. https://www.who.int. Accessed 13 July 2020

12. FDA. Pregnancy and lactation labeling final rule; 2014. https://www.fda.gov. Accessed 20 July 2020
13. Matsui D. Adherence with drug therapy in pregnancy. Obstet Gynecol Int. 2012;2012:796590. https://doi.org/10.1155/2012/796590.
14. Olesen C, Søndergaard C, Thrane N, et al. Do pregnant women report use of dispensed medications? Epidemiology. 2001;12(5):497–501. https://doi.org/10.1097/00001648-200109000-.
15. de Jonge L, de Walle HE, de Jong-van den Berg LT, et al. Actual use of medications prescribed during pregnancy: a cross-sectional study using data from a population-based congenital anomaly registry. Drug Saf. 2015;38(8):737–47. https://doi.org/10.1007/s40264-015-0302-z.
16. Kayhan Tetik B, Gedik Tekinemre I. Emziren annelerde ilaç kullanımı. Jour Turk Fam Phy. 2017;8(3):83–9. (in Turkish). https://doi.org/10.15511/tjtfp.17.00383.
17. Akkoca AN, Özler GS, Keskin Kurt R, et al. Ear, nose and throat changes observed during three trimester of pregnancy. Sci J Clin Med. 2014;3(3):52–6.
18. Mgbe RB, Umana AN, Adekanye AG. Ear nose and throat changes observed in pregnancy in Calabar-Nigeria. Offiong Global J Pure Appl Sci. 2017;23:355–9. https://doi.org/10.4314/gjpas.v23i2.16.
19. Schmidt PM, Flores Fda T, Rossi AG, et al. Hearing and vestibular complaints during pregnancy. Braz J Otorhinolaryngol. 2010;76(1):29–33.
20. Bhagat DR, Chowdhary A, Verma S, et al. Physiological changes in ENT during pregnancy. Indian J Otolaryngol Head Neck Surg. 2006;58(3):268–70. https://doi.org/10.1007/BF03050836.
21. Stanley AY, Durham CO, Sterrett JJ, et al. Safety of over-the-counter medications in pregnancy. MCN Am J Matern Child Nurs. 2019;44(4):196–205. https://doi.org/10.1097/NMC.0000000000000537.
22. Kayaalp SO. Akılcıl Tedavi Yönünden Tıbbi Farmakoloji, 13. Basım. Pelikan Kitapevi, Ankara; 2018 (ın Turkish).
23. Bookstaver PB, Bland CM, Griffin B, et al. Review of antibiotic use in pregnancy. Pharmacotherapy. 2015;35(11):1052–62.
24. Briggs GG, Freeman RK. Drugs in pregnancy and lactation: a reference guide to fetal and neonatal risk. 11th ed. Philadelphia: Lippincott Williams & Wilkins; 2007.
25. Crider KS, Cleves MA, Reefhuis J, et al. Antibacterial medication use during pregnancy and risk of birth defects: national birth defects prevention study. Arch Pediatr Adolesc Med. 2009;11:978–85. https://doi.org/10.1001/archpediatrics.2009.188.
26. Mungan MT. Gebelikte Antibiyotik Kullanımı. Turkiye Klinikleri J Gynecol Obst. 2001;11(6):451–60. (in Turkish)
27. Guinto VT, De Guia B, Festin MR, et al. Different antibiotic regimens for treating asymptomatic bacteriuria in pregnancy. Cochrane Database Syst Rev. 2010;8(9):CD007855. https://doi.org/10.1002/14651858.CD007855.pub2.
28. Muanda FT, Sheehy O, Bérard A. Use of antibiotics during pregnancy and risk of spontaneous abortion. CMAJ. 2017;189(17):E625–33. https://doi.org/10.1503/cmaj.161020.
29. Bush K, Bradford PA. β-lactams and β-lactamase inhibitors: an overview. Cold Spring Harb Perspect Med. 2016;6(8):a025247. https://doi.org/10.1101/cshperspect.a025247.
30. Khanna NR, Gerriets V. Beta lactamase inhibitors. StatPearls [Internet], Treasure Island, FL; 2020. https://www.ncbi.nlm.nih.gov/books/NBK557592/
31. Lee QU. Use of cephalosporins in patients with immediate penicillin hypersensitivity: cross reactivity revisited. Hong Kong Med J. 2014;20:428–36.
32. Blaskovich MAT, Hansford KA, Butler MS, et al. Developments in glycopeptide antibiotics. ACS Infect Dis. 2018;4(5):715–35. https://doi.org/10.1021/acsinfecdis.7b00258.
33. Reyes MP, Ostrea EM Jr, Cabinian AE, et al. Vancomycin during pregnancy: does it cause hearing loss or nephrotoxicity in the infant? Am J Obstet Gynecol. 1989;161(4):977–81.
34. Dijkmans AC, Zacarías NVO, Burggraaf J, et al. Fosfomycin: pharmacological, clinical and future perspectives. Antibiotics (Basel). 2017;6(4):24.

35. Trimble MJ, Mlynárčik P, Kolář M, et al. Polymyxin: alternative mechanisms of action and resistance. Cold Spring Harb Perspect Med. 2016;6(10):a025288. https://doi.org/10.1101/cshperspect.a025288.

36. Roemer H, Martinez, MT, Katz VL, et al. ENT issues in pregnancy; 2013. https://www.acep-now.com/article/ent-issues-pregnancy/

37. Dinos GP. The macrolide antibiotic renaissance. Br J Pharmacol. 2017;174:2967–83.

38. Seifert R. Basic knowledge of pharmacology. Switzerland: Springer; 2019.

39. Bulska M, Szcześniak P, Pięta-Dolińska A, et al. The placental transfer of erythromycin in human pregnancies with group B streptococcal infection. Ginekol Pol. 2015;86(1):33–9. https://doi.org/10.17772/gp/1896.

40. Heikkinen T, Laine K, Neuvonen PJ, et al. The transplacental transfer of the macrolide antibiotics erythromycin, roxithromycin and azithromycin. BJOG. 2000;107(6):770–5. https://doi.org/10.1111/j.1471-0528.2000.tb13339.x.

41. Bahat Dinur A, Koren G, Matok I, et al. Fetal safety of macrolides. Antimicrob Agents Chemother. 2013;57(7):3307–11. https://doi.org/10.1128/AAC.01691-12.

42. Källén BAJ, Olausson PO. Maternal drug use in early pregnancy and infant cardiovascular defect. Reprod Toxicol. 2003;17(3):255–61.

43. Albert RK, Schuller JL. COPD clinical research network. Macrolide antibiotics and the risk of cardiac arrhythmias. Am J Respir Crit Care Med. 2014;189(10):1173–80.

44. Patel PH, Hashmi MF. Macrolides. StatPearls [Internet], Treasure Island, FL; 2020. https://www.ncbi.nlm.nih.gov/books/NBK551495/

45. Woodhead JL, Yang K, Oldach D, et al. Analyzing the mechanisms behind macrolide antibiotic-induced liver injury using quantitative systems toxicology modeling. Pharm Res. 2019;36(3):48. https://doi.org/10.1007/s11095-019-2582-y.

46. Fernandes P, Martens E, Pereira D. Nature nurtures the design of new semi-synthetic macrolide antibiotics. J Antibiot. 2017;70(5):527–33. https://doi.org/10.1038/ja.2016.137.

47. Smieja M. Current indications for the use of clindamycin: a critical review. Can J Infect Dis. 1998;9(1):22–8. https://doi.org/10.1155/1998/538090.

48. Avent ML, Rogers BA, Cheng AC. Current use of aminoglycosides: Indications, pharmacokinetics and monitoring for toxicity. Intern Med J. 2011;41:441–9.

49. Krause KM, Serio AW, Kane TR, et al. Aminoglycosides: an overview. Cold Spring Harb Perspect Med. 2016;6(6):a027029. https://doi.org/10.1101/cshperspect.a027029.

50. McWilliams CJ, Smith CH, Goldman RD. Acute otitis externa in children. Can Fam Physician. 2012;58(11):1222–4.

51. Heikkila AM. Antibiotics in pregnancy—a prospective cohort study on the policy of antibiotic prescription. Ann Med. 1993;5:467–71.

52. Sharma CP, Jain A, Jain S. Fluoroquinolone antibacterials: a review on chemistry, microbiology and therapeutic prospects. Acta Poloniae Pharmaceutica ñ Drug Research. 2009;66(6):587–604.

53. Wall GM, Stroman DW, Roland PS, et al. Ciprofloxacin 0.3%/dexamethasone 0.1% sterile Otic suspension for the topical treatment of ear infections: a review of the literature. Pediatr Infect Dis J. 2009;28(2):141–4. https://doi.org/10.1097/INF.0b013e31818b0c9c.

54. Acuin J, Smith A, Mackenzie I. Interventions for chronic suppurative otitis media. Cochrane Database Syst Rev. 2000;(2):CD000473. https://doi.org/10.1002/14651858.CD000473.

55. Yefet E, Schwartz N, Chazan B. The safety of quinolones and fluoroquinolones in pregnancy: a meta-analysis. BJOG. 2018;125(9):1069–76. https://doi.org/10.1111/1471-0528.15119.

56. de Clercq E. Molecular targets for antiviral agents. J Pharmacol Exp Therap. 2001;297(1):1–10.

57. Paintsil E, Cheng YC. Antiviral agents. Encyclopedia Microbiol. 2009;2009:223–57. https://doi.org/10.1016/B978-012373944-5.00178-4.

58. Chaudhuri S, Symons JA, Deval J, et al. Innovation and trends in the development and approval of antiviral medicines: 1987-2017 and beyond. Antiviral Res. 2018;155:76–88. https://doi.org/10.1016/j.antiviral.2018.05.005.

59. Louie JK, Acosta M, Jamieson DJ. Severe 2009 H1N1 influenza in pregnant and postpartum women in California. N Engl J Med. 2010;362:27–35.
60. Qiu S, Shen Y, Pan H, et al. Effectiveness and safety of oseltamivir for treating influenza: an updated meta-analysis of clinical trials. Infect Dis (Lond). 2015;47(11):808–19. https://doi.org/10.3109/23744235.2015.1067369.
61. Hayashi M, Yamane R, Tanaka M, et al. Pregnancy outcome after maternal exposure to oseltamivir phosphate during the first trimester: a case series survey [Japanese]. Nihon Byoin Yakuzaishi Gakkai Zasshi. 2009;45:547–50.
62. Meijer WJ, van Noortwijk AG, Bruinse HW, et al. Influenza virus infection in pregnancy: a review. Acta Obstet Gynecol Scand. 2015;94(8):797–819. https://doi.org/10.1111/aogs.12680.
63. Graner S, Svensson T, Beau AB, et al. Neuraminidase inhibitors during pregnancy and risk of adverse neonatal outcomes and congenital malformations: population based European register study. BMJ. 2017;356:j629. https://doi.org/10.1136/bmj.j629.
64. Svensson T, Granath F, Stephansson O. Birth outcomes among women exposed to neuraminidase inhibitors during pregnancy. Pharmacoepidemiol Drug Saf. 2011;20(10):1030–4. https://doi.org/10.1002/pds.2194.
65. Wentges-van Holthe N, van Eijkeren M, van der Laan JW. Oseltamivir and breast-feeding. Int J Infect Dis. 2008;12:451.
66. Ison MG. Clinical use of approved influenza antivirals: therapy and prophylaxis. Influenza Other Respir Viruses. 2013;7(Suppl 1):7–13. https://doi.org/10.1111/irv.12046.
67. Morris DJ. Adverse effects and drug interactions of clinical importance with antiviral drugs. Drug Saf. 1994;10(4):281–91. https://doi.org/10.2165/00002018-199410040-00002.
68. Eviston TJ, Croxson G, Kennedy PGE, et al. Bell's palsy: aetiology, clinical features and multidisciplinary care. J Neurol Neurosurg Psychiatry. 2015;86:1356–61.
69. Hussain A, Charles Nduka C, Moth P, et al. Bell's facial nerve palsy in pregnancy: a clinical review. J Obstet Gynaecol. 2017;37(4):409–15.
70. Pasternak B, Hviid A. Use of acyclovir, valacyclovir, and famciclovir in the first trimester of pregnancy and the risk of birth defects. JAMA. 2010;304(8):859–66. https://doi.org/10.1001/jama.2010.1206.
71. Anwar K, Gohar MS. Otomycosis; clinical features, predisposing factors and treatment implications. Pak J Med Sci. 2014;30(3):564–7. https://doi.org/10.12669/pjms.303.4106.
72. Vennewald I, Klemm E. Otomycosis: diagnosis and treatment. Clin Dermatol. 2010;28:202–11.
73. Moudgal VV, Sobel JD. Antifungal drugs in pregnancy: a review. Expert Opin Drug Saf. 2003;2(5):475–83.
74. Thompson GR III, Patterson TF. Mycosis of the maxillary fungal disease of the nose and paranasal sinuses. J Allergy Clin Immunol. 2012;129(2):321–6.
75. Seidman MD, Gurgel RK, Lin SY, et al. Clinical practice guideline: allergic rhinitis. Otolaryngol Head Neck Surg. 2015;152(1 Suppl):S1–S43. https://doi.org/10.1177/0194599814561600.
76. Caparroz FA, Gregorio LL, Bongiovanni G, et al. Rhinitis and pregnancy: literature review. Braz J Otorhinolaryngol. 2016;82(1):105–11. https://doi.org/10.1016/j.bjorl.2015.04.011.
77. Ellegård EK. Clinical and pathogenetic characteristics of pregnancy rhinitis. Clinic Rev Allerg Immunol. 2004;26:149–59. https://doi.org/10.1385/CRIAI:26:3:149.
78. Derendorf H, Meltzer EO. Molecular and clinical pharmacology of intranasal corticosteroids: clinical and therapeutic implications. Allergy. 2008;63(10):1292–300. https://doi.org/10.1111/j.1398-9995.2008.01750.x.
79. Sastre J, Mosges R. Local and systemic safety of intranasal corticosteroids. J Investig Allergol Clin Immunol. 2012;22(1):1–12.
80. NHS, Hull & East Riding Prescribing Committee. Prescribing guideline for rhinitis; 2020. https://www.hey.nhs.uk. Accessed 13 July 2020
81. Alhussien AH, Alhedaithy RA, Alsaleh SA. Safety of intranasal corticosteroid sprays during pregnancy: an updated review. Eur Arch Otorhinolaryngol. 2018;275(2):325–33. https://doi.org/10.1007/s00405-017-4785-3.

82. Ridolo E, Caminati M, Martignago I, et al. Allergic rhinitis: pharmacotherapy in pregnancy and old age. Expert Rev Clin Pharmacol. 2016;9(8):1081–9. https://doi.org/10.1080/1751243 3.2016.1189324.
83. Keles N. Treatment of allergic rhinitis during pregnancy. Am J Rhinol. 2004;18(1):23–8.
84. Mazzotta P, Loebstein R, Koren G. Treating allergic rhinitis in pregnancy. Safety considerations. Drug Saf. 1999;20(4):361–75. https://doi.org/10.2165/00002018-199920040-00005.
85. Drugs and Lactation Database (LactMed). Mometasone, nasal; 2020. https://www.ncbi.nlm. nih.gov. Accessed 13 July 2020
86. Cobanoglu B, Toskala E, Ural E, et al. Role of leukotriene antagonists and antihistamines in the treatment of allergic rhinitis. Curr Allergy Asthma Rep. 2013;13:203–8.
87. Hoecke HV, Vandenbulcke L, Van Cauwenberge P. Histamine and leukotriene receptor antagonism in the treatment of allergic rhinitis. Drugs. 2007;67(18):2717–26.
88. Church MK, Church DS. Pharmacology of antihistamines. Indian J Dermatol. 2013;58(3):219–24. https://doi.org/10.4103/0019-5154.110832.
89. McParlin C, O'Donnell A, Robson SC, et al. Treatments for hyperemesis gravidarum and nausea and vomiting in pregnancy: a systematic review. JAMA. 2016;316(13):1392–401. https://doi.org/10.1001/jama.2016.14337.
90. Poluzzi E, Diemberger I, De Ridder M, et al. Use of antihistamines and risk of ventricular tachyarrhythmia: a nested case-control study in five European countriesfrom the ARITMO project. Eur J Clin Pharmacol. 2017;73:1499–510.
91. Gilbert C, Mazzotta P, Loebstein R, et al. Fetal safety of drugs used in the treatment of allergic rhinitis. Drug-Safety. 2005;28:707–19.
92. Seto A, Einarson T, Koren G. Pregnancy outcome following first trimester exposure to antihistamines: meta-analysis. Am J Perinatol. 1997;14(3):119–24. https://doi. org/10.1055/s-2007-994110.
93. Kar S, Ajay Krishnan A, Preetha K. A review of antihistamines used during pregnancy. J Pharmacol Pharmacother. 2012;3(2):105–8.
94. Pali-Schöll I, Namazy J, Jensen-Jarolim E. Allergic diseases and asthma in pregnancy, a secondary publication. World Allergy Organ J. 2017;10(1):10. https://doi.org/10.1186/ s40413-017-0141-8.
95. Devillier P, Roche N, Faisy C. Clinical pharmacokinetics and pharmacodynamics of desloratadine, fexofenadine and levocetirizine: a comparative review. Clin Pharmacokinet. 2008;47(4):217–30. https://doi.org/10.2165/00003088-200847040-00001.
96. Golembesky A, Cooney M, Boev R, et al. Safety of cetirizine in pregnancy. J Obstet Gynaecol. 2018;38(7):940–5. https://doi.org/10.1080/01443615.2018.1441271.
97. Wang XY, Lim-Jurado M, Prepageran N, et al. Treatment of allergic rhinitis and urticaria: a review of the newest antihistamine drug bilastine. Ther Clin Risk Manag. 2016;12:585–97. https://doi.org/10.2147/TCRM.S105189.
98. Andersson NW, Torp-Pedersen C, Andersen JT. Association between fexofenadine use during pregnancy and fetal outcomes. JAMA Pediatr. 2020;174(8):e201316. https://doi.org/10.1001/ jamapediatrics.2020.1316.
99. Salib RJ, Howarth PH. Safety and tolerability profiles of intranasal antihistamines and intranasal corticosteroids in the treatment of allergic rhinitis. Drug Saf. 2003;26(12):863–93. https://doi.org/10.2165/00002018-200326120-00003.
100. Namazy J, Schatz M. The treatment of allergic respiratory disease during pregnancy. J Investig Allergol Clin Immunol. 2016;26(1):1–7.
101. Lipworth BJ. Leukotriene-receptor antagonists. Lancet. 1999;353(9146):57–62. https://doi. org/10.1016/S0140-6736(98)09019-9.
102. Wilson AM, O'Byrne PM, Parameswaran K. Leukotriene receptor antagonists for allergic rhinitis: a systematic review and meta-analysis. Am J Med. 2004;116(5):338–44. https://doi. org/10.1016/j.amjmed.2003.10.030.
103. Choi J, Azmat CE. Leukotriene receptor antagonists. StatPearls [Internet], Treasure Island, FL; 2020. https://www.ncbi.nlm.nih.gov/books/NBK554445/

104. Wang H, Li N, Huang H. Asthma in pregnancy: pathophysiology, diagnosis, whole-course management, and medication safety. Can Respir J. 2020; https://doi.org/10.1155/2020/9046842.
105. Cavero-Carbonell C, Vinkel-Hansen A, Rabanque-Hernández MJ, et al. Fetal exposure to montelukast and congenital anomalies: a population based study in Denmark. Birth Defects Res. 2017;109(6):452–9. https://doi.org/10.1002/bdra.23621.
106. Bakhireva LN, Jones KL, Schatz M, et al. Safety of leukotriene receptor antagonists in pregnancy. J Allergy Clin Immunol. 2007;119(3):618–25. https://doi.org/10.1016/j.jaci.2006.12.618.
107. Tamada T, Ichinose M. Leukotriene receptor antagonists and antiallergy drugs. In: Page C, Barnes P, editors. Pharmacology and therapeutics of asthma and COPD. Handbook of experimental pharmacology, vol 237. Switzerland: Springer; 2016. https://doi.org/10.1007/164_2016_72.
108. Gluck JC, Gluck PA. Asthma controller therapy during pregnancy. Am J Obstet Gynecol. 2005;192(2):369–80. https://doi.org/10.1016/j.ajog.2004.07.056.
109. Wahid NWB, Shermetaro C. Rhinitis Medicamentosa. StatPearls [Internet], Treasure Island, FL; 2020. https://www.ncbi.nlm.nih.gov/books/NBK538318/.
110. Passàli D, Salerni L, Passàli GC, et al. Nasal decongestants in the treatment of chronic nasal obstruction: efficacy and safety of use. Expert Opin Drug Saf. 2006;5(6):783–90. https://doi.org/10.1517/14740338.5.6.783.
111. Gonzalez-Estrada A, Geraci SA. Allergy medications during pregnancy. Am J Med Sci. 2016;352(3):326–31. https://doi.org/10.1016/j.amjms.2016.05.030.
112. Torfs CP, Katz EA, Bateson TF, et al. Maternal medications and environmental exposures as risk factors for gastroschisis. Teratology. 1996;54(2):84–92. https://doi.org/10.1002/(SICI)1096-9926(199606)54:2<84::AID-TERA4>3.0.CO;2-4.
113. Werler MM, Mitchell AA, Shapiro S. First trimester maternal medication use in relation to gastroschisis. Teratology. 1992;45(4):361–7. https://doi.org/10.1002/tera.1420450407.
114. Werler MM, Sheehan JE, Mitchell AA. Maternal medication use and risks of gastroschisis and small intestinal atresia. Am J Epidemiol. 2002;155(1):26–31. https://doi.org/10.1093/aje/155.1.26.
115. Aljazaf K, Hale TW, Ilett KF, et al. Pseudoephedrine: effects on milk production in women and estimation of infant exposure via breastmilk. Br J Clin Pharmacol. 2003;56(1):18–24. https://doi.org/10.1046/j.1365-2125.2003.01822.x.
116. Bandoli G, Palmsten K, Forbess Smith CJ, et al. A review of systemic corticosteroid use in pregnancy and the risk of select pregnancy and birth outcomes. Rheum Dis Clin North Am. 2017;43(3):489–502. https://doi.org/10.1016/j.rdc.2017.04.013.
117. Vlastarakos PV, Nikolopoulos TP, Manolopoulos L. Treating common ear problems in pregnancy: what is safe? Eur Arch Otorhinolaryngol. 2008;265(2):139–45. https://doi.org/10.1007/s00405-007-0534-3.
118. Källén BAJ. Maternal drug use and infant cleft lip/palate with special reference to corticoids. Cleft Palate Craniofac J. 2003;40(6):624–8. https://doi.org/10.1597/02-077.
119. Bjørn AM, Ehrenstein V, Nohr EA, et al. Use of inhaled and oral corticosteroids in pregnancy and the risk of malformations or miscarriage. Basic Clin Pharmacol Toxicol. 2015;116(4):308–14. https://doi.org/10.1111/bcpt.12367.
120. Hviid A, Mølgaard-Nielsen D. Corticosteroid use during pregnancy and risk of orofacial clefts. CMAJ. 2011;183(7):796–804. https://doi.org/10.1503/cmaj.101063.
121. Powrie RO, Larson L, Miller M. Managing asthma in expectant mothers. Treat Respir Med. 2006;5(1):1–10. https://doi.org/10.2165/00151829-200605010-00001.
122. El-Qutob D. Off-label uses of omalizumab. Clinic Rev Allerg Immunol. 2016;50:84–96.
123. Tsabouri S, Tseretopoulou X, Priftis K, et al. Omalizumab for the treatment of inadequately controlled allergic rhinitis: a systematic review and meta-analysis of randomized clinical trials. J Allergy Clin Immunol Pract. 2014;2(3):332–40. https://doi.org/10.1016/j.jaip.2014.02.001.
124. Kelly W, Massoumi A, Lazarus A. Asthma in pregnancy: physiology, diagnosis, and management. Postgrad Med. 2015;127(4):349–58. https://doi.org/10.1080/00325481.2015.1016386.

125. Namazy J, Cabana MD, Scheuerle AE, et al. The Xolair pregnancy registry (EXPECT): the safety of omalizumab use during pregnancy. J Allergy Clin Immunol. 2015;135(2):407–12. https://doi.org/10.1016/j.jaci.2014.08.025.
126. Labrador-Horrillo M, Ferrer M. Profile of omalizumab in the treatment of chronic spontaneous urticaria. Drug Design Dev Ther. 2015;9:4909–15.
127. Pakes GE, Brogden RN, Heel RC, et al. Ipratropium bromide: a review of its pharmacological properties and therapeutic efficacy in asthma and chronic bronchitis. Drugs. 1980;20(4):237–66. https://doi.org/10.2165/00003495-198020040-00001.
128. Sur DKC, Plesa ML. Chronic nonallergic rhinitis. Am Fam Physician. 2018;98(3):171–6.
129. Niggeschulze A, Palmer AK. Reproduktionstoxikologische Untersuchungen mit Ipratropiumbromid [Reproductive toxicological investigations with ipratropiumbromide (author's transl)]. Arzneimittelforschung. 1976;26(5a):989–92.
130. Egan M, Bunyavanich S. Allergic rhinitis: the "Ghost Diagnosis" in patients with asthma. Asthma Res and Pract. 2015;1:8. https://doi.org/10.1186/s40733-015-0008-0.
131. Sankaran P, Brockwell C, Wilson A. The effect of theophylline in patients with allergic rhinitis: a double-blind, randomised, crossover study. Eur Respir J. 2014;44:4666.
132. Basnet RM, Zizioli D, Guarient M, et al. Methylxanthines induce structural and functional alterations of the cardiac system in zebrafish embryos. BMC Pharmacol Toxicol. 2017;18(1):72. https://doi.org/10.1186/s40360-017-0179-9.
133. Park BK, Kitteringham NR. Assessment of enzyme induction and enzyme inhibition in humans: toxicological implications. Xenobiotica. 1990;20(11):1171–85. https://doi.org/10.3109/00498259009046837.
134. Rosa F. Databases in the assessment of the effects of drugs during pregnancy. J Allergy Clin Immunol Pract. 1999;103(2):S360–1. https://doi.org/10.1016/S0091-6749(99)70264-2.
135. Stenius-Aarniala BS, Hedman J, Teramo KA. Acute asthma during pregnancy. Thorax. 1996;51(4):411–4. https://doi.org/10.1136/thx.51.4.411.
136. Schatz M. Asthma treatment during pregnancy what can be safely taken? Drug Safety. 1997;16(5):342–50.
137. Bonham CA, Patterson KC, Strek ME. Asthma outcomes and management during pregnancy. Chest. 2018;153(2):515–27. https://doi.org/10.1016/j.chest.2017.08.029.
138. Carter BL, Driscoll CE, Smith GD. Theophylline clearance during pregnancy. Obstet Gynecol. 1986;68(4):555–9.
139. Magnan J, Özgirgin ON, Trabalzini F, et al. European position statement on diagnosis, and treatment of Meniere's disease. J Int Adv Otol. 2018;14(2):317–21. https://doi.org/10.5152/iao.2018.140818.
140. Buharalioglu CK, Acar S, Erol-Coskun H, et al. Pregnancy outcomes after maternal betahistine exposure: a case series. Reprod Toxicol. 2018;79:79–83. https://doi.org/10.1016/j.reprotox.2018.06.004.
141. Babaei AH, Foghaha MH. A randomized comparison of vitamin B6 and dimenhydrinate in the treatment of nausea and vomiting in early pregnancy. Iran J Nurs Midwifery Res. 2014;19(2):199–202.
142. Shiny Sherlie V, Varghese A. ENT changes of pregnancy and its management. Indian J Otolaryngol Head Neck Surg. 2014;66(Suppl 1):6–9. https://doi.org/10.1007/s12070-011-0376-6.
143. Boelig RC, Barton SJ, Saccone G, et al. Interventions for treating hyperemesis gravidarum: a Cochrane systematic review and meta-analysis. J Matern Fetal Neonatal Med. 2018;31(18):2492–505. https://doi.org/10.1080/14767058.2017.1342805.
144. Fejzo MS, Trovik J, Grooten IJ, et al. Nausea and vomiting of pregnancy and hyperemesis gravidarum. Nat Rev Dis Primers. 2019;5:62. https://doi.org/10.1038/s41572-019-0110-3.
145. Mazzotta P, Magee LA. A risk-benefit assessment of pharmacological and nonpharmacological treatments for nausea and vomiting of pregnancy. Drugs. 2000;59:781–800. https://doi.org/10.2165/00003495-200059040-00005.
146. Danielsson B, Webster WS, Ritchie HE. Ondansetron and teratogenicity in rats: evidence for a mechanism mediated via embryonic hERG blockade. Reprod Toxicol. 2018;81:237–45.

147. Lavecchia M, Chari R, Campbell S, et al. Ondansetron in pregnancy and the risk of congenital malformations: a systematic review. J Obstet Gynaecol Can. 2018;40(7):910–8. https://doi.org/10.1016/j.jogc.2017.10.024.

148. Huybrechts KF, Hernández-Díaz S, Straub L, et al. Association of maternal first-trimester ondansetron use with cardiac malformations and oral clefts in offspring. JAMA. 2018;320(23):2429–37. https://doi.org/10.1001/jama.2018.18307.

149. Murthy JM, Saxena AB. Bell's palsy: treatment guidelines. Ann Indian Acad Neurol. 2011;14(Suppl 1):S70–2. https://doi.org/10.4103/0972-2327.83092.

150. Sullivan FM, Swan IR, Donnan PT, et al. Early treatment with prednisolone or acyclovir in Bell's palsy. N Engl J Med. 2007;357(16):1598–607. https://doi.org/10.1056/NEJMoa072006.

151. Engström M, Berg T, Stjernquist-Desatnik A, et al. Prednisolone and valaciclovir in Bell's palsy: a randomised, double-blind, placebo-controlled, multicentre trial. Lancet Neurol. 2008;7(11):993–1000. https://doi.org/10.1016/S1474-4422(08)70221-7.

152. Bajalan M, Biggs TC, Jayaram S, et al. A guide to new anticoagulant medications for ENT surgeons. J Laryngol Otol. 2015;129(12):1167–73. https://doi.org/10.1017/S0022215115002765.

153. Onishi A, St Ange K, Dordick JS, et al. Heparin and anticoagulation. Front Biosci (Landmark Ed). 2016;21:1372–92. https://doi.org/10.1016/j.reprotox.2018.08.018.

154. Fogerty AE. Management of venous thromboembolism in pregnancy. Curr Treat Options Cardiovasc Med. 2018;20(8):69. https://doi.org/10.1007/s11936-018-0658-3.

155. Devis P, Knuttinen MG. Deep venous thrombosis in pregnancy: incidence, pathogenesis and endovascular management. Cardiovasc Diagn Ther. 2017;7(Suppl 3):S309–19. https://doi.org/10.21037/cdt.2017.10.08.

156. Toyoda K. Antithrombotic therapy for pregnant women. Neurol Med Chir (Tokyo). 2013;53(8):526–30. https://doi.org/10.2176/nmc.53.526.

157. Burnett AE, Mahan CE, Vazquez SR, et al. Guidance for the practical management of the direct oral anticoagulants (DOACs) in VTE treatment. J Thromb Thrombolysis. 2016;41(1):206–32. https://doi.org/10.1007/s11239-015-1310-7.

158. Piccioni MG, Derme M, Salerno L, et al. Management of severe epistaxis during pregnancy: a case report and review of the literature. Case Reports Obstet Gynecol. 2019; https://doi.org/10.1155/2019/5825309.

159. Wu PH, Cheng PW, Young YH. Inner ear disorders in 68 pregnant women: a 20-year experience. Clin Otolaryngol. 2016;42:844–950.

160. Xie S, Wu X. Clinical management and progress in sudden sensorineural hearing loss during pregnancy. J Int Med Res. 2019; https://doi.org/10.1177/0300060519870718.

161. Conlin AE, Parnes LS. Treatment of sudden sensorineural hearing loss: I. A systematic review. Arch Otolaryngol Head Neck Surg. 2007;133(6):573–81. https://doi.org/10.1001/archotol.133.6.573.

162. Richter JE. Gastroesophageal reflux disease during pregnancy. Gastroenterol Clin North Am. 2003;32(1):235–61. https://doi.org/10.1016/s0889-8553(02)00065-1.

163. Pasternak B, Hviid A. Use of proton-pump inhibitors in early pregnancy and the risk of birth defects. N Engl J Med. 2010;363(22):2114–23. https://doi.org/10.1056/NEJMoa1002689.

164. Black E, Khor KE, Kennedy D, et al. Medication use and pain management in pregnancy: a critical review. Pain Pract. 2019;19(8):875–99. https://doi.org/10.1111/papr.12814.

165. Antonucci R, Zaffanello M, Puxeddu E, et al. Use of non-steroidal anti-inflammatory drugs in pregnancy: impact on the fetus and newborn. Curr Drug Metab. 2012;13(4):474–90. https://doi.org/10.2174/138920012800166607.

166. Flint J, Panchal S, Hurrell A, et al. BSR and BHPR guideline on prescribing drugs in pregnancy and breastfeeding-Part II: analgesics and other drugs used in rheumatology practice. Rheumatology (Oxford). 2016;55(9):1698–702. https://doi.org/10.1093/rheumatology/kev405.

167. Källén B, Reis M. Ongoing pharmacological management of chronic pain in pregnancy. Drugs. 2016;76(9):915–24. https://doi.org/10.1007/s40265-016-0582-3.

Herpes Simplex Viral Infections in Pregnancy

29

Fatih Öner, Cemal Cingi, and William Reisacher

29.1 Introduction

The herpes simplex viruses (HSV) are responsible for acute infections of the cutaneous system. Infection presents as groups of vesicles with basal erythema. The genome of the HSV consists of linear, double-stranded DNA. Most infections are relatively mild, but occasionally HSV may produce a severe illness with the potential to harm a pregnancy. The majority of HSV infections exhibit the feature of multiple recurrences, usually at the same location each time. The most frequent manifestation is herpes labialis secondary to HSV-1 (herpes simplex type 1). Herpetic infections of the genitals are generally secondary to HSV-2. It is possible for herpes to cause other forms of illness, but this rarely occurs [1].

Shedding of virus may happen when infection first occurs, when the infection recurs or even when no symptoms are evident. For transmission to occur, mucous membranes must come into contact or skin which is damaged must be exposed. The primary herpetic infection occurs at the location where contact first occurred. The lipid and glycoprotein envelope of the virus joins to the outer plasma membrane of the epithelium (skin or mucosa), following which the viral genome becomes

F. Öner (✉)
Otorhinolaryngology Section, Erzurum Regional Training and Research Hospital,
Erzurum, Turkey
e-mail: fatihoner.ent@gmail.com

C. Cingi
Department of Otorhinolaryngology, Medical Faculty, Eskisehir Osmangazi University,
Eskisehir, Turkey
e-mail: cemal@ogu.edu.tr

W. Reisacher
Department of Otolaryngology—Head & Neck Surgery, Weill Cornell Medical College/New
York-Presbyterian Hospital, New York, NY, USA

C. Cingi et al. (eds.), *ENT Diseases: Diagnosis and Treatment during Pregnancy
and Lactation*, https://doi.org/10.1007/978-3-031-05303-0_29

integrated into the nuclear DNA of the host [2]. Herpes simplex bears the C glycoprotein, which stabilizes the envelope of the virus and assists with entry into the host cell [3]. When toll-like receptors of the host recognize viral DNA, both the innate and adaptive branches of immune defence are triggered into action and interferon is synthesized [2]. There are complex interactions between the viral proteins and the host immune system, as a result of which, HSV is able to shut down the immune response and evade destruction. A key molecule which acts in this way is the virion host shutoff protein (VHS), synthesized early on in infection and acting to prevent cellular immunity responses from occurring [2]. The viral glycoprotein C attaches to the complement factor C3b, preventing a response mediated through the complement system, and this helps to suppress the action of immunoglobulins targeting HSV [3]. HSV is then free to enter nerve cells and begin replicating itself. It does the same in cells of the epidermis and dermis. The virions migrate from the location where primary infection first occurred to the dorsal root ganglion of the sensory nerves and the virus then enters a latent phase. This latency comes about because the HSV genes are not being expressed. However, when the host is subject to stress, the virus may emerge from its latency and become active again [1].

As the virus replicates itself within the dorsal ganglia, clinically this presents as a recurrent episode. There are a variety of events which may cause viral reactivation, including trauma, exposure to ultraviolet light, extreme cold or heat, stress, suppression of the immune system, a surgical operation (including laser surgery) and endocrine alterations. It appears that CD8+ T lymphocytes with specificity for HSV are key to controlling the extent to which the virus can become active again and produce infection [3]. These CD8+ T lymphocytes are brought into action by both branches of the immune response at the point when primary infection occurs. These lymphocytes express a higher than usual level of CXCR3 and CCR10, which are receptors for the chemokines. It is likely these receptors influence movement of the T lymphocytes to the area where HSV is active and help to orchestrate the inflammatory response [4].

29.2 Aetiology

The two variants of HSV, HSV-1 and HSV-2, are together responsible for herpetic infections of the facial lips, the genitals, mat herpes, herpetic whitlow, herpetic keratoconjunctivitis, eczema herpeticum, herpes folliculitis, lumbosacral herpes, disseminated herpes, herpetic infections in newborns and encephalitis [5]. HSVs are also sometimes implicated in patients with erythema multiforme, being found in 18% of children with this condition [6]. Pyrexia, UV irradiation, traumatic injury, and infection of the upper respiratory tract or psychological stress may all trigger a recurrence of herpes labialis due to HSV-1 [1].

29.3 Clinical Features

The prevalence of HSV-1 infection varies geographically, socioeconomically and with age range. For HSV-2, serological evidence of infection shows the highest prevalence in female sex workers, gay men and patients infected with HIV [1].

29.3.1 Orolabial Herpes

Herpes labialis presents with cold sores/fever blisters. It is usually the result of infection with HSV-1, although in some cases HSV-2 has been implicated. In such cases, transmission generally occurs through oral sex. The primary infection by HSV-1 frequently takes place while the patient is still a child and generally does not result in symptoms [1].

29.3.1.1 Primary Infection

The onset of symptomatic primary infection of the mouth and lips by HSV may be preceded by prodromal pyrexia, after which pharyngitis and stomatitis develop, accompanied by submandibular or cervical lymph gland enlargement. Paediatric cases may additionally feature gingivostomatitis, and children may find swallowing painful. There is formation of labial, gingival, palatal or lingual vesicles, which are painful and often surrounded by an erythematous, swollen area. The vesicles may coalesce and become pustular, then become ulcerous. In the ulcerated form, they have a scalloped margin. Resolution occurs after 2–3 weeks [1].

29.3.2 Recurrences

HSV maintains latency for differing lengths of time. If HSV-1 becomes reactivated within the sensory ganglia of the fifth cranial nerve, vesicles reappear over the face, mouth, lips and mucosal surfaces of the eye. Before the appearance of vesicles, the patient may complain of pain, a burning sensation, pruritus or pins and needles. When the vesicles appear, they form an ulcer after a while or become crusted. The lesions have a predilection for the junction of the lips with the skin. Without intervention, symptomatic duration is typically around seven days. Recurrent infections of the mouth and lips by HSV-1 sometimes result in a recurrence of erythema multiforme. A study investigating the shedding of virus by HSV-1 found that the median length of time for which this occurred was from 48 to 60 h after symptoms first occurred. Once 96 h had elapsed from the first symptoms, virus shedding could no longer be detected [7].

29.3.3 Genital Herpes

The most frequent cause of genital herpetic infection is HSV-2. Nonetheless, primary infection of the genitalia with HSV-1 is becoming detected at ever greater rates, up to 80% in some populations [8]. These infections probably result from oral sex. Indeed, HSV-1 is implicated in a third of primary herpetic infections of the genitals. It is most frequent in individuals below the age of 30, those of Caucasian ethnicity and in men who engage in sexual activity with other men [9]. Herpetic genital infections of recurrent type, nonetheless, are virtually always the result of HSV-2 infection [1].

29.3.3.1 Primary Infection

The primary episode of genital herpetic infection takes place between 2 days and 2 weeks after viral transmission occurs. Primary episodes are more severe than recurrent episodes and in general have a duration of between two and three weeks.

Male patients typically develop vesicles on the penis. These lesions are surrounded by erythema and undergo ulceration. Less commonly, they are found in the anal and perineal regions. Female patients with a primary herpetic genital infection have vesicles that ulcerate on the cervix as well as on both sides of the vulva. These lesions cause pain. The occurrence of herpetic vesicles has also been noted within the vagina, on the perineum, the buttocks and, occasionally, the legs, where they follow the distribution of the sacral nerve. In both sexes, the symptomatic presentation includes pyrexia, a feeling of being unwell, swelling, enlarged inguinal lymph nodes, painful urination and a discharge from the penis or vagina.

A potential complication in women is a lumbosacral radiculopathy. Up to a quarter of female patients in whom a primary infection with HSV-2 occurs may develop aseptic meningitis [1].

29.3.3.2 Recurrences

Following the primary infection, viral latency may last for several months or years. Eventually, the virus undergoes reactivation. The HSV-2 resides in the lumbosacral ganglia; hence reactivation produces symptoms below the level of the waist. When recurrence occurs, the clinical picture is less severe. The initial indications of recurrence are prodromal pain, pruritus, tingling, a burning sensation or pins and needles.

There are certain patients whose initial exposure to HSV does result in infection but no symptoms are noted. The first time that symptoms occur may be several months or even years after the initial infection occurred. In such cases, the symptoms will be less severe than those in a true primary infective episode.

Above 50% of patients with serological evidence of infection with HSV-2 do not show any other evidence of infection, in other words, they are asymptomatic. Nonetheless, the virus is still shed on occasion by such patients and therefore they present a risk of transmission to individuals with whom they engage in sexual contact [1].

29.4   HSV During Pregnancy

Other than during a primary infective episode, the risk of transmission from a pregnant woman to her foetus is low. Nonetheless, up to 50% of foetuses may be infected if the primary infection occurs during pregnancy [10]. It is not appropriate to screen pregnant women as a matter of course for HSV, but diagnostic investigations are called for if herpes genitalis is the putative diagnosis [10, 11]. The clinician should manage herpes genitalis on the basis of a thorough history and careful physical examination. This especially applies at the delivery stage. Unless there are indications of an active herpetic infection at the time of delivery, vaginal delivery is not contraindicated [11]. In cases where there is either a primary episode of HSV infection or recurrence of latent HSV, delivery should occur by Caesarean section, since this renders vertical transmission less likely [11]. Antiviral agents are safe to administer systemically during pregnancy and may allow a normal delivery to proceed [11]. Even with the use of antivirals, transmission to the foetus remains a possibility [11].

The treatment recommendations to suppress an outbreak of herpes genitalis in a pregnant woman are listed below [1]:

- Acyclovir 400 mg by mouth TID (beginning when the pregnancy reaches 36 weeks' gestation)
- Valaciclovir 500 mg by mouth BID (beginning when the pregnancy reaches 36 weeks' gestation)

29.4.1 Vertical Transmission

Generally speaking, the way HSV is transmitted from the mother to the foetus is by the foetus coming directly into contact with shed virus at the time of delivery and labour. The virus may be shed from the cervical, vaginal, vulvar or perianal epithelia [12].

There are a number of facts about how HSV is transmitted to the infant that must be noted to understand the way cases present [13]:

In the majority of cases where a neonate is infected with HSV perinatally, there is no corresponding maternal history of symptoms or signs of herpetic genital infection [14].

Transmission is most likely to occur if the mother had the primary episode of herpes genitalis shortly before the time of birth. In cases where the first clinically apparent episode does not coincide with the time of initial infection with HSV, there is a somewhat reduced likelihood of transmission. This risk is even lower where HSV episodes are recurrent. The authors of two case series [15, 16] performed viral culture on specimens obtained from women brought to the labour ward for delivery. From those cases where maternal viral culture identified HSV, there were different rates of neonatal infection, depending on the maternal characteristics, as follows:

- If the mother was undergoing a primary infective episode, the rate of transmission in one study was 40% (2 out of 5 cases) [16], while in the other study the rate was 44% (4 out of 9 cases) [15].
- In mothers where the first clinically apparent episode did not coincide with the time of initial infection with HSV, the rate of transmission was reported as 31% (4 out of 13) [16] or 24% (4 out of 17) [15].
- Where there were recurrent episodes, the rate was either 3% (1 out of 34) [16] or 1.3% (2 out of 151) [15].

A probable explanation for the data showing that transmission is more probable when the mother is experiencing a primary or non-primary initial HSV episode is that in such cases the mother has not yet seroconverted and the shedding of virus is at its maximum, both in terms of number of particles shed and length of time over which this occurs.

The immune system typically begins expressing immunoglobulins with a specificity for HSV no later than 12 weeks following infection. Initially, IgM is produced, indicating acute infection, followed by the production of IgG, which confirms prior infection status. These immunoglobulins continue to be expressed indefinitely [17]. The fact that transmission occurs at a lower rate in mothers whose HSV infection is recurrent than in those with a primary episode most likely relates to greater protection provided by specific immunoglobulins and the fact that viral shedding from the genital tract is less intense or long-lasting when the virus is reactivated [18]. It is noteworthy that women infected with HSV who seroconvert following a primary or nonprimary initial episode at an earlier stage of pregnancy seemingly also transmit HSV at a lower rate to the foetus [19].

Even where there are non-clinically evident vesicles and no symptoms, virus may still be shed [13, 20–22]. Research conducted into viral shedding in patients who were not pregnant [22] found that 13% of those with a symptomatic lesion were shedding virus, whilst in asymptomatic individuals, the rate was still 9%. This study recruited individuals who were seropositive for immunoglobulins targeting HSV-2. The samples were obtained by swabbing the genitalia. Detection of viral shedding was accomplished by performing the polymerase chain reaction for viral DNA.

Shedding of virus occurs more often in herpes genitalis secondary to HSV-2 than HSV-1. This affects the rate of vertical transmission and thus the risk of complications for the newborn. However, clinical management does not differ according to whether HSV-1 or HSV-2 is the cause.

There are anecdotal reports indicating that HSV has been transmitted to the foetus before labour and delivery by crossing the placenta or ascending through the uterine cervix. Such an infection may lead to spontaneous abortion, development of congenital defects (such as ventricular enlargement or central nervous anomalies), premature delivery and/or restricted ability of the foetus to grow *in utero* [19, 23–26]. There appears to be no association between recurrent type HSV infection and pregnancy complications [27]. If a neonate appears infected with HSV at an early stage even though delivery occurred via caesarean section and the foetal membranes were not disturbed, there is a possibility that infection had actually already occurred *in utero* [15, 28].

29.4.2 Evidence

There are a number of studies which have played a key role in identifying the risk factors involved in vertical transmission and in quantifying the risks involved. One of these studies employed a prospective design and ran from 1982 to 1999 [15]. In this study, 58,000 pregnant women were enrolled. They were divided into cases considered primary, non-primary or recurrent infections by HSV. This division was made on the basis of serology, viral culture and amplification of viral DNA [15]. In 202 participants, representing 0.5% of the sample, HSV was detected in swabs of the vulva or cervix at the point when they entered labour. The study identified the following outcomes concerning transmission to the newborn [12]:

- The existence of shed virus at the time of labour strongly correlated with the risk that the newborn would be infected with HSV (odds ratio: 346). Transmission to the newborn was identified in some 5% (10 patients out of 202) of those individuals where HSV was cultured, whereas this only occurred in 0.02% (6 women out of 39,821) where HSV was not cultured.
- The maximum likelihood of vertical transmission occurred in women who had recently acquired a primary infection with herpes genitalis, as evidenced by positivity for HSV, but non-detectable specific immunoglobulins. In these cases, the rate of transmission was 54 per 100,000 live births. This is higher than where the mother produced antibodies to HSV-1 (26 in 100,000 live births) or to HSV-2 (22 in 100,000 live births).

These studies also identified other risk factors. Isolation of cervical HSV raised the risk (odds ratio:33), as did shed virus of type HSV-1 rather than HSV-2 (odds ratio:17). Some indirect factors also indicated a higher risk, namely invasive monitoring of the foetus (odds ratio:7), premature delivery (i.e. earlier than 38 weeks' gestation; odds ratio:4) and mothers age 21 years and under (odds ratio:4).

29.4.3 Management During Pregnancy

There are two ways in which the risk of vertical transmission of HSV can be reduced in pregnant women. The first is to commence antiviral pharmacotherapy from 36 weeks' gestation onwards to minimize the chance of the infection becoming reactivated at the time of giving birth. The second intervention is to offer Caesarean section to certain at-risk women. These two strategies are insufficient to entirely remove the possibility of the neonate becoming infected with HSV. One approach, which reflects the recommendations of the American College of Obstetricians and Gynecologists, involves classifying cases according to whether HSV infection of the genitalia is primary, non-primary or recurrent, how severely affected the woman is and the length of interval between symptoms and the expected due date [29].

If a woman who has not previously had an episode of herpes genitalis develops *de novo* ulceration of the genitalia whilst pregnant, the authors recommend an empirical trial of an antiviral agent and virological investigation. A new episode of herpes genitalis usually recovers spontaneously, but therapeutic intervention may shorten the episode, alleviate symptoms and reduce the length of time over which viruses are being shed. Acyclovir 400 mg p.o. TID is a suitable treatment. If HSV infection features complications, such as involvement of the brain and spinal cord, other organs or is disseminated around the body, this agent will need to be administered intravenously at first [17].

Treatment is usually administered for between 7 and 10 days, but may be needed for a longer period if there is no total resolution following a 10-day course. Acyclovir needs to be re-introduced at 36 weeks' gestation to inhibit viral reactivation around the time of delivery [12].

29.4.3.1 Suppressive Therapy at 36 weeks

The authors' recommendation is to administer antiviral therapy from 36 weeks' gestation until labour to any woman who develops herpes genitalis during pregnancy. This recommendation applies whatever the timing of the infection and regardless of whether the infection is primary, non-primary or recurrent. A suitable regime involves acyclovir 400 mg TID. Note that the renal clearance of this agent is increased during pregnancy and therefore a higher dose is called for than in non-pregnant patients [12].

29.4.3.2 Topical Antivirals

There is also a topical preparation available, in the form of an ointment or cream containing 5% acyclovir. This preparation may be used either five or six times daily and the course lasts between 4 and 7 days. It is suitable for both herpes labialis and herpes genitalis. However, the cream is not suitable for application to the genital area. Topical acyclovir offers only a moderate degree of benefit in HSV infection, as noted in real world settings, despite clinical trial data indicating a statistically significant degree of efficacy. One trial [30] compared a cream containing 5% acyclovir with placebo to treat orolabial HSV infection and recorded a reduction in symptomatic duration of one-half day. A topical preparation containing acyclovir 5% and hydrocortisone 1% may be used 5 times daily, being initiated as soon as symptoms of a recurrence occur. This preparation demonstrated an advantage in stopping the episode from progressing when compared with acyclovir alone, or with placebo [31]. A further topical preparation that may be used for orolabial HSV infections is penciclovir 1% cream. It may be applied once every two hours and benefits from comparable efficacy to acyclovir. An over-the-counter product to consider is docosanol 10% cream, which may be administered five times daily for a maximum of ten days. A study in which docosanol competed against placebo found that cases where docosanol was used resolved on average after around four days, whereas those where placebo was used lasted a further 18 hours [32]. However, all topical preparations used as antivirals in cases of HSV infection have a considerably lower efficacy than when administered orally or parenterally. Accordingly, the US Centers for Disease Control do not support their use, citing low clinical efficacy [11].

29.4.4 Drug Selection, Dosage and Safety

There are three antiviral agents available which work against HSV, acyclovir, famciclovir and valaciclovir. The agent about which the most is known in pregnancy, however, is acyclovir, at a dosage of 400 mg p.o. TID. In an acute infective episode, the course lasts for between 7 and 10 days, or longer if the symptoms persist. For use as an inhibitor of viral reactivation, it is administered from the 36th week of pregnancy up to the time the child has been delivered [12].

An alternative to acyclovir in either indication is valaciclovir. However, this agent generally costs more than acyclovir, even as a generic, and the evidence base for its safety and clinical benefit is less well-established [33]. One situation in which valaciclovir may be a better choice is where patients may not be fully concordant, as this agent requires BID dosing, which may be easier to ensure than TID dosing, as needed with acyclovir.

The evidence on teratogenicity of acyclovir gathered from animal testing and in humans indicates this agent is non-teratogenic throughout pregnancy, including during organogenesis [33]. The evidence for valaciclovir is less extensive, but has not thus far highlighted any concerns. The evidence for the safety of famciclovir in pregnant women is extremely limited.

29.5 Postpartum and Neonatal Management

If either the parents or anyone else looking after an infant has an active herpetic infection, caution is needed when touching the child. The vesicles or ulcers must be covered and strict handwashing observed. Between 5 and 15% of HSV infections in newborns are actually transmitted by a relative after the birth [34].

There is no contraindication to breastfeeding an infant, provided the mother has no signs of infection on the breasts. Maternal treatment with acyclovir or valaciclovir is also not a reason to stop breastfeeding [35, 36].

It is vital that a paediatrician be consulted for advice in any neonate who has been exposed to HSV. If the newborn has been or is at risk, it is vital to observe the infant for clinical indications of herpetic infection.

References

1. McGregor SP. Dermatologic manifestations of herpes simplex treatment & management. In: James WD, editor. Medscape. Updated: 17 Mar 2020. https://emedicine.medscape.com/article/1132351-treatment#d7. Accessed online 1 April 2021.

2. Roizman B, Whitley RJ. An inquiry into the molecular basis of HSV latency and reactivation. Annu Rev Microbiol. 2013;67:355–74.

3. Komala Sari T, Gianopulos KA, Nicola AV. Glycoprotein C of herpes simplex virus 1 shields glycoprotein B from antibody neutralization. J Virol. 2020;94(5)

4. Hensel MT, Peng T, Cheng A, De Rosa SC, Wald A, Laing KJ, et al. Selective expression of CCR10 and CXCR3 by circulating human herpes simplex virus-specific CD8 T cells. J Virol. 2017;91(19)

5. Weinberg JM, Mysliwiec A, Turiansky GW, Redfield R, James WD. Viral folliculitis. Atypical presentations of herpes simplex, herpes zoster, and molluscum contagiosum. Arch Dermatol. 1997;133(8):983–6.

6. Zoghaib S, Kechichian E, Souaid K, Soutou B, Helou J, Tomb R. Triggers, clinical manifestations, and management of pediatric erythema multiforme: a systematic review. J Am Acad Dermatol. 2019;81(3):813–22.

7. Boivin G, Goyette N, Sergerie Y, Keays S, Booth T. Longitudinal evaluation of herpes simplex virus DNA load during episodes of herpes labialis. J Clin Virol. 2006;37(4):248–51.

8. James SH, Kimberlin DW. Neonatal herpes simplex infection: epidemiology and treatment. Clin Perinatol. 2015;42:47–59.

9. Dabestani N, Katz DA, Dombrowski J, Magaret A, Wald A, Johnston C. Time trends in first-episode genital herpes simplex virus infections in an urban sexually transmitted disease clinic. Sex Transm Dis. 2019;46(12):795–800.

10. Subramaniam A, Britt WJ. Herpesviridae infection: prevention, screening, and management. Clin Obstet Gynecol. 2018;61(1):157–76.

11. (Guideline) Centers for Disease Control and Prevention. 2015 Sexually transmitted diseases treatment guidelines. https://www.cdc.gov/std/tg2015/default.htm. January 25, 2017. Accessed 5 Dec 2017.

12. Riley LE, Wald A. Genital herpes simplex virus infection and pregnancy. In: Hirsch MS, Lockwood CJ, Mitty J, Barss VA, editors. UpTodate. Last updated: 10 Jun 2020.

13. Wald A, Zeh J, Selke S, et al. Reactivation of genital herpes simplex virus type 2 infection in asymptomatic seropositive persons. N Engl J Med. 2000;342:844.

14. Pinninti SG, Kimberlin DW. Maternal and neonatal herpes simplex virus infections. Am J Perinatol. 2013;30:113.

15. Brown ZA, Wald A, Morrow RA, et al. Effect of serologic status and cesarean delivery on transmission rates of herpes simplex virus from mother to infant. JAMA. 2003;289:203.

16. Brown ZA, Benedetti J, Ashley R, et al. Neonatal herpes simplex virus infection in relation to asymptomatic maternal infection at the time of labor. N Engl J Med. 1991;324:1247.

17. Workowski KA, Bolan GA, Centers for Disease Control and Prevention. Sexually transmitted diseases treatment guidelines, 2015. MMWR Recomm Rep. 2015;64:1.

18. Johnston C, Magaret A, Selke S, et al. Herpes simplex virus viremia during primary genital infection. J Infect Dis. 2008;198:31.

19. Brown ZA, Selke S, Zeh J, et al. The acquisition of herpes simplex virus during pregnancy. N Engl J Med. 1997;337:509.

20. Corey L, Wald A, Patel R, et al. Once-daily valacyclovir to reduce the risk of transmission of genital herpes. N Engl J Med. 2004;350:11.

21. Wald A, Corey L, Cone R, et al. Frequent genital herpes simplex virus 2 shedding in immunocompetent women. Effect of acyclovir treatment. J Clin Invest. 1997;99(1092)

22. Tronstein E, Johnston C, Huang ML, et al. Genital shedding of herpes simplex virus among symptomatic and asymptomatic persons with HSV-2 infection. JAMA. 2011;305:1441.

23. Brown ZA, Benedetti J, Selke S, et al. Asymptomatic maternal shedding of herpes simplex virus at the onset of labor: relationship to preterm labor. Obstet Gynecol. 1996;87:483.

24. Nahmias AJ, Josey WE, Naib ZM, et al. Perinatal risk associated with maternal genital herpes simplex virus infection. Am J Obstet Gynecol. 1971;110:825.

25. Brown ZA, Vontver LA, Benedetti J, et al. Effects on infants of a first episode of genital herpes during pregnancy. N Engl J Med. 1987;317:1246.

26. Fa F, Laup L, Mandelbrot L, et al. Fetal and neonatal abnormalities due to congenital herpes simplex virus infection: a literature review. Prenat Diagn. 2020;40:408.
27. Harger JH, Amortegui AJ, Meyer MP, Pazin GJ. Characteristics of recurrent genital herpes simplex infections in pregnant women. Obstet Gynecol. 1989;73:367.
28. Stone KM, Brooks CA, Guinan ME, Alexander ER. National surveillance for neonatal herpes simplex virus infections. Sex Transm Dis. 1989;16:152.
29. Management of Genital Herpes in Pregnancy. ACOG practice bulletinacog practice bulletin, number 220. Obstet Gynecol. 2020;135:e193.
30. Spruance SL, Nett R, Marbury T, Wolff R, Johnson J, Spaulding T. Acyclovir cream for treatment of herpes simplex labialis: results of two randomized, double-blind, vehicle-controlled, multicenter clinical trials. Antimicrob Agents Chemother. 2002;46(7):2238–43.
31. Hull CM, Harmenberg J, Arlander E, Aoki F, Bring J, Darpö B, et al. Early treatment of cold sores with topical ME-609 decreases the frequency of ulcerative lesions: a randomized, double-blind, placebo-controlled, patient-initiated clinical trial. J Am Acad Dermatol. 2011;64(4):696.e1–696.e11.
32. Sacks SL, Thisted RA, Jones TM, Barbarash RA, Mikolich DJ, Ruoff GE, et al. Clinical efficacy of topical docosanol 10% cream for herpes simplex labialis: a multicenter, randomized, placebo-controlled trial. J Am Acad Dermatol. 2001;45(2):222–30.
33. Briggs GG, Freeman RK, Yaffe, SJ. Acyclovir. In: Drugs in pregnancy and lactation, 8th ed., e-book; 2021.
34. Caviness AC, Demmler GJ, Selwyn BJ. Clinical and laboratory features of neonatal herpes simplex virus infection: a case-control study. Pediatr Infect Dis J. 2008;27:425.
35. LactMed.   Acyclovir.   http://toxnet.nlm.nih.gov/cgi-bin/sis/search/f?./temp/~aVoLKr:1. Accessed 01 March 2021.
36. LactMed.   Valacyclovir.   http://toxnet.nlm.nih.gov/cgi-bin/sis/search/f?./temp/~aVoLKr:2. Accessed 10 March 2021.

Headache During Pregnancy and Lactation

30

Deniz Avcı, Yücel Kurt, and Francesco Maria Passali

30.1 Introduction

Treating and managing pregnant women with headache is a challenging task. Women who were already prone to headache before becoming pregnant may find headaches worsen, a headache may impact the pregnancy itself, and pharmacotherapy needs to be evaluated in the light of safety concerns both for the mother and the foetus. Any pregnant or postpartum woman presenting with a headache for the first time needs to undergo a diagnostic work-up, including assessment of pregnancy-related conditions that may produce a headache. A woman who is over 20 weeks pregnant and presents with a headache must be carefully assessed to exclude the possibility of underlying pre-eclampsia [1].

The type of headaches that pregnant women may suffer from, whether secondary or primary in nature, frequently differ from those in non-pregnant individuals. Around 2 out of 3 pregnant women with a predisposition to migraine do actually find that migraine symptoms improve whilst they are pregnant. However, for those women whose migraine continues to be troublesome or who have other types of headache, clinicians need to adopt an appropriate clinical strategy, encompassing

D. Avcı (✉)
Department of Otorhinolaryngology, Nevsehir State Hospital, Nevşehir, Turkey
e-mail: deniz.avci@hotmail.com

Y. Kurt
Section of Otorhinolaryngology, Ministry of Health, Finike State Hospital,
Finike, Antalya, Turkey

F. M. Passali
Department of Clinical Sciences and Translational Medicine, University Tor Vergata,
Rome, Italy

C. Cingi et al. (eds.), *ENT Diseases: Diagnosis and Treatment during Pregnancy and Lactation*, https://doi.org/10.1007/978-3-031-05303-0_30

diagnostic investigations, provision of advice on what to expect whilst pregnant and breastfeeding and adjustments to treatment as dictated by the need to reduce potential harms to the foetus or breastfeeding infant [2].

30.2 Aetiology

30.2.1 Primary Headaches

The majority of instances of headache in pregnant women are primary in nature. Amongst women seeking help for the condition, migraines and tension-type headaches (TTH) feature most prominently. A number of studies have used an observational design to investigate how primary headaches progress whilst the patient is pregnant [3]. It has been noted that primary headaches tend to change in type after the woman becomes pregnant. Thus, migraine that usually does not involve an aura now develops one or *vice versa*, and a simple migraine may transform into a TTH, or the other way round. A study in Italy [4] identified that 9% of women who usually complained of TTH developed a migraine without an aura, and the opposite change occurred in 10%. So far, no study has linked TTH to negative outcomes in pregnant patients, although the small number of participants in the studies conducted so far preclude a definitive conclusion that no link exists [5].

30.2.2 Migraine

The studies which have examined migraine in pregnant women over the last two decades have reached conclusions similar to the earlier studies [6, 7]. The newer studies adopted both prospective and retrospective designs. From 50% to 75% of women migraine sufferers have a noticeable decrease in how often attacks occur and how severe they are, even sometimes finding no attacks occur at all [8–18]. In those individuals whose migraine does continue, the average intensity of pain and the length of the attack both decrease over the course of the pregnancy [13, 17]. In line with this trend, the annual frequency of headaches, both migraine and others, is lower in pregnant women expecting their first child than in women who are not pregnant [19].

The incidence of *de novo* migraine without accompanying aura (migraine only, MO) in pregnant women is reported to range from 1 to 10% [5, 15–17, 20], with retrospective data indicating an ever higher rate than this—approaching 16.7% [13]. The classical presentation of *de novo* MO is within the initial trimester [5–7, 20]. The severity of migraine may also actually increase, particularly within the initial trimester. The reported frequency of increased severity is 8% of cases [5, 8–16].

Research into how alterations in oestrogen level affect migraine with aura (MA) is less common. It is more usual for MA than MO to have its onset or to deteriorate, whilst a woman is pregnant. MA first occurs in pregnancy between 10.7 and 14% of the time [5, 11]. In 8.4% of cases, symptoms of MA deteriorated during pregnancy, but the most frequent situation was for there to be no alteration in the pattern of symptoms. Approaching 50% of women prone to MA still experience attacks during pregnancy [11]. Data generally show that it is more common for the clinical features to improve in MO than in MA [5, 13, 14], although sometimes the converse applies [16]. This difference may be attributable to the greater degree of reactivity by the endothelium in cases of MA than in cases of MO [21]. It is possible for pregnant women to experience aura for the first time [22, 23], which may occur in isolation, without an accompanying headache [24]. In certain cases, which are generally somewhat rare, diagnosing a hemiplegic migraine may be complex, particularly where this occurs in the final trimester of pregnancy [25, 26].

The frequency of headache of any type in women postpartum is approximately 30–40% [6, 9, 13]. The peak incidence of headache was in the first week postpartum, with attacks not seeming to occur on the day of actually giving birth. The average pain intensity, length and need for painkillers all went up during the puerperium, according to a prospective study (MIGRA) which enrolled large numbers of women [17]. The same study [17], however, also found that attacks became less common five weeks postpartum. It is not expected that pregnant women whose headaches remit entirely within the first two trimesters will have a migrainous attack in the third trimester [13], although there is other evidence suggesting that headaches become more troublesome to women with multiple children in the month prior to giving birth, giving rise to a curve of frequency of migraine *vs* time in pregnancy that is U-shaped [9].

30.2.3 Tension-type Headache

TTH accounts for 26% of cases of headache in pregnant women [27]. On endocrine grounds, it would be anticipated that pregnancy will result in an improvement in TTH, since the endorphins and 5-hydroxytryptamine, which play a major role in the disorder, are under the control of female hormones [5]. However, what has been observed is no alteration in symptoms for 17.9% of pregnant women, greater severity in 5% and the expected improvement only occurs in one-in-four cases [27, 28]. It has been demonstrated in one study [4], however, that the rate of remission and symptomatic improvement is higher than that seen in MO.

30.2.4 Cluster Headache

Cluster headaches occur somewhat infrequently as a primary headache disorder, and are more common in males than females. The pain is of high severity, stabbing in nature, has a significantly debilitating effect and may occur alongside symptoms of autonomic dysfunction. There are no large-scale trials involving high numbers of pregnant participants, which may be due to the low frequency in pregnancy, i.e. below 0.3%.

30.2.5 Secondary Headaches

Pregnancy increases the risk that a secondary headache disorder will occur. There are numerous factors which may render secondary headaches more common, including endocrine alterations, prothrombotic adaptations and the use of anaesthesia during delivery [3].

Robbins et al., in a recent study, evaluated acute headaches in 140 pregnant patients. Secondary headaches accounted for 35% of these presentations, of which 51% were attributable to a hypertensive disorder of pregnancy (i.e. around 18% of the total cases), predominantly pre-eclampsia. The other disorders involved were posterior leukoencephalopathy syndrome (PRES, eclampsia), reversible cerebral vasoconstriction syndrome (RCVS) or acute arterial hypertension [29]. The frequency of occurrence of secondary headaches in this study lies between two previous estimates—14.3% [16] and 52.6% [30]. In pregnant women who have a pre-existing primary headache syndrome, the presenting feature most suggestive of a secondary, rather than primary, headache syndrome as the cause, is greater than usual length. This difference was statistically significant in one study [29], and nearly so in another [30].

30.2.6 Ischaemic Stroke

In around 33% of cases of ischaemic stroke, particularly when one of the posterior vessels is occluded, headache is a symptom. However, typically there are obvious localising signs or obtundation of conscious level, which means that it is unlikely a cerebrovascular accident (CVA) would be misdiagnosed as a primary headache. When the United States (US) Nationwide Inpatient Sample from the Healthcare Cost and Utilization Project of the Agency for Healthcare Research and Quality was queried, it was noted that the risk of an ischaemic CVA was higher in sufferers from migraine [31].

30.2.7 Subarachnoid Haemorrhage

Typically a severe headache is the most obvious indication of subarachnoid haemorrhage (SAH). This type of headache comes on abruptly and is of high severity, reaching maximum intensity within a few seconds or minutes ("thunderclap headache"), after which the patient often vomits and becomes unconscious [32]. SAH is a grave emergency. Between 40 and 50% of cases of SAH result in death. Indeed, between 10 and 20% of associated mortality occurs outside the hospital. The key distinguishing feature of SAH is how quickly it begins and the fact that it may come on whilst exercising or during sexual activity. The risk of SAH is twenty times higher during the puerperium, where it always manifests with thunderclap headache [27].

30.2.8 Idiopathic Intracranial Hypertension

Idiopathic intracranial hypertension (IIH) generally affects pregnant women in the first trimester who also suffer from obesity. In these patients, there is a headache that occurs every day, worsening each time, the severity of which is increased by changing position or performing the valsalva manoeuvre. On examination, there is papilloedema and marked visual field loss, ringing in the ears and an abducens nerve palsy [27, 33, 34]. Patients often describe the headache as in the region of the forehead or behind the eyes and resembling an explosion or a build-up of pressure. On occasion, the headache may resemble a migraine.

30.3 Diagnostic Evaluation

Any pregnant woman over 20 weeks gestation who complains of a headache must be assessed for possible preeclampsia. 1 in 3 pregnant women who complain of a headache for the first time or who have a different type of headache from usual is found to be suffering from preeclampsia [16].

Headaches are seen in severe cases of preeclampsia and may herald the onset of eclampsia (i.e. preeclampsia plus fitting) [35]. Headaches are usually over the whole head, present continuously, throbbing in character and have any type of intensity. Sometimes there is blurring of vision and photophobia, or the patient becomes disorientated and obtundation of consciousness is observed. The clinical picture bears similarity to a migraine, although migraine often only affects one side. In some women, there may be a competing diagnosis of mild hypertension secondary to pain. However, in a pre-eclamptic patient, there are usually other signs, such as blind spots, blurry vision, diplopia, photophobia, amaurosis or hemianopsia, accompanied by pain in the epigastrium. Laboratory investigations may reveal a low platelet count, abnormal liver function tests, evidence of haemolysis and a high creatinine level [1].

Typically there are no abnormalities detected in the neurological examination of a woman with pre-eclampsia. Where there are signs of a neurological focus, they may be interpreted as evidence of a complication (such as CVA) or suggest a different diagnostic possibility, such as migraine plus aura or an unrelated CVA. Fitting is essential to diagnosing eclampsia, but a number of other neurological conditions may also provoke a seizure, such as cerebral venous thrombosis, an intracranial bleed and a mass lesion [1].

30.3.1 Women at Risk of a Severe Underlying Condition Require Thorough Assessment Without Delay

If headache occurs in conjunction with any of the following signs or symptoms, the risk of a severe underlying condition is raised and clinicians must be prepared to intervene rapidly. The underlying condition may be a result of pregnancy, or be unrelated. The frequency of some severe neurological conditions is raised in pregnancy, in particular CVA or thrombus formation in the central veins [1].

- Headache associated with a change in mental state, papilloedema, visual system alterations, nuchal rigidity or indications of a neurological focus.
- Abruptly beginning extremely intense headache ("the worst headache I have ever had").
- *De novo* presentation of a migraine syndrome.
- Headache in a patient with immunosuppression.
- Headache which differs in some aspect (pain quality, pattern, intensity) from the patient's usual experience.
- Headache accompanied or preceded by pyrexia, traumatic injury to the head, drug misuse, being exposed to toxins, coughing, exerting oneself, engaging in sexual activity or performing the valsalva manoeuvre.
- A new headache of sufficient intensity to wake a sleeping patient.
- Headache where painkillers are ineffective.

30.3.2 General Principles When Assessing a Pregnant Woman with a Headache

The majority of pregnant patients in whom headaches are primary do not present for the first time during pregnancy. Examples of primary headaches are TTH, migraine or cluster headaches [16]. It is possible for a pregnant woman who was previously prone to primary headaches to keep on having them, and provided pre-eclampsia has been excluded as a cause, there is no indication for undertaking a complex diagnostic work-up.

30.3.3 Assessment of Women During the Postpartum Interval

Women undergo multiple physiological and endocrine alterations during the postpartum, and are frequently sleep-deprived, unable to eat regularly, are greatly tired and under psychological pressure. Furthermore, many of these patients are recovering from spinal or epidural anaesthesia given to ease labour and may have been administered drugs that act on blood vessels to suppress bleeding, such as the ergotderivatives. This combination of factors makes headaches considerably more likely than usual. In assessing a woman with a headache at this stage, the following factors need to be taken into consideration [36, 37]:

- The key diagnosis to exclude in a postpartum woman who is hypertensive is preeclampsia, since this condition can present after delivery, generally no more than two days after delivery, but, occasionally, up to a week later.

Where the patient's blood pressure is normal and a neuraxial anaesthetic technique was used for labour, the possibility of postdural puncture headache (PDPH) must be considered and referral to an anaesthetic or neurologist colleague should be made for advice on management. In cases of PDPH, the onset of the headache is usually no more than 48 h after the procedure and standing up or lifting the bed head usually makes the headache more intense, whereas lying supine and resting usually brings relief. It is unusual for other neurological signs, such as tinnitus, nausea, vomiting or a palsy of the cranial nerves to develop [1].

Where there are no localising neurological signs and no features suggestive of pre-eclampsia, the probable diagnosis is TTH. It is also not unusual for postpartum women with a previous history of migraine to experience a migraine, which may or may not involve an aura [1].

30.4 Treating Headaches in Patients Who Are Pregnant or Lactating

When treating pregnant women, the potential to harm the foetus through administration of a teratogen needs to be carefully considered [38, 39]. The fact that the majority of patients do not know that drugs may cause foetal malformations and that they should only be used after consideration of their risk and benefit is an unfortunate reality [40].

This being the case, wherever possible, treatment of headaches in pregnant and lactating women should be attempted without the need for medication. However, if a headache is not treated appropriately, the patient may suffer unnecessary levels of distress, interference with sleep, low mood and loss of appetite, and these consequences may impact negatively on both the mother and infant. Hence, where non-drug treatment is unsatisfactory, pharmacotherapy needs to be considered following a comprehensive risk-benefit analysis for both the mother and infant [4]. The key principle to observe is that any medication used should be at the lowest dose that provides the effect and for no longer than is absolutely necessary.

The medications used to treat women who are not breastfeeding their infants are identical to those used in non-pregnant women and are chosen according to the condition producing the headache. However, in a lactating patient, the use of agents which are secreted in high concentration in breast milk and where there is the potential for harm to the baby is not permissible. Examples of unsuitable agents to use in lactating women are ergotamine, which may make the child vomit, suffer loose stools, become weak and lose control of blood pressure, and codeine, which may depress the infant's central nervous system [1].

The reason to treat headache in pregnant women is to reduce maternal discomfort. There is no evidence from trials involving significant numbers of women with headache during pregnancy which would allow formulation of evidence-based treatment guidelines. The key precept to be borne in mind is *"primum non nocere"* (avoidance of harm) as headaches *per se* have no apparent negative impact on the outcomes of pregnancy [5, 41, 42].

Medications with established teratogenicity, as well as those that may interfere with the pregnancy (such as ecbolic agents or those with a vasoconstrictive action), are contraindicated. Once these agents have been excluded, therapy follows the same principles as in non-pregnant headache sufferers, with the proviso that the medication should have the most favourable safety profile from the point of view of the foetus. The dose should be as low as possible and polypharmacy should be avoided. Other considerations are the patient's previous drug treatment history, other comorbidities and the stage of the pregnancy. The first trimester encompasses organogenesis and is higher risk than later trimesters [1].

It is important to manage patient expectations about what is achievable by treatment, but provided the woman has been fully informed about the risks involved to the foetus, a request for more aggressive treatment should be responded to with the provision of a more aggressive treatment plan.

30.4.1 Acute Migraine Treatment

The strategy in treating migraine during pregnancy differs from that adopted at other times due to the need to avoid teratogenicity. Paracetamol is a suitable first agent to use on account of its possessing favourable safety characteristics for the mother and foetus. Where paracetamol lacks sufficient efficacy, other agents may be tried, which are listed in order of preference. In a pregnant women with a migraine persisting for several days and failing to remit with pharmacotherapy by mouth, there should be an evaluation of factors that may be triggering the attack and a more aggressive approach will be called for [1].

If monotherapy using paracetamol does not provide relief in migraine, other agents may be added, as detailed below [1]:

- Paracetamol (dose range 650–1000 mg) plus metoclopramide 10 mg
- Paracetamol plus codeine 30 mg
- Combined preparations with paracetamol, butalbital and caffeine

The safety profile of these agents in pregnancy is satisfactory in general [1].

The dosage of caffeine in combination products for migraine is between 40 and 50 mg. There is a low risk to the pregnancy provided the combined caffeine consumption (including drinks, etc.) is not above 200 mg.

Butalbital and codeine may both cause withdrawal symptoms in a neonate if administered for lengthy periods.

Neonates may suffer from vitamin K-dependent haemostatic deficiencies following long-term maternal use of barbiturates; however, it is routine practice for all US neonates to be administered vitamin K1 (phylloquinone) prophylactically shortly post delivery as a means of stopping haemorrhage caused by deficient vitamin K. There is no evidence showing butalbital has teratogenic potential [1].

How safe it is for women in the initial trimester to use opioids for brief periods has not been fully established. There are some data (albeit limited) which appear to link opioids with neonatal nervous system anomalies [1].

30.4.2 Preeclampsia

The only definitive way to treat pre-eclampsia is to deliver the child, thus preventing complications in the foetus or mother. To limit the risk of CVA and bring down the blood pressure, antihypertensive pharmacotherapy is required. The use of magnesium sulphate is to guard against an eclamptic fit or to prevent a second fit from occurring. The headaches associated with pre-eclampsia generally respond to pharmacotherapy using paracetamol [1].

References

1. Lee M-J, Guinn D, Hickenbottom S. Headache in pregnant and postpartum women. In: Lockwood CJ, Swanson JW, Barss VA, editors. UpToDate. Last updated 02 Dec 2020.
2. Marcus DA. Managing headache during pregnancy and lactation. Expert Rev Neurother. 2008;8(3):385–95. https://doi.org/10.1586/14737175.8.3.385.
3. Negro A, Delaruelle Z, Ivanova TA, Khan S, Ornello R, Raffaelli B, Terrin A, Reuter U, Mitsikostas DD, European Headache Federation School of Advanced Studies (EHF-SAS). Headache and pregnancy: a systematic review. J Headache Pain. 2017;18(1):106. https://doi.org/10.1186/s10194-017-0816-0.
4. Maggioni F, Alessi C, Maggino T, Zanchin G. Headache during pregnancy. Cephalalgia. 1997;17(7):765–9. https://doi.org/10.1046/j.1468-2982.1997.1707765.x.
5. Dixit A, Bhardwaj M, Sharma B. Headache in pregnancy: a nuisance or a new sense? Obstet Gynecol Int. 2012;2012:697697.
6. Callaghan N. The migraine syndrome in pregnancy. Neurology. 1968;18(2):197–9. https://doi.org/10.1212/WNL.18.2.197.
7. Somerville BW. A study of migraine in pregnancy. Neurology. 1972;22(8):824–8. https://doi.org/10.1212/WNL.22.8.824.
8. Granella F, Sances G, Zanferrari C, Costa A, Martignoni E, Manzoni GC. Migraine without aura and reproductive life events: a clinical epidemiological study in 1300 women. Headache. 1993;33(7):385–9. https://doi.org/10.1111/j.1526-4610.1993.hed3307385.x.
9. Scharff L, Marcus DA, Turk DC. Headache during pregnancy and in the postpartum: a prospective study. Headache. 1997;37(4):203–10. https://doi.org/10.1046/j.1526-4610.1997.3704203.x.
10. Marcus DA, Scharff L, Turk D. Longitudinal prospective study of headache during pregnancy and postpartum. Headache. 1999;39(9):625–32. https://doi.org/10.1046/j.1526-4610.1999.3909625.x.
11. Granella F, Sances G, Pucci E, Nappi RE, Ghiotto N, Nappi G. Migraine with aura and reproductive life events: a case control study. Cephalalgia. 2000;20(8):701–7. https://doi.org/10.1046/j.1468-2982.2000.00112.x.
12. Mattsson P. Hormonal factors in migraine: a population-based study of women aged 40 to 74 years. Headache. 2003;43(1):27–35. https://doi.org/10.1046/j.1526-4610.2003.03005.x.

13. Sances G, Granella F, Nappi RE, Fignon A, Ghiotto N, Polatti F, Nappi G. Course of migraine during pregnancy and postpartum: a prospective study. Cephalalgia. 2003;23(3):197–205. https://doi.org/10.1046/j.1468-2982.2003.00480.x.

14. Kelman L. Women's issues of migraine in tertiary care. Headache. 2004;44(1):2–7. https://doi.org/10.1111/j.1526-4610.2004.04003.x.

15. Ertresvåg JM, Zwart JA, Helde G, Johnsen HJ, Bovim G. Headache and transient focal neurological symptoms during pregnancy, a prospective cohort. Acta Neurol Scand. 2005;111(4):233–7. https://doi.org/10.1111/j.1600-0404.2005.00350.x.

16. Melhado EM, Maciel JA Jr, Guerreiro CA. Headache during gestation: evaluation of 1101 women. Can J Neurol Sci. 2007;34(2):187–92. https://doi.org/10.1017/S0317167100006028.

17. Kvisvik EV, Stovner LJ, Helde G, Bovim G, Linde M. Headache and migraine during pregnancy and puerperium: the MIGRA-study. J Headache Pain. 2011;12(4):443–51. https://doi.org/10.1007/s10194-011-0329-1.

18. Macgregor EA. Migraine in pregnancy and lactation. Neurol Sci. 2014;35(Suppl 1):61–4. https://doi.org/10.1007/s10072-014-1744-2.

19. Aegidius K, Zwart JA, Hagen K, Stovner L. The effect of pregnancy and parity on headache prevalence: the head-HUNT study. Headache. 2009;49(6):851–9. https://doi.org/10.1111/j.1526-4610.2009.01438.x.

20. Aubé M. Migraine in pregnancy. Neurology. 1999;53(4 Suppl 1):S26–8.

21. Contag SA, Mertz HL, Bushnell CD. Migraine during pregnancy: is it more than a headache? Nat Rev Neurol. 2009;5(8):449–56. https://doi.org/10.1038/nrneurol.2009.100.

22. Wright GD, Patel MK. Focal migraine and pregnancy. Br Med J (Clin Res Ed). 1986;293(6561):1557–8. https://doi.org/10.1136/bmj.293.6561.1557.

23. Goadsby PJ, Goldberg J, Silberstein SD. Migraine in pregnancy. BMJ. 2008;336(7659):1502–4. https://doi.org/10.1136/bmj.39559.675891.AD.

24. Bending JJ. Recurrent bilateral reversible migrainous hemiparesis during pregnancy. Can Med Assoc J. 1982;127(6):508–9.

25. Barbour PJ, Castaldo JE, Shoemaker EI. Hemiplegic migraine during pregnancy: unusual magnetic resonance appearance with SPECT scan correlation. Headache. 2001;41(3):310–6. https://doi.org/10.1046/j.1526-4610.2001.111006310.x.

26. Turner DP, Smitherman TA, Eisenach JC, Penzien DB, Houle TT. Predictors of headache before, during, and after pregnancy: a cohort study. Headache. 2012;52(3):348–62. https://doi.org/10.1111/j.1526-4610.2011.02066.x.

27. Pearce CF, Hansen WF. Headache and neurological disease in pregnancy. Clin Obstet Gynecol. 2012;55(3):810–28. https://doi.org/10.1097/GRF.0b013e31825d7b68.

28. Menon R, Bushnell CD. Headache and pregnancy. Neurologist. 2008;14(2):108–19. https://doi.org/10.1097/NRL.0b013e3181663555.

29. Robbins MS, Farmakidis C, Dayal AK, Lipton RB. Acute headache diagnosis in pregnant women: a hospital-based study. Neurology. 2015;85(12):1024–30. https://doi.org/10.1212/WNL.0000000000001954.

30. Ramchandren S, Cross BJ, Liebeskind DS. Emergent headaches during pregnancy: correlation between neurologic examination and neuroimaging. AJNR Am J Neuroradiol. 2007;28(6):1085–7. https://doi.org/10.3174/ajnr.A0506.

31. Wabnitz A, Bushnell C. Migraine, cardiovascular disease, and stroke during pregnancy: systematic review of the literature. Cephalalgia. 2015;35(2):132–9. https://doi.org/10.1177/0333102414554113.

32. Linn FH, Rinkel GJ, Algra A, van Gijn J. Headache characteristics in subarachnoid haemorrhage and benign thunderclap headache. J Neurol Neurosurg Psychiatry. 1998;65(5):791–3. https://doi.org/10.1136/jnnp.65.5.791.

33. Wells RE, Turner DP, Lee M, Bishop L, Strauss L. Managing migraine during pregnancy and lactation. Curr Neurol Neurosci Rep. 2016;16(4):40. https://doi.org/10.1007/s11910-016-0634-9.

34. Schoen JC, Campbell RL, Sadosty AT. Headache in pregnancy: an approach to emergency department evaluation and management. West J Emerg Med. 2015;16(2):291–301. https://doi.org/10.5811/westjem.2015.1.23688.

35. Witlin AG, Saade GR, Mattar F, Sibai BM. Risk factors for abruptio placentae and eclampsia: analysis of 445 consecutively managed women with severe preeclampsia and eclampsia. Am J Obstet Gynecol. 1999;180:1322.
36. Goldszmidt E, Kern R, Chaput A, Macarthur A. The incidence and etiology of postpartum headaches: a prospective cohort study. Can J Anaesth. 2005;52:971.
37. Stella CL, Jodicke CD, How HY, et al. Postpartum headache: is your work-up complete? Am J Obstet Gynecol. 2007;196:318.e1.
38. Marcus DA. Pregnancy and chronic headache. Expert Opin Pharmacother. 2002;3(4):389–93. https://doi.org/10.1517/14656566.3.4.389.
39. Fox AW, Chambers CD, Anderson PO, Diamond ML, Spierings EL. Evidence-based assessment of pregnancy outcome after sumatriptan exposure. Headache. 2002;42:8–15. https://doi.org/10.1046/j.1526-4610.2002.02007.x.
40. Bohio R, Brohi ZP, Bohio F. Utilization of over the counter medication among pregnant women; a cross-sectional study conducted at Isra University hospital, Hyderabad. J Pak Med Assoc. 2016;66:68–71.
41. MacGregor EA. Headache in pregnancy. Neurol Clin. 2012;30:835.
42. Aromaa M, Rautava P, Helenius H, Sillanpää ML. Prepregnancy headache and the well-being of mother and newborn. Headache. 1996;36(409)

Oral Health During Pregnancy and The Lactation

31

Zeynep Çukurova Yılmaz and Nurcan Altaş

31.1 Introduction

Oral health is an integral part of overall health, and its deterioration negatively affects the general health and the quality of human life. Therefore, the relationship between pregnancy and oral health has been frequently investigated, and possible mechanisms are discussed. The purpose of this chapter is to briefly discuss this relationship and shed light on the importance of preserving oral health during pregnancy.

31.2 Periodontal Diseases and Adverse Pregnancy Outcomes

Periodontal and peri-implant diseases, affecting more than 90% of the world population, [1] occur in response to microbial plaque deposits on teeth, implants, and/or prostheses and destroy tooth and implant supporting tissues [2, 3]. Periodontal diseases include many stages, from easily treatable and reversible gingivitis to irreversible, severe periodontitis.

Periodontal diseases have been associated with many diseases or conditions such as cardiovascular diseases, diabetes, chronic liver disease, obesity, metabolic syndrome, and cancer [4]. This relationship is mainly based on inflammatory cytokines,

Z. Ç. Yılmaz (✉)
Oral and Maxillofacial Surgery Department, Faculty of Dentistry, Istanbul Medipol University, Istanbul, Turkey
e-mail: zeynepcukurova@gmail.com

N. Altaş
Periodontology Department, Faculty of Dentistry, Istanbul Medipol University, Istanbul, Turkey
e-mail: nurcanaksaka@gmail.com

C. Cingi et al. (eds.), *ENT Diseases: Diagnosis and Treatment during Pregnancy and Lactation*, https://doi.org/10.1007/978-3-031-05303-0_31

pathogenic bacteria, and/or their virulence factors into the circulation, thus initiating the systemic inflammatory response [5]. All bacteria and/or their products, such as lipopolysaccharide (LPS) that can initiate the systemic inflammatory response, can cross the placental barrier and adversely affect pregnancy outcomes [6, 7]. *F. nucletaum,* a highly invasive oral pathogen, and *P. gingivalis* can be found in placental and fetal tissues in cases of preterm birth. Although uncertain, there may be a relationship between periodontal diseases and adverse pregnancy outcomes such as preterm birth, low birth weight, preeclampsia, gestational diabetes, and spontaneous abortion. In this case, maintaining oral health before and during pregnancy can protect the newborn and mother from the following risks:

31.2.1 Preterm Birth (PB) and Low Birth Weight (LBW) of Neonates

Preterm birth and low birth weight are defined as delivery before 37 weeks of gestation and low delivery weight less than 2500 g of a newborn. With a prevalence of 6–10%, PB constitutes 75–80% of perinatal mortality globally [8]. Besides, it has been shown that neonates with LBW have a 40 times more risk of mortality in the neonatal period compared to neonates with normal birth weight. Moreover, it has been reported that congenital anomalies, respiratory system disorders, and neurological anomalies can occur in newborns with LBW [9].

Risk factors for PB and LBW include gestational age, smoking, alcohol use, hypertension, diabetes, multiple pregnancies, and PB and LBW history. Bacterial infections that spread to the uterus and amniotic fluid initiate the inflammation and cause PB. Infection and inflammation account for dominance in the etiology of PBS [10]. It has been reported that most women who delivered before the 30th gestational week had signs of infection in the amniotic fluid and/or membranes, and this rate was much lower in those who gave birth after the 37th week. Inflammatory mediators produced by maternal periodontal bacteria and products that may occur after some infections such as intrauterine, urinary tract, or cervical infections may be responsible for the unexplained part of this adverse outcome [11].

Studies have reported that patients with periodontitis have higher rates of PB and LBW than gingivally healthy patients. In periodontitis, cytokines such as TNF-α, IL-1, IL-6, prostaglandins, and endotoxins of bacteria can spread from the oral cavity hematogenously or along the genitourinary tract to the fetal-placental unit. Also, these mediators may reach the liver and increase cytokine production and acute phase protein response, thereby exacerbating inflammation in the fetal-placental unit [12].

It has been observed that amniotic fluid infected by oral microorganisms such as *Streptococcus* spp., *Eikenella corrodens, F. nucleatum,* and *P. gingivalis* may cause PB in some cases. There may be a relationship between the increase in the number of bacteria that will spread to the bloodstream and adverse pregnancy outcomes. Some periodontal pathogens such as *F. nucleatum* can allow other bacteria to enter the circulation by making the endothelium permeable, may increase the risk of bacteremia, and cause PB and LBW [13, 14].

31.2.2 Pregnancy Hypertension and Preeclampsia

Hypertensive diseases of pregnancy are the most common medical complication during pregnancy and a significant cause of maternal mortality and morbidity. According to The Committee on Terminology of the American College of Obstetricians and Gynecologists (ACOG), for the diagnosis of hypertension in pregnancy, the two blood pressure values obtained with an interval of 6 h should be 140/90 mmHg or more. Additionally, over the 20th gestational week, systolic >30 mmHg or diastolic >15 mmHg from the previously measured blood pressure value should be detected [15].

Preeclampsia, which develops after 20 weeks of gestation, is characterized by hypertension and proteinuria. Although the exact etiology is not known well, endothelial dysfunction of the maternal vascularity may play a role in developing this multi-organ disease. Studies, diseases, or conditions that can cause low-grade inflammation such as periodontal diseases, diabetes, cardiovascular diseases, or obesity have been investigated and associated with preeclampsia. However, evidence-based results are needed with larger-scale studies that provide standardization [16, 17].

31.2.3 Gestational Diabetes Mellitus (GDM)

GDM defines the impaired glucose tolerance that first begins and diagnose in the second or third trimester of pregnancy. Advanced maternal age, obesity, polycystic ovary syndrome, and previous are the main risk factors for GDM. Evidence supports the association between GDM and chronic low-grade inflammation, which can be seen during periodontal diseases. Constant high IL-6 and TNF-α can inhibit carbohydrate metabolism, and glucose intolerance may develop, resulting in GDM [18].

31.2.4 Spontaneous Abortion (SA)

SA or miscarriage refers to the involuntary termination of pregnancy for any reason before the 20th gestational week or before the baby reaches 500 g of weight. Various risk factors, including genetic disorders, hormonal diseases, smoking, and a history of miscarriage, can cause SA in the first or second trimester of pregnancy. Poor periodontal health can be one of the contributing factors to miscarriage [19].

31.3 Dental Caries and Adverse Pregnancy Outcomes

Caries formation starts with the fermentation of dietary carbohydrates by microorganisms and inorganic acids. A decrease in pH level below 5.5, which is the critical value for enamel, may cause the hydroxylapatite crystals to dissolve. *Streptococcus mutans* is the most cariogenic bacteria known [20].

Although there are conflicting results between caries and adverse pregnancy outcomes, *S. mutans* can pass from the mother to the newborn by vertical transmission immediately before or after birth. Therefore, this transmission poses a significant risk for developing dental caries in the future for the baby [21].

31.4 Dental Management Guideline During Pregnancy

Protecting the mother's oral health during pregnancy contributes to a healthy life and indirectly to the baby. For example, risky situations such as premature delivery and preeclampsia can occur due to physiological changes during pregnancy and adversely affects oral health condition.

Lack of awareness and knowledge about oral health and pregnancy outcomes of pregnant women, absence of communication between gynecologists and dentists, and sometimes the unwillingness and fear of the dentist to treat pregnant patients affect the quality of life of the pregnant patient and the baby.

Physiological changes arise in both the mother's body and the oral mucosa during pregnancy. When medically assessing these improvements, this situation can be handled and monitored if the proper procedures are followed.

Some pregnant women are reluctant to seek dental care before delivery. Recent studies have shown that many dental procedures such as impacted or erupted and asymptomatic tooth removal, appropriate local anesthetic administration with gynecologist consultation, treatment of the root canals, root scaling, and smoothing can be performed safely during pregnancy [22, 23]. The timing of treatments can affect what a specialist should do before, during, and after dental treatment and how it should be done. Dental care and treatment for a pregnant patient can be categorized into four groups based on physiological changes and timing of pregnancy:

31.4.1 Emergency Treatment

Medical situations are requiring immediate attention and treatment before definitive surgical or interventional treatment. It may cover practices that may require first aid or other emergency intervention not to risk the mother's life. In emergency cases, current infections may have a much more significant negative impact on a baby's health than the detrimental consequences of dental care. As a result, dental treatment should be carried out with the advice of her gynecologist. Oral emergencies include massive oral hemorrhage, abscesses or cellulitis spread over broad anatomical areas, Ludwig's angina, or traumatic injuries to the head, neck, and maxillofacial structures that may interfere with breathing and need airway management.

31.4.2 Urgent Treatment

This term is used for accidents, critical or urgent medical problems that need immediate attention, but not severe enough to necessitate the use of an emergency room. However, it requires medical attention within 24 h. Urgent dental conditions include mainly endodontic treatment, a cracked tooth, teeth where inflammation and pain are severe, irreversible pulpitis, and abscess.

31.4.3 Necessary Treatment

It is required for enhancing the health of the mother and the fetus during the all-pregnancy period. It includes the diagnosis and dental treatment to prevent and treat orofacial disease, infection, and pain, restore dental structure (including materials, instruments, and devices), and follow-up care and function [24]. Examples include caries that are already symptomatic or exacerbated throughout the pregnancy period, fractured and cracked tooth, painful or not, teeth with mild periodontal disease, and asymptomatic not painful pulpitis. Also, since the pregnant mother will receive general anesthesia during cesarean delivery, if there is a mobile tooth after being intubated, it can be pulled out because of the risk of aspiration.

31.4.4 Elective Treatment

An elective treatment is one that the patient or practitioner chooses (elects) because it is beneficial to the patient but not urgent. The procedure is applicable, but it is not completely necessary at the moment. Tooth polishing or whitening, orthodontic therapy, lingual braces or orthodontic aligners, amalgam restoration replacement with tooth-colored composite restorations and the replacement of esthetically damaged anterior crowns are examples for elective treatment [25]. Although the procedure is beneficial, it is not a necessary treatment. The mother's *urgent* and *emergency* dental needs must be provided at any time of her pregnancy to stay on the safe side [26, 27]. Depending on the patient's clinical history and the type of diagnosis, the doctor must determine whether dental care will be done in a hospital or an outpatient clinic [28].

31.5 Dental Treatment Timings in Pregnant Patients

All dental therapies are prohibited in the first trimester of pregnancy, according to old-fashioned, conventional treatment protocols, in order to protect the fetus during organogenesis. However, with the advancement of science and knowledge, there is no longer sufficient reason to disregard dental care, even during the first trimester of pregnancy. Attempts at emergency dentistry are often advised through pregnancy and thus might be performed at any time during each trimester, bearing in mind that delaying appropriate care can put both the mother and the fetus at risk.

The beginning of the second trimester is appropriate for the total dental care of a pregnant woman for elective dental procedures. There is no threat of teratogenesis at this interval. Nausea and vomiting that disturb the oral care have stopped, and the baby is not huge enough to cause any discomfort to the mother.

Dental scaling, teeth polishing, and root planning are recommended at every pregnancy period to protect and improve oral health [29, 30]. Extensive and complicated dental therapies should be postponed till after delivery.

31.5.1 Treatment for the First Trimester (1–12 weeks)

The first trimester is not an appropriate timing for performing complicated dental procedures. Organogenesis is the process by which the baby's organs develop during the first trimester. Radiation and chemicals are more sensitive at this period. In two ways, dental care during the first trimester of pregnancy is risky. First, teratogens pose the greatest danger to the developing child during organogenesis, and second, one of every five pregnancies is known to result in spontaneous abortions during the first trimester. Dental operations conducted close to the time of spontaneous abortion may be the cause, and the doctor should be alert [31, 32].

The most common recommended protocols for the first trimester are as follows:

- Patients should be informed and enlightened about the oral changes that occur during pregnancy.
- Highlight the importance of following specific oral hygiene guidelines, including using plaque control methods.
- Restrain your dental care to oral health and gum prophylaxis.
- Possible to perform emergency treatments.
- Elective dental operations should be avoided.
- For diagnostic purposes, avoid regular radiographs. They should be used cautiously and only when necessary.

31.5.2 Treatment for the Second Trimester (13–24 weeks)

Since organogenesis is completed in the second trimester, there would be a slight risk to the fetus. The mother gets used to the physiological effects of pregnancy. The fetus has not evolved to an improbably disturbing size that would make it difficult for her to stay immobile for an extended period of time. The dental chair position should be managed and monitored while doing the dental treatment. It is essential to ensure that pregnant patients are appropriately seated and comfortable when conducting chairside procedures. High venous pressure in the lower limbs, decreased blood return to the heart, decreased cardiac output due to obstruction of the inferior vena cava, a rapid increase in venous pressure that may lead to placental separation, and a reduction in kidney function are all symptoms of pregnancy. Both of these problems can result from lying in the supine position late in pregnancy, which can cause the uterus to compress the inferior vena cava [33]. Suppose the mother is placed supine during the dental procedures. In that case, the weight of the gravid uterus can exert enough pressure to obstruct blood flow to the inferior vena cava, the femoral vessels, and the aorta, resulting in supine hypotension. As a result of the obstructed blood flow, blood pressure decreases, resulting in a syncopal or near-syncopal episode. This condition can be easily corrected by placing the patient on her left side and elevating the chair's head which helps in venous circulation relief. In the dental chair, the ideal position for a pregnant patient is left lateral decubitus with the right buttock and hip raised by 15° (Fig. 31.1) [34]. If the patient's hypotension does not improve, she should be placed in an entire left lateral position.

The most common recommended protocols for the second trimester are as follows:

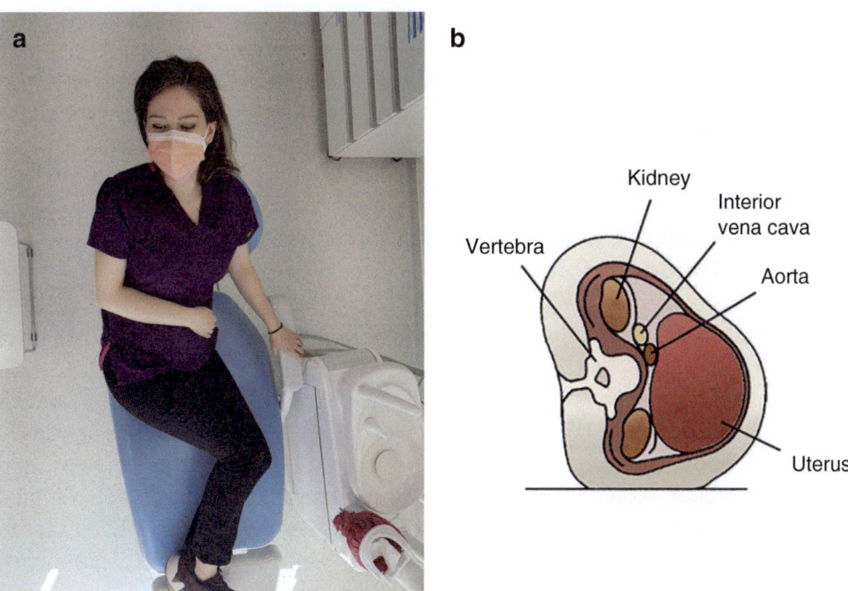

Fig. 31.1 Ideal positioning for a pregnant patient; left lateral decubitus with the right buttock and hip raised by 15° (**a**). Schematic representation of uterus and relation with anatomical structures (**b**)

- Oral hygiene should be provided, and also maintenance and plaque control.
- If required, periodontal treatments covering root scaling, polishing, and curettage can be done.
- Whether any active oral diseases exist, they must be treated.
- Elective procedures are safe, but elective dental treatment should be avoided during the second half of the third trimester.
- Avoid regular radiographs. They should be used cautiously and only when necessary [28].

31.5.3 Treatment for the Third Trimester (13–24 weeks)

During this stage, fetal development continues, and the primary concern now is the imminent delivery process and the pregnant woman's protection and comfort. Routine dental operations are safe to undergo in the early stages of the third trimester, but they should be stopped by the middle of the third trimester. Root scaling (in the first and second trimesters) and oral prophylaxis can help to maintain oral health by minimizing hormonal gingival alteration in this period [35]. Patients who are pregnant must be appropriately positioned, particularly in the third trimester. The uterus grows to accommodate the expanding fetus and placenta.

The most common recommended protocols for the third trimester are as follows:

- Oral hygiene should be provided, and also maintenance and plaque control.
- If required, root scaling, polishing, and curettage can be performed.
- If there are any active oral diseases, they must be managed.
- Procedures should not be performed after the mid-time of the third trimester.
- Elective procedures are secure, but elective dental treatment should be avoided during the 20–24 weeks interval.

31.6   Dental Care and Oral Health Recommendations for Pregnant Patients

In the dental clinic, appointments should be 15–30 min long. Pregnant women must keep their stress levels low.

Suppose a radiograph is required for emergency cases. In that case, the amount of ionizing radiation may be minimized by wearing lead gowns and aprons covering the overall body, using high-speed films, using well-calibrated instruments, and using a collimator would not cause harm to the fetus. According to the National Radiation Protection Committee, the overall amount of radiation should be kept to a minimum and not exceed 0.20 Gy, as doses of greater magnitude can cause microcephaly and mental incapacity [36, 37].

The use of amalgam restorations in pregnant women is debatable due to mercury release. Since mercury has been linked to congenital malformations, these restorative materials should be avoided. Because of the potential for adverse effects on fetal development, pregnant women should avoid even minimal contact with mercury [38]. Low-level prenatal mercury exposure is linked to an increased risk of attention-deficit/hyperactivity disorder (ADHD)-related behaviors [39]. It was declared that 1 µg/day of mercury exposure during the pre-pregnancy period is related to ADHD in infants.

Local anesthetics such as lidocaine and prilocaine are free from side effects when used following the Food and Drug Administration's (FDA) recommendations during this period [37, 40].

31.7   Oral Health Management

A combination of personal and clinical care is critical and plays a significant role in promoting oral health. Corrective and preventive procedures administered during pregnancy were positively associated with plaque accumulation and caries prevalence [41]. During pregnancy, it is recommended that the patient's current dental health be assessed. Then, she will be educated about the possible changes during pregnancy and preventative measures that may help her avoid pain and discomfort. The fetus is not harmed by dental examination and routine dental care that can be done in the second and third trimesters. If the problem, such as dental decay, is not treated, it can lead to infant caries at a later stage [42]. According to recommendations, oral hygiene and dental treatment should be practiced daily. A comprehensive oral examination must be completed early in pregnancy to ensure optimum oral health and develop the habit of maintaining it, as there is a connection between hormonal imbalances linked with gingival diseases. Dental soft brushes and dental floss should be used at least twice a day for effective dental treatment. It is essential to use fluoridated alcohol-free mouthwashes (Fig. 31.2, Table 31.1).

31.8   Dietary Guidelines and Food Recommendations to Provide Essential Oral Health During Pregnancy

A good and balanced diet is vital for maintaining general health. The nutritional requirements increase considerably during pregnancy, and malnutrition during this particular process adversely affects maternal and infant health. Vitamins A, B6, C, D, E and minerals such as folic acid, iron, zinc, and iodine should be taken from foods in sufficient amounts daily. Vitamin and mineral supplements may be recommended when necessary by the gynecologist. Green leafy vegetables and milk and dairy products to provide sufficient daily calcium intake are also crucial for bone development during this period. Consumption of cariogenic foods such as sugar, chocolate, and acidic beverages should be avoided as much as possible to avoid caries formation.

Especially in the first trimester of pregnancy, 50–90% of pregnant women suffer from nausea and vomiting. Hyperemesis gravidarum (HG) is a severe condition characterized by severe nausea and vomiting during pregnancy and can lead to

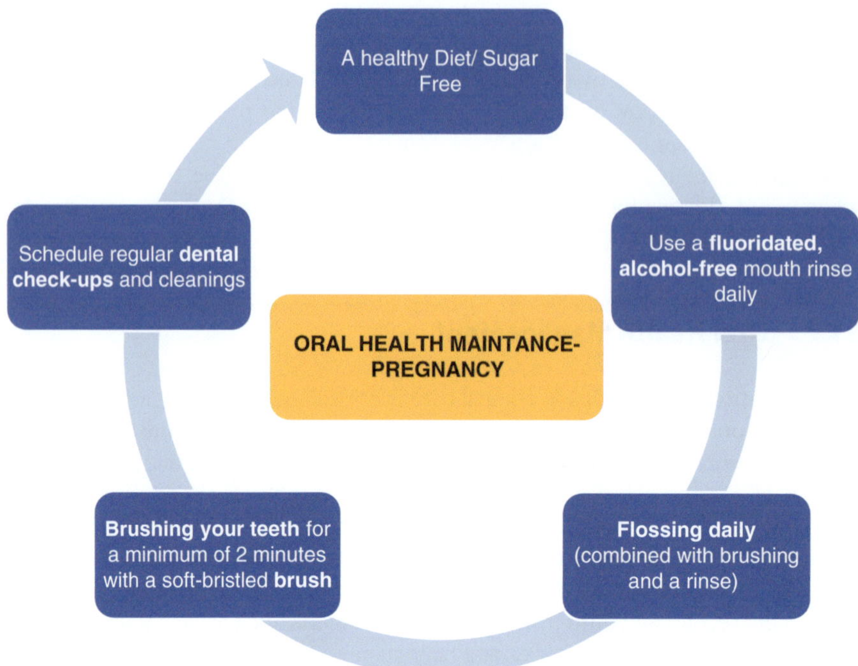

Fig. 31.2 All treatment modalities should emphasize oral disease prevention, regular monitoring, and dental checkups. (Adopted from Ref. [63])

electrolyte and fluid imbalance, weight loss, and nutrition deficiency [44]. The acid that occurs after vomiting can cause erosion on the tooth surface (perimylolysis). Teeth should not be brushed immediately after vomiting to reduce the severity of the enamel destruction. The mouth can be rinsed with carbonated water to balance the pH.

31.9 Nicotine, Tobacco, and Alcohol Consumption During Pregnancy

The mother's oral health problems have an indirect impact on the infant. Cigarette smoke contains over 4000 different chemicals. Acids, aldehydes, ketones, cyanide, and carbon monoxide, to name a few, are all directly poisonous. Carbon monoxide, which constitutes 4% of cigarette smoke by binding to hemoglobin in red blood cells, has been shown to inhibit oxygen transport. The ability of smokers' hemoglobin to transport oxygen is decreased by 2.5 percent to 15%. Also, the embryo's oxygen capacity, as well as the mother's organs, decreases. Smokers are more likely to have an abortion or a stillbirth. Besides, the baby's birth weight is lower than expected when the baby is born. Premature or neonatal mortalities are much more common in babies whose mothers smoke [45, 46]. Nicotine is also a neurological

Table 31.1 Evaluation of dental considerations during the pregnancy period (adopted from Ref. [64])

Department	Dental evaluation and treatment management
Prosthodontic treatment	• Not an emergency treatment • It can be postponed after the delivery takes place • Gagging may disturb the mother while taking impressions • An esthetically damaged tooth can be restored
Periodontal treatment	• Routine periodontal screening can be done in every period • Supragingival scaling, teeth polishing, and root planning—safe • Non-surgical periodontal therapy • Gingivectomy—second-mid-third trimester—safe • Consultation with gynecologist • Be aware of pregnancy tumors granuloma of pregnancy, lobular capillary hemangioma, and pregnancy epulides [43]—especially they exist in the second trimester • Inadequate nutrition or systemic hormonal stimulation may affect periodontal health
Endodontic treatment	• Second trimester—an ideal period to undertake endodontic treatment • Asymptomatic cases can be postponed • Always use a rubber dam • Amalgam restoration—avoided • Glass ionomer and composite restorations can be applied
Oral surgery	• Emergency and urgent treatment—with the consultation • Second and half of the third trimester—safe • Hyperplasia of the gingival tissues, also defined as pregnancy epulides, may be caused by inadequate oral hygiene
Orthodontic treatment	• Long time supine positions should be avoided • Oral hygiene maintenance and continuous education • The presence of fixed oral orthodontic appliances could increase dental plaque accumulation
Oral diagnostic treatment	• Radiographs should not be taken in the ovum and embryogenic period • In emergency cases—preventive measures should be followed

teratogen since it crosses the placental barrier and can activate nicotine receptors on acetylcholine, affecting the nervous tissue system negatively [47].

Sudden infant death syndrome (SIDS) is characterized as an unexpected death in the first year of life, and the cause remains unknown despite thorough investigation, including autopsy, death scene investigation, and analysis of previous symptoms [48]. The main risk factor for postpartum deaths is maternal smoking.

In infants, excessive alcohol intake is teratogenic and can result in fetal alcohol syndrome. Epithelial growth factor receptors regulate dental proliferation and differentiation. Dental anomalies may lead to alterations in these receptors caused by alcohol consumption. In a study, tiny teeth, structural degradation of the enamel, and delayed tooth eruption were observed in newborn rats when pregnant rats were given alcohol at various doses. It may also damage the mother's hepatic and oral systems and have an indirect impact on the baby's condition in the placenta [49–52]. While not even all children of mothers who consume alcohol during pregnancy exhibit all of the signs of FAS, there is growing evidence that even low levels of alcohol during pregnancy can trigger developmental issues in the future life [53, 54].

Mothers who smoked and drank both before and during pregnancy had a lower gestational age and birth weight, as well as growth retardation, respiratory deficiency, central nervous system disorders, and behavioral and cognitive problems later in life [55]. Therefore, gynecologists should warn pregnant women and women considering pregnancy to abstain from alcohol entirely for future baby's potential quality of life.

31.10 Mother of Infant-Lactation Period and Breastfeeding

Breastfeeding may affect two major oral health issues: malocclusions and dental caries. It facilitates the development of facial bones and muscles by affecting the sucking mechanism. Lactating children have more adequate craniofacial growth and jaw development than bottle-fed children. As a result, there is a higher risk of insufficient growth of these anatomical components, and, consequently, tooth eruption is absent in bottle-fed children [56]. Furthermore, the nipple of an infant feeding bottle is generally made of a less flexible material, which may press against the interior of the oral cavity, causing improper tooth alignment and interfering with proper palate development [57]. Another advantage of breastfeeding is that the mother's nipple adapts to the internal shape of the oral cavity, allowing for a perfect oral seal and, as a result, adequate nasal breathing growth. Babies who breathe through their noses are less likely to develop open-mouth posture, leading to an increase in vertical facial dimension [58].

Especially in underdeveloped countries, frequent use of sugary bottles while sleeping or between meals is harmful to tooth development and overall health. To fix dietary intake under a common risk factor strategy, the WHO demands "no sugars before two years." Breastfeeding is recommended exclusively for 6 months and until two years or beyond in tandem with adequate complementary feeding for a child's optimum growth and development [59]. Starting with the eruption of the first tooth, the mother should brush the baby's teeth. Due to the routine removal and control of the biofilm, daily tooth brushing with fluoride toothpaste is essential for preventing oral diseases [60, 61]. Fluoride kinds of toothpaste facilitate tooth mineralization. Regular follow-ups allow adequate preventive care to be administered. Preventive strategies include maternal counseling on diet and oral hygiene, plaque removal, and competent fluoride varnish application [62].

References

1. Pihlstrom BL, Michalowicz BS, Johnson NW. Periodontal diseases. Lancet. 2005;366:1809–20.
2. Caton JG, Armitage G, Berglundh T, Chapple ILC, Jepsen S, Kornman KS, Mealey BL, Papapanou PN, Sanz M, Tonetti MS. A new classification scheme for periodontal and peri-implant diseases and conditions—introduction and key changes from the 1999 classification. J Clin Periodontol. 2018;45(Suppl 20):S1–8.
3. Papapanou PN, Sanz M, Buduneli N, Dietrich T, Feres M, Fine DH, Flemming TF, Garcia R, Giannobile WV, Graziani F, Greenwell H, Herrera D, Kao RT, Kebschull M, Kinane DF,

Kirkwood KL, Kocher T, Kornman KS, Kumar PS, Loos BG, Mattei E, Meng H, Mombelli A, Needleman I, Offenbacher S, Seymour GJ, Teles R, Tonetti MS. Periodontitis: consensus report of workgroup 2 of the 2017 world workshop on the classification of periodontal and peri-implant diseases and conditions. J Periodontol. 2018;89(Suppl 1):S173–82.

4. Linden GJ, Lyons A, Scannapieco FA. Periodontal systemic associations: review of the evidence. J Clin Periodontol. 2013;40(14):8–19.

5. Hajishengallis G. Periodontitis: from microbial immune subversion to systemic inflammation. Nat Rev Immunol. 2015;15(1):30–44.

6. Bobetsis YA, Barros SP, Offenbacher S. Exploring the relationship between periodontal disease and pregnancy complications. J Am Dental Assoc. 2006;137:7–13.

7. Figuero E, Han YW, Furuichi Y. Periodontal diseases and adverse pregnancy outcomes: mechanisms. Periodontol 2000. 2020;83(1):175–88. https://doi.org/10.1111/prd.12295.

8. Puertas A, Magan-Fernandez A, Blanc V, Revelle's L, O'Valle F, Pozo E, León R, Mesa F. Association of periodontitis with preterm birth and low birth weight: a comprehensive review. J Matern Fetal Neonatal Med. 2018;31(5):597–602.

9. Goldenberg RL, Culhane JF, Johnson DC. Maternal infection and adverse fetal and neonatal outcomes. Clin Perinatol. 2005;32(3):523–59.

10. Goldenberg RL, Culhane JF, Iams JD, Romero R. Epidemiology and causes of preterm birth. Lancet. 2008;371(9606):75–84.

11. Goldenberg RL, Hauth JC, Andrews WW. Intrauterine infection and preterm delivery. N Engl J Med. 2000;342(20):1500–7.

12. Tettamanti L, Lauritano D, Nardone M, Gargari M, Silvestre-Rangil J, Gavoglio P, Tagliabue A. Pregnancy and periodontal disease: does exist a two-way relationship? Oral Implantol (Rome). 2017;10(2):112–8.

13. Bui FQ, Almeida-da-Silva CLC, Huynh B, Trinh A, Liu J, Woodward J, Asadi H, Ojcius DM. Association between periodontal pathogens and systemic disease. Biomed J. 2019;42(1):27–35.

14. Fischer LA, Demerath E, Bittner-Eddy P, Costalonga M. Placental colonization with periodontal pathogens: the potential missing link. Am J Obstet Gynecol. 2019;221(5):383–392.e3.

15. ACOG Committee on Obstetric Practice. ACOG practice bulletin. Diagnosis and management of preeclampsia and eclampsia. Number 33, January 2002. American College of Obstetricians and Gynecologists. Int J Gynaecol Obstet. 2002;77(1):67–75.

16. Kunnen A, van Doormaal JJ, Abbas F, Aarnoudse JG, van Pampus MG, Faas MM. Periodontal disease and pre-eclampsia: a systematic review. J Clin Periodontol. 2010;37(12):1075–87.

17. Pralhad S, Thomas B, Kushtagi P. Periodontal disease and pregnancy hypertension: a clinical correlation. J Periodontol. 2013;84(8):1118–25.

18. Kumar A, Sharma DS, Verma M, Lamba AK, Gupta MM, Sharma S, Perumal V. Association between periodontal disease and gestational diabetes mellitus—a prospective cohort study. J Clin Periodontol. 2018;45(8):920–31.

19. Daalderop LA, Wieland BV, Tomsin K, Reyes L, Kramer BW, Vanterpool SF, Been JV. Periodontal disease and pregnancy outcomes: overview of systematic reviews. JDR Clin Trans Res. 2018;3(1):10–27.

20. Cho GJ, Kim SY, Lee HC, Kim HY, Lee KM, Han SW, Oh MJ. Association between dental caries and adverse pregnancy outcomes. Sci Rep. 2020;10(1):5309.

21. Thakur DV, Thakur DR, Kaur DM, Kaur DJ, Kumar DA, Virdi DD, Jassal DS. Pregnancy & oral health and dental management in pregnant patient. J Curr Med Res Opin. 2020;3(11):724–31.

22. Silk H, Douglass AB, Douglass JM, Silk L. Oral health during pregnancy. Am Fam Physician. 2008;77:1139–44.

23. George A, Dahlen HG, Reath J, Ajwani S, Bhole S, Korda A, et al. What do antenatal care providers understand and do about oral health care during pregnancy: a cross-sectional survey in New South Wales, AustraliaAustralia. BMC Pregnancy Childbirth. 2016;16:382.

24. American Academy of Pediatric Dentistry. Policy on medically-necessary care. The Reference Manual of Pediatric Dentistry. Chicago, Ill: American Academy of Pediatric Dentistry; 2020. p. 22–7.

25. Christensen GJ. Elective vs. mandatory dentistry. J Am Dental Assoc (1939). 2000;131(10):1496–8.
26. American College of Obstetricians and Gynecologists, Committee 506 on Obstetric Practice. Guidelines for diagnostic imaging during 507 pregnancy. ACOG Committee opinion, 1995. Oral Health Care During Pregnancy Expert Workgroup.
27. Oral health care during pregnancy: a national consensus statement. Washington, DC: National Maternal and Child Oral Health Resource Center; 2012.
28. Management of severe odontogenic infections in pregnancy. Aust Dent J 2012 dental management of the pregnant patient, 1st ed. John Wiley & sons; 2018.
29. Trivedi S, Lal N, Singhal R. Periodontal diseases and pregnancy. J Orofacial Sci. 2015;7:67.
30. Huda S, Doering H, Tenenbaum HC, Whittle W, Sigal MJ, Glogauer M. Oral neutrophil levels: a screening test for oral inflammatory load in pregnancy in a medical setting. J Periodontol. 2015;86:72–81.
31. Chaveli Lopez B, Sarrion Perez MG, Jimenez SY. Dental considerations in pregnancy and menopause. J Clin Exp Dent. 2011;3(2):e135–44.
32. Nayak AG, Denny C, Veena KM. Oral health care considerations for the pregnant woman. Dent Update. 2012;39(1):51–4.
33. Scott DB, Kerr MG. Inferior vena cave pressure in late pregnancy. BJOG. 1963;70(6):1044–9.
34. Kurien S, Kattimani VS, Sriram RR, Sriram SK, Rao VKP, Bhupathi A, Bodduru RR, Patil N. Management of pregnant patient in dentistry. J Int Oral Health. 2013;5(1):88–97.
35. Soni UN, Baheti MJ, Toshniwal NG, Jethliya AR. Pregnancy and orthodontics: the interrelation. Int J App Den Sci. 2015;1(3):15–9.
36. ADA Council on Scientific Affairs. An update on radiographic practices: information and recommendations. ADA Council on Scientific Affairs. J Am Dent Assoc. 2001;132:234–8.
37. Brunick A, Clark MS. Nitrous oxide and oxygen sedation: an update. Dent Assist. 2013;82:12–4.
38. Vigeh M, Nishioka E, Ohtani K, et al. Prenatal mercury exposure and birth weight. Reprod Toxicol. 2018;76:78–83.
39. Sagiv SK, Thurston SW, Bellinger DC, Amarasiriwardena C, Korrick SA. Prenatal exposure to mercury and fish consumption during pregnancy and attention-deficit/hyperactivity disorder–related behavior in children. Arch Pediatr Adolesc Med. 2012;166:1123–31.
40. Dörtbudak O, Eberhart R, Ulm M, Persson GR. Periodontitis, a marker of risk in pregnancy for preterm birth. J Clin Periodontol. 2005;32:45–52.
41. Seow WK. Early childhood caries. Pediatr Clin North Am. 2018;65:941–54.
42. George A, Johnson M, Blinkhorn A, Ellis S, Bhole S, Ajwani S. Promoting oral health during pregnancy: current evidence and implications for Australian midwives. J Clin Nurs. 2010;19:3324–33.
43. Rader C, Piorkowski J, Bass DM, Babigian A. Epulis gravidarum manum: pyogenic granuloma of the hand occurring in pregnant women. J Hand Surg Am. 2008;33(2):263–5.
44. Altas N, Boyama BA, Çakmak BD. The association between hyperemesis gravidarum and periodontal disease in pregnancy. Eur J Gen Dent. 2020;9:108–12.
45. Christensen LB, Jeppe-Jensen D, Petersen PE. Self reported gingival conditions and self-care in the oral health of danish women during pregnancy. J Clin Periodontol. 2003;30:949–53.
46. Anderson ME, Johnson DC, Batal AH. Sudden infant death syndrome and prenatal maternal smoking: risk attributed in the back to sleep era. BMC Med. 2005;3:4.
47. Dwyer JB, Broide RS, Leslie FM. Nicotine and brain development. Birth Defects Res C Embryo Today. 2008;84:30–44.
48. Willinger M, James LS, Catz C. Defining the sudden infant death syndrome (SIDS): Deliberations of an expert panel convened by the National Institute of Child Health and Human Development. Pediatr Pathol. 1991;11(5):677–84.
49. Jiménez-Farfán D, Guevara J, Zenteno E, Malagón H, Hernández-Guerrero JC. EGF-R and erB-2 murine tooth development after ethanol exposure. Birth Defects Res A Clin Mol Teratol. 2005;73:65–71.

50. Bhalla S, Kaur K, Mahmood A, Mahmood S. Postnatal development of alcohol dehydrogenase in liver and intestine of rats exposed to ethanol in utero. Indian J Med Res. 2005;121:39–45.

51. Hoang M, Kim JJ, Kim Y, Tong E, Trammell B, Liu Y, et al. Alcohol-induced suppression of KDM6B dysregulates the mineralization potential in dental pulp stem cells. Stem Cell Res. 2016;17:111–21.

52. Pinto GDS, Costa FDS, Machado TV, Hartwig A, Pinheiro RT, Goettems ML, Demarco FF. Early-life events and developmental defects of enamel in the primary dentition. Community Dent Oral Epidemiol. 2018;46:511–7.

53. Sood B, Delaney-Black V, Covington C, Nordstrom-Klee B, Ager J, Templin T, et al. Prenatal exposure and childhood behavior at age 6 to 7 years: 1. Dose-response effect. Pediatrics. 2001;108:e34.

54. Flak AL, Su S, Bertrand J, Denny CH, Kesmodel US, Cogswell ME. The association of mild, moderate, and binge prenatal alcohol exposure and child neuropsychological outcomes: a meta-analysis. Alcohol Clin Exp Res. 2014;38:214–26.

55. Lanting CI, van Dommelen P, van der Pal-de KM, Gravenhorst JB, van Wouwe JP. Prevalence and pattern of alcohol consumption during pregnancy in the Netherlands. BMC Public Health. 2015;15(1):1–5.

56. Degano MP, Degano RA. Breastfeeding and oral health. A primer for the dental practitioner. N Y State Dent J. 1993;59(2):30–2.

57. Inoue N, Sakashita R, Kamegai T. Reduction of masseter muscle activity in bottle-fed babies. Early Hum Dev. 1995;42(3):185–93.

58. Henderson E, Mackillop L. Prescribing in pregnancy and during breastfeeding: using principles in clinical. Postgrad Med J. 2011;87(1027):349–54. https://doi.org/10.1136/pgmj.2010.103606.

59. WHO Expert Consultation on Public Health Intervention Against Early Childhood Caries: Report of a Meeting, Bangkok, Thailand, 26–28 January 2016, World Health Organization, Geneva, 2017 (WHO/NMH/PND/17.1) Licence: CC BY-NC-SA 3.0 IGO.

60. European Academy of Pediatric Dentistry (EAPD), Hrsg, Guidelines on prevention of early childhood caries—an EAPD policy document; 2008. http://www.eapd.gr/dat/1722F50D/file.pdf.

61. Wright JT, Hanson N, Ristic H, Whall CW, Estrich CG, Zentz RR. Fluoride toothpaste efficacy and safety in children younger than 6 years: a systematic review. J Am Dent Assoc. 2014;145(2):182–9.

62. Wagner Y, Heinrich-Weltzien R. Evaluation of an interdisciplinary preventive programme for early childhood caries: findings of a regional German birth cohort study. Clin Oral Investig. 2016;20(8):1943–52.

63. Naseem M, Khurshid Z, Khan HA, Niazi F, Zohaib S, Zafar MS. Oral health challenges in pregnant women: Recommendations for dental care professionals. Saudi J Dental Res. 2016;7(2):138–46.

64. Rao PK. Oral health care guidelines for gestating patients: a review. Surg Clin J. 2020;2:1026.

## Part III

Otology, Neurotology and Skull Base Surgery During Pregnancy and the Postpartum Period

The Management of Hearing Loss During Pregnancy and the Postpartum Period

32

Fatma Ceyda Akın Öçal, Yavuz Fuat Yılmaz, and Emmanuel P. Prokopakis

32.1 Introduction

Pregnancy is a physiological process in which changes occur in the entire biological system to meet the needs of the growing and developing fetus. Before prescribing any medication, it is very significant to be aware of its potential impacts on the fetus and mother. The American Food and Drug Commission (FDA) divides the drugs used by pregnant women into five different classes according to their effects on the fetus (A, B, C, D, and X) (Table 32.1) [1].

During pregnancy, it is ideal to avoid any medication, particularly during the first 3 months. In practice, nevertheless, roughly 85% of women will have at least one medicinal prescription throughout their pregnancy. Furthermore, 6% of pregnant women get at least one drug in the first trimester [2].

Various metabolic, endocrinological, and physiological changes during pregnancy can cause otorhinolaryngological complaints including ear and hearing problems. In this section, approach to diseases that cause hearing loss in pregnant women and postpartum period will be discussed. These diseases will be mentioned in the list below respectively.

F. C. A. Öçal (✉) · Y. F. Yılmaz
Department of Otorhinolaryngology, University of Health Sciences, Gülhane Training and Research Hospital, Ankara, Turkey
e-mail: fceydaakin@gmail.com; yfyilmaz@gmail.com

E. P. Prokopakis
Department of Otorhinolaryngology, University of Crete School of Medicine, Heraklio, Crete, Greece
e-mail: eprokopakis@gmail.com

C. Cingi et al. (eds.), *ENT Diseases: Diagnosis and Treatment during Pregnancy and Lactation*, https://doi.org/10.1007/978-3-031-05303-0_32

Table 32.1 A, B, C, D, and X classes of drugs according to their effects on the fetus by FDA

Category	Description
Category A	They are the most reliable drugs for pregnant women. These drugs have not been shown to be harmful to the fetus in controlled studies.
Category B	Although studies in animals show that the drug does not have a teratogenic effect on the fetus, controlled studies in humans or animal studies have not shown a teratogenic effect on the fetus, but no risk of teratogenic impact on the fetus has been found in controlled studies in humans.
Category C	Teratogenic effects have been demonstrated in experimental animals, but clinical experience in pregnant women is insufficient or medication has not been examined in pregnant women and experimental animals. Drugs in this category can be used if the therapeutic benefit to meet the potential risk is anticipated.
Category D	Although there is clear evidence of the risk of teratogenic effects on the fetus, they are drugs that can be used in pregnant women if safer drugs cannot be used in life-threatening diseases or if they are ineffective.
Category X	Studies in experimental animals and pregnant women showed that the drug is definitely harmful to the fetus (teratogenic). The therapeutic benefit in pregnant women can be neglected according to the harm to the fetus. The drugs in this category are not used in any way in pregnant women and those who are likely to become pregnant.

1. Hearing changes due to hormonal changes
2. Otosclerosis
3. Sudden hearing loss
4. Meniere's disease
5. Otitis media and otitis externa

32.2　Hearing Changes Due To Hormonal Changes

Gender impact of hearing loss has been investigated in the past, and the higher incidence of hearing loss in women has been attributed to hormonal changes and differences in the anatomical length of the auditory pathway [3].

Pregnancy can also pose a risk for hearing loss because it is one of the most intense periods of hormonal changes for women. Alteration in the level of sex hormones can affect the hearing thresholds and affect the hearing system.

It has been shown that there is a reduction in pure tone averages at 125, 250 and 500 Hz from the first trimester to the third trimester that cannot be considered as hearing loss in accordance with the American National Standards Institute (ANSI), as well as a decrease in uncomfortable level (UCL) and return to normal in the postpartum period. The high-frequency hearing level is not affected, and there is no difference observed between all three trimesters of pregnancy, the postpartum period, and the control group in ABR. This situation is thought to be due to excessive water and salt retention [3, 4].

Progesterone and estrogen are two significant hormones which may affect the hearing system at different levels. Estrogen receptors (ER) are found in the cochlea in both humans and animal models. ER receptors can be found in spiral ganglia, outer hair cells, inner hair cells, stria vascularis, and cochlear vessels [5]. These can regulate auditory transmission in the cochlea, fluid-electrolyte balance, and blood supply in the cochlea. Additionally, estrogen can affect auditory function at various levels of the central nervous system (CNS) by modifying the GABA-ergic, serotonergic, and glutamatergic systems. Throughout pregnancy, levels of these two hormones are higher than normal, and some other changes arise, such as the risk of thrombosis and increased blood volume. These modifications can affect circulation in the cochlea and cochlear fluid homeostasis, leading to fluid retention and impaired circulation.

These hormones cause an increase in both intracellular and extracellular fluid during pregnancy. This fluid retention and shift in osmolality has an effect on the inner ear and bring about hearing loss, particularly at low frequencies like Meniere [3]. A worsening of complaints during pregnancy in a patient with Meniere's disease has been also reported [6]. This is attributed to the fact that the two conditions are with a similar pathophysiological mechanism. Sudden hearing loss during pregnancy is attributed to hypercoagulability due to increased sex hormones during pregnancy. This situation is thought to affect cochlear microcirculation.

As a result, pregnancy may cause low hearing thresholds, which are evident at low frequencies, and loud sound intolerance that mimics cochlear pathology. It starts in the first trimester and increases in the second and third trimesters. However, this situation does not reach pathological thresholds, and returns to normal in the postpartum period. Speech audiometry is also normal throughout pregnancy. Therefore, no additional intervention is required.

32.3 Otosclerosis

Otosclerosis is an idiopathic disease of the otic capsule with stapes fixation due to new bone formation in focus. The cause is multifactorial, and multiple factors such as genetics, water fluoridation, vitamin D deficiency, measles exposure, and hormonal conditions like pregnancy are indicated in its development [7]. It is frequently seen in women of childbearing age. Genetic transmission is a well-known situation and familial cases of otosclerosis are frequently reported in the literature. It is thought that there are at least three gene foci in this autosomal dominant type of otosclerosis. Fluoride deficiency in water can affect the incidence density of otosclerosis, and fluoride supplements for these patients are recommended. Deficiency of vitamin D can also exacerbate hearing loss in the otoscleroticapatient. Vitamin D supplementation has been found to be effective in stabilizing hearing levels, or even a correction. The contribution of the measles virus in the improvement of otosclerosis is not clear. An inflammatory reaction to the viral state has been reported, while it seems that measles virus in bone samples of otosclerotic patients are not included [7]. Hormonal conditions such as puberty, pregnancy, and menopause may be related with increased hearing loss in patients with pre-existing otosclerosis. Estrogen receptors on otosclerotic cells have been found, however the particular regulatory mechanism of these receptors is still uncertain. The relationship between otosclerosis and pregnancy continues to be an issue of debate. While the common belief is that there is a relationship between otosclerosis and pregnancy or postpartum period, there are publications indicating that there is no such relationship in recent years [7, 8].

For years, women have been informed that when they are diagnosed with otosclerosis, pregnancy may put their hearing at risk, while breastfeeding in the postpartum period is also harmful. In 1951, Pearson recommended termination and sterilization of pregnancy as a treatment in progressive cases of otosclerosis and pregnancy. In 1939, 69 women with otosclerosis in Germany were given abortion and sterilization according to a published guideline [9].

The relationships between pregnancy and otosclerosis progression are based on clinical observations. No objective audiological evaluation has been performed so far.

Despite it being generally believed that otosclerosis arises throughout pregnancy or the postpartum period, the effect of pregnancy on hearing level is not fully known. In otorhinolaryngology literature, there is a lack of information about the impact of pregnancy on hearing in women with otosclerosis. Perhaps pregnancy is an accidental event because the disease usually occurs in young women and does not aggravate the disease.

The role of endocrine factors in the etiopathogenesis of otosclerosis has been recognized because the symptoms of the disease often appear during pregnancy or in the postpartum period. It has been observed that between 30% and 60% of women with otosclerosis who have had at least one pregnancy develop or progress to hearing loss. Precechtel evaluated 100 pregnant women with otosclerosis and observed that more than a third of them had aggravated symptoms [10].

Otosclerosis is common in women in their fertile period. This situation brings to mind the question of whether the disease is triggered by hormonal changes during pregnancy or whether it is coincidental. The hormonal effect of oral contraceptives does not cause a predisposition to otosclerosis in women. Despite the established role of estrogen in osteoblastic function, the effect of osteoblasts and sex hormones in the pathogenesis of otosclerosis is still uncertain.

A study conducted in 1974 indicated that out of 1341 women with otosclerosis, only 107 (8 percent) had their disease aggravated throughout pregnancy [11]. Assuming that pregnancy accelerates the otosclerotic process, women with children would have been expected to undergo stapedectomy at a younger age. In another study conducted in 2005, no side effect on hearing was reported in otosclerotic women with children compared to women without children, and no difference was observed between the two groups in terms of stapedectomy age. In the same study, there was no difference between breastfeeding women and non-breastfeeding women in terms of hearing loss [7]. An additional evidence supports the hypothesis that pregnancy can accelerate the progression of otosclerosis in at least some of the women [12]. As a result, the relationship between otosclerosis and pregnancy is controversial.

Conductive hearing loss (CHL) is seen clinically due to stapes fixation. Sometimes it can cause sensorineural hearing loss and vestibular symptoms due to bone destruction and release of proteolytic enzymes by involving cochlea or labyrinth structures. Usually the involvement is bilateral (70–80%), but it can rarely begin unilaterally. Hearing loss, dizziness, and tinnitus are the three main symptoms.

32.3.1 Treatment Approach

Otosclerosis treatment includes follow-up, amplification, medical treatment, and surgical treatment.

32.3.1.1 Follow-up

If the hearing loss does not affect the work or school performance or social relations of the patient, it can be followed during pregnancy. The patient's personality, profession, and age are important factors when making a follow-up decision.

32.3.1.2 Amplification (Hearing Aids)

Hearing aids are recommended for patients who cannot undergo stapes surgery or have sensorineural hearing loss. Hearing aids amplify sound and increase sound transmission to the inner ear. It can be recommended for patients with a hearing loss of more than 25 dB. Hearing aid is recommended if the patient has difficulty communicating in daily life. Since the speech discrimination rate is very good in patients with otosclerosis, patients with mild or moderate hearing loss benefit greatly from hearing aids. Therefore, it is a very good alternative for pregnant women [13].

32.3.1.3 Medical Treatment

Pharmacological options are not the main treatment for otosclerosis. Sodium fluoride is the most commonly used agent. However, the evidence supporting the use of sodium fluoride is limited and contradictory. Sodium fluoride acts as an antagonist to bone reformation and osteoclast activation throughout the skeletal system. The dosage of sodium fluoride required for the otic capsule to stop bone reformation is unknown. Sodium fluoride, which causes delayed bone resorption in the meanwhile accelerating calcification, is contraindicated in pregnancy by the reason of perverse fetal effects [13, 14].

32.3.1.4 Surgical Treatment (Stapedotomy-Stapedectomy)

Surgery is recommended for the patient in the postpartum period. Therefore, information should be given in terms of stapedectomy [13].

32.4 Sudden Hearing Loss

Sudden hearing loss (SHL) is defined as a sensorineural hearing loss of more than 30 dB that develops in less than three days, in at least three consecutive frequencies without any cause. It is an otological emergency. SSNHL (sudden sensorineural hearing loss) may occur at a low incidence rate during pregnancy, and it has been reported with a rate of 2.71 per 100000 pregnancies [15]. Since SSNHL that develops during pregnancy is a rare event, there is little research on the subject. Therefore, there is a lack of information in the literature about the cause of its occurrence, clinical features, treatment, and recovery.

The basis of the theories indicating the expectative relationship between hearing loss and pregnancy is the increase in hormone levels during pregnancy. During pregnancy, the hormones estrogen and progesterone increase significantly, high estrogen concentration causes an electrolyte imbalance that conduces to an enhancement in the extracellular fluid volume. In the inner ear, this situation may result in the deterioration of the chemical composition of both endolymph and perilymph and the emergence of SSHNL by affecting the cochlea similar to Meniere's disease [4, 16]. Despite all this, it is not known whether the sudden hearing loss that develops during pregnancy is due to the direct effects of estrogen on the auditory pathway [17]. Another theory is that the increase in coagulation factors VII, VIII, IX, X, XII, and fibrinogen during pregnancy and the decrease in factor XI create a hypercoagulable state, which increases the risk of thromboembolism, thus disrupting microcirculation and SSNHL during pregnancy [18]. In addition, other etiologies such as acoustic neurinoma occurring with SSNHL during pregnancy have been defined [17].

SSNHL during pregnancy usually occurs in the second or third trimester and in older pregnant women. This situation can be explained by the fact that the maternal physiological state is affected more strongly by sex hormones in the last months of pregnancy [15, 19, 20].

32.4.1 Treatment Approach

There is no unity of ideas on the treatment of sudden hearing loss during pregnancy. While the treatment given is aimed at improving the hearing of the pregnant patient, the necessity of not harming the fetus in the womb makes the treatment difficult. In addition, SSNHL is a disease that can recover spontaneously, but its course in pregnancy is unknown, so medical treatment should be recommended [20].

The only successful treatment agent reported so far is dextran 40, a form of colloid solution used as a plasma expander [21]. Dextran 40 decreases blood viscosity and increases microcirculation and thus reduces cochlear hypoxia. However, dextran 40 has side effects such as renal impairment, coagulopathy, and non-cardiogenic pulmonary edema. Accordingly, possible benefits and risks need to be weighed before starting treatment.

Systemic steroid therapy (category C) is the most commonly used and recommended therapy for SSNHL. It reduces inflammation and directly affects the inner ear neuroepithelium. However, this treatment has never been examined on pregnant SSNHL and it should be kept in mind that excessive prenatal steroid exposure may lead to alteration of the metabolic and endocrine balance of the fetal system, and especially the development of oral cleft. However, the common belief is that it is not used in the first trimester, and it can be used safely in the second and especially third trimesters [2, 21, 22]. Both prednisone and prednisolone can be used.

In the postpartum period, less than 0.1% of prednisolone can pass into milk when taken orally, which corresponds to less than 10% of infant cortisol production. Corticosteroid exposure at these levels is considered to be ineffective on infant development [23]. The time for corticosteroids to reach the maximum level in milk is in the second hour. However, if prolonged high-dose CS treatment is required, it should be taken 3–4 h before breastfeeding to minimize corticosteroid exposure of the infant. When systemic corticosteroids are used, H2 receptor antagonists or proton pump inhibitors should be used to protect the gastric mucosa. Both H2 receptor antagonists and proton pump inhibitors can be safely administered as they are category B drugs.

Another treatment proposed is ***intratympanic steroids***. This treatment is recommended by some otologists as the initial treatment for severe and profound SSNHL [24, 25]. Topical intratympanic treatments provide the annular ligament of the oval window through the round membrane and provide high-dose drug concentration to the perilymph via the otic capsule [24, 26]. Intratympanic steroid therapy only provides therapeutic impacts in the affected ear, thus it can also prevent the detrimental side reactions of systemic steroid concentration. Therefore, it is indicated in the treatment of SSNHL in pregnant women [20]. Since it can be applied under local anesthesia, it is well tolerated by patients. Generally, dexamethasone and methylprednisolone are used for intratympanic injection, yet methylprednisolone (US FDA category B) can be more convenient for pregnant patients than dexamethasone (US FDA category C). It is known that pregnant patients with SSNHL acquire complete or partial recovery after intratympanic corticosteroid injection without any side effects [22, 27].

Although acyclovir pregnancy category B is another therapeutic agent that can be used, it should be carefully considered while administering it. The dosage schema should be tapered during pregnancy for both intravenous and oral administration. However, it should be noted that unless active viral infection is proven, the potential benefit to the mother is no more important than the potential harm to the fetus, because acyclovir is a drug with anti-DNA properties [2].

The use of ***hyperbaric oxygen (HBO)*** therapy as adjuvant therapy for SSNHL is also recommended. However, HBO therapy during pregnancy is controversial due to its potential adverse effects such as premature retinopathy, teratogenicity, and cardiovascular side effects in the fetus. During HBO therapy, it has been shown that short-term hyperoxygenation can be allowed by the fetus in whole periods of pregnancy. No harmful result has been observed in 2 atmospheres for a period of 2 h as HBO therapy [22, 28].

Data on the safety of **vasodilator agents** are lacking and their use during pregnancy is not supported.

32.5 Meniere's Disease

Meniere's disease is an inner ear disease described by episodic attacks of spontaneous vertigo, fluctuating hearing loss, feeling of fullness/pressure in the ear and tinnitus.

Although the Barany Society published new diagnostic criteria for Meniere's disease based on clinical symptoms in 2015, there is still no gold standard test to confirm the diagnosis (Table 32.2) [29]. It has been suggested that Meniere's disease is an immune-mediated endolymphatic sac disorder.

It can sometimes be difficult to differentiate vertigo attacks in pregnant women from the very common bouts of nausea and vomiting, especially in the first trimester of pregnancy. In such cases, the presence of nystagmus may aid the diagnosis.

Estrogen receptors are found in inner and outer hair cells as well as spiral ganglion cells. These receptors provide a possible way to clarify the impacts of pregnancy on hearing. Other possible mechanisms are changes in the balance between inner ear fluids and immunomodulation. There is a relationship between endolymphatic hydrops and serum osmolarity. Patients with low serum osmolarity experience more frequent attacks of vertigo. There is also a decrease in serum osmolarity in the early period in pregnant women [6]. Estrogen has serious impacts on fluid regulation by means of its effects on arginine vasopressin (AVP), the renin-angiotensin-aldosterone system, and the atrial natriuretic peptide. The inner ear can contain aquapine receptors that are the target of AVP, allowing estrogen to influence the intension of endolymphatic hydrops [30].

Pregnancy also affects immune system functions for the maternal body to tolerate the semiallogenic fetus. Complex pathways conduce to down-regulation of the immune system through estrogen inhibiting hematopoiesis. Meniere's disease responds to immunosuppressive steroids, thought to be through immunomodulation [31].

Table 32.2 Diagnostic criteria for Meniere's disease

CERTAIN	2 or more spontaneous episodic vertigo attacks, each lasting between 20 min and 12 h
	Identification of the affected ear with low-mid frequency sensorineural hearing loss audiometrically at least once during or after a vertigo attack
	Fluctuating aural symptoms (hearing, tinnitus, or fullness) in the affected ear
	Not explained by another vestibular disease
PROBABLE	2 or more episodes of vertigo or dizziness, each lasting between 20 min and 24 h
	Fluctuating aural symptoms (hearing, tinnitus, or fullness) in the affected ear
	Not explained by another vestibular disease

32.5.1 Treatment Approach

Conservative treatment is suitable for Meniere's disease during pregnancy. Salt restriction should be recommended.

H1 antihistamines are antiemetics that can be applied in vertigo attacks, and **meclizine** and **dimenhydrinate** (dramamine) (belonging to category B) are the ones with the lowest risk of teratogenicity. Systemic **metoclopramide** (category B) is also known to be effective and safe in persistent vomiting. **Isosorbide** has also been found effective in the control of Meniere disease and can be used safely during pregnancy [6]. The use of **betahistine** is contraindicated during pregnancy. Intramuscular injection of low-dose **diazepam** is very effective against vertigo attacks. However, pregnancy category is D and it is generally recommended not to be used. **Diuretics** should be avoided during pregnancy as they cause hypotension, hypovolemia, and decrease cardiac output, but low doses can be used as maintenance therapy in the first trimester. However, their use in severe attacks is not recommended due to possible hyponatremia, hyperbilirubinemia, thrombocytopenia, placental hypoperfusion, and preeclampsia. Considering all of these, the combination of **dimenhydrinate and B6** (category B) appears to be safer during attacks of Meniere's disease than the above-mentioned drugs with potential risks to the fetus [2].

Symptoms of Meniere's disease can be improved with steroid administration, an effect that can be mediated by the same receptors as sex steroids such as estrogen [31].

Another treatment option is **intratympanic steroids**. It is thought that the intratympanic steroid crosses the blood-labyrinth barrier and reaches the perilymph primarily through the membrane of the round window, but also through the lacunar mesh and oval window membrane surrounding the labyrinth.

It is estimated that the concentration of steroids in perilymph is 260-fold higher intra-tympanically compared to oral administration [32]. The incidence of side effects is quite low. It is also believed that the intratympanic route is a safe application with few complications. The most common complications are temporary dizziness, pain, burning sensation, tinnitus, post-injection vertigo, numbness of the tongue, and small perforation of the tympanic membrane. Intratympanic dexamethasone is effective and safe in pregnant women.

In a study, salt restriction, isosorbide, and intramuscular diazepam were administered to a 10-week pregnant patient of Meniere, and a decrease in the frequency of attacks was observed [6].

32.6   Otitis Media and External Otitis

Respiratory mucosal edema or a subsequent infection, which is common in pregnant women, can cause otitis media.

32.6.1 Treatment Approach

Otitis media treatment consists of the administration of antibiotics together with nasal decongestants and/or H1 receptor antagonists (antihistamines) in non-pregnant women. Beta-lactam antibiotics are the safest choice during pregnancy (category B) and can be used in all three trimesters [2]. As an alternative to beta-lactam, macrolides (category B) can be used. At the same time, although these antibiotics are generally considered safe during pregnancy, the risk of congenital malformations such as cardiovascular defects should be kept in mind after erythromycin therapy. This negative result may occur in any period of pregnancy [33].

In addition, there is a possible relationship between erythromycin administration in early pregnancy and infant pyloric stenosis. The use of clarithromycin (category C) is not recommended. Newer macrolide members, such as roxithromycin, can be used alternatively, but larger studies are needed to fully assess their safety.

It may be recommended to wash the nose with a saline solution. Nasal decongestants (pregnancy category C) can be used to relieve obstruction and facilitate the administration of other topical treatments such as nasal corticosteroids. However, their use should be in less than seven days due to the potential rhinitis medicamentosa caused by their long-term administration. Although the use of nasal decongestants in pregnant women has been suggested in several articles, there are few studies evaluating their safety in pregnancy. Therefore, they should be used carefully. Oral decongestants are not recommended due to their proven teratogenicity in animals. A relationship has been found between pseudoephedrine used in the first trimester and gastroschisis.

Intranasal corticosteroids appear to be safe during pregnancy. Budesonide, which can be used both intranasally and inhaled and is in category B, is a suitable treatment option [34]. Again, beclomethasone and fluticasone propionate may be preferred.

H1 receptor antagonists are typically prescribed to facilitate nasal decongestion. However, it is not recommended for use in the first trimester of pregnancy. First-generation antihistamines are preferred to second-generation ones. In pregnant women who cannot tolerate first-generation antihistamines, cetirizine (third trimester) or loratadine (second and third trimester), both listed as category B drugs, may be considered.

Otitis externa can also arise during pregnancy, especially during the summer months. Systematic absorption of local aminoglycosides has been demonstrated, with the exception of streptomycin, which is absolutely contraindicated in pregnancy. Therefore, it should only be given when the anticipated benefit preponderates the possible risk [2].

If non-steroidal anti-inflammatory drugs (NSAIDs) administered orally during pregnancy are discontinued 8 weeks before delivery, potential adverse effects (narrowing of ductus arteriosus, permanent fetal circulation and renal dysfunction or pregnancy, delivery and prolongation of bleeding) are protected. At the same time, although there is no evidence of the teratogenicity of conventional non-selective

NSAIDs, including low-dose aspirin, in humans, aspirin and ibuprofen use should be avoided because of their association with gastroschisis.

The development of orofacial clefts was observed after the administration of naproxen in the first trimester of pregnancy. The use of selective COX-2 inhibitors is contraindicated during pregnancy. Paracetamol (acetaminophen) can be given as an alternative analgesic throughout pregnancy, but it does not have any anti-inflammatory properties.

Otomycosis can also occur during pregnancy and it is essential to clear the hyphae. Clotrimazole drops can be used in pregnancy for topical treatment [2].

References

1. Sachdeva P, Patel BG, Patel BK. Drug use in pregnancy; a point to ponder. Indian J Pharm Sci. 2009;71:1–7. https://doi.org/10.4103/0250-474X.51941.
2. Vlastarakos PV, Nikolopoulos TP, Manolopoulos L, et al. Treating common ear problems in pregnancy: what is safe? Eur Arch Otorhinolaryngol. 2008;265:139–45. https://doi.org/10.1007/s00405-007-0534-3.
3. Kwatra D, Kumar S, Singh GB, et al. Can pregnancy lead to changes in hearing threshold? Ear Nose Throat J:145561319871240. https://doi.org/10.1177/0145561319871240.
4. Sennaroglu G, Belgin E. Audiological findings in pregnancy. J Laryngol Otol. 2001;115:617–21. https://doi.org/10.1258/0022215011908603.
5. Stenberg AE, Wang H, Fish J 3rd, et al. Estrogen receptors in the normal adult and developing human inner ear and in Turner's syndrome. Hear Res. 2003;182:19–23.
6. Uchide K, Suzuki N, Takiguchi T, et al. The possible effect of pregnancy on Meniere's disease. ORL J Otorhinolaryngol Relat Spec. 1997;59:292–5.
7. Lippy WH, Berenholz LP, Schuring AG, et al. Does pregnancy affect otosclerosis? Laryngoscope. 2005;115:1833–6. https://doi.org/10.1097/01.MLG.0000187573.99335.85.
8. Qian ZJ, Alyono JC. Effects of pregnancy on otosclerosis. Otolaryngol Head Neck Surg. 2020;162:544–7. https://doi.org/10.1177/0194599820907093).
9. Tange RA. Some historical facts on otosclerosis in pregnancy. Int Adv Otol. 2013;9:395–402.
10. Precechteˇl A. Determination of the effect of pregnancy on the activation of otosclerosis [in French]. Acta Otolaryngol. 1967;63:121–7.
11. Hall JG. Otosclerosis in Norway, a geographical and genetical study. Acta Otolaryngol Suppl. 1974;324:1–20.
12. Crompton M, Cadge BA, Ziff JL, et al. The epidemiology of otosclerosis in a British cohort. Otol Neurotol. 2019;40:22–30. https://doi.org/10.1097/MAO.0000000000002047.
13. Shiny Sherlie V, Varghese A. ENT changes of pregnancy and its management. Indian J Otolaryngol Head Neck Surg. 2014;66:6–9. https://doi.org/10.1007/s12070-011-0376-6.
14. Batson L, Rizzolo D. Otosclerosis: An update on diagnosis and treatment. JAAPA. 2017;30:17–22. https://doi.org/10.1097/01.JAA.0000511784.21936.1b.
15. Yen TT, Lin CH, Shiao JY, et al. Pregnancy is not a risk factor for idiopathic sudden sensorineural hearing loss: a nationwide population-based study. Acta Otolaryngol. 2016;136:446–50.
16. Sharma K, Sharma S, Chander D. Evaluation of audio-rhinological changes during pregnancy. Indian J Otolaryngol Head Neck Surg. 2011;63:74–8.
17. Goh AY, Hussain SS. Sudden hearing loss and pregnancy: a review. J Laryngol Otol. 2012;126:337–9.
18. Hou ZQ, Wang QJ. A new disease: pregnancy-induced sudden sensorineural hearing loss? Acta Otolaryngol. 2011;131:779–86.
19. Zeng XL, He JC, Li P, et al. Sudden sensorineural hearing loss during pregnancy: a 21 cases report. Chin J Otol. 2014;12:207–10.

20. Ming X, Jiang Q, Tang H. Sudden sensorineural hearing loss during pregnancy: clinical characteristics, management and outcome. Acta Otolaryngol. 2019;139:38–41. https://doi.org/10.1080/00016489.2018.1535192.
21. Wang YP, Young YH. Experience in the treatment of sudden deafness during pregnancy. Acta Otolaryngol. 2006;126:271–6.
22. Xie S, Wu X. Clinical management and progress in sudden sensorineural hearing loss during pregnancy. J Int Med Res. 2019:300060519870718. [Published online ahead of print, 2019 Aug 27]. https://doi.org/10.1177/0300060519870718.
23. Greenberger PA. Pharmacokinetics of prednisolone transfer tobreastmilk. Clin Pharmacol Ther. 1993;53:324–8.
24. Qiang Q, Wu X, Yang T, et al. A comparison between systemic and intratympanic steroid therapies as initial therapy for idiopathic sudden sensorineural hearing loss: a metaanalysis. Acta Otolaryngol. 2017;137:598–605.
25. Demirhan H, Gokduman AR, Hamit B, et al. Contribution of intratympanic steroids in the primary treatment of sudden hearing loss. Acta Otolaryngol. 2018;138:648–51.
26. Tsounis M, Psillas G, Tsalighopoulos M, et al. Systemic, intratympanic and combined administration of steroids for sudden hearing loss. A prospective randomized multicenter trial. Eur Arch Otorhinolaryngol. 2018;275:103–10. https://doi.org/10.1007/s00405-017-4803-5. Epub 2017 Nov 22.
27. Fu Y, Jing J, Ren T, Zhao H. Intratympanic dexamethasone for managing pregnant women with sudden hearing loss. J Int Med Res. 2019;47:377–82. https://doi.org/10.1177/0300060518802725.
28. Elkharrat D, Raphael JC, Korach JM, et al. Acute carbon monoxide intoxication and hyperbaric oxygen in pregnancy. Intensive Care Med. 1991;17:289–92. https://doi.org/10.1007/BF01713940.
29. Lopez-Escamez JA, Carey J, Chung WH, et al. Diagnostic criteria for Meniere's disease. J Vestib Res. 2015;25:1–7.
30. Stachenfeld NS, Keefe DL. Estrogen effects on osmotic regulation of AVP and fluid balance. Am J Physiol Endocrinol Metab. 2002;283:E711–21. https://doi.org/10.1152/ajpendo.00192.2002.
31. Stevens MN, Hullar TE. Improvement in sensorineural hearing loss during pregnancy. Ann Otol Rhinol Laryngol. 2014;123:614–8. https://doi.org/10.1177/0003489414525590.
32. Devantier L, Djurhuus BD, Hougaard DD, et al. Intratympanic steroid for Menière's disease: a systematic review. Otol Neurotol. 2019;40:806–12. https://doi.org/10.1097/MAO.0000000000002255.
33. Källén BA, Otterblad Olausson P. Maternal drug use in early pregnancy and infant cardiovascular defect. Reprod Toxicol. 2003;17:255–61. https://doi.org/10.1016/s0890-6238(03)00012-1.
34. Osur SL. The management of asthma and rhinitis during pregnancy. J Womens Health (Larchmt). 2005;14:263–76. https://doi.org/10.1089/jwh.2005.14.263.

Sudden Sensorineural Hearing Loss During Pregnancy and the Postpartum Period

33

Ramazan Gündoğdu, Halil Erdem Özel, and Vedat Topsakal

33.1 Introduction

Sudden sensorineural hearing loss (SSNHL) is defined as a hearing loss of at least 30 dB that occurs within 72 h at three contiguous frequencies. Although this is the general acceptance, there is no consensus regarding the degree of hearing loss and the duration of its occurrence [1]. Bilateral involvement is rare. Accompanying symptoms may include fullness in the affected ear, varying degrees of tinnitus, dizziness, and impaired balance [2, 3]

SSNHL is extremely rare in pregnant women. Pregnancy causes many physiological changes in hormonal, hematological, and cardiovascular systems. The relationship of these physiological changes to sudden hearing loss is not entirely clear. The treatment of this disease is challenging due to the risks for both mother and fetus.

SSNHL reaches its peak incidence in the sixth decade in the normal population. There are different rates regarding the incidence of SSNHL. Byl [4] stated that this rate was 5–20/100,000 per year in the normal population in the report in which he shared his 8-year experience. Alexander et al. [5] stated this rate as 27/100,000 per year. In a study conducted in Germany, it was reported that this rate could reach 160/100,000 per year [6].

Tsunoda et al. reported that pure tone audiometry was within normal limits in pregnant patients presenting with ear problems [7]. In another study, it was reported

R. Gündoğdu (✉) · H. E. Özel
Department of Otorhinolaryngology, Derince Training and Research Hospital, Faculty of Medicine, Health Sciences University, Kocaeli, Turkey
e-mail: gundogduramazan@yahoo.com; heozel@yahoo.com

V. Topsakal
Department of Otorhinolaryngology, Head and Neck Surgery, Vrije Universiteit Brussel (VUB), University Hospital UZ Brussel, Brussels Health Campus, Brussels, Belgium
e-mail: lazvedat@icloud.com

C. Cingi et al. (eds.), *ENT Diseases: Diagnosis and Treatment during Pregnancy and Lactation*, https://doi.org/10.1007/978-3-031-05303-0_33

that there is non-pathological hearing loss at low frequencies (at 125, 250, and 500 Hz) starting from the first trimester in healthy pregnants. This reduction in low tones was similar to Meniere's disease and improved in the postpartum period [8]. The incidence of SSNHL in pregnant women is low. In the study conducted by Yen et al. in Taiwan, this rate was reported to be 2.71/1,000,000 and had a lower incidence than the normal population [9]. In the study conducted by Lee et al., the rate of SSNHL in pregnant women was found to be 19.5/100,000, while it was found to be 60.7/100,000 in the control group [10].

In pregnant women, SSNHL commonly occurs in the second or third trimester, and the incidence increases with age. The reason attributed SSNHL to be observed more frequently in the last trimester is the prominence of maternal physiological changes in the last months of pregnancy due to sex hormones [9, 11, 12]

Seasonal changes and urbanization seem to not affect SSNHL in pregnant women [13]. The incidence of SSNHL increases in high-income pregnant women. It is known that high-income people are exposed to higher work-related stress, heavy alcohol consumption, and less time to exercise [9]. The risk of SSNHL may increase due to unhealthy lifestyle choices and the negative impact of stress on quality of life.

33.2 Audiological Findings

Audiological findings of SSNHL in pregnant women vary. Hearing loss usually occurs in a moderate to profound spectrum. Audiograms can be in the form of high-tone, low-tone, flat type, and profound hearing loss [11]. Profound hearing loss is not uncommon. Zeng et al. found profound hearing loss in 37% and Xu et al. in 80% in their study [11, 12].

33.3 Etiopathogenesis

Although many etiologic factors have been suggested, most of the patients are idiopathic. Trauma, neoplasm, autoimmune diseases, toxicity, vascular pathologies, neurological, and metabolic diseases may be responsible for the etiology [14]. Although the pathophysiology is not clear, some hypotheses have been proposed. During pregnancy, some physiological changes occur affecting the hormonal system, cardiovascular system, and hematological system. Estrogen and progesterone production increases greatly during pregnancy and causes sodium and water retention, leading to electrolyte imbalance. The increase in the sodium and water content of endolymph may cause hearing loss by creating a state similar to endolymphatic hydrops [15–17]. Extracellular and intracellular fluid volume increases during pregnancy. All these changes have significant effects on the cardiovascular system. Peripheral edema is frequently observed in pregnancy due to peripheral resistance reducing the role of progesterone, decrease in venous flow due to the uterus, increased plasma volume, increased vascular permeability, and decreased colloid volume. The cochlea may be affected, as a similar increase in edema also occurs in the labyrinth [18].

Some authors state that disruption of cochlear circulation due to excessive increase of hormones during pregnancy and causing cochlear fluid imbalance may cause SSNHL. However, there are also authors who advocate the opposite. Estrogen receptors in the cochlea are thought to play an important role in the hemostasis of the auditory system. Estrogen receptors can be found in spiral ganglion, outer hair cells, inner hair cells, stria-vascularis, and cochlear vessels [16]. Estrogen has a stimulating effect on the hearing system. Estrogen is thought to modulate auditory conduction, regulate fluid-electrolyte balance, and regulate the blood flow of the cochlea. In addition, it has effects on the central nervous system by modulating GABAergic, serotonergic, and glutamatergic systems [19, 20]. Because of all these regulatory effects, estrogen is thought to have a protective effect on hearing. Hearing loss was found in mice with estrogen β receptor deficiency. This suggests that estrogen has a positive effect on hearing [20, 21]. From this point of view, the lower incidence of SSNHL during pregnancy compared to the normal population can be attributed to the protective effect of estrogen. However, progesterone has an inhibitory effect on the auditory system in general, but there is no specific progesterone receptor defined in the auditory system [15, 22]. From another point of view, changes that occur with the excessive increase or fluctuations of these two hormones during pregnancy may cause changes in cochlear circulation and cochlear fluid balance, leading to the development of SSNHL.

Impairment of cochlear microcirculation may be a factor causing hearing loss. Decreased erythrocyte deformability, increased plasma viscosity, and erythrocyte aggregation are hemodynamic changes observed in pregnant women [23]. In addition, factors VII, VIII, IX, X, XII, fibrinogen increase, and decrease in factor XI level are observed during pregnancy. These changes predispose pregnant women to hypercoagulability. This may cause vascular occlusion of the cochlea due to microembolisms [18, 24]. It has been reported that the risk of venous thromboembolism increases 4.29 times during pregnancy and postpartum period. Moreover, it has been reported that the risk of deep vein thrombosis increases even more in the postpartum period [25]. Although systemic venous thrombosis has been reported, the effect of this on the cochlea has not been fully elucidated. Arterial blood supply of the cochlea is provided by the antero-inferiorcerebellar artery. Occlusion of this artery can cause SSNHL. However, it is not known to what extent pregnancy-related hypercoagulation will cause occlusion problems in the arteries. There are studies indicating that there is no relation between myocardial ischemia and SSNHL [26]. Therefore, the role of ischemia in SSNHL remains to be elucidated.

There are some authors stating that SSNHL is closely related to pregnancy. Kenny et al. [27] published a case who developed SSNHL in two consecutive pregnancies and went into spontaneous remission after birth. It has been stated that the cause of SSNHL during pregnancy is different from the SSNHL seen in the normal population. During pregnancy, metabolic, anatomical, and hormonal changes may be the main factors that may predispose to SSNHL. In the presence of anatomical variations such as partial or full patent cochlear aquaduct, cerebrospinal fluid pressure changes may have a more noticeable effect [28]. Chemical composition of perilymph and endolymph may deteriorate with hormonal changes. The possible asymmetric structure of cochlear aquaduct may play an important role in the pathogenesis of SSNHL by contributing to the deterioration of the chemical composition. It can be argued that anatomical variations are a good hypothesis to explain the unilateral nature of hearing loss.

33.4 Acoustic Neurinoma

Acoustic neuroma is included in the etiology of SSNHL in pregnant women, as in the normal population. Acoustic neurinoma is a benign tumor originating from the Schwann cells of the vestibular nerve (myelin sheath). Tumors tend to grow during pregnancy due to hormones. With the growth, symptoms such as hearing loss and tinnitus may occur. In the first trimester, due to the toxic effects of anesthesia on the fetus and causing spontaneous abortion, the general approach is to postpone the surgery related to acoustic neuroma until after delivery [29]. There are case reports that meningiomas, the second most common tumor in the cerebellopontine angle, cause SSNHL in pregnant women [30]. The week of gestation and whether the pregnant woman has neurological complications is important in the management of the treatment. In the absence of neurological complications, surgical approach can be recommended after pregnancy.

33.5 Sudden Sensorineural Hearing Loss in the Postpartum Period

SSNHL is extremely rare in the postpartum period. A small number of cases with SSNHL after spinal anesthesia during delivery have been reported [31]. Hearing losses developing after spinal anesthesia and lumbar puncture have also been reported in non-pregnant patient groups [32, 33]. In a study conducted with pregnant women on this subject, Finegold et al. found that spinal anesthesia did not cause hearing loss in both low and high frequencies [34]. The existence of a patent cochlear aquaduct is an entity that should be kept in mind in cases with temporary and permanent hearing loss.

In a study comparing antepartum and postpartum hearing losses, it was reported that postpartum hearing loss was observed less than in the antepartum period [35]. In the postpartum period, an increase in upper respiratory tract infections is observed due to decreased cellular immunity. Therefore, viral pathogenesis may be more prominent in postpartum hearing loss [36]. In addition, patients with superior semicircular canal dehiscence and perilymph fistula presenting with hearing loss and balance problems in the postpartum period have also been reported [37, 38].

33.6 Immune-Mediated Disorders

Although the cause of SSNHL has not been fully elucidated, viral agents and vascular etiologies are the most blamed. In addition to these, there are many publications stating that autoimmune diseases may cause SSNHL [39, 40]. The formation of reactive autoantibodies may play a role in the pathogenesis in patients with SSNHL.

Antiphospholipid syndrome can cause SSNHL and recurrent miscarriages in pregnant women. It may occur primarily or secondary to other autoimmune diseases. Changes caused by antiphospholipid or anticardiolipin antibodies in tissues and cells can cause recurrent vascular thrombosis. Thrombotic events in the utero-placental unit and inner ear may cause SSNHL and recurrent miscarriages [41].

33.7 The Relationship of Sudden Sensorineural Hearing Loss and Morbidity

Hormones have important effects on glucose and lipid metabolism, especially in the last trimester. These physiological changes are very important in terms of the nutritional support of the fetus. As a result of these changes, both insulin resistance and lipolytic hormones increase. After all, energy use shifts in favor of fat rather than carbohydrate. Total serum cholesterol and triglycerides increase significantly in the last period of pregnancy [27]. These metabolic changes may also cause other pregnancy-related complications such as gestational diabetes, preeclampsia, gestational hypertension, fetal hydrops, fetal growth retardation, abortions, placenta previa, premature labor, spontaneous abortion, and fetal stress [42].

While some authors state that patients with SSNHL during pregnancy have a higher incidence of complications related to pregnancy and childbirth, some authors argue that there is no difference. Lee et al. [43] stated that cerebral ischemia developed in 4 out of 12 pregnant women who developed SSNHL. Lin et al. [44] stated that SSNHL increased the risk of stroke. Yen et al. compared the rates of complications in pregnant women with SSNHL compared with healthy pregnant women, and they reported that there was no significant difference [9].

33.8 Treatment

Treatment of SSNHL in pregnant women is challenging due to insufficient clinical experience. Clinicians should consider the profit/loss ratio while creating treatment plans, and avoid procedures that will endanger the health of the mother and fetus. Although cases with spontaneous recovery after the termination of pregnancy have been reported, hearing-related sequelae may remain in most of the cases [12, 45]. Follow-up without treatment can be performed because of the possibility of spontaneous recovery of the disease and avoiding the side effects of drugs on the baby and mother. However, for ethical and medical-legal reasons, most clinicians choose to treat SSNHL [11, 46]. Moreover, studies show that it is important to treat pregnant women having SSNHL appropriately. In the study of Zhang et al. improvement was observed in 7 of 8 patients in the treated group, while spontaneous recovery was observed in only one of eight patients in the untreated group [35].

In general, treatment initiated within 10 days after the onset of hearing loss is considered to be satisfactory. The optimum treatment plan is controversial. Commonly used treatment agents are intratympanic steroid (ITS), hyperbaric oxygen, systemic steroid, dextran 40, and carbogen. These treatments can be used alone or in combination. Although systemic steroids, which act by reducing inflammation and immune response, are the most commonly used therapeutic agent in the treatment of SSNHL, they are rarely used in pregnancy due to their adverse effects on the pregnant and fetus (pregnancy category C). Since the fetus is in a teratogenically sensitive period, especially in the first trimester of pregnancy, the use of systemic steroids during this period is not recommended. In addition, there are publications stating that systemic steroids do not have a negative effect on the health of the mother and baby in the last trimester and significantly improve the hearing loss. Significant improvement in hearing was observed in studies in which dextran and oral steroids were used together [12, 35].

Intratympanic steroids, which are believed to be more targeted and have few side effects, are ideal for pregnants. Pregnancy category of ITS is B. These drugs can reach therapeutic concentration in the inner ear through the round window. Local application to the affected ear allows avoiding the systemic effects of the steroids. In the study of Fu et al. [46] using only ITS, they found that the average hearing loss in 6 patients decreased from 90.5 db ± 18.8 to 42.5 ± 14.5 dB. Significant improvement in hearing was also observed in patients where Chen et al. [47] applied ITS with an endoscope. In studies in which ITS and other agents were combined, improvement in hearing was also observed [11, 48].

There are studies indicating that dextran 40 molecule used in thrombotic diseases and flap transposition may also be useful in the treatment of SSNHL (US FDA Category C). Dextran 40 can reduce cochlear hypoxia by reducing blood viscosity and increasing cochlear microcirculation. Xu et al. concluded that Dextran-40 is a safe and beneficial therapy for SSNHL patients during pregnancy and adjuvant ITS increases the probability of hearing recovery [11]. In their study Wang et al. used dextran 40 in 6 pregnant women with SSNHL, and 16.7% complete recovery and 16.7% partial recovery were observed [49]. Dextran is a drug to be carefully used because of its side effects such as coagulopathy, acute renal failure, and noncardiogenic pulmonary edema [50]. Nevertheless, many researchers do not mention any negative effects of dextran in the studies they performed on pregnant women with SSNHL [11, 35, 48].

Hyperbaric oxygen and carbogen therapy was also used in the treatment of SSNHL [35, 51–53]. Hyperbaric oxygen therapy should be used cautiously due to retinopathy of prematurity, teratogenicity, and possible cardiovascular effects. No adverse effects have been reported in the short-term use of this treatment [54].

33.9 Conclusion

SSNHL is rare in pregnant women and is usually seen unilaterally, and most frequently in the second or third trimester. Profound hearing loss is not uncommon. The exclusion of the causes other than idiopathic SSNHL is important. The treatment is challenging due to the risks for both mother and fetus. Early-onset of treatment increases the chance of success. Commonly used treatment agents are ITS, systemic steroid, hyperbaric oxygen, dextran, and carbogen. These treatments can be used alone or in combination. Especially in the first trimester of pregnancy, the use of systemic steroids is not recommended. Intratympanic steroids, which are believed to be more targeted and have few side effects, are ideal for pregnants. Hyperbaric oxygen therapy and dextran should be used cautiously due to possible side effects.

References

1. Schreiber BE, Agrup C, Haskard DO, Luxon LM. Sudden sensorineural hearing loss. The Lancet. 2010;375(9721):1203–11.
2. Mattox DE, Lyles CA. Idiopathic sudden sensorineural hearing loss. Otol Neurotol. 1989;10(3):242–7.
3. Shaia FT, Sheehy JL. Sudden sensori-neural hearing impairment: a report of 1,220 cases. Laryngoscope. 1976;86(3):389–98.
4. Byl FM Jr. Sudden hearing loss: eight years' experience and suggested prognostic table. Laryngoscope. 1984;94(5):647–61.
5. Alexander TH, Harris JP. Incidence of sudden sensorineural hearing loss. Otol Neurotol. 2013;34(9):1586–9.
6. Klemm E, Deutscher A, Mösges R. A present investigation of the epidemiology in idiopathic sudden sensorineural hearing loss. Laryngo-rhino-otologie. 2009;88(8):524.
7. Tsunoda K, Takahashi S, Takanosawa M, Shimoji Y. The influence of pregnancy on sensation of ear problems–ear problems associated with healthy pregnancy. J Laryngol Otol. 1999;113(4):318–20.
8. Sennaroglu G, Belgin E. Audiological findings in pregnancy. J Laryngol Otol. 2001;115(8):617–21.
9. Yen T-T, Lin C-H, Shiao J-Y, Liang K-L. Pregnancy is not a risk factor for idiopathic sudden sensorineural hearing loss: a nationwide population-based study. Acta Oto-Laryngol. 2016;136(5):446–50.
10. Lee SY, Lee SW, Kong IG, Oh DJ, Choi HG. Pregnancy does not increase the risk of sudden sensorineural hearing loss: a national cohort study. Laryngoscope. 2020;130(4):E237–E42.
11. Xu M, Jiang Q, Tang H. Sudden sensorineural hearing loss during pregnancy: clinical characteristics, management and outcome. Acta Oto-Laryngol. 2019;139(1):38–41.
12. Zeng X, He J, Li P. Sudden sensorineural hearing loss during pregnancy: a 21 cases report. Chin J Otol Chinese. 2014;12:207–10.
13. Lin H-C, Lee H-C, Chao P-Z, Wu C-S. The effects of weather on the incidence of sudden sensorineural hearing loss: a 5-year population-based study. Audiol Neurotol. 2006;11(3):165–71.
14. Stew B, Fishpool S, Williams H. Sudden sensorineural hearing loss. Br J Hosp Med. 2012;73(2):86–9.
15. Al-Mana D, Ceranic B, Djahanbakhch O, Luxon L. Hormones and the auditory system: a review of physiology and pathophysiology. Neuroscience. 2008;153(4):881–900.

16. Lee JH, Marcus DC. Estrogen acutely inhibits ion transport by isolated stria vascularis. Hearing Res. 2001;158(1-2):123–30.

17. Goh A, Hussain S. Sudden hearing loss and pregnancy: a review. J Laryngol Otol. 2012;126(4):337.

18. Hou Z-Q, Wang Q-J. A new disease: Pregnancy-induced sudden sensorineural hearing loss? Acta Oto-Laryngol. 2011;131(7):779–86.

19. Guimaraes P, Zhu X, Cannon T, Kim S, Frisina RD. Sex differences in distortion product otoacoustic emissions as a function of age in CBA mice. Hearing Res. 2004;192(1-2):83–9.

20. Woolley CS, Weiland NG, McEwen BS, Schwartzkroin PA. Estradiol increases the sensitivity of hippocampal CA1 pyramidal cells to NMDA receptor-mediated synaptic input: correlation with dendritic spine density. J Neurosci. 1997;17(5):1848–59.

21. Simonoska R, Stenberg AE, Duan M, Yakimchuk K, Fridberger A, Sahlin L, et al. Inner ear pathology and loss of hearing in estrogen receptor-b deficient mice. J Endocrinol. 2009;201(3):397.

22. Katzenellenbogen BS. Mechanisms of action and cross-talk between estrogen receptor and progesterone receptor pathways. J Soc Gynecol Investig JSGI. 2000;7(1):S33–S7.

23. Bollini A, Hernandez G, Bravo Luna M, Cinara L, Rasia M. Study of intrinsic flow properties at the normal pregnancy second trimester. Clin Hemorheol Microcirc. 2005;33(2):155–61.

24. Lavy J. Sudden onset deafness: two cases associated with pregnancy. Int J Clin Pract. 1998;52(2):129–30.

25. Heit JA, Kobbervig CE, James AH, Petterson TM, Bailey KR, Melton LJ III. Trends in the incidence of venous thromboembolism during pregnancy or postpartum: a 30-year population-based study. Ann Intern Med. 2005;143(10):697–706.

26. Kim SY, Sim S, Kim H-J, Choi HG. Sudden sensory neural hearing loss is not predictive of myocardial infarction: a longitudinal follow-up study using a national sample cohort. Sci Rep. 2018;8(1):1–7.

27. Kenny R, Patil N, Considine N. Sudden (reversible) sensorineural hearing loss in pregnancy. Irish J Med Sci. 2011;180(1):79–84.

28. Rajasekaran A, Kirk P, Varshney S. Transient hearing loss with labour epidural block. Anaesthesia. 2003;58(6):613–4.

29. Gaughan RK, Harner SG. Acoustic neuroma and pregnancy. Otol Neurotol. 1993;14(1):88–91.

30. Liang Y, Fang B, Chen D, Zhang S, Wu X, Zeng X. Sudden hearing loss and vertigo caused by a transitional meningioma in pregnancy. Ear Nose Throat J. 2020:0145561320901401.

31. Kilickan L, Gürkan Y, Ozkarakas H. Permanent sensorineural hearing loss following spinal anesthesia. Acta Anaesthesiol Scand. 2002;46(9):1155–7.

32. Walsted A, Salomon G, Olsen K. Hearing loss after spinal anesthesia. An audiological controlled trial. Ugeskrift for Laeger. 1993;155(38):3009–11.

33. Michel O, Brusis T, Loennecken I, Matthias R. Inner ear hearing loss following cerebrospinal fluid puncture: a too little appreciated complication? HNO. 1990;38(2):71–6.

34. Finegold H, Mandell G, Vallejo M, Ramanathan S. Does spinal anesthesia cause hearing loss in the obstetric population? Anesthesia Analgesia. 2002;95(1):198–203.

35. Zhang B-Y, Young Y-H. Sudden deafness during antepartum versus postpartum periods. ORL. 2017;79(5):274–81.

36. Gjerdingen DK, Froberg DG, Chaloner KM, McGovern PM. Changes in women's physical health during the first postpartum year. Arch Fam Med. 1993;2(3):277–83.

37. Watters KF, Rosowski JJ, Sauter T, Lee DJ. Superior semicircular canal dehiscence presenting as postpartum vertigo. Otol Neurotol. 2006;27(6):756–68.

38. van Ophoven M, Schmäl F, Stoll W. Differential perilymph fistula diagnosis. HNO. 2001;49(9):750–3.

39. Bachor E, Kremmer S, Kreuzfelder E, Jahnke K, Seidahmadi S. Antiphospholipid antibodies in patients with sensorineural hearing loss. Eur Arch Oto-Rhino-Laryngol Head Neck. 2005;262(8):622–6.

40. Toubi E, Halas K, Ben-David J, Sabo E, Kessel A, Luntz M. Immune-mediated disorders associated with idiopathic sudden sensorineural hearing loss. Ann Otol Rhinol Laryngol. 2004;113(6):445–9.
41. Yin T, Huang F, Ren J, Liu W, Chen X, Li L, et al. Bilateral sudden hearing loss following habitual abortion: a case report and review of literature. Int J Clin Exp Med. 2013;6(8):720.
42. Homko CJ, Sivan E, Reece EA, Boden G. Fuel metabolism during pregnancy. Seminars in reproductive endocrinology: Copyright© 1999 by Thieme Medical Publishers, Inc.; 1999, pp 119–25.
43. Lee H, Sohn S-I, Jung D-K, Cho Y-W, Lim J-G, Yi S-D, et al. Sudden deafness and anterior inferior cerebellar artery infarction. Stroke. 2002;33(12):2807–12.
44. Lin H-C, Chao P-Z, Lee H-C. Sudden sensorineural hearing loss increases the risk of stroke: a 5-year follow-up study. Stroke. 2008;39(10):2744–8.
45. Xie S, Wu X. Clinical management and progress in sudden sensorineural hearing loss during pregnancy. J Int Med Res. 2019:0300060519870718.
46. Fu Y, Jing J, Ren T, Zhao H. Intratympanic dexamethasone for managing pregnant women with sudden hearing loss. J Int Med Res. 2019;47(1):377–82.
47. Chen Y, Wen L, Hu P, Qiu J, Lu L, Qiao L. Endoscopic intratympanic methylprednisolone injection for treatment of refractory sudden sensorineural hearing loss and one case in pregnancy. J Otolaryngol Head Neck Surg Le Journal d'oto-rhino-laryngologie et de chirurgie cervico-faciale. 2010;39(6):640–5.
48. Dazhi S, Juan X, Li Y. Clinical characteristics and prognosis of sudden sensorineural hearing loss during pregnancy. J Audiol Speech Pathol. 2019;27:156–9.
49. Wang Y-P, Young Y-H. Experience in the treatment of sudden deafness during pregnancy. Acta Oto-Laryngol. 2006;126(3):271–6.
50. Kuo S-T, Hsu W-C, Young Y-H. Dextran-induced pulmonary edema in patients with sudden deafness. Otol Neurotol. 2002;23(5):661–4.
51. Chon K-M, Goh E-K, Kong S-K, Kim Y-W, Koo H-J. Sudden sensorineural hearing loss during pregnancy and puerperium. Korean J Audiol. 2007;11(1):9–16.
52. Cinamon U, Bendet E, Kronenberg J. Steroids, carbogen or placebo for sudden hearing loss: a prospective double-blind study. Eur Arch Oto-Rhino-Laryngol. 2001;258(9):477–80.
53. Hender KM, Anderson JN, Vallance NA. Carbogen gas for treatment of sudden deafness. Med J Austr. 2002;176(8):387–8.
54. Van Hoesen KB, Camporesi EM, Moon RE, Hage ML, Piantadosi CA. Should hyperbaric oxygen be used to treat the pregnant patient for acute carbon monoxide poisoning?: A case report and literature review. JAMA. 1989;261(7):1039–43.

Vestibular Disorders During Pregnancy and the Postpartum Period

34

Gökçe Aksoy Yıldırım, Nagihan Bilal, and Mario Milkov

34.1 Introduction

Pregnancy is a special period in a woman's life. Although it is a physiological process, many changes are seen in the body at this time. Physiological and physical changes occur, such as hormonal, anatomic, cardiovascular, pulmonary, musculoskeletal system changes, weight gain affecting posture, and oedema, and the pregnant woman is affected physically, physiologically, emotionally, and psychologically by this process [1].

Oestrogen and progesterone, which are female sex hormones, do not just have an effect on the female genital system. These hormones have an effect on the whole body. The menstrual cycle, pregnancy, menopause, the usage of oral contraceptives, and hormone replacement therapy affect the whole body because of hormonal changes. Directly or indirectly, the inner ear can also be affected. The presence of oestrogen receptor has been shown in the inner ear in mice, rats, and humans [2]. Neurotransmitters expressed during pregnancy can cause an increase in neuro-otological symptoms by changing the biochemical control of the inner ear. There may be effects associated with changes in osmotic fluid [1].

G. A. Yıldırım (✉)
Department of Otorhinolaryngology, University of Health Sciences, Bozyaka Training and Research Hospital, Izmir, Turkey
e-mail: gokceaksoy79@yahoo.com

N. Bilal
Department of Otorhinolaryngology, Kahramanmaras Sutcu Imam University, Faculty of Medicine, Kahramanmaraş, Turkey
e-mail: nagihanyazan@gmail.com

M. Milkov
Department of Otorhinolaryngology, Varna University, Faculty of Medicine, Varna, Bulgaria
e-mail: mario.milkov@gmail.com

C. Cingi et al. (eds.), *ENT Diseases: Diagnosis and Treatment during Pregnancy and Lactation*, https://doi.org/10.1007/978-3-031-05303-0_34

Hearing and vestibular disorders can develop in the inner ear affected by hormonal disruptions. Vestibular disorders in particular have a negative effect on the individual as daily routine and social relationships may be affected, they can lead to loss of concentration and performance, and a subsequent loss of confidence and disappointment can result in depression. Vestibular symptoms experienced in pregnancy can place the pregnant woman under stress, which in turn may trigger vertigo, and a vicious cycle can develop. With concerns of an adverse situation related to the infant or that the infant could be negatively affected by what the mother is experiencing, the pregnant woman may come under more stress. This stress and anxiety disorder can trigger depression in the pregnant woman.

Although there are few studies in literature, there is thought to be a relationship between hormones and vestibular disorders. Meniere syndrome, migraine, autoimmune diseases, and vestibular schwannoma, which are seen more often in females, are evaluated as diseases related to hormonal disorders [3].

The inner ear and vestibular system can be affected by reasons such as changes in circulation in pregnancy, hypercoagulability status, increasing sensitivity to viral infections, an increase in hormones, and increased sensitivity to allergens [4]. In the third trimester of pregnancy, there is an increase in body fluid, which decreases in the postpartum period.

Vestibular disorders such as vertigo and dizziness are often seen during pregnancy. However, surprisingly, there are few studies in the literature related to this [1].

In a study by Schmidt et al., the frequency of hearing and vestibular complaints was investigated in 82 pregnant women, and the most frequent vestibular complaint was found to be dizziness. This complaint was seen at a higher rate in women in the first two trimesters and at a lower rate in women in the third trimester, which suggested that it was secondary to labyrinth habituation. In addition, nausea, which was found to be the main symptom related to vertigo in these patients, was seen most often in the first trimester and decreased with progression of the pregnancy [1]. Nausea and vomiting in pregnancy are very frequently seen and affect the majority of pregnant women. It is thought that nausea and vomiting in pregnancy are related to motion sickness, which is a part of vestibular diseases [5].

Nausea and vomiting are often seen in acute vestibular disorders (e.g. vestibular neuritis) and acute attacks of episodic vestibular disorders (e.g. Meniere syndrome). Most patients who have a vestibular disease also suffer from motion sickness. Pregnant patients have most complaints of nausea and vomiting in the first trimester.

The vestibular system can be affected by symptoms of nausea and vomiting during pregnancy. An asymptomatic woman with a previous disorder in vestibular function may become more sensitive to hormonal triggering of nausea and vomiting, or in those with a normal vestibular system, symptoms may emerge as a result of the strong hormonal effect. In a study of 1000 pregnant women by Whitehead et al., nausea was determined in 85% and vomiting in 52%, and there was found to be a significantly higher frequency of vomiting during pregnancy in the women with a history of motion sickness compared to those with no such history [6].

In pregnancy, there is hyperventilation and a predisposition to hyperventilation, which is thought to form as a result of progesterone stimulating the central nervous system [7]. Hyperventilation will also trigger vertigo, nausea, and vomiting in some vestibular disorders [5]. All these conditions are a marker that the whole body, and especially the inner ear, has been affected by hormonal disorders.

The vestibular system diseases seen during pregnancy and in the postpartum period should be examined in detail.

34.2 Meniere Syndrome

Women with chronic vestibular disorder usually show a worsening at various stages of the menstrual cycle. Andrews et al. determined that symptoms were increased in the late luteal phase of the menstrual cycle in women with Meniere syndrome, and this was confirmed with audiological and vestibular tests [8]. These hormonal changes may cause similar changes in the vestibular system in the early pregnancy period.

Oestrogen and progesterone are chemically and structurally similar to adrenocortical hormones. These hormones cause sodium and water to be held in the renal tubules. Moreover, it is thought that in pregnancy these hormones cause vestibular symptoms by affecting the thyroid [8].

In the early stage of pregnancy, a sudden fall in serum osmolarity causes free fluid to enter the endolymphatic area by inducing an osmotic gradient between the inner and outer endolymphatic sacs and the development of hydrops, or the exacerbation of existing hydrops, causing a worsening of Meniere disease. Chemical changes occurring in pregnancy affect the inner ear fluid balance, thereby resulting in the emergence of various vestibular symptoms [3]. Uchide et al. reported that pregnant patients with Meniere syndrome experienced frequent attacks associated with a fall in osmolarity in the early stage of pregnancy, and the frequency of attacks decreased in the advanced stages of pregnancy when osmolarity normalized [9].

Small fluctuations in plasma osmolarity may also cause severe vestibular-mediated nausea and vomiting in women with endolymphatic hydrops. The period of the onset of nausea and vomiting in pregnancy is characterized by a significant decrease in plasma osmolarity. Vestibular-mediated nausea and vomiting may be due to the hormonal change in osmolarity in the early stage of pregnancy [10].

In brief, pre-existing Meniere disease may become worse in pregnancy and patients may experience more attacks while they are pregnant. Vertigo attacks can increase with a fall in serum osmolarity in pregnancy. Sennaroglu et al. reported that this finding revealed labyrinth or inner ear involvement in pregnancy [11, 12].

Conservative treatment should be preferred for a pregnant Meniere patient, and they should be recommended to avoid stress and salt, caffeine, and alcohol intake. In an acute attack, dimenhydrinate, meclizine, and metoclopramide can be used [12]. Betahistine, diazepam, and vasodilator agents are contraindicated in pregnancy [13].

34.3　Benign Paroxysmal Positional Vertigo (BPPV)

BPPV is the most commonly seen peripheral vestibular vertigo and is seen more in females than males. Although the aetiology is idiopathic in 50–70% of cases, trauma, infection, Meniere syndrome, a history of surgery, prolonged bed rest, and vascular and metabolic pathologies may cause this disease [14]. Hormonal changes during the menstrual cycle, pregnancy, and menopause cause various hemostatic and metabolic effects. Oestrogen receptors have been determined in mice, rat, and human inner ears [2]. There are two types of oestrogen receptors, namely, alpha and beta. Oestrogen receptors alpha and beta have been determined in the spiral ganglion [2]. The stria vascularis regulates hemostasis of the inner ear. It is thought that changes in oestrogen or disruptions in the endolymphatic fluid electrolyte balance lead to degeneration in the otoconial fibres or induce endolymphatic pH causing otoconial degeneration [15]. It has also been hypothesized that oestrogen induces macula and otoconia vascular feeding because of various glucose and lipid metabolisms [14].

Giacomini et al. reported that BPPV developed secondary to oral contraceptive use. It was suggested that BPPV could form with otoconial degeneration and otoconia detachment as a result of altered endolymphatic pH and impaired glucose/lipid metabolism caused by oral contraceptive treatment disrupting the fluid and electrolyte balance [15]. Following termination of oral contraceptive use, the symptoms of all these patients in that study recovered. Therefore, it was concluded that hormonal impairments in females could trigger some forms of BPPV, and the increased prevalence seen in females compared to males could be related to hormonal changes [15].

Coban et al. reported four cases diagnosed with BPPV for the first time during pregnancy [14]. It was claimed that in addition to hormonal effects the general recommendation to sleep on the left side during pregnancy could be another risk factor for BPPV [14]. Impairments in calcium and vitamin D metabolism are also thought to be a risk factor for BPPV [16]. As the foetus grows rapidly in the third trimester, calcium and vitamin D metabolism can be affected in pregnancy, which may constitute a risk factor for pregnant women developing BPPV [14].

Ogun et al. discussed the increased tendency for BPPV associated with hormonal fluctuations in menopause. However, it was emphasized that in addition to hormonal fluctuations symptoms could develop as a result of ageing, leading to otoconial degeneration [17].

BPPV may be recurrent. Factors which could affect disease recurrence include female gender and comorbid Meniere disease [15].

In the treatment of BPPV, it is appropriate to apply repositioning manoeuvres if they can be applied without forcing the pregnant patient. It is recommended to apply the Epley manoeuvre and Brandt–Daroff exercises to BPPV in the posterior and superior semicircular canals, and the barbecue manoeuvre to BPPV in the lateral semicircular canal [17].

34.4   Vestibular Neuritis

Vestibular neuritis, which is a peripheral vestibular disease, is thought to be caused by neurotropic viruses. Gokgoz et al. published the case of a patient who developed vestibular neuritis in pregnancy. It was reported that vestibular neuritis may be seen because of the increased susceptibility to viral infections in pregnancy [13].

34.5   Migraine and Migraine-Associated Vertigo

Migraine has a reported prevalence of 15–20% in females and 7–8% in males [18, 19]. The female sex hormones, oestrogen and progesterone, with PGR and ESR1 receptors, are known to play significant roles in the central nervous system [18]. The menstrual cycle, oral contraceptive use, pregnancy and birth, and the use of hormone replacement therapy are known to be associated with migraine attacks [20]. Migraine-associated vertigo (MAV) is a migraine syndrome that is seen more commonly in females than in males. Studies by Lee et al. showed a relationship between MAV and progesterone receptor (PGR) [18]. Hormonal changes occurring in pregnancy may trigger nausea, vomiting, dehydration, sleep disorders, and stress migraine attacks [20]. As a migraine subtype, MAV is affected by these particular conditions in the same way.

34.6   Superior Semicircular Canal Dehiscence (SSCD)

SSCD, which is characterized by dizziness or vertigo triggered by a sudden change in pressure or high-volume noise, conductive-type hearing loss, aural fullness, and autophony, was defined for the first time by Minor in 1998 [21, 22]. In situations such as lifting a heavy weight, the Valsalva manoeuvre, sneezing or coughing, and dizziness or vertigo may develop (Hennebert sign). Vestibular symptoms may also develop with loud noise (Tullio phenomenon). This condition is thought to be caused by dehiscence of the bone in the superior semicircular canal. In a study of 1000 temporal bones by Carey et al., it was reported that the superior semicircular canal was covered with a very fine bone structure in 1.3% of cases, with dehiscence determined at the rate of 0.7% [23]. During pregnancy, and especially during the birth, symptoms may develop secondary to an increase in intracranial or inner ear pressure. In women with vestibular complaints in the postpartum period and a record in the anamnesis that these complaints started after the birth, SSCD must be kept in mind in the differential diagnosis.

34.7   Perilymph Fistula (PLF)

PLF is described as an abnormal opening causing passage of perilymph between the inner and middle ears. Generally, perilymph leaks from a round or oval window from the inner ear to the middle ear, related to a sudden pressure change. It manifests with hearing loss and vestibular symptoms. PLF can develop association with a sudden increase in intracranial or inner ear pressure, generally during birth. In three patients with PLF examined by Whitehead [24], stapes fracture was determined. From the anamneses, it was learned that sudden hearing loss and vertigo had developed after sneezing in two cases and after giving birth in one case [24]. PLF may develop in conditions where there is a sudden pressure change such as in the Valsalva manoeuvre, lifting a heavy weight, sneezing, coughing, or giving birth.

34.8   Vestibular Schwannoma (Acoustic Neuroma)

Vestibular schwannomas are benign tumours arising from the eighth cranial nerve sheath, which manifest with hearing loss and vestibular symptoms [25]. They are seen more often in females than in males and tend to be larger and more vascular in females [26]. In an experimental study on a rat model, Stidham et al. determined that vestibular schwannoma grew statistically significantly more rapidly in the group administered with oestrogen compared to the group not given oestrogen [27]. Brown et al. found an increase in oestrogen receptors in samples of sporadic vestibular schwannoma compared to normal nerve samples [28]. It has been reported that these tumours grow rapidly during pregnancy, and that this mechanism can be explained by the role of increased hormone receptors and increased blood volume [25].

34.9   Meningioma

Meningioma is the second most commonly seen tumour of the pontocerebellar corner after vestibular schwannoma [29]. It is seen more in females than in males and is thought to be related to female sex hormones [30]. Rapid growth has been reported in pregnancy and the luteal phase of the menstrual cycle [31]. There are hormone receptors on tumour cells, and this rapid growth occurring in pregnancy is thought to be associated with hormonal changes, fluid retention, vascular congestion, and increased oedema [32].

34.10   Otosclerosis

Otosclerosis is one of the most common reasons for acquired hearing loss. There is known to be hormone sensitivity in otosclerosis and progression in pregnancy [12]. Although it is generally seen with symptoms of hearing loss and tinnitus, dizziness and vertigo are complaints that may also be seen in otosclerosis. In a pregnant patient with conductive-type hearing loss and vestibular symptoms, otosclerosis should be considered in the differential diagnosis.

34.11 Conclusion

Vestibular complaints are seen in pregnancy and postpartum breastfeeding period. It is extremely important that a good anamnesis is taken first in women presenting with vestibular complaints in these periods. A detailed physical examination must be made, and tests should be requested accordingly. Treatment should be planned taking into consideration the benefit–harm risk for both mother and infant of the treatment to be applied, and whenever possible treatment should be conservative.

References

1. Schmidt PM d S, Flores F d T, Rossi AG, da Silveira AF. Hearing and vestibular complaints during pregnancy. Braz J Otorhinolaryngol [Internet]. 2010;76(1):29–33. https://doi.org/10.1590/S1808-86942010000100006.
2. Stenberg AE, Wang H, Sahlin L, Stierna P, Enmark E, Hultcrantz M. Estrogen receptors α and β in the inner ear of the "turner mouse" and an estrogen receptor β knockout mouse. Hear Res. 2002;166(1–2):1–8.
3. Haybach BPJ. Hormones and vestibular disorders. Vestibular Disorders Association (503), pp 1–9.
4. Kumar R, Hayhurst KL, Robson AK. Ear, nose, and throat manifestations during pregnancy. Otolaryngol Head Neck Surg. 2011;145(2):188–98.
5. Black FO. Maternal susceptibility to nausea and vomiting of pregnancy: is the vestibular system involved? Am J Obstet Gynecol. 2002;186(5):204–9.
6. Whitehead SA, Andrews PLR, Chamberlain GVP. Characterisation of nausea and vomiting in early pregnancy: a survey of 1000 women. J Obstet Gynaecol (Lahore). 1992;12(6):364–9.
7. Med JP, Fadel HE, Northrop G, Misenhimer HR, Harp RJ. Original articles normal pregnancy: a model of sustained respiratory alkalosis curriculum vitae HOSSAM E. FADEL 1 Mater Methods. 1979;3
8. Andrews JC, Ator GA, Honrubia V. The exacerbation of symptoms in Meniere's disease during the premenstrual period. Arch Otolaryngol Neck Surg. 1992;118(1):74–8.
9. Uchide K, Suzuki N, Takiguchi T, Terada SIM. The possible effect of pregnancy on Meniere's disease. ORL. 1997;59:292–5.
10. Murphy GT. Nausea and vomiting of pregnancy: an obstetric syndrome. Am J Obstet Gynecol. 2002;186(5):184–9.
11. Sennaroglu G, Belgin E. Main articles audiological ndings in pregnancy. 2001; 115(February):617–21.
12. Swain SK, Pati BK, Mohanty JN. Otological manifestations in pregnant women—a study at a tertiary care hospital of eastern India. J Otol [Internet]. 2020;15(3):103–6. https://doi.org/10.1016/j.joto.2019.11.003.
13. Gökgöz MC, Binar M, Arslan F, Satar B. Vestibular neuritis presenting in pregnancy: case report of rare entity and treatment options. Eur Res J. 2018;5(5):909–12.
14. Coban K, Yigit N, Aydin E. Benign paroxysmal positional vertigo in pregnancy. Turk Otolarengoloji Arsivi/Turkish Arch Otolaryngol. 2017;55(2):83–6.

15. Giacomini PG, Napolitano B, Alessandrini M, Di Girolamo S, Magrini A. Recurrent paroxysmal positional vertigo related to oral contraceptive treatment. Gynecol Endocrinol. 2006;22(1):5–8.
16. Talaat HS, Abuhadied G, Talaat AS, Abdelaal MSS. Low bone mineral density and vitamin D deficiency in patients with benign positional paroxysmal vertigo. Eur Arch Oto-Rhino-Laryngol. 2015;272(9):2249–53.
17. Ogun OA, Büki B, Cohn ES, Janky KL, Lundberg YW. Menopause and benign paroxysmal positional vertigo. Menopause. 2014;21(8):886–9.
18. Lee JH, Marcus DC. Estrogen acutely inhibits ion transport by isolated stria vascularis. Hear Res. 2001;158(1–2):123–30.
19. Lipton RB, Bigal ME, Diamond M, Freitag F, Reed ML, Stewart WF. Migraine prevalence, disease burden, and the need for preventive therapy. Neurology. 2007;68(5):343–9.
20. Todd C, Lagman-Bartolome AM, Lay C. Women and migraine: the role of hormones. Curr Neurol Neurosci Rep. 2018;18(7):1–6.
21. Minor LB, Solomon D, Zinreich JS, Zee DS. Sound- and/or pressure-induced vertigo due to bone dehiscence of the superior semicircular canal. Arch Otolaryngol Head Neck Surg. 1998;124(3):249–58.
22. Watters KF, Rosowski JJ, Sauter T, Lee DJ. Superior semicircular canal dehiscence presenting as postpartum vertigo. Otol Neurotol. 2006;27(6):756–68.
23. Carey JP, Minor LB, Nager GT. Dehiscence or thinning of bone overlying the superior semicircular canal in a temporal bone survey. Arch Otolaryngol Head Neck Surg. 2000;126(2):137–47.
24. Whitehead E. Sudden sensorineural hearing loss with fracture of the stapes footplate following sneezing and parturition. Clin Otolaryngol Allied Sci. 1999;24(5):462–4.
25. Akella SS, Mattson JN, Moreira NN. Vestibular Schwannoma growth during pregnancy: case report of neurofibromatosis type 2 in pregnancy right cavernous sinus meningioma with involvement of right trigeminal nerve Vestibular Schwannoma growth during pregnancy. Proc Obstet Gynecol. 2019;9(1):1–9.
26. Kasantikul V, Netsky MGGM. Acoustic neurilemmoma: clinicoanatomical study of 103 patients. J Neurosurg. 1980;52:28–35.
27. Stidham KR, Roberson J. Effects of estrogen and tamoxifen on growth of human vestibular schwannomas in the nude mouse. Otolaryngol Head Neck Surg. 1999;120(2):262–4.
28. Brown CM, Ahmad ZK, Ryan AF, Doherty JK. Estrogen receptor expression in sporadic vestibular schwannomas. Otol Neurotol. 2011;32(1):158–62.
29. Liang Y, Fang B, Chen D, Zhang S, Wu X, Zeng X. Sudden hearing loss and vertigo caused by a transitional meningioma in pregnancy. Ear, Nose Throat J. 2020:1–3.
30. Schrell UMH, Adams EF, Fahlbusch R, Greb R, Jirikowski G, Prior R, et al. Hormonal dependency of cerebral meningiomas. Part 1: female sex steroid receptors and their significance as specific markers for adjuvant medical therapy. J Neurosurg. 1990;73(5):743–9.
31. Gurcay AG, Bozkurt ISS. Diagnosis, treatment, and management strategy of meningioma during pregnancy. Asian J Neurosurg. 2018;13:86–9.
32. Kanaan I, Jallu A, Kanaan H. Management strategy for meningioma in pregnancy: a clinical study. Skull Base. 2003;13(4):197–202.

Meniere's Disease During Pregnancy and The Postpartum Period

35

Sinem Daşlı, Selahattin Genç, and Bert Schmelzer

35.1 Introduction

Meniere's disease (MD) is a syndrome characterized by attacks of recurrent spontaneous vertigo, sensorineural hearing loss, tinnitus, and aural fullness. Clinically, we can divide the course of the disease into three periods: initial, active, and final. However, pregnancy is of particular importance in female patients in terms of the course of the disease. Hormones such as human chorionic gonadotropin (HCG) secreted during pregnancy and increased estrogen and progesterone levels can increase vertigo attacks in Meniere's disease by various mechanisms. In particular, it has been shown that estrogen increases endolymphatic hydrops (EH) by affecting the aquaporin receptors in the inner ear through the arginine vasopressin (AVP) system. In addition, it is thought that decreased body osmolality during pregnancy due to the effect of these hormonal changes also triggers vertigo. In the postpartum period, it is said that prolactin can worsen Meniere's symptoms by increasing anxiety and depression.

S. Daşlı (✉) · S. Genç
Department of Otorhinolaryngology, Health Sciences University, Faculty of Medicine, Derince Research and Training Hospital, Kocaeli, Turkey
e-mail: yagmur_sd@hotmail.com; drsgenc@yahoo.com

B. Schmelzer
Ziekenhuis Netwerk Antwerpen (ZNA), Section of Otorhinolaryngology, Head and Neck Surgery, Antwerpen, Belgium
e-mail: bertschmelzer@outlook.com

C. Cingi et al. (eds.), *ENT Diseases: Diagnosis and Treatment during Pregnancy and Lactation*, https://doi.org/10.1007/978-3-031-05303-0_35

35.2 Meniere's Disease

MD is a syndrome caused by unusual diseases influencing the inner ear and characterized by attacks of recurrent spontaneous vertigo, sensorineural hearing loss (SNHL), tinnitus, and aural fullness. Meniere is a chronic disease and usually affects one ear. However, in the later stages of the disease, 45% of the patients who were followed for 20 years were affected in the opposite ear and the disease became bilateral. MD usually occurs in adults, but it is estimated that 3% of cases are under 18 years of age. The disease occurs in population often between the ages of 40 and 60 and is more common in women than in men [1, 2]. Its prevalence and incidence vary by ethnicity and region around the world, but range from 3 to 513 per 100,000 people [1].

The etiology of MD includes genetics, autoimmunity, allergic factors, hormonal factors, and viral infections. MD shows a familial relation, and familial MD has been noticed with an autosomal-dominant inheritance pattern in 10% of cases [3]. The prevalence of autoimmune diseases such as rheumatoid arthritis (RA), systemic lupus erythematosus (SLE), Hashimoto thyroiditis, and psoriasis is increased in MD compared to the general population [1, 4]. The improvement in vertigo symptoms after allergy treatment in patients with environmental or food allergies confirms the role of allergy in the etiology [1]. In addition, MD patients associated with vestibular migraine, which shows a common pathophysiology with MD, have been described. Otherwise, MD has been associated with other disorders such as benign paroxysmal positional vertigo, trauma, structural diversity, and psychological factors such as stress or anxiety, but these factors are thought to increase attacks more [1].

In two different studies by Frejo et al., unilateral and bilateral Meniere's disease was examined in five clinical subtypes, which differ according to etiological factors [5, 6]:

- Type 1: classic unilateral MD; metachronic SNHL in bilateral MD without migraine
- Type 2: delayed unilateral MD (history of SNHL >1 month prior to vertigo onset); synchronic onset in bilateral MD with no autoimmune disease
- Type 3: familiar history without autoimmune disease (unilateral and bilateral MD patients)
- Type 4: migraine history and sporadic MD (uni−/bilateral MD patients)
- Type 5: history of autoimmune disease without migraine (uni−/bilateral MD patients)

In the first 2–3 years of the disease, vertigo attacks, SNHL, tinnitus (classical triad), and ear fullness are seen in patients. The most common initial symptom is vertigo. Acute attacks usually occur 5–10 times a year and continue with remission phases with variable month and year periods. Hearing loss is progressive, fluctuant, and often affects low frequencies. Tinnitus is at low frequencies and is narrow band noise [1].

In the active phase of the disease, progression begins in SNHL. With fluctuation, hearing loss begins to affect higher frequencies. Vertigo attacks persist and tend to decrease in remission periods for up to several months [1].

There is no active vertigo in the last stage of the disease, but there is a feeling of imbalance in the patients. The hearing loss has become permanent, and the tinnitus has increased [1].

Hearing tests (audiometry, tympanometry, acoustic reflexes, otoacoustic emissions, electrocochleography) and vestibular function tests (caloric tests, vestibular evoked myogenic potentials, video head impulse test) are useful in diagnosis. MRI is useful in both diagnosis and differential diagnosis by showing endolymphatic hydrops with intravenous gadolinium [1].

The earliest diagnostic criterion was recommended by the American Academy Otolaryngology–Head and Neck Surgery (AAO-HNS) in 1995 in which the diagnosis of MD was classified into four categories: certain MD, definite MD, probable MD, and possible MD [7].

The diagnostic criteria were improved in a coordinated work with the AAO-HNS, European Academy of Otology and Neurotology, Japan Society for Equilibrium Research, Korean Balance Society, and Bárány Society in 2015, considering two categories [8] as follows.

35.2.1 Definite MD

(a) Two or more spontaneous episodes of vertigo, lasting 20 min to 12 h
(b) Audiometrically documented low- to medium-frequency SNHL in one ear, defining the affected ear on at least one occasion before, during, or after one of the episodes of vertigo
(c) Fluctuating aural symptoms (hearing, tinnitus, or fullness) in the affected ear
(d) Not better accounted for by another vestibular diagnosis

35.2.2 Probable MD

(a) Two or more episodes of vertigo or dizziness, lasting 20 min to 24 h
(b) Fluctuating aural symptoms (hearing, tinnitus, or fullness) in the affected ear
(c) Not better accounted for by another vestibular diagnosis

35.3 Treatment

35.3.1 Acute Attack (Early 48 h)

Benzodiazepines, H1 antihistamine receptors, antidopaminergic agents, and anticholinergics are administered generally. These drug deliveries should not last longer than 48–72 h due to slowing down vestibular compensation and side effects of the drugs.

Table 35.1 First-line and second-line therapy for MD

	DIETARY MODIFICATION	DRUGS ADMINISTRATION
FIRST-LINE TREATMENT	Low salt diet Abundan water intake Alcohol and caffeine restriction Gluten-free diet Specially processed cereals	Diuretics Steroids Betahistine Dimenhydrinate Benzodiazepines
	CONSERVATIVE PROCEDURES	ABLATIVE PROCEDURES
SECOND-LINE TREATMENT	intratympanic steroids Endolymphatic sac surgery Pressure pulse treatment	intratympanic gentamicin Vestibular neurectomy Labyrinthectomy

Source: De Luca P, Cassandro C, Ralli M, et al. [9] Dietary Restriction for The Treatment of Meniere's Disease. *Transl Med UniSa*. 2020;22:5–9. Published 2020 May 31

35.3.2 Prevention of Attacks

Diet restriction, steroids, diuretics, betahistine, intratympanic treatments (corticosteroid, gentamicin), surgery (endolymphatic sac decompression, vestibular neurectomy, semicircular canal occlusion, labyrinthectomy), vestibular rehabilitation, audiological rehabilitation, and Meniett device (Table 35.1).

35.4 Pregnancy

The pregnant woman has a unique position in medicine. Pregnancy-related metabolic, endocrinological, and physiological changes affect every organ system to some extent [10]. Otological symptoms are usually seen in pregnant women due to changes in hormonal levels, including estrogen and progesterone [11].

HCG is secreted in the course of pregnancy. Estrogen and progesterone are at their minimal blood levels along the first 8 weeks of pregnancy. Their levels increase greatly between the 12th and 24th weeks. These high estrogen and progesterone levels persist from 24th week to parturition [12].

The production rates of these hormones in nonpregnant women, whose production rates are estrogen 0.02–0.1 mg/24 h and progesterone 0.1–40 mg/24 h, are up to 50–100 mg/24 h estrogen and 250–600 mg/24 h in early pregnant women increases. While these hormonal changes create optimal conditions for pregnancy, they cause an increase of 6.5 L in extracellular fluids and 1.25 L in intracellular fluids [13]. As a result of these osmotic changes in the body, water and salt retention occurs. This change in sex hormones affects the sensory nervous system and hearing system by causing fluid retention in the labyrinth [11, 13].

Estrogen has strong effects on fluid regulation owing to its effects on arginine vasopressin (AVP), the renin–angiotensin–aldosterone system, and the atrial natriuretic peptide. It can alter the severity of endolymphatic hydrops by affecting the aquaporin receptors, which are the targets of AVP in the inner ear [14].

Although the increase of endolymphatic fluid during pregnancy is not at a pathological level, an analogous situation that consists in MD can also be aforesaid in preggers [15].

During pregnancy, a sensorineural type of hearing loss that involves low frequencies mimicking cochlear pathology may occur. This hearing loss is at frequencies of 125, 250, and 500 Hz, and the loss occurs in the first trimester and progresses in the second and third trimesters. Generally, it returns to normal in the postpartum period [11]. This hearing loss mimicking MD is generally within physiological borders [10]. However, symptoms of preexisting Meniere's disease may worsen. Vertigo attacks may increase with the decrease in serum osmolality during pregnancy. This indicates inner ear involvement also during pregnancy [10, 11]. The fullness and ringing of the ears in pregnant women are caused by Eustachian tube dysfunction or changes in the inner ear fluid or auditory pathway [10].

The cause of reversible sensorineural hearing loss in preggers is the conclusion of increased mechanical compression on hair cells in the inner ear and changes in tissues. Mechanical pressure disappears after pregnancy and hearing thresholds return to their normal levels [15]. Pregnancy has no particular effect at high frequencies, resulting in hearing loss at low frequencies, and this decrement rises from the early 3 months to the last 3 months of pregnancy. Weight gain throughout pregnancy does not appear to be directly connected to hearing loss at low frequencies. Edema could be a major component in lowering hearing levels at low frequencies [15].

In a study by Schmidt et al., conducted on pregnant patients in the normal population without a diagnosis of Meniere, it was observed that the most common auditory complaint in preggers was tinnitus. It has been noticed that dizziness occurs in more than half of preggers and is more common in the early 6 months. Nausea was the primary symptom connected with dizziness in preggers, which was more common in the first trimester of pregnancy, and was connected with gravidity perpetuation. The evidence of this research indicates that a potential vestibular change due to hormonal change causes vertigo in the early 3 months, and this complaint decreases in the following months due to labyrinthine habituation. The increase in imbalance complaints seen in the next trimester and the gradient down in the last trimester could be explained by the increase in body weight and the increasing postural change that occurs with the progress of pregnancy [16]. This study shows that, independent of Meniere, vestibular symptoms increase in the first trimester in pregnant patients.

Vertigo attacks increased statistically in the early pregnancy period in a case with Meniere's disease known to be described by Uchide et al. Serum osmolality decreased to 268 mosm/kg (N: 278–295 mosm/kg). Normally, this change starts at the fifth week of pregnancy and decreases to 10 mosm/kg below normal values until the tenth week. In this case, they reported that there was a decrease in osmolality in the early pregnancy period, and after the fourth week of gestation, the patient's serum osmolality increased to normal levels and at this point the patient's vertigo attacks decreased. According to their hypotheses, due to the sudden decrease in serum osmolality during pregnancy, there is a change in the internal and external osmotic gradient of the endolymphatic sac, so fluid passes into the sac and hydrops occurs, which worsens the symptoms of Meniere. However, there was no change in osmolality in the postpartum period, and they attributed the deterioration in this period to the stress experienced by the patient (mother). In this case, 90 mL/day isosorbide and low-dose diazepam (total dose 25 mg) were administered in the first trimester, and no side effects were observed [17]. However, the hearing values of the case during pregnancy were not reported.

In the early gestational period (5–8 weeks), body tonicity decreases with the change of osmotic thresholds as a result of AVP release and thirst. Posmol and thresholds both remain at these new lows for the remainder of the pregnancy, but there is an increase in Posmol late in the pregnancy. The HCG secreted during pregnancy may play an important role in decreasing osmolality by increasing AVP secretion. In a study in which HCG injections were applied to rats with intact ovaries, it was shown that osmolality decreased [18].

There is substantial evidence that the homeostasis of the fluids in the inner ear is partially regulated by the vasopressin-aquaporin-2 (VP-AQP2) system [19, 20]. During sodium chloride loading, acute vertigo attacks occur in the sodium diuresis phase; the cause of the attack is said to be closely related to hormones such as vasopressin (VP) and aldosterone, which are in the water and salt balance [19]. This finding suggests that excessive AVP levels may be pathophysiological, and a new physiological function of AVP in the inner ear may be to retain water in the endolymphatic area [19, 21]. It is thought that AVP exerts its effects through stria vascularis in the cochlea. Studies conducted with electron microscopy have shown that AVP administered acutely causes vacuole formation in strial cells and enlargement of the intrastrial space. Progressive damage to the SV tissue can increase fluid flow from perilymph to endolymph, and ultimately EH may occur following AVP administration [20]. Significantly higher vasopressin type 2 receptor (V2R) levels were observed in the endolymphatic sac of Meniere's patients. Maekawa et al. reported that mRNA and AQP2 protein expression was significantly higher in Meniere's patients [22]. In studies on psychosomatic conditions in MD, it has been shown that stress increases plasma VP levels in patients with MD [19]. Increased plasma VP levels exacerbate endolymphatic hydrops in Meniere's disease, causing vertigo and hearing loss attacks [19, 21].

Increasing HCG and estrogen levels during pregnancy, especially in the first trimester, may lead to endolymphatic hydrops by increasing AVP release. This may aggravate the symptoms of existing Meniere's disease.

Stevens et al. reported that a pregnant woman with Meniere's disease and vestibular migraine at the same time explained the temporary improvement they detected in hearing values during the two pregnancies that they experienced as estrogen may be autoprotective in the inner ear. Previous studies also have shown that estrogen is autoprotective in noise-induced auditory trauma and presbycusis. The presence of estrogen receptors in spiral ganglion cells as well as inner and outer hair cells explains this situation. In the reported case, hearing values were reverted in the last period of pregnancy as estrogen levels decreased [14].

In addition, estrogen can adversely affect the immune system by inhibiting the hematopoiesis of B cells through complex means. Several proofs suggest that MD responds to treatment with immunosuppressive steroids, putting forward the immunomodulation caused by pregnancy may have an effect on hearing improvement in the reported case [14].

In a study by Kilicdag et al., examining the effects of estrogen replacement therapy on hearing in postmenopausal women, better hearing results were obtained at lower frequencies in the group receiving estrogen therapy alone compared to those receiving estrogen and progesterone treatment. The hearing results of the estrogen and progesterone group were better than the control group. Estrogen receptors have been shown in the inner ears of mice. They have been identified in the spiral ganglion and stria vascularis, which are particularly important in hearing conduction and inner ear homeostasis [23].

In patients with migraine, decreases in estrogen levels during the late luteal phase are associated with worsening symptoms, while high estrogen levels disposed to decrease the frequency and violence of migraines in the course of pregnancy. They reported that Meniere's symptoms worsen in the late luteal phase, as in their own patients, and those hearing values return to their normal state in the last period of pregnancy as estrogen levels decrease [17].

The fluctuation of symptoms during the menstrual cycle in some patients with Meniere's disease could mean that changes in hormones associated with reproduction or stress may be involved in the pathophysiology of this disease. The typical effect of menopause on the onset or worsening of Meniere's disease when there is a sharp decline in reproductive hormones has not been reported in the literature, but the fact that the peak incidence of the disease covers the menopausal age range indicates a possible link [24].

In a study by Andrews et al., they showed that symptoms exacerbated in the late luteal phase (premenstrual period) of the menstrual cycle in a group of female patients with Meniere and objectively proved this with audiometric and vestibular test results [25]. There is evidence to suggest that edema formation in some women in the late luteal phase of the menstrual cycle may have a direct effect on the pattern of endolymphatic hydrops or MD [26].

Aldosterone secretion increases during premenstrual period like estrogen levels. Increasing aldosterone and estrogen raises fluid level in the inner ear and elicits vestibular symptoms [12].

Increased blood viscosity (thickening) before menstruation can damage blood flow to the inner ear and changes the fluid stability; this may be the reason for having auditory and/or vestibular symptoms [12].

Increasing quantity of cerebrospinal fluid during the premenstrual cycle may increase the pressure in the head. This pressure is transmitted to the inner ear by the cochlear aqueduct, which is an inherent tube binding the inner ear to the subarachnoid area in the brain; this may be the reason for having pressure, balance, and/or hearing symptoms [12].

Progesterone can induce dizziness, faintness, drowsiness, and depression. The depressant nature of progesterone can cause decompensation, leading to vestibular symptoms [12]. During pregnancy, progesterone causes hyperventilation by stimulating the central respiratory center. Hyperventilation causes respiratory alkalosis and provokes vomiting and vertigo in vestibular diseases [27].

Another hypothesis could explicate the aggravation of vestibular symptoms due to hormonal changes [12]:

- The alike factors induce motion sickness during pregnancy of healthy preggers and also could exacerbate vestibular symptoms in women having vestibular impairment.
- Increased triglycerides caused by increased estrogen levels can lead to balance and hearing signs.
- Except for the fluctuation in fluid balance, estrogen's and/or progesterone's chemical attributes can cause symptoms.
- Increased estrogen can induce an autoimmune response, which could be the reason for having vestibular and hearing symptoms.
- The increase in estrogen causes an increase in appetite and food. Women who are allergic may eat or drink substances that alter the fluid balance in the inner ear and cause auditory and/or vestibular symptoms.
- High estrogen levels can lead to edema around the Eustachian tube, which impedes middle ear function. This, still unspecified, can affect inner ear function and cause vestibular and/or auditory symptoms [12].

35.5 Postpartum Period

In the last period of pregnancy, prolactin and oxytocin hormones start to increase in the mother, and this increase continues after birth.

The main function of prolactin is lactogenesis, but more than 300 different functions, including osmoregulation, have been reported. Prolactin release in animals and humans is linked to psychological stress. Patients with hyperprolactinemia often have emotional problems such as anxiety and depression. Obsession and anxiety scores were found to be high in these individuals according to personality tests performed on Meniere's patients [28]. Based on this, we can say that the stress and anxiety experienced by the mother during the lactation period can provoke the current Meniere's disease. On the other hand, based on the available data, it is not possible to determine whether the elevated prolactin controls inner ear pathology or, conversely, plays a protective role. However, prolactin binding sites have been identified in the cochlear duct of late gestational fetal rats [28].

Prolactin causes breast swelling and general edema in the body during pregnancy and premenstrual period, perhaps also causing the increased inner ear symptoms that women may experience during these times [12]. In addition, the appearance of vertigo in patients with hyperprolactinemia indicates that there may be a connection between prolactin and the inner ear [28].

Oxytocin secreted toward the termination of pregnancy also releases prostaglandins that can lead to hearing and/or balance symptoms. If a woman only has complaints about balance or hearing while breastfeeding, then perhaps the cause is oxytocin [12].

35.6 Treatment

The use of small doses of dimenhydrinate (Dramamine) and meclizine hydrochloride (Antivert) in the acute period in the treatment of Meniere attacks during pregnancy has been reported to be safe (category B) [11, 17, 29, 30]. Benzodiazepines are very successful agents in the treatment of acute attacks in Meniere's patients, but their use in pregnant women is not recommended (category D) [30]. Isosorbide is effective in correcting endolymphatic hydrops and can be used safely in pregnant women [17]. Metoclopramide can be used safely in pregnant women having persistent nausea and vomiting (category B) [11]. Histamines and diuretics should be avoided, especially in the first trimester, as they cause hypovolemia and hypotension and lower cardiac output [11, 29].

Systemic corticosteroids are not recommended for use in pregnant women (category C) [30]. It is known that they have teratogenic effects on fetal organs especially in the first trimester. However, according to the prescribing guideline of Ambro et al., It has been reported that the use of corticosteroids in the third trimester is safe [31]. However, intratympanic corticosteroid administration should be preferred instead of systemic steroids during pregnancy. Thus, we can achieve a topical high-dose effect and avoid the harmful side effects of corticosteroids. Traditionally, dexamethasone and methylprednisolone have been used in intratympanic injection, but methylprednisolone (US FDA category B) may be more suitable for pregnant patients than dexamethasone (US FDA category C) [32].

Despite its controversial therapeutic use in Meniere's disease, betahistine is indicated for the prophylaxis of vertigo attacks and is not recommended for the treatment of any chronic/persistent symptoms that may be associated with MD and/or EH [29]. Studies with betahistine in pregnant rabbits have failed to show any teratogenic effects, and evidence in humans is currently very limited. Betahistine has been assigned to category B in the FDA risk categories, which has been declared to be replaced by the new pregnancy and breastfeeding labeling rule [33].

References

1. Perez-Carpena P, Lopez-Escamez JA. Current understanding and clinical management of Meniere's disease: a systematic review. Semin Neurol. 2020;40(1):138–50. https://doi.org/10.1055/s-0039-3402065.
2. Basura GJ, Adams ME, Monfared A, et al. Clinical practice guideline: Ménière's disease executive summary. Otolaryngol Head Neck Surg. 2020;162(4):415–34. https://doi.org/10.1177/0194599820909439.
3. Requena T, Espinosa-Sanchez JM, Cabrera S, Trinidad G, Soto-Varela A, Santos-Perez S, Teggi R, Perez P, Batuecas-Caletrio A, Fraile J, Aran I, Martin E, Benitez J, Pérez-Fernández N, Lopez-Escamez JA. Familial clustering and genetic heterogeneity in Meniere's disease. Clin Genet. 2014;85(3):245–52. https://doi.org/10.1111/cge.12150.
4. Ralli M, Di Stadio A, De Virgilio A, Croce A, de Vincentiis M. Autoimmunity and Otolaryngology Diseases. J Immunol Res. 2018;2018:2747904. Published 2018 Oct 4. https://doi.org/10.1155/2018/2747904.
5. Frejo L, Soto-Varela A, Santos-Perez S, Aran I, Batuecas-Caletrio A, Perez-Guillen V, Perez-Garrigues H, Fraile J, Martin-Sanz E, Tapia MC, Trinidad G, García-Arumi AM, González-Aguado R, Espinosa-Sanchez JM, Marques P, Perez P, Benitez J, Lopez-Escamez JA. Clinical subgroups in bilateral Meniere disease. Front Neurol. 2016;24(7):182. https://doi.org/10.3389/fneur.2016.00182.
6. Frejo L, Martin-Sanz E, Teggi R, Trinidad G, Soto-Varela A, Santos-Perez S, Manrique R, Perez N, Aran I, Almeida-Branco MS, Batuecas-Caletrio A, Fraile J, Espinosa-Sanchez JM, Perez-Guillen V, Perez-Garrigues H, Oliva-Dominguez M, Aleman O, Benitez J, Perez P, Lopez-Escamez JA. Meniere's disease Consortium (MeDiC). Extended phenotype and clinical subgroups in unilateral Meniere disease: a cross-sectional study with cluster analysis. Clin Otolaryngol. 2017;42(6):1172–80. https://doi.org/10.1111/coa.12844. Epub 2017 Feb 26.
7. Liu Y, Yang J, Duan M. Current status on researches of Meniere's disease: a review. Acta Otolaryngol. 2020:1–5. [Published online ahead of print, 2020 Jun 21]. https://doi.org/10.1080/00016489.2020.1776385.
8. Lopez-Escamez JA, Carey J, Chung WH, Goebel JA, Magnusson M, Mandalà M, Newman-Toker DE, Strupp M, Suzuki M, Trabalzini F, Bisdorff AM. Diagnostic criteria for Menière's disease according to the Classification Committee of the Bárány Society. HNO. 2017;65(11):887–93. German. https://doi.org/10.1007/s00106-017-0387-z.
9. De Luca P, Cassandro C, Ralli M, et al. Dietary restriction for the treatment of Meniere's disease. Transl Med UniSa. 2020;22:5–9. Published 2020 May 31.
10. Bhagat DR, Chowdhary A, Verma S, Jyotsana. Physiological changes in ENT during pregnancy. Indian J Otolaryngol Head Neck Surg. 2006;58(3):268–70. https://doi.org/10.1007/BF03050836.
11. Kumar Swain S, Kumar Pati B, Mohanty JN. Otological manifestations in pregnant women—a study at a tertiary care hospital of eastern India. J Otol. 2019; https://doi.org/10.1016/j.joto.2019.11.003.
12. Haybach PJ, RN, MS. Hormones and vestibular disorders. 1999, 2006 Vestibular Disorders Association. www.VESTIBULAR.ORG.
13. Sharma K, Sharma S, Chander D. Evaluation of audio-rhinological changes during pregnancy. Indian J Otolaryngol Head Neck Surg. 2011;63(1):74–8. https://doi.org/10.1007/s12070-010-0103-8.
14. Stevens Madelyn N, Hullar TE. Improvement in sensorineural hearing loss during pregnancy. Ann Otol Rhinol Laryngol. 2014;123(9):614–8. https://doi.org/10.1177/0003489414525590.
15. Dag EK, Gulumser C, Erbek S. Decrease in middle ear resonance frequency during pregnancy. Audiol Res. 2016;6(1):147. Published 2016 Apr 20. https://doi.org/10.4081/audiores.2016.147.
16. Schmidt PM, Flores Fda T, Rossi AG, Silveira AF. Hearing and vestibular complaints during pregnancy. Braz J Otorhinolaryngol. 2010;76(1):29–33.

17. Uchide K, Suzuki N, Takiguchi T, Terada S, Inoue M. The possible effect of pregnancy on Ménière's disease. ORL J Otorhinolaryngol Relat Spec. 1997;59(5):292–5. https://doi.org/10.1159/000276956.
18. Davison JM, Shiells EA, Philips PR, Lindheimer MD. Serial evaluation of vasopressin release and thirst in human pregnancy. Role of human chorionic gonadotrophin in the osmoregulatory changes of gestation. J Clin Invest. 1988;81(3):798–806. https://doi.org/10.1172/JCI113386.
19. Takeda T, Takeda S, Kakigi A, et al. Hormonal aspects of Ménière's disease on the basis of clinical and experimental studies. ORL J Otorhinolaryngol Relat Spec. 2010;71(Suppl 1):1–9. https://doi.org/10.1159/000265113.
20. Jiang L, He J, Chen X, Chen H. Effect of electroacupuncture on arginine vasopressin-induced endolymphatic hydrops. J Tradit Chin Med. 2019;39(2):221–8.
21. Kumagami H, Loewenheim H, Beitz E, et al. The effect of anti-diuretic hormone on the endolymphatic sac of the inner ear. Pflugers Arch. 1998;436(6):970–5. https://doi.org/10.1007/s004240050731.
22. Maekawa C, Kitahara T, Kizawa K, Okazaki S, Kamakura T, Horii A, Imai T, Doi K, Inohara H, Kiyama H. Expression and translocation of aquaporin-2 in the endolymphatic sac in patients with Meniere's disease. J Neuroendocrinol. 2010;22(11):1157–64. https://doi.org/10.1111/j.1365-2826.2010.02060.x.
23. Kilicdag EB, Yavuz H, Bagis T, Tarim E, Erkan AN, Kazanci F. Effects of estrogen therapy on hearing in postmenopausal women. Am J Obstet Gynecol. 2004;190(1):77–82. https://doi.org/10.1016/j.ajog.2003.06.001.
24. Al-Mana D. Ovarian steroid hormones and auditory function. The Ear Institute University College London A thesis presented to UCL for the degree of Doctor of Philosophy 2013 Feb. www.researchgate.net.
25. Andrews JC, Honrubia V. Premenstrual exacerbation of Meniere's disease revisited. Otolaryngol Clin N Am. 2010 Oct;43(5):1029–40. https://doi.org/10.1016/j.otc.2010.05.012.
26. Kenny R, Patil N, Considine N. Sudden (reversible) sensorineural hearing loss in pregnancy. Ir J Med Sci. 2011;180(1):79–84. https://doi.org/10.1007/s11845-010-0525-z.
27. Black FO. Maternal susceptibility to nausea and vomiting of pregnancy: is the vestibular system involved? Am J Obstet Gynecol. 2002;186(5 Suppl Understanding):S204–9. https://doi.org/10.1067/mob.2002.122602.
28. Falkenius-Schmidt K, Rydmarker S, Horner CK. Hyperprolactinemia in some Ménière patients even in the absence of incapacitating vertigo. Hearing Res. 2005;203(1–2):154–8. https://doi.org/10.1016/j.heares.2004.11.015.
29. Bächinger D, Eckhard AH, Röösli C, Veraguth D, Huber A, Dalbert A. Endolymphatic hydrops mimicking obstructive Eustachian tube dysfunction: preliminary experience and literature review. Eur Arch Otorhinolaryngol. 2020. [Published online ahead of print, 2020 Jun 24]; https://doi.org/10.1007/s00405-020-06139-9.
30. Vlastarakos PV, Nikolopoulos TP, Manolopoulos L, Ferekidis E, Kreatsas G. Treating common ear problems in pregnancy: what is safe? Eur Arch Otorhinolaryngol. 2008;265(2):139–45. https://doi.org/10.1007/s00405-007-0534-3.
31. Ambro BT, Scheid SC, Pribitkin EA. Prescribing guidelines for ENT medications during pregnancy. Ear Nose Throat J. 2003;82(8):565–8.
32. Xie S, Wu X. Clinical management and progress in sudden sensorineural hearing loss during pregnancy. J Int Med Res. 2019:300060519870718. [published online ahead of print, 2019 Aug 27]. https://doi.org/10.1177/0300060519870718.
33. Buharalioglu CK, Acar S, Erol-Coskun H, et al. Pregnancy outcomes after maternal betahistine exposure: a case series. Reprod Toxicol. 2018;79:79–83. https://doi.org/10.1016/j.reprotox.2018.06.004.

Management of Chronic Otitis Media and Its Complications During Pregnancy and the Postpartum Period

36

Nurcan Yurtsever Kum and Slobodan Spremo

36.1 Introduction

Pregnancy is a miraculous process that causes significant alterations in female physiology. It is desirable for the mother and baby to complete this process healthfully. The organism's oxygen consumption, cardiac output, and blood volume increase during pregnancy, and mucosal edema develops in parallel with an increase in total body fluid. Mucosal edema in the upper respiratory tract may lead to middle ear hypoventilation and otitis media [1]. In addition, serum estrogen, progesterone, and cortisol levels increase during pregnancy. Alterations in the levels of these hormones may result in suppression of the immune system, paving the way for bacterial and viral infections [1]. Otorhinolaryngological disorders are frequent conditions; therefore, they are also frequently encountered during pregnancy and breastfeeding periods. Various metabolic, endocrinological, and physiological alterations occurring during pregnancy may manifest as the conditions affecting the ear.

During pregnancy and breastfeeding, the treatment approach should not harm the mother or the fetus/baby. It is best for the mother not to take any medications, particularly in the first 3 months of gestation. However, approximately 85% of women are prescribed at least once during their pregnancies [2, 3]. Teratogenicity, defined as structural or functional dysgenesis of fetal organs, is an important consideration when prescribing to pregnant women. The otorhinolaryngologist must have information on capability of the medications to be secreted in the breast milk, as well as

N. Y. Kum (✉)
Department of Otorhinolaryngology, Ankara City Hospital, Ankara, Turkey
e-mail: nurcanyurtsever@hotmail.com

S. Spremo
University Clinic Center Banja Luka, Department for Otorhinolaryngology,
Faculty of Medicine, University of Banja Luka, Banja Luka, Bosnia and Herzegovina
e-mail: spremosl@gmail.com

© The Author(s), under exclusive license to Springer Nature
Switzerland AG 2022
C. Cingi et al. (eds.), *ENT Diseases: Diagnosis and Treatment during Pregnancy
and Lactation*, https://doi.org/10.1007/978-3-031-05303-0_36

their teratogenic potential. It is necessary to avoid teratogenic drugs, particularly in the first trimester, during organogenesis. Otherwise, grave adverse effects leading to spontaneous abortion or congenital anomalies may be encountered.

36.2 Chronic Otitis Media

Otitis media is the infectious inflammation of the middle ear. It may progress into chronic otitis media associated with tympanic membrane (TM) perforation and purulent discharge, despite appropriate treatment. Chronic otitis media is more prevalent in people with poor socioeconomic status in the developing countries. *Pseudomonas aeruginosa*, *Staphylococcus aureus*, *Klebsiella* sp., *Proteus* sp., *Haemophilus influenzae*, *Moraxella catarrhalis*, and *Streptococcus pneumonia* are the most frequent causative agents [4–6]. Chronic otitis media may be a stable and nonprogressive condition affecting TM, middle ear, and mastoid cavity, or it may manifest as an active and progressive disease accompanied by cholesteatoma, with or without ear discharge. With invention and widespread use of antibiotics, chronic otitis media and its complications are not encountered as frequent as pre-antibiotic era; however, management of chronic otitis media should be well known due to its potentially severe complications [7]. Intracranial complications such as brain abscess and meningitis are the most common causes of death in patients with chronic otitis media [8]. In this chapter, the management of chronic otitis media during pregnancy and breastfeeding period will be reviewed, without detailing the definition and classification of the disease.

During pregnancy, patients may consult a physician with various signs and symptoms of chronic otitis media, including TM perforation, hearing loss, ear discharge, ear pain, retraction pockets, polyps in the external auditory canal, inflamed middle ear mucosa, and keratin debris and cholesteatoma. Uju et al. investigated the prevalence of otorhinolaryngological disorders in 150 pregnant women and detected chronic otitis media in 4% of them [9]. If TM is perforated but there is no infection or discharge in the middle ear, medical or surgical management is not necessary, and surgery may be postponed after the delivery or the end of breastfeeding. The middle and inner ears may remain stable for years as long as the ear remains dry. Suggesting protection of the ear while bathing and routine external auditory canal care would be sufficient. However, if there is otorrhea or other symptoms such as pain or fever, treatment may be necessary by taking the gestation trimester into account. Surgery may be required if medical treatment fails or in case of complications. The complications of chronic otitis media mostly arise due to the spread of the current pathological process (infection and/or cholesteatoma) beyond the limits of the middle ear and the mastoid into the adjacent organs and tissues. Chronic otitis media complications are classified into extracranial and intracranial ones, and the extracranial complications are classified into intratemporal and extratemporal complications [9]. Intratemporal complications include mastoiditis, mastoid abscess, facial palsy, labyrinthitis, and petrositis, whereas extratemporal complications are postauricular abscess, zygomatic abscess, Bezold's abscess, Luc's abscess, and

Citelli's abscess. Intracranial complications include extradural abscess, subdural abscess, brain abscess, sigmoid and lateral sinus thrombophlebitis, meningitis, and otitic hydrocephalus [7, 10]. Albeit rarely, the aforementioned complications may appear during pregnancy and may have a dramatic course.

36.3   Medication Classification

The US Food and Drug Administration (FDA) has made a classification on the use of medications in pregnancy in the light of the evidence provided by the research and classified medications into five categories (Table 36.1) [10, 11].

The patient's history, complaints, and otoscopic examination are usually sufficient in the diagnosis of chronic otitis media during pregnancy. However, if complications are suspected, and there is a need for a high-resolution temporal bone computed tomography (Temporal HRCT), concerns arise about the teratogenic and carcinogenic effects of ionizing radiation on the developing fetus. In a standard CT scan, the fetus is exposed to about 25 mGy or less radiation. This dose has no risk of teratogenic effects on the fetus; however, it leads to a small increase in the risk of cancer for the fetus. Iodinated contrast agents may be administered through intravenous or oral routes during pregnancy. Intravenous iodinated contrast is an FDA category B agent for pregnant women [12, 13]. CT imaging is performed only in the presence of life-threatening complications and if the pregnant woman accepts the risks. Magnetic resonance imaging (MRI), another radiological imaging modality, is safe in all trimesters of pregnancy at 1.5 T or lower magnetic field strengths, and

Table 36.1 US Food and Drug Administration (FDA) classification for medication risk during pregnancy and management strategies [10, 11]

Category	Definition
A	Adequate and well-controlled studies on pregnant women have failed to demonstrate a risk to the fetus in the first trimester of pregnancy.
B	Animal reproduction studies have failed to demonstrate a risk to the fetus, but there are no adequate and well-controlled studies on pregnant women. *Or* animal studies demonstrate a risk, and adequate and well-controlled studies on pregnant women have not been done during the first trimester.
C	Animal reproduction studies have shown an adverse effect on the fetus, but there are no adequate and well-controlled studies on humans. The benefits of the use of the drug in pregnant women might be acceptable despite its potential risks. *Or* animal studies have not been conducted and there are no adequate and well-controlled studies on humans.
D	There is positive evidence of human fetal risk based on adverse reaction data from investigational or marketing experience or studies of humans, but the potential benefits of the use of the drug in pregnant women might be acceptable despite its potential risks.
X	Studies in animals or humans have demonstrated fetal abnormalities or there is positive evidence of fetal risk based on adverse reaction reports from investigational or marketing experience, or both. The risk involved in the use of the drug in pregnant women clearly outweighs any possible benefits.

may be used for differential diagnosis in case of complications or life-threatening situations. The safety of 3.0 T and above magnetic fields has not been proven in pregnant women. Pregnant patients should have MRI using 1.5 T or lower magnetic field strengths [12, 13]. When these imaging methods are necessary, the obstetrician of the patient should be informed, and the physician should behave according to the trimester of pregnancy and the presentation of the mother.

Proper and regular cleaning of the ear canal and use of topical antimicrobials are the current primary treatment methods for chronic otitis media in pregnancy. However, topical agents may pass into the systemic circulation and cause adverse effects in pregnant women and fetus as a result of local absorption as well as ingestion since they pass through TM perforation and the Eustachian tube into the nasopharynx and are ingested. Therefore, the benefit–harm balance should be considered when administering topical agents to a pregnant woman.

Ofloxacin ear drop is a category C agent. Although it has been supposed that a very small amount passes into the systemic circulation after its topical use, its exact effect is not known during breastfeeding (Table 36.2). In animals, its use during pregnancy has been shown to cause cartilage disorders in the fetus [14]. Teratogenicity has not been observed in humans after its topical application, although controlled clinical trials are lacking. Ofloxacin otic solution 0.3% should be used during pregnancy and breastfeeding only if the potential benefit outweighs the potential risk to the fetus. It is administered as 5–10 drops b.i.d. to the affected ear. The obstetrician should be consulted whenever necessary.

Ciprofloxacin is a category C agent during pregnancy. There are no controlled studies on pregnant women (Table 36.2). No harmful effects are expected after its use during pregnancy since systemic exposure is negligible when used as a topical ear drop [15]. Systemic administration of ciprofloxacin to breastfeeding women leads to secretion of the agent in the breast milk. However, maternal use of ciprofloxacin ear drops carries negligible risk for breastfed babies, although its effects on the breastfed babies are not known. It should be administered by considering the benefit–harm balance for the mother and fetus, and after consulting with the obstetrician.

Table 36.2 Ototopical agents that can be administered in pregnancy and lactation [16]

Antibiotics	Pregnancy	Lactation
Ofloxacin	Category C	Unknown
Ciprofloxacin + dexamethasone	Category C	Probably safe
Antifungals		
Clotrimazole (1% Cream, solution)	Category B	Probably safe
Miconazole (2% cream)	Category C	Probably safe
Ketoconazole (2% cream)	Category C	Safety unknown

Beta-lactam antibiotics are the safest choices during pregnancy (category B) and may be administered in all three trimesters when there is a need for systemic antibiotics [17, 18].

Uncomplicated, chronic otitis media-related mastoiditis during pregnancy and breastfeeding may be treated with oral or parenteral antibiotics, depending on the patient's presentation. It is usually controlled with medical treatment. Surgery is not considered unless it is complicated. If necessary, mastoidectomy may be considered after delivery. Beta-lactam antibiotics can be used empirically. Extracranial–extra-temporal abscesses may be drained under local anesthesia, and systemic antibiotics should be prescribed. The decision whether to suspend breastfeeding is made in consultation with the obstetrician, depending on the medical agent to be administered. The benefit–harm balance should always be considered in preference of the therapeutic agents.

Facial paralysis due to chronic otitis media is rare, and it is usually seen in cases with cholesteatoma. Surgery is recommended as early as possible in nonpregnant patients. However, if facial paralysis due to chronic otitis media is encountered during pregnancy, the decision should be made by considering the benefits to the mother and fetus. After obtaining the opinion of the obstetrician and the consent of the mother, and if the gestational age of the fetus is suitable, surgical treatment may be considered following Cesarean section.

Although rare, bacterial meningitis during pregnancy carries significant mortality risk for both mother and child. Meningitis is the most frequent intracranial complication of chronic otitis media [19]. Otitis media is the most frequent source of meningitis in gestational period [20]. The most common causative agents are Gram-positive cocci (*S. pneumoniae*) followed by *Listeria monocytogenes*, *Neisseria meningitidis*, *Haemophilus influenzae*, and Group A streptococci [21–24]. Meningitis should be suspected when symptoms such as fever, headache, neck stiffness, and confusion are observed in addition to findings of otitis. In diagnosis, brain CT and lumbar puncture to enable a CSF analysis are performed in addition to the physical examination and blood tests. Antibiotics are chosen depending on the causative agent; however, empirical treatment with parenteral third-generation cephalosporins (ceftriaxone) may be preferred. If meningitis is complicated with brain herniation, multiorgan failure, or septic shock, it threatens the life of the mother, and therefore, the fetus. In this case, considering the gestational week, it may be decided to terminate pregnancy by taking the opinion of the obstetrician. Dexamethasone may be used for treating brain edema [25]. Physicians may hesitate to administer dexamethasone to pregnant women as cleft lip/palate is associated with its administration in the first trimester [26]. Few side effects have been reported in late pregnancy, and corticosteroids are frequently administered to improve fetal lung maturation in case of premature birth. Dexamethasone seems suitable for use in pneumococcal meningitis of pregnant women due to its beneficial effects on survival and limited adverse effects [20]. Maternal mortality rate due to meningitis during pregnancy has been reported as 28%, whereas abortion, stillbirth, or neonatal mortality rates are 37%. In addition, it has been reported that maternal mortality is less when pneumococcal meningitis occurs in the first trimester [20].

One case with lateral sinus thrombophlebitis due to meningitis during pregnancy has been reported [27]. Presentation is similar to clinical signs of meningitis. In addition, pain over the mastoid area, intermittent high fever, anemia, and poor general medical condition are evident. MR venography is useful in the diagnosis. Evacuation of the fetus may be decided by taking the gestational trimester into account. Similar to treatment of meningitis, parenteral high-dose third-generation cephalosporins (ceftriaxone) are preferred. Low-molecular-weight heparin should also be added to the treatment [27].

Brain abscess due to otitis media may develop during pregnancy. The symptoms of brain abscess include headache, nausea, and localized neurological signs. MRI is a safe and highly sensitive diagnostic imaging modality during pregnancy, and diagnosis is made by taking clinical, laboratory, and imaging findings into account. Care should be taken since the clinical signs of brain abscess may be confused with preeclampsia [28]. The antibiotics administered to treat brain abscess should be able to effectively cross the blood–brain barrier, and an antibiogram should be obtained. Corticosteroids are also recommended to prevent a high intracranial pressure and development of brain edema [29]. However, their effects on the fetus are of great concern as treatment for a severe brain abscess with antibiotics and corticosteroids takes 6–8 weeks [30]. The benefit/harm consideration is necessary for the use of betamethasone and dexamethasone, particularly in the first trimester, due to their possible teratogenic effects. In addition, administration of antiepileptic agents is recommended early in the course of the disease since epilepsy is encountered in 70% of the patients with brain abscess. Treatment decisions should be made by consulting with an obstetrician, by taking gestational age and the condition of the mother into account during the entire treatment period. Current risks should be well explained to the patients and their relatives. Neurosurgeons, obstetricians, and otorhinolaryngologists should be in coordination while deciding treatment, and if there is a life-threatening brain abscess, it should be surgically drained.

It is easier to decide the management of postpartum chronic otitis media and its complications compared to the pregnancy period. Breastfeeding may be suspended until the end of the treatment in cases with life-threatening conditions in case the medications to be used are secreted in the breast milk. If the clinical condition is not life-threatening and the medications are not secreted or secreted in small amounts in the breast milk, a pediatrician may be consulted and the patient may be treated without any interruption of breastfeeding.

The benefit/harm balance of the mother and fetus should always be considered while treating chronic otitis media and its complications encountered during pregnancy and breastfeeding. A multidisciplinary approach is essential in the management of pregnant patients, and obstetricians, neurosurgeons, and pediatricians should be consulted whenever necessary.

References

1. Torsiglieri AJ Jr, Tom LW, Keane WM, Atkins JP Jr. Otolaryngologic manifestations of pregnancy. Otolaryngol Head Neck Surg. 1990;102:293–7.
2. Holt GR, Mabry RL. ENT medications in pregnancy. Otolaryngol Head Neck Surg. 1983;91:338–6.
3. Ambro BT, Scheid SC, Pribitkin EA. Prescribing guidelines for ENT medications during pregnancy. Ear Nose Throat J. 2003;82:565–8.
4. Kim SH, Kim MG, Kim SS, et al. Change in detection rate of methicillin-resistant Staphylococcus aureus and Pseudomonas aeruginosa and their antibiotic sensitivities in patients with chronic Suppurative otitis media. J Int Adv Otol. 2015;11:151–6.
5. Rath S, Das SR, Padhy RN. Surveillance of bacteria Pseudomonas aeruginosa and MRSA associated with chronic suppurative otitis media. Braz J Otorhinolaryngol. 2017;83:201–6.
6. Mittal R, Lisi CV, Gerring R, et al. Current concepts in the pathogenesis and treatment of chronic suppurative otitis media. J Med Microbiol. 2015;64:1103–16.
7. Dubey SP, Larawin V. Complications of chronic suppurative otitis media and their management. Laryngoscope. 2007;117:264–7.
8. Sun J, Sun J. Intracranial complications of chronic otitis media. Eur Arch Otorhinolaryngol. 2014;271:2923–6.
9. Uju IM, Semenitari AD. Ear nose and throat conditions seen in pregnant women attending antenatal Clinic in a Tertiary Hospital in Port Harcourt. J Global Biosci. 2020;9:7019–33.
10. Boothby LA, Doering PL. FDA labeling system for drugs in pregnancy. Ann Pharmacother. 2001;35:1485–9.
11. Law R, Bozzo P, Koren G, Einarson A. FDA pregnancy risk categories and the CPS: do they help or are they a hindrance? Can Fam Physician. 2010;56:239–6.
12. Chen MM, Coakley FV, Kaimal A, Laros RK. Guidelines for computed tomography and magnetic resonance imaging use during pregnancy and lactation. Obstet Gynecol. 2008;112:333–40.
13. Patel SJ, Reede DL, Katz DS, et al. Imaging the pregnant patient for nonobstetric conditions: algorithms and radiation dose considerations. Radiographics. 2007;27:1705–22.
14. Takayama S, Watanabe T, Akiyama Y, et al. Reproductive toxicity of ofloxacin. Arzneimittelforschung. 1986;36:1244–8.
15. Mosges R, Nematian-Samani M, Eichel A. Treatment of acute otitis externa with ciprofloxacin otic 0.2% antibiotic ear solution. Ther Clin Risk Manag. 2011;7:325–36.
16. Lee DJ, Roberts D. Topical therapies for external ear disorders. In Flint PW, Haughey BH, Robbins KT et al. (eds): Cummings otolaryngology-head and neck surgery. 6th ed. Philadelphia: Elsevier Health Sciences 2014; 2136–2137.
17. Leophonte P. Antibiotics during pregnancy and breast feeding: consequences for the treatment of respiratory infections. Rev Mal Respir. 1988;5:293–8.
18. Vlastarakos PV, Nikolopoulos TP, Manolopoulos L, et al. Treating common ear problems in pregnancy: what is safe? Eur Arch Otorhinolaryngol. 2008;265:139–45.
19. Osma U, Cureoglu S, Hosoglu S. The complications of chronic otitis media: report of 93 cases. J Laryngol Otol. 2000;114:97–100.
20. Adriani KS, Brouwer MC, van der Ende A, van de Beek D. Bacterial meningitis in pregnancy: report of six cases and review of the literature. Clin Microbiol Infect. 2012;18:345–51.
21. Polayes SH, Ohlbaum C, Winston HB. Meningococcus meningitis with massive hemorrhage of the adrenals' (Waterhouse-Friderichsen syndrome) complicating pregnancy with pre-eclamptic toxemia. Am J Obstet Gynecol. 1953;65:192–6.
22. Williams M. Meningitis and encephalitis in pregnancy. Nurs Mirror Midwives J. 1969;129:33–6.
23. Ferrazzini G, Peduzzi R, Balestra B. Group A beta-hemolytic streptococcal meningitis in a pregnant woman. Schweiz Med Wochenschr. 1996;126:1842–4.
24. Braun TI, Pinover W, Sih P. Group B streptococcal meningitis in a pregnant woman before the onset of labor. Clin Infect Dis. 1995;21:1042–3.

25. Brouwer MC, Tunkel AR, van de Beek D. Epidemiology, diagnosis, and antimicrobial treatment of acute bacterial meningitis. Clin Microbiol Rev. 2010;23:467–92.
26. Carmichael SL, Shaw GM, Ma C, et al. Maternal corticosteroid use and orofacial clefts. Am J Obstet Gynecol. 2007;197:585 e1–7; discussion 683–4, e1–7.
27. Konya P, Demirtürk N. Bacterial meningitis complicated by venous sinus thrombosis: a case of a pregnant woman. Infect Dis Clin Microbiol. 2020:168–70.
28. Jendoubi A, Aissa S, Dridi R, et al. Brain abscess during pregnancy mimicking eclampsia: a diagnostic and therapeutic challenge. Anaesth Crit Care Pain Med. 2016;35:365–7.
29. Lu CH, Chang WN, Lui CC. Strategies for the management of bacterial brain abscess. J Clin Neurosci. 2006;13:979–85.
30. Yoshida M, Matsuda H, Furuya K. Successful prognosis of brain abscess during pregnancy. J Reprod Infertil. 2013;14:152–5.

Otosclerosis During Pregnancy and The Postpartum Period

37

Sebla Çalışkan, Adin Selçuk, and Klara Van Gool

37.1 Introduction

Otosclerosis is a human-specific otic capsule disease. First, in 1741, Valsalva, the Italian anatomist and surgeon, caught the attention of the lesion of otosclerosis in a deaf person's temporal dissection [1]. He observed that the ankylose of footplate occurred due to annular ligament ossification. In 1860, Toynbee first described stapes footplate ankyloses in his cadaveric studies [2]. Politzer, in 1894, described the otosclerotic temporal bone in the final stage of disease [3]. Siebenmann also first defined and used the term "otospongiosis" to show the active stage of disease [4].

Hearing loss due to otosclerosis is variable. It may cause usually a conductive hearing loss or a mixed conductive-sensorineural hearing loss and sometimes pure sensorineural hearing loss. The disease is bilateral in 70% of cases, and the hearing loss begins during the third decade of life. It occurs two times more often in women than in men [5]. The disease has a distinctly racial distinction. In blacks, the

S. Çalışkan (✉)
Department of Otorhinolaryngology, Faculty of Medicine, Health Sciences University, Derince Training and Research Hospital, Kocaeli, Turkey
e-mail: seblakumas@hotmail.com

A. Selçuk
Department of Otorhinolaryngology, Faculty of Medicine, Medical Park Göztepe Hospital, Bahçeşehir University, Istanbul, Turkey
e-mail: sadin27@yahoo.com

K. Van Gool
Department of Otorhinolaryngology, Head & Neck Surgery, University Hospital Antwerp, Antwerp, Belgium
e-mail: Klara.VanGool@uza.be

C. Cingi et al. (eds.), *ENT Diseases: Diagnosis and Treatment during Pregnancy and Lactation*, https://doi.org/10.1007/978-3-031-05303-0_37

incidence of clinical otosclerosis is almost zero or rare in Asians and Native Americans. However, whites and mostly Caucasians have 10 times higher histological otosclerosis than clinical otosclerosis. The rate of histological otosclerosis is about 10% [6–9].

37.2 Etiology

Numerous studies have shown that there is a genetic inheritance. The chromosomal loci associated with otosclerosis have about nine possible genes: COL1A1, OTSC1, OTSC2, OTSC3, OTSC4, OTSC5, OTSC6, OTSC7, and OTSC8 [10–17] (Table 37.1). According to the literature review, the most possible theory about the genetic inheritance is the autosomal-dominant character with incomplete penetrance and variable expressivity [18].

Persistent measles virus infection has been blamed for years, and some studies support this theory [19–21]. In spite of vaccination of children in developed countries, otosclerosis is still common; however, in developing countries such as Africa, the prevalence of otosclerosis is very low and measles is highly endemic. Also, some endocrine factors have been researched, but there is no evidence to indicate that they play a role in the etiology of otosclerosis [22].

37.3 Histopathology

The most commonly involved area of the otic capsule is the area anterior to the oval window, fissula ante fenestram. The disease has early- and late-phase findings. The early phase is called otospongiotic phase. Multinuclear osteoclastic cells resorb the vessels around the normal lamellar bone of the otic capsule and perivascular spaces are formed. In the late phase, these spaces are replaced with a new bone by osteocytes, and this new bone takes up a larger space than before. In the following period, the new bone turns into lamellar bone, which is acellular and highly dense. Both active and inactive phases may act together at the same place [23].

The type of hearing loss depends on which part of the otic capsule is involved. The lesion begins from the anterior (most common) or posterior part of the oval

Table 37.1 Genetic studies associated with otosclerosis inheritance

Study	Year	Locus	Position
McKenna et al. [10]	1998	COL1A1	17q21.31–q21.32
Tomek et al. [11]	1998	OTSC1	15q25–q26
Van Den Bogaert et al. [12]	2001	OTSC2	7q34–q36
Chen et al. [13]	2002	OTSC3	6p21.3–22.3
Brownstein et al. [14]	2006	OTSC4	16q22.1–23.1
Van Den Bogaert et al. [15]	2004	OTSC5	3q22–24
Not published	–	OTSC6	–
Thys et al. [16]	2007	OTSC7	6q13–16.1
Bel Hadj Ali et al. [17]	2007	OTSC8	9p13.1–9q21

window around the margin of the stapes footplate and involves the anterior and posterior annular ligament so that it may result in stapedial fixation, thereby causing conductive hearing loss. Sometimes, otosclerosis may involve round window or other region in otic capsule and causes sensorineural hearing loss due to toxic fluids in the inner ear.

37.4 Symptoms, Signs, and Audiogram

Hearing loss is the most presenting symptom and usually begins in the 20s and progresses slowly. The disease is generally bilateral, and most of the patients have conductive hearing loss. Patients with otosclerosis hear well in noisy surroundings, and it is known as the Paracusis of Willis. Tinnitus and vertigo may accompany. Family history is frequent in most of the cases.

Otoscopic examination is quite normal and mobile. In some cases, a reddish spot may be seen, which is an active angiomatous otospongiotic focus reflection named as the Schwartze sign.

In tuning fork tests, with 512 Hz Weber test lateralizes to the ear with conductive or greater conductive (in bilateral cases) hearing loss and negative Rinne test with 256 Hz, later 512 Hz and 1026 Hz when the stapedial fixation is settled.

The immittance audiometry battery must consist of tympanometry, static compliance, and acoustic reflex testing. Tympanometry shows generally type A or later flattened curve As. Diphasic or absent stapedial reflex can be seen.

Pure tone audiometry shows loss of air conduction, more for lower frequencies when bone conduction is normal. Sometimes, there is an artificial depression in the bone conduction line centered on 2 kHz called Carhart's notch. After a successful stapes surgery, this notch disappears (Figs. 37.1, 37.2, 37.3, 37.4).

37.5 Otosclerosis and Pregnancy

Otosclerosis is more common in women than in men, and the ages of women getting the disease are their reproductive years. So, whether there is an endocrine factor or whether pregnancy is having any effects on the disease still remains unclear. In his study, Wakwick mentioned the role of pregnancy as the inhibition of the ovaries causing an increase in calcium metabolism. İnhibiting the ovaries made removal of the inhibiting effect of the ovarian secretion on the pituitary and thyroid glands, which, when not thus inhibited, normally cause an increase in the calcium content of the blood. He assumed that pituitary and thyroid glands had an active role in the process of deposition of calcium salts in various embryonic cartilaginous residues like labyrinthine capsule and in the footplate of the stapes in prepuberty [24]. Contrary to what is believed when the literature is reviewed from the past to present, it does not appear that pregnancy has a definite effect on reducing hearing in patients with otosclerosis. Because of the lack of successful surgical treatment prevention and later influenced by the popularity of eugenics, sterilization and abortion were the options to treat otosclerosis in pregnancy in the first half of the twentieth century [25].

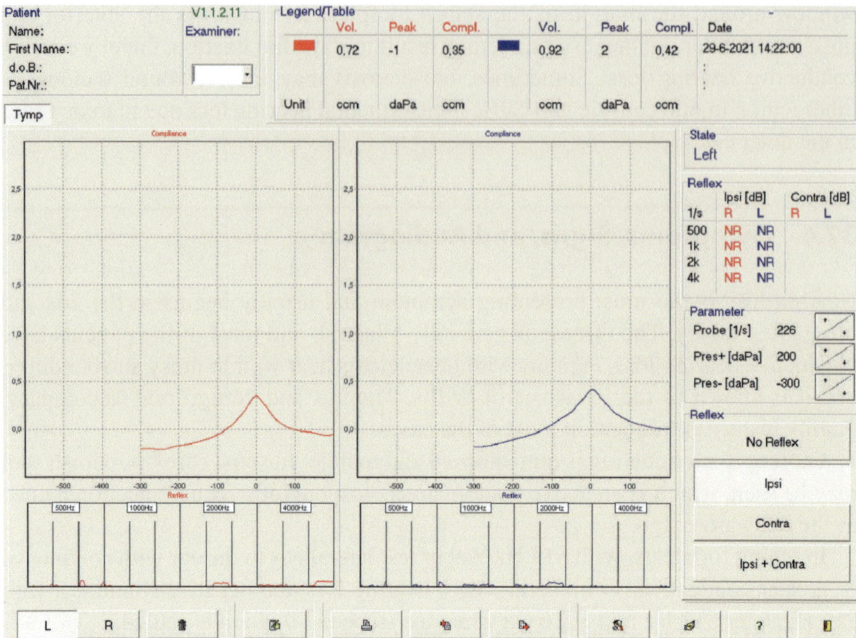

Fig. 37.1 Tympanometry shows generally type A. Acoustic reflex testing shows bilateral absent stapedial reflex

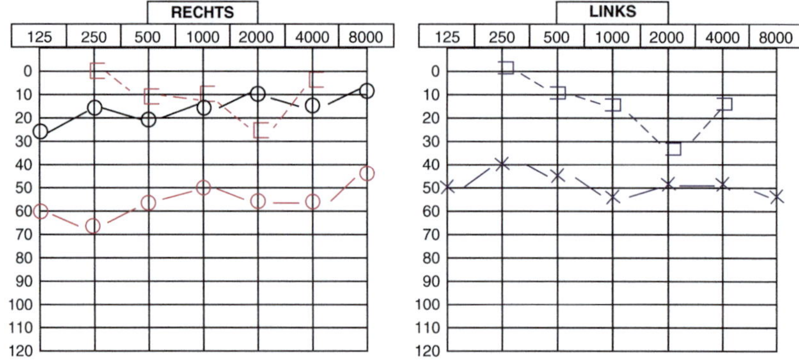

Fig. 37.2 Blue: conductive hearing loss in the left ear with Carhart's notch on 2 kHz in the bone conduction line. Red: conductive hearing loss on the right side with Carhart's notch: preoperative measurement. Black: 3 months after successful stapes surgery, the "artificial" Carhart's notch disappears

In the nineteenth century, eugenic science and social movement were quite fashionable. It was accepted that eugenic sterilization or abortion was the solution for genetic disorders that had inheritance for the following generation. In 1918, Arturo Blohmke did a survey of different German clinics to find out whether pregnancy had a negative effect on hearing and whether it ending of pregnancy was indicated or not [26].

Fig. 37.3 Cone beam CT scan of the right ear. Oblique reconstruction: fenestral otosclerosis with stapedial fixation; hypodensity in contact with the ottic capsule

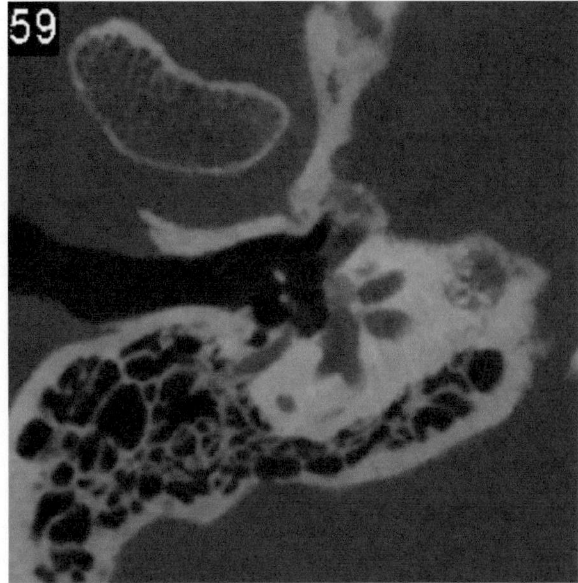

Fig. 37.4 Cone beam CT scan of the right ear. Oblique reconstruction: Teflon piston centered in oval window

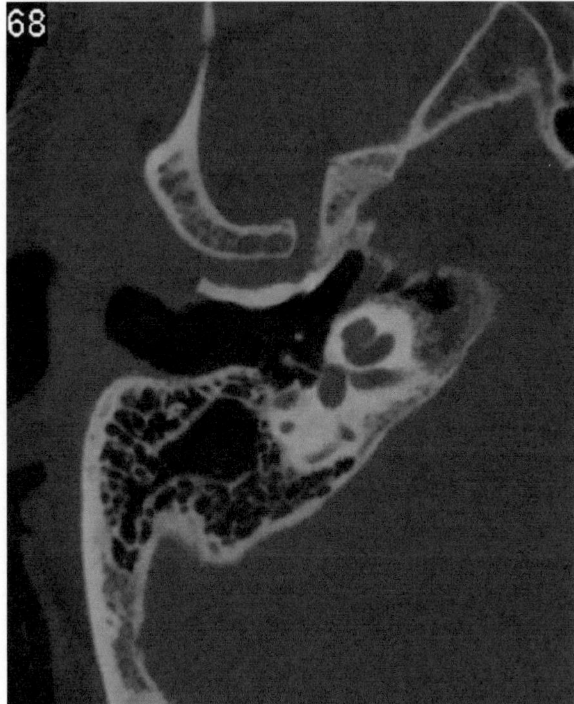

The answers to this survey were many case reports on hearing loss and severe tinnitus due to pregnancy. Some abortions were done to stop hearing loss. Guggenheim stated that over 50% of otosclerotic women had hearing loss following childbirth and during the latter half of pregnancy [27]. In Germany, in 1933, there was a sterilization law written by Ernst Rüdin, the president of the International Federation of Eugenics Societies, named in English as the "Law on the prevention of offspring with hereditary diseases," that had been modeled before in 1922 in the United States by Laughlin [28, 29]. During the Nazi regime, it was assumed that there were hundreds or thousands of pregnant women who were treated by sterilization and/or abortion. After about 10 years later, the abortion or sterilization treatment argument for the otosclerotic women began to change. In 1945, Allen reported in an article that he collected the cases from the literature and personal communication and analyzed the data on their age, family history about deafness, and obstetric history. He concluded that if a therapeutic abortion was decided the patient had to be informed that this disease is progressive even without pregnancy and the patient would have to learn lip reading and need to wear hearing aids [30]. In 1948, Smith reported in a study that he collected 73 cases. The data for each patient were the age at the time of examination; the age at the onset of symptoms; the presence or absence of a history of familial deafness; the number of term pregnancies; the number of incomplete gestations; and whether the deafness was associated with, or increased by, pregnancy, or was not associated with, or increased by, pregnancy. He found that 37% (28 women) of deafness was associated with, or increased by, pregnancy, but 63% women reported that pregnancy had no effect on their hearing loss. The average age of the patients at the time deafness was first noted was 25 [31]. Till the 1950s, all studies were based on patients' discourses. Walsh had reviewed 243 consecutive cases that had otosclerosis with pregnancy history, of which 139 described no effect but 104 (43%) stated having worse hearing in pregnancy. He needed more reliable information about the subject, meaning audiogram. In 1954, Walsh found great worsening hearing thresholds in two operated patients and 7 of 40 patients' hearing loss progressed in the unoperated ear after pregnancy in 3–5 years verified with audiograms. Hence, he concluded this situation to be the nature of the disease [32]. A survey by Goethals at Mayo Clinic was also remarkable. He found that 211 of 375 patients (56.2%) had loss of hearing initiated or increased by pregnancy. In total, 158 of 211 patients' hearing loss were at the initiation or during pregnancy (42.1%). Of these, the first pregnancy experience number was 106, the second was 35, and the third was 17. The number of patients having hearing loss prior to gestation and increased by pregnancy was 53 (14.1%). Of these, 35 patients had the first gestation experience, whereas the remaining 18 patients had second pregnancy and 8 had association with it [33]. There were no audiograms done.

Podoshin et al. reported oral contraceptives (OC) and otosclerosis communication. They reviewed 600 women between the ages 16 and 30 using OCs during 12–36 months. There were three cases pointing to otosclerosis with pathological audiometry after excluding the other ear disease. They did not find a correlation between the chemical composition of the OC, age of the women, duration of OC use, and clinical otosclerosis [34]. In 1983, Gristwood and Venables' studied 362 female patients with otosclerosis who had at least one pregnancy, according to the

Table 37.2 Studies on hearing loss in pregnancy

Author	Year	Hearing loss	
		Cases	%
Allen [30]	1945	72	48
Smith [31]	1948	73	37
Walsh [32]	1954	243	43
Goethals [33]	1960	375	56.2
Gristwood [35]	1983	362	43.3

laterality of conductive deafness and its aggravation by pregnancy. This was also a study done without using audiograms. They found that at least one pregnancy caused 33% hearing impairment in bilateral cases, reaching up to 63% after the sixth pregnancy [35]. All these studies had poor strength of evidence, and most did not include appropriate control groups or were without statistical analyses. Lippy's study in 2005 was a milestone on this topic. It included 94 patients and two groups as having children or not. Due to the fact that some cases were bilateral, a total of 128 ears were investigated. All the patients underwent stapedectomy. Women with children were paired with each other according to their ages with childless women, and their preoperative and postoperative tests were compared. They found no deleterious effect of pregnancy on otosclerosis [36]. Like Lippy's findings, Marchese et al. obtained similar findings [37]. Qian's study is the most recent study done on this topic. Qian's hypothesis states that if pregnancy progresses the hearing loss and then gender affect the relationship between the number of children and age of stapedectomy. They found that the age at initial stapedectomy was significantly lower in females than males, women with children than childless women, and males with children than childless males. They concluded that the initial stapedectomy age is getting younger with parenthood [38].

In conclusion, the negative effect of pregnancy on hearing loss in patients with otosclerosis was supported in the nineteenth and twentieth centuries with political reasons and by some studies that had low-level evidence. In the twenty-first century, this hypothesis seems to have expired. Studies with a large-size cohort and statistical analyses and high-level evidence show that pregnancy has no negative effect on hearing loss in patients with otosclerosis. So, further prospective studies need to be done (Table 37.2).

37.6 Treatment

Medical curative treatment of otosclerosis is not possible today. Sodium fluoride and bisphosphonates have been used for this purpose. Studies on treatment using sodium fluoride showed that it slows down the progression of sensorineural hearing loss by neutralization of enzymes that have a toxic effect on hair cells. It does not make any change such as converting an active spongiotic focus to an inactive focus [39]. Because of its teratogenic adverse condition, it is contraindicated in pregnancy. Although the mechanism is unknown and controversies exist in bisphosphonate therapy, the current prospective randomized studies have found safety for the proper management of this therapy in cases of otosclerosis [40].

Surgical treatments of otosclerosis include stapedotomy or stapedectomy. Patient choice is important. Air conduction hearing threshold should be 30 dB or worse. Average air–bone gap should be at least 15 dB with Rinne test and negative for 256 and 512 Hz. Speech discrimination score should be 60% or more. Although it is a low risk, the patient must be informed about total sensorineural hearing loss and also other complications such as vertigo, facial paralysis, tinnitus, taste disturbance, tympanic membrane perforation, and perilymph fistula.

Stapedectomy was first described by Shea and House. In the Shea technique, total stapedectomy is performed and oval window is covered with a vein graft and interposition of a polyethylene strut [41]. Similarly, in the House technique, after a total stapedectomy is performed a gel foam and steel wire prosthesis are replaced [42]. More recently, stapedotomy has become common. This procedure includes only a small fenestra in the footplate [43–45]. Stapedotomy technique shows slightly better results in early and late postoperative air conduction thresholds at 4 kHz than stapedectomy [46].

37.6.1 Steps of Stapedotomy

1. Local anesthesia of four quadrants of external ear.
2. Incision and elevation of tympanomeatal flap.
3. Exposure of stapedial area. If there is a posterosuperior bony overhang canal, it must be removed (Fig. 37.5).
4. Ossicular chain palpation.
5. Making a small fenestration hole in the footplate (Fig. 37.6).
6. Incision of stapedial tendon.
7. Removal of the suprastructure.
8. Replacing the titanium, Teflon, or nitinol piston prosthesis (Fig. 37.7).
9. Supporting the footplate hole small amount of blood.
10. Replacing the tympanomeatal flap.

Since stapedotomy is more preferred, some other techniques have been developed. Classical operation has been performed under local anesthesia and microscopy for years, and although it is still performed, mostly authors prefer general anesthesia and endoscopic stapes surgery. Current studies support that endoscopic stapes surgery is a good alternative technique compared to microscopic ones in regard to operating time, chorda tympani nerve injury, and postoperative audiological results [47–49].

To make a small fenestration, a vehicle-like microdrill, fine pick, or laser use is needed. Generally, two types of laser are used: visible green light lasers such as the argon or potassium-titanyl-phosphate (KTP-532) and infrared carbon dioxide (CO_2) lasers [5]. Perkins first described argon laser as multiple small vaporized holes forming a rosette in the footplate [50]. When KTP laser can be carried through the

Fig. 37.5 Stapes footplate with otosclerosis (star). Circle shows the incus

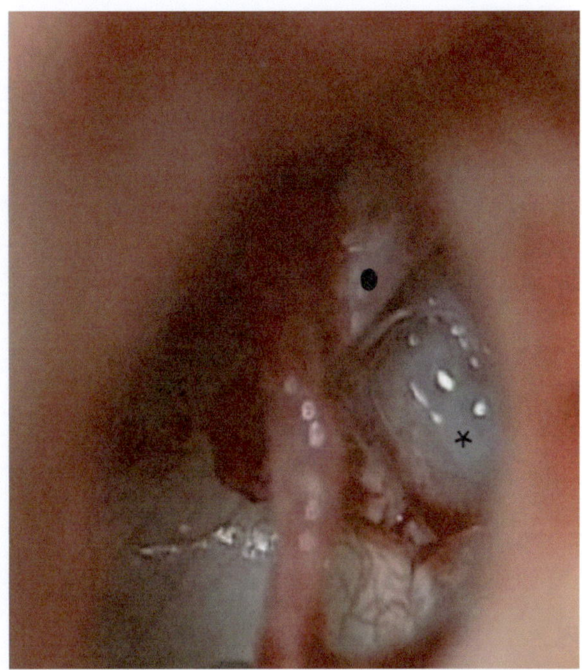

Fig. 37.6 Drilling the footplate

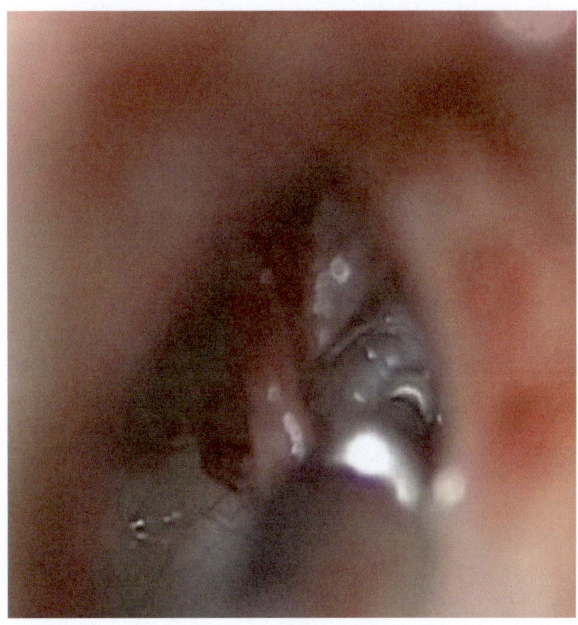

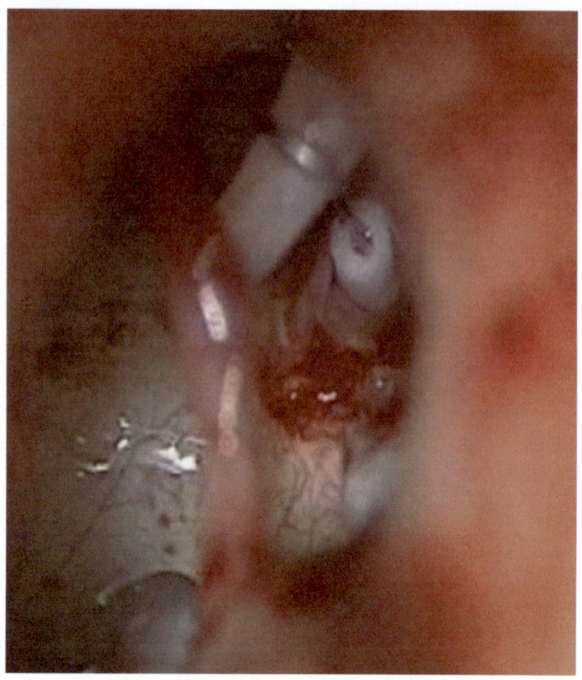

Fig. 37.7 Replacement of titanium prosthesis

fiber optic cables, CO_2 laser needs mirrors and lenses. Lesinski and Palmer [51] published CO_2 laser system that could be used for stapes surgery. Both lasers seem to be safe, but Vincent et al. reported in their study that postoperative air–bone gap closure within 10 dB was more effective in CO_2 laser than KTP laser [52]. Another alternative method for fenestration is micro drill technique. The latest meta-analysis study shows that there is no clinical or statistically significant difference between the use of drills or lasers in regard to postoperative hearing outcomes [53].

37.7 Hearing Aids

Hearing aids as always can be used in patients with conduction hearing loss due to otosclerosis. In patients not willing to be operated or having failed stapes surgery and in cochlear otosclerosis causing sensorineural hearing loss, hearing aids are quite an effective alternative option.

References

1. Valsalva A. Valsalvae opera et Morgagni epistolae. Venetiis, Italy: Francescus Pitteri:Venetiis. Francescus Pitteri, Italy; 1741.
2. Toynbee J. Diseases of the ear. Philadelphia: Blanchard &Lea; 1860.
3. Politzer A. Uber primare erkrankung der knockernen labyrinthkapsel. Zeitschrift Fur Ohrenheilkunde. 1894;25:309–27.

4. Siebenman F. Totaler knocherner verschluss beider labyrinthfester und labyrinthitis serosa infolge progessiver spongiosierung. Verhanlungen Deutschen Otologischenn Gesellschaft. 1912;6:267–83.

5. Flint PW. Cummings otolaryngology-head & neck surgery. 6th ed. Philadelphia: Elsevier; 2015. p. 2211.

6. Morrison AW. Genetic factors in otosclerosis. Ann R Coll Surg Engl. 1967;41(2):202–37.

7. Hueb MM, Goycoolea MV, Paparella MM, Oliveira JA. Otosclerosis: the University of Minnesota temporal bone collection. Otolaryngol Head Neck Surg. 1991;105(3):396–405.

8. Ohtani I, Baba Y, Suzuki T, Suzuki C, Kano M, Deka RC. Why is otosclerosis of low prevalence in Japanese? Otol Neurotol. 2003;24(3):377–81.

9. Levin G, Fabian P, Stahle J. Incidence of otosclerosis. Am J Otol. 1988;9:299.

10. McKenna MJ, Kristiansen AG, Bartley ML, Rogus JJ, Haines JL. Association of COL1A1 and otosclerosis: evidence for a shared genetic etiology with mild osteogenesis imperfecta. Am J Otol. 1998;19(5):604–10.

11. Tomek MS, Brown MR, Mani SR, et al. Localization of a gene for otosclerosis to chromosome 15q25–q26. Hum Mol Genet. 1998;7(2):285–90.

12. Van Den Bogaert K, Govaerts PJ, Schatteman I, et al. A second gene for otosclerosis, OTSC2, maps to chromosome 7q34-36. Am J Hum Genet. 2001;68(2):495–500.

13. Chen W, Campbell CA, Green GE, et al. Linkage of otosclerosis to a third locus (OTSC3) on human chromosome 6p21.3-22.3. J Med Genet. 2002;39(7):473–7.

14. Brownstein Z, Goldfarb A, Levi H, et al. Chromosomal mapping and phenotypic characterization of hereditary otosclerosis linked to the OTSC4 locus. Arch Otolaryngol Head Neck Surg. 2006;132(4):416–24.

15. Van Den Bogaert K, De Leenheer EM, Chen W, et al. A Wfth locus for otosclerosis, OTSC5, maps to chromosome 3q22–24. J Med Genet. 2004;41(6):450–3.

16. Thys M, Van Den Bogaert K, Iliadou V, et al. A seventh locus for otosclerosis, OTSC7, maps to chromosome 6q13-16.1. Eur J Hum Genet. 2007;15(3):362–8.

17. Bel Hadj Ali I, Thys M, Beltaief N, et al. A new locus for otosclerosis, OTSC8, maps to the pericentromeric region of chromosome 9. Hum Genet. 2008;123(3):267–72.

18. Markou K, Goudakos J. An overview of the etiology of otosclerosis. Eur Arch Otorhinolaryngol. 2009;266:25–35.

19. McKenna MJ, Mills BG. Immunohistochemical evidence of measles virus antigens in active otosclerosis. Otolaryngol Head Neck Surg. 1989;101:415–21.

20. McKenna MJ, Kristiansen AG, Haines J. Polymerase chain reaction amplification of a measles virus sequence from human temporal bone sections with active otosclerosis. Am J Otol. 1996;17:827–30.

21. Niedermeyer H, Arnold W, Neubert WJ, et al. Evidence of measles virus RNA in otosclerotic tissue. ORL J Otorhinolaryngol Relat Spec. 1994;56:130–2.

22. Schrauwen I, Van Camp G. The etiology of otosclerosis: a combination of genes and environment. Laryngoscope. 2010;120(6):1195–202. https://doi.org/10.1002/lary.20934.

23. Quesnel AM, Ishai R, McKenna MJ. Otosclerosis: temporal bone pathology. Otolaryngol Clin N Am. 2018;51(2):291–303.

24. Wakwick HL, Stevenson HM. Is there an endocrine factor in otosclerosis? Acta Oto-Laryngol. 1926;9(1):317–24.

25. Tange RA. Some historical facts on otosclerosis in pregnancy. Int Adv Otol. 2013;9:395–402.

26. Blohmke A. Otosklerose und Schwangerschaft. Archiv für Ohren-, Nasen- und Kehlkopfheilkunde. 1918;102:1–41.

27. Guggenheim LK. On the diagnosis and treatment of otosclerosis. Am J Surg. 1938;43:156.

28. Laughlin HH. Eugenical sterilization in the United States. Chicago, Ill: Municipal Court. Psychiatric Institute Psychopathic Laboratory of the Municipal Court of Chicago; 1922. p. 1–502.

29. Gütt A, Rüdin E, Ruttke F. Zur Verhütung erbkranken Nachwuchses. München: J.F. Lehmanns Verlag; 1934.

30. Allen ED. Pregnancy and otosclerosis. Am J Obstet Gynecol. 1945;49:2–48.
31. Smith HW. Effect of pregnancy on otosclerosis. Arch Otolaryngol. 1948;48(2):159–70.
32. Walsh TE. The effect of pregnancy on the deafness due to otosclerosis. J Am Med Assoc. 1954;154(17):1407–9.
33. Goethals PL, Banner EA, Hedgecock LD. Effect of pregnancy on otosclerosis. Am J Obstet Gynecol. 1963;86(4):522–9.
34. Podoshin L, Gertner R, Fradis M, et al. Oral contraceptive pills and clinical otosclerosis. Int J Gynaecol Obstet. 1978;15(6):554–5.
35. Gristwood RE, Venables WN. Pregnancy and otosclerosis. Clin Otolaryngol Allied Sci. 1983;8(3):205–10.
36. Lippy WH, Berenholz LP, Schuring AG, et al. Does pregnancy affect otosclerosis? Laryngoscope. 2005;115(10):1833–6. https://doi.org/10.1097/01.MLG.0000187573.99335.85.
37. Marchese MR, Conti G, Cianfrone F, et al. Predictive role of audiological and clinical features for functional results after stapedotomy. Audiol Neurootol. 2009;14(5):279–85. https://doi.org/10.1159/000212105.
38. Qian ZJ, Alyono JC. Effects of pregnancy on otosclerosis. Otolaryngol Head Neck Surg. 2020;162(4):544–7. https://doi.org/10.1177/0194599820907093.
39. Parahy C, Linthicum FH Jr. Otosclerosis and otospongiosis: clinical and histological comparisons. Laryngoscope. 1984;94(4):508–12. https://doi.org/10.1288/00005537-198404000-00015.
40. de Oliveira PN, de Oliveira VA. Medical management of otosclerosis. Otolaryngol Clin N Am. 2018;51(2):441–52. https://doi.org/10.1016/j.otc.2017.11.006.
41. Shea JJ Jr. Fenestration of the oval window. Ann Otol Rhinol Laryngol. 1958;67:932.
42. House HP. The prefabricated wire loop-Gelfoam stapedectomy. Arch Otolaryngol. 1962;76(298)
43. Marquet J. "Stapedotomy" technique and results. Am J Otol. 1985;6:63–7.
44. Fisch U. Comment on stapedotomy versus stapedectomy, 1982. Otol Neurotol. 2009; 30(8):1166–7.
45. Vincent R, Sperling NM, Oates J, et al. Surgical findings and long term hearing results in 3,050 stapedotomies for primary otosclerosis: a prospective study with the otology-neurotology database. Otol Neurotol. 2006;27(8 Suppl 2):S25–47.
46. House HP, Hansen MR, Al Dakhail AA, et al. Stapedectomy versus stapedotomy: comparison of results with long-term follow-up. Laryngoscope. 2002;112(11):2046–50. https://doi.org/10.1097/00005537-200211000-00025.
47. Kojima H, Komori M, Chikazawa S, et al. Comparison between endoscopic and microscopic stapes surgery. Laryngoscope. 2014;124(1):266–71. https://doi.org/10.1002/lary.24144.
48. Koukkoullis A, Tóth I, Gede N, et al. Endoscopic versus microscopic stapes surgery outcomes: a meta-analysis and systematic review. Laryngoscope. 2020;130(8):2019–27. https://doi.org/10.1002/lary.28353.
49. Nassiri AM, Yawn RJ, Dedmon MM, et al. Primary endoscopic stapes surgery: audiologic and surgical outcomes. Otol Neurotol. 2018;39(9):1095–101. https://doi.org/10.1097/MAO.0000000000001958.
50. Perkins RC. Laser stepedotomy for otosclerosis. Laryngoscope. 1980;90(2):228–40. https://doi.org/10.1288/00005537-198002000-00007.
51. Lesinski SG, Palmer A. Lasers for otosclerosis: CO2 vs. Argon and KTP-532. Laryngoscope. 1989;99(6 Pt 2 Suppl 46):1–8.
52. Vincent R, Bittermann AJ, Oates J, et al. KTP versus CO2 laser fiber stapedotomy for primary otosclerosis: results of a new comparative series with the otology-neurotology database. Otol Neurotol. 2012;33(6):928–33. https://doi.org/10.1097/MAO.0b013e31825f24ff.
53. Bartel R, Huguet G, Cruellas F, et al. Laser vs drill for footplate fenestration during stapedotomy: a systematic review and meta-analysis of hearing results. Eur Arch Otorhinolaryngol. [Published online ahead of print, 2020 Jun 13]. 2020; https://doi.org/10.1007/s00405-020-06117-1.

Facial Nerve Disorders During Pregnancy and the Postpartum Period

Duygu Ayhan Başer, Fatih Özdoğan, and Ulugbek Khasanov

38.1 Introduction

Facial nerve disorders in pregnancy and the postpartum period are uncommon; however, they are important diseases. In most studies, higher incidence of Bell's palsy in pregnant and postpartum women was reported. The etiology of facial palsy in pregnancy is not well known. Same symptoms are observed in pregnant and postpartum women in general population. Bell's palsy is mainly diagnosed clinically, and imaging is not recommended initially. The prognosis of Bell's palsy in pregnant women is worse. Management of facial nerve palsy in pregnancy can be categorized into medical, physiotherapy, and surgical options. A multidisciplinary approach is required in the ideal management of pregnant and postpartum women with Bell's palsy.

"Facial nerve disorders" exhibit variable levels of facial dysfunction and cover many diseases and causes: viral infections, strokes, trauma, surgery, tumors, etc. [1]. One of the most common facial nerve disorders is Bell's palsy, and in disease,

D. Ayhan Başer (✉)
Department of Family Medicine, Faculty of Medicine, Hacettepe University, Ankara, Turkey
e-mail: dr.duyguayhan@gmail.com

F. Özdoğan
Department of Otorhinolaryngology, Faculty of Medicine, Health Sciences University, Derince Training and Research Hospital, Ankara, Turkey
e-mail: ozdogan.fatih@gmail.com

U. Khasanov
Department of Otorhinolaryngology and Stomatology, Tashkent Medical Academy, Tashkent, Uzbekistan
e-mail: ukhasanov@yahoo.com

C. Cingi et al. (eds.), *ENT Diseases: Diagnosis and Treatment during Pregnancy and Lactation*, https://doi.org/10.1007/978-3-031-05303-0_38

severe facial muscle weakness or paralysis occurs due to viral infection of the facial nerve. Bell's palsy can emerge at any age, which is the most common cause of facial paralysis seen in pregnancy [1–3]. Charles Bell was the first scientist who detected higher incidence of Bell's palsy in pregnant and postpartum patients; [4] however, not much is still known about the relationship between them. Although there is information that Bell's palsy is more common during pregnancy in previous studies [5–9], recent studies have reported that the incidence does not increase during pregnancy [10]. In addition, there is a strong evidence of the lower rates of early diagnosis, treatment, and full recovery of Bell's palsy, higher progression to complete facial nerve paralysis during pregnancy and the postpartum period, and regardless of the incidence, being aware of the diagnosis, close monitoring, and good management of pregnant/postpartum women is very important. So, Bell's facial palsy in pregnancy and the postpartum period is an uncommon but important disease.

38.2 Epidemiology and Etiology

In most studies, the incidence of Bell's palsy is mentioned more often (three times higher) during pregnancy and postpartum interval [5, 6]. Most of the cases are seen in the third trimester and early postpartum interval [8]. There are various hypotheses to define this higher incidence [4, 11]. The most commonly cited causes are viral causes [9, 12, 13]. It has been stated that herpes simplex virus (HSV) is more common in pregnant women. High cortisol levels may cause immunosuppression in the third trimester, and therefore, increased susceptibility to viral infections and HSV reactivation can be seen [14]. Other hypothesis is a result of the toxemia of pregnancy, high levels of estrogen and progesterone [15, 16], and increased interstitial fluid volume in pregnancy leading to compression of the facial nerve and ischemia in the Fallopian canal [17]. On the other hand, no relationship was reported between perinatal outcomes and spontaneous facial nerve paralysis during pregnancy [18, 19].

38.3 Clinic Course

Clinically, the biggest part of the patients with Bell's palsy has a viral prodrome. Sound sensitivity, impaired taste, and ear pain are the prodromal symptoms. Symptoms in the order of frequency are tearing, postauricular pain, taste disturbances, and hyperacusis. Other accompanying symptoms include smoothed nasolabial folds, smoothing of wrinkles on the occupied side, flagging mouth corner, inability to lift the eyelid, show teeth, and whistle [20, 21]. Symptoms of facial nerve paralysis in pregnant and postpartum women are the same as others [20]. The course of the disease may include exposing the upper part of the sclera when closing the eyelid, dry eyes, changes in taste in the anterior 2/3 of the tongue, and sensitivity to noise. Typical symptoms of acute facial nerve palsy develop within 24–48 h. After the paralysis develops, if it takes longer than 7–10 days, it should be evaluated for progression to complete paralysis [22]. Gilman et al. mentioned that progression to complete facial paralysis is more often seen in pregnant and postpartum women [9].

38.4 Diagnosis

Bell's palsy is mainly diagnosed clinically, and imaging is not recommended initially for diagnosis [23]. CT and MRI can be used to exclude other etiologies of facial paralysis if there are concerns of symptoms associated with Bell's paralysis such as

- Complication of chronic ear disease
- Progression after 3 weeks
- Recurrent facial paralysis
- Surgical intervention
- Functions that cannot be restored within 3 months
- Asymmetrical facial weakness
- Additional focal neurological deficits

There is no clear explanation for diagnostic imaging methods during pregnancy and postpartum interval, and both patients and clinicians are concerned. The American College of Obstetricians and Gynecologists' Committee on Obstetric Practice (ACGCOP) has recently recommended diagnostic imaging methods during pregnancy and the postpartum period; the recommended method is MRI, and other methods are not recommended [24]. Electrophysiological stimulation tests are recommended after the fourth day of onset of complete paralysis and are useful for diagnosis and early referral, and this test has no special risk for pregnant or postpartum women [2].

38.5 Prognosis

The prognosis is worse in pregnant women and the postpartum period with Bell's palsy; one study reported that pregnant women regained facial muscle function at a lower rate compared to nonpregnant women of similar ages [9]. Prognosis is good for pregnant women with incomplete facial nerve palsy, but functional deficiencies may remain in case of complete paralysis, in this case the prognosis is worse [22]. Pregnant women with Bell's palsy have a risk of preeclampsia, who require appropriate prenatal follow-up and strict blood pressure monitoring.

38.6 Treatment

Management of facial nerve palsy in pregnancy can be categorized into medical, physiotherapy, and surgical options. Medical options consist of corticosteroid therapy and antiviral therapy.

38.6.1 Eye Protection

It is very important to protect corneal damage (dry/red eyes, gritty/burning sensation in the eyes,) which is the most important side effect of treatments. It is recommended to apply moisturizing, sterile eye drops several times a day and refer the patient to an ophthalmologist [6].

38.6.2 Corticosteroid Therapy

Steroids have become the classic treatment method for Bell's paralysis due to their anti-inflammatory and immunosuppressive effects. Early corticosteroid therapy is suggested by recent guidelines (AAO-HNSF) within 72 h of symptom onset with a 10-day course of oral steroids. The most commonly used corticosteroids during pregnancy are prednisolone, dexamethasone, and betamethasone. Dexamethasone and betamethasone pass through the placental barrier much more easily [6, 25]. There are some risks of the antenatal corticosteroid usage:

- Maternal comorbidities
- Fetal comorbidities
- Gestational age
- Age of mother
- Drug type
- Dosage
- Treatment duration [26, 27]

The first trimester is the most critical period for the complications. Early corticosteroid usage (from 48 to 72 h) is stated as 17–20% improvement in total recovery in some studies [28–30].

At the beginning of the treatment of Bell's palsy, oral prednisolone 1 mg/kg body weight for 5 days is applied with next dose reduction. Other treatment options include

- Prednisolone 25 mg, two times a day for 10 days.
- Prednisolone 60 mg for 5 days, then reduction of dose to 10 mg for 5 days.

Breastfeeding can be continued on steroid therapy in the postpartum period [31]. Steroid use in pregnant and postpartum women should always be consulted with the responsible obstetrician/gynecologist, and frequent monitoring of blood glucose and blood pressure, maternal and fetal weight, and fetal parameters is important.

38.6.3 Antiviral Therapy

There are some suggestions for the use of antiviral drugs in facial nerve palsy during pregnancy. Some studies show that combined therapy of antiviral agents with corticosteroids gives better results than corticosteroids alone [22, 32, 33]. The purpose is to prevent the HSV reactivation. The American Academy of Neurology (AAN) also recommends adding antivirals to corticosteroid therapy. Antiviral therapy is classified as having the B pregnancy category. There are insufficient data on the use of these drugs in pregnant women; valaciclovir and famciclovir are more recommended for maternal and fetal health.

38.6.4 Physiotherapy

The use of physiotherapy such as exercises or electrostimulation has no proven efficiency in the treatment of facial nerve palsy [33]. Especially therapeutic ultrasound can be used in the treatment of facial paralysis from the early stages, and it is possible to reduce edema, increase blood circulation, and facilitate the repair of the nerve sheath. It has been demonstrated that coupling physiotherapy and botulinum toxin therapy provides benefits in terms of both function and quality of life in cases of synkinesis, hypertonicity, and residual weakness [34].

38.6.5 Surgical Treatments

In addition to medical treatment after diagnosis, it is important to apply the right surgical treatment at the right time. Surgical treatments can be divided into dynamic and static surgical procedures. While dynamic surgeries are performed with the aim of restoring function in the early period, static surgical procedures are aimed at preserving the orbit and providing oral sphincter function. The urgent surgical treatment of facial nerve palsy is composed of surgical decompression or reconstruction of normal eyelid protective function.

Tarsorrhaphy is considered as a static surgical method for lagophthalmos, where the eyelids are partially stitched together to prevent them from being open. Temporary suture tarsorrhaphies are better techniques for quick eyelid closure.

Dynamic techniques for restoring function in the early period contain platinum weight or chain insertion, and palpebral springs. Current methods are composed of

- Placement of punctual plugs to increase lubrication
- Temporary or permanent eyelid closure methods
- Horizontal eyelid-tightening methods
- Temporary (botulinum toxin) or permanent (upper lid weight) procedures improving blink and eyelid closure
- Planned reconstruction of normal blink reflex and function

Glucocorticosteroids should be administered first in pregnant women; however, in cases of severe class dysfunction or delay in recovery, surgical treatment may be considered after consulting the responsible gynecologist.

38.7 Conclusions

Pregnancy and the postpartum period are difficult periods for women with many biopsychosocial changes. Facial paralysis of pregnant and postpartum women can cause functional and psychosocial problems. Treatment of pregnant/postpartum women diagnosed with Bell's palsy should be initiated with early corticosteroid therapy in collaboration with the responsible obstetrician/gynecologist. Antiviral therapy may be recommended for patients with complete paralysis. Topical ophthalmologic care should be offered to all patients with inadequate eyelid closure. Surgical treatment can be considered by obtaining the opinion of the obstetrician/gynecologist in case of unresponsiveness to medical treatment. A multidisciplinary approach is required in the optimal management of pregnant and postpartum women with Bell's palsy.

References

1. Davies J, Al-Hassani F, Kannan R, et al. Facial nerve disorder: a review of the literature. Int J Surg Oncol. 2018;3(7):e65.
2. Baugh RF, Basura GJ, Ishii L, et al. Clinical practice guideline: Bell's palsy executive summary. Otolaryngol Head Neck Surg. 2013;149(5):656–63.
3. Hilsinger RL, Adour KK, Doty HE, et al. Idiopathic facial paralysis, pregnancy, and the menstrual cycle. Ann Oto Rhinol Laryngol. 1975;84:433–42.
4. Cohen Y, Lavie O, Granovsky-Grisaru S, et al. Bell palsy complicating pregnancy: a review. Obstet Gynecol Surv. 2000;55:184–8.
5. McGregor JA, Guberman A, Amer J, et al. Idiopathic facial nerve paralysis (Bell's palsy) in late pregnancy and the early puerperium. Obstet Gynecol. 1987;69:435–8.

6. Hussain A, Nduka C, Moth P, et al. Bell's facial nerve palsy in pregnancy: a clinical review. J Obstet Gynaecol. 2017;37(4):409–15.

7. Phillips KM, Heiser A, Gaudin et al (2017) Onset of bell's palsy in late pregnancy and early puerperium is associated with worse long-term outcomes. Laryngoscope 127:2854–2859.

8. Shapiro JL, Yudin MH, Ray JG, et al. Bell's palsy and tinnitus during pregnancy: predictors of pre-eclampsia? Three cases and a detailed review of the literature. Acta Otolaryngol. 1999;119:647–51.

9. Gillman GS, Grant S, Schaitkin B, et al. Bell's palsy in pregnancy: a study of recovery outcomes. Otolaryngol Head Neck Surg. 2002;126:26–30.

10. Choi HG, Hong SK, Park S-K, et al. Pregnancy does not increase the risk of Bell's palsy. Otol Neurotol. 2020;41:e111–7.

11. Mylonas I, Kästner R, Sattler C, et al. Idiopathic facial paralysis (Bell's palsy) in the immediate puerperium in a patient with mild preeclampsia: a case report. Arch Gynecol Obstet. 2005;272:241–3.

12. Lambert M. Bassman E, Talavera, et al. Bell's Palsy. (serial online) 2005 (cited 2005; 11); 1(1): (10 screens). Available from: http://www.emedicine.com/emerg/topic56.htm.

13. Al Ghamdi SA. Idiopathic facial nerve paralysis (Bell's palsy) in the Asir region. Ann Saudi Med. 1997;17(6):609–12.

14. Naib ZM, Nahmias AJ, Josey WE, et al. Relation of cytohistopathology of genital herpes virus infection to cervical anaplasia. Cancer Res. 1973;33:1452–63.

15. Falco NA, Eriksson E. Idiopathic facial palsy in pregnancy and the puerperium. Surg Gynecol Obstet. 1989;169:337–40.

16. Ben David Y, Tal J, Podoshin L. Brain stem auditory evoked potentials: effects of ovarian steroids correlated with increased incidence of Bell's palsy in pregnancy. Otolaryngol Head Neck Surg. 1995;113:32–5.

17. Selesnick SH, Patwardhan A. Acute facial paralysis: evaluation and early management. Am J Otolaryngol. 1994;15(6):387–408.

18. Fawale MB, Owolabi MO, Ogunbode O. Bell's palsy in pregnancy and the puerperium: a report of five cases. Afr J Med Med Sci. 2010;39:147–51.

19. Katz A, Sergienko R, Dior U, et al. Bell's palsy during pregnancy: is it associated with adverse perinatal outcome? Laryngoscope. 2011;121:1395–8.

20. Aditya V. Facial palsy in pregnancy: an opportunity to predict preeclampsia–report and review. Case Reports in Obstetrics and Gynecology; 2014.

21. Hussain A, Nduka C, Moth P, et al. Bells facial nerve palsy in pregnancy: a clinical review. J Obstet Gynaecol. 2017;37(4):409–15.

22. Vrabec JT, Isaacson B, Van Hook JW. Bell's palsy and pregnancy. Otolaryngol Head Neck Surg. 2007;137:858–61.

23. Fuzi J, Spencer S, Seckold E. Bell's palsy during pregnancy and the post-partum period: a contemporary management approach. Am J Otolaryngol. 2021;42(3):845–6.

24. Committee Opinion. Guidelines for diagnostic imaging during pregnancy and lactation. Obstet Gynecol. 2017;130:e210–6.

25. Van Runnard Heimel PJ, Franx A, Schobben AF, et al. Corticosteroids, pregnancy, and HELLP syndrome: a review. Obstet Gynecol Surv. 2005;60:57–70.

26. Gregersen TL, Ulrik CS. Safety of bronchodilators and corticosteroids for asthma during pregnancy: what we know and what we need to do better. J Asthma Allergy. 2013;6:117–25.

27. Park-Wyllie L, Mazzotta P, Pastuszak A. Birth defects after maternal exposure to corticosteroids prospective cohort study and meta-analysis of epidemiological studies. Teratology. 2000;62:385–92.

28. Ramsey MJ, Der Simonian R, Holtel MR, et al. Corticosteroid treatment for idiopathic facial nerve paralysis: a meta-analysis. Laryngoscope. 2000;110:335–41.
29. Sullivan FM, Swan IR, Donnan PT, et al. Early treatment with prednisolone or acyclovir in Bell's palsy. N Engl J Med. 2007;357:1598–607.
30. Engström M, Berg T, Stjernquist-Desatnik A, et al. Prednisolone and valaciclovir in Bell's palsy: a randomised, double-blind, placebo-controlled, multicentre trial. Lancet Neurol. 2008;7:993–1000.
31. Kunze M, Arndt S, Zimmer A, et al. Idiopathic facial palsy during pregnancy. HNO. 2012;2012(60):98–101.
32. Adour KK, Ruboyianes JM, Von Doersten PG, et al. Bell's palsy treatment with acyclovir and prednisone compared with prednisone alone: a double-blind, randomized, controlled trial. Ann Otol Rhinol Laryngol. 1996;105:371–8.
33. Hato N, Yamada H, Kohno H. Valacyclovir and prednisolone treatment for Bell's palsy: a multicenter, randomized, placebo-controlled study. Otol Neurotol. 2007;28:408–13.
34. Van Landingham SW, Diels J, Lucarelli MJ. Physical therapy for facial nerve palsy: applications for the physician. Curr Opin Ophthalmol. 2018;29:469–75.

Infections of the External Ear During Pregnancy and the Postpartum Period

39

Ferit Bayakır, Selahattin Genç, and Khassan M. Diab

39.1 Introduction

Otitis externa (OE) is an inflammatory process that affects the external auditory canal and occasionally the tragus, pinna, and even the tympanic membrane. Symptoms usually appear within the first 48 hours and can last up to 3 weeks. In cases of inflammation exceeding 3 months, it is defined as chronic otitis externa [1–4].

Eighty percent of the cases are seen during the summer season. It is more common in hot and humid environments. The annual incidence of OE in the United States is determined as four per thousand. However, the lifetime incidence of OE is 10%. The rate of bilaterality is around 10%. Between the ages of 5 and 12, the OE rate increases up to five times. In cases with anatomical or iatrogenic causes that result in obstruction of the external auditory canal, excessive hygienic ear cleaning, hearing aid use, disruptions in the delicate flora, and epithelial integrity of the external auditory canal may initiate the inflammatory process [1–5].

F. Bayakır (✉)
Department of Otolaryngology—Head and Neck Surgery, İnegol State Hospital, Bursa, Turkey
e-mail: ord.dr.ferit@hotmail.com

S. Genç
Department of Otorhinolaryngology, Health Sciences University, Faculty of Medicine, Derince Training and Research Hospital, Kocaeli, Turkey
e-mail: drsgenc@yahoo.com

K. M. Diab
Scientific and Clinical Center of Otorhinolaryngology of the Medico-Biological Agency, and Ministry of Health, Federal State Budgetary Institution, Pirogov Russian National Research Medical University, Moscow, Russia
e-mail: hasandiab@mail.ru

C. Cingi et al. (eds.), *ENT Diseases: Diagnosis and Treatment during Pregnancy and Lactation*, https://doi.org/10.1007/978-3-031-05303-0_39

523

39.2 Pathophysiology

The external auditory canal is an "S"-shaped canal that ends with the tympanic membrane. It is approximately 25 mm long. The outer third of the canal consists of cartilage, and the rest consists of bone. Under the keratinized epithelium that lines the cartilage of external auditory canal, there are hair follicles and glands that produce serum. Serum has the property of making the outer ear canal slightly acidic (pH 5–5.7). Apart from that, it has a bacteriostatic feature with its lysozyme content [2, 3]. The inflammatory process begins with the change of acidic balance in the external ear canal and disruption of the epithelial integrity. During this period, inflammation develops in the epithelium and subepithelial tissue, and pain, swelling, discharge in the ear, sensitivity in the tragus and pinna, fullness, and conductive hearing loss can be seen accordingly [4]. Regional lymphadenitis may be observed in some patients. Ninety-eight percent of the causative pathogens are bacterial. The most common pathogens are *Pseudomonas aeruginosa* (20–60%) and *Staphylococcus aureus* (10–70%) [2, 3]. They are due to fungal and viral reasons, and they develop more sporadically [1, 4, 6]. Chronic OE is a different disease process, and its etiological causes are completely different.

Staphylococcus epidermidis (9%), other *Staphylococcus* species (8%), diphtheroids (9%), other Gram-negative rods (e.g., *Enterobacter, Klebsiella, Proteus, Escherichia coli*) (9%), *Streptococcus-Enterococcus* strains (4%), and *Aspergillus-Candida* strains (2%) are the other most common causative pathogens [4].

39.3 Clinical Presentation

Patients usually present with complaints such as severe ear pain, fullness, hearing loss, and itching and pain spreading to the jaw in the last 3 weeks.

The diagnosis of the disease is made clinically. Symptoms can range from mild pain and swelling to severe pain, edema, and discharge, leading to conductive hearing loss. Typical findings are pain by pressing the tragus or stretching the pinna. External auditory canal edema may be too high to prevent the tympanic membrane from being visible. The tympanic membrane may be hyperemic [2, 5].

39.4 Treatment

The classical treatment steps of OE are pain control, elimination of the causative pathogen, and elimination of predisposing factors. For this purpose, the first approach should be careful cleaning of the ear. The mainstay of treatment is topical antimicrobial and anti-inflammatory drops. These drops must reach the epithelial surface in order to affect the ear. In order to ensure this, cerumen, debris, and foreign body should be cleaned first. In addition, edema that develops in the external ear canal should be removed so that topical drops can reach the target area [2, 7]. Edema is sometimes so severe that topical drops administered cannot reach the external auditory canal. Foam pad made of gelfoam or polyvinyl alcohol to be

Table 39.1 FDA drug categories [8]

Category A
Category A is the safest drug category.
Category B
If necessary, category B drugs can be used.
Category C
The potential benefits may justify the use of the drug in pregnant women despite the potential risks.
Category D
The drug can be used with caution if the mother and fetus face greater risks from not using the drug.
Category X
The risks of the drug outweigh the potential benefits of its use during pregnancy. Its use is not recommended.

placed in the external auditory canal will help both the topical drops to remain constant in that area and the regression of edema with their mechanical effect. The United States Food and Drug Administration (FDA) drug categories related to safe drug use in pregnant women are given in Table 39.1.

OE can rarely cause a severe painful disease that may require parenteral analgesics. Oral nonsteroidal anti-inflammatory drugs (NSADs) often provide adequate analgesia. However, the use of these drugs during pregnancy varies depending on the dose and trimester. For example, while some NSADs are category B in the first trimester, they can be C or even D in the last trimester. Systemic use of NSADs during pregnancy can increase mortality and dead birth by three times. However, the use of systemic paracetamol is recommended as category B in pain control [9–11].

Topical antibiotic drops form the basis of treatment. There are a variety of topical drops available on the market. However, the ideal drop should be effective against pathogenic bacteria, partially acidic, easily accessible, and affordable; on the other hand, it should not be ototoxic, cause allergies, or leave any deposit [3, 4, 7, 12].

There is not yet an ideal topical drop that contains all of the above properties. With the topical use of antibiotics, much higher titration values are achieved in the ear compared to systemic use. This also allows overcoming the bacterial resistance mechanism, so there is not much difference between antibiotic classes in terms of efficacy [4].

Combination of polymyxin, neomycin, and hydrocortisone is effective in eradication of *Pseudomonas aeruginosa* and *Staphylococcus aureus* strains. However, it is not recommended to use neomycin in patients with perforated tympanic membrane due to its ototoxic properties. In addition, considering the 15% development of contact dermatitis due to neomycin, it limits the use of this combination [7].

The quinolones are effective drugs for both *Pseudomonas aeruginosa* and *Staphylococcus aureus*. In addition, they do not have ototoxic effects and do not develop contact dermatitis. However, ciprofloxacin may form deposits in the external auditory canal. Another disadvantage of topical use of quinolones is that their pregnancy category is C. However, there is no evidence that quinolones increase the risk of congenital anomalies or fetal death [8, 12–14].

The steroid ear drops are effective in controlling inflammation, relieving edema and pain control. These drugs make it easier for antibiotics to reach the epithelium. They play an auxiliary role in treatment by partially acidifying the environment. The effect of topical corticosteroids on the fetus is unknown. The teratogenic effects of corticosteroids have been demonstrated in animal studies but have not been confirmed in humans. The categories of topical corticosteroids are designated as C [8, 11, 13, 15].

Systemic antibiotic use is unnecessary in uncomplicated cases. Their use is limited due to increasing bacterial resistance, side effects, and cost. Nevertheless, it has been determined that the topical and systemic antibiotic prescriptions were given together to 44% of the patients by general practitioners in the United Kingdom [5]. Generally, this antibiotic is an ineffective choice against *Pseudomonas aeruginosa.* Systemic antibiotics should generally be preferred in immunosuppressive patients, diabetics, patients receiving radiotherapy, or complicated OE cases [2, 3, 5]. Since the antibiotic to be chosen will get into the systemic circulation and pose a risk for pregnant women, more attention should be given to topical drops. Also, this antibiotic should have a broad spectrum to include *Pseudomonas aeruginosa* and *Staphylococcus aureus* strains.

In the treatment of OE, some topical mixtures may be useful to restore the impaired pH value of the external auditory canal. Mixtures with acidic and antiseptic properties such as boric acid, acetic acid, and aluminum acetate can be given as examples [2–4]. These mixtures can help to relieve the inflammation and pain. They can be used alone or in combination with other topical drops. There is not enough data in terms of the safety of these drops in pregnant women. However, they can be considered in cases where there is no other option left [8, 11, 13].

Fungal hyphae and debris should be carefully cleaned in OE due to fungi. The acidic environment of the external auditory canal must be restored [2–4]. Antifungal creams containing pregnancy category B terbinafine can be used.

Finally, the patient should be advised to stay away from the factors that predispose them to EO. For example, it is necessary to minimize the contact of the ear with water during the illness. In addition, irritating and traumatizing activations such as cotton swabs and the use of earphones should be avoided [2–4].

39.5 Complications

OE can spread to surrounding tissues, resulting in cellulite, perichondritis, and chondritis. External auditory canal stenosis may develop due to recurrent and chronic infections. The tympanic membrane may be perforated. Fatal malignant OE may develop in diabetic patients with poor immune system. Serious complications such as meningitis, cranial abscess, dural sinus thrombosis, and cranial nerve paralysis may develop. In the presence of complications, the causative microorganism should be tried to be identified at first. Then, profit and loss assessment should be made in pregnant patients and systemic antibiotherapy should be started according to the antibiogram result [1–4].

References

1. Roland PS, Stroman DW. Microbiology of acute otitis externa. Laryngoscope. 2002;112:1166–77.
2. Rosenfeld RM et al. Clinical practice guideline: acute otitis externa. Otolaryngol Head and Neck Surgery. 2006; 134: S4-S23.
3. Wipperman J. Otitis externa. Prim Care Clin Office Pract. 2014;41(1):1–9.
4. Cummings CW, Flint PW, Harker L, et al. (eds). Cummings otolaryngology: head and neck surgery. 4th ed. Elsevier Mosby: Philadephia, USA; 2005. pp. 2979–87.
5. Pabla L, Jindal M, Latif K. The management of otitis externa in UK general practice. Eur Arch Otorhinolaryngol. 2012;269:753–6.
6. Ghanpur AD, Nayak DR, Chawla K, Shashidhar V, Rohit S. Comparison of microbiological flora in the external auditory canal of normal ear and an ear with acute otitis externa. J Clin Diagn Res. 2017;11(9):MC01–4.
7. Amani S, Moeini M. Comparison of boric acid and combination drug of polymyxin, neomycin and hydrocortisone (polymyxin NH) in the treatment of acute otitis externa. J Clin Diagn Res. 2016;10(7):MC01–4.
8. Yenerel NM, Küçümen RB. Pregnancy and eye. Turk J Ophthalmol. 2015;45(5):213–9.
9. Swain SK, Pati BK, Mohanty JN. Otological manifestations in pregnant women—a study at a tertiary care hospital of eastern India. J Otol. 2020;13(3):103–6.
10. Özbudak H, Ünal AZ, Sabuncuoğlu S. The evaluation of the use of non-steroidal anti-inflammatory drugs in pregnancy. Marmara Pharm J. 2016;20:64–71.
11. Bozkurt M, Uçar D. Rheumatoid arthritis treatment in pregnancy: a review. Konuralp Med J. 2013;5:62–9.
12. Mösges R, Nematian-Samani M, Eichel A. Treatment of acute otitis externa with ciprofloxacin otic 0.2% antibiotic ear solution. Ther Clin Risk Manag. 2011;7:325–36.
13. Chung CY, Kwok AKH, Chung KL. Use of ophthalmic medications during pregnancy. Hong Kong Med J. 2004;10:191–5.
14. Bomford JA, Ledger JC, O'keeffe BJ, Reiter CH. Ciprofloxacin use during pregnancy. Drugs. 1993;45(Suppl 3):461–2.
15. Schaefer C, Amoura-Elefant E, Vial T, et al. Pregnancy outcome after prenatal quinolone exposure. Evaluation of a case registry of the European network of teratology information services (ENTIS). Eur J Obstet Gynecol Reprod Biol. 1996;69:83–9.

Acute Otitis Media and Otitis Media with Effusion During Pregnancy and the Postpartum Period

40

Kemal Koray Bal, Talih Özdaş, and Hesham Negm

40.1 Introduction

Otitis media (OM) refers to inflammation within the middle ear, which occurs in response to infection by a virus affecting the respiratory tract, or a pathogenic bacterium.

Both acute otitis media (AOM) and otitis media with effusion (OME) occur very frequently, particularly in children. Four out of ten children suffer from an episode of AOM at least once between their third and seventh birthday [1].

The mucosal linings of the respiratory tract frequently become oedematous during pregnancy or after a respiratory tract infection. This may reduce ventilation to the middle ear space, including its mucosal surfaces, and thus provoke an inflammatory response [2].

To treat an episode of AOM or otitis media with effusion (OME), the condition needs first to be accurately diagnosed. There is no perfect way to identify a case of OME or AOM other than on the basis of the clinical features, particularly the onset and course of the illness. Examination of the middle ear must involve sufficient visualisation to permit a diagnosis of otitis media. Thus, the clinician should make use of the biggest speculum that can be comfortably accommodated within the ear canal as this then permits the widest range of views to be obtained. The speculum

K. K. Bal (✉)
Faculty of Medicine, Department of Otorhinolaryngology, Mersin University, Mersin, Turkey
e-mail: dr.kemalkoraybal@gmail.com

T. Özdaş
Department of Otorhinolaryngology, Faculty of Medicine, Health Sciences University, Adana City Training and Research Hospital, Adana, Turkey
e-mail: talih02@gmail.com

H. Negm
Department of Otorhinolaryngology, Faculty of Medicine, Cairo University, Cairo, Egypt
e-mail: drnegment@hotmail.com

C. Cingi et al. (eds.), *ENT Diseases: Diagnosis and Treatment during Pregnancy and Lactation*, https://doi.org/10.1007/978-3-031-05303-0_40

chosen must be a snug fit within the cartilaginous portion of the external auditory meatus. The curvature of the meatus may tend to prevent adequate views, but if the auricle is gently retracted backwards, the speculum may sit more comfortably within the canal. Healthy tympanic membranes appear pearly grey in colour and exhibit translucency, with the handle and short process of the malleus clearly visible. Usually, it is also possible to visualise other components within the middle ear through the membrane. When the tympanic membrane loses these normal appearances, the most frequent causes are AOM or OME. Familiarity with what a clinician is seeing on otoscopy makes for clearer communication with ENT specialists. The appearance of the tympanic membrane in case of otitis media differs considerably from the normal appearances. Furthermore, a patient with OME may describe feeling the ear is full and indicate auditory problems, although in some cases there are actually no symptoms, neither otalgia nor otorrhoea [1, 3].

When performing an otoscopic examination in a patient with OME, the membrane may be in its usual position or have a degree of retraction. The colour tends to be between yellow and creamy white. The membrane will be less mobile than usual and an air-fluid level or bubbles of air may be visible through the membrane.

An effusion that lasts less than 3 weeks is classified as acute, whereas a duration exceeding 3 months qualifies the effusion as chronic.

There are a number of identifiable risk factors for the development of otitis media, particularly a history of acute middle ear infections, infections of the upper airways, adenoid vegetations, congenital abnormalities in anatomy, being bottle-fed, wintertime, exposure to others' smoking, and disorders affecting the nose or sinuses. The disorders of the nose and sinuses that raise the risk of otitis media include sinus inflammation, a deviated septum, atretic or stenotic choanae, nasopharyngeal neoplasms, a poorly pneumatised mastoid, and certain previous medical procedures, especially radiotherapy and stenosis following removal of the adenoids [2].

It has been estimated that the Eustachian tubes function abnormally in between 5% and 30% of women in pregnancy. The dysfunction may arise due to blockage or widening. When the mucosae swell, OME may develop alongside Eustachian blockage and thus dysfunction. This condition generally presents in the second or third trimester. A woman whose Eustachian tubes are blocked may describe feeling her ears are stuffed up. If obstruction is highly severe, sound perception may be altered and OME may occur [4].

If a disorder of the nose or nasopharynx is suspected to underlie a case of OME, endoscopy (rigid or flexible) may be used to obtain detailed views. In this way, an infection, tumour, allergic reaction, or hypertrophied adenoidal tissue may be identified.

There are different findings in patients with AOM from in patients with OME. Otalgia may be present. On otoscopy, the tympanic membrane may be erythematous and the vessels within the membrane stand out. There may be an effusion within the middle ear space, which is recognisable as pus, whilst the eardrum may swell up or be in its usual position. The eardrum is less able to move than in the healthy state.

Accuracy in diagnosing otitis media is vital since treatment is guided by the diagnosis. The 2013 Clinical Practice Guideline: AOM Diagnosis and Management from the American Academy of Pediatrics (AAP) is a further development of the criteria for diagnosis which were originally detailed within the AAP guidelines dating from 2004, but are more detailed. The more recent document stresses the need for the clinician to examine the tympanic membrane using an otoscope before a correct diagnosis can be given.

The key pathogenic bacteria implicated in AOM and OME are *Streptococcus pneumoniae*, *Haemophilus influenzae*, and *Moraxella catarrhalis*. The viruses that are most often identified are rhinovirus, adenovirus, parainfluenza, or influenza virus and respiratory syncytial virus (RSV).

40.2   Tympanometry

Tympanometry and pneumatic otoscopy both enjoy widespread use in paediatric assessment of cases of suspected otitis media. Currently, the majority of primary care settings employ probe frequencies at the lower end of the range, that is, 220–226 Hz. The resulting tympanogram can be classified into one of three types, Jerger A, Jerger B, or Jerger C. A normal tympanogram is Jerger type A. Type C shows maximum middle ear compliance at a negative ear canal pressure, and type B is flat, without a clear peak. Pneumatic otoscopy has greater precision than tympanometry, but the latter has the greatest utility for excluding a case of OME [5].

There are a number of other investigations that may be used to assess the middle ear, in cases where otitis media is suspected, such as high-frequency (1000 Hz) tympanometry, multifrequency tympanometry and wideband acoustic transmission functions, particularly wideband reflectance (WBR) tympanometry. Experimental evidence confirms the utility of these techniques in ruling in or out an effusion of the middle ear. 1 kHz frequency tympanograms are useful to screen babies under 1 year of age and to ascertain wideband reflectance. However, there is a need for further studies to delineate the precise part they should play in diagnosis. A further investigation of value in suspected middle ear effusion is acoustic reflectometry. This latter is almost as sensitive and specific as pneumatic otoscopy or tympanometry in diagnosing a middle ear effusion [6, 7].

40.3   Audiological Testing

Audiometric evaluation is suitable for the assessment of auditory function in cases of OM. However, an abnormal result should only be attributed to a middle ear effusion where the effusion has been present for at least 3 months, otherwise another cause should be suspected in a child who speaks late or has difficulty learning. Audiometry may reveal auditory loss of up to 55 dB in a patient with OM. The mean auditory loss is 25 dB, and around one in five cases has a loss above 35 dB. The type of hearing loss is conductive and occurs due to the presence of an effusion occupying the middle ear space or because the tympanic membrane is being retracted. It is usual for the very-low-frequency sounds to be lost to a greater extent than higher pitched sounds because of the way the sound is transmitted via the eardrum and ossicles [7, 8].

OM is amongst the most frequently occurring conditions to affect very young children or the paediatric age group in general. Although antibiotic therapy has been extensively researched in OM, there is no consensus as to the optimum treatment. There were guidelines issued in 2013 to update the earlier suggested treatment for OME, which dates from 2004. In 2014 the new recommendations covered treatment in paediatric patients who have grommets in situ [9, 10].

In fact, antibiotics offer only partial benefit in cases of AOM, unless it is severe. However, many clinicians prefer to use antibiotics in this condition out of fear that AOM is complicated by mastoiditis or meningitis. There is also evidence indicating that timely administration of antibiotic therapy in cases of AOM does actually shorten the period needed for symptoms to begin resolving.

Prior to administering antibiotics, or any other medication, to a pregnant woman, the clinician should be aware of any potential harm to the mother or foetus and should seek an obstetric opinion first [11].

If the decision to prescribe antibiotic therapy has been made, and provided there is no penicillin allergy, it is recommended in the guidelines that amoxicillin be employed at a dose of 80–90 mg/kg/day in total, administered b.d. The patient should also not have received amoxicillin within the preceding 30 days. Where amoxicillin has been used in this period or there have been previous repeated episodes of AOM where amoxicillin was ineffective, co-amoxiclav is suitable. The dose recommendation is 90 mg/kg/day in total, administered b.d. (i.e., at the high end of the dose range). Choice of medication should be guided by the FDA categorisation of medications for use in pregnancy. Virtually all pharmacological agents administered to the mother are capable of crossing the placenta, and the level in the foetal circulation may range from half the mother's serum level to the same level. The FDA has categorised the following antibiotic agents as category B: azithromycin, cephalosporins, erythromycin, clindamycin, and penicillins (including co-amoxiclav, ampicillin-sulbactam). The recommendation is to avoid employing antibiotics as prophylaxis for AOM. If an analgesic is required, paracetamol or aspirin is currently thought safe up to the third trimester. Nonetheless, aspirin, which falls under category C, does entail a risk of prolonged bleeding in both the woman and the foetus [12–14].

Amongst the NSAIDs, ibuprofen and naproxen do not raise the risk of a congenital malformation, but the former has been linked to a lower volume of amniotic fluid. Additionally, there is a theoretical risk that these agents may make the ductus arteriosus close prematurely, given their known action of inhibiting prostaglandin synthetase. The FDA classifies ibuprofen and naproxen as category B. The more recently marketed agents which inhibit COX-2, for example, celecoxib or rofecoxib, are classified as category C [15].

In theory, decongestants given orally may lead to a reduction in arterial supply to the uterus, but this has so far not been reported to actually occur. Nonetheless, pregnant women who may have placental insufficiency or hypertension due to pregnancy may not receive systemic agents causing vasoconstriction. Pseudoephedrine is classified by the FDA as a category C agent, but, despite this, it is still recommended as a decongestant when taken orally [16].

Xylometazoline is used topically for decongestion. It is under category C. There is an associated risk of rhinitis medicamentosa [16].

The anti-histamines that fall under category B are chlorpheniramine, cetirizine, loratadine, and diphenhydramine [17].

Myringotomy or tympanocentesis undertaken during an acute episode of OM is associated with less pain and has the additional benefit of permitting a sample to be sent to microbiology for culture and sensitivity testing. Nonetheless, neither the duration of the effusion nor the risk of recurrence is lessened by either operation [18].

Several studies have proven that grommet insertion has the benefit of making recurrence less frequent in cases of recurrent AOM [19].

Turning to the subject of adjunctive treatments, neither anti-histamine nor decongestant pharmacotherapy in cases of OME has any proven clinical advantage. Guidelines issued in 2004 deprecate the use of either class of agent. Furthermore, administration of corticosteroids by mouth is also not recommended since any benefit is of relatively brief duration and comes at the cost of a large number of potential adverse effects.

It has been established that topical nasal steroids have a low systemic absorption and thus a lower incidence of adverse effects, but the review published by the Cochrane Collaboration in 2010 failed to find any benefit from the use of topical nasal steroids in OME, whether used as monotherapy or alongside antibiotics, and regardless of the length of follow-up [20].

References

1. Preciado D, editor. Otitis media: state of the art concepts and treatment. Heidelberg: Springer; 2015.
2. Vlastarakos PV, Nikolopoulos TP, Manolopoulos L, et al. Treating common ear problems in pregnancy: what is safe? Eur Arch Otorhinolaryngol. 2008;265(2):139–45.
3. Lieberthal AS, Carroll AE, Chonmaitree T, et al. The diagnosis and management of acute otitis media. Pediatrics. 2013;131(3):964–99.
4. Weissman A, Nir D, Shenhav R, et al. Eustachian tube function during pregnancy. Clin Otolaryngol Allied Sci. 1993;18(3):212–4.
5. Jerger JF. Clinical experience with impedence audiometry. Arch Otolaryngol. 1970;92:311–24.
6. Hızalan MI. Effüzyonlu otitis media. In: Çelik O, editor. Kulak Burun Boğaz Hastalıkları ve Baş Boyun Cerrahisi. Istanbul: Turgut Yayıncılık; 2002.
7. Akyıldız N. Kulak Hastalıkları ve Mikrocerrahisi Cilt-1. Ankara: Bilimsel Tıp Kitapevi; 1998.
8. Stach BA. Audiologic evaluation of otologic/neurotologic disease. In: Gulya AJ, Minor LB, Poe DS, editors. Glasscock-Shambaugh's surgery of the ear. 6th ed. Shelton, CT: People's Medical Publishing House; 2010. p. 189–221.
9. American Academy of Pediatrics Subcommittee on Management of Acute Otitis Media. Diagnosis and management of acute otitis media. Pediatrics. 2004;113(5):1451–65.
10. Rosenfeld RM, Culpepper L, Doyle KJ, et al. Clinical practice guideline: otitis media with effusion. Otolaryngol Head Neck Surg. 2004;130:95–118.
11. Cavanaugh SJ. Pregnant pause. Johns Hopkins Magazine. 2001;53(4):50–7.
12. Grijalva CG, Nuorti JP, Griffin MR. Antibiotic prescription rates for acute respiratory tract infections in US ambulatory settings. JAMA. 2009;302(7):758–66.

13. Koc C, Muluk NB. Otitis Media'da Tanıya Gidiş. Türkiye Klinikleri J Surg Med Sci. 2005;1(7):15–9.
14. McCaig LF, Besser RE, Hughes JM. Trends in antimicrobial prescribing rates for children and adolescents. JAMA. 2002;287(23):3096–102.
15. Hickok DE, Hollenbach KA, Reilley SO, et al. The association between decreased amniotic fluid volume and treatment with nonsteroidal anti-inflammatory agents for preterm labor. Am J Obstet Gynecol. 1989;160:1525–30; discussion 1530–1.
16. Ambro BT, Scheid SC, Pribitkin EA. Prescribing guidelines for ENT medications during pregnancy. Ear Nose Throat J. 2003;82(8):565–8.
17. Schatz M, Petitti D. Antihistamines and pregnancy. Ann Allergy Asthma Immunol. 1997;78:157–9.
18. Kaleida PH, Casselbrant ML, Rockette HE, et al. Amoxicillin or myringotomy or both for acute otitis media: results of a randomized clinical trial. Pediatrics. 1991;87(4):466–74.
19. Gebhart DE. Tympanostomy tubes in the otitis media prone child. Laryngoscope. 1981;91(6):849–66.
20. Simpson SA, Lewis R, van der Voort J, et al. Oral or topical nasal steroids for hearing loss associated with otitis media with effusion in children. Cochrane Database Syst Rev. 2011, 2011;(5):CD001935. https://doi.org/10.1002/14651858.CD001935.pub3.

## Part IV

Rhinology and Allergy During Pregnancy and the Postpartum Period

Gözde Orhan Kubat, Caner Şahin, and Nuray Bayar Muluk

41.1 Introduction

Rhinitis and sinusitis are common diseases in which everyone may be affected at least once or more. Rhinitis is a condition that causes loss of efficiency and large economic expenses in patients [1].

Rhinitis has a wide range, which includes different inflammatory phenotypes. There are allergic, infectious, and nonallergic noninfectious subgroups [2].

Although clinical features, diagnosis, and treatment of respiratory tract infections are similar in pregnant and nonpregnant patients, an increased susceptibility to infection during pregnancy and changes in female physiology should be considered. The effects of infection and treatment on the fetus should be considered.

Acute respiratory infections, including acute uncomplicated bronchitis, pharyngitis, RS, and colds, are caused by viruses and do not require antibiotic therapy.

Also, 20–40% of women stated that they had rhinitis and sinonasal disease during their fertility years. About 10–30% said their complaints worsened during pregnancy [3].

Nasal reactive conditions and increased blood volume induced by maternal hormones are accused of rhinitis in pregnant women. In a study of a group selected randomly from pregnancies, 30% of patients were shown to report symptoms of

G. O. Kubat (✉) · C. Şahin
Department of Otorhinolaryngology, Faculty of Medicine, Alaattin Keykubat University, Alanya, Turkey
e-mail: drgkubat@gmail.com; caner.sahin@alanya.edu.tr

N. Bayar Muluk
Department of Otorhinolaryngology, Faculty of Medicine, Kırıkkale University, Kırıkkale, Turkey
e-mail: nbayarmuluk@yahoo.com

C. Cingi et al. (eds.), *ENT Diseases: Diagnosis and Treatment during Pregnancy and Lactation*, https://doi.org/10.1007/978-3-031-05303-0_41

rhinitis and rhinosinusitis (RS). This rate may be higher in patients with a history of atopy [4].

Causes of rhinitis that frequently require treatment in pregnant women include pregnancy rhinitis, allergic rhinitis, rhinitis medicamentosa, RS, and vasomotor rhinitis [4, 5].

The frequency of sinusitis can be as high as 1.5% in pregnancy, which indicates a sixfold increase compared to the nonpregnant population [4].

41.2 Respiratory System Physiology in Pregnancy

During pregnancy, there are important anatomical, physiological, and biochemical adaptations in respiratory, cardiac, and other systems. The changes start with fertilization and continue throughout pregnancy [6].

Most adaptations are affected by hormonal or mechanical stimulus that occurs with the growth of the uterus. Increasing estrogen and progesterone increases mucosal vacuity, edema, and incidence of rhinitis and epistaxis. The incidence of gastroesophageal reflux disease (GERD) and pregnancy rhinitis increases. GERD also causes postnasal drip [4, 6].

The nasal mucosal histology of pregnant women differs from those who are not pregnant [4]. In the first and second trimesters of pregnancy, blood volume and plasma increase in circulation. In the upper respiratory tract mucosa, the extravascular area is plasma cured in the third trimester. Estrogen has a direct cholinergic effect on the nasal mucosa, which causes vascular dilation; glandular hypersecretion, increased phagocytic activity, and increased mucopolysaccharide content are observed. This situation decreases within 5 days in the postpartum period [3, 7].

Most women with gestational rhinitis are affected in different ways by physiological changes [4].

Physiological dyspnea is a common condition seen in 60–70% of women as of 30 weeks of pregnancy. In physiological changes, blood volume changes, central hemodynamic, and pulmonary vascular changes are seen. Variable parameters are shown in Table 41.1 [7].

Knowing the changes in respiratory physiology during pregnancy is important in the diagnosis and treatment of respiratory diseases. It is necessary to pay attention to some points while evaluating:

Table 41.1 Hemodynamic changes in pregnancy

Parameters	%
Cardiac output	30–50 increase
Heart rate	15–20 increase
Stroke volume	20–30 increase
Main arterial pressure	0–5 decrease
Systemic vascular resistance	20–30 increase
Pulmonary vascular resistance	30 decrease

- Although physiological dyspnea is common in pregnancy, no change in the number of breaths is expected.
- In pregnant women, hypoxia and acidosis develop faster than in nonpregnant women.
- It may increase the risk and severity of infection due to changes in the immune system during pregnancy.

41.3 Rhinitis Symptoms and Signs

Rhinitis is a symptomatic inflammatory disease of the nasal mucosa with at least two nasal symptoms [8]. Rhinitis symptoms are written below:

41.3.1 Nasal Congestion and Difficulty Breathing through the Nose

Structural disorders of the septum (turbinate hypertrophy, septum deviation, foreign body in the nose, nasal polyp, tumor), gastroesophageal reflux [9, 10], nasal reflexes (postural reflex, warm–cold skin temperature reflex, light reflex, bronchionasal reflex, ovulatory reflex) [11], in diseases such as allergic rhinitis, pregnancy rhinitis, infectious rhinitis, and as a side effect of some medications (aspirin, antihypertensive drugs, nonsteroidal anti-inflammatory drugs) [12], they should be kept in mind in differential diagnosis since nasal obstruction may be complained.

Smoking, allergic rhinitis, infection, and long-term topical vasoconstrictor spray use are among the causes of nonhormonal nasal obstruction during pregnancy [7].

41.3.2 Itching in the Nose

41.3.3 A Discharge from the Anterior or Posterior of the Nose

41.3.4 Odor Disorder

Odor disorder is a frequent finding in chronic RS (CRS) patients and decreases the quality of life [13]. CRS disease is reported as the most common cause of odor disorder [14]. There is a decrease in smell in rhinitis, pregnancy, and the postpartum period [15].

41.4　Clinical Approach

In the evaluation of a pregnant woman, there is anamnesis, physical examination, and differential diagnosis similar to a nonpregnant patient. It should be determined whether the diagnostic and treatment approaches bear any risk for the patient or fetus. Potential fetal risks of the disease, diagnosis, and treatment should be taken into consideration, with the increased susceptibility of the pregnant patient to the disease and its susceptibility to complications. Alternative diagnosis and treatment methods should be explored and explained to the patient.

41.5　Pregnancy Rhinitis

Gestational rhinitis has been defined as nasal congestion, seen in the last 1–2 months of pregnancy, without respiratory infection symptoms and a known history of allergy, disappearing completely within 2 weeks after birth [16]. Although the etiology of pregnancy rhinitis is not known clearly, hormonal changes are blamed, and estrogen increases the production of mucosal acetylcholine, causing edema and hypersecretion [17]. Placental growth hormone (PGH) was found to be high in pregnancy rhinitis [12].

In 18–42% [18–20] of pregnant women, symptomatic nasal congestion and serous secretion are observed during pregnancy. Mouth breathing should be done due to nasal congestion. Obstructive sleep apnea syndrome (OSAS) and associated poor quality sleep, daytime sleepiness, headache, and lack of concentration are observed [20, 21]. OSAS negatively affects the growth of the fetus and gestational hypertension [22], and can trigger the development of other diseases such as gestational hypertension and sinusitis [7].

Symptoms and signs may not be correlated in pregnancy rhinitis. Although nasal congestion is observed in the early period of the first trimester, complaints peak in the late stages of pregnancy. Increased blood volume in pregnancy also plays a role in etiology [7].

Smoking and allergic factors have been accused in etiology, but they have not been confirmed [22]. Other causes of rhinitis should be excluded from diagnosis [18].

41.6　Treatment

There is no obvious treatment. Firstly, nonpharmacological treatment methods are recommended. From pharmacological treatments, short-term nasal decongestants and long-term topical nasal steroids may be useful [12].

Oral decongestants contain pseudoephedrine, although these preparations are not recommended in the first trimester and in pregnant women with hypertension, although they can rarely be used in the second and third trimesters with severe rhinitis [23].

41.6.1 Common Cold

Similar to nonpregnant patients, cold symptoms are mild in pregnant women and do not require treatment. However, many pregnant patients resort to clinicians for treatment. In a cold, symptoms disappear in about 10 days, but cough complaints can last longer. There are no reliable data on randomized controlled trials and teratogenic risks in the treatment of colds in pregnant women. Drug therapy can alleviate symptoms, but it does not shorten the duration. Therefore, treatment should be started after the effects of the disease and the side effects of the treatments on pregnancy and fetus are explained [24].

The use of acetaminophen for sore throat and headache and inhalation of heated, humidified air for nasal congestion is the most reliable and effective treatment method. Nasal ipratropium bromide nasal spray can be used in patients with severe rhinorrhea; teratogenic effects have not been observed in animal studies, but no study on humans. Other options for patients with severe cold symptoms include intranasal chromoline sodium spray for nasal congestion, and drugs containing dextromethorphan or guaifenesin for cough suppression. Caution should be exercised in asthmatic patients as inhaled cromolyn preparations can cause temporary bronchospasm, throat irritation, and cough. Antibiotics are not indicated for treatment in the common cold except for the group of patients who develop secondary bacterial infection. The pregnancy of the patient does not constitute an indication for the use of antibiotics [24].

In an epidemiological study, the association of colds or colds with fever with the risk of preterm birth and congenital anomaly has been shown, but this relationship has not been shown in patients without fever [25].

41.6.2 Rhinosinusitis

Due to the vasculary, nervous and anatomical connections of the nose and sinuses, inflammation and congestion occur together in the nasal structure and sinuses in the upper respiratory tract infections, and therefore the infection is called RS [26]. In the diagnosis of RS, complaints of nasal obstruction or nasal discharge (anterior or posterior discharge), pressure on the face, and loss of smell are found [26].

When rhinosinusitis is classified by time:

- In acute RS, which takes less than 4 weeks.
- In subacute RS, which takes between 4 and 12 weeks.
- In chronic RS, there are symptoms that last longer than 12 weeks.
- Recurrent acute RS has four or more acute sinusitis attacks per year with a full recovery period in between [24].

41.6.3 Acute Rhinosinusitis (ARS)

Its annual prevalence is in the range of 6–15% and is mostly seen after viral colds. ARS symptoms last less than 4 weeks [27]. It is classified according to etiology and clinical findings [27].

<u>Acute viral rhinosinusitis (AVRS)</u>: Viruses are involved in the etiology.

<u>Uncomplicated acute bacterial rhinosinusitis (ABRS)</u>: Bacteria are involved in the etiology. There is no extension outside the paranasal sinus and nasal cavity.

<u>Complicated acute bacterial RS</u> (ABRS): The cause is bacteria, leading to complications (neurological, ophthalmological, or soft tissue) by extending out of the paranasal sinus and nasal cavity [27].

Its incidence is high in adults aged 45–64 years. Age, smoking, air travel, atmospheric pressure change (e.g., diving), swimming, concomitant history of asthma and allergies, dental disease, and immune deficiency are risk factors for ARS [28].

41.6.4 Acute Viral RS

It begins with the inoculation of viruses into the nasal mucosa or conjunctiva. Symptoms begin approximately 1 day after inoculation. Rhinovirus, influenza, and parainfluenza viruses are the most common viruses in AVRS. Symptoms pass between 7 and 10 days on average [26].

Viral rhinitis spreads to the paranasal sinuses systemically or directly. Applying positive intranasal pressure pushes nasal discharge, which is contaminated by virus, from the nasal cavity to the sinuses. An increase in inflammation causes an increase in vascular permeability and an increase in secretion in the nasal cavity and paranasal sinuses. Viruses also disrupt nasal mucociliary clearance. Sinuses become obliterated due to increased secretion and impaired mucociliary activity [27].

41.6.5 Acute Bacterial RS

Some of the ARS cases are of bacterial origin. It develops secondary to sinus mucosa inflammation. ABRS is also associated with impaired mucociliary clearance conditions such as nasal congestion, impaired local or systemic immune function, impaired mucociliary clearance conditions such as allergic nonallergic rhinitis, nasal structural disorders, dental infection, cystic fibrosis, and ciliary dysfunction syndrome [27].

The most common bacterial agents are *Streptococcus pneumoniae*, *Haemophilus influenzae*, and *Moraxella catarrhalis*. Anaerobic bacteria can be detected in dental infections [29]. Although there are studies indicating that ABRS infection is more common in pregnant patients than nonpregnant patients [30], this issue was not supported in large-scale studies [31]. Since many pregnant women do not have classic symptoms and signs of sinusitis, the diagnosis of sinusitis should always be kept in mind during pregnancy [32].

41.6.6 Chronic Rhinosinusitis

Chronic rhinosinusitis is a complex disease consisting of various variants, with different underlying pathophysiological mechanisms. Limited information is available in terms of CRS pathophysiology and treatment approaches [26]. CRS is characterized by inflammation of the paranasal sinus mucosa. It is divided into two main clinical groups according to nasal endoscopic examination: CRS with nasal polyp and CRS without nasal polyp [33]. In the literature, the information on the diagnosis and treatment of rhinosinusitis disease during pregnancy is very low. This makes it difficult to approach the treatment of rhinosinusitis in pregnant women [34].

The effectiveness of imaging methods, the similarity of clinical symptoms and findings in upper respiratory diseases, and treatment and clinical approaches are still controversial issues [26]. The American Academy of Otorhinolaryngology, Head and Neck Surgery and the European Society of Rhinology cannot offer finalized guideline for use in pregnant patients in the treatment of chronic rhinosinusitis [34].

41.7 Symptoms

Among the symptoms of ARS are nasal congestion, purulent runny nose, maxillary toothache, feeling of fullness in the sinuses when bent forward, localized facial pain, or pressure. These also include fever, weakness, cough, hyposmia or anosmia, ear pressure or fullness, headache, and bad breath. Patients may also have signs and symptoms of Eustachian tube dysfunction (e.g., ear pain, fullness or pressure, hearing loss, or tinnitus) [27].

Purulent nasal discharge can also be seen in AVRS, and purulent discharge is a symptom of sinus inflammation. In a few days, it becomes serous secretion. Fever is usually absent. When there is a fever, it passes within 24–48 hours [35].

In order to diagnose ABRS, the criteria supported by the American Society of Infectious Diseases and the American Academy of Otorhinolaryngology and Head and Neck Surgery should be evaluated [27]:

Symptoms and symptoms last at least 10 days and the clinic does not worsen.

Having a fever, purulent runny nose, or facial pain >39 °C from the beginning of the disease, continuing for at least 3–4 consecutive days.

The person has had viral upper respiratory disease in the anamnesis, her existing complaints worsened, or she has complaints of new fever, headache, and runny nose.

At least two clinical findings should be supported by objective and radiological findings in the diagnosis of CRS. At least one finding should be one of nasal secretion or nasal congestion. Other findings may be pain and smell disorders on the face [26].

The majority of RS cases are of viral origin, secondary bacterial infection occurs in a small population of patients. In uncomplicated VRS patients, complaints pass on average 7–10 days. Some pregnant patients do not have nasal congestion, purulent runny nose, maxillary toothache, odor loss, facial pain, and pressure sensation, with classic RS complaints and signs. In pregnant patients, with the effect of congestion of the nasal mucosa caused by hormonal changes, there is a high risk of developing RS and Eustachian tube dysfunction after a cold [30].

41.8 Physical Examination Findings

Erythema or edema in the periorbital region, sensitivity in the cheek area, upper teeth, increased facial pain with sinus percussion and pressure sensation, and purulent discharge in the nose or posterior pharynx [27]. Physical examination findings are not sensitive and specific for RS. Transillumination of the sinuses can be examined in endoscopic examination, but this method can only be used to examine the maxillary and frontal sinuses, and it does not have high sensitivity or specificity in diagnosis [36].

In anterior rhinoscopic examination, diffuse mucosal edema, narrowing of the middle meatus, lower turbinate hypertrophy, and nasal purulent discharge may be observed. Polyps or septum deviation are anatomical risk factors in the development of ABRS [27]. Endoscopic examination is important in showing mucosal edema, secretion, and polyp structure, especially in osteomeatal complex or sphenoethmoidal recess [26].

In endoscopic examination, nasal polyps, mucopurulent discharge, moderate meatus edema, or mucosal obstruction, and changes in paranasal sinus mucosa in tomography imaging are objective diagnostic criteria of CRS [26].

41.9 Complications

ARS is generally a self-limiting disease, but life-threatening and even death-threatening complications have also been described [37].

Complications occur when bacterial infection spreads from the paranasal sinuses and nasal cavity to the central nervous system, orbit, or surrounding anatomical structures. Complications directly from adjacent anatomical structures, bone dehiscences, and cavities also can spread through diploic veins (Breschet veins), thrombophlebitis, and osteitis [37].

Complications are classified as local or systemic. Local complications are mucocele, pre-septal cellulitis, orbital cellulitis, subperiosteal abscess, orbital abscess, osteomyelitis, meningitis, brain abscess, subdural empyema, and sinus vein thrombosis [37]. Pre-septal cellulitis, orbital cellulitis, subperiosteal abscess, and orbital abscess are the most common complications [38].

Orbital complications are divided into five stages according to the Chandler classification:

Stage 1: inflammatory edema and pre-septal cellulitis.
Stage 2: orbital cellulitis.
Stage 3: subperiosteal abscess.
Stage 4: orbital abscess.
Stage 5: cavernous sinus thrombosis [39].

Pre-septal (periorbital) cellulitis: There is eyelid edema and pain in the eyes. Increased pain with proptosis, double vision, and eye movements are absent at this stage.

Orbital cellulitis: It is a clinic of infection that occurs in the soft tissues posterior to the orbital septum. Ocular pain, eyelid edema, and erythema are present in patients with orbital cellulitis. Proptosis and diplopia can be seen.

Subperiosteal abscess: When orbital cellulitis progresses, abscess formation develops. Proptosis, pain that increases with eye movements, diplopia, decrease in visual acuity, limitation of eye movements, and the mass effect of abscess are exophthalmos.

Osteomyelitis: A few days after the onset of symptoms of ARS, pain, tension, warmth, erythema, and edema occur suddenly on the affected sinus side. There may be fever and restlessness complaints.

Meningitis: Fever, neck stiffness, and change in consciousness are seen in meningitis.

Intracranial abscess: The complaint of headache that does not respond to medical treatment. Fever, neck stiffness, mental change, nausea, and vomiting often accompany.

Septic cavernous sinus thrombosis: Although it has nonspecific symptoms, it should be kept in mind in the differential diagnosis in the presence of cranial nerve palsy.

When complications develop, the patient should be evaluated urgently, and radiological imaging and microbiological tests should be performed.

Treatment of complications varies depending on the stage and orbital involvement. Chandler 1–3 stages are treated with broad-spectrum antibiotics. If visual impairment occurs, it may be necessary to treat it surgically. Surgery and medical treatment should be applied together in Chandler 4–5 stages. Anticoagulant therapy is still controversial in cavernous sinus thrombosis, but it can be added. Penicillin and amoxicillin-lavulanate are antibiotics that should be given in the first step. While oral treatment can be given at an early stage, parenteral treatment should be applied at stages 2–5 [39].

Intracranial complications usually develop secondary to ethmoidal or frontal sinusitis. High fever, nausea–vomiting, mental status changes, meningeal irritation findings, and headache are the main symptoms. Neurological findings such as behavior or movement change may be seen in the development of intracranial abscess. Emergency drainage and long-term use of antibiotics are required for abscess development [39].

If frontal sinusitis causes vascular necrosis in the frontal bone and osteitis in the anterior–posterior tabula of the frontal sinus, it causes a palpable mass under the skin and is called a Pott's puffy tumor. Posterior tabula osteitis can cause meningitis, peridural abscess, or brain abscess. Surgical drainage, debridement of necrotic tissues, and broad-spectrum antibiotics are the main treatment methods [38].

41.10 Radiological Imaging

The damages of ionizing radiation in the fetus depend on the dose of radiation and the weeks of gestation. The most sensitive period of the fetal nervous system is between the tenth and 17th weeks of pregnancy, and it is necessary to avoid radiation as much as possible during this period [3]. The maximum cumulative dose of ionizing radiation that can be taken during pregnancy is 5 rad [40]. Ionizing radiation may cause spontaneous abortion and malformation development with cumulative dose effect [41].

Paranasal sinus MRI does not contain radiation, but most of the diagnoses require contrast and contrast material is harmful to the fetus. CT is superior to MRI in operation planning. The patient should be discussed with the contrast agent, the ionizing radiation dose of CT, and all the risks the disease may cause [3].

Radiological imaging has no place in the diagnosis of uncomplicated sinusitis cases [35]. In CT, air-fluid level in the sinuses and mucosal edema suggests ARS, but they are not specific findings [26].

Radiological imaging should be performed using the pelvic shield in pregnant women in the presence of symptoms and findings suggestive of complications such as decreased visual acuity, diplopia, periorbital edema, severe headache, and change in mental status [42]. Although the sensitivity and specificity of direct radiographs are low, direct radiographs should be preferred before CT because the radiation dose is lower [42]. CT and MRI should be preferred before complicated, treatment-resistant or surgical procedures.

While CT and MRI are taken with contrast in nonpregnant women, contrast material should be avoided in pregnant patients [42].

The risk of ionizing radiation (diagnostic X-ray) during breastfeeding has not been demonstrated [42].

41.11 Microbiological Tests

When the complications have been developed, culture should be taken from the middle meatus or maxillary sinus with the help of an endoscope. The blind swab technique is not suitable for taking aspirate culture.

S. pneumoniae, H. influenzae, and *Moraxella catarrhalis* have been shown to be the bacteria most commonly grown in ABRS in cultures taken from the maxillary sinus [27]. In a study, in the sinus aspirate, 20–43% *S. pneumoniae,* 22–35% *H. influenzae,* 2–10% *M. catarrhalis,* and 10% *Staphylococcus aureus* were detected [27].

41.12 Treatment

Although the treatment approach in pregnant patients is similar to nonpregnant patients, there are main differences. Different algorithms are followed in acute RS and chronic RS patients [43]. When using drugs in a pregnant woman, the potential risks of the drugs and the risks of untreated diseases should be evaluated together. It is known that drug use during pregnancy has harm potential, but less than 1% of drugs have been associated with congenital malformations [44]. However, from an ethical point of view, it is not possible to prove that any drug is safe for a pregnant woman.

In pregnant patients who are immunocompetent, in good general condition, and uncomplicated, a wait-and-see approach with close follow-up is recommended and antibiotic treatment will be initiated in case of worsening of the clinical picture. Antibiotics should be initiated in the presence of acute rhinosinusitis symptoms such as fever, nasal congestion, purulent runny nose, and severe headache. High fever is closely related to the serious disease picture [34]. It should not be used in pregnant women due to the negative effects of fluoroquinolones and tetracyclines on fetus cartilage, bone, and dental structures. Correct diagnosis and treatment are important for rational antibiotic use [1].

As an adjunct to antibiotic therapy, saline nasal spray or saline nasal irrigation, acetaminophen and steroid nasal sprays (e.g., beclomethasone or budesonide) may be given for patients who cannot tolerate nasal obstruction and pain [34]. Nasal steroids provide limited symptomatic benefits in patients with sinusitis; they will be more useful in patients with underlying allergic rhinitis. Antihistamines have not been shown to be effective in the symptomatic treatment of acute bacterial sinusitis in nonatopic patients. Treatment of rhinosinusitis during pregnancy has not been adequately described in the literature. The American Academy of Otorhinolaryngology Head and Neck Surgery and the European Rhinology Association does not provide reliable guidelines on the treatment of rhinosinusitis in pregnant patients [34].

The US Food and Drug Administration (FDA) divided drugs into five categories (A, B, C, D, and X) based on their potential to cause adverse effects during pregnancy and required drugs introduced after 1980 to be classified according to these categories in their package insert [45]. The categories are prepared by looking at the results of animal studies, human data, and whether the benefit of the drug during pregnancy outweighs the risk.

In treatments, it is recommended to choose B class to C class (risk cannot be neglected) drugs based on reliable animal studies. Oral steroids and decongestants are in class C and should be avoided in the first trimester. Topical steroids have minimal systemic absorption, and although the risk of adverse effects on the fetus is low, they are in class C, except budesonide [3] (Table 41.2).

According to the US FDA five-letter pregnancy risk classification [46]:

Category A: In controlled studies on pregnant women, there was no risk for the fetus in the first trimester of pregnancy (no risk evidence for subsequent trimesters).

Category B: Animal studies have not demonstrated a risk to the fetus, and there are no controlled studies on pregnant women.

Category C: There are no controlled studies on pregnant women, and animal studies have shown an adverse effect on the fetus. It is stated that the use of the drug is acceptable despite the potential risks of its benefits in pregnant women.

Table 41.2 Risk classification

	Class B	Classes C and D
Antimicrobial agents	Penicillins (including sulbactam and clavulanate), cephalosporin, clindamycin, erythromycin, azithromycin	Clarithromycin, fluoroquinolone, aminoglycoside, sulfonamide, tetracycline, vancomycin
Antihistamine agents	Chlorpheniramine, loratadine, cetirizine	Brompheniramine, fexofenadine
Intranasal steroids	Budesonide	Mometasone, beclomethasone, fluticasone
Decongest		Neo-synephrine, oxymetazoline

Category D: According to research and marketing experiences and studies in humans, there is evidence that there is a risk of adverse reactions in the fetus, but the potential benefits of using the drug in pregnant women are acceptable despite the potential risks.

Category X: Based on research marketing experience, abnormalities in the animal or human fetus have been demonstrated. Reports state that although there is positive evidence about fetal risk the risk of using the drug in a pregnant woman clearly outweighs any benefit [46].

41.12.1 Nonpharmacological Treatments

Nonpharmacological treatments should be recommended first in pregnant patients.

Hypertonic nasal sprays or nasal irrigation: It is a safe, nonpharmacological, effective treatment method. It can be applied to many diseases such as pregnancy rhinitis, allergic rhinitis, and acute rhinosinusitis [34].

Exercise: Exercise at regular intervals can help relief by making nasal vasoconstriction. Controlled exercise during pregnancy is beneficial for the mother and fetus, helping to reduce the risk of gestational diabetes and preeclampsia. During exercise, nasal resistance decreases, which starts at 30 seconds and reaches maximum effect in the fifth minute, and this effect continues for another 30 minutes after exercise [11].

External valve opening bands or intranasal apparatuses and raising the bed head 30–45 degrees are not a permanent solution, but they can relieve patients while they sleep at night [47].

41.12.2 Pharmacological Treatments

Oxymetazoline HCL drops or sprays should be used in the minimum dose and for 3–5 days when needed. There is a risk of developing rhinitis medicamentosa with the use of oxymetazoline for more than 5 days [4, 12]. Systemic absorption of topical oxymetazoline is negligible. Hypertension, rebound hypotension, shock development, and placental insufficiency may develop due to overdose use of topical imidazoline [21].

Oral corticosteroids: It can be used for a short time after the first trimester. It is more useful in chronic RS cases causing asthma exacerbation. Oral CKS has been associated with a low rate of cleft lip (with or without cleft palate), preeclampsia, preterm delivery, and low birth weight [34].

The risk of untreated asthma, the risks that may be experienced due to chronic RS, and the risks of CCS should be evaluated and decided according to the patient's clinic. It may have teratogenic effects in the first trimester. Hyperglycemia and diabetes may occur or cause diabetes to worsen. This may lead to additional maternal–fetus risks. If long-term CCS is to be initiated in the pregnant woman, diabetes research should be done first [34]. The American Academy of Pediatrics stated that the mother can use oral CCS while breastfeeding.

Nasal topical corticosteroids: New-generation nasal CSSs should be used at recommended doses during pregnancy and the postpartum period for safety. New-generation nasal sprays have negligible systemic absorption, but there is no evidence that unwanted side effects during pregnancy will not occur [34].

As in the treatment of allergic rhinitis, nasal topical CSRs are considered effective in the treatment of acute and chronic rhinosinusitis [1].

Although there are no adequate clinical studies on intranasal CCS used during pregnancy, the use of fluticasone furoate, mometasone, and budesonide within the recommended therapeutic dose range is considered to be safe [21]. Intranasal budesonide is the only topical CCS accepted in group B according to the FDA category [48].

Minimal local side effects such as nasal dryness, stinging, and burning sensation can be seen. There is no evidence of using osteoporosis due to the use of intranasal CKS or growth retardation in children [49, 50].

Oral antibiotics: Penicillin and cephalosporin group antibiotics that will not harm the fetus can be used in acute exacerbations of ARS and CRS. Long-term use of macrolide and doxycycline group antibiotics is not recommended. Tetracycline, aminoglycoside, trimethoprim -sulfamethoxazole, and fluoroquinolone group antibiotics should not be used during pregnancy [34].

Amoxicillin is the first-line antibiotic treatment to be used in ABRS cases because it is safe, effective, and cheap. In case of amoxicillin resistance, amoxicillin-clavulanate treatment should be preferred [27].

Although the role of bacterial infection in chronic RS cases is not clearly determined, there is resistance to many antibiotics in CRS cases. Macrolide group and doxycycline are used in the normal population because of their antibacterial and anti-inflammatory activities [51]; however, these drugs are in group C in pregnant patients [3].

Leukotriene antagonist: Leukotriene antagonists should be avoided during pregnancy [34]. Montelukast passes into breast milk, and there is no information about the side effects that may occur in the breastfed baby [34].

Oral decongestants, antihistamines: Oral decongestants should not be used during pregnancy. First-generation antihistamines should not be used due to their sedative and anticholinergic side effects [34]. Among the second-generation antihistamines, loratadine (10 mg once a day) and cetirizine (10 mg once a day) can be preferred during pregnancy. This group of drugs is classified in category B. Levocetirizine is also included in group B, but there are few published data [52].

Hypertonic nasal irrigation and topical CKS sprays are applications that can be recommended for CRS treatment during pregnancy [34].

Although the studies, workshops, and reviews show that the symptoms of allergic rhinitis and rhinosinusitis increase during pregnancy, no significant study has been shown for CRS. No specific algorithm has been demonstrated in the treatment of rhinosinusitis. There are considerable deficiencies in the process of CRS disease, approach to the patient, diagnosis, and treatment during pregnancy [34].

41.12.3 Surgical Treatment

Surgical treatment should be considered as a last-line treatment when other medical treatments failed. Some studies have shown an increase in preterm deliveries after receiving general anesthesia in the first two trimesters. The effect of inhaled anesthetics and narcotics on the fetus is not fully understood [53].

41.12.4 Postpartum Infection Control

Women who have given birth to respiratory tract infection should rarely be separated from their babies, but handwashing, mask use, and hygiene rules should be observed in order to minimize the risk of transmission [54]. Recommendations for the control of prenatal and postnatal respiratory infections are available on the US Centers for Disease Control and Prevention (CDC) website (https://www.cdc.gov/flu/professionals/infectioncontrol/peri-post-settings.htm).

41.12.5 Breastfeeding

Breastfeeding is the preferred feeding method for newborn babies and provides passive immunization. Breastfeeding should not be abandoned due to the infection in the mother. All of the drugs used in pregnancy can also be used in breastfeeding mothers. Quinolone and tetracycline group antibiotics should also be avoided during breastfeeding.

Almost all medicines pass into breast milk. However, since many drugs will not be absorbed or destroyed in the gut of the baby, it is generally assumed to have a negative effect on the newborn [4].

Newborn babies, especially those who are premature, are more exposed to the negative effects of therapeutic agents because the blood–brain barrier is more permeable, the enzyme conjugation capacity is weak, and the protein binding ability and glomerular filtration rate are less [55].

Both the UpToDate drug database and the United States National Library of Medicine's Drugs and Lactation Database (LactMed) provide information on drug levels in milk and possible drug effects on breastfed babies (https://www.ncbi.nlm.nih.gov/books/NBK501922/).

References

1. Fokkens WJ, Lund VJ, Hopkins C, Hellings PW, Kern R, Reitsma S, et al. European position paper on rhinosinusitis and nasal polyps 2020. Rhinology. 2020;58(Supplement 29):1–464.
2. Papadopoulos NG, Bernstein J, Demoly P, Dykewicz M, Fokkens W, Hellings P, et al. Phenotypes and endotypes of rhinitis and their impact on management: a PRACTALL report. Allergy. 2015;70(5):474–94.
3. Goldstein G, Govindaraj S. Rhinologic issues in pregnancy. Allergy Rhinol. 2012;3(1):ar. 2012.3. 0028.
4. Incaudo GA. The diagnosis and treatment of rhinosinusitis during pregnancy and lactation. Immunol Allergy Clin N Am. 2000;20(4):807–30.
5. Gümüşsoy M, Gümüşsoy S, Çukurova İ. Gebelik döneminde sık karşılaşılan rinolojik sorunlar: Tanı ve tedavide uygun yaklaşımlar. İzmir Tepecik Eğitim ve Araştırma Hastanesi Dergisi. 27(1):13–9.
6. Mehta N, Chen K, Hardy E, Powrie R. Respiratory disease in pregnancy. Best Pract Res Clin Obstet Gynaecol. 2015;29(5):598–611.
7. Hegewald MJ, Crapo RO. Respiratory physiology in pregnancy. Clin Chest Med. 2011;32(1):1–13.
8. Hellings PW, Fokkens WJ, Akdis C, Bachert C, Cingi C, Dietz de Loos D, et al. Uncontrolled allergic rhinitis and chronic rhinosinusitis: where do we stand today? Allergy. 2013;68(1):1–7.
9. Kahrilas PJ, Talley N, Grover S. Clinical manifestations and diagnosis of gastroesophageal reflux in adults. UpToDate, Basow DS, editor. UpToDate, Waltham, MA; 2008.
10. Dagli E, Yüksel A, Kaya M, Ugur KS, Turkay FC. Association of oral antireflux medication with laryngopharyngeal reflux and nasal resistance. JAMA Otolaryngol Head Neck Surg. 2017;143(5):478–83.
11. Baraniuk JN, Merck SJ. Nasal reflexes: implications for exercise, breathing, and sex. Curr Allergy Asthma Rep. 2008;8(2):147–53.
12. Cingi C, Ozdoganoglu T, Songu M. Nasal obstruction as a drug side effect. Ther Adv Respir Dis. 2011;5(3):175–82.
13. Rombaux P, Huart C, Levie P, Cingi C, Hummel T. Olfaction in chronic rhinosinusitis. Curr Allergy Asthma Rep. 2016;16(5):41.
14. Holbrook EH, Leopold DA. An updated review of clinical olfaction. Curr Opin Otolaryngol Head Neck Surg. 2006;14(1):23–8.
15. Fornazieri MA, Prina DMC, Favoreto JPM, KRE S, Ueda DM, de Rezende Pinna F, et al. Olfaction during pregnancy and postpartum period. Chemosens Percept. 2019;12(2):125–34.
16. Ellegård E, Karlsson G. Nasal congestion during pregnancy. Clin Otolaryngol Allied Sci. 1999;24(4):307–11.
17. Sobol SE, Frenkiel S, Nachtigal D, Wiener D, Teblum C. Clinical manifestation of sinonasal pathology during pregnancy. J Otolaryngol. 2001;30(1)
18. Shushan S, Sadan O, Lurie S, Evron S, Golan A, Roth Y. Pregnancy-associated rhinitis. Am J Perinatol. 2006;23(07):431–3.
19. Gilbey P, McGruthers L, Morency A-M, Shrim A. Rhinosinusitis-related quality of life during pregnancy. Am J Rhinol Allergy. 2012;26(4):283–6.
20. Ellegård E, Hellgren M, Karlsson N. Fluticasone propionate aqueous nasal spray in pregnancy rhinitis. Clin Otolaryngol Allied Sci. 2001;26(5):394–400.

21. Alhussien AH, Alhedaithy RA, Alsaleh SA. Safety of intranasal corticosteroid sprays during pregnancy: an updated review. Eur Arch Otorhinolaryngol. 2018;275(2):325–33.
22. Demir UL, Demir BC, Oztosun E, Uyaniklar OO, Ocakoglu G, editors. The effects of pregnancy on nasal physiology. International forum of allergy & rhinology. Wiley Online Library; 2015.
23. Yau W-P, Mitchell AA, Lin KJ, Werler MM, Hernández-Díaz S. Use of decongestants during pregnancy and the risk of birth defects. Am J Epidemiol. 2013;178(2):198–208.
24. Larson L, Powrie R, File T. Treatment of respiratory infections in pregnant women. UpToDate, Rose BD, editor, UpToDate, Waltham, MA; 2008.
25. Waller DK, Hashmi SS, Hoyt AT, Duong HT, Tinker SC, Gallaway MS, et al. Maternal report of fever from cold or flu during early pregnancy and the risk for noncardiac birth defects, National Birth Defects Prevention Study, 1997–2011. Birth Defects Res. 2018;110(4):342–51.
26. Akdis CA, Bachert C, Cingi C, Dykewicz MS, Hellings PW, Naclerio RM, et al. Endotypes and phenotypes of chronic rhinosinusitis: a PRACTALL document of the European Academy of Allergy and Clinical Immunology and the American Academy of Allergy, Asthma & Immunology. J Allergy Clin Immunol. 2013;131(6):1479–90.
27. Rosenfeld RM, Piccirillo JF, Chandrasekhar SS, Brook I, Ashok Kumar K, Kramper M, et al., editors. Clinical practice guideline (update): adult sinusitis. Otolaryngol Head Neck Surg. 2015;152(2_suppl):S1–S39.
28. Wilson J. Correction: In the clinic: acute sinusitis. Ann Internal Med. 2010;153(12)
29. Küçükcan NE, Bafaqeeh SA, Sallavaci S. Microbiology of rhinosinusitis and antimicrobial resistance. All around the nose. Springer. 2020:193–7.
30. Incaudo GA. Diagnosis and treatment of allergic rhinitis and sinusitis during pregnancy and lactation. Clin Rev Allergy Immunol. 2004;27(2):159–77.
31. Namazy JA, Schatz M, Yang S-J, Chen W. Antibiotics for respiratory infections during pregnancy: prevalence and risk factors. J Allergy Clin Immunol Pract. 2016;4(6):1256–7.e2.
32. Sorri M, Hartikainen-Sorri AL, Kärjä J. Rhinitis during pregnancy. Rhinology. 1980;18(2):83–6.
33. Jutel M, Agache I, Bonini S, Burks AW, Calderon M, Canonica W, et al. International consensus on allergy immunotherapy. J Allergy Clin Immunol. 2015;136(3):556–68.
34. Lal D, Jategaonkar AA, Borish L, Chambliss LR, Gnagi SH, Hwang PH, et al. Management of rhinosinusitis during pregnancy: systematic review and expert panel recommendations. Rhinology. 2016;54(2):99.
35. DeCastro A, Mims L, Hueston WJ. Rhinosinusitis. Prim Care. 2014;41(1):47–61.
36. Low DE, Desrosiers M, James McSherry M, Garber G, Williams JW Jr, Rémy H, et al. A practical guide for the diagnosis and treatment of acute sinusitis. Can Med Assoc J. 1997;156(6):S1.
37. Erdem D, Arıcıgil M, Chua D. Complications of rhinosinusitis. All around the nose. Springer; 2020. p. 221–8.
38. Thiagarajan B. Complications of sinusitis. http://otolaryngology.wdfiles.com/local--files/rhinology/sinusitis_comp.pdf. Accessed online at May 27, 2022.
39. Chandler JR, Langenbrunner DJ, Stevens ER. The pathogenesis of orbital complications in acute sinusitis. Laryngoscope. 1970;80(9):1414–28.
40. McCollough CH, Schueler BA, Atwell TD, Braun NN, Regner DM, Brown DL, et al. Radiation exposure and pregnancy: when should we be concerned? Radiographics. 2007;27(4):909–17.
41. Applegate K. Pregnancy screening of adolescents and women before radiologic testing: does radiology need a national guideline? J Am Coll Radiol. 2007;4(8):533–6.
42. Obstetricians ACo. Gynecologists. Guidelines for diagnostic imaging during pregnancy and lactation. Committee Opinion No. 723. Obstet Gynecol. 2017;130:e210–6.
43. Hellings PW, Akdis CA, Bachert C, Bousquet J, Pugin B, Adriaensen G, et al. EUFOREA Rhinology Research Forum 2016: report of the brainstorming sessions on needs and priorities in rhinitis and rhinosinusitis. Rhinology. 2017;55:202–10.
44. Scialli A, Lione A. Pregnancy effects of specific medications used to treat asthma and immunological diseases. Lung Biol Health Dis. 1998;110:157–228.
45. Metzger WJ, Turner E, Patterson R. The safety of immunotherapy during pregnancy. J Allergy Clin Immunol. 1978;61(4):268–72.

46. Ramoz LL, Patel-Shori NM. Recent changes in pregnancy and lactation labeling: retirement of risk categories. Pharmacotherapy. 2014;34(4):389–95.
47. Dinardi RR, de Andrade CR, da Cunha Ibiapina C. External nasal dilators: definition, background, and current uses. Int J General Med. 2014;7:491.
48. Caparroz FA, Gregorio LL, Bongiovanni G, Izu SC, Kosugi EM. Rhinitis and pregnancy: literature review. Braz J Otorhinolaryngol. 2016;82(1):105–11.
49. Allen DB. Systemic effects of intranasal steroids: an endocrinologist's perspective. J Allergy Clin Immunol. 2000;106(4):S179–S90.
50. Corren J. Intranasal corticosteroids for allergic rhinitis: how do different agents compare? J Allergy Clin Immunol. 1999;104(4):s144–s9.
51. Fokkens WJ, Lund VJ, Mullol J, Bachert C, Alobid I, Baroody F, et al. European position paper on rhinosinusitis and nasal polyps 2012. Rhinol Suppl. 2012;23:3 p preceding table of contents, 1–298.
52. Källén B. Use of antihistamine drugs in early pregnancy and delivery outcome. J Matern Fetal Neonatal Med. 2002;11(3):146–52.
53. Kuczkowski KM. The safety of anaesthetics in pregnant women. Expert Opin Drug Saf. 2006;5(2):251–64.
54. Palmore TN. Infection control measures for prevention of seasonal influenza. In: Hirsch MS, Baron EL, editors. UpToDate. last updated: Jan 21, 2022.
55. Koletzko B, Poindexter B, Uauy R. Nutritional care of preterm infants: scientific basis and practical guidelines. Karger Medical and Scientific Publishers; 2014.

The Management of Nasal Obstruction During Pregnancy and the Postpartum Period

42

Erdem Köroğlu, Fatih Özdoğan, and Michael B. Soyka

42.1 Introduction

Nasal congestion affects a large part of the population and is one of the most common symptoms in otolaryngological practice. A detailed history and physical examination are important to reach the diagnosis. Endoscopic examination of the nose is the most valuable examination method in the evaluation of nasal obstruction. In endoscopic examination, nasal mucosa and its features, pathologies of anatomical structures (septal deviation, septal perforation, turbinate hypertrophy etc.), nasal discharge and its characteristics, intranasal masses (polyp, tumor, etc.), and the nasopharynx are evaluated.

Nasal obstruction during pregnancy is a common complaint and may be caused by different pathologies (Table 42.1). Preexisting conditions may deteriorate and become evident during pregnancy (allergic rhinitis, septal deviation, etc.) or become newly diagnosed during pregnancy (gestational rhinitis, rhinosinusitis, nasal granuloma gravidarum, etc.).

Sufficient nasal airflow requires open nasal passages, normal functioning receptors of airflow (trigeminal), intact mucociliary function, and lack of mucosal inflammation [1]. A disorder in any of these factors can lead to nasal congestion. Nasal obstruction has substantial impact on quality of life and can cause sleep disturbance and xerostomia.

E. Köroğlu (✉) · F. Özdoğan
Department of Otorhinolaryngology, Faculty of Medicine, Health Sciences University, Derince Training and Research Hospital, Kocaeli, Turkey
e-mail: erdemkoroglu1907@gmail.com; ozdogan.fatih@gmail.com

M. B. Soyka
Department of Otorhinolaryngology, Head and Neck Surgery, University Hospital and University of Zurich, Zurich, Switzerland
e-mail: michael@soyka.ch

C. Cingi et al. (eds.), *ENT Diseases: Diagnosis and Treatment during Pregnancy and Lactation*, https://doi.org/10.1007/978-3-031-05303-0_42

Table 42.1 Causes of nasal obstruction

Dynamic	Architectural	Inflammatory	Tumors
– Nasal cycles – Positional – Hormonal (Pregnancy rhinitis) – Exercise – Physiologic	– Septal deviation – Turbinate hypertrophy – Alar collapse – Narrow nasal valve – Adenoid hypertrophy	– Upper respiratory tract infections – Rhinitis – Chronic rhinosinusitis	– Benign masses – Malign masses – Malformations

42.2 Dynamic Causes

Nasal congestion may be perceived on both sides of the nasal cavity due to the synchronous increase in nasal resistance or present variable on both sides. The duration of physiological unilateral turbinate swelling, called the nasal cycle, varies between 30 min and 6 h and is not present in every individual [2].

Positional nasal congestion may occur as a result of the formation of congestion in the lower nose with the pregnant woman lying on her side. Lying with the head elevated 30 degrees reduces airway obstruction [3].

Depending on the activation of the sympathetic system in exercise and cold weather, the nasal cycle is disrupted and nasal congestion may occur [4]. Emotional factors such as anxiety, stress, and irritability can cause nasal congestion [5].

42.3 Structural Causes

Preexisting anatomical changes may become symptomatic during pregnancy. The most common anatomical variations that cause nasal obstruction in pregnant women are septal deviations and inferior turbinate hypertrophy (due to various reasons). However, nasal congestion can also be seen caused by alar collapse and valve problems. While the treatment approach in alar collapse is to support the collapsed using different techniques, surgery should be avoided during pregnancy. External nasal splits are the preferred treatment in pregnant women for dilation of this area.

42.3.1 Septal Deviation

The nasal septum is a structure that divides the nasal cavity, provides central support to the nose, and also plays an important role in the regulation of nasal airflow. Septal deviation is the most common cause of nasal obstruction in adults. Deviation can involve the septal cartilage, bone, or both (Fig. 42.1). Classical submucosal resection, septoplasty, and open techniques are the preferred surgical approaches for the correction of the deviated septum. It is advisable to either solve this problem before pregnancy or postpone it to postpartum or even later, when breastfeeding is terminated. Otherwise, a troublesome breathing impairment during pregnancy may be

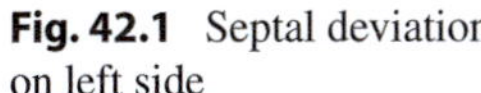

Fig. 42.1 Septal deviation on left side

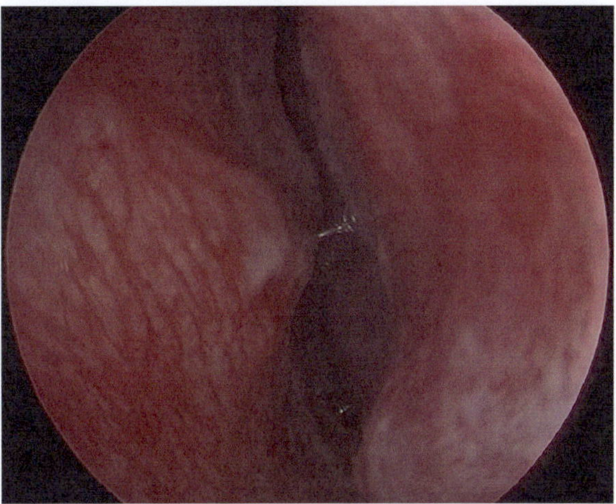

encountered, which is characterized by sleep disorders, snoring, and a decrease in quality of life, anxiety, and psychological problems [6–8].

In pregnant women, local anesthetics may pass to the fetus through the placenta [9]. Its importance increases in terms of fetal teratogenicity especially in the first 3 months of pregnancy. Other effects of local anesthetics on the fetus are that they may cause bradycardia. However, it is generally accepted that the use of local anesthetics is safe during pregnancy, and high doses of adrenaline should be avoided due to systemic effects.

Septal deviation operations during pregnancy are not preferred by physicians due to possible side effects of general anesthesia and long recovery. Postponing surgery requires pregnant women to bear with this negative situation until the end of pregnancy [10, 11].

42.3.2 Turbinate Hypertrophy

The most common inferior turbinate pathology is turbinate hypertrophy and may have different causes affecting the soft tissue and bone. Inferior turbinate hypertrophy represents the main cause of symptomatic nasal obstruction, besides septal deviations [12]. Perennial allergic rhinitis and nonallergic rhinitis are the most common noninfectious causes of lower turbinate mucosal swelling leading to a temporary reduction in nasal airflow [13]. However, it may occur as compensatory mechanism in patients with septal deviations.

Most of the cases with turbinate hypertrophy respond well to medical treatment with topical corticosteroids. However, in some patients, these nasal inflammatory processes result in chronic nasal obstruction due to enlargement of the venous sinuses or fibrosis. In this case, surgical methods such as turbinate lateralization, radiofrequency ablation, or turbinoplasty may be applied.

It should be borne in mind that rhinitis of pregnancy resolves spontaneously after a limited period of time. These surgical methods should be carefully considered only in severe cases, for example, in women with rhinitis and sleep apnea during pregnancy, if other treatments of the nose have failed and sustained positive airway pressure is not tolerated.

42.4 Rhinitis

Rhinitis is an inflammatory disease of the nasal mucosa characterized by two or more of the symptoms such as nasal congestion, runny nose, itchy nose, and sneezing. It can be classified as allergic and nonallergic rhinitis [14].

42.4.1 Allergic Rhinitis

Allergic rhinitis (AR) is a type 1 hypersensitivity inflammation of the nasal mucosa mediated by IgE after exposure to the allergens. Patients present with nasal obstruction, a runny nose and sneezing complaints, and serous nasal discharge often combined with ophthalmological complaints. Edematous and hypertrophic turbinates are observed on physical examination. AR management includes prevention of exposure to allergens, pharmacological treatments, and immunotherapy.

AR affects about 30% of women of childbearing age and may worsen during pregnancy [15]. The first recommendation for treatment in a pregnant woman with AR is allergen avoidance. However, sometimes this is not feasible or not enough to control symptoms.

Histamine is the major mediator of AR symptoms. Antihistamines are needed to suppress rhinitis and allergic symptoms. Second-generation antihistamines can be used safely during pregnancy [16]. Loratadine and cetirizine are antihistamines recommended in guidelines [17, 18]. Both of them are in group B according to the Food and Drug Administration (FDA) risk categories. Cetirizine also has an antiemetic effect that is beneficial during pregnancy [19]. Intranasal antihistamines should be avoided during pregnancy. No safety data are available in humans, and adverse effects in the fetus have been observed in animal studies [20].

Topical decongestants (phenylephrine, naphazoline, oxymetazoline, xylometazoline) are in the "C" category according to the FDA. There are studies showing that oxymetazoline can be used at the lowest possible dose, preferably after the first trimester, in patients with severe nasal congestion that can interfere with the patient's sleep [21]. It should not be used close to birth.

Intranasal corticosteroids (INCS) are commonly used drugs in AR. Only trace amounts of INCS pass into the systemic circulation, and they do not cause nasal mucosal atrophy in long-term use. INCS reach a high concentration on the receptor in the nasal mucosa. These drugs have pronounced antiallergic and anti-inflammatory effects. Improvements in all nasal symptoms of allergic rhinitis such as discharge, postnasal drip, congestion, and itching were noted after INCS treatment.

Due to insufficient human studies, the FDA has not included any INCS in category A in the course of pregnancy. Budesonide is the only INCS in category B. First-generation INCS (triamcinolone acetonide, flunisolide, beclomethasone) have high bioavailability. Therefore, they are not preferred during pregnancy. Second-generation INCSs (fluticasone furoate, mometasone, fluticasone propionate) are safer than older agents. Because of their low bioavailability (less than 1%), the risk of systemic side effects and the possibility of affecting the fetus are low. Triamcinolone should not be used due to the association with congenital respiratory defects [22].

Immunotherapy initiated before pregnancy can be continued in pregnancy if maintenance doses are reached, no side effects have occurred, and clearly benefit is seen. However, immunotherapy should not be started during pregnancy [23] due to the risk of anaphylaxis in the early stages of immunotherapy and during dose increase. Therefore, there is a risk of death for the mother and the unborn. Cromolyn is reported to be safe in pregnancy [24].

In their study, Garavello et al. revealed that nasal irrigation with hypertonic saline is an effective option in the treatment of pregnant women with seasonal allergic rhinitis [25]. No harmful effects on the fetus are expected with this treatment.

42.4.2 Hormonal Rhinitis/Pregnancy-Induced Rhinopathy

Nasal mucosa cycle and mucociliary transport are negatively affected due to the increase in pregnancy hormones, especially the increase in the amount of estrogen. In the pathophysiology of pregnancy-induced rhinitis, (i) increased estrogen and progesterone levels, (ii) increased mucosal acetylcholine receptors, (iii) decreased alpha-adrenergic response and related vascular enlargement in smooth muscles, (iv) increased blood volume in the extravascular space, and (v) increased placental growth hormone are thought to play a role [26]. The clinical picture with nasal obstruction is described as pregnancy-induced rhinitis or rhinopathy (PIR). In a study of 599 patients, the incidence of PIR was found to be 22% [27]. PIR is a non-allergic rhinitis lasting 6 or more weeks and resolves within 2 weeks after labor [28]. PIR is a subgroup of rhinitis characterized by nasal congestion without any other clinically diagnosed reason. The turbinates are the regions where congestion is most common. Significant inferior turbinate hypertrophy is seen in nasal examination. In cases of congestion, there is often a watery or viscous clear discharge from the nose. Especially in the third trimester, rhinitis findings increase even more [29]. Smoking and nasal hyperreactivity are among the risk factors for PIR [30].

Snoring is a common complaint in PIR because nasal congestion increases in the supine position. Adverse effects such as maternal hypertension, preeclampsia, intra-uterine growth retardation, and low Apgar scores may occur due to snoring [31]. Ellegard also mentioned the importance of a possible connection between PIR and preeclampsia in her study [32].

The first step in treatment is patient education. It is especially important to prevent unnecessary and wrong drug use and possible complications. Saline irrigation (isotonic or hypertonic), raising the headrest (30 or 45 degrees), and nasal external dilators, as well as nasal splints (to increase the nasal valve angle), are safe and effective conservative treatment methods. Studies have shown that the effect of nasal external dilator used in pregnant women on sleep quality and snoring during the 6-month follow-up period is as significant as the effects of local decongestants [33].

A limited number of studies have shown that oxymetazoline may be safer when used in limited doses than other local decongestants. However, since there is a risk of rhinitis medicamentosa, it is unfavorable to use it for more than 5 days [34]. Systemic (oral) decongestants should be avoided especially during the first trimester [35].

Nasal steroids, whose efficacy in PIR could not be clearly demonstrated yet, are recommended in PIR in terms of providing nasal patency and reducing the frequency of using local decongestants. Second-generation INCS with low bioavailability should be preferred and approval by the obstetrician should be sought.

Radiofrequency ablation can be applied for marked hypertrophic lower turbinates in case of severe deterioration in sleep quality and snoring due to nasal obstruction in PIR.

PIR needs to be distinguished from allergic rhinitis. The presence of allergic complaints before pregnancy, a history of a positive skin prick test, or the presence of drugs used for allergic rhinitis may be helpful hints in the diagnosis. The problem is the increase in allergic symptoms and aggravation of the picture during pregnancy that is thought to be caused by increase in eosinophil migration into the nasal mucosa due to progesterone and estrogen levels [36]. In addition to PIR findings, Eustachian tube dysfunction, cough, and headache symptoms may accompany AR.

42.4.3 Acute Infectious Rhinitis

Viral or bacterial upper respiratory tract infections can cause nasal congestion in pregnant women. The diagnosis can be made easily with the patient's symptoms and physical examination. Spontaneous recovery occurs in a short time, but some patients may require treatment to reduce symptoms. The use of topical decongestants during a short period of time can be discussed with the treating obstetrician. Depending on the exact cause, topical steroids and antibiotics may also be required. Infrequently acute rhinitis can progress into acute bacterial rhinosinusitis, which is discussed below.

42.5　Rhinosinusitis

Rhinosinusitis is a symptomatic inflammation of the paranasal sinuses, defined as a complex of symptoms, including nasal blockage, rhinorrhea, and decreased sense of smell and pain along with objective finding. Diagnosing rhinosinusitis can become a difficult issue, even in nonpregnant patients, and the presence of nasal obstruction lacks specificity in this regard. Purulent secretion and nasal polyposis are strong diagnostic signs for rhinosinusitis, but these findings are much more specific than sensitive. In addition, nasal congestion during pregnancy may be the only symptom of sinusitis [32]. Imaging may be required and should be done with adequate precautions when ionizing radiation is used such as in DVT or CT scanning. MRI may be an adequate alternative.

In the treatment of viral rhinosinusitis and uncomplicated acute bacterial rhinosinusitis, analgesics, topical corticosteroids, and/or saline should be recommended first. Oral antibiotics that are nontoxic to the fetus can be used in acute rhinosinusitis or acute exacerbation of chronic rhinosinusitis (CRS). Long-term use of macrolides or doxycyclines is not recommended for CRS during pregnancy [37]. Cephalosporin and penicillin are the safest classes and can be given in severe cases, when purulent inflammation is present on endoscopic examination.

Topical INCS spray and saline nasal rinses are likely appropriate maintenance therapy for CRS during pregnancy. Saline irrigation provides physical cleansing by removing thick mucus and air pollutants. In some cases, hypertonic solutions have been shown to be more beneficial than isotonic solutions [38].

42.5.1 Chronic Rhinosinusitis with Nasal Polyps

Chronic rhinosinusitis with nasal polyps may become bothersome during pregnancy, though preexistent. This chronic inflammation with characteristic benign hyperplastic muscosal growth is usually observed bilaterally and needs to be discerned from other similarly looking tumors. On endoscopic examination, they appear as pale, transparent, and smooth-surfaced mass lesions (Fig. 42.2). While it may be asymptomatic, patients can present with symptoms of nasal congestion,

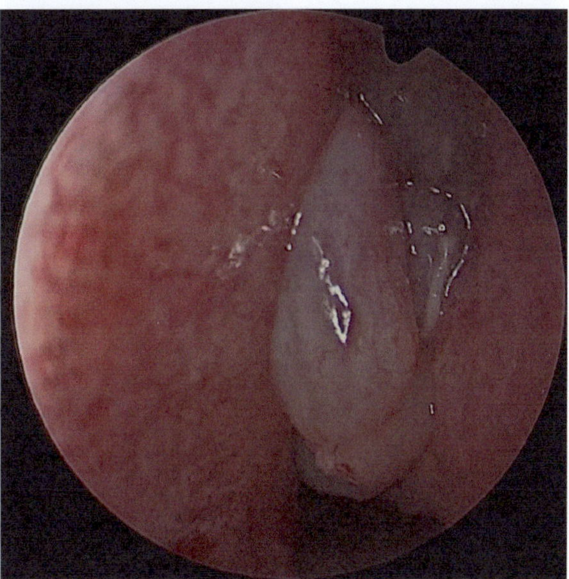

Fig. 42.2 Endoscopic finding of nasal polyps in primary diffuse CRS

runny nose, odor disorders, and more infrequently headaches. Topical steroids provide benefit in symptom control during pregnancy. Systemic steroids may be used after a thorough discussion with the treating obstetrician. Surgery and imaging should be postponed to after pregnancy. The safety of biologics, including dupilumab, mepolizumab, and omalizumab, during pregnancy is not completely proven and should thus be avoided.

42.6 Neoplasias

Tumors of the nose and paranasal sinuses are rare. Benign and malignant tumors are seen in the general population. Inverted papilloma is the most common benign epithelial tumor in the sinonasal region. . It usually originates from the lateral wall of the nose or the middle meatus (Fig. 42.3). Despite the benign histological features of inverted papilloma, they can show locally aggressive behavior and progression to malignancy. Endoscopic nasal examination and imaging, preferably using MRI, helps in evaluating the dignity of the tumor. However, malignant neoplasm may occur during pregnancy and treatment should not be deferred to later time points. Biopsies in local anesthesia should be avoided due to false-negative results. In the third trimester, preterm delivery by Cesarean section followed by sinonasal surgery in general anesthesia needs to be evaluated to obtain adequate histological material. In earlier pregnancy, surgery may be performed after thorough counseling and discussion with the obstetrician and anesthesiologist.

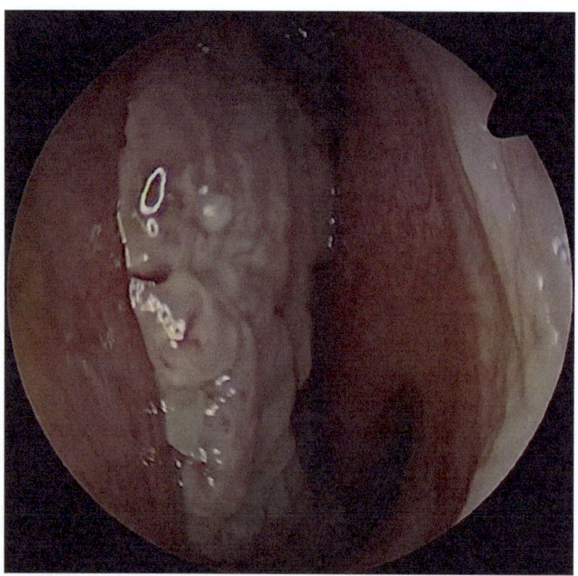

Fig. 42.3 Endoscopic view of an inverted sinonasal papilloma

The most common nasal mass seen during pregnancy is nasal granuloma gravidarum, which is discussed below.

42.6.1 Nasal Granuloma Gravidarum

It is a rapidly growing benign tumor that causes nasal congestion, also known as pregnancy granuloma. Histology is identical to a pyogenic granuloma. It is almost always unilateral and tends to cause recurrent nosebleeds. It is commonly seen during late pregnancy. Examination of the nasal cavity reveals a well-vascularized lesion that bleeds easily when touched. It can even protrude and occupy the nasal vestibule and may be visible from the outside. When small, imaging of the lesion usually is unnecessary, otherwise MRI is the method of choice. Excisional biopsy is the treatment of choice in order to stop nasal bleeding and obtain adequate histology, although it may disappear spontaneously after giving birth [39].

42.7　Conclusion

Different causes of nasal breathing impairment may manifest during pregnancy and affect the quality of life. Most are self-limited and may be treated symptomatically. Careful evaluation of potential side effects for both the mother and unborn child needs to be performed, and treatment initiation should be closely discussed with the treating obstetrician.

References

1. Hsu DW, Suh JD. Anatomy and physiology of nasal obstruction. Otolaryngol Clin N Am. 2018;51:853–65.
2. Kahana-Zweig R, Geva-Sagiv M, Weissbrod A, et al. Measuring and characterizing the human nasal cycle. PLoS One. 2016;11:e0162918.
3. Souza FJF d B, Genta PR, de Souza Filho AJ, et al. The influence of head-of-bed elevation in patients with obstructive sleep apnea. Sleep Breath. 2017;21(4):815–20.
4. Baraniuk JN, Merck SJ. Nasal reflexes: implications for exercise, breathing, and sex. Curr Allergy Asthma Rep. 2008;8(2):147–53.
5. Pendolino AL, Lund VJ, Nardello E, Ottaviano G. The nasal cycle: a comprehensive review. Rhinology. 2018;1(1):67–76.
6. Kumar R, Hayhurst KL, Robson AK. Ear, nose, and throat manifestations during pregnancy. Otolaryngol Head Neck Surg. 2011;145(2):188–98.
7. Shiny Sherlie V, Varghese A. ENT changes of pregnancy and its management. Indian J Otolaryngol Head Neck Surg. 2014;66:6–9.
8. Singla P, Gupta M, Matreja PS, Gill R. Otorhinolaryngological complaints in pregnancy: a prospective study in a tertiary care Centre. Int J Otorhinolaryngol Head Neck Surg. 2015;1(2):75–80.
9. Lee JM, Shin TJ. Use of local anesthetics for dental treatment during pregnancy; safety for parturient. J Dent Anesth Pain Med. 2017;17:81–90.

10. Steinbrook RA. Anaesthesia, minimally invasive surgery and pregnancy. Best Pract Res Clin Anaesthesiol. 2002;16:131–43.
11. Cheek TG, Baird E. Anesthesia for nonobstetric surgery: maternal and fetal considerations. Clin Obstet Gynecol. 2009;52:535–45.
12. Dursun E, Terzi S, Demirci M. Alt Konka Cerrahi Teknikleri. Turkiye Klinikleri J ENT-Special Topics. 2015;8(4):9–26.
13. Passàli D, Passàli FM, Damiani V, et al. Treatment of inferior turbinate hypertrophy: a randomized clinical trial. Ann Otol Rhinol Laryngol. 2003;112(8):683–8.
14. Wallace DV, Dykewicz MS, Bernstein DI, et al. The diagnosis and management of rhinitis: an updated practice parameter. J Allergy Clin Immunol. 2008;122:S1–84.
15. Ridolo E, Caminati M, Martignago I, et al. Allergic rhinitis: pharmacotherapy in pregnancy and old age. Expert Rev Clin Pharmacol. 2016;9:1081–9.
16. Gilboa SM, Ailes EC, Rai RP, et al. Antihistamines and birth defects: a systematic review of the literature. Expert Opin Drug Saf. 2014;13:1667–98.
17. Einarson A, Bailey B, Jung G, et al. Prospective controlled study of hydroxyzine and cetirizine in pregnancy. Ann Allergy Asthma Immunol. 1997;78:183–6.
18. Moretti ME, Caprara D, Coutinho CJ, et al. Fetal safety of loratadine use in the first trimester of pregnancy: a multicenter study. J Allergy Clin Immunol. 2003;111:479–83.
19. Einarson A, Levichek Z, Einarson TR, Koren G. The antiemetic effect of cetirizine during pregnancy. Ann Pharmacother. 2000;34:1486–7.
20. Gonzalez-Estrada A, Geraci SA. Allergy medications during pregnancy. Am J Med Sci. 2016;352:326–31.
21. Incaudo GA, Takach P. The diagnosis and treatment of allergic rhinitis during pregnancy and lactation. Immunol Allergy Clin N Am. 2006;26:137–54.
22. Bérard A, Sheehy O, Kurzinger ML, et al. (2016) intranasal triamcinolone use during pregnancy and the risk of adverse pregnancy outcomes. J Allergy Clin Immunol. 2016 Jul;138(1):97–104.e7.
23. Oykhman P, Kim HL, Ellis AK. Allergen immunotherapy in pregnancy. Allergy, Asthma Clin Immunol. 2015;11:31.
24. Ratner PH, Ehrlich PM, Fineman SM, et al. Use of intranasal cromolyn sodium for allergic rhinitis. Mayo Clin Proc. 2002;77(4):350–4.
25. Garavello W, Somigliana E, Acaia B, et al. Nasal lavage in pregnant women with seasonal allergic rhinitis: a randomized study. Int Arch Allergy Immunol. 2010;151:137–41.
26. Gumussoy M, Gumussoy S, Cukurova İ. The most frequently encountered rhinologic problems during pregnancy: appropriate approaches toward diagnose and therapy. J Tepecik Educ Res Hosp. 2017;27:13–9.
27. Ellegård E, Hellgren M, Torén K, Karlsson G. The incidence of pregnancy rhinitis. Gynecol Obstet Investig. 2000;49(2):98–101.
28. Baudoin T, Šimunjak T, Bacan N, et al. Redefining pregnancy-induced rhinitis. Am J Rhinol Allergy. 2021;35:315–22.
29. Bende M, Hallgårde U, Sjögren C. Occurrence of nasal congestion during pregnancy. Am J Rhinol. 1989;3:217–9.
30. Shushan S, Sadan O, Lurie S, et al. Pregnancy-associated rhinitis. Am J Perinatol. 2006;23:431–3.
31. Franklin KA, Holmgren PA, Jönsson F at al (2000) Snoring, pregnancy-induced hypertension, and growth retardation of the fetus. Chest 117(1):137–141.
32. Ellegård EK. Pregnancy rhinitis. Immunol Allergy Clin N Am. 2006;26:119–35.
33. Dinardi RR, de Andrade CR, Ibiapina C da C (2014) External nasal dilators: definition, background, and current uses. Int J Gen Med 7:491–504.
34. Caparroz FA, Gregorio LL, Bongiovanni G, et al. Rhinitis and pregnancy: literature review. Braz J Otorhinolaryngol. 2016;82:105–11.
35. Dykewicz MS, Wallace DV, Amrol DJ, et al. Rhinitis 2020: a practice parameter update. J Allergy Clin Immunol. 2020;146(4):721–67.

36. Wei J, Gerlich J, Genuneit J, Nowak D, et al. Hormonal factors and incident asthma and allergic rhinitis during puberty in girls. Ann Allergy Asthma Immunol. 2015;115(1):21–27.e2.
37. Lal D, Jategaonkar AA, Borish L, et al. Management of rhinosinusitis during pregnancy: systematic review and expert panel recommendations. Rhinology. 2016;54(2):99–104.
38. Kanjanawasee D, Seresirikachorn K, Chitsuthipakorn W, Snidvongs K. Hypertonic saline versus isotonic saline nasal irrigation: systematic review and meta-analysis. Am J Rhinol Allergy. 2018;32:269–79.
39. Oakes RE, Frampton SJ, Scott PMJ. Granuloma gravidarum: management. J Obstet Gynaecol. 2012;32:805.

Smell and Taste Disorders During Pregnancy and the Postpartum Period

43

Bilal Sizer, Aylin Gül, and Michael Rudenko

43.1 Introduction

The senses of smell and taste are two senses that complement each other. The flavor is a term that combines taste and smell. Retronasal olfaction occurs when the odor molecules that emerge during chewing, ingestion, and swallowing of food reach the olfactory epithelium. Therefore, some patients who experience smell problems may also complain about taste problems; however, this usually reflects the loss of smell perception rather than real taste disturbance.

Pregnancy is an exceptional condition that affects all physiology of women. The effects of pregnancy on the sense of smell have not been fully illuminated yet. There are some anecdotal reports and questionnaire studies, but there is a lack of consistent scientific information in this field. Some studies reported that there might be an increase in olfactory sensitivity, particularly in the early months of pregnancy that may be defined as the presence of hyperosmia in pregnancy. Odor test studies did not support this data. Saltiness is preferred during pregnancy, and the perceived intensity of salty taste decreases as the pregnancy progresses. This may be due to a

B. Sizer (✉)
Department of Otorihinolaryngology, Istanbul Arel University Faculty of Medicine, Istanbul, Turkey
e-mail: bilalsizer@arel.edu.tr

A. Gül
Department of Otorihinolaryngology, Medical Park Gaziantep Hospital, Gaziantep, Turkey
e-mail: draylingul@gmail.com

M. Rudenko
Section of Pediatric Allergy and Immunology, The London Allergy and Immunology Centre, London, UK
e-mail: rudenko_michael@yahoo.com

C. Cingi et al. (eds.), *ENT Diseases: Diagnosis and Treatment during Pregnancy and Lactation*, https://doi.org/10.1007/978-3-031-05303-0_43

physiological need to meet the increased salt requirement. While drinks that are low in sugar are preferred, sweet snacks are consumed more in the second trimester, possibly due to increased energy needs in this period.

43.2   Sense of Smell

Sense of smell is an essential element of normal physiological functioning. It is closely related to life quality and plays a role in many vital functions such as nutrition, sexual attraction, safety, and mother–infant attachment [1–4]. The occurrence of life-threatening situations due to the lack of perception caused by the loss of smell shows the importance of a strong sense of smell [5].

43.2.1 Anatomy and Physiology

The olfactory epithelium, which we use as the basis for olfactory function, is of pseudostratified columnar epithelium type. It is located in the upper septum, cribriform layer, superior turbinate, and middle turbinate part [6]. The transport of the airflow to the olfactory epithelium initiates the process of detecting odor molecules. The signal begins to be transmitted after odor molecules dissolved in mucus bind to olfactory receptors. Olfactory molecules can reach the olfactory area both through nasal and retronasal routes. The retronasal route, which is a different pathway, has been commonly associated with the sense of taste. The signal initiated by olfactory molecules at one end of the olfactory cells is carried to the olfactory bulb following the synapsis made by the other ends of olfactory cells through which the cribriform plate was passing with secondary neurons. The signal is transmitted from the olfactory tract to the olfactory sulcus. The transmission pathway is divided into lateral, intermediate, and medial striae in front of the anterior perforated substance and synapses with the parts of the primary olfactory cortex (olfactory tubercle, piriform cortex, amygdala, peri-amygdaloid complex, and entorhinal complex). There is a secondary olfactory cortex in the orbitofrontal area of the brain, and it has many connections with the primary cortex, mediated by the medial dorsal nucleus of the thalamus [7].

43.2.2 Evaluation of the Sense of Smell

In recent years, psychophysical and electrophysiological tests have been used to evaluate the sense of smell.

43.2.2.1   Psychophysical Tests

Psychophysical tests are subjective tests that can direct the individuals as their results are based on self-report statements. The results may further vary depending on the person's communication or perceptual impairment to whom the test is applied [8]. The most crucial advantage of psychophysical odor tests is that they can be easily prepared without advanced technology and can be applied under polyclinic conditions. Psychophysical tests are used to measure the odor threshold, discrimination, and identification. Sniffin' Sticks test has been frequently applied to patients with smell disorders since it is a practical and reliable method. The interaction of taste and smell is essential in the formation of the perception of taste. This interaction occurs when the odor molecules released from the food contents during chewing or swallowing reach the olfactory mucosa through the retronasal route. Whereas the evaluation is made through the orthonasal route in the tests similar to Sniffin' Sticks, Candy Smell test evaluates the sense of smell through the retronasal route [9–12].

Threshold Test: Odor value at the most minimal concentration that can be detected by a human nose.
Discrimination Test: The patient is asked to discriminate the odors.
Odor Identification Test: The patient is asked to identify the odor.

43.2.2.2 Electrophysiological Tests

Electro-olfactography: An electrode is placed in the olfactory area. If the receptor is stimulated with the given stimulation, a negative wavelength occurs. It is used to differentiate olfactory mucosal diseases from central diseases [13].

Olfactory-Evoked Potentials: It was designed based on the idea that olfactory stimulation may cause electroencephalography changes. It is based on the measurement of brainstem potentials against odorous substances with the help of electrodes placed percutaneously [14].

43.2.3 Smell Disorders

Smell disorders can be examined under two headings, namely, qualitative and quantitative disorders. The odor is perceived more in quantitative smell disorders and can be expressed in number by some tests. Conditions such as stimulation of the olfactory epithelium or the presence of odor molecules in the medium are not required to develop qualitative odor disorders (Table 43.1). The situation where odor thresholds

Table 43.1 Smell disorders (adapted from Ref. [18])

Quantitative smell disorders	Qualitative smell disorders
1. Anosmia: It describes the lack of ability to smell or odor thresholds below a certain value	1. Troposmia: It is the smell disorder that occurs although the olfactory system is intact
2. Hyposmia: Odor is detected but the ability to detect odors reduces	2. Parosmia: It refers to the inability to fully recognize the odor or wrong perception of odors
3. Hyperosmia: It is an increased olfactory acuity	3. Phathosmia: It is the perception of odor when there is no odor stimulus in the environment
	4. Cacosmia: It is the perception of unpleasant odor when there are no preconditions for recognizing an unpleasant odor in the environment

Table 43.2 Quantitative thresholds for the three commonly preferred odor tests (adapted from the Refs. [15–17])

	Anosmia	Hyposmia	Normosmia
Sniffin' sticks test	<16	16–30	>30
UPSIT	<19	19–33	$\geq$34
CCCRC	<3	4–6	>6

UPSIT The University of Pennsylvania Smell Identification Test, *CCCRC* Connecticut Chemosensory Clinical Research Center

are above an absolute value is called normosmia. The tests created for the evaluation of odor are used. However, performing a validity study of the test in the population to be tested is of great importance due to cultural differences in odor. Table 43.2 summarizes some tests frequently used to assess quantitative smell disorder [15–17].

43.2.4 Etiology of Smell Disorders

The etiology of smell disorders can be examined in three groups: conductive defects due to the obstruction of orthonasal or retronasal pathway, sensorineural defects due to the lack of olfactory neuroepithelium, and defects related to the central nervous system. Olfactory dysfunction may be caused by many reasons, including chemical agents, various drugs, surgical interventions, traumas, some congenital diseases, endocrinological disorders, infectious events, benign–malignant masses that prevent the transmission of odor molecules to the olfactory area, some psychiatric and neurological diseases, pregnancy, and aging [19].

The relationship between pregnancy and olfactory dysfunction will be discussed in more detail in the following sections.

43.3 Sense of Smell During Pregnancy and the Postpartum Period

According to the studies, including questionnaire studies, most pregnant women rate their smell higher than usual. However, the effects of pregnancy on the sense of smell have not been fully illuminated yet [20]. Understanding pregnancy's effect on the sense of smell may lead to a better understanding of maternal nutritional status [21].

Studies have shown an increase in olfactory sensitivity, particularly in the early months of pregnancy. This olfactory sensitivity reported by pregnant women has been significantly more intense in certain scents [22, 23]. In a study by Nordin et al., compared to nonpregnant women, pregnant women were reported to have an increased smell identification of particular ones, such as coffee, spoiled or freshly baking food, eau de cologne, oriental spices, and cigarettes smoke [24].

Considering that self-reported data based on questionnaires and anecdotal reports indicate hyperosmia in pregnancy, it seems to be not supported by studies using the odor test [25–28]. In other words, the increase in olfactory sensitivity reported by the pregnant may not correspond to the same meaning as the hyperosmia term used by the rhinology specialists. Disgust and hedonic ratings during pregnancy and the postpartum period will be evaluated in the light of literature data with olfactory thresholds, odor identification, and intensity parameters.

43.3.1 Olfactory Thresholds During Pregnancy and the Postpartum Period

According to the literature data, pregnant women showed a similar odor detection threshold with nonpregnant women. Even pregnant women's thresholds have been higher than those of nonpregnant women [22, 25, 26, 29]. In a study by Laska et al., they followed 20 pregnant women during the whole pregnancy and 2–3 months after delivery, and included 20 nonpregnant women as the control group. Mostly they had higher thresholds in the first trimester. In comparison, they had much lower thresholds in the last trimester. A significant sensitivity was reported in the third trimester compared to the first two trimesters and the postpartum period [30]. The studies reporting lower smell detection thresholds in the first 3 months are scarce [20]. There is no sufficient clue for a general change of smelling during pregnancy indicated by self-report and questionnaire studies.

43.3.2 Identification Thresholds During Pregnancy and the Postpartum Period

Examining the effects of pregnancy on odor identification has shown that pregnancy does not significantly affect odor identification. Some studies comparing pregnant women with odor identification controls have reported that pregnant women identify clove, strawberry, and watermelon odors better than controls [26, 30–33]. In a study by Cameron et al., 20 pregnant women were examined in each trimester and evaluated in the postpartum period, and pregnant women were compared with 20 nonpregnant women. The idea that pregnancy did not have a general effect on odor identification stood out [23].

43.3.3 Odor Intensity Ratings During Pregnancy and the Postpartum Period

Pregnant women's odor intensity ratings may be higher for selected odors, although their overall odor intensity ratings are not higher than those of nonpregnant women.

Swallow et al. reported that melon was statistically significantly more robust by pregnant women than nonpregnant women and men. Laska et al. reported that pregnant women significantly rated galaxolide and androstenone more intense than others.

Similarly, Cameron et al. reported that pregnant women rated these three (lemon, leather, and natural gas) among the tested 39 odors as statistically significantly more intense than controls [23, 25, 30, 34, 35].

43.3.4 Hedonics, Disgust, and Nausea-Vomiting During Pregnancy

The majority of studies have demonstrated that there are changes in odor hedonics during pregnancy and that the rating of the pleasantness of odor reduces, although it varies according to the origin of the odor. Some authors reported that cigarettes, coffee, rum, clove, coffee, orange, and natural gas were defined as unpleasant by pregnant participants [23, 25, 33]. Fornazieri et al. reported that pregnant women rated coffee as less pleasant, particularly in the first trimester, than other trimesters and rated cloves less pleasant in the second trimester [28]. On the contrary, studies on which odors are perceived as pleasant by women during pregnancy are somewhat limited. Acetic acid was rated as significantly more acceptable or even pleasant after the first trimesters of pregnancy by Ochsenbein-Kölble et al. Interestingly, androstenone was more pleasant in Gilbert and Wysocki's study (lit).

In contrast, Cameron reported that fruit punch was accepted more pleasant in the first 3 months of pregnancy [23, 32, 33]. In a study in which pregnant women were asked to identify odors that they evaluate as pleasant or just the opposite, pregnant women declared that food odors such as fish, meat, and eggs are pleasant and harmful smells like fumes, cigarettes, and garbage as unpleasant [23]. As it is understood, there is no consensus about which odors are perceived as pleasant and unpleasant during pregnancy, indicating that it is challenging to produce generally accepted evidence regardless of differences such as geographical region, culture, sociodemographic characteristics, and belief.

The fact that odors disgusted by pregnant women are some food smells besides smells of cigarette smoke. The idea behind it may be pregnant women's consideration of these odors as harmful [20]. In a study in which the Disgust Scale was applied to pregnant women, it was found that pregnant women in the first 3 months had significantly higher scores from this scale compared to the rest of their pregnancy period [36].

Nausea and vomiting affect nearly 75% of pregnant women. Several studies have emphasized that odors cause nausea during pregnancy, reported by pregnant women, and that the severity of nausea and vomiting is higher in those who are adversely affected by odors [34, 37]. Although the idea of establishing a causal link between nausea and vomiting and the increase in odor detection sensitivity, particularly in the first trimester, emphasized in self-report studies seems reasonable, it is required to document the increased odor detection sensitivity.

43.3.5 Possible Underlying Causes of Changes in the Sense of Smell During Pregnancy

Embryo protective hypothesis is based on the notion that the heightened sense of smell, particularly in the early pregnancy, which leads to nausea and vomiting in the first trimester, the most crucial phase of intrauterine growth and development, provides a protective function for the embryo by preventing the pregnant woman from ingesting teratogens [38]. However, according to the odor test results, the evidence for hyperosmia in pregnancy is weak, as demonstrated before. Therefore, based on the current knowledge, it seems unlikely that hyperosmia underlies nausea and vomiting that would protect the embryo [20].

Gradually increasing progesterone and estrogen hormones causes significant hormonal changes in pregnant women. Although changes in the sense of smell during pregnancy are thought to be related to this [39], the hCG hormone's course during pregnancy can be considered the underlying cause of the olfactory perception of odor hedonics variation. Nausea and vomiting also appear to be related to hCG levels in pregnancy. The nasal blockage usually occurs mainly during the last months of pregnancy with the contribution of hormonal changes and the changing physiology, and thus airflow is reduced, which reduces the ability to perceive odors [20].

43.4 Sense of Taste

The sense of taste allows us to distinguish and identify the substances swallowed during feeding. Although the sense of taste emerges with taste buds, the olfactory system must be healthy to perceive the flavor created by the combination of smell and taste [19].

Pregnancy is a natural physiological process. However, the nutritional status of pregnant women is of great importance for healthy intrauterine growth and development. Therefore, knowing the changes in the sense of taste during pregnancy and the postpartum period, in preferred flavors, and taste intensity will contribute to a healthier pregnancy process [40].

43.4.1 Anatomy and Physiology

Sense of taste occurs after signals that occur following the stimulation of taste receptors in taste receptor cells with a limited life span reach the central nervous system through afferent pathways. Taste receptor cells, which have a life span of about 10 days, are continually being replaced by basal cells. Taste receptor cells are found in taste buds, mostly in the tongue and in the palate, epiglottis, and esophagus. Flavors reach the receptor cells in the taste buds through the taste pores located at the epithelium's surface [41, 42].

Taste buds are found in structures called papillae that give the tongue its characteristic rough texture. Papillae are divided into four groups. Filiform papillae, which are found in large numbers, have no role in the taste function. Fungiform papillae are mostly located on the anterior part of the tongue and cover its anterior two-thirds. Foliate papillae are located near the tongue's root, and circumvallate papillae are located on the tongue's dorsal surface in an inverted V-shape [43, 44].

There are five tastes perceived by humans: umami, which was first described by K. Ikeda in 1908, and basic sweet, bitter, sour, and salty tastes [45, 46]. The tongue map is a misconception, which was inspired by Haenig's study and created in Wilhelm Wundt's laboratory in 1901, and expresses that every taste is perceived in different parts of the tongue. Basic tastes can be detected anywhere; there are taste buds [19].

A solution is formed in the mouth with the salivary secretion stimulated when foods are put in the mouth. Taste receptor cells are first stimulated by the solutions formed in the mouth through microvilli. Sweet and bitter substances interact with the microvilli membrane receptors, while salty and sour stimuli interact with ion channels in the membrane [41, 47] (Table 43.3).

Three different cranial nerves innervate the areas containing the taste bud. The chorda tympani branch of the facial nerve transmits the taste buds on the anterior 2/3 of the tongue, whereas the superficial petrosal branch transmits taste buds on the palate. The taste buds located on the posterior part of the tongue, covering the circumvallate papillae, are transmitted by the glossopharyngeal nerve, and the vagus nerve is responsible for the transmission of taste buds in the pharynx and the larynx. Primary taste neurons synapse in the nucleus of the solitary tract. Taste information is transferred from here to the thalamus and from there to the cortex [48].

43.4.2 Evaluation of the Sense of Taste

There are two types of tests used to evaluate taste function: chemical tests and electrogustometry. Chemical tests are carried out using sweet, bitter, salty, and sour flavors. Umami is generally not preferred in chemical tests. In general, sucrose, sodium chloride, quinine hydrochloride or caffeine, citric acid, and monosodium L

Table 43.3 Flavors and their receptor stimuli (adapted from Refs. [41, 46])

Flavor	Receptor stimulus
Salty	Sodium ions
Sweet	Sucrose, maltose, lactose, glucose, some alcohols and ketones, chloroform, beryllium salts, and various amides of aspartic acid
Sour	Hydrogen ions
Bitter	Quinine sulfate, strychnine hydrochloride, morphine, nicotine, caffeine, urea, and inorganic salts of magnesium, ammonium, calcium
Umami	Glutamate (monosodium)

glutamate are used for sweet, salty, bitter, sour, and umami, respectively. Taste tablets, taste bands, and taste discs are used to evaluate threshold. They are applied in increasing concentrations until the correct taste is determined. The concentration correctly detected by the patient is determined as the threshold value. The perceived taste intensity is assessed using concentrations above the taste threshold value [49–51].

In the test performed with electrogustometry, a weak electric current is applied to the tongue surface with the help of a stimulator. The first perceived taste value is considered as the threshold value. This stimulus is generally perceived as a sour taste [52].

43.4.3 Taste Disorders

Although the sense of taste is not deemed necessary, particularly as sight and hearing, taste disorders can significantly negatively affect life quality. Taste disorders can be classified as quantitative and qualitative disorders [42, 53] (Table 43.4).

43.4.4 Etiology of Taste Disorders

Poor oral hygiene, excessive smoking, and excessive alcohol consumption are the most common conditions affecting the sense of taste. Deficiency in certain vitamins and minerals and dry mouth can also cause loss of taste. Sense of taste can be further adversely affected by liver and kidney pathologies, endocrinological disorders, depression, central nervous system disorders, surgical interventions around the nerves involved in the transmission of taste, and antineoplastic agents. Moreover, people may experience taste dysfunctions in physiological processes such as aging, menopause, and pregnancy [54–56]. It is emphasized that pregnancy affects taste function, and women tend to develop hypoxia during pregnancy. Therefore, recognizing a possible change in taste function is essential for a healthy pregnancy [40].

Table 43.4 Taste disorders (adapted from Refs. [42, 53])

Quantitative disorders	Qualitative disorders
1. Ageusia: Absence of the sense of taste, inability to taste	1. Parageusia: Misperception of the taste stimulus
2. Hypogeusia: Decreased sensitivity in the sense of taste	2. Cacogeusia: Perceiving flavors as unpleasant
3. Dysgeusia: Impaired sense of taste	3. Phantom taste: Perception of a constant taste that occurs in the absence of a taste stimulus
4. Hyperguesia: Increased sense of taste	4. Aliageusia: Perceiving a typically pleasant-tasting food or drink as an unpleasant taste

43.5 Sense of Taste During Pregnancy and the Postpartum Period

The pregnancy process can be examined in three trimesters, where the nutritional requirement is different depending on the intrauterine growth and development of the baby. Compared to the second and third trimesters, the nutritional energy requirement is less in the first trimester, whereas the energy requirement increases, particularly in the third trimester when the baby starts to overgrow. Cultural perceptions and beliefs and the physical and physiological changes brought by the pregnancy can also affect food choices, and the amount of food consumed [40, 57].

Women are thought to be more conscious and careful about their food choices and consumption during pregnancy. Studies indicate that behaviors such as avoiding the consumption of potentially harmful foods are related to safety concerns. It is further believed that women's taste perception changes during pregnancy, which affects their dietary preference and food consumption [58, 59] (Fig. 43.1).

43.5.1 Taste Thresholds During Pregnancy and the Postpartum Period

Studies have reported that pregnant women have higher sweet taste thresholds and are more sensitive to odor than nonpregnant women, whereas studies report no difference in sweet taste thresholds in the first-trimester nonpregnant controls and the

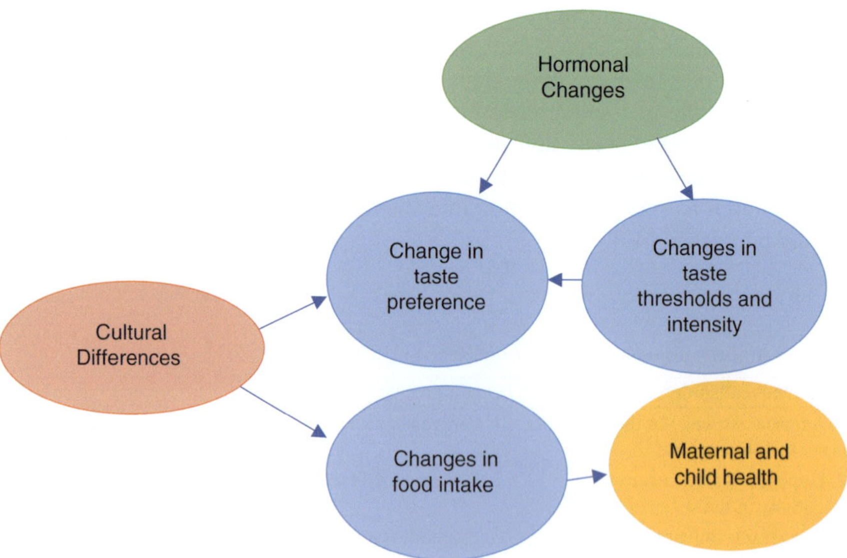

Fig. 43.1 Model of the causes and possible consequences of changing taste perception during pregnancy. (Adapted from Ref. [57])

postpartum period [25, 35, 60, 61]. Sweet taste thresholds were reported to decrease after the first trimester and late pregnancy, suggesting that sweet taste sensitivity increased during pregnancy [60, 61].

In a study by Kuga et al., in which pregnant women were compared with controls for sour and salty taste, it was reported that the sour and salty taste thresholds of pregnant women were higher during the first trimester than in nonpregnant controls and that pregnant women were more sensitive to salty taste in the first trimester compared to the second and third trimesters [60]. In another study, no significant difference was reported in sour and salty taste thresholds between nonpregnant women, pregnant women, and women in the postpartum period [35].

Kölble et al. and Kuga et al. emphasized that the bitter taste thresholds of pregnant women in the first trimester were higher than those of nonpregnant women [25, 60]. Another study found that pregnant women's bitter taste thresholds were higher during pregnancy and 7 weeks after pregnancy than nonpregnant controls [35] (Table 43.5).

Table 43.5 Taste threshold changes during pregnancy and the postpartum period (adapted from Ref. [57])

Author (year)	Sweet	Salty	Sour	Bitter
Kolble et al. (2001)	No significant difference between pregnant women in the first trimester and controls.	No difference between pregnant women in the first trimester and controls.	No difference between pregnant women in the first trimester and controls.	The taste function scores of pregnant women in the first trimester were lower than nonpregnant controls.
Kuga et al. (2002)	Pregnant women in the first trimester had a higher sweet taste threshold compared to controls. The taste threshold of women in the first trimester was higher than that of women in the second and third trimesters.	Pregnant women in the first trimester had a higher salty taste threshold compared to controls. The taste threshold of women in the first trimester was higher than that of women in the second and third trimesters.	Pregnant women in the first trimester had a higher sour taste threshold compared to controls.	Pregnant women in the first trimester had a higher bitter taste threshold compared to controls.
Ochsenbein-Kolble et al. (2005)	Postpartum period and controls versus pregnant women in the first trimester: No difference.	Postpartum period and controls versus pregnant women in the first trimester: No difference.	Postpartum period and controls versus pregnant women in the first trimester: No difference.	Compared to nonpregnant controls, pregnant women had lower taste function scores in the first trimester and 7 weeks after delivery.

43.5.2 Changes in Perceived Taste Intensity During Pregnancy and the Postpartum Period

Koble et al. reported no difference between women in any trimester of pregnancy, those in the postpartum period, and nonpregnant controls in terms of sweet taste intensity perception [25, 57].

The literature review showed that the intensity of the perceived salty taste decreased during pregnancy. Bowen et al. reported that the three salty foods were rated less salty in the third trimester and the postpartum period than the first and second trimesters [62]. Similarly, Duffy et al. found that the perceived salty taste intensity decreased from the first to the second trimester and from the first to the third trimester [63].

It is thought that there is no difference in perception of sour taste intensity in pre-pregnancy, pregnancy, and the postpartum period [25, 35, 63].

In three cross-sectional studies evaluating the bitter taste intensity perception, no difference was reported between pregnant women and nonpregnant controls in terms of bitter taste intensity. Two of these studies emphasized no significant difference in bitter taste perception intensity during pregnancy [25, 35, 64]. However, the study by Duffy et al. is the only longitudinal study on pain intensity. In their study, the perception of pain intensity was higher in the first trimester than in the pre-pregnancy period, and it was stated that the intensity of pain decreased during the three trimesters [63]. This notion suggests that there may be a slight increase in bitter taste perception intensity during the first trimester and a decrease in bitter taste perception intensity throughout pregnancy. However, it should be supported by other studies since it is based on a single study.

43.5.3 Changes in the Sense of Taste during Pregnancy and the Postpartum Period

When the pregnancy period is evaluated in terms of sweet taste, drinks low in sugar are preferred, while sweet snacks are preferred in the second trimester when energy needs are high [62, 64]. Studies showed that pregnant women favored salty taste when compared to nonpregnant women. It was further observed that salty snacks were consumed more during pregnancy than during the postpartum period. Based on this data, pregnancy does not significantly affect sour and bitter taste preferences [57].

43.6 Treatment

The treatment approach for smell and taste disorders discussed in this section has not been presented only for pregnancy and the postpartum period; it is aimed to provide a general approach.

There is no standard treatment for taste and smell disorders. A careful head and neck examination, endoscopic examination, and testing of the sense of taste and smell should be performed since the underlying cause of the current situation in both smell and taste disorders may be a disease. There is no effective treatment method for the changes in smell and taste perception during pregnancy since it is a physiological process [65]. Although not specific to pregnancy, treating smell and taste disorders generally includes treating the underlying disease and providing support to patients to cope with the current situation.

Zinc, steroids, and various antioxidants are recommended in smell disorders; however, their effects are not predictable for all situations. In recent years, odor exercises have been tried to treat smell disorders, and promising outcomes have been obtained [66–69]. Methods such as taking zinc supplements, alpha-lipoic acid, clonazepam, and oral ice cube application have effectively treated taste disorders [70–73]. It is recommended to consume light foods such as chicken, milk, and eggs for unpleasant tastes and low taste thresholds. Furthermore, it is thought that cooling the foods before eating can reduce unpleasant tastes and smells [74].

References

1. Jacob S, McClintock MK, Zelano B, et al. Paternally inherited HLA alleles are associated with women's choice of male odor. Nat Genet. 2002;30(2):175–9.
2. Doucet S, Soussignan R, Sagot P, et al. The secretion of areolar (Montgomery's) glands from lactating women elicits selective, unconditional responses in neonates. PLoS One. 2009;4(10):e7579.
3. Mennella JA, Jagnowm CP, Beauchamp GK. Prenatal and postnatal flavor learning by human infants. Pediatrics. 2001;107(6):e88.
4. Murphy C, Schubert CR, Cruickshanks KJ, et al. Prevalence of olfactory impairment in older adults. JAMA. 2002;288(18):2307–12.
5. Santos DV, Reiter ER, DiNardo LJ, et al. Hazardous events associated with impaired olfactory function. Arch Otolaryngol Head Neck Surg. 2004;130(3):317–9.
6. Hummel T, Welge-Lüssen A, editors. Taste and smell: an update. Switzerland: Karger Medical and Scientific Publishers; 2006.
7. Gottfried JA, Deichmann R, Winston JS, et al. Functional heterogeneity in human olfactory cortex: an event-related functional magnetic resonance imaging study. J Neurosci. 2002;22(24):10819–28.
8. Guducu C, Oniz A, Ikiz AO, et al. Chemosensory function in congenitally blind or deaf teenagers. Chemosens Percept. 2016;9(1):8–13.
9. Hummel T, Sekinger B, Wolf SR, et al. Sniffin' sticks': olfactory performance assessed by the combined testing of odor identification, odor discrimination and olfactory threshold. Chem Senses. 1997;22(1):39–52.
10. Altundag A, Salihoglu M, Cayonu M, et al. The effect of anatomic clearance between tongue and soft palate on retronasal olfactory function. Chemosens Percept. 2014;7(1):40–5.
11. Bojanowski V, Hummel T. Retronasal perception of odors. Physiol Behav. 2012;107(4):484–7.
12. Renner B, Mueller CA, Dreier J, et al. The candy smell test: a new test for retronasal olfactory performance. Laryngoscope. 2009;119(3):487–95.
13. Seiden AM, Duncan HJ (2001) The diagnosis of a conductive olfactory loss. Laryngoscope 111(1): 9–14.

14. Nordin S, Murphy C, Davidson TM, et al. Prevalence and assessment of qualitative olfactory dysfunction in different age groups. Laryngoscope. 1996;106(6):739–44.
15. Muirhead N, Benjamin E, Saleh H. Is the University of Pennsylvania Smell Identification Test (UPSIT) valid for the UK population. Otorhinolaryngol. 2013;2:99–103.
16. Cain WS, Goodspeed RB, Gent JF, et al. Evaluation of olfactory dysfunction in the Connecticut chemosensory clinical research center. Laryngoscope. 1988;98(1):83–8.
17. Oniz A, Erdogan I, Ikiz AO, et al. The modified Sniffin' Sticks test in Turkish population based on odor familiarity survey. J Neurol Sci. 2013;30(2):270–80.
18. Leopold D. Distortion of olfactory perception: diagnosis and treatment. Chem Senses. 2002;27(7):611–5.
19. Bailey BJ, editor. Head & neck surgery--otolaryngology. Lippincott Williams & Wilkins; 2011.
20. Cameron EL. Pregnancy and olfaction: a review. Front Psychol. 2014;5:67–78.
21. Lacroix R, Eason E, Melzack R. Nausea and vomiting during pregnancy: a prospective study of its frequency, intensity, and patterns of change. Am J Obstet Gynecol. 2000;182(4):931–7.
22. Nwankwo U, Fasunla AJ, Oladokun A, et al. Comparison between olfactory function of pregnant women and non-pregnant women in reproductive age group in Ibadan, Nigeria. Niger J Clin Pract. 2017;20(5):610–5.
23. Leslie Cameron E. Measures of human olfactory perception during pregnancy. Chem Senses. 2007;32(8):775–82.
24. Nordin S, Broman DA, Olofsson JK, et al. A longitudinal descriptive study of self-reported abnormal smell and taste perception in pregnant women. Chem Senses. 2004;29(5):391–402.
25. Kölble N, Hummel T, von Mering R, et al. Gustatory and olfactory function in the first trimester of pregnancy. Eur J Obstet Gynecol Reprod Biol. 2001;99(2):179–83.
26. Savović SN, Ninčić DP, Lemajić SN, et al. Olfactory perception in women with physiologically altered hormonal status (during pregnancy and postmenopause). Med Pregl. 2002;55(9–10):380–3.
27. Simsek G, Muluk NB, Arikan OK, et al. Marked changes in olfactory perception during early pregnancy: a prospective case-control study. Eur Arch Otorhinolaryngol. 2015;272(3):627–30.
28. Fornazieri MA, Prina DMC, Favoreto JPM, et al. Olfaction during pregnancy and postpartum period. Chemosens Percept. 2019;12(2):125–34.
29. Gül A, Yılmaz B, Karababa S, et al. Gebelikte koku fonksiyon değişiminin değerlendirilmesi. Kulak Burun Bogaz Ihtis Derg. 2015;25(2):92–6.
30. Laska M, Koch B, Heid B, et al. Failure to demonstrate systematic changes in olfactory perception in the course of pregnancy: a longitudinal study. Chem Senses. 1996;21(5):567–71.
31. Kim HJ, Park HJ, Park JY, et al. The possibility of morning sickness from olfactory hypersensitivity during pregnancy. Korean J Otorhinolaryngol-Head Neck Surg. 2011;54(7):473–6.
32. Gilbert AN, Wysocki CJ. Quantitative assessment of olfactory experience during pregnancy. Psychosom Med. 1991;53(6):693–700.
33. Ochsenbein-Kölble N, Von Mering R, Zimmermann R, et al. Changes in olfactory function in pregnancy and postpartum. Int J Gynecol Obstet. 2007;97(1):10–4.
34. Swallow BL, Lindow SW, Masson EA. Women with nausea and vomiting in pregnancy demonstrate worse health and are adversely affected by odours. J Obstet Gynaecol. 2005;25(6):544–9.
35. Ochsenbein-Kölble N, Von Mering R, Zimmermann R, et al. Changes in gustatory function during the course of pregnancy and postpartum. BJOG. 2005;112(12):1636–40.
36. Fessler DM, Eng SJ, Navarrete CD. Elevated disgust sensitivity in the first trimester of pregnancy: evidence supporting the compensatory prophylaxis hypothesis. Evol Hum Behav. 2005;26(4):344–51.
37. Cantoni P, Hudson R, Distel H, et al. Changes in olfactory perception and dietary habits in the course of pregnancy: a questionnaire study. Chem Senses. 1999;24(58):111.
38. Profet M. Pregnancy sickness as adaptation: a deterrent to maternal ingestion. In: Barkow JH, Cosmides L, Tooby J, editors. The adapted mind: evolutionary psychology and the generation of culture. New York: Oxford University Press; 1995.
39. Doty RL, Cameron EL. Sex differences and reproductive hormone influences on human odor perception. Physiol Behav. 2009;97(2):213–28.

40. Fasunla AJ, Nwankwo U, Onakoya PA, et al. Gustatory function of pregnant and non-pregnant women in a tertiary health institution. Ear Nose Throat J. 2019;98(3):143–8.
41. Breslin PA, Huang L. Human taste: peripheral anatomy, taste transduction, and coding. Taste Smell. 2006;63:152–90.
42. Mann NM, Lafreniere D. Overview of taste and olfactory disorders in adults https://www.uptodate.com/contents/overview-of-taste-and-olfactory-disorders-in-adults. Accessed 17 Aug 2020.
43. Cheng LHH, Robinson PP. The distribution of fungiform papillae and taste buds on the human tongue. Arch Oral Biol. 1991;36(8):583–9.
44. Miller IJ Jr. Variation in human fungiform taste bud densities among regions and subjects. Anat Rec. 1986;216(4):474–82.
45. Bromley SM. Smell and taste disorders: a primary care approach. Am Fam Physician. 2000;61(2):427–36.
46. Yamaguchi S, Ninomiya K. Umami and food palatability. J Nutr. 2000;130(4):921–6.
47. Mistretta CM. Developmental neurobiology of the taste system. In: Getchell TV, Bartoshuk LM, Doty RL, Snow Jr JB, editors. Smell and taste in health and disease. New York: Raven; 1991.
48. Landis BN, Welge-Luessen A, Brämerson A, et al. "Taste Strips"—a rapid, lateralized, gustatory bedside identification test based on impregnated filter papers. J Neurol. 2009;256(2):242–8.
49. Ahne G, Erras A, Hummel T, Kobal G. Assessment of gustatory function by means of tasting tablets. Laryngoscope. 2000;110:1396–401.
50. Schiffman SS, Frey AE, Luboski JA, et al. Taste of glutamate salts in young and elderly subjects: role of inosine 5′-monophosphate and ions. Physiol Behav. 1991;49(5):843–54.
51. Stillman JA, Morton RP, Hay KD, et al. Electrogustometry: strengths, weaknesses, and clinical evidence of stimulus boundaries. Clin Otolaryngol Allied Sci. 2003;28(5):406–10.
52. Fark T, Hummel C, Hähner A, Nin T, et al. Characteristics of taste disorders. Eur Arch Otorhinolaryngol. 2013;270(6):1855–60.
53. Ng K, Woo J, Kwan M, et al. Effect of age and disease on taste perception. J Pain Symptom Manag. 2004;28(1):28–34.
54. Nelson GM. Biology of taste buds and the clinical problem of taste loss. Anat Rec. 1998;253(3):70–8.
55. Torpet LA, Kragelund C, Reibel J, et al. Oral adverse drug reactions to cardiovascular drugs. Crit Rev Oral Biol Med. 2004;15(1):28–46.
56. Weenen H, Olsen A, Nanou E, et al. Changes in taste threshold, perceived intensity, liking, and preference in pregnant women: a literature review. Chemosens Percept. 2019;12(1):1–17.
57. Hill AJ, Cairnduff V, McCance DR. Nutritional and clinical associations of food cravings in pregnancy. J Hum Nutr Diet. 2016;29(3):281–9.
58. Verbeke W, De Bourdeaudhuij I. Dietary behaviour of pregnant versus non-pregnant women. Appetite. 2007;48(1):78–86.
59. Kuga M, Ikeda M, Suzuki K, et al. Changes in gustatory sense during pregnancy. Acta Otolaryngol. 2002;122(4):146–53.
60. Sonbul H, Ashi H, Aljahdali E, et al. The influence of pregnancy on sweet taste perception and plaque acidogenicity. Matern Child Health J. 2017;21(5):1037–46.
61. Bowen DJ. Taste and food preference changes across the course of pregnancy. Appetite. 1992;19(3):233–42.
62. Duffy VB, Bartoshuk LM, Striegel-Moore RU. Taste changes across pregnancy a. Ann N Y Acad Sci. 1998;855(1):805–9.
63. Nanou E, Brandt S, Weenen H, et al. Sweet and bitter taste perception of women during pregnancy. Chemosens Percept. 2016;9(4):141–52.
64. Dikici O, Muluk NB, Şahin E, Altıntoprak N. Effects of pregnancy on olfaction. ENT Updates. 2017;7(2):104–7.
65. Reden J, Herting B, Lill K, et al. Treatment of postinfectious olfactory disorders with minocycline: a double-blind, placebo-controlled study. Laryngoscope. 2011;121(3):679–82.
66. Altundag A, Cayonu M, Kayabasoglu G, et al. Modified olfactory training in patients with postinfectious olfactory loss. Laryngoscope. 2015;125(8):1763–6.

67. Henkin R, Schecter PJ, Friedewald WT, et al. A double-blind study of the effects of zinc sulfate on taste and smell dysfunction. Am J Med Sci. 1976;272(3):285–99.
68. İkeda K, Sakurada T, Takasaka T, et al. Anosmia following head trauma: preliminary study of steroid treatment. Tohoku J Exp Med. 1995;177(4):343–51.
69. Fujiyama R, Ishitobi S, Honda K, et al. Ice cube stimulation helps to improve dysgeusia. Odontology. 2010;98(1):82–4.
70. Takaoka T, Sarukura N, Ueda C, et al. Effects of zinc supplementation on serum zinc concentration and ratio of apo/holo-activities of angiotensin-converting enzyme in patients with taste impairment. Auris Nasus Larynx. 2010;37(2):190–4.
71. Femiano F, Scully C, Gombos F. Idiopathic dysgeusia; an open trial of alpha-lipoic acid (ALA) therapy. Int J Oral Maxillofac Surg. 2002;31(6):625–8.
72. Grushka M, Epstein J, Mott A. An open-label, dose-escalation pilot study of the effect of clonazepam in burning mouth syndrome. Oral Surg Oral Med Oral Pathol Oral Radiol Endodontol. 1998;86(5):557–61.
73. Hong JH, Omur-Ozbek P, Stanek BT, et al. Taste and odor abnormalities in cancer patients. J Support Oncol. 2009;7(2):58–65.

Yunus Kantekin and Ali Bayram

44.1 Introduction

Epistaxis is one of the most frequent otolaryngological emergency that presents in up to 60% of the general population. Approximately 10% of epistaxis necessitates medical attention, whereas 0.16% will require hospitalization [1–3]. Peaks in incidence demonstrate a bimodal distribution with children under 10 years of age and in adults over 50 years [4, 5]. Age is one of the significant factors that affect the severity of the epistaxis. Epistaxis in young adults tends to arise from anterior nasal septum and more minor, whereas more severe epistaxis originated from posterior part of the nasal cavity tends to occur in older adults.

Nasal cavity has an extensive vascular supply originated from external and internal carotid arteries with frequent anastomotic connections. External carotid artery provides vascular supply to the nasal cavity by the facial artery and internal maxillary artery. Facial artery gives off the superior labial artery that supplies the anterior nasal septum. Internal maxillary artery enters into the posterolateral nasal cavity as sphenopalatine artery through the sphenopalatine foramen. Sphenopalatine artery gives off two major branches (nasal septal branch and the posterior lateral nasal artery), which provides blood supply to 90% of the nasal mucosa [6]. Greater palatine and posterior pharyngeal arteries also contribute to the vascular supply of nasal cavity. The internal carotid artery majorly provides vascular supply to the superior portion of the nasal cavity via the anterior and posterior ethmoid arteries that arise from the ophthalmic artery. There are also two main sites in the nasal cavity that harbor plexus of vessels: Kiesselbach's plexus (also known as Little's area) and Woodruff plexus. Kiesselbach's plexus is located at the entrance of the nasal cavity and involves terminal branches of the anterior and posterior ethmoidal arteries,

Y. Kantekin (✉) · A. Bayram
Department of Otorhinolaryngology, Kayseri City Hospital, Kayseri, Turkey
e-mail: ykantekin@yahoo.com; dralibayram@gmail.com

C. Cingi et al. (eds.), *ENT Diseases: Diagnosis and Treatment during Pregnancy
and Lactation*, https://doi.org/10.1007/978-3-031-05303-0_44

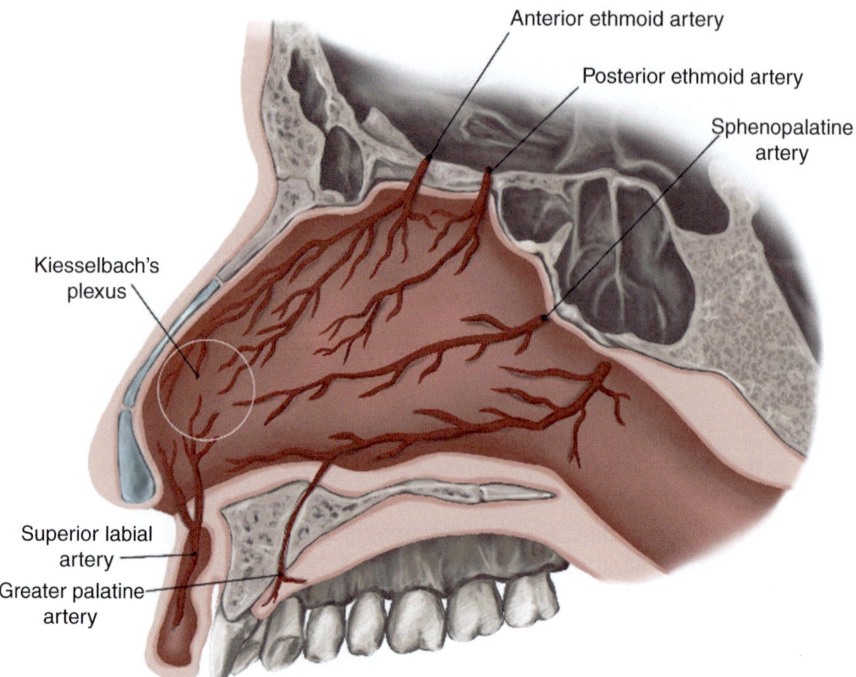

Fig. 44.1 Vascular anatomy of the nasal septum

Table 44.1 Causes of secondary epistaxis

Local	Systemic
Trauma (e.g., blunt, digital)	Coagulopathy (e.g., anticoagulation, hemophilia)
Infectious/inflammatory	
Structural (e.g., septal deviation, spur)	Hypertension
Sinonasal tumors	Hematologic malignancy (e.g., leukemia)
Granulomatous diseases (e.g., Wegener, sarcoidosis	Hepatobiliary disease
Environmental irritants (e.g., smoke, chemicals)	von Willebrand disease
Iatrogenic	Hereditary hemorrhagic telangiectasia
Foreign bodies	Vascular/connective tissue disorders
Drugs (e.g., topical steroids, cocaine abuse)	Malnutrition

superior labial, sphenopalatine, and greater palatine arteries (Fig. 44.1). Woodruff plexus consists of the anastomoses between the sphenopalatine and posterior pharyngeal arteries and is located at the posterior end of the inferior turbinate. The venous drainage of the nasal cavity usually follows the arteries within the mucosa.

Epistaxis can be classified as primary (or idiopathic) and secondary according to its etiological factor. Primary epistaxis accounts for the majority of the cases, whereas secondary epistaxis occurs due to several local or systemic factors (Table 44.1). Epistaxis has also two common types according to the site of origin: anterior and posterior epistaxis. Anterior epistaxis mostly arises from the anterior nasal septum (90%), especially within Kiesselbach's plexus. Posterior epistaxis usually occurs from the vascular sources that supply posterior nasal septum and lateral nasal wall (sphenopalatine artery and terminal branches of the maxillary artery). Although posterior epistaxis is seen more rarely, their diagnosis and management are often more difficult and require hospitalization, referral to otolaryngology, and posterior nasal packing [7].

The management of the epistaxis has classically been divided into conservative and surgical treatment. It should be noted that the vast majority of epistaxis are self-limited and require no medical intervention. Moisturizing or humidifying agents such as nasal saline mist and gels, petrolatum-based ointments, and room humidifiers are conservative treatment options mostly utilized for chronic recurrent epistaxis. The management of acute hemorrhagic conditions necessitates securing the patient's airway and hemodynamic stability as an initial step. Systemic etiological factors that contribute to nasal bleeding such as hypertension, thrombocytopenia, and coagulopathies should be examined and treated to facilitate bleeding control. Localizing the origin of the epistaxis is of the utmost importance, and the basic treatment should be occluding the vessel near its bleeding point. Nasal packing should be avoided as an initial option for the treatment of the epistaxis since it causes further trauma to the nasal mucosa. Therefore, nasal packing should be reserved in cases without an identified bleeding site. Absorbable hemostatic agents are favorable materials for nasal packing since they cause minimal trauma to the nasal mucosa. Nonabsorbable nasal packs such as layered ribbon gauze and expandable polyvinyl acetate can be used if absorbable packing is ineffective or unavailable [8]. For posterior epistaxis, posterior nasal packing with nasal balloons or 14 Fr Foley catheter inflated with 15 mL of saline may be required to tamponade the entire nasal cavity and nasopharynx. Endovascular embolization and surgical interventions such as ligation of the ethmoid, internal maxillary, or the external carotid arteries can be employed when conservative treatment options have failed to stop the bleeding. More recently, endoscopic vascular ligations have been introduced as a surgical treatment modality for patients with epistaxis. Endoscopic sphenopalatine artery ligation with clipping or diathermy is currently recommended as the first-line surgical intervention in epistaxis that is not relieved with conservative approaches [9, 10].

The prevalence of epistaxis in pregnancy is increased, although most of them do not require a medical attention. In a study conducted with 1470 pregnant and 275 nonpregnant women, Dugan-Kim et al. [11] reported that the prevalence of epistaxis was significantly higher in pregnant women than nonpregnant women (20.3% versus 6.2%). Numerous predisposing factors may contribute to the tendency of epistaxis in pregnancy. The cardiovascular system experiences significant changes during pregnancy and maternal blood volume increases by 30–50%. Progesterone provokes an increase in blood volume and nasal vascular congestion. Placental growth hormone has systemic effects, including vasodilation [12]. Rhinitis during pregnancy is an alteration in nasal physiology, including nasal mucosal congestion, edema, and rhinitis driven by elevated hormonal levels [13]. Rhinitis during pregnancy is classified as a hormonal rhinitis according to nonallergic rhinitis: position paper of the European Academy of Allergy and Clinical Immunology [14]. It typically manifests in the second or third trimester of the pregnancy without any known allergic causes and lasts at least 6 weeks. More typically, it subsides entirely within 2 weeks after delivery. Hormonal changes during pregnancy may cause indirect effects that interact with the receptors of the nasal mucosa and exert nasal hyperreactivity. Hamano et al. [15] reported evidence regarding the presence of hormonal activity through histamine receptors by increasing the expression of H1 receptors in nasal epithelium and microvascular endothelial cells. Cytokines may also contribute to nasal hyperreactivity during pregnancy.

During pregnancy, epistaxis may also occur due to the granuloma gravidarum and coagulopathies associated with pregnancy, including idiopathic thrombocytopenic purpura, HELLP syndrome, gestational thrombocytopenia, and vitamin K deficiency induced by hyperemesis gravidarum [16]. Granuloma gravidarum is a benign, rapidly growing, fibrovascular lesion with extensive endothelial proliferation [17]. Since these lesions represent a lobular capillary hemangioma, the nomenclature of "granuloma" is not accurate. The gross appearance of the lesion is a red, solitary, friable, and pedunculated papule that frequently has an ulcerated surface. Microscopically, the lesion involves lobular aggregates of capillary-sized vessels and a variable amount of inflammatory cell infiltrate within highly vascular granulation tissue. The microscopic characteristics of the granuloma gravidarum resemble those in pyogenic granuloma; nevertheless, the presence of foamy histiocytes is usually found more frequently in granuloma gravidarum [18]. Granuloma gravidarum usually appears in the second and third trimesters of the pregnancy with a prevalence of 0.5–5% of all pregnancies. Although the exact cause of this entity is unclear, it is hypothesized that the lesion occurs due to the inflammatory responses to the hyper-hormonal status of pregnancy [19]. It usually arises from the intraoral mucosa in the head and neck region, most commonly from gingiva, and termed also as epulis gravidarum and granuloma of pregnancy. However, granuloma gravidarum may rarely occur in the nasal mucosa and may cause nasal obstruction and epistaxis during pregnancy. Management of the granuloma gravidarum depends on the severity of the symptoms. Small and painless lesions without recurrent bleeding should be managed with clinical observation and follow-up since granuloma gravidarum usually regresses after pregnancy. However, surgical excision is an ideal treatment method in cases with severe epistaxis [20].

Although severe epistaxis is uncommon during pregnancy, acute blood loss with a large volume can be life-threatening both for the mother and fetus. Severe epistaxis during pregnancy necessitates hospitalization with a rapid multidisciplinary medical approach managed by obstetricians, otolaryngologists, and anesthesiologists. Nevertheless, treatment options are limited due to absolute or relative contraindications during pregnancy. Blood transfusion should be made if necessary with caution for hemolytic reactions, isoimmunization, and infection transmission [21]. The first-line therapy should involve conservative management options such as intravenous tranexamic acid administration, nasal packing, silver nitrate, and bipolar cautery. Anterior nasal packing with Merocel or Rapid Rhino packs can be used in pregnancy, but bismuth iodoform paraffin paste (BIPP)-soaked ribbon gauze is contraindicated. Also, posterior nasal packs with nasal balloon or Foley catheter are suitable for using in pregnant individuals. However, local anesthetic and topical vasoconstrictor agents should be used with the consideration of their increased risk of systemic absorption, which decreases uterine blood flow. If the conservative management fails, surgical management with vessel ligation and termination of the pregnancy should be considered by the medical team. If the gestational age is near to term, delivery induction or cesarean section should be evaluated by the obstetrician. Vaginal delivery is theoretically contraindicated because of the efforts and pushes that may induce epistaxis during labor and emergent or elective cesarean section should be performed to ensure maternal and fetal safety. Sphenopalatine artery, anterior ethmoidal artery, and posterior ethmoidal artery ligations can be performed to terminate epistaxis in pregnant individuals; nevertheless, the risk of general anesthetics should be considered cautiously. Intravenous and inhaled anesthetics for any surgical procedures such as cesarean section or vessel ligation are known to increase the risk of preterm labor, especially during the first two trimesters of pregnancy [16]. Also, a rapid sequence induction is required to prevent gastric aspiration with a left lateral tilt on the operating table to prevent aortocaval compression [10]. The risk of radiological embolization is unquantified in the treatment of epistaxis during pregnancy, whereas the intravenous contrast substances have a potential for contrast-induced neonatal hypothyroidism [22].

References

1. Chaaban MR, Zhang D, Resto V, Goodwin JS. Demographic, seasonal, and geographic differences in emergency department visits for epistaxis. Otolaryngol Head Neck Surg. 2017;156:81–6.
2. Cooper SE, Ramakrishnan VR. Direct cauterization of the nasal septal artery for epistaxis. Laryngoscope. 2012;122:738–40.
3. Viehweg TL, Roberson JB, Hudson JW. Epistaxis: diagnosis and treatment. J Oral Maxillofac Surg. 2006;64:511–8.
4. Tomkinson A, Roblin DG, Flanagan P, Quine SM, Backhouse S. Patterns of hospital attendance with epistaxis. Rhinology. 1997;35:129–31.
5. Fishpool SJ, Tomkinson A. Patterns of hospital admission with epistaxis for 26,725 patients over an 18-year period in Wales, UK. Ann R Coll Surg Engl. 2012;94:559–62.
6. Loughran S, Hilmi O, McGarry GW. Endoscopic sphenopalatine artery ligation—when, why and how to do it. An on-line video tutorial. Clin Otolaryngol. 2005;30:539–43.
7. Womack JP, Kropa J, Jimenez SM. Epistaxis: outpatient management. Am Fam Physician. 2018;98:240–5.
8. Corbridge RJ, Djazaeri B, Hellier WP, Hadley J. A prospective randomized controlled trial comparing the use of merocel nasal tampons and BIPP in the control of acute epistaxis. Clin Otolaryngol Allied Sci. 1995;20:305–7.
9. Gede LL, Aanaes K, Collatz H, Larsen PL, von Buchwald C. National long-lasting effect of endonasal endoscopic sphenopalatine artery clipping for epistaxis. Acta Otolaryngol. 2013;133:744–8.
10. Kumar S, Shetty A, Rockey J, Nilssen E. Contemporary surgical treatment of epistaxis. What is the evidence for sphenopalatine artery ligation? Clin Otolaryngol Allied Sci. 2003;28:360–3.
11. Dugan-Kim M, Connell S, Stika C, Wong CA, Gossett DR. Epistaxis of pregnancy and association with postpartum hemorrhage. Obstet Gynecol. 2009;114:1322–5.

12. Sobol SE, Frenkiel S, Nachtigal D, Wiener D, Teblum C. Clinical manifestations of sinonasal pathology during pregnancy. J Otolaryngol. 2001;30:24–8.
13. Piccioni MG, Derme M, Salerno L, Morrocchi E, Pecorini F, Porpora MG, et al. Management of severe epistaxis during pregnancy: a case report and review of the literature. Case Rep Obstet Gynecol. 2019;2019:5825309.
14. Hellings PW, Klimek L, Cingi C, Agache I, Akdis C, Bachert C, et al. Non-allergic rhinitis: position paper of the European Academy of Allergy and Clinical Immunology. Allergy. 2017;72:1657–65.
15. Hamano N, Terada N, Maesako K, Ikeda T, Fukuda S, Wakita J, et al. Expression of histamine receptors in nasal epithelial cells and endothelial cells--the effects of sex hormones. Int Arch Allergy Immunol. 1998;115:220–7.
16. Crunkhorn RE, Mitchell-Innes A, Muzaffar J. Torrential epistaxis in the third trimester: a management conundrum. BMJ Case Rep. 2014;2014:bcr2014203892.
17. Shemen L, Falkowski O. Giant nasal granuloma gravidarum. BMJ Case Rep. 2020;13:e237612.
18. Skau NK, Pilgaard P, Neilsen G. Granuloma gravidarum of the nasal mucous membrane. J Laryngol Otol. 1987;101:1286–8.
19. Hugoson A. Gingival inflammation and female sex hormones. A clinical investigation of pregnant women and experimental studies in dogs. J Periodontal Res Suppl. 1970;5:1–18.
20. Ginat DT, Schatz CJ. Nasal septum granuloma gravidarum. Ear Nose Throat J. 2017;96:412–4.
21. Bukar M, Audu BM, Bako BG, Garandawa HI, Kagu MB, et al. Idiopathic thrombocytopaenic purpura in pregnancy presenting with life-threatening epistaxis. J Obstet Gynaecol. 2009;29:439–40.
22. Hardy JJ, Connolly CM, Weir CJ. Epistaxis in pregnancy—not to be sniffed at! Int J Obstet Anesth. 2008;17:94–5.

Allergic Rhinitis During Pregnancy

45

Nuray Bayar Muluk, Cemal Cingi, and Glenis Scadding

45.1 Introduction

Whilst she is pregnant, a woman may develop an atopic disorder for the first time, such as rhinitis, urticaria, angioedema, or allergic eczema, or she may already have such a condition. However, whereas there has been extensive investigation of asthma during pregnancy, other atopic conditions during this period have been somewhat neglected by researchers [1].

In most cases, allergic rhinitis (AR) is already present before a woman conceives, albeit it may not yet have presented or been diagnosed. The usual symptomatic complaints in cases of AR are a noticeable tendency to sneeze, itching of the nose, and a clear nasal discharge. This is sometimes accompanied by conjunctival irritation and pruritus. The allergens causing symptoms are usually house dust mites (*Dermatophagoides pteronyssinus and D. farinae*), animal dander, molds, or pollen [1].

It has been proven that being pregnant affects and alters the functioning of particular factors involved in the immediate phase allergic reaction. The circulating histamine level is significantly reduced during the first trimester of pregnancy in

N. Bayar Muluk (✉)
Department of Otorhinolaryngology, Faculty of Medicine, Kırıkkale University, Kırıkkale, Turkey
e-mail: nbayarmuluk@yahoo.com

C. Cingi
Department of Otorhinolaryngology, Medical Faculty, Eskisehir Osmangazi University, Eskisehir, Turkey
e-mail: cemal@ogu.edu.tr

G. Scadding
Consultant Allergist & Rhinologist, RNENT Hospital, University College Hospital, London, UK
e-mail: gscadding@gmail.com

© The Author(s), under exclusive license to Springer Nature Switzerland AG 2022
C. Cingi et al. (eds.), *ENT Diseases: Diagnosis and Treatment during Pregnancy and Lactation*, https://doi.org/10.1007/978-3-031-05303-0_45

women suffering from atopic disorders compared to the period after birth. The placenta synthesizes the enzyme histaminase, which may explain this [2]. In theory, this lower level should result in an improvement in AR symptoms, but there is no experimental evidence at present to confirm the theory. From a clinical point of view, the key observation is that pregnancy potentially causes endocrine alterations, resulting in the mucosal lining of the nose becoming more congested. The higher circulating volume in all pregnant women and more active mucosae in the nose lead to edema and a hypersecretory state [3]. Rhinitis of pregnancy is dealt with in Chap. 46.

Just as occurs in cases of asthma, pregnancy may have a worsening effect on long-standing persistent rhinitis, improve the situation, or have no noticeable effect. More precisely, the reported rate of symptomatic improvement in pregnant women with AR is 34%, some 15% of cases become more severe and the remaining cases are unaltered in severity [4]. Pregnant patients with AR frequently complain of autophony, the abnormal sound of one's own voice, related to the ear feeling full. This is typically the result of the Eustachian tubes being congested [5].

Since AR can affect sleep and well-being, it is important to make an accurate diagnosis and treat it effectively but safely.

45.2 Signs and Symptoms

The usual presenting symptoms of AR are as follows [6]:

- Sneezing, itching (nasal, ocular, otic, or palatal)
- Nasal discharge
- Postnasal discharge
- Nasal blockage
- Impaired ability to smell
- Headache otalgia
- Excess lacrimation
- Ocular erythema
- Periocular edema
- Lethargy
- Sleepiness
- Poor concentration
- Feeling generally unwell

45.3 Diagnosis

45.3.1 History

AR diagnosis is based largely on the patient's history, backed up by examination findings and by tests for the relevant specific IgE. Details of symptoms, where and when they occur, what worsens or improves them, what treatment has been taken, and whether or not it worked are needed. Since nonallergic rhinitis during pregnancy can occur, special attention should be paid to possible indications of allergy such as eye involvement, nasal itching, and itching of the palate, which are more likely in AR [7].

45.3.2 Examination

AR may be complicated by [6].

- Acute or persistent sinus inflammation
- Nonfunctioning Eustachian tubes
- Middle ear inflammation
- Insomnia or apnea
- Worsening of concurrent asthma

Therefore, a full ENT and chest examination should be undertaken, including an objective lower airways measurement such as spirometry or peak flow.

The following features should be sought [6]:

- Mouth breathing.
- Dark circles under eyes.
- Allergic salute, whereby the patient keeps pushing up the nose in response to itching.
- Allergic crease, a horizontal crease running from side to side on the inferior portion of the bridge of the nose as a result of the allergic salute.
- Clear, non-viscous rhinorrhea.
- Pale swollen nasal mucosa.
- The septum of the nose may deviate to one side or have been perforated. This may be due to a number of conditions.
- If present since childhood, AR may result in a high arched palate and dental malocclusion.

AR also produces ocular, otic, and oropharyngeal signs as follows [6]:

- On otoscopy, the eardrum may be retracted and have altered mobility.
- The conjunctival vessels may be swollen and erythematous around the lids, and there is hyper lacrimation. The vessels around the eyes may have been persistently dilated, related to the congestion in the nose, and this may lead to Dennie–Morgan lines (seen under the lower lid, a noticeable crease) and "allergic shiners," that is, darkening of the skin periorbitally.
- Lymphoid tissue may take on a cobblestone-like appearance in the posterior oropharyngeal region. The tonsils may be hypertrophied. There may be some degree of malocclusion, and the palate is more raised than normal.
- Chest examination may reveal wheezing, and objective airway measurements may reveal outflow obstruction.

45.3.3 Tests for Specific IgE

In pregnancy, it is preferable to perform laboratory-based tests for specific IgE to isolate which specific aeroallergens are the likely culprits, if no previous cutaneous testing results are available [1].

There is widespread availability of in vitro serological quantification of specific IgE to particular allergens.

Since both false-positive and false-negative results occur, it is important to relate the test result to the history.

If tests fail to confirm that a specific allergen or allergens are responsible for symptoms, an empirical trial of treatment is appropriate, rather than undertaking nasal allergen challenge in pregnancy [1]..

45.4 Treatment

A key principle to consider when treating pregnant patients with AR is the balance of risk between failing to treat and any harm that the medication may do to the mother and fetus. Although in theory there is considerable potential for teratogenicity to occur, in practice less than 1 in 100 congenital malformations is ascribable to the use of medication [8]. In the United States, the Food and Drugs Administration (FDA) employs a scheme with five categories/classes to classify the teratogenic potential of pharmacological agents. The five categories are named A, B, C, D, and X. Any drug licensed since 1980 must state within the product insert to which class it belongs to [9]. A number of agents that are frequently employed in treating atopic disease fall under category B, namely, budesonide (both inhaler and nasal spray), cromolyn sodium, cetirizine, levocetirizine, loratadine, and omalizumab [1].

The first-line treatment is avoidance of the allergen (including environmental modification) where the allergenic trigger has been identified. This approach may be sufficient, provided symptoms are not especially troubling. Other environmental exacerbators such as pollutants like cigarette smoke should also be avoided and nasal saline sprays or drops can be used to clear the nose if and allergen or exacerbator has been encountered [8].

45.4.1 Cromolyn Sodium Nasal Spray

Cromolyn sodium nasal spray has been identified as possessing excellent safety characteristics when used as initial monotherapy in AR of mild degree in pregnant patients. This profile is related to the very low circulating plasma level when it is used topically on mucosae [10]. The pooled results of three trials, involving 600 pregnancies, and where the agent was administered even in the initial trimester, indicated no additional risk of any congenital anomaly with this agent, when taken via inhaler. However, the data do not extend to when this agent is used intranasally or as an eye drop and the need for repeated nasal use some three or four times daily renders it unsuitable for most busy women [11].

45.4.2 Glucocorticoid Nasal Sprays

Glucocorticoid nasal sprays possess high efficacy in AR, especially in symptomatic relief from a blocked nose and postnasal discharge. If a pregnant patient has AR that is of at least moderate degree, these agents are the most appropriate treatment. In such circumstances, the dose needs to be the minimum at which benefit is observed [1].

The deduction that intranasal steroids are safe to employ in pregnant patients with AR is extrapolated from the data on their use in pregnant patients with asthma. In asthma, the dosage exceeds that used in AR [12]. Safety data on the use of nasal steroids come from a trial involving in excess of 140,000 pregnant women, with 2502 individuals prescribed nasal steroids within the initial trimester. These data are from 2016 [13, 14]. The rate of congenital anomaly or miscarriage did not differ between those exposed and those not exposed to nasal steroids. The sole agent of this class that may have an association with malformations is triamcinolone. There was a raised incidence of congenital respiratory anomalies [adjusted odds ratio (OR) = 2.71 (95% CI 1.11–6.64)], but the actual instances of anomaly were few, consisting, as they did, of two instances where there was a congenital malformation of the respiratory tract NOS, one instance of laryngeal anomaly, two instances of tracheal or bronchial anomaly, and a single instance of choanal atresia. No other steroid produced a signal. There is a preference among prescribers for budesonide as the initial agent in a pregnant woman with AR newly starting treatment. This preference appears based on the FDA categorization of budesonide as a class B agent, a judgment informed by data gathered by the Medical Birth Registry in Sweden, favoring the use of budesonide. The majority of other nasal steroid agents fall under FDA class C [15].

45.4.3 Oral Antihistamines

Taking an antihistamine by mouth is less efficacious in treating AR than topical nasal steroids, especially in terms of alleviating a blocked nose and preventing postnasal discharge. A number of studies have been conducted in which safety aspects of antihistamine use in pregnant women were assessed [16–20]. In pregnant patients who do need an antihistamine, in the majority of cases, the newer (second generation) antihistamines are a better choice than the older agents, which have a more severe range of adverse effects due to their action on cholinergic transmission, and produce more sedation [1].

There are also some differences among individual drugs within the second generation. The two agents that are most suitable for pregnant women are loratadine (at a dose of 10 mg od) and cetirizine (also 10 mg od). These two agents have both been extensively evaluated in many women and fall under category B of the FDA scheme [20]. While levocetirizine is also a class B agent, the amount of data available is significantly less. Fexofenadine lacks sufficient safety data and falls under category C [1].

If the patient complains of intermittent problems and symptoms are of mild degree, an antihistamine of the second generation may be prescribed on a regular or PRN basis.

45.4.4 Antihistamine Nasal Sprays

Azelastine has US FDA pregnancy category C. Animal reproduction studies have shown an adverse effect on the fetus, and there are no adequate and well-controlled studies in humans. However, the FDA states that potential benefits may warrant use of the drug in pregnant women despite potential risks [21, 22]. Olopatadine is not recommended "during pregnancy and in women of childbearing potential not using contraception." Available data in animals have shown "excretion of olopatadine in milk following oral administration." A risk to the newborn/infants cannot be excluded [23].

Given this gap in our safety knowledge, the authors recommend not employing either agent except where a patient has only been able to obtain symptomatic relief with these agents prior to conceiving [1].

Fixed-dose combination sprays with intranasal corticosteroid plus intranasal antihistamine should also be avoided unless absolutely necessary and with the full informed consent of the pregnant woman and her partner.

45.4.5 Decongestants

Decongestant agents act by constricting nasal blood vessels and exist in both an oral and topical intranasal form. Their ability to cross the placenta remains a matter of conjecture [24]. One study concluded that oxymetazoline and xylometazoline may be linked to a number of congenital anomalies [24].

Gastroschisis occurs spontaneously in 1 in 10,000 births. According to the results of two studies employing a case–control methodology, pseudoephedrine may increase the risk of this anomaly [24, 25]. It is also noted in the literature that gastroschisis in infants may be linked to the mother taking phenylpropanolamine [26], which raises the possibility the association may apply to all members of the class. Moreover, taking pseudoephedrine during the first 3 months of pregnancy may result in limb reduction defects [24].

In the light of the risk that decongestants may be linked to a number of otherwise unusual congenital anomalies, they should not be prescribed at all during pregnancy [24].

45.4.6 Montelukast

Montelukast has a marketing authorization for the indication of AR, and so far safety studies in both animal and human subjects reveal no concerns about resulting birth defects [27–29]. This agent, nonetheless, possesses lower efficacy in AR than nasal steroids [30] and thus use should be confined to those women where a trial preceding the pregnancy resulted in significant benefit, or where nasal steroids and antihistamine pharmacotherapy have failed to manage the symptoms of AR [1].

45.4.7 Allergen Immunotherapy

This can be given by two routes: subcutaneous injection (SCIT) and sublingual tablets or drops (SLIT).

Subcutaneous allergen immunotherapy (SCIT) should not be newly started in pregnant women. There are various reasons for this including [1]

- The risk of a systemic reaction has not been quantified.
- The benefit can occur earlier, especially with SLIT.

Persevering with preexisting SCIT in a pregnant patient does seem to be a safe practice, albeit a systemic reaction is still possible. There are two studies involving the use of injection immunotherapy in pregnancy. There were 171 women enrolled, and 230 pregnancies in total. Comparison with a group of pregnant women with atopic disease not receiving immunotherapy showed no additional risk of miscarriage, perinatal mortality, premature birth, toxemia, or birth defects. Neither was the risk raised compared to the background population risk [9, 15].

- Bearing these data in mind, the authors suggest that SCIT should not be halted if the patient is pregnant and the following conditions apply [31]:
- There is evidence of existing benefit from SCIT.
- The patient has no demonstrable tendency toward systemic allergic reactions to the treatment.
- The patient is on the maintenance dose, or as a minimum, on a dose that affords actual benefit.

Sublingual immunotherapy (SLIT) may be managed in a similar fashion to SCIT in pregnant patients. In research involving 185 pregnant women, the rate of pregnancy-related complications was no higher in those receiving SLIT than control patients or the background population risk [29]. The authors concluded that SLIT was safe in pregnancy, even when initiated for the first time in a pregnant patient [32].

Our advice is that with SCIT, SLIT should not be freshly started if a patient is pregnant unless absolutely necessary; however, where treatment is already underway and benefit is being derived, it should be continued [1].

In the COVID pandemic, it makes sense to switch patients from SCIT to SLIT in order to avoid the need for frequent clinic visits [33].

45.5 Conclusions

AR can preexist or arise during pregnancy. Given its known complications and multimorbidities, it warrants accurate diagnosis and effective treatment. Avoidance of relevant allergens and exacerbating factors plus nasal saline are initial measures that can safely be supplemented by pharmacotherapeutic measures with good safety ratings such as budesonide, loratadine, and cetirizine. Allergen-specific immunotherapy, both SCIT and SLIT, can be continued if started prior to pregnancy and proves effective. The patient and her partner should always be clearly informed about the risks and benefits of AR treatment in pregnancy.

References

1. Schatz M. Recognition and management of allergic disease during pregnancy. In: Lockwood CJ, Feldweg AM, editors. UpToDate. Last updated: Dec 16, 2019.
2. Beeley L. Adverse effects of drugs in later pregnancy. Clin Obstet Gynecol. 1981;8:275–90.
3. Sorri M, Bortikanen-Sorri AL, Karja J. Rhinitis during pregnancy. Rhinology. 1980;18:83–6.
4. Schatz M, Zeiger RS. Diagnosis and management of rhinitis during pregnancy. Allergy Proc. 1988;9:545–54.
5. Mazzotta P, Loebstein R, Koren G. Treating allergic rhinitis in pregnancy. Drug Safety Apr. 1999;20(4):361–75.
6. Sheikh J. Allergic rhinitis. In: Kaliner MA, editor. Medscape. https://emedicine.medscape.com/article/134825-overview. Accessed online at June 25, 2020.
7. Scadding GK, Kariyawasam H, Scadding G, et al. BSACI guideline for the diagnosis and management of allergic and non-allergic rhinitis (Revised Edition 2017; First edition 2007). Clin Exp Allergy. 2017;47:856–89. Available at www.bsaci.org (Accessed online at July 5, 2021).
8. Scialli A, Lone A. Pregnancy effects of specific medications used to treat asthma and immunological diseases. In: Schatz M, Zeiger RS, Claman HN, editors. Asthma and immunological diseases in pregnancy and early infancy. New York: Marcel Dekker; 1998.
9. Metzger WJ, Turner E, Patterson R. The safety of immunotherapy during pregnancy. J Allergy Clin Immunol. 1978;61:268.
10. National Asthma Education and Prevention Program: Expert panel report III: Guidelines for the diagnosis and management of asthma. Bethesda, MD: National Heart, Lung, and Blood Institute, 2007. (NIH publication no. 08-4051). www.nhlbi.nih.gov/guidelines/asthma/asthgdln.htm. Accessed 23 February 2010.
11. Wilson J. Use of sodium cromoglycate during pregnancy. J Pharm Med. 1982;8:45.
12. National Heart, Lung, and Blood Institute, National Asthma Education and Prevention Program Asthma and Pregnancy Working Group. NAEPP expert panel report. Managing asthma during pregnancy: recommendations for pharmacologic treatment-2004 update. J Allergy Clin Immunol. 2005;115:34.
13. Bérard A, Sheehy O, Kurzinger ML, Juhaeri J. Intranasal triamcinolone use during pregnancy and the risk of adverse pregnancy outcomes. J Allergy Clin Immunol. 2016;138:97.
14. Namazy JA, Schatz M. The safety of intranasal steroids during pregnancy: a good start. J Allergy Clin Immunol. 2016;138:105.
15. Shaikh WA. A retrospective study on the safety of immunotherapy in pregnancy. Clin Exp Allergy. 1993;23:857.
16. Schatz M, Petitti D. Antihistamines and pregnancy. Ann Allergy Asthma Immunol. 1997;78:157.

17. Diav-Citrin O, Shechtman S, Aharonovich A, et al. Pregnancy outcome after gestational exposure to loratadine or antihistamines: a prospective controlled cohort study. J Allergy Clin Immunol. 2003;111:1239.
18. Moretti ME, Caprara D, Coutinho CJ, et al. Fetal safety of loratadine use in the first trimester of pregnancy: a multicenter study. J Allergy Clin Immunol. 2003;111:479.
19. Gilbert C, Mazzotta P, Loebstein R, Koren G. Fetal safety of drugs used in the treatment of allergic rhinitis: a critical review. Drug Saf. 2005;28:707.
20. Källén B. Use of antihistamine drugs in early pregnancy and delivery outcome. J MaternFetal Neonatal Med. 2002;11:146.
21. Somoskövi A, Bártfai Z, Tamási L, et al. Population-based case-control study of allergic rhinitis during pregnancy for birth outcomes. Eur J ObstetGynecolReprodBiol. 2007;131:21.
22. https://www.drugs.com/pregnancy/azelastine-nasal.html. Accessed 5 July 2021.
23. https://www.medicines.org.uk/emc/medicine/11776/spc#gref. Accessed 5 July 2021.
24. Yau WP, Mitchell AA, Lin KJ, et al. Use of decongestants during pregnancy and the risk of birth defects. Am J Epidemiol. 2013;178:198.
25. Werler MM, Mitchell AA, Shapiro S. First trimester maternal medication use in relation to gastroschisis. Teratology. 1992;45:361.
26. Torfs CP, Katz EA, Bateson TF, et al. Maternal medications and environmental exposures as risk factors for gastroschisis. Teratology. 1996;54:84.
27. Sarkar M, Koren G, Kalra S, et al. Montelukast use during pregnancy: a multicentre, prospective, comparative study of infant outcomes. Eur J Clin Pharmacol. 2009;65:1259.
28. Nelsen LM, Shields KE, Cunningham ML, et al. Congenital malformations among infants born to women receiving montelukast, inhaled corticosteroids, and other asthma medications. J Allergy Clin Immunol. 2012;129:251.
29. Cavero-Carbonell C, Vinkel-Hansen A, Rabanque-Hernández MJ, et al. Fetal exposure to Montelukast and congenital anomalies: a population based study in Denmark. Birth Defects Res. 2017;109:452.
30. Dykewicz MS, Wallace DV, Baroody F, et al. Treatment of seasonal allergic rhinitis: an evidence-based focused 2017 guideline update. Ann Allergy Asthma Immunol. 2017;119:489.
31. Dombrowski MP, Schatz M. ACOG Committee on Practice Bulletins-Obstetrics. ACOG practice bulletin: clinical management guidelines for obstetrician-gynecologists number 90, February 2008: asthma in pregnancy. Obstet Gynecol. 2008;111(457). Reaffirmed 2019.
32. Shaikh WA, Shaikh SW. A prospective study on the safety of sublingual immunotherapy in pregnancy. Allergy. 2012;67:741.
33. Scadding GK, Hellings PW, Bachert C, et al. Allergic respiratory disease care in the COVID-19 era: a EUFOREA statement. World Allergy Organ J. 2020;5:100124. https://doi.org/10.1016/j.waojou.2020.100124.

Gestational Rhinitis

46

Harun Soyalıç, Elvan Evrim Ünsal Tuna,
Toppila-Salmi Sanna, and Annina Lyly

46.1 Introduction

Nonallergic rhinitis (nAR) is characterized by mucosal inflammation with the occurrence of a minimum of two nasal symptoms such as nasal obstruction, rhinorrhea, sneezing, and/or itchy nose. These symptoms occur with no clinical endonasal infection or evidence of inhalant allergen sensitization. Nonallergic rhinitis has a wide severity range and frequently presents or is induced by hyperresponsive/nonspecific environmental causes. Nasal hyperresponsiveness is a feature of both allergic and nonallergic rhinitis. nAR involves different subgroups (Table 46.1) and is classified below.

H. Soyalıç (✉)
Faculty of Medicine, Department of Otolaryngology, Head and Neck Surgery, Ahi Evran University, Kırşehir, Turkey
e-mail: harun_soyalic@hotmail.com

E. E. Ü. Tuna
Faculty of Medicine, Department of Otolaryngology, Head and Neck Surgery, Health Sciences University, Ankara City Research and Training Hospital, Ankara, Turkey
e-mail: e_unsal@yahoo.com

T.-S. Sanna
Skin and Allergy Hospital, Helsinki University Hospital and University of Helsinki, Helsinki, Finland
e-mail: sanna.salmi@helsinki.fi

A. Lyly
Skin and Allergy Hospital, Helsinki University Hospital, Inflammation Centre, University of Helsinki, Helsinki, Finland

Department of Otorhinolaryngology-Head and Neck Surgery, Helsinki University Hospital, University of Helsinki, Helsinki, Finland

C. Cingi et al. (eds.), *ENT Diseases: Diagnosis and Treatment during Pregnancy and Lactation*, https://doi.org/10.1007/978-3-031-05303-0_46

Table 46.1 Types and causes of rhinitis [1]

Rhinitis: common types and etiologies of noninfectious rhinitis
Allergic rhinitis
Seasonal
Perennial
Nonallergic rhinitis
Pregnancy
Vasomotor
Gustatory
NARES (nonallergic rhinitis with eosinophilia syndrome)
Atrophic
CPAP-associated rhinitis
Rhinitis medicamentosa
Nasal decongestant sprays
Intranasal cocaine
Systemic medication-induced rhinitis
Oral contraceptives
Erectile dysfunction drugs
Alpha-blockers
Some hypertensives
Aspirin and other NSAIDS
Some antidepressants
Some benzodiazepines
Systemic diseases
Hypothyroidism
Granulomatosis with polyangiitis (Wegener's granulomatosis)
Midline granuloma
Sarcoidosis
Cystic fibrosis
Immotile cilia syndrome (Kartagener)
Mixed rhinitis
Noninfectious rhinitis during pregnancy
Nonallergic rhinitis
Gestational rhinitis
Pregnancy vasomotor rhinitis
Rhinitis medicamentosa
Allergic rhinitis

46.2 Gestational Rhinitis

Gestational rhinitis (GR), or pregnancy rhinitis, is characterized by nasal obstruction during pregnancy [2]. It normally presents idiopathically in the second/third trimester, lasts 6 weeks or longer, and resolves by 2 weeks following the pregnancy. There is much debate about GR terms. Some highlight an important difference between "during pregnancy" rhinitis and GR. During pregnancy, rhinitis encompasses all types (allergic rhinitis, nonallergic rhinitis, mixed rhinitis) and may not be specifically identified during the second or third trimester [2].

46.2.1 GR History

Several reports speculated on an association with the female genitals and the nose in the nineteenth century. MacKenzie was the first to report on menstrual/sexual stimulation resulting in nasal symptom worsening [3]. Soon after, Endriss showed epistaxis exacerbation and nasal complications during menstruation or pregnancy [4].

In 1943, Mohun showed a relationship with vasomotor rhinitis during pregnancy, worsening in the last trimester, and recovery following delivery. His conclusion was that pregnancy-induced estrogen expression resulted in vasomotor rhinitis development [5].

46.2.2 Incidence and Prevalence

Women have been documented to report symptoms of rhinitis during childhood/adolescence (20–40%), and some (10–30%) have stated worsening of symptoms while pregnant [6].

Small cohort studies consistently struggle to differentiate GR from other rhinitis with an occurrence of 18–30% for all types during pregnancy [7].

A large cohort study from Sweden, including 599 patients on GR occurrence during pregnancy, revealed 22% prevalence [8]. However, a study that assessed 109 pregnant women using questionnaires and anterior rhinoscopy only showed a 9% GR occurrence during pregnancy. This finding is consistent with another study [9]. It has been observed that the duration of pregnancy is directly proportional to the severity of nasal obstruction. In a study conducted by Bende and Gredmark, nasal congestion and obstruction were evaluated as 27% at 12th week, 37% at 20th week, and 40% at 39th week. In particular, rhinitis findings increased even more during third trimester [10, 11].

46.2.3 Etiology and Physiopathology

While many etiological factors have been suggested, our understanding of GR physiopathology is lacking [6, 7]. GR has been associated with changes in hormones during pregnancy [12]. Etiology and physiopathology of GR are summarized in Table 46.2.

Table 46.2 Suggested etiology and physiopathology of gestational rhinitis

Increased circulating estrogen and progesterone
Increased mucous acetylcholine receptors
Decreased alpha-adrenergic response and associated vascular enlargement of smooth muscle
Fullness and congestion with increased blood volume in the extravascular area
Increased placental growth hormone

Throughout pregnancy, observations of augmented estrogen and progesterone levels have been linked to nasal mucosal hyperreactivity and have been shown to contribute to mucosal swelling, nasal obstruction, and worsening of symptoms [13–15]. Furthermore, estrogen may complicate symptoms by enhancing histamine receptors in the epithelium and microvasculature [16]. On the other hand, progesterone may contribute to local nasal vasodilation and augmentation of circulating blood volume (CBV), which transpires during pregnancy [17]. Placental growth hormone may also contribute to nasal congestion. Physiological deviations during pregnancy may increase the severity of symptoms. The CBV associated with pregnancy (and 40% of pre-pregnancy) has been linked to enhanced nasal airway resistance [15].

46.3 Pregnancy Hormones and Nasal Physiology

During pregnancy, alterations in hormones impact nasal physiology by multiple means and cause changes to the nasal mucosa [18].

46.3.1 Estrogen

Estrogen levels are intensely elevated during pregnancy [12]. It is known that estrogen can block acetylcholine esterase, resulting in acetylcholine production, and induced parasympathetic activity. This phenomenon affects vasodilatation and swelling of the nasal mucosa [19, 20].

Estrogen can also affect vascular permeability, glandular function, protein biosynthesis, and vasomotor sensitivity of the autonomic nervous system. Increased biosynthesis of proteins and glycosaminoglycans (i.e., hyaluronic acid) in the nasal mucosa results in thickened mucus and alterations in mucociliary clearance [19, 20]. Additionally, estrogen hormone causes an increase in blood pooling by decreasing of alpha adrenergic smooth muscle tension or edema due to the vascular hyperpermeability [12].

Increased plasma volume in pregnant women has been shown to take place throughout the 6–8-week gestation period and peak at the 32nd week [12]. Volume has been shown to increase to 4.7–5.2 L, which is a 45% rise compared to the nonpregnant. This is caused by the induction of the renin–angiotensin–aldosterone system and high estrogen hormone levels causing sodium and water retention. Water retention can cause mucosal edema, leading to nasal congestion [21].

Estrogen can activate immune responses via mast cell α-estrogen receptor signaling [12]. The activation peak happens throughout menstruation, pregnancy, consumption of oral contraceptive, and/or hormone therapy. It is possible that estrogen and progesterone regulate Th2 cell differentiation and production. These cells are known to regulate IgE and other antibody synthesis. Antibodies that regulate mast cells can result in their degranulation, and thus release histamine, cytokines, and leukotrienes [22, 23].

46.3.2 Progesterone

No differences have been reported in circulating progesterone levels in pregnant and nonpregnant women with rhinitis [14]. Other studies have shown enhanced blood volume and nasal congestion, which is most likely from vasodilatation due to increased progesterone levels in pregnant women [12]. Nasal vascular pooling, from smooth muscle relaxation, has been shown to be linked to increased progesterone [12]. Augmentation of vasoactive intestinal peptide release may result in increased nasal congestion and is related to progesterone and oxytocin [12]. Fibroblast-associated progesterone may impact the extracellular matrix lining the nasal mucosa [20].

46.3.3 Prolactin

Prolactin production via the pituitary gland has been shown to be enhanced throughout pregnancy and may be linked to the pathogenesis of pregnancy rhinitis [14]. Nevertheless, the absence of rhinitis and nasal congestion contradicts this phenomenon in patients suffering from prolactinoma tumors [14]. Moreover, bromocriptine and quinagolide decrease the production of prolactin and have nasal congestion as a known side effect [12].

46.3.4 Neuropeptides

The parasympathetic nerve (PN) induces acetylcholine, norepinephrine, and vasoactive intestinal peptide (VIP) release. Postganglionic PN innervates serous–mucous glands, arterial and venous smooth muscle, and arteriovenous anastomoses [24]. VIP induces nasal serous secretion, nasal vasodilatation, and can dominate mucociliary clearance [24]. VIP has been linked to rhinitis and during pregnancy, potentially mediating nasal mucosa vasodilation that is responsible for nasal congestion [12]. Investigators asserted that the role of estrogen on the nasal mucosa is facilitated by VIP and substance P (SP) via increased nasal mucosal gland secretion, mucosal vasodilatation, and reduction of vasoconstriction caused by neuropeptide Y (NPY) [12]. VIP has been shown to relax blood vessels in the upper airways, trachea, bronchi, and pulmonary vessels.

SP is synthesized by the trigeminal nerve of the afferent sensory neurons within the nasal mucosa. Neurotransmitters stimulate vasodilatation, enhanced permeability of blood vessels, and hypersecretion of submucosal glands, which result in multiple symptoms. The exact molecular mechanisms in GR are unclear [25].

46.3.5 Placental Growth Hormone

Human growth hormone (hGH) is released in bursts between peaks [14]. Later, hGH secretion is replaced with placental growth hormone (PGH) following the first gestational trimester. PGH has been shown to be augmented throughout pregnancy and in greater amounts in women with GR [12, 14]. Presumably, PGH triggers nasal mucosal infection similar to progesterone and causes peripheral vasodilatation, increased extracellular volume, and thus, GR. The mechanism still remains unknown, and future studies are needed to uncover these details [26].

46.4 Risk Factors

Smoking was the only risk factor recognized in the progression GR [7, 27]. This same report showed that IgE to house dust mites predisposes to the advancement of the complication [27]. No association has been determined between GR and preexisting asthma [28]. In addition, no link has been observed between maternal and gestational age, gender, and/or parity [7, 10, 14]. In comparison to AR, electron microscopy observations in pregnant women with GR showed very similar results to AR [4]. Based on this and literature supporting evidence of patients with GR having dust mite sensitivity, it was determined that GR patients present similarly to an AR subgroup. However, there is spontaneous resolve following delivery [7]. Furthermore, serum markers for allergies such as soluble intercellular adhesion molecule-1 (sICAM-1) are not increased in GR [14].

46.5 Diagnosis and Clinical Significance

Diagnosis of GR is based on typical symptoms (nasal obstruction) and the exclusion of other causes of nasal congestion. Women with GR often describe continuous nasal congestion accompanied by watery/viscous nasal secretions [7, 14, 28]. These symptoms have been shown to disrupt night mouth breathing sleep quality [29].

Diagnosis of GR is clinical, and often the conditions worsen due to nasal obstruction. Caution should be regarded when considering the criteria for nasal obstruction during pregnancy and should include only those with impacted life quality [30]. Identification of GR is done through medical history, recording symptoms, and physical examination. This is done to exclude other nasal complications. Currently, differentiating allergic versus nonallergic rhinitis is difficult and is contingent on determining the triggering factors [12].

Head and neck analysis using rhinoscopy or nasoendoscopy should be performed before and after nasal decongestants to exclude other complications. The nasal mucosa and turbinates can present as swollen and/or shielded with serous-to-seromucoid discharge. Currently, other methods do not exist to diagnose GR [12].

46.6 Impact on Quality of Life

GR may have a remarkable impact on quality of life such as worse sleep in pregnant women [31]. In particular, snoring and obstructive sleep apnea can present during this time and may also be linked to pregnancy weight gain [30]. Oral breathing complications are also a consequence of GR and cause reduced nitric oxide inhalation, decreased vascular resistance, and limited oxygenation. Reduced nitric oxide in lungs can severely affect the fetus and result in hypertension and preeclampsia in the mother as well as intrauterine growth retardation and lower Apgar scores in newborns. Moreover, nasal blockage and sleep complications can contribute to overuse of nasal decongestants, and further nonresolving rhinitis even following childbirth. Even still, there is limited data to support the relationship between GR and poor pregnancy outcomes [2].

46.7 Differential Diagnosis

Differential diagnosis for GR includes distinguishing between sinusitis, allergic rhinitis (AR), rhinitis medicamentosa, acute/subacute upper airway infection, anatomical variation, and pregnancy granuloma (Table 46.3) [2].

Rhinitis medicamentosa has often been associated with GR, and typically patients do not disclose their history of persistent nasal decongestant usage. Thus, it is helpful to gather this medical information. Often, individuals with rhinitis medicamentosa lose their nasal congestion complications within 2 days of halting decongestant use. If congestion persists for more than a week following reduced nasal spray use, then diagnosis should be GR in pregnant women [12].

Acute viral and/or bacterial rhinosinusitis (ARS) may be a consequence of GR [14, 32]. Acute rhinosinusitis in adults is defined as sudden onset of two or more symptoms, one of which should be either nasal blockage, obstruction, congestion or nasal discharge (anterior/posterior nasal drip), facial pain or pressure, and reduction or loss of smell for less than 12 weeks [32]. GR and AR have similar symptoms; however, in AR the symptoms are caused by specific IgE-mediated inflammation in presensitized individual. Typical AR symptoms include, in addition to nasal congestion, watery discharge, sneezing, and itching after allergen challenge that is not observed in GR. Yet, house dust allergy may present predominantly with nasal congestion. Mixed rhinitis, such as co-existing AR and GR, is also common in pregnancy.

AR diagnosis is based on serum allergen-specific IgE, whereas pregnant women should only have skin prick testing if detection of an allergy and subsequent treatment outweighs the risks in rare cases, and uterine contractions may occur as a result of a systemic reaction [33]. Diagnosis of AR is important during pregnancy if it affects treatment and self-education instructions (such as allergen avoidance) [12, 14, 34].

Table 46.3 Differential diagnosis of gestational rhinitis

Rhinitis medicamentosa
Chronic rhinosinusitis
Acute rhinosinusitis
Allergic rhinitis
Nasal granuloma gravidarum

Nasal granuloma gravidarum (also known as pregnancy tumor, pregnancy granuloma, telangiectatic polyp) is a type of benign tumor that results in nasal blockage [35]. The histology is similar to pyogenic granuloma. In contrast to GR, it is typically unilateral and results in recurrent epistaxis [35]. Following nasal cavity inspection, a well-vascularized lesion can be observed that is sensitive to bleeding upon touching. The polyp may present as a protrusion that occupies the vestibulum of the nose, which is easily visualized externally. If blockages or nosebleeds lessen the patient's quality of life, excision of these granulomas can be done under local anesthesia; however, overtime they may dissolve by themselves following childbirth [35].

## 46.8	Treatment

Treatment is summarized in Table 46.4, and it includes conservative medical and nonmedical therapies, and other treatment such as surgery.

### 46.8.1	Conservative Treatment

Conservative approach to pregnant women suffering from gestational rhinitis is very important. Doctors should explain to patients that nasal congestion is a common physiological condition during pregnancy. This information and suggested treatment options should be explained to the patient with gestational rhinitis during the first prenatal examination [12, 28].

#### 46.8.1.1	Physical Exercise
Physical exercise is known to reduce congestion in GR patients. A 30–45° elevation of the head when lying down can reduce the likelihood of vena cava syndrome and snoring. Another option is to use a dilator that enlarges the nostrils. This device dilates

Table 46.4 Treatment options

General
Information, patient education
Physical exercise
Head and neck elevation during sleep
Mechanical dilation
Nasal saline irrigation
Special indications
Decongestants
Nasal corticosteroid sprays
CPAP
Surgery (such as noninvasive inferior turbinate reduction) for rare cases
Not indicated
Systemic corticosteroids
Oral decongestants
Antibiotics

the nasal valve, which is the narrowest part of the upper airways. The external-type dilator can reduce nasal congestion associated with nocturnal breathing in pregnant women, while the internal-type dilator can reduce snoring as much as nasal decongestants in men. Dilators may lead to local irritation of the skin from the pressure [36].

46.8.1.2　Nasal Saline Irrigation

Nasal saline irrigation has been shown to be an effective treatment for reducing nasal symptoms, such as congestion [32]. Nasal saline irrigation improves mucociliary clearance, reduces mucosal edema, reduces inflammatory mediators, and removes mucus and triggering agents from the nasal mucosa symptoms, such as congestion [32]. Nasal irrigation is performed using 30–500 mL (average 200–250 mL) of isotonic saline solution with a pH range of 6.2–8.4. The higher volume of saline irrigates a larger area in the nasal cavity. Hypertonic solution (3.0% NaCl solution) has major effect on removing dense mucus [37]. In accordance with the device and saline volume, nasal irrigation is applied to the nasal cavity with a compression pressure ≥ 120 mbar and for an average of 1 min [38].

46.8.2　Pharmacological Treatment

Drugs can be used as an option if other holistic therapies fail to alleviate the GR.

46.8.2.1　Decongestant

Decongestants are vasoconstrictors that effectively work to temporarily reduce nasal blockage. Most systemic decongestants, including phenylephedrine, pseudoephedrine, and phenylpropanolamine, are classified as category C by the United States Food and Drug Administration (US FDA) [12]. A previous study showed that acquired gastroschisis anomaly in 206 infants was due to the use of these category C drugs during pregnancy, even though there are limited reports on the usefulness of systemic decongestant for GR [2, 14]. In most subjects that use decongestants, systemic side effects have been documented, including hypertension, palpitations, anorexia, tremors, and sleep disorders [19].

Topical decongestants, such as phenylephrine and oxymetazoline, reduce congestion in a short time. During pregnancy, these decongestants often are misused because GR is an unceasing complication and results in unresolved rhinitis medicamentosa following childbirth. The nasal sprays overstimulate the α-adrenergic responses and cause recurrent mucosal edema and worse/sustained nasal congestion [20, 21]. Benzalkonium chloride, a typical preserving agent found in these decongestants, can also increase congestion and complications. Continued use of these decongestants for more than 5–10 days increases the risk of rebound nasal congestion, nasal crusting, and development of rhinitis medicamentosa [39]. Thus, it is recommended to use for the short term at a lower dosage [14, 32].

46.8.2.2　Glucocorticoids

Glucocorticoids are steroids that are effective for managing all types of rhinitis. Intranasal steroids reduce the need for a systemic steroid and have been shown to have a significant effect on GR. A randomized controlled trial study found that results upon the use of fluticasone propionate given 8 weeks to GR patients [28]. This study showed that intranasal steroids have no impact on maternal cortisol levels and fetal growth by prenatal ultrasound.

Nevertheless, the FDA classifies triamcinolone acetonide, fluticasone furoate, fluticasone propionate, and mometasone furoate as category C drugs [2, 12, 14]. According to the Swedish Medical Birth Registry, there have been no reports of increased incidence of congenital malformation in patients with gestational rhinitis using budesonide inhalation in the first trimester of pregnancy. Therefore, it has been classified in category B [14, 28, 33].

Long-term, repeated oral–parenteral usage of corticosteroids by pregnant women should be hindered because of the link to adrenal suppression and other side effects. To use corticosteroids for less than 2 weeks may be safe and effective.

Higher doses of corticosteroids are hazardous in the first trimester and have been linked to fetal blindness, lung edema, uterine contraction inhibition, and fluid overload [3]. Therefore, it is recommended that corticosteroids be avoided throughout pregnancy, except in severe conditions. Oral corticosteroids are contraindicated as a treatment of GR due to their risk of side effects [2, 12].

46.8.2.3 Antibiotics

Antibiotics are not recommended for GR, even though some cases such as bacterial sinusitis are more widely prescribed. In pregnant women, higher antibiotic doses are needed and are often increased by 50% due to higher renal clearance throughout pregnancy [14].

46.8.2.4 Antihistamine

Antihistamines should be used when it is necessary. Antihistamines are effective for sneezing and nasal itching [14, 15]. They have been well documented to have no harmful effects on the fetus. Nevertheless, some of the first-generation antihistamines (e.g., diphenhydramine triprolidine, chlorpheniramine) have some adverse effects, including drowsiness, dry mouth, and increase appetite [39]. These first-generation drugs have also been linked to cleft lip and palate. The second-generation antihistamines (i.e., cetirizine, loratadine, desloratadine, levocetirizine, fexofenadine) may, with caution, be used in pregnancy [12, 34]. The systemic decongestants (usually as a combination treatment of antihistamines) are contraindicated during pregnancy due to their teratogenic risks, such as endocardial cushion defect, ear defects, and pyloric stenosis [40].

46.8.3 Other Treatments

46.8.3.1 Nasal Continuous Positive Airway Pressure (CPAP)

CPAP has been used for GR with OSA. For normal OSA patients, CPAP has been regarded as effective and has been shown to improve sleep quality. The pressure can be adjusted to a pregnant woman's needs. A previous report has shown that CPAP can lower nighttime blood pressure in preeclamptic women [14].

46.8.3.2 Surgery

GR is an usually self-limiting disease for a relatively short period, and thus surgery is not recommended as a treatment for GR. Noninvasive surgical procedures (such as radiofrequency, electrocautery, and cryotherapy) could be considered in rare cases in which GR causes remarkable problems with daily activities and sleep despite maximal conservative therapy (including nasal lavage, pharmacological treatment, and CPAP) [12, 14]. Table 46.4 summarizes the treatment options for the control of gestational rhinitis.

46.8.3.3 Nonallergic Rhinitis in Pregnancy

nAR symptoms may mimic AR symptoms but can be distinguished by lack of allergen-specific IgE-mediated inflammation and symptoms varying based on allergen challenge. Vasomotor rhinitis is a part of nAR. Vasomotor rhinitis is characterized by hyperresponsiveness to stimuli, yet without allergen sensitization [41]. Its physiopathology is not clearly understood, and the condition has been characterized by nasal hyperactivity and nasal discharge that starts with exposure to hot and cold factors.

The relative increase in parasympathetic activity of the nasal mucosa, along with nasal vasodilation, congestion, and secretion, is among the top symptoms. Exposure to hot and cold, hormonal changes (pregnancy, oral contraceptives containing high estrogen), thyroid pathologies (mixed edema), and drugs [antihypertensives (guanethidine-alpha adrenergic blockade)] are critical in the etiology. Although similar to gestational rhinitis, it is characterized by the persistence of symptoms after delivery [42–45].

Ipratropium bromide (category B), an anticholinergic nasal sprays, has been shown to be effective in the treatment of rhinorrhea symptoms related to nAR (or vasomotor rhinitis) [46].

Another disorder of nAR group is rhinitis medicamentosa. It is also known as rebound rhinitis or chemical rhinitis and is caused by long-term use of local nasal decongestants to relieve nasal congestion. The most common precipitant is over-the-counter decongestant nasal sprays containing oxymetazoline. The thought is that these drugs are safer than oral drugs and are widely used by pregnant women. Several days of using these nasal decongestant sprays can cause rebound and chronic nasal congestion as the medication wears off, can prompt patients to increase the dose in an effort to obtain relief of symptoms, and can elicit a perpetual cycle of nasal congestion and escalating medication use [29].

Local nasal decongestants should be used to provide temporary relief of nasal congestion, preferably within 3–5 days (in cases like acute sinusitis), and should never be preferred in the treatment of nasal obstruction [46].

Current therapies are termination of nasal decongestants and treatment with intranasal glucocorticoids [29].

Consequently, both GR and rhinitis during pregnancy are similar complications that have gained popularity over the years. Several factors may be a reason for this. First, the identification of the maternal obstructive sleep apnea syndrome (OSAS) and the potentially unfavorable consequences to the fetus are warranted. Lastly, there was an important suggestive impact on pregnant women's quality of life [2, 7, 31]. The otorhinolaryngologist as well as the obstetrician should work together to help determine GR and adequate treatment using safety measures and medications.

References

1. Carroll MP, Bulkhi AA, Lockey RF. Rhinitis and sinusitis. In: Namazy J, Schatz M, editors. Asthma, allergic and immunologic diseases during pregnancy. Cham: Springer; 2019.
2. Caparroz FA, Gregorio LL, Bongiovanni G, Izu SC, Kosugi EM. Rhinitis and pregnancy: literature review. Braz J Otorhinolaryngol. 2016;8:105–11.
3. MacKenzie J. The physiological and patholical relations between the nose and the sexual apparatus of man. Aliens Neurol. 1898;19:219–39.
4. Toppozada H, Michaels L, Toppozada M, El-Ghazzawi I, Talaat M, Elwany S. The human respiratory nasal mucosa in pregnancy. An electron microscopic and histochemical study. J Laryngol Otol. 1982;96:613–26.
5. Mohun M. Incidence of vasomotor rhinitis during pregnancy. Arch Otolaryngol. 1943;37:699–709.
6. Namazy JA, Schatz M. Diagnosing rhinitis during pregnancy. Curr Allergy Asthma Rep. 2014;14:458.
7. Orban N, Maughan E, Bleach N. Pregnancy-induced rhinitis. Rhinology. 2013;51:111–9.
8. Ellegard E, Hellgren M, Toren K, Karlsoon T. The incidence of pregnancy rhinitis. Gynecol Obstet Invest. 2000;49:98–101.
9. Shushan S, Sadan O, Lurie S, Evron S, Golan A, Roth Y. Pregnancy-associated rhinitis. Am J Perinatol. 2006;23:431–3.
10. Bende M, Gredmark T. Nasal stuffiness during pregnancy. Laryngoscope. 1999;109:1108–10.
11. Bende M, Hallgarde U, Sjogren C. Occurance of nasal congestion during pregnancy. Am J Rhinol. 1999;3:217–9.
12. Poerbonegoro NL. Nasal congestion and its Management in Pregnancy Rhinitis. Indones J Obstet Gynecol. 2019;7:318–26.
13. Demoly P, Piette V, Daures J-P. Treatment of allergic rhinitis during pregnancy. Drugs. 2003;63:1813–20.
14. Ellegård EK. Pregnancy rhinitis. Immunol Allergy Clin North Am. 2006;26:119–35.
15. Keles N. Treatment of allergic rhinitis during pregnancy. Am J Rhinol. 2004;18:23–8.
16. Hamano N, Terada N, Maesako K, Ikeda T, Fukuda S, Wakita J, et al. Expression of histamine recepetors in nasal epithelial cellsand endothelial cells—the effect of sex hormones. Int Arch Allergy Appl Immunol. 1998;115:220–7.
17. Schatz M, Zeiger RS. Asthma and allergy in pregnancy. Clin Perinatol. 1997;24:407–32.
18. Akkoca AN, Özler GS, Kurt RK, Karapınar OS, Özdemir ZT, Yanık S. Ear, nose and throat changes observed during three trimesters of pregnancy. Sci J Clin Med. 2014;3:52–6.
19. Lekas MD. Rhinitis during pregnancy and rhinitis medicamentosa. Otolaryngol Head Neck Surg. 1992;107:845–9.
20. Philpott CM, Conboy P, Al-Azzawi F, Murty G. Nasal physiological changes during pregnancy. Clin Otolaryngol Allied Sci. 2004;29:343–51.
21. Indirani B, Raman R, Omar SZ. Hormonal changes causing rhinitis in pregnancy among Malaysian women. J Laryngol Otol. 2013;127:876–81.
22. Bonds RS, Midoro-Horiuti T. Estrogen effects in allergy and asthma. Curr Opin Allergy Clin Immunol. 2013;13(1):92–9.
23. Shah S. Hormonal link to autoimmune allergies. ISRN Allergy. 2012;2012:910437.

24. Kim D-H, Park I-H, Cho J-S, Lee Y-M, Choi H, Lee H-M. Alterations of vasoactive intestinal polypeptide receptors in allergic rhinitis. Am J Rhinol Allergy. 2011;25:e44–7.
25. Chaen T, Watanabe N, Mogi G, Mori K, Takeyama M. Substance P and vasoactive intestinal peptide in nasal secretions and plasma from patients with nasal allergy. Ann Otol Rhinol Laryngol. 1993;102(1 Pt 1):16–21.
26. Ellegård EK, Oscarsson J, Bougoussa M, et al. Serum level of placental growth hormone is raised in pregnancy rhinitis. Arch Otolaryngol Head Neck Surg. 1998;124:439–43.
27. Ellegard E, Karlson G. IgE-mediated reactions and hyperreactivity in pregnancy rhinitis. Arch Otolaryngol Head Neck Surg. 1999;37:50–5.
28. Ellegard EK. Clinical and pathogenetic characteristics of pregnancy rhinitis. Clin Rev Allergy Immunol. 2004;26:149–59.
29. Namazy JA, Schatz M. Asthma and rhinitis during pregnancy. Mt Sinai J Med. 2011;78:661–70.
30. Goanta CM, Cirpaciu D, Tuşaliu M, Budu VA. Pregnancy rhinitis. Arch Balk Med Union. 2018;53:114–6.
31. Gilbey P, McGruthers L, Morency AM, Shrim A. Rhinosinusitis-related quality of life during pregnancy. Am J Rhinol Allergy. 2012;26:283–6.
32. Fokkens WJ, Lund VJ, Hopkins C, et al. European position paper on rhinosinusitis and nasal polyps 2020. Rhinology. 2020;58(Suppl S29):1–464.
33. The Joint Council of Allergy, Asthma & Immunology (JCAAI). Practice parameters for allergy diagnostic testing. www.jcaai.org. Accessed Oct 2011.
34. Bousquet J, Anto JM, Bachert C, et al. Allergic rhinitis. Nat Rev Dis Primers. 2020;6:95.
35. Park YW. Nasal granuloma gravidarum. Otolaryngol Head Neck Surg. 2002;126:591–2.
36. Ellegård EK. Special considerations in the treatment of pregnancy rhinitis. Womens Health. 2005;1(1):105–14.
37. Tapiala J, Hyvärinen A, Toppila-Salmi S. Nasal saline irrigation: prescribing habits and attitudes of physicians and pharmacists. Scand J Prim Health Care. 2021;39:35–43.
38. Bastier PL, Lechot A, Bordenave L, Durand M, de Gabory L. Nasal irrigation: from empiricism to evidence-based medicine. A review. Eur Ann Otorhinolaryngol Head Neck Dis. 2015;132:281–5.
39. Ellegård EK. Etiology and management of pregnancy rhinitis. Am J Respir Med. 2003;2:469–75.
40. Yau WP, Mitchell AA, Lin KJ, Werler MM, Hernández-Díaz S. Use of decongestants during pregnancy and the risk of birth defects. Am J Epidemiol. 2013;178(2):198–208.
41. Dykewicz MS, et al. Rhinitis 2020: a practice parameter update. J Allergy Clin Immunol. 2020;146(4):721–67.
42. Cauwenberge P, Bachert C, Passalacgua G, et al. Consensus statement on the treatment of allergic rhinitis. Allergy. 2000;55:116–34.
43. Hallén H, Enerdal J, Graf P. Fluticasone propionate nasal spray is more effective and has a faster onset of action than placebo in treatment of rhinitis medicamentosa. Clin Exp Allergy. 1997;27:552–8.
44. Bachert C. Persistent rhinitis-allergic or nonallergic? Allergy. 2004;59(suppl 76):11–5; discussion 15.
45. Hellings PW, Klimek L, Cingi C, et al. Non-allergic rhinitis: position paper of the European Academy of Allergy and Clinical Immunology. Allergy. 2017;72:1657–65.
46. Gümüşsoy M, Gümnüşsoy S, Çukurova İ. The most frequently encountered rhinologic problems during pregnancy: appropriate approaches in diagnosis and therapy. J Tepecik Educ Res Hosp. 2017;27(1):13–9.

Nasal Polyposis During Pregnancy and the Postpartum Period

47

Nevreste Didem Sonbay Yılmaz, Özer Erdem Gür, and Andrey Lopatin

47.1 Introduction

Pregnancy is a physiological process in which the mother's body is prepared to meet the needs of the growing and developing foetus [1]. It is necessary to be very careful when using medication during pregnancy because drugs or their metabolites can pass to the foetus via the placenta and cause anomalies in foetal growth and development, known as teratogenicity [2].

Five categories of drug use during pregnancy have been reported by the Food and Drug Administration (FDA) (Table 47.1) [3].

Very few drugs belong to the A category in the FDA classification. Therefore, it is necessary to be very careful when using drugs during pregnancy [4]. Medication should be prescribed during pregnancy only when the apparent benefit of the drug is greater than its apparent risk [2].

During pregnancy, the most sensitive period in terms of drug use is the organogenesis phase, which covers the 18th–21st and 56th–60th days following conception [1, 5]. It is considered the riskiest period in terms of teratogenicity because the rate of cell division is very high and there is differentiation in tissues and organs [5]. The teratogenicity of drugs is related to their dose, duration of use, specific effect on tissues, passage through the placenta and metabolism, in addition to the age and

N. D. S. Yılmaz (✉) · Ö. E. Gür
Department of Otorhinolaryngology, Antalya Training and Research Hospital, Antalya, Turkey
e-mail: didem_ece@yahoo.com; erdemkaptan@yahoo.com

A. Lopatin
Medical Department, Business Administration of the President of Russian Federation, Policlinic №1, Moscow, Russia
e-mail: lopatin.andrey@inbox.ru

C. Cingi et al. (eds.), *ENT Diseases: Diagnosis and Treatment during Pregnancy and Lactation*, https://doi.org/10.1007/978-3-031-05303-0_47

Table 47.1 Categories of pharmaceutical agents assessing risk for use in pregnancy

Category	Description
A	Adequate, well-controlled studies on pregnant women have not shown an increased risk of foetal abnormalities
B	Animal studies have revealed no evidence of harm to the foetus; however, there are no adequate and well-controlled studies on pregnant women Or Animal studies have shown an adverse effect, but adequate and well-controlled studies on pregnant women have failed to demonstrate a risk to the foetus
C	Animal studies have shown an adverse effect, or no animal studies have been conducted, and there are no adequate and well-controlled studies on pregnant women
D	Adequate, well-controlled, or observational studies on pregnant women have demonstrated a risk to the foetus. However, the benefits of therapy may outweigh the potential risk
X	Adequate, well-controlled, or observational studies on animals or pregnant women have demonstrated positive evidence of foetal abnormalities. The use of the product is contraindicated in women who are or may become pregnant

weight of the mother. A low-molecular-weight, fat-soluble, non-polar and non-protein-binding substance can easily cross the placenta [6].

Attention should also be paid to the use of medication during the lactation period after pregnancy because drug metabolites can reach the infant through breast milk and cause side effects in the infant [5]. Resources on drug use during lactation can be confusing. There are no exact criteria for drug use during lactation. Publications of the American Academy of Paediatricians (AAP) serve as an important guide when using medication during lactation [7].

It is necessary to be very careful in the treatment of nasal polyposis during pregnancy, especially in the third trimester, when increased hormonal activity and disruption of the nasal mucosal cycle and mucociliary transport cause nasal congestion [5]. This condition, also called pregnancy rhinitis, results in nasal congestion in pregnant women and causes more serious problems in pregnant women diagnosed with nasal polyposis. It can seriously impair the quality of life of pregnant women by negatively affecting their eating and sleeping patterns and emotional well-being [2, 8]. Therefore, it needs to be treated. However, it is important to prevent unnecessary and wrong drug use in order to prevent possible complications during pregnancy [8].

47.2 Medical Treatment

47.2.1 Nasal Saline Irrigation

Nasal saline irrigation is perhaps the most reliable first-line treatment for nasal polyposis during pregnancy and lactation. Through this process, the mucus, crust, cell debris, pathogens inhaled from the air, allergens, and airborne particles are mechanically cleaned and mucociliary clearance is increased [9]. Nasal saline irrigation decreases the local concentrations of pro-inflammatory mediators and moisturises the nasal mucosa in patients with many chronic sinonasal pathologies [10].

However, there is little consensus regarding the best method of irrigation, the tonicity (concentration) of the saline solution, and the volume (low or high), pressure (low or high), frequency, devices, and head position when rinsing [11].

High-volume devices include droppers, atomisers, and nebulisers, while low-volume devices include sprays, squeeze bottles, and sinus wash kits. The use of high-volume devices results in better distribution of the solution to the nasal cavity and skull base and better penetration, especially into the sinuses [12]. Regardless of the device used, fitting the nosepiece tightly to the nostril and inserting it into the nasal entrance at an upward angle of 45° ensures optimal washing of the entire nasal cavity and minimises the loss of the lavage solution [13].

The lavage solutions used include solutions containing electrolytes, sterile saline solutions, Ringer's lactate, and ionised seawater. Home-made solutions containing water, salt, and sodium bicarbonate mixed in various proportions can also be used. However, the composition and sterility of such solutions cannot be controlled. Moreover, they are not reproducible and reliable [13].

For a long time, isotonic saline solution has been the preferred lavage solution. However, the use of hypertonic saline solution has gradually increased recently [14]. Hypertonic saline solutions reduce oedema, improve mucociliary clearance, and relieve nasal breathing by affecting the osmotic pressure [15]. In recent studies, no difference has been found between the effects of isotonic and hypertonic saline solutions on mucociliary clearance [14]. However, hypertonic saline solutions should be used considering their side effects, such as nasal irritation and burning sensation [16].

The pH values of the used solutions have been found to be between 4.5 and 8 [17]. Isotonic saline solutions have a pH of 4.5–7, Ringer's lactate has a pH of 6–7.5, and seawater has a pH around 8. Solutions with slightly alkaline pH have the maximum effect on mucociliary clearance.

Nasal irrigation is recommended as the first-line treatment for patients diagnosed with nasal polyposis during pregnancy, especially if there is a history of allergic rhinitis and rhinosinusitis. Nasal irrigation relieves the symptoms and increases the effectiveness of intranasal corticosteroids. In some cases, it also alleviates the need for oral treatment [15, 16].

47.2.2 Antibiotics

Antibiotics are not used individually in patients diagnosed with nasal polyposis. They should be used in the case of acute rhinosinusitis attacks in patients with nasal polyposis. The increase in the plasma volume and decrease in plasma protein levels, especially in the first 5 months of pregnancy, cause changes in the pharmacokinetics of the drugs used. This change is most pronounced in the case of antibiotics. It is recommended to shorten the dose interval or increase the dose level during pregnancy [18].

The first choice is a combination of penicillin and β-lactam antibiotics. Clavulanic acid, which is used as a penicillin-type and β-lactam antibiotic, is classified into pregnancy category B [18]. Antibiotic treatment should be initiated when purulent discharge is detected during endoscopic examination, and treatment should be completed as soon as possible (7–10 days) [4].

Cephalosporin antibiotics are classified into pregnancy category B. However, it is recommended to use this antibiotic group when resistance develops against the penicillin group [19].

If a pregnant woman is allergic to penicillin or β-lactam antibiotics, macrolide antibiotics may be preferred [4]. Macrolide antibiotics are also preferred for treating nasal polyposis because of their anti-inflammatory effects [20]. Erythromycin is classified into pregnancy category B; however, its use in the treatment of sinusitis is limited because *Haemophilus influenzae* type b is erythromycin resistant [4]. Azithromycin and clarithromycin (category B) may be preferred when a patient is allergic to penicillin. The long-term use of clarithromycin during pregnancy is not recommended because of its cardiac side effects, such as Q-T prolongation [21].

Although studies have shown that doxycycline treatment also reduces the polyp size and inflammation [22], the use of antibiotics such as tetracyclines, aminoglycosides, trimethoprim–sulfamethoxazole, and fluoroquinolones or the long-term use of macrolide or doxycycline is not recommended during pregnancy.

47.2.3 Intranasal Antibiotics

The absorption of drugs directly applied to the nasal mucosa is much faster than that of oral and transdermal drugs because the nasal mucosa has a large surface area and a high blood supply [23]. After a drug is administered intranasally, it is absorbed by diffusion through the mucosa [24].

Many antibiotics can be administered intranasally. Mupirocin is the most common intranasal antibiotic; however, it may not reach all parts of the nasal mucosa as it is applied as an ointment [25]. Antibiotics that are frequently administered via nebulisers include quinolone antibiotics, such as ciprofloxacin, levofloxacin, and moxifloxacin. In addition, various antibiotics, such as tobramycin, ceftazidime, and gentamicin, have been used according to the sensitivity of the pathogens [26].

Although intranasal antibiotic therapy seems to be effective in patients with chronic rhinosinusitis after surgery and acute exacerbations, there is still no consensus regarding the method of administration and the antibiotic to be used [27]. While the use of topical antibiotics in patients with nasal polyposis remains controversial, no topical antibiotics belonging to categories A and B have been used [4].

47.3   Histamine Receptor Antagonists

Histamines are endogenous amines stored in mast cells and basophils [28]. Histamines have specific cell receptors in the target tissue (H1, H2, H3). Moreover, they have a neurotransmitter effect on the central nervous system (CNS) [29].

Histamines released as a result of antigen–antibody reaction may cause varying degrees of different pharmacological effects depending on the receptor density in the target cell [29]. The degree of these effects can vary from mild irritation and itching to anaphylaxis [28].

H1 receptor antagonists are used for treating nasal polyposis and allergic rhinitis [30]. H1 receptor antagonists reversibly and competitively inhibit H1 receptors [28]. First-generation H1 receptor antagonists can stimulate as well as suppress CNS functions. Symptoms of CNS stimulation are less common but can occur even with therapeutic doses [29].

All first-generation H1 receptor antagonists have an atropine-like effect [31]. Therefore, they can cause dry mouth, urination problems, and impotence. In addition, they can result in decreased vision, diplopia, euphoria, increased blood pressure, anorexia, constipation or diarrhoea, and epigastric disorders [32]. Newer second-generation H1 receptor antagonists (loratadine and fexofenadine) have lesser anticholinergic activity [27]. H1 receptor antagonists are metabolised in the liver. The duration of action of first-generation H1 receptor antagonists is 4–6 h, while that of second-generation H1 receptor antagonists is around 12–24 h [33].

Antihistaminic drugs are particularly effective in treating sneezing and rhinorrhoea that develop due to allergies [4]. However, they have no significant effect on nasal polyposis [30]. The pregnancy classification of antihistamines is shown in Table 47.2. Because of their central effects, first-generation H1 receptor antagonists are not recommended during pregnancy [4]. Second-generation H1 receptor antagonists are not recommended during the first trimester [30]. Moreover, antihistamines are not recommended during lactation because they can pass into breast milk and cause side effects in the infant [30]. If antihistamines are used for certain reasons, such as anaphylaxis, their use should be discontinued 3–4 days before delivery [34].

Table 47.2 FDA classification of antihistamines

First generation	FDA	Second generation	FDA
Alkylamines		Astemizole	C
Brompheniramine	C	Azelastine	C
Chlorpheniramine	B	Cetirizine	B
Triprolidine	C	Fexofenadine	C
Dexchlorpheniramine	B	Terfenadine	C
Ethylenediamine		Loratadine	B
Tripelennamine	B	Desloratadine	C
Piperazines			
Hydroxyzine	C		
Ethanolamines			
Diphenhydramine	B		
Clemastine	C		
Carbinoxamine	C		
Phenothiazines			
Promethazine	C		

47.4 Intranasal Antihistamines

Azelastine (trade name, Astelin) was the first antihistamine developed as a topical nasal spray. Azelastine and olopatadine are available as nasal sprays [4]. They can be used to treat nasal congestion due to allergic and nonallergic rhinitis because of their anti-inflammatory effect [34]. Their action starts faster (less than 15 min) than that of intranasal corticosteroids. They may be systemically absorbed and cause sedation [35].

47.5 Corticosteroids

Glucocorticoid (hydrocortisone) secreted from the adrenal cortex is a hormone that can effectively regulate protein, lipid, and carbohydrate metabolism. It is used in many areas of otolaryngology because of its extremely powerful anti-inflammatory effect [36]. It is used both systemically and intranasally in patients with nasal polyposis.

Corticosteroids (prednisone, dexamethasone, prednisolone, and methyl prednisolone), which are synthetic derivatives of hydrocortisone, are used clinically [37]. The duration of action of corticosteroids is shown in Table 47.3 [38]. Although these agents are used because of their powerful anti-inflammatory effect, it should be kept in mind that they also have a glucocorticoid structure [36]. Therefore, these agents increase gluconeogenesis and decrease the efficacy of insulin in peripheral tissues, delay wound healing, and cause immunosuppression. As the mineralocorticoid effects of these agents are relatively low, their water and salt retention efficiency is very low.

The short-term use of systemic corticosteroids (7–21 days) in patients with nasal polyposis decreases the size of the nasal polyp and reduces its inflammatory response [38]. It may also have tolerable side effects, such as insomnia, mood change, and gastrointestinal side effects. It is usually used with intranasal corticosteroids. As a general treatment plan, if there is no response to topical corticosteroid therapy for 4–6 weeks, short-term systemic steroid therapy is initiated for 7–10 days. If there is no response to this as well, surgical treatment is planned. However, if there is a response to systemic therapy, topical therapy is continued [39].

Table 47.3 Duration of action of corticosteroids

Betamethasone	Long-acting
Dexamethasone	Long-acting
Methylprednisolone	Intermediate-acting
Triamcinolone	Intermediate-acting
Prednisone	Intermediate-acting
Prednisolone	Intermediate-acting
Hydrocortisone	Short-acting
Cortisone	Short-acting

The use of corticosteroids in pregnant women remains controversial. The potential neurological effects of oral glucocorticoids on the developing brain tissue have been demonstrated in animal studies; however, the results of human studies are conflicting [4]. Therefore, the benefit–damage ratio should be well evaluated when administering corticosteroids [28]. The use of oral corticosteroids during the first trimester should be restricted to life-threatening conditions [40]. Although no study has associated the use of oral steroids with a major teratogenic risk and major congenital malformations, an increased association with the development of oral clefts has been reported [41].

The use of glucocorticoids is not recommended during lactation; however, if they are used in emergencies, breastfeeding should be delayed for 3–4 h. In addition, if the dose needs to exceed 20 mg/day, prednisolone should be preferred as its passage to breast milk is less [7].

47.5.1 Intranasal Corticosteroids

Intranasal corticosteroids have been shown to be effective in treating nasal polyposis. These preparations decrease the oeosinophilic inhibition in the nasal epithelium and cytokine production by T lymphocytes and vasoconstriction by affecting arachidonic acid metabolism [42]. In addition, they enable the paranasal sinus ostium to remain open due to their anti-inflammatory and membrane-stabilising effects. They significantly improve the quality of life and sleep quality of patients, especially those with allergic rhinitis [43]. Beclomethasone (beconase, vancenase), budesonide (rhinocort), dexamethasone (dexacort), flunisolide (nasalide), fluticasone (flonase), triamcinolone (nasacort), and mometasone furoate (nasonex) are intranasal steroid preparations.

Comparative studies have reported that intranasal corticosteroids are more effective than oral antihistamines in controlling nasal symptoms and that there is no difference in terms of ocular symptoms [44].

No systemic side effect or adrenal suppression is observed when using intranasal corticosteroids [45]. Their side effects are limited to the nasal region. Nasal burning, epistaxis, and sneezing are the most common side effects. In fact, nasal burning is thought to be caused by the active substance in the spray other than corticosteroids; this problem is usually solved by using incandescent substances in preparations [42]. Epistaxis is mostly caused by the incorrect use of the spray and by positioning the pump on the septum. However, epistaxis may occur with chronic use because corticosteroids increase capillary fragility. Albeit very rare, septal perforation may occur [46].

For a full therapeutic effect, the spray should be used regularly for several weeks; however, symptomatic relief occurs within hours [43]. Prior nasal decongestant spray application increases the effectiveness of the spray by allowing the steroid to reach the mucosa more easily.

According to the US FDA classification of drugs used in pregnancy by their teratogenic effects, all intranasal corticosteroids, except for budesonide (which belongs to pregnancy category B), belong to pregnancy category C [47].

The injection of long-acting corticosteroids into the inferior turbinate is no longer recommended because the long-term results are not satisfactory and very serious side effects, such as amaurosis, can occur due to microembolic vascular occlusion resulting from the particle size [46].

47.6　Antileukotrien Drugs

Leukotrienes, which are products of arachidonic acid metabolism, are biologically active structures [48]. Phospholipase A2 causes the release of arachidonic acid from the phospholipid layer of the cell membrane. Following this, arachidonic acid metabolises into cysteinyl leukotrienes by oxidative metabolism (the 5-lipoxygenase pathway) or into prostaglandins, prostacyclin, and thromboxane via cyclooxygenase [49].

Antileukotriene drugs are divided into two groups: leukotriene antagonists and leukotriene receptor antagonists [50]. Zileuton is the only leukotriene antagonist in use [51]. Zafirlukast and montelukast are leukotriene receptor antagonists [50], with montelukast being the most commonly used leukotriene receptor antagonist [47]. However, leukotriene antagonists are used for treating allergic rhinitis rather than nasal polyposis [38]. It has been shown that the use of leukotriene antagonists alone or in combination in patients with nasal polyposis does not cause any change in the polyp size [4]. However, if a patient has allergic rhinitis or allergic asthma together with nasal polyposis, leukotriene antagonists can be added to the treatment. Montelukast is classified into pregnancy category B [46]. It is not recommended during pregnancy because of its low effectiveness in treating nasal polyposis. However, montelukast may be continued or be initiated in patients with persistent asthma during pregnancy, especially in those with a previous response.

47.7　Surgical Treatment

Elective surgery should be postponed in pregnant women. The use of anaesthetic substances during pregnancy may induce labour and cause premature birth or miscarriage [52]. It may also cause intrauterine growth retardation and teratogenicity. If necessary, the most appropriate period is the second trimester [53]. Premedication is not recommended before anaesthesia.

Local anaesthetic agents, especially lidocaine, can pass through the placenta within a few minutes even if very low doses are administered. While local anaesthetic agents increase the risk of teratogenicity, especially in the first trimester, they cause foetal bradycardia in the second and third trimesters [54].

References

1. Donati S, Baglio G, Spinelli A. Drug use in pregnancy among women. Eur J Clin Pharmacol. 2000;56:323–8.
2. Sachdeva P, Patel BG, Patel BK. Drug use in pregnancy; a point to ponder. Indian J Pharm Sci. 2009;71:1–7.

3. Summary of proposed rule on pregnancy and lactation. www.fda.gov/Drugs/DevelopmentApprovalProcess/DevelopmentResources/Labeling/ucm093310.htm2009.
4. Incaudo GA. Diagnosis and treatment of allergic rhinitis and sinusitis during pregnancy and lactation. Clin Rev Allergy Immunol. 2004;27(2):159–77. https://doi.org/10.1385/CRIAI:27:2:159.
5. Syme MR, Paxton JW, Keelan JA. Drug transfer and metabolism by the human placenta. Clin Pharmacokinet. 2004;43:487–514.
6. Conley JM, Richards SM. Teratogenesis. In: Jorgensen S, editor. Ecotoxicology. San Diego: Academic; 2008. p. 3528.
7. American Academy of Pediatrics Committee on Drugs. Transfer of drugs and other chemicals into human milk. Pediatrics. 2001;108:776–89.
8. Bhagat DR, Chowdhary A, Verma S. Physiological changes in ENT during pregnancy. Indian J Otolaryngol. 2006;58:268–70.
9. Fokkens WJ, Lund VJ, Mullol J, et al. European position paper on rhinosinusitis and nasal polyps. Rhinol Suppl. 2012;20:1–136.
10. Talbot AR, Herr TM, Parsons DS. Mucociliary clearance and buffered hyper tonic saline solution. Laryngoscope. 1997;107(4):500–3.
11. Fokkens WJ, Lund VJ, Hopkins C, et al. European position paper on rhinosinusitis and nasal polyps. Rhinology. 2020;58(Suppl S29):1–464. https://doi.org/10.4193/Rhin20.600.
12. Principi N, Esposito S. Nasal irrigation: an imprecisely defined medical procedure. Int J Environ Res Public Health. 2017;14(5):516. https://doi.org/10.3390/ijerph14050516.
13. Bastier PL, Lechot A, Bordenave L, et al. Nasal irrigation: from empiricism to evidence based medicine. A review. Eur Ann Otorhinolaryngol Head Neck Dis. 2015;132:281–5.
14. Unal M, Seymen HO. Effect of ringer-lactate and isotonic saline solutions on mucociliary clearance of tracheal epithelium: an experimental study in rats. J Laryngol Otol. 2002;116:536–8.
15. Keojampa BK, Nguyen MH, Ryan MW. Effects of buffered saline solution on nasal mucociliary clearance and nasal airway patency. Otolaryngol Head Neck Surg. 2004;131:679–82.
16. Woods CM, Tan S, Ullah S, et al. The effect of nasal irrigation formulation on the antimicrobial activity of nasal secretions. Int Forum Allergy Rhinol. 2015;5:1104–10.
17. Tomooka LT, Murphy C, Davidson TM. Clinical study and literature review of nasal irrigation. Laryngoscope. 2000;110:1189–93.
18. Norwitz ER, Greenberg JA. Antibiotics in pregnancy: are they safe? Rev Obstet Gynecol. 2009;2(3):135–6. https://doi.org/10.3909/riog0092.
19. Berkovitch M, Segal-Socher I, Greenberg R, et al. First trimester exposure to cefuroxime: a prospective cohort study. Br J Clin Pharmacol. 2000;50:161–5.
20. Peric AV, Baletic N, Milojevic M, et al. Effects of preoperative clarithromycin administration in patients with nasal polyposis. West Indian Med J. 2014;63:721–7.
21. Root AA, Wong AY, Ghebremichael-Weldeselassie Y, et al. Evaluation of the risk of cardiovascular events with clarithromycin using both propensity score and self-controlled study designs. Br J Clin Pharmacol. 2016;82:512–21.
22. Van Zele T, Gevaert P, Holtappels G, et al. Oral steroids and doxycycline: two different approaches to treat nasal polyps. J Allergy Clin Immunol. 2010;125:1069–1076.e4.
23. Ishikawa F, Katsura M, Tamai I, et al. Improved nasal bioavailability of elcatonin by insoluble powder formulation. Int J Pharm. 2001;224:105–14.
24. Fortuna A, Alves G, Serralheiro A, et al. Intranasal delivery of systemic-acting drugs: small molecules and biomacromolecules. Eur J Pharm Biopharm. 2014;88(1):8–27.
25. Desrosiers M, Bendouah Z, Barbeau J. Effectiveness of topical antibiotics on Staphylococcus aureus biofilm in vitro. Am J Rhinol. 2007;21:149–53.
26. Dhand R. The role of aerosolized antimicrobials in the treatment of ventilator-associated pneumonia. Respir Care. 2007;52:866–84.
27. Lim M, Citardi MJ, Leong J. Topical antimicrobials in the management of chronic rhinosinusitis: a systematic review. Am J Rhinol. 2008;22:381–9.
28. Gonzalez-Estrada A, Geraci SA. Allergy medications during pregnancy. Am J Med Sci. 2016;352(3):326–31. https://doi.org/10.1016/j.amjms.2016.05.030.
29. Gilbert C, Mazzotta P, Loebstein R, et al. Fetal safety of drugs used in the treatment of allergic rhinitis: acritical review. Drug Saf. 2005;28(8):707–19.

30. Haye R, Aanesen JP, Burtin B, et al. The effect of cetirizine on symptoms and signs of nasal polyposis. J Laryngol Otol. 1998;112:1042–6.
31. Gray SL, Anderson ML, Dublin S, et al. Cumulative use of strong anticholinergics and incident dementia: a prospective cohort study. JAMA Intern Med. 2015;175(3):401–7.
32. Schatz M, Petitti D. Antihistamines and pregnancy. Ann Allergy Asthma Immunol. 1997;78:157–9.
33. Seresirikachorn K, Khattiyawittayakun L, Chitsuthipakorn W, et al. Antihistamines for treating rhinosinusitis: systematic review and meta-analysis of randomised controlled studies. J Laryngol Otol. 2018;132:105–10.
34. Cheng LH, Lee JC, Wu PC, et al. Azelastine nasal spray inhibiting sympathetic function on human nasal mucosa in patients with allergy rhinitis. Rhinology. 2019;57(4):268–72. https://doi.org/10.4193/Rhin18.274.
35. Bernstein JA. Azelastine hydrochloride: a review of pharmacology, pharmacokinetics, clinical efficacy and tolerability. Curr Med Res Opin. 2007;23(10):2441–52. https://doi.org/10.1185/030079907X226302.
36. Van Camp C, Clement PA. Results of oral steroid treatment in nasal polyposis. Rhinology. 1994;32:5–9.
37. Kondo H, Nachtigal D, Frenkiel S, et al. Effects of steroids on nasal inflammatory cells and cytokine profile. Laryngoscope. 1999;109:91–6.
38. Xu Z, Luo X, Xu L, et al. Effect of short-course glucocorticoid application on patients with chronic rhinosinusitis with nasal polyps. World Allergy Organ J. 2020;13(6):100131. https://doi.org/10.1016/j.waojou.2020.100131. eCollection 2020 Jun.
39. Woodworth BA, Joseph K, Kaplan AP. Alterations in eotaxin, monocyte chemoattractant protein-4, interleukin-5, and interleukin-13 after systemic steroid treatment for nasal polyps. Otolaryngol Head Neck Surg. 2004;131(5):585–9.
40. Mullol J, Obando A, Pujol L, et al. Corticosteroid treatment in chronic rhinosinusitis: the possibilities and the limits. Immunol Allergy Clin North Am. 2009;29(4):657–68. https://doi.org/10.1016/j.iac.2009.07.001.
41. Rodriguez-Pinilla E, Martinez-Frias ML. Corticosteroids during pregnancy and oral clefts. A case control study. Teratology. 1998;58(1):2–5.
42. Schenkel EJ, Skoner DP, Bronsky EA, et al. Absence of growth retardation in children with perennial allergic rhinitis after one year of treatment with mometasone furoate aqueous nasal spray. Pediatrics. 2000;105(2):E22. https://doi.org/10.1542/peds.105.2.e22.
43. Rosenblut A, Bardin PG, Muller B, et al. Long-term safety of fluticasone furoate nasal spray in adults and adolescents with perennial allergic rhinitis. Allergy. 2007;62:1071–7.
44. Weiner JM, Abramson MJ, Puy RM. Intranasal corticosteroids versus oral H1 receptor antagonists in allergic rhinitis: systematic review of randomized controlled trials. BMJ. 1998;31:1624–9.
45. Wei CC, Adappa ND, Cohen NA. Use of topical nasal therapies in the management of chronic rhinosinusitis. Laryngoscope. 2013;123:2347–59.
46. Lanier B, Kai G, Marple B, et al. Pathophysiology and progression of nasal septal perforation. Ann Allergy Immunol. 2007;99:473–80.
47. Caparroz FA, Gregorio LL, Bongiovanni G, et al. Rhinitis and pregnancy: literature review. Braz J Otorhinolaryngol. 2016;82(1):105–11.
48. Nayak AS, Philip G, Lu S, et al. Efficacy and tolerability of montelukast alone or in combination with loratadine in seasonal allergic rhinitis: a multicenter randomized double blind placebo controlled trial performed in the fall. Ann Allergy Asthma Immunol. 2002;88:592–60.
49. Price DB, Swern A, Tozzi CA, et al. Effect of montelukast on lung function in asthma patients with allergic rhinitis: analysis from the COMPACT trial. Allergy. 2006;61:737–42.
50. Cingi C, Ozlugedik S. Effects of montelukast on quality of life in patients with persistent allergic rhinitis. Otolaryngol Head Neck Surg. 2010;142:654–8.
51. Scow DT, Luttermoser GK, Dickerson KS. Leukotriene inhibitors in the treatment of allergy and asthma. Am Fam Physician. 2007;75:65–70.

52. Steinbrook RA. Anaesthesia for minimally invasive surgery and pregnancy. Best Pract Res Clin Anaesthesiol. 2002;16:131–43. https://doi.org/10.1053/bean.2001.0212.
53. Van De Welde M, De Buck F. Anesthesia for nonobstetric surgery in the pregnant patient. Minerva Anestesiol. 2007;73:235–40.
54. Cheek TG, Baird E. Anesthesia for nonobstetric surgery: maternal and fetal considerations. Clin Obstet Gynecol. 2009;52:535–45. https://doi.org/10.1097/GRF.0b013e3181c11f60.

Pregnancy Rhinorrhoea

48

Ali Seyed Resuli, Muhammet Dilber, and Cemal Cingi

48.1 Introduction

Rhinorrhoea refers to a greater volume than the usual discharge of fluid from the nose. Patients complain of a runny nose. The liquid may be of varying viscosity, translucent or opaque, and may be discharged intermittently or continuously [1].

Pregnancy rhinitis (PR) is a type of persistent non-unfavourably susceptible rhinitis not present before pregnancy that shows itself during pregnancy with complete goal of manifestations after conveyance. Pregnancy rhinitis is characterised as nasal blockage in the last at least a month and a half of pregnancy, without different indications of respiratory plot disease and with no known hypersensitive reason, with complete goal of side effects inside about 14 days after conveyance. Pregnancy rhinitis happens in around one-fifth of pregnancies, can show up at practically any gestational week, and influences the lady and perhaps at the same time the baby [2].

The pathogenesis of pregnancy rhinitis is not clear, yet placental development chemical is recommended to be included. Smoking and refinement to house dust bugs are plausible danger factors. It is normally hard to make a differential analysis of sinusitis: endoscopy of a decongested nose is the symptomatic technique for

A. S. Resuli (✉)
Faculty of Medicine, Department of Otorhinolaryngology, İstanbul Yeni Yüzyıl University, İstanbul, Turkey
e-mail: a.s.resul@hotmail.com

M. Dilber
The Dilber Ear, Nose, and Throat Diseases and Surgery Clinic, İstanbul, Turkey
e-mail: muhammetdilber@hotmail.com

C. Cingi
Department of Otorhinolaryngology, Eskisehir Osmangazi University, Medical Faculty, Eskisehir, Turkey
e-mail: cemal@ogu.edu.tr

C. Cingi et al. (eds.), *ENT Diseases: Diagnosis and Treatment during Pregnancy and Lactation*, https://doi.org/10.1007/978-3-031-05303-0_48

decision. At times ultrasound or x-beam might be essential. Sinusitis ought to be dealt with forcefully with expanded portions of beta-lactam anti-infection agents and antral water system. Nasal decongestants give great transitory alleviation from pregnancy rhinitis, yet they will in general be abused, prompting the advancement of rhinitis medicamentosa. Corticosteroids have not been demonstrated to be powerful in pregnancy rhinitis, and their foundational organisation ought to be stayed away from during pregnancy. Nasal corticosteroids might be controlled in pregnant ladies when demonstrated for different kinds of rhinitis. Nasal alar dilators and saline washings are protected intending to calm nasal blockage; however, a definitive treatment for pregnancy rhinitis still needs to be found [2].

48.2 Causes

The nose and paranasal sinuses are anatomically and physiologically a unified whole, somewhat resembling a bungalow, where there are a number of rooms opening off each other. The meati may be likened to doors connecting the rooms. There is a continuous epithelial lining throughout the nasal interior and adjacent sinuses. An insult to any part of this epithelium usually provokes a response throughout the epithelium. Such insults may arise from a coryzal viral illness, an allergen, such as pet dander, or an irritant substance, such as tobacco fumes. Because these structures are all interconnected, treating rhinitis or nasal discharge may call for consideration of the entire sinonasal unit [3].

Rhinosinusitis of both an allergic and non-allergic type is often worsened by viral pharyngitis or viral infection of the proximal airway if it keeps returning. Such infective episodes can cause bronchitis or asthma, especially where sinusitis is persistent or there is polyposis within the nose. The co-occurrence of asthma, nasal polyposis, and sensitivity to aspirin, the so-called Samter Triad (Samter and Beers), is a familiar situation to clinicians [3]. Chronic rhinosinusitis has a frequent association with hyposmia or anosmia. Sufferers may notice a nasal quality to their voice or have become hoarse. This arises when the resonating sinuses become inflamed or there is inflammation of the vocal cords. Rhinosinusitis is also commonly accompanied by coughing and postnasal drip, as well as strident snoring. Where snoring occurs, this is frequently accompanied by sleep disorder, including, potentially, sleep apnoea. This problem most often occurs in males who are advancing in age and prone to obesity. Bacteria may produce an infection if there is blockage of the meati by oedema or pooling of secretions [3].

In healthy individuals, there is production of mucus to maintain the moisture of the nasal lining. This mucus moves posteriorly towards the pharynx, before being swallowed. Numerous different disorders produce excessive nasal discharge, such as [1]

- *Coryza and influenza*: Mucous build-up may physically obstruct the nose for a particular period.
- *Lacrimation*: Tears pass into the lacrimal ducts, which empty into the nasal interior and pass out as a discharge.

- *Cold weather*: The nose may react to cold temperatures by excessive mucous secretion.
- *Sinusal or adenoidal infections*: Mucus containing trapped pathogens may pool within the sinuses, provoking sinusitis. The adenoids, located within the nasopharynx, are also prone to infections in a child, which may also lead to pooled mucus with entrapped pathogens.
- *Allergic rhinitis*: An allergic reaction to, for example, pollen or animal dander, may provoke excess mucus formation.
- *Non-allergic rhinitis*: The nose may respond to an irritant (e.g. tobacco fumes or polluted air), pungent substances (e.g. spicy food), or a physical stimulus (e.g. cold temperatures) by producing extra mucus.
- *Hypertrophied or oedematous turbinates*: This may result from nasal responses to infection or allergens and may obstruct the nasal passages.
- *Hypertrophied adenoids*: This condition affects children.
- *Polyp formation within the nose*: Polyps grow outwards into the nasal passages. Their shape resembles grapes.
- *Foreign body*: A young child may sometimes insert a foreign body into the nasal cavity, such as a peanut or a bead, which then blocks the nose and produces a malodorous mucous nasal discharge.
- *Nasal cysts or neoplasia*: Although uncommon, unilateral (usually) nasal obstruction may result from a neoplasm (whether benign or malignant) or cyst formation.
- *Choanal atresia or piriform aperture stenosis*: In choanal atresia, the nasopharynx is obstructed from birth onwards. The blockage may be bony or soft tissue type. Bilateral choanal atresia typically presents at birth if bilateral, whereas unilateral atresia may present at a later stage. Stenosis of the piriform aperture is another way in which partial nasal obstruction occurs.
- *Deviation of the nasal septum*: The nasal septum divides the nasal interior into right and left halves. It consists of bony and cartilaginous portions. Where deviation occurs, the side to which the septum bends may obstruct that nasal passage. Cases may be congenital or occur due to trauma later in life.

48.3 History

The history should cover the patient's general state of health. Pyrexia needs to be asked about. Symptoms which exhibit a seasonal pattern may suggest allergic rhinitis, as may pruritus affecting the nose. A personal history of allergic dermatitis or asthma or a family history of atopic disorders points towards allergic rhinitis. If symptoms coincide with stopping a nasal decongestant, this may indicate a drug withdrawal effect.

The length of time for which symptoms are present may also provide clues that help distinguish between a neoplasm, a polyp, or sinusitis. Malodorous discharge points towards a foreign body. A history of facial injury should raise the suspicion of CSF rhinorrhoea. Consider whether symptoms coincide with starting a new drug, such as an oral contraceptive pill or blood pressure controlling agent [4].

48.4   Differential Diagnosis in a Case of Rhinorrhoea

The likely causes can be divided into those conditions featuring inflammation and those that do not. Inflammatory conditions include infections, which may be bacterial or viral, and non-infectious, that is, hay fever, year-round rhinitis (allergic or non-allergic) and non-allergic rhinitis with eosinophilia. Non-inflammatory conditions include vasomotor rhinitis and cerebrospinal fluid leakage [2].

48.4.1 Cerebrospinal Fluid (CSF) Rhinorrhoea

CSF rhinorrhoea is predominantly the result of trauma either through accidental injury or surgery. A mere 3–4% is from other causes [4–9], but where this does occur, diagnosing the cause may be highly complicated.

CSF rhinorrhoea occurs whenever there is a fistulous communication between the dura mater and the base of the skull. As noted above, cases may be traumatic or non-traumatic in origin [10, 11]. Non-traumatic CSF rhinorrhoea affects individuals above the age of 30. It begins slowly and may be mistaken for allergic rhinitis. In non-traumatic CSF rhinorrhoea, hyposmia/anosmia or pneumocephalus is rarely seen. These features are more associated with traumatic cases. Erosive tumours (cholesteatoma, tuberculoma), defective anatomy of the skull base from the time of birth, and meningocele or meningoencephalocele are likely to underlie non-traumatic CSF rhinorrhoea. Head trauma gives rise to around 80% of instances of CSF rhinorrhoea, whilst a further 16% arise from operations that affect the base of the skull [7, 12].

Although CSF rhinorrhoea rarely occurs, it is a condition prone to potentially grave complications, including death. The leakage occurs because the protective barriers interposed between the sinuses, the nose, and the intracranial fossae (anterior and middle) are breached. Because this presents a portal of entry to pathogenic organisms, CSF rhinorrhoea is associated with severe infective complications and possibly catastrophic neurological problems in the future [12].

The composition of CSF includes water, inorganic ions (Na^+, K^+, Mg^{2+}, Ca^{2+}, Cl^-, and HCO_3^-), glucose (at a concentration between 0.6 and 08× blood glucose), amino acids, and a variety of proteins (22–38 mg/dL). CSF is colourless, non-turbid, and usually has no cellular contents. If cells are present, they are polymorphonucleocytes or mononucleocytes (<5/μL) [13].

CSF is mainly (50–80%) produced by the choroid plexus. The remaining volume is produced by the ependyma, which can produce at most 30%, and ultrafiltration from the capillaries, at most 20%, of the total volume. CSF is the final stage of a process whereby plasma is ultrafiltered by the choroidal plexus epithelium, which lines the ventricular spaces of the central nervous system. Sodium ions are actively transported across the epithelial base layer by a Na^+/K^+ATPase channel, which sets up a gradient favourable to water entering the epithelium. HCO_3^- ions are formed by intracellular carbonic anhydrase. An apically located sodium-potassium ion exchange channel then excretes sodium into the ventricular lumen. Water movement also occurs in the same direction to minimise the osmotic gradient. Thus, CSF forms in the ventricular lumen [13].

Synthesis of CSF is continuous, with formation of around 20 mL hourly, giving a total daily volume produced of around 500 mL. The circulating volume of CSF through the entire CNS is in the range 90–150 mL. The usual pattern of circulation is for CSF to pass from its points of formation within the lateral ventricles, through the cerebral aqueduct into the third ventricle, whence it passes into the fourth ventricle and then through the foramen of Magendie and foramen of Luschka into the subarachnoid space. From the subarachnoid space, reabsorption into the blood occurs at the arachnoid villi [13].

The CSF circulates thanks to a pressure gradient set up between the sites of formation and the arachnoid villi. The usual pressure is between 10 and 15 mmHg. A CSF intracranial pressure exceeding 20 mmHg is considered abnormally elevated [13].

The most suitable pathology test available at present to diagnose CSF in sinonasal discharge is a β2-transferrin assay. However, this test cannot tell the clinician where the fluid is leaking from, nor even from which side. Fluorescein can be used to localise the point where leakage is coming from. For this purpose, fluorescein needs to be injected intrathecally [13].

The optimal technique for diagnosing a defect in the basal skull leading to CSF rhinorrhoea is computed tomography (CT) imaging at high resolution. CT imaging can reveal defects at the base of the skull produced by trauma (in an accident or during surgical procedures), anatomical or developmental anomalies, and destructive lesions affecting the skull base, for example, a tumour [13].

It has been suggested that conservative management is appropriate for instances in which CSF rhinorrhoea begins immediately following an accident since such leakage tends to spontaneously resolve. The approach involves confining the patient to bed for between 7 and 10 days, with the head end raised by around 15–30° [13].

There are a number of possible operative techniques that may be employed to repair CSF leaks arising from the basal skull. In the past, it was common for leakage from the anterior cranial fossa to be approached intracranially, and this technique still finds favour in particular cases. Frontal craniotomy was used to gain access to the anterior fossa [13].

On the other hand, a leak that affects the posterior wall of the frontal sinus can be accessed by a coronal incision and the creation of an osteoplastic flap. Creating this flap allows the clinician to visualise the posterior table of the frontal sinus in its entirety, which is of particular value if the leak occurs at a point higher than 2 cm above the floor and with the lamina papyracea on the medial aspect [13].

Endoscopic repair enjoys a number of advantages over open repair. These include being able to see more of the surgical field, better lighting, and having a magnified view. The scope can also be angled to reach awkward crevices. Using an endoscope, grafts, both under- and overlay types, can be positioned with superior accuracy. Endoscopic repair succeeds in closing defects within the basal skull in 90–95% of cases, as has been repeatedly shown by researchers [14–19].

48.4.1.1   CSF Rhinorrhoea Due to Trauma

Ninety per cent of instances where CSF leakage occurs are produced by penetrating or closed trauma to the skull. If CSF rhinorrhoea starts within 48 h of trauma, this is classified as 'immediate'. If not, it is 'delayed'. The bulk of cases where accidental trauma (e.g. road traffic accident) results in CSF rhinorrhoea are of the immediate type. The majority (95%) of cases of delayed CSF leakage are observed less than 3 months after the initiating trauma occurs [13].

48.4.1.2   Iatrogenic CSF Rhinorrhoea

Unlike CSF rhinorrhoea following accidental trauma, CSF rhinorrhoea secondary to surgical trauma is seen in the first 7 days post-surgery in only half of the cases. Thus, for the majority, CSF rhinorrhoea will only become apparent after returning home from hospital. Accordingly, it is vital that at-risk patients are warned to look out for a salty or metallic taste in their mouth, which might indicate CSF leakage [13].

All types of surgery involving the base of the skull are associated with a risk of iatrogenic injury leading to CSF leakage. Iatrogenic trauma ranges from a straightforward crack in the bone to defects above 1 cm across that may rupture the dura mater and possibly even damage the brain itself [13].

ENT surgical operations, for example, functional endoscopic sinus surgery (FESS) or septoplasty, may damage the integrity of the basal skull and result in CSF rhinorrhoea. There are particular operations used in neurosurgery, for example, craniotomy or transsphenoidal resection of the pituitary, which are frequently found to cause leakage of CSF via the nose [13].

The area most prone to iatrogenic injury during FESS is the lateral lamella of the cribriform plate. This is the point at which the bone forming the base of the skull is at its most slender. The rear fovea ethmoidalis and the rear portion of the frontal recess are also areas where iatrogenic injury is not uncommon [13].

48.4.1.3   CSF Rhinorrhoea Related to a Tumour

Benign neoplasms rarely cause discharge of CSF from the nose. In contrast, tumours that are locally destructive, for example, an inverted papilloma or a malignancy, may cause osteolysis of the anterior cranial fossa. These lesions release enzymes which degrade and lyse the osseous tissues, provoking an inflammatory response and potentially also damaging the dural matter. A tumour may not in itself be responsible for discharge of CSF through the nose. However, when the lesion is excised, immediate-type CSF rhinorrhoea may occur. Surgical planning for such resections needs to encompass how to repair any potential CSF leaks, whether by a transcranial or endoscopic approach [13].

48.4.1.4   Congenital CSF Rhinorrhoea

The anterior neuropore may fail to close completely in early development, resulting in nervous tissue herniating through the anterior cranial fossa. On rare occasions, this gives rise to CSF rhinorrhoea. The usual embryological anomaly is a patent fonticulus frontalis or foramen caecum. The usual presentation of a meningo-encephalocoele is as a mass within or exterior of the nose that can be transilluminated and increases in size when the baby cries, the so-called Furstenberg sign. Any mass which occurs within the nose in a child should provoke suspicion, even more so if the mass is central. Biopsy is absolutely contraindicated before a thorough radiological investigation has been undertaken [13].

48.4.1.5 Spontaneous CSF Rhinorrhoea

CSF discharge through the nose can occur seemingly spontaneously. Calling CSF 'spontaneous' tends to suggest that the real cause is unknown, but in fact it has recently become apparent that spontaneous CSF nasal discharge may be the consequence of raised intracranial pressure (ICP). ICP may become raised for a number of reasons, but, in the case of spontaneous CSF rhinorrhoea, the cause is idiopathic intracranial hypertension. ICP may also become raised if the patient suffers from obstructive sleep apnoea [2].

48.5 Treatment Options

The differential diagnosis of rhinorrhoea can, in the majority of cases, be reached on the sole basis of the patient's account. This dependence on the history has several consequences in terms of how quickly treatment can be initiated and with what degree of efficacy, and to the cost of caring for such patients. In the majority of cases, few investigations will be called for. For example, skin pinprick tests and a full blood count plus nasal smear to test for eosinophilia may be sufficient. Paranasal imaging is not generally indicated if a focus for disease within a particular sinus is not suspected. In such circumstances, the history and physical examination, which reveals pain in a particular area when touched, indicating an air–fluid level, provide the diagnosis. However, it is worth noting that in some cases the history indicates rhinorrhoea or nasal congestion, but with no focus apparent either from the history or examination. Nonetheless, subsequent x-radiography reveals an air–fluid level. Where treatment failure occurs on first-line agents, such as H1-specific antihistamines and intranasal steroid sprays, more intensive and costly investigations may be warranted, that is, CT or MRI studies [2].

If the clinicians think that a bacterial pathogen is also present, the nasal discharge may be sent for laboratory culture. Bacterial superinfection occurs at a late stage in sinusitis, which means antibiotic treatment is not appropriate at the beginning of symptoms. In any case, viral pathogens will be unaffected by antibiotic treatment [2].

References

1. Chronic rhinorrhea (runny nose). https://www.stanfordchildrens.org/en/service/ear-nose-throat/conditions/chronic-rhinorrhea. Accessed 5 Jan 2020.
2. Baudoin T, Šimunjak T, Bacan N, Jelavić B, Kuna K, Košec A. Redefining pregnancy-induced rhinitis. Am J Rhinol Allergy. 2021;35(3):315–22. https://doi.org/10.1177/1945892420957490. Epub 2020 Sep 9. PMID: 32903019.
3. Knight A. The differential diagnosis of rhinorrhea. J Allergy Clin Immunol. 1995;95:1080–3.

4. Runny nose. https://www.urgentcarepeds.org/clinical/runny-nose/. Accessed 5 Jan 2020.

5. O'Conell JF. Primary spontaneous cerebrospinal fluid rhinorrhea. J Neurol Neurosurg Psychiatry. 1964;27(3):241–6.

6. Raghavan U, Mujumdar S, Jones NS. Spontaneous CSF rhinorrhea from separate defects of the anterior and middle cranial fossa. J Laryngol Otol. 2002;116(7):546–7.

7. Ahmad FU, Sharma BS, Garg A, Chandra PS. Primary spontaneous CSF rhinorrhea through the clivus: possible etiopathology. J Clin Neurosci. 2008;15(11):1304–8.

8. Loew F, Pertuiset B, Chaumier EE, Jaksche H. Traumatic, spontaneous and post-operative CSF rhinorrhea. Adv Tech Stand Neurosurg. 1984;11:169–207.

9. Ruiz-Huidobro E, Khan D. Subacute rhinorrhea in a 42 year-old man. Ann Allergic Asthma Immunol. 2000;85(1):23–7.

10. Silva LR, Santos RP, Zymberg ST. Endoscopic endonasal approach for cerebrospinal fluid fistulae. Minim Invasive Neurosurg. 2006;49(2):88–92.

11. Tóth M, Selivanova O, Schaefer S, Mann W. Spontaneous cerebrospinal fluid rhinorrhea: a clinical and anatomical study. Laryngoscope. 2010;120(9):1724–9.

12. Ozdogan S, Gergin YE, Gergin S, Tatarli N, Hicdonmez T. Spontaneous Rhinorrhea mimicking sinusitis. Pan Afr Med J. 2015;20:97. https://doi.org/10.11604/pamj.2015.20.97.5748.

13. Oakley GM, Alt JA, Schlosser RJ, Harvey RJ, Orlandi RR. Diagnosis of cerebrospinal fluid rhinorrhea: an evidence-based review with recommendations. Int Forum Allergy Rhinol. 2016;6(1):8–16. https://doi.org/10.1002/alr.21637.

14. Lal D, Jategaonkar AA, Borish L, Chambliss LR, Gnagi SH, Hwang PH, Rank MA, Stankiewicz JA, Lund VJ. Management of rhinosinusitis during pregnancy: systematic review and expert panel recommendations. Rhinology. 2016;54(2):99–104. https://doi.org/10.4193/Rhino15.228.

15. Weinstein L. Cerebrospinal fluid rhinorrhea complicating pregnancy. South Med J. 1979;72(8):1026–7. https://doi.org/10.1097/00007611-197908000-00045.

16. Shofty B, Gonen L, Avraham S, Abergel A, Umansky D, Margalit N. Postoperative cerebrospinal fluid rhinorrhea in puerperal women following transcranial resection of tuberculum sella meningiomas. J Neurosurg Sci. 2019;63(2):233–35. https://doi.org/10.23736/S0390-5616.17.04143-1.

17. Mishra SK, Mathew GA, Paul RR, Asif SK, John M, Varghese AM, Kurien M. Endoscopic Repair of CSF Rhinorrhea: An Institutional Experience. Iran J Otorhinolaryngol. 2016;28(84):39–43. PMID: 26878002; PMCID: PMC4735615.

18. Ibrahim AA, Okasha M, Elwany S. Endoscopic endonasal multilayer repair of traumatic CSF rhinorrhea. Eur Arch Otorhinolaryngol. 2016;273(4):921–6. https://doi.org/10.1007/s00405-015-3681-y. Epub 2015 Jun 6. PMID: 26048356.

19. Ruggiero J, Zocchi J, Gallo S, Pietrobon G, De Bernardi F, Bignami M, Locatelli D, Castelnuovo P. Congenital Anterior Skull Base Encephaloceles: Long-Term Outcomes After Transnasal Endoscopic Reconstruction. World Neurosurg. 2020;143:e324–e333. https://doi.org/10.1016/j.wneu.2020.07.128.

Part V

Laryngology

Laryngopharyngeal Reflux During Pregnancy and Lactation

49

Saffet Kılıçaslan, Masaany Binti Mansor, and Nergis Salman

49.1 Introduction

Gastro-oesophageal reflux is a condition that occurs even in normal, healthy people. It should be distinguished, however, from gastro-oesophageal reflux disease (GORD), in which the stomach contents are refluxed to an extent that troublesome signs and symptoms are produced and the patient's quality of life suffers. Koufman wrote the first description of laryngopharyngeal reflux (LPR) in 1991 [1]. LPR refers to a situation wherein the stomach contents are refluxed back up the oesophagus to a level higher than the superior oesophageal sphincter [2]. There is a high frequency of both GORD and LPR in general populations. Pregnant women are particularly prone to GORD, especially in the last trimester of pregnancy. Up to four out of five women have this issue [3]. LPR and GORD have several features in common, but they represent separate disease entities (see Table 49.1) [4]. Ten percent of the US population are thought to suffer from heartburn each day, whilst 20% have symptoms at least once a week and between 30 and 60% report heartburn from time to time [5]. In pregnant women, the principal complaint is heartburn, which becomes increasingly frequent over the course of the pregnancy, but resolves following

S. Kılıçaslan (✉)
Department of Otorhinolaryngology, Düzce Ataturk State Hospital, Düzce, Turkey
e-mail: saffet82@yahoo.com

M. B. Mansor
Department of Otolaryngology—Head and Neck Surgery, Universiti Teknologi MARA Selangor Branch, Sungai Buloh Campus, Sungai Buloh, Selangor, Malaysia
e-mail: masaanymansor@yahoo.com

N. Salman
Department of Otorhinolaryngology, Private Saygı Hospital, İstanbul, Turkey
e-mail: nergissalman@hotmail.com

© The Author(s), under exclusive license to Springer Nature Switzerland AG 2022
C. Cingi et al. (eds.), *ENT Diseases: Diagnosis and Treatment during Pregnancy and Lactation*, https://doi.org/10.1007/978-3-031-05303-0_49

Table 49.1 Differences between GERD and LPR (Adopted from reference [4])

GERD	LPR
Accompanied by esophagitis and/or heartburn	Oesophagitis or heartburn is rarely present
Reflux is nocturnal or in supine position	Reflux during daytime or in upright position
Abnormal oesophageal motility and prolonged oesophageal acid exposure	Intermittent episodes of reflux
Dysfunction of the lower oesophageal sphincter	Dysfunction of the upper oesophageal sphincter
Throat-related symptoms are sometimes present	Leads to throat-related symptoms and damage to the laryngopharyngeal epithelium

delivery [6]. There is an inverse correlation between the age of the mother and the likelihood of suffering heartburn whilst pregnant [7].

49.2 Epidemiology

Gastro-oesophageal reflux generally affects between 30 and 50% of women during pregnancy; however, the prevalence may reach 80% in certain populations [8, 9]. There is a paucity of data to indicate just how common LPR is in pregnant women and the lack of an agreed absolute standard for diagnosing the condition adds to the difficulty of calculating the precise frequency [10].

49.3 Pathophysiology

The elevated level of progesterone in pregnant women leads to a lower muscle tone in the sphincter of the oesophagus. The uterine volume is greater, and this raises the pressure within the abdominal cavity. Furthermore, food passes more slowly through the gut as a result of endocrine alterations, and this may predispose the patient towards reflux [11].

The refluxate comes into contact with the cilia-bearing respiratory epithelial mucosa, injuring it and preventing the mucus from being cleared. There are both direct and indirect mechanisms by which LPR produces symptoms affecting the upper respiratory tract. Direct action occurs when the upper aerodigestive tract is irritated by the corrosive chemicals contained within refluxed stomach contents, such as hydrochloric acid and digestive enzymes, including pepsin. An indirect action occurs if the refluxed stomach contents do not rise as high as the upper aerodigestive tract, but still trigger reflex action by the larynx or bronchi. These reflexes include laryngospasm, apnoea, coughing, and constriction of the bronchi

Table 49.2 Laryngeal conditions reported to be associated with LPR (Adopted from reference [12])

Subglottic stenosis
Carcinoma of the larynx
Endotracheal intubation injury
Contact ulcers and granuloma
Posterior-glottic stenosis
Arytenoid-cartilage fixation
Paroxysmal laryngospasm
Globus pharyngeus
Vocal nodules
Polypoid degeneration
Laryngomalacia
Pachydermia laryngitis
Recurrent leucoplakia
Sudden infant death syndrome

similar to that which occurs in asthma. These reflexes are mediated by the tenth cranial nerve [10].

The various symptoms that LPR may trigger, namely, dysphonia, persistent tickly cough, repeated spasm of the larynx, and the sensation of globus, have a negative impact on the sufferer's quality of life. Furthermore, LPR has an association with a broad range of disorders affecting the respiratory system, such as chronic laryngitis, paradoxical action of the vocal cords, stenotic narrowing of the larynx and trachea, laryngomalacia, sudden infant deaths, abnormal sleep, sleep apnoea, cricoarytenoid fixation, chronic rhinosinusitis, asthma, and malignant neoplasms of the larynx (see Table 49.2) [12].

49.4 Clinical Presentation

In around 20% of cases, LPR is asymptomatic. The usual reason for such a case to attend an otorhinolaryngology appointment is a complaint of dysphonia. Where symptoms are present, they usually involve a hoarse voice, coughing, globus sensation in the throat, mucus build-up in the pharynx, the need to keep clearing the throat, and mild difficulties with swallowing (see Table 49.3) [12]. LPR may result in recurrent and chronic pharyngitis, particularly on waking, a burning pain in the pharynx, coughing, clearing the throat, offensive breath odour, feeling something is stuck in the throat, and dysphonia. These symptoms may also be due to other disorders, such as postnasal discharge, allergic rhinitis, infections of the upper respiratory tract, clearing the throat as a habit, smoking, alcohol consumption, overuse of the voice, alterations in temperature or type of weather, emotional problems, and exposure to air pollution, amongst others [10].

Table 49.3 ENT symptoms related to LPR (Adopted from reference [12])

Laryngeal symptoms	Pharyngeal symptoms
Hoarseness	Globus pharyngeus
Dysphonia	Sore throat
Voice fatigue	Dysphagia
Difficulty in producing high-frequency voice	Odynophagia
Chronic or frequent recurrent irritating cough	
Excessive throat clearing	
Excessive mucus in the throat	
Laryngospasm/cough syncope	

Table 49.4 Reflux Symptom Index (RSI) (Adopted from reference [15])

Item	Symptom[a]	Score[b]					
1	Hoarseness or a problem with your voice	0	1	2	3	4	5
2	Clearing your voice	0	1	2	3	4	5
3	Excess throat mucous or postnasal drip	0	1	2	3	4	5
4	Difficulty swallowing food, liquids, or pills	0	1	2	3	4	5
5	Coughing after you ate or after lying down	0	1	2	3	4	5
6	Breathing difficulties or choking episodes	0	1	2	3	4	5
7	Troublesome or annoying cough	0	1	2	3	4	5
8	Sensations or something sticking in your throat	0	1	2	3	4	5
9	Heartburn, chest pain, indigestion, or stomach pain	0	1	2	3	4	5

Laryngopharyngeal reflux is considered if RSI > 13
[a] Patients are asked to determine how the associated problems affect them within the last month
[b] 0–5 rating scale with 0 = no problem and 5 = severe

49.5 Diagnosis

Diagnosis of LPR during pregnancy involves an approach that does not greatly differ from that taken in adults generally. To diagnose the condition reliably, the clinician should obtain a clear symptomatic history and establish that the symptoms abate following appropriate alterations to lifestyle and the use of medication for GORD [12–14]. The Reflux Symptom Index (RSI), which was created by Belafsky and colleagues, is a clinical questionnaire consisting of nine items answered directly by the patient, the purpose of which is to aid the initial diagnosis in cases of LPR and to grade how severe the disorder is. This questionnaire has the limitation that it does not ask about how often symptoms occur or how long they have been present (see Table 49.4) [15].

For assessment of mucosal integrity and pathological changes secondary to LPR, endoscopic laryngoscopy is suitable. The classical findings in cases of LPR are inflammation and mucosal thickening of the posterior portion of the larynx, together with mucosal thickening of the posterior commissure and the postcricoid. In addition to the RSI, Befalsky et al. also created the Reflux Finding Score (RFS), consisting of eight items to be assessed during flexible laryngoscopic examination, which then indicate clinical severity. These items include the presence of a pseudosulcus due to swelling below the level of the glottis and extending from the anterior to the

Table 49.5 Reflux Finding Score (RFS) (Adopted from reference [16])

Item	Symptom	Score
1	Subglottic oedema (pseudosulcus)	0 = absent, 2 = present
2	Ventricular obliteration	0 = none, 2 = partial, 4 = complete
3	Erythema/hyperaemia	0 = none, 2 = arytenoids only, 4 = diffuse
4	Vocal fold oedema	0 = none, 1 = mild, 2 = moderate, 3 = severe, 4 = polypoid
5	Diffuse laryngeal oedema	0 = none, 1 = mild, 2 = moderate, 3 = severe, 4 = obstructing
6	Posterior commissure hypertrophy	0 = none, 1 = mild, 2 = moderate, 3 = severe, 4 = obstructing
7	Granuloma/granulation	0 = absent, 2 = present
8	Thick endolaryngeal mucus	0 = absent, 2 = present

Laryngopharyngeal reflux is considered if RFS > 7

posterior commissure, loss of visualisation of the ventricle, erythema and hyperaemia, swelling of the vocal cords, widespread oedema within the larynx, hypertrophied posterior commissure, formation of granulation tissue, and oversecretion of mucus within the lumen of the larynx (see Table 49.5) [16].

The efficacy of treatment can be reliably assessed through use of the RFS and RSI.

More invasive assessment methods are typically unnecessary and rarely undertaken. X-rays are not needed and mean the foetus is exposed to radiation. Although they are not often needed, manometric analysis and acidity measurements of the oesophagus may be undertaken without undue risk [11]. Where symptoms due to reflux demonstrate treatment resistance or complications develop, endoscopic examination is undertaken. It is considered safe, provided the blood pressure and oxygen levels are diligently monitored during the procedure. A conscious sedation technique should also be used as applicable. For sedation, midazolam is likely to be safe for the foetus from the second trimester onwards. If foetal monitoring is also instigated, this may render the procedure even safer [17].

49.6 Treatment

A key principle in the treatment of heartburn in pregnant and breastfeeding mothers is to start by modifying contributory lifestyle factors. A further essential element is to consider any teratogenic potential from different pharmacological treatments.

The potential management of LPR involves alterations to diet and lifestyle, after which there may remain a need for pharmacotherapy.

49.6.1 Dietary and Lifestyle Modification

A gap of 3 h should be left between meals, and the portion size should not be excessive. The patient should eat slowly and masticate carefully. Drinking water while eating is to be discouraged. Water may be consumed between meals. The patient should not eat anything within 3 h of lying down to sleep. The following food items and beverages are best avoided: chocolate, greasy or highly spiced food, food or drinks that are acidic, caffeine, citrus fruits, tomatoes, ketchup, and carbonated beverages. If the woman sits up straight and takes a measured walk for 1 h after eating, this reduces symptoms. Clothing should be comfortable; weight gain should be avoided and the consumption of yoghurt or warm milk lessens symptoms. Chewing gum, if sugar free, also helps as this promotes the flow of saliva, which may neutralise oesophageal acidity. There are several food items and beverages that have a low potential to worsen reflux and thus may be suggested to the patient, namely, apples, bananas, jacket potatoes, broccoli, cabbages, carrots, green beans, garden peas, steak, chicken breast, egg albumen, fish, cheese, goat's cheese, bran, oats, corn bread, rice, mineral water, and salad without dressing [18, 19].

As a beverage, chamomile tea or warm milk with the addition of honey may be helpful. Complementary therapies (such as yoga) may be advised at the physician's discretion. Lifting up the head of the bed and adopting a sleeping posture lying on the left side may help to alleviate symptoms [11].

49.6.2 Pharmacotherapy

The usual approach to medical therapy is a proton pump inhibitor (PPI), an alginic acid derivative, drugs that promote gut motility, and histamine H2 receptor blockers. The choice of agent to use is affected by whether the patient is pregnant or not. Greater caution and deliberation is required in treating pregnant women, so that the benefits can be weighed against potential harms to the mother or foetus. The teratogenic potential of the particular medication needs to be considered when prescribing. The suitable agents to use during pregnancy are the H2 blockers and PPIs [3].

The H2 blockers with current US marketing authorisation are cimetidine, ranitidine, famotidine, and nizatidine. They fall under category B of the FDA teratogenicity scheme. Nizatidine was moved from category C to category B. Use of nizatidine should only be where absolutely required.

Cimetidine is the first, and ranitidine the second, choice if an H2 blocker is needed for a pregnant patient. Use of these drugs in a pregnant patient should be carefully documented. One study exists showing that neither of these medications caused negative outcomes in pregnancy nor produced drug reactions [20]. Another study, this time undertaken in the southern district of Israel, and involving the Clalit Health Organisation, involved 117,960 babies between 1998 and 2007. A total of 1148 neonates had had exposure to H2 blockers whilst in the initial trimester, but without any corresponding increase in the incidence of congenital malformation, perinatal death, premature birth, being underweight at birth, or an Apgar score that was low [21].

A meta-analysis brought together the results of four studies providing data on how safe H2 blockers are in pregnancy. The rates of spontaneous abortion, premature birth, and being small for date were compared in 2398 pregnant women who received H2 blockers and 119,892 who had no such exposure. No increase in the risk of adverse events of these types was found [22].

Medications which promote motility have been employed to treat reflux occurring during pregnancy. Metoclopramide is a dopamine antagonist used in this indication. Metoclopramide is beneficial in reducing GORD-associated symptoms, but the principal action is to reduce vomiting and nausea. Cisapride is classified as a category C agent from the point of view of teratogenic potential. It is known to be severely cardiotoxic, as revealed in animal experiments. Domperidone is another agent that promotes gut motility and is anti-emetic. It is an unresolved question how safe domperidone is in pregnant women, and thus it, too, is a category C drug [3].

The use of proton pump inhibitors in pregnancy is acceptable from a safety viewpoint as they fall under category B.

Lechien et al. [23] undertook a systematic review of 76 studies, dating from January 1990 to February 2019 and involving 6457 individuals. The review showed that mostly treatment for LPR involved PPI pharmacotherapy on an o.d. or b.d. basis, with the course lasting from 4 to 24 weeks. Currently, the therapeutic option chosen by the majority of clinicians is a PPI on an o.d. or b.d. basis [23, 24].

Omeprazole is the only PPI classified by the FDA as a category C agent, the others (dexlansoprazole, esomeprazole, lansoprazole, pantoprazole, and rabeprazole) falling under category B. Provided adjustments to lifestyle and pharmacotherapy employing antacids or H2 blockers have failed to alleviate symptoms, treatment should proceed with a PPI. There are no reports of foetal injury or teratogenicity associated with lansoprazole, pantoprazole, or esomeprazole. Despite the fact that the data on the use of PPĪs in pregnancy are still incomplete, the rationale for treatment is a reduction in the risk of maternal aspiration [25].

A meta-analysis has been published [26] in which the outcomes in 1530 pregnant women with exposure to PPIs in the first trimester or early on in pregnancy were compared to 133,410 pregnant women without such exposure. The study authors advised that the use of PPI pharmacotherapy in early pregnancy was acceptable.

Another study of Danish origin, using a cohort design, collected data from all live births from January 1996 to September 2008. The aim was to examine any correlation between exposure to PPIs from up to 4 weeks prior to conception to early pregnancy. In more than 840,000 cases, there was no evidence to support a link between PPI and congenital malformations [27].

In contrast, however, a meta-analysis which pooled the results of 26 individual studies did discover a raised incidence of congenital defects where PPIs had been used, mostly from studies with a case–control design. This risk was not found if the agent used was an H2 blocker. The use of PPĪ did not raise the risk of abortion, stillbirth, newborn mortality, prematurity or low weight at birth, whereas H2 blockers did have an association with premature delivery [28].

Alginic acid derivatives act by coalescing as a layer protecting the oesophagus or larynx from acidity-related damage if the gastric contents are refluxed. This action is useful in providing symptomatic relief in cases of LPR [29]. This class of agent benefits from safety and high efficacy when used for heartburn or the symptoms of GORD in pregnant women [30]. It has been suggested that alginic acid derivatives are suitable as the initial treatment of heartburn and symptomatic GORD in pregnant women since their risk profiles are favourable and their cost is low [31].

In treating pregnant women with symptoms of reflux, a stepped approach is essential, given that the majority of cases where symptoms are no more than mild can be successfully managed by dietary and lifestyle changes, without the need for medication. If symptoms are of moderate intensity, medication may be added, particularly an alginic acid derivative or H2 blocker. In the general adult population, the therapy with the highest efficacy in reflux disorder is PPI treatment. However, their use should be confined to cases of treatment resistance or where complications develop [10].

## 49.7	Treatment in Breastfeeding Women

Although it is common for symptoms of reflux to cease after the woman has given birth, in certain women the problem persists whilst they are still breastfeeding [25]. Following birth, women should be advised to keep going with the alterations to diet and lifestyle which aim to reduce symptoms. Since the majority of drugs are found within breast milk and thus may lead to adverse effects in neonates, it is safest not to prescribe any medication to breastfeeding mothers unless absolutely required. There is a paucity of specific data on treating LPR in breastfeeding women, although a limited number of cases reports do detail adverse outcomes from pharmacotherapy for GORD given to breastfeeding mothers. Accordingly, lifestyle and dietary manipulations are the essential first step to take. The known side effects of H2 blockers are gynaecomastia and galactorrhoea, resulting from prolactin release, plus potential interaction with other agents, arising from competitive inhibition of hepatic cytochromes. Amongst H2 blockers, the agent with the highest concentration in breast milk is cimetidine, which is also the most potent hepatic cytochrome inhibitor. Famotidine is the weakest inhibitor of hepatic mixed function oxidases and thus the least objectionable H2 blocker for use in lactating mothers. With the use of this medication, there are no specific precautions which need to be taken during lactation.

However, where there is treatment resistance or complications develop, the use of PPIs is warranted. What data do exist on the use of PPIs during breastfeeding are confined to pantoprazole and omeprazole. This underlies the reasoning for making pantoprazole and omeprazole the PPIs to choose for breastfeeding mothers [32]. However, a review [33] concerning PPIs failed to recommend they be used in this situation.

As occurs with H2 blockers, PPIs may result in prolactinaemia. There are multiple case reports of gynaecomastia that resolved when treatment was stopped, together with reports of galactorrhoea. These cases were mainly with omeprazole, although esomeprazole, lansoprazole, and rabeprazole have also been implicated [34].

49.8 Laryngitis During Pregnancy and Lactation

Laryngitis is any condition in which the larynx becomes inflamed [35]. If the inflammation has a duration of under 3 weeks, laryngitis is classified as acute, whereas inflammation that lasts longer than this is considered chronic [36]. The majority of cases of laryngitis are acute and resolve spontaneously within 3 weeks, but a proportion of cases go on to become chronic. There are both infectious and non-infectious causes of acute laryngitis, as listed in Tables 49.6 and 49.7 [37].

Although laryngitis in a pregnant woman may cause discomfort, spontaneous recovery without complications for the foetus is the norm. Thus, the majority of cases do not entail high risk. However, laryngitis should be treated as a potential emergency since, in a minority of cases, the airway may rapidly become severely compromised.

Pregnancy leads to a state of relative immunosuppression [38]. The circulating level of cortisol rises, and this then leads to gestational immune suppression. Dormant viral infections may then become active. Furthermore, the higher circulating progesterone level and the greater pressure within the abdomen caused by the increase in uterine size may lead to symptomatic LPR and the consequences of LPR [39].

49.8.1 Acute Laryngitis

Acute laryngitis most frequently results from a viral infection of the upper respiratory tract. The usual pathogens are rhinovirus, parainfluenza virus, respiratory

Table 49.6 Causes of infectious laryngitis (Adopted from reference [37])

Infectious laryngitis	
Acute laryngitis	Chronic laryngitis
Acute Viral Laryngitis – Rhinovirus, parainfluenza, paramyxovirus – Laryngotracheobronchitis (croup)	Chronic Viral Laryngitis – Post-viral vagal neuropathy – Varicella zoster – Idiopathic ulcerative laryngitis – Chronic cough
Acute Bacterial Laryngitis – Group A streptococcus, *S. pneumonia*, *S. aureus*, *H. influenzae* type B – Epiglottitis (acute supraglottitis) – Diphtheria	Chronic Bacterial Laryngitis – *S. aureus* – Tuberculosis – Syphilis – Leprosy – Actinomycosis – Rhinoscleroma
Acute Fungal Laryngitis – Candidiasis	Chronic Fungal Laryngitis – Histoplasmosis – Blastomycosis – Paracoccidioides

Table 49.7 Causes of non-infectious laryngitis (Adopted from reference [37])

Non-infectious laryngitis	
Acute laryngitis	Chronic laryngitis
1. Phonotrauma	1. Reflux laryngitis
2. Irritants (exogenous, endogenous, or iatrogenic: smoking, chemical irritants, allergy, inhaled corticosteroids, intubation trauma)	2. Pseudomyxomatous laryngitis
	3. Irritants (exogenous, endogenous, or iatrogenic: smoking, chemical irritants, allergy, inhaled corticosteroids, intubation trauma)
	4. Autoimmune diseases • Pemphigoid and pemphigus Granulomatosis with polyangiitis • Relapsing polychondritis • Connective tissue diseases (rheumatoid arthritis, systemic lupus erythematosus, scleroderma, Sjögren's syndrome
	5 Laryngitis associated with systemic inflammatory disease • Sarcoidosis • Amyloidosis
	6 Radiation-related laryngitis

syncytial virus, coronavirus, adenovirus, or influenza. Laryngitis may also follow on from respiratory tract infections (both upper and lower), for example, adenotonsillitis, pharyngitis, or a chest infection. The typical presentation is dysphonia with indications of coryza. In particular individuals, a bacterial superinfection may occur, which increases the severity of laryngitis. The pathogen in such cases is most likely to be *Streptococcus pneumoniae, Haemophilus influenzae,* or *Moraxella catarrhalis* [35, 36].

The usual cause for acute laryngitis is an infection. However, it may also result from phonotrauma (damage to the cords, misusing the voice), GORD, an allergic reaction, asthma, air pollution, cigarette fumes, injury due to inhalation, and psychological factors (such as a conversion disorder). Phonotrauma may be due to improper use of the voice (shouting for too long, too loudly, etc.). Misuse/abuse of the voice may be recent, such as laryngitis after shouting for only 1 or 2 days. This phonotrauma makes the vocal cords become swollen and bleed [40]. If the patient is also dehydrated, phonotraumatic injury may be worsened due to alteration in the pressure required to produce phonation [41]. A number of factors render individuals at greater risk of developing laryngitis, particularly during the colder months of the year. These factors include stress, immunodeficiency, irritation by cigarette fumes, alcohol misuse, and allergenic substances [42].

Laryngitis principally presents with voice problems. Symptoms which may indicate pharyngeal or laryngeal involvement include dysphonia (hoarse voice), loss of the voice (at an advanced stage), painful throat, difficulty or pain in swallowing, feeling something is stuck in the throat, repetitive clearing of the throat, a nonproductive cough, pharyngeal lymphadenopathy, and a generalised muscular ache (i.e. myalgia) [35, 36]. Shortness of breath or stridor rarely occurs, but is an indication of respiratory distress.

To diagnose laryngitis, clinicians rely on the pattern of presenting complaint(s), a thorough, targeted history and a detailed physical examination, with use of the laryngoscope. The patient should be asked about symptoms affecting the throat, when the problem began, any previous illnesses, what treatment has been attempted already, whether any other drugs are in use, smoking status, and the patient's employment history. The inside of the mouth and oropharyngeal region should be examined, and visualisation of the larynx will then permit a definitive diagnosis. Flexible laryngoscopy allows the larynx to be seen directly and photographic records may be taken if required. There are no particular problems associated with using the flexible laryngoscope in pregnant patients. The appearance of the larynx is variable, depending on the grade of laryngeal inflammation.

In the early stages of laryngitis, the epiglottis, aryepiglottic folds, arytenoids, and vocal folds are reddened and swollen. As laryngitis worsens, the erythema becomes more pronounced. There may be viscous secreted substances between the vocal folds or between the arytenoids. Pus within the interior of the larynx is more likely to represent laryngitis secondary to a bacterial than a viral pathogen [36]. In cases of acute trauma sustained to the voice, there may be bleeding in the submucosal layer. Reinke's oedema is frequently noted in laryngitis cases, whether acute or chronic [35, 36].

49.8.2 Therapy in Pregnant Patients

Pregnant patients present particular challenges in their treatment since there exists the possibility of harm to both the mother and unborn child. Since drug treatment may carry a risk of teratogenicity, clinicians need to consider both maternal and foetal effects of any medication before use.

Therapy for laryngitis in pregnant patients typically consists of support and entails alleviating symptoms. In a few cases, infections occurring at a level above the glottis will result in admission to hospital, parenteral antimicrobial therapy, and use of supplementary oxygen [39]. In potentially fatal infections, clinicians should be ready to intubate and aggressively manage the airway as the risk to life is very real.

At the other end of the spectrum of severity, where treatment aims to provide support, the measures to be initiated involve resting the voice, humidifying the atmosphere and ensuring adequate fluid intake. Menthol or eucalyptus may be taken by steam inhalation, and the patient should drink adequate amounts of water. Symptoms may be alleviated by pain killers and mucolytic agents. In cases where pain is no more than moderate, pregnant women may take acetaminophen or non-steroidal anti-inflammatory drugs (NSAIDs) [43, 44]. Where non-pharmacological measures fail to alleviate pain in pregnancy, the most suitable initial drug is acetaminophen, the use of which has been found not to raise the risk of congenital malformations when used in the initial trimester of pregnancy [45]. A review from

2019 advises that acetaminophen not be used above a daily total of 4 g and not over lengthy periods [44].

In the final trimester of pregnancy, NSAIDs should not be employed since their use after 30 weeks gestation is associated with premature closure of the ductus arteriosus, inadequate amniotic fluid, and difficulty controlling bleeding in the foetus [46, 47].

Mucolytic agents render the respiratory tract more capable of clearing excess mucus. Where fluids by mouth or alternative (non-pharmacological) treatments have failed, the initial agents recommended in pregnant patients are N-acetylcysteine, ambroxol, and bromhexine. Mucolytic agents that contain iodine must not be used, particularly from the second trimester onwards, as this may result in the foetal thyroid being inappropriately suppressed [48].

Pregnant women who suffer from a chronic cough may be prescribed an antitussive agent, with codeine or dextromethorphan being suitable throughout the pregnancy if the cough is troublesome and long term. Nonetheless, if high doses are administered for a prolonged period, or the agent is used towards the end of the pregnancy, the neonate may suffer from symptoms of withdrawal and respiration may be depressed [49, 50].

Under normal circumstances, acute laryngitis resolves spontaneously. On occasion, however, its severity may be high enough to cause respiratory distress. Where acute laryngitis is of this degree of severity, it may be necessary to administer adrenaline by injection and via nebuliser, a beta-2-agonist (i.e. salbutamol) also via nebuliser and systemic corticosteroids, consisting of either prednisolone or its prodrug form, prednisone. These measures collectively dampen down the inflammatory response and reduce airway swelling, thus maintaining patency in the airway [39]. The use of systemic steroid treatment is acceptable after the end of the first trimester, especially in the last trimester [51].

Since in the majority of cases the pathogen responsible for acute laryngitis is a virus, antibiotic treatment is not advocated for this condition. A Cochrane Database Review dating from 2013 noted no apparent benefit when antibiotics were administered and therefore their use at the beginning of acute laryngitis is not recommended since there is no benefit in doing so. There is evidence to suggest that patients self-rate their voice as less affected after 1 week and cough less severe after 2 weeks when given erythromycin [52].

If there are definite indications of a bacterial infection, namely, pus within the endolarynx and symptoms, indicating a high degree of severity, antibiotic treatment may be warranted. The agents suitable for this situation include a cephalosporin of the third generation, such as ceftriaxone, a second-generation cephalosporin, or a broad-spectrum penicillin. In all cases, the dose is administered intravenously [53]. Efficacy has also been demonstrated for macrolide antibiotics, namely, erythromycin and clarithromycin. In these cases, the pathogen may have been *Moraxella catarrhalis* [54]. A cohort study conducted between 1990 and 2016 looked at maternal use of macrolide monotherapy with erythromycin, clarithromycin, or azithromycin or penicillin monotherapy, administered between week 4 of gestation and the end of pregnancy. The conclusions were that macrolide treatment in the initial trimester raised the incidence of major congenital anomalies, and specifically cardiac anomalies, more than penicillin treatment. Macrolide therapy at any point in the pregnancy raised the risk of anomalies affecting the genitalia. Thus, prescription of macrolides in pregnant women should involve caution [55].

49.8.3 Advice for Preventing Laryngitis During Pregnancy and Lactation

- Avoid voice abuse and preferably rest the voice
- Try not to shout or sing loudly for an extended period
- Quit smoking and alcohol
- Avoid irritants. Dust, allergens, and pollutants can cause laryngitis.
- Humidify the air. Adding moisture to the air can help to reduce irritation
- Drink plenty of fluids to prevent dehydration
- Drink warm drinks and avoid cold drinks
- Avoid throat clearing. This can irritate the larynx and cause laryngitis. Try swallowing instead.
- Avoid decongestants as they can dry out the throat
- Evade eating 3 h before sleep and raise the head with pillows when sleeping. This can help to prevent acid reflux that may cause laryngitis.
- Try not to shout or sing loudly for long periods. Rest the voice.
- Avoid decongestants as they can dry out the throat
- Avoid food or drinks that can cause laryngopharyngeal reflux (LPR), for example, caffeinated beverages such as coffee or tea, carbonated drinks, sour fruits or food, spicy and oily food.
- Avoid people who have respiratory infections like the common cold or flu.
- Good personal hygiene. Viral infections usually cause laryngitis. These can sometimes be prevented by washing hands with warm, soapy water and disinfecting surfaces in the home.

49.9 Acute Epiglottitis (Supraglottitis)

Acute epiglottitis is an acute infection of the supraglottis characterized by inflammation of the supraglottic mucosa, including epiglottis, ventricular folds, and aryepiglottic folds. Hemophilus influenzae type B is the most common causative organism, even though its incidence has dramatically decreased since the initiation of childhood vaccination programs with Hib-conjugated vaccines in the late 1980s [56]. Other common pathogens are Streptococcus pneumoniae, Staphylococcus aureus, β-hemolytic Streptococci, and Klebsiella pneumoniae [57] Acute epiglottitis is more common in children though there have been a few reports of epiglottitis during pregnancy [58]. Acute epiglottitis should be considered to be an emergency condition due to the potential rapid and progressive airway obstruction. The main complaint is of a painful throat with associated odynophagia. Dyspnoea, fever, and drooling may also be seen but are not always present [59]. Diagnosis may be confirmed by directly examining the larynx using a transnasal fiber-optic laryngoscopy, which may reveal an erythematous and congested epiglottis with inflammation of the surrounding supraglottic structures [60].

The most important part of treatment involves securing the airway. Patients should be hospitalized due to the potential rapid and progressive airway obstruction. Acute epiglottitis may require endotracheal intubation to protect the airway. Tracheal intubation can be difficult due to distorted anatomy and profuse secretions. Acute epiglottitis rarely requires tracheostomy since endotracheal intubation is commonly sufficient to secure the airway. However, during an emergency, a tracheostomy should be performed if intubation fails. Systemic corticosteroids and nebulized adrenaline may be used in patients with significant airway compromise. Intravenous antibiotics are recommended especially broad-spectrum antibiotics against β-lactamase positive H influenzae such as second- or third-generation cephalosporins (cefuroxime or ceftriaxone) or ampicillin-sulbactam [61]. Most patients will respond to medical treatment, showing an improvement within 24–48 h. This can be evaluated by examination with trans-nasal fiber-optic laryngoscopy and monitoring clinical and biochemical parameters [59].

49.9.1 Treatment During Lactation

During the lactation period, treatment begins with supportive measures. Supportive measures include voice rest, humidification, and hydration in mild cases. Steamy inhalations of menthol or eucalyptus and plenty of water are helpful. Medication should be considered as benefits and risks because most drugs are excreted into breast milk. Thus, this can cause side effects and harm to the baby. Symptomatic treatment includes analgesics and mucolytics.

Paracetamol is considered the safest analgesic for nursing mothers [62]. The excreted amounts of paracetamol into breast milk are much less than doses usually given to infants [63]. Adverse effects in breastfed infants are rarely reported. A maculopapular rash on a 2-month-old infant attributed to paracetamol in breast milk was reported [64].

The American Academy of Pediatrics has evaluated that ibuprofen, naproxen, diclofenac, indomethacin, ketorolac, piroxicam, mefenamic acid, and flufenamic acid are all compatible with breastfeeding [65]. Among the NSAIDs during breastfeeding, ibuprofen is the drug of the first choice [48]. Ibuprofen has a short half-life (2 h). The excreted amounts of ibuprofen into breast milk are deficient [66]. No adverse events related to exposure via breast milk have been reported [67]. A review searching the most common anti-migraine drugs and their lactation risks revealed that ibuprofen and paracetamol were safe during lactation and diclofenac ketoprofen, naproxen was compatible with breastfeeding but warranting caution [62].

Mucolytic drugs increase and ease the clearance of mucus in the respiratory tract. N-acetylcysteine, ambroxol, and bromhexine are the choice of mucolytics during lactation if (oral) fluid therapy and other nonmedical treatment are not sufficiently effective [48].

With severe dry coughing, single doses of dextromethorphan or codeine are approved during breastfeeding [48]. Many cases report adverse effects in breastfed infants following maternal codeine use, such as apnea, lethargy, infant drowsiness, central nervous system depression [68]. There is also a death report in an infant following maternal codeine use during breastfeeding [69]. The use of codeine should be avoided during the lactation period [68].

Most cases of acute laryngitis are viral agents; therefore, antibiotic medication is not recommended. Antibiotics can be given in the presence of bacterial infection, as evident by actual purulent endolaryngeal discharge and severe laryngitis symptoms. The excreted amounts of antibiotics can cause adverse effects in breastfed infants, such as rash and disruption of the infant's gastrointestinal flora, resulting in diarrhea or thrush [68]. Third-generation cephalosporin (ceftriaxone), a second-generation cephalosporin (cefuroxime axetil), broad-spectrum penicillins (amoxicillin) should be used during the lactation period [53]. Macrolides are acceptable in nursing mothers because of the low levels in breastmilk and safe administration directly to infants [48]. The primary concern associated with the use of macrolides in nursing mothers is related to numerous cases of pyloric stenosis in children treated with macrolides [70, 71]. A systematic review and meta-analysis study revealed that the use of macrolides during breastfeeding showed no significant association with infantile hypertrophic pyloric stenosis in infants [72]. In a prospective, controlled observational study, fifty-five infants exposed to macrolide antibiotics were compared to a control cohort of 36 infants exposed to amoxicillin. The study revealed that seven (12.7%) infants in the macrolide group experienced adverse reactions (rash, diarrhea, loss of appetite, and somnolence) versus three infants (8.3%) in the amoxicillin group rashes and somnolence and rates and types of minor adverse reactions in breastfed infants exposed to a macrolide or amoxicillin in breastmilk were comparable [73].

Acute laryngitis is a self-limiting condition. However, it can become severe and may cause respiratory distress. In more severe cases, epinephrine (systemic and nebulized), nebulized B2 agonist (salbutamol), and systemic steroids (prednisone and its metabolite prednisolone) may be required to reduce inflammation and edema in order to sustain a patent airway [39].

Both prednisone and prednisolone are found in breast milk in low concentrations. No adverse effects have been reported in breastfed infants with maternal use of any corticosteroid during breastfeeding [74].

References

1. Koufman JA. The otolaryngologic manifestations of gastroesophageal reflux disease (GERD): a clinical investigation of 225 patients using ambulatory 24-hour pH monitoring and an experimental investigation of the role of acid and pepsin in the development of laryngeal injury. Laryngoscope. 1991;101(4 Pt 2 Suppl 53):1–78. https://doi.org/10.1002/lary.1991.101.s53.1.

2. Lechien JR, Saussez S, Karkos PD. Laryngopharyngeal reflux disease: clinical presentation, diagnosis and therapeutic challenges in 2018. Curr Opin Otolaryngol Head Neck Surg. 2018;26(6):392–402. https://doi.org/10.1097/MOO.0000000000000486.

3. Thelin SC, Richter JE. Review article: the management of heartburn during pregnancy and lactation. Aliment Pharmacol Ther. 2020;51(4):421–34. https://doi.org/10.1111/apt.15611.

4. Kuo CL. Laryngopharyngeal reflux: an update. Arch Otorhinolaryngol Head Neck Surg. 2019;3(1):1–7. https://doi.org/10.24983/scitemed.aohns.2019.00094.

5. Locke GR, Talley NJ, Fett SL, et al. Prevalence and clinical spectrum of gastroesophageal reflux: a population-based study in Olmsted County, Minnesota. Gastroenterology. 1997;112(5):1448–56. https://doi.org/10.1016/s0016-5085(97)70025-8.

6. Bor S, Kitapcioglu G, Dettmar P, et al. Association of heartburn during pregnancy with the risk of gastroesophageal reflux disease. Clin Gastroenterol Hepatol. 2007;5(9):1035–9.

7. Habr F, Raker C, Lin CL, et al. Predictors of gastroesophageal reflux symptoms in pregnant women screened for sleep disordered breathing: a secondary analysis. Clin Res Hepatol Gastroenterol. 2013;37(1):93–9.

8. Ramya RS, Jayanthi N, Alexander PC, et al. Gastroesophageal reflux disease in pregnancy: a longitudinal study. Trop Gastroenterol. 2014;35(3):168–72.

9. Ramu B, Mohan P, Rajasekaran MS, et al. Prevalence and risk factors for gastroesophageal reflux in pregnancy. Indian J Gastroenterol. 2011;30(3):144–7.

10. Vejvechaneyom W. Laryngopharyngeal reflux in pregnancy. Thai J Obstet Gynaecol. 2011;19(2):40–4.

11. Vedat G. Ideal approach to gastroesophageal reflux in pregnancy. Mathews J Gastroenterol Hepatol. 2018;3(1):011.

12. Wackym PA, Snow JB. Ballenger's otorhinolaryngolgy head and neck surgery. In: Altman KW, Koufman JA, editors. Laryngopharyngeal reflux, infections and manifestations of systemic diseases. Shelton: People's Medical Publishing House; 2016. p. 1154–7.

13. Medication during pregnancy: an intercontinental cooperative study. Collaborative Group on Drug Use in Pregnancy (C.G.D.U.P.). Int J Gynaecol Obstet. 1992;39(3):185–196.

14. Vlastarakos PV, Nikolopoulos TP, Monolopoulus L, et al. Treating common ear problems in pregnancy: what is safe? Eur Arch Otorhinolaryngol. 2007;265(2):139–45. https://doi.org/10.1007/s00405-007-0534-3.

15. Befalsky PC, Postma NG, Kofman JA. Validity and reliability of the reflux symptom index (RSI). J Voice. 2002;16(2):274–7. https://doi.org/10.1016/s0892-1997(02)00097-98.

16. Befalsky PC, Postma NG, Kofman JA. The validity and reliability of the reflux finding score (RFS). Laryngoscope. 2001;111(8):1313–7. https://doi.org/10.1097/00005537-200108000-00001.

17. Capell MS. The safety and efficacity of gastrointestinal endoscopy during pregnancy. Gastroenterol Clin North Am. 1998;27(1):37–71.

18. MacFarlane B. Management of gastroesophageal reflux disease in adults: a pharmacist's perspective. Integr Pharm Res Pract. 2018;7:41–52. https://doi.org/10.2147/IPRP.S142932.

19. Van der Woude CJ, Metselaar HJ and Danese S. (2014). Management of gastrointestinal and liver diseases during pregnancy. Gut. 63(6): 1014-1023.

20. Young A, Kumar MA, Thota PN. GERD: a practical approach. Cleve Clin J Med. 2020;87(4):223–30. https://doi.org/10.3949/ccjm.87a.19114.

21. Matok I, Gorodicher R, Koren G. The safety of H(2)-blockers use during pregnancy. J Clin Pharmacol. 2010;50(1):81–7. https://doi.org/10.1177/0091270009350483.

22. Gill SK, O'Brien L, Koren G. The safety of histamine 2 (H_2) blockers in pregnancy: a meta-analysis. Dig Dis Sci. 2010;54(9):1835–8. https://doi.org/10.1007/s10620-008-0587-1.

23. Lechien JR, Mouvad F, Barillari MR, et al. Treatment of laryngopharyngeal reflux disease: a systematic review. World J Clin Cases. 2019;7(19):2995–3011. https://doi.org/10.12998/wjcc.v7.i19.2995.

24. Lechien JR, Akst LM, Al H, et al. Evaluation and management of laryngopharyngeal reflux disease: state of the art review. Otolaryngol Head Neck Surg. 2019;160(5):762–82. https://doi.org/10.1177/0194599819827488.

25. Richter JE. Gastroesophageal reflux disease during pregnancy. Gastroenterol Clin North A. 2003;32(1):235–61.
26. Gill SK, O'Brien L, Einarson T, et al. The safety of proton pump inhibitors (PPIs) in pregnancy: a meta-analysis. Am J Gastroenterol. 2009;104(6):1541–5.
27. Pasternak B, Hviid A. Use of proton-pump inhibitors in early pregnancy and the risk of birth defects. N Engl J Med. 2010;363(22):2114–23. https://doi.org/10.1056/NEJMoa1002689.
28. Li CM, Zhernakova A, Engstrand C, et al. Systematic review with meta-analysis: the risks of proton pump inhibitors during pregnancy. Aliment Pharmacol Ther. 2020;1(4):410–20. https://doi.org/10.1111/apt.15610.
29. McGlashan JA, Johnstone LM, Sykes J, et al. The value of a liquid alginate suspension (Gaviscon advance) in the management of laryngopharyngeal reflux. Eur Arch Otorhinolaryngol. 2009;266(2):243–51.
30. Vicki S, Bassin J, Swales SV, et al. Assessment of the safety and efficacy of a raft-forming alginate reflux suppressant (liquid Gaviscon) for the treatment of heartburn during pregnancy. ISRN Obstet Gynecol. 2012;2012:481870. https://doi.org/10.5402/2012/481870.
31. Powell J, O'Hara J, Wilson JA. Are persistent throat symptoms atypical features of gastric reflux and should they be treated with proton pump inhibitors? BMJ. 2014;349:g5813.
32. Anderson PO. Treating gastroesophageal reflux and heartburn while breastfeeding. Breastfeed Med. 2018;13(7):463–4. https://doi.org/10.1089/bfm.2018.0124.
33. Majithia R, Johnson DA. Are proton pump inhibitors safe during pregnancy and lactation? Evidence to date. Drugs. 2012;72(2):171–9. https://doi.org/10.2165/11597290-000000000-0000.
34. Carvajal A, Macias D, Gutierrez A, et al. Gynaecomastia associated with proton pump inhibitors: a case series from the Spanish pharmacovigilance system. Drug Saf. 2007;30(6):527–31. https://doi.org/10.2165/00002018-200730060-00006.
35. Jaworek AJ, Earasi K, Lyons KM, et al. Acute infectious laryngitis: a case series. Ear Nose Throat J. 2018;97(9):306–13. https://doi.org/10.1177/0145561318097000920.
36. Dworkin JP. Laryngitis: types, causes and treatments. Otolaryngol Clin North Am. 2008;41(2):419–36. https://doi.org/10.1016/j.otc.2007.11.011.
37. Yigit O, Kara CO. Kulak Burun Bogaz ve Bas Boyun Cerrahisi Uzmanlık Egitimi. In: Sirin S, editor. Larenjit (Laryngitis). Istanbul: Logos Yayıncılık; 2018. p. 709.
38. Mor G, Cardenas I. The immune system in pregnancy: a unique complexity. Am J Reprod Immunol. 2010;63(6):425–33. https://doi.org/10.1111/j.1600-0897.2010.00836.x.
39. Kumar R, Hayhurst KL, Robson AK. Ear nose and throat manifestation during pregnancy. Otolaryngol Head Neck Surg. 2011;145(2):188–98. https://doi.org/10.1177/0194599811407572.
40. Verdolini K, Rosen CA, Branski RC, et al. Shifts in biochemical markers associated with wound healing in laryngeal secretions following phonotrauma: a preliminary study. Ann Otol Rhinol Laryngol. 2003;112(12):1021–5. https://doi.org/10.1177/000348940311201205.
41. Verdolini K, Min Y, Titze IR, Lemke J, et al. Biological mechanisms underlying voice changes due to dehydration. J Speech Lang Hear Res. 2002;45(2):268–81. https://doi.org/10.1044/1092-4388(2002/021).
42. Danielides V, Nousia CS, Patrikakos G, et al. Effect of meteorological parameters on acute laryngitis in adults. Acta Otolaryngol. 2002;122(6):655–60. https://doi.org/10.1080/000164802320396358.
43. Hultzsch S, Schaefer C. Analgesic drugs during pregnancy. Schmerz. 2016;30(6):583–93. https://doi.org/10.1007/s00482-016-0167-9.
44. Black A, Khor KE, Kennedy D, et al. Medication use and pain management in pregnancy: a critical review. Pain Pract. 2019;19(8):875–99. https://doi.org/10.1111/papr.12814.
45. Feldkamp ML, Meyer RE, Krikov S, et al. Acetaminophen use in pregnancy and risk of birth defects: findings from the National Birth Defects Prevention Study. Obstet Gynecol. 2010;115(1):109–15. https://doi.org/10.1097/AOG.0b013e3181c52616.
46. Kennedy D. Analgesics and pain relief in pregnancy and breastfeeding. Aust Prescr. 2011;34(1):8–10. https://doi.org/10.18773/austprescr.2011.007.

47. Koren G, Florescu A, Costei AM, et al. Nonsteroidal antiinflammatory drugs during third trimester and the risk of premature closure of the ductus arteriosus: a meta-analysis. Ann Pharmacother. 2006;40(5):824–9. https://doi.org/10.1345/aph.1G428.

48. Schaefer C, Peters P, and Miller RK, editors. Drugs during pregnancy and lactation treatment options and risk assessment. Elsevier; 2007.

49. Nezvalová-Henriksen K, Spigset O, Nordeng H. Effects of codeine on pregnancy outcome: results from a large population-based cohort study. Eur J Clin Pharmacol. 2011;67(12):1253–61. https://doi.org/10.1007/s00228-011-1069-5.

50. Martinez-Frias ML, Rodriguez-Pinilla E. Epidemiologic analysis of prenatal exposure to cough medicines containing dextromethorphan: no evidence of human teratogenicity. Teratology. 2001;63(1):38–41.

51. Ambro BT, Scheid SC, Pribitkin EA. Prescribing guidelines for ENT medications during pregnancy. ENT J. 2003;82(8):565–8.

52. Reveiz L, Cardona AF. Antibiotics for acute laryngitis in adults. Cochrane Database Syst Rev. 2013;(3):CD004783. https://doi.org/10.1002/14651858.CD004783.pub4.

53. Fairbanks DNF. Pocket guide to antimicrobial therapy in otolaryngology-head and neck surgery, 11th ed. American Academy of Otolaryngology-Head and Neck Surgery Foundation; 2003.

54. Hol C, Scahlen C, Verduin CM, et al. Moraxella catarrhalis in acute laryngitis: infection or colonization? J Infect Dis. 1996;174(3):636–8.

55. Fan H, Gilbert R, O'Callaghan F. Associations between macrolide antibiotics prescribing during pregnancy and adverse child outcomes in the UK: population based cohort study. BMJ. 2020;368:m331. https://doi.org/10.1136/bmj.m331.

56. Wenger JD. Epidemiology of Hemophilus influenzae type b disease and impact of Hemophilus influenzae type b conjugate vaccines in the United States and Canada. Pediatr Infect Dis J. 1998;17(9 Suppl):S132–6. https://doi.org/10.1097/00006454-199809001-00008;17(9Suppl):S132-6.

57. Stroud RH, Friedman NR. An update on inflammatory disorders of the pediatric airway: epiglottitis, croup, and tracheitis. Am J Otolaryngol. 2001;22(4):268–75. https://doi.org/10.1053/ajot.2001.24825.

58. Glock JL, Morales WJ. Acute epiglottitis during pregnancy. South Med J. 1993;86(7):836–8. https://doi.org/10.1097/00007611-199307000-00026.

59. Hebert PC, Ducic Y, Boisvert D, et al. Adult epiglottitis in a Canadian setting. Laryngoscope. 1998;108(1 Pt 1):64–9. https://doi.org/10.1097/00005537-199801000-00012.

60. Katori H, Tsukuda M. Acute epiglottitis: analysis of factors associated with airway intervention. J Laryngol Otol. 2005;119(12):967–72. https://doi.org/10.1258/0022215505775010823.

61. Tulunay OE. Laryngitis-diagnosis and management. Otolaryngol Clin North Am. 2008;41(2):437–51.

62. Davanzo R, Bua J, Facchina G, et al. Breastfeeding and migraine drugs. Eur J Clin Pharmacol. 2014;70(11):1313–24. https://doi.org/10.1007/s00228-014-1748-0.

63. Bitzen PO, Gustafsson B, Jostell KG, et al. Excretion of paracetamol in human breast milk. Eur J Clin Pharmacol. 1981;20(2):123–5. https://doi.org/10.1007/BF00607148.

64. Matheson I, Lunde PKM, Notarianni L. Infant rash caused by paracetamol in breast milk? Pediatrics. 1985;76(4):651–2.

65. American Academy of Pediatrics Committee on Drugs. The transfer of drugs and other chemicals into human milk. Pediatrics. 2001;108(3):776–89. https://doi.org/10.1542/peds.108.3.776.

66. Townsend RJ, Benedetti TJ, Erickson SH, et al. Excretion of ibuprofen into breast milk. Am J Obstet Gynecol. 1984;149(2):184–6. https://doi.org/10.1016/0002-9378(84)90195-9.

67. Ito S, Blajchman A, Stephenson M, et al. Prospective follow-up of adverse reactions in breast-fed infants exposed to maternal medication. Am J Obstet Gynecol. 1993;168(5):1393–9. https://doi.org/10.1016/s0002-9378(11)90771-6.

68. Andersen JT, Futtrup TB. Drugs during lactation. Adv Drug React Bull. 2020;323(1):1251–4. https://doi.org/10.1097/fad.0000000000000049.

69. Koren G, Cairns J, Chitayat D, et al. Pharmacogenetics of morphine poisoning in a breastfed neonate of a codeine-prescribed mother. Lancet. 2006;368(9536):704. https://doi.org/10.1016/S0140-6736(06)69255-6.
70. Honein MA, Paulozzi LJ, Himelright IM, et al. Infantile hypertrophic pyloric stenosis after pertussis prophylaxis with erythromycin: a case review and cohort study. Lancet. 1999;354(9196):2101–5. https://doi.org/10.1016/s0140-6736(99)10073-4.
71. Lozada LE, Royall MJ, Nylund CM, et al. Development of pyloric stenosis after a 4-day course of oral erythromycin. Pediatr Emerg Care. 2013;29(4):498–9. https://doi.org/10.1097/PEC.0b013e31828a3663.
72. Abdellatif M, Ghozy S, Kamel MG, et al. Association between exposure to macrolides and the development of infantile hypertrophic pyloric stenosis: a systematic review and meta-analysis. Eur J Pediatr. 2019;178(3):301–14. https://doi.org/10.1007/s00431-018-3287-7.
73. Goldstein LH, Berlin M, Tsur L, et al. The safety of macrolides during lactation. Breastfeed Med. 2009;4(4):197–200. https://doi.org/10.1089/bfm.2008.0135.
74. Ryu RJ, Easterling TR, Caritis SN, et al. Prednisone pharmacokinetics during pregnancy and lactation. J Clin Pharmacol. 2018;58(9):1223–32. https://doi.org/10.1002/jcph.1122.

Voice Disorders and Therapy During Pregnancy and the Postpartum Period

İbrahim Hıra, Murat Doğan, and Ljiljana Jovancevic

50.1 Introduction

Voice production is a complex mechanism that starts with healthy breathing and release of air with appropriate subglottic pressure and occurs with faultless harmonization of vocal cords and resonator mechanisms to this process. A disruption in any part of this process will affect voice quality. Many systemic diseases such as hormonal dysregulation, neurological disorders, respiratory diseases, and gastrointestinal disorders can impair the process. Although pregnancy is a physiological process, it is associated with many multisystemic alterations.

Human gestation starts with last menstrual period in an obstetric manner while it starts after ovulation in an embryonic manner. There are anatomic, physiological, metabolic, and psychological changes occurring in a woman during pregnancy and during the postpartum period; thus, these alterations affect voice structure. The changes in pregnancy vary among trimesters. Therefore, the effects of pregnancy on voice should be evaluated based on these changes.

The causes of voice disorders during pregnancy and the postpartum period can be classified into four topics:

İ. Hıra (✉)
Department of Otorhinolaryngology, Ankara Şereflikoçhisar State Hospital, Ankara, Turkey
e-mail: dr.ibrahimhira@gmail.com

M. Doğan
Department of Otorhinolaryngology, Private Acıbadem Kayseri Hospital, Kayseri, Turkey
e-mail: drmdogan@hotmail.com

L. Jovancevic
Faculty of Medicine, Department of Otorhinolaryngology, Head and Neck Surgery,
University of Novi Sad, Clinical Centre of Vojvodina, Novi Sad, Serbia
e-mail: jovancevicljiljana@gmail.com

C. Cingi et al. (eds.), *ENT Diseases: Diagnosis and Treatment during Pregnancy and Lactation*, https://doi.org/10.1007/978-3-031-05303-0_50

1. Hormonal changes
2. Anatomic and physiological changes
3. Metabolic changes
4. Psychological changes

50.2 Etiological Factors

50.2.1 Hormonal Changes

Larynx structures are similar in male and female individuals until puberty; however, they begin to change with onset of puberty via influences by sex hormones. In women, vocal cords are shorter with narrower infra-glottic space and lower vital capacity. In addition, the distance between cartilage laminae of thyroid is wider [1]. In addition to gross differences, steroid sex hormones also have influences mediated by receptors [2]. It is known that there are androgen, estrogen, and progesterone receptors in the larynx and that their expression levels are affected by blood hormone levels in a reversible manner [2]. During pregnancy, estrogen and progesterone levels are elevated, which directly act on genital system, mucosa, musculoskeletal tissues, cerebral cortex, and larynx [3]. The larynx is highly sensitive to sex hormones and considered as a secondary sexual organ [4].

The elevated estrogen level leads to an increase in the thickness of vocal fold epithelial barrier while elevated progesterone levels mainly affect intermediate layer, resulting in increased tissue viscosity. In studies during menstrual cycle, it was shown that the highest voice quality is seen during ovulation period where peak estrogen levels are seen in women [5]. In addition, during the premenstrual period when estrogen levels are lowest, voice is more fatigue and hoarse with loss in higher tones [4].

Vascular permeability is increased with fluid leakage to interstitial space due to elevated sex steroids. Vocal cords become edematous and hyperemic and vibrator amplitude is decreased [3]. The voice produced at vocal cord is modified by resonator and articulator structures in supraglottic, oropharyngeal, and nasal regions. Since the nineteenth century, it has been well known that there are several changes in upper airway and larynx during pregnancy. Although etiology has not been fully elucidated, estrogen theory is the most commonly accepted one [6]. It was shown that estrogen leads to vascular dilatation and enhanced secretions from mucosal glands through anticholinergic effect and that it causes sinonasal symptoms in a histological manner [7]. During pregnancy, elevated progesterone levels lead to smooth muscle relaxation, vascular dilation, and pooling by influencing nasal mucosa. This results in sinonasal changes affecting voice quality [8, 9].

Demirci et al. showed that upper airway resistance is increased and nasalance scores are lower in pregnancy by rhinometry compared to normal population [10]. Thus, alterations in upper airway change voice quality affect voice resonance in particular.

50.2.2 Anatomic and Physiological Changes

In pregnancy, all organs develop several adaptation mechanisms to provide needs for fetal development and to adopt changes in the mother. Total blood volume is increased, reaching peak level at gestational week 34. In addition, a weight gain of approximately 12.5 kg is seen in normal pregnancy as a result of fetus, placenta, uterus, maternal fat accumulation, and changes in breast tissue. Airflow is affected by breathing pattern and laryngeal structure. During pregnancy, intra-abdominal pressure is increased, resulting in changes in breathing pattern. In particular, diaphragm is elevated due to the mechanical effect of fetus and weight gain in the third trimester. Total respiratory volume is increased and respiratory alkalosis develops as a result of increased respiratory rate. Thus, breathing becomes more challenging; supraglottic air pressure is decreased and phonation time is shortened.

In addition to esophageal dysmotility resulting from the effect of gestational hormones, gastroesophageal reflux (GER) becomes more incident after the second trimester due to increased uterine volume. This is a predominant cause of hoarseness seen during the pregnancy.

GER is a common factor in prolonged hoarseness. It is thought that GER affects larynx in two ways. Firstly, more commonly accepted theory is chronic mucosal inflammation developing after direct contact of larynx with gastric content (acid, pepsin, trypsin, biliary salt, and gastroduodenal proteins). Second theory is cough and clearance movement via chemoreceptor activation following contact of distal esophagus with gastric content [11, 12].

In pregnancy, laryngopharyngeal reflux (LPR) symptoms are more commonly seen, particularly in the first and third trimesters [13]. This results in higher incidence of nausea and vomiting in the first trimester and mechanical effect of fetus and weight gain in the third trimester. In a study by Salturk et al., it was demonstrated that reflux symptom score (RSS) was highest in the first and third trimesters [14]. At this period, erythema and edema are the most common findings in larynx endoscopy.

In a study by Cassiraga et al., it was reported that GER and clavicular respiration are more common in the third trimester of pregnancy [15]. Again, in that study, it was found that complaints of dyspnea (31.82%), hoarseness (11.96%), and dyspnea plus hoarseness (15.91%) were more common in the study group compared to controls; however, there was no significant difference in F0 (primary frequency), shimmer, jitter, and noise-to-harmonics ratio (NHR).

In conclusion, fatigue and changes (mainly decreased phonation time) in voice occur due to multiple factors in pregnancy [14].

50.2.3 Metabolic Changes

In pregnancy, cardiac output is increased by 30–40% with a slight decrease in blood pressure. Minute ventilation is increased and diaphragm is elevated in the third trimester as a result of fetus. The infrasternal angle becomes wider. The functional residual capacity and residual volume are decreased with increased oxygen consumption during rest. Gastric and intestinal motilities are decreased. Lower sphincter pressure is decreased in esophagus, resulting in increased GER symptoms and frequency.

Such alterations lead to changes in breathing pattern and negatively affects voice quality by causing chronic laryngeal inflammation and decreased subglottic air pressure.

Moreover, some endocrine disorders that may lead to mortality and/or morbidity in both mother and infant can be seen or become evident during pregnancy. These patients can initially present with voice disorder. For instance, high human chorionic hormone (hCG) concentrations in early pregnancy can cause hyperthyroidism while apparent hypothyroidism may develop in pregnant women positive for thyroid peroxidase and thyroglobulin antibodies [16, 17].

There are thyroid hormone receptors in the larynx; thus, even mild deficiency may cause important voice alterations such as hoarseness, roughness, low voice range, and fatigue [18]. In addition, hyperthyroidism can lead also to voice disorder. The most common change in voice is decreased fundamental frequency (F0) in hyperthyroidism [19, 20]. In conclusion, it should be kept in mind that thyroid hormone disorders can affect voice and even vocal changes can be the first sign, and that voice quality can be improved by medical therapy.

Another important change during pregnancy occurs in glucose metabolism. In a normal pregnancy, insulin resistance and postprandial glucose levels are increased by the second trimester. In particular, it was shown that the risk for gestational diabetes mellitus (GDM) is increased by two- to ninefold in correlation with weight gain [21]. Diabetes mellitus (DM) leads to several disorders by affecting neuromuscular and vascular systems. In the literature, effects of type 2 DM on voice have been investigated and many causes have been demonstrated, including xerostomia secondary to neuropathy, GER, high-volume speaking to compensate hearing loss, or neuromuscular involvement [22–25]. Although the majority of complications develop in long term, it should be kept in mind that viscosity and mucosal dryness can impair voice quality via interaction with vibrator and resonator components localized at larynx and upper respiratory tract.

The DM should be suspected in pregnant women with hoarseness if there is no laryngeal lesion. In particular, pregnant women at risk should be monitored for GDM.

50.2.4 Psychological Changes

All expectant mothers can experience a negative mood termed as anxiety during pregnancy due to several factors, including both physical and physiological changes and infant's health, impending delivery, and concerns about competence [14]. This may vary according to many parameters, including undesired pregnancy, preterm labor, first pregnancy, socioeconomic status of family, and psychological status of mother before pregnancy. In addition, several psychological problems can be observed after delivery, including persistent anxiety, which was aggravated before delivery and postpartum psychosis. In the literature, it was reported that acute-onset voice disorders (also termed as psychogenic voice disorder [PVD]) are defined as conversion dysphonia, psychological functional dysphonia, phononeuroses, or hysteric aphonia/dysphonia [26, 27]. PVD can develop as a result of psychological diseases such as anxiety, depression, personality disorder, somatization, and conversion reaction [28].

PVD diagnosis can be made by ruling out organic disorders and recovery of noncommunication voices (coughing, crying, laughing, etc.) in voice disorders such as aphonia and dysphonia. In differential diagnosis, insufficient glottic closure, muscular tension dysphonia (MTD), some hyper-functional voice disorders, and vocal cord atrophy. Diagnosis can be challenging as they have variable clinic presentation and can be confused with functional voice disorders. In general, the patients have a history of psychological disorders.

50.3 Treatment Methods

Although voice therapies are the main treatment options used in the voice disorders, they are used in combination with surgery or medical treatment modalities in some cases. However, in voice disorders occurring during pregnancy and the postpartum period caused by the abovementioned problems, therapy and medical treatment options come to the forefront. The voice therapies can be discussed in two groups using a multifaceted, multilayer approach based on the method used to change phonation pattern of technique (way of using voice muscles). The voice therapies are mainly classified as direct and indirect therapies. The indirect methods include measures and behavioral changes targeting the removal of factors affecting voice indirectly. In direct methods, it is aimed to change vocal behavior based on motor learning principles by influencing muscle contractions forming phonation. These methods are classified into subgroups as general and specific approaches. In general approaches, phonation system is changed holistically rather than addressing subsystems (respiration, vibration, resonance). In specific methods, subsystems of phonation mechanisms are individually addressed; these methods are structured based on the type and etiology of voice disorders [29].

Table 50.1 presents direct and indirect therapy methods [30]. In voice problems occurring during pregnancy and/or the postpartum period, etiology should be addressed primarily as voice disorders seen in nonpregnant patients. An algorithm for voice therapy should be outlined by comparing voice problem with voice before pregnancy and assessing patient perception with acoustic assessment if needed. In addition, physiological voice problems occurring in distinct hormonal and diaphragmatic changes throughout pregnancy (from the first to the third trimester) should be evaluated holistically for voice comfort of patient. Certainly, diaphragmatic changes will become more prominent later on during pregnancy, resulting in apparent changes in parameters such as maximum phonation time and phonation threshold pressure. At this period, treatment plans should avoid exercises that

Table 50.1 Classification of voice therapy methods

Indirect therapy methods	Direct therapy methods	
	Holistic approaches	Specific approaches
Counseling	Resonance voice therapy	**Techniques used in hyper-functional**
Audiophonic arrangement	Vocal function exercises	
Voice rest	Emphasis method	Yawn-sigh
Voice hygiene	Semi-occluded vocal tract exercises	Inhalation voice therapy
Elimination of mechanical trauma		Chewing method
Addressing laryngopharyngeal reflux	Artificial vocal tract elongation	Stretching–blowing technique
Prevention of irritant substance inhalation	Combined semi-occluded vocal tract elongation approach (LaxVox, DoctorVox)	Glottal attack and damping techniques
Hydration- humidification		Register sliding
Other factors		Circumlaryngeal massage
Respiratory support	Estill approach	Slow-motion technique
Abdominodiaphragmatic respiration	Voice focusing (muscle-specific voice exercises)	**Techniques used in hypo-functional voice disorders**
Schlaffhorst Andersen Method		Isometric contraction (pulling-pushing)
Prozodi approach	Phonetic manipulation	
Respiratory coordination approach	Formant accord	Hard glottal attack
s/z exercise	Messa di Voce exercise	Lee Silverman voice therapy technique
Posture	Register phonation exercise	
General measures		PhoRTE voice therapy technique
Alexander technique	Vegetative guidance	
Feldenkrais	Arrangement of vertical larynx position	Masking
Yoga and Qi-gong	Interview-based voice therapy	Phonation with swallow
Relaxation		Lateral compression
Jacobson-progressive relaxation		Laryngeal rotation with head rotation
Wolpe-reciprocal inhibition		Twang (nasal voice) therapy
Stretching-relaxation exercises		Explosive consonants
Scene formation technique		Phonation with smelling
Feedback		**Voice pitch-directed approaches**
Auditory feedback		Manual manipulation
Visual feedback		Voice pitch shifting-movement—new tone formation
Vibrotactile/kinesthetic-proprioceptive feedback		Ear education for tone awareness
Cognitive feedback		Vegetative function use
Verbal feedback		Registration with head hyper-extension/anteflexion
Device-assisted feedback		Phonation against high reverse pressure
Environmental feedback		**Techniques for psychogenic aphonia**
Psycho-emotional approach		**Episodic paroxysmal laryngospasm therapy**
Psychotherapy		**Vocal granuloma therapy**
Emotional guidance		**Inhalation phonation**
Reverse exercise		**Transsexual voice therapy**
Complementary and traditional medicine		**Pediatric voice therapy**
Acupuncture-acupressure		**Perioperative voice therapy**
Conscious medical hypnosis		**Spasmodic dysphonia**
Phytotherapy		**Alaryngeal voice therapy**
Apitherapy		
Homeopathy		
Music therapy		
Laryngeal osteopathy		
Electro-stimulation		
Kinesio taping		
Local vibration therapy		

increase intra-abdominal pressure and provide glottic-diaphragmatic adaptation. The therapy process should be started with a detailed history, including previous habits, lifestyle, and voice data of pregnant woman; it should continue with standard measures and appropriate therapy technique should be recommended. Preferentially, voice hygiene should be ensured in pregnant or postpartum women with voice disorder. Open, short, and simple recommendations should be given on an individual basis. Alcohol consumption, active or passive smoking, and high-volume voice (intentionally or unintentionally) should have to be prohibited. Increasing fluid intake and avoiding throat clearance and dry, dusty environments (BRAT: Basic practical principles of behavior readjustment voice therapy). Naso-oral abdomino-diaphragmatic breathing should be recommended for breathing patterns affected by fetal volume and weight gain. In pregnancy, other specific therapy techniques, including breathing, phonation, and posture exercises, should be employed based on anatomic and physiological changes. The lax-vox technique is one of the methods that can be preferred to relieve edema at vocal cord level during pregnancy and the postpartum period. During pregnancy, technique is initiated with 3–5 cmH$_2$O and can be maintained at 7–8 cmH$_2$O, providing glottic-diaphragmatic adaptation for patients. Again, breathing exercises improve voice quality by providing relaxation during pregnancy and decreasing muscular tension. In addition, resonance therapy can level glottic pressure via oral vibration in the postpartum period and can be used as an appropriate therapy method to elevate voice. Given stress factor during pregnancy, circumlaryngeal massage should be attempted [31]. By this technique, the short, stiff, and strained muscle is elongated; thus, relaxation can be achieved. The goal is to lower larynx level and reduce supralaryngeal muscle tension. This improves the range of movement in the larynx, thyrohyoid space is enlarged, and phonation is improved.

For GER, diet and lifestyle modifications can lead to marked symptomatic improvement in the majority of patients. However, antacid agents, H2 receptor antagonists, and proton pump inhibitors (PPI) should be used when the abovementioned measures fail. Medical treatment and voice therapy should be used in combination. In a study, it was shown that PPI plus voice therapy was more beneficial compared to PPI alone [32].

Appropriate medical treatment should be initiated as soon as possible in case of known metabolic disease (GDM, hypothyroidism, hyperthyroidism, etc.). This is not only important for voice quality but also fetal and maternal health.

In conversion/psychogenic voice disorders, etiology should be identified if possible. Psychiatric assessment should be ordered to eliminate stress factor. Secondary gain should be kept in mind. Psychotherapy in combination with voice therapy is preferred [33, 34].

References

1. Aronson AE, Bless DM. Normal voice development. In: Aronson AE, Bless DM, editors. Clinical voice disorders. 4th ed. New York: Thieme; 2009.
2. Newman SR, Butler J, Hammond EH, et al. Preliminary report on hormone receptors in the human vocal fold. J Voice. 2000;14:72–81.
3. Hamdan AL, Mahfoud L, Sibai A, et al. Effect of pregnancy on the speaking voice. J Voice. 2009;23:490–3.
4. Abitbol J, Abitbol P, Abitbol B. Sex hormones and the female voice. J Voice. 1999;13:424–46.
5. Raj A, Gupta B, Chowdhury A, et al. A study of voice changes in various phases of menstrual cycle and in postmenopausal women. J Voice. 2010;24:363–8.
6. Toppozada H, Michaels L, Toppozada M, et al. The human respiratory nasal mucosa in pregnancy. An electron microscopic and histochemical study. J Laryngol Otol. 1982;96:613–26.
7. Bende M, Gredmark T. Nasal stuffiness during pregnancy. Laryngoscope. 1999;109:1108–10.
8. Schatz M, Zeiger RS. Diagnosis and management of rhinitis during pregnancy. Allergy Proc. 1988;9:545–54.
9. Incaudo GA, Takach P. The diagnosis and treatment of allergic rhinitis during pregnancy and lactation. Immunol Allergy Clin North Am. 2006;26:137–54.
10. Demirci Ş, Tüzüner A, Küçük Z, et al. The impact of pregnancy on nasal resonance. Kulak Burun Bogaz Ihtis Derg. 2016;26:7–11.
11. Jiang A, Liang M, Su Z, et al. Immunohistochemical detection of pepsin in laryngeal mucosa for diagnosing laryngopharyngeal reflux. Laryngoscope. 2011;121:1426–30.
12. Johnston N, Yan JC, Hoekzema CR, et al. Pepsin promotes proliferation of laryngeal and pharyngeal epithelial cells. Laryngoscope. 2012;122:1317–25.
13. Ali RA, Egan LJ. Gastroesophageal reflux disease in pregnancy. Best Pract Res Clin Gastroenterol. 2007;21:793–806.
14. Saltürk Z, Kumral TL, Bekiten G, et al. Objective and subjective aspects of voice in pregnancy. J Voice. 2016;30:70–3.
15. Cassiraga VL, Castellano AV, Abasolo J, et al. Pregnancy and voice: changes during the third trimester. J Voice. 2012;26:584–6.
16. Medici M, de Rijke YB, Peeters RP, et al. Maternal early pregnancy and newborn thyroid hormone parameters: the Generation R Study. J Clin Endocrinol Metab. 2012;97:646–52.
17. De Leo S, Pearce EN. Autoimmune thyroid disease during pregnancy. Lancet Diabetes Endocrinol. 2018;6:575–86.
18. Altman KW, Haines GK, Vakkalanka SK, et al. Identification of thyroid hormone receptors in the human larynx. Laryngoscope. 2003;113:1931–4.
19. Watt T, Groenvold M, Rasmussen AK, et al. Quality of life in patients with benign thyroid disorders. A review. Eur J Endocrinol. 2006;154:501–10.
20. Kadakia S, Carlson D, Sataloff RT. The effect of hormones on the voice. J Sing. 2013;69:571–4.
21. Yessoufou A, Moutairou K. Maternal diabetes in pregnancy: early and long-term outcomes on the offspring and the concept of "metabolic memory". Exp Diabetes Res. 2011;2011:218598. https://doi.org/10.1155/2011/218598.
22. Hamdan AL, Jabbour J, Nassar J, et al. Vocal characteristics in patients with type 2 diabetes mellitus. Eur Arch Otorhinolaryngol. 2012;269:1489–95.
23. Kumar K, Garg A, Chandra N, et al. Voice and endocrinology. Indian J Endocrinol Metab. 2016;20:590–4.
24. Sreebny LM, Yu A, Green A, et al. Xerostomia in diabetes mellitus. Diabetes Care. 1992;15:900–4.
25. Hamdan AL, Jabbour J, Barazi R, et al. Prevalence of laryngopharyngeal reflux disease in patients with diabetes mellitus. J Voice. 2013;27:495–9.
26. Guardino CM, Dunkel Schetter C. Understanding pregnancy anxiety: concepts, correlates, and consequences. Zero to Three. 2014;34:12–21.

27. Andresson K, Schalén L. Etiology and treatment of psychogenic voice disorder: results of a follow-up study of thirty patients. J Voice. 1998;12:96–106.
28. Baker J. Psychogenic voice disorders—heroes or hysterics? A brief overview with questions and discussion. Logoped Phoniatr Vocol. 2002;27:84–91.
29. Verdolini-Marston K, Burke MK, Lessac A, et al. Preliminary study of two methods of treatment for laryngeal nodules. J Voice. 1995;9:74–85.
30. Denizoğlu İ. Ses Terapisi (Direkt Yöntemler). Türkiye Klinikleri Kulak Burun Boğaz-Özel Konular. 2019;3:89–96.
31. Roy N, Bless DM, Heisey D, et al. Manual circumlaryngeal therapy for functional dysphonia: an evaluation of short- and long-term treatment outcomes. J Voice. 1997;11:321–31.
32. Ezzeldin H, Hasseba AA. Effect of proton pump inhibitor and voice therapy on reflux-related laryngeal disorders. Tanta Med J. 2015;43:127–33.
33. Elias A, Raven R, Butcher P, et al. Speech therapy for psychogenic voice disorder: a survey of current practice and training. Br J Disord Commun. 1989;24:61–76.
34. Tezcaner ZÇ, Gökmen MF, Yıldırım S, et al. Clinical features of psychogenic voice disorder and the efficiency of voice therapy and psychological evaluation. J Voice. 2019;33:250–4.

Benign and Premalignant Lesions of the Larynx During Pregnancy and the Postpartum Period

Rezarta Taga Senirli, Omer Tarik Selcuk, and Eugenio De Corso

51.1 Introduction

Laryngeal tumors may be benign, premalign, or malignant often presenting with progressive voice hoarseness and upper airway obstruction. Theoretically, these lesions can be seen at any age, though it is known that vocal fold nodules are mostly seen in young boys and middle-aged women; polyps are commonly seen in both males and females, especially in the 40–50 age bracket [1], similarly premalignant lesions are mostly seen in older ages.

Common complaints are hoarseness, vocal fatigue, foreign body sensation in throat, throat irritation, difficulty in breathing, or some kind of painful voice production. Many factors like pulmonary, gastrointestinal, hormonal, or even some psychosocial factors, in the absence of any organic pathology, can affect the voice [2]. Therefore, the clinician must always consider both organic disorders and psychogenic problems.

Patients presenting voice disorders usually firstly consult Ear Nose and Throat (ENT) surgeon. About 50% of these patients will have benign vocal fold changes [3, 4] and in their treatment, conservative and interventional measurements are often combined.

R. T. Senirli (✉) · O. T. Selcuk
Faculty of Medicine, Department of Otolaryngology—Head and Neck Surgery, Health Sciences University, Antalya Research and Training Hospital, Antalya, Turkey
e-mail: rezartats@gmail.com; omertarikselcuk@yahoo.com

E. De Corso
Department Head and Neck Surgery, Catholic University of Sacred Heart, Institute of Otorhinolaryngology, Rome, Italy
e-mail: eugenio.decorso@policlinicogemelli.it

C. Cingi et al. (eds.), *ENT Diseases: Diagnosis and Treatment during Pregnancy and Lactation*, https://doi.org/10.1007/978-3-031-05303-0_51

In this chapter, we will discuss laryngeal lesions during pregnancy and postpartum period in two subheadings:

1. Benign laryngeal lesions of the larynx
2. Premalignant lesions of the larynx

51.2 Benign Lesions of the Larynx During Pregnancy and Postpartum Period

Benign neoplasms of the larynx constitute an interesting spectrum of lesions. These have been defined as "An abnormal mass of tissue in the larynx, the growth of which exceeds and is uncoordinated with that of normal tissue and persists in the same excessive manner after cessation of stimuli, which evoked the change." [5] In everyday clinics, we see these lesions in different shapes and localizations;

Vocal fold epithelium	Laryngeal papillomatosis
	Hyperkeratosis
Lamina Propria	Reinke's edema
	Pseudocyst
	Vascular malformations
	Vocal fold nodules
	Vocal fold polyp
	Vocal fold cyst
	Vocal fold scarring
Arytenoid	Vocal fold process granuloma
	Postintubation granuloma

51.2.1 Laryngeal Papillomatosis

The incidence of laryngeal papillomatosis is approximately 1.8 per 100,000 [6]. It is usually transmitted vertically through vaginal birth. Human papilloma virus (HPV) is the etiologic agent and subtypes 6 and 11 are chiefly responsible. There are two forms that have been described: the adult-onset form and the more aggressive juvenile-onset recurrent respiratory papillomatosis (RRP). Although histologically benign, the clinical behavior, and the propensity for recurrence makes laryngeal papillomatosis a dangerous disease. Endoscopically, these lesions are exophytic and show a "raspberry"-like growth.

There are no specific reports on the effects of RRP in pregnancy, because only a few cases have been reported. However, we know that RRP is associated with hypoxia. On the other hand, it is supposed that estrogen plays a role in RRP, since it has been discovered that it exhibits increased binding of estrogen [7], an important regulator hormone known to show higher levels in the second and third trimesters of pregnancy. One reported maternal death has been attributed to laryngeal papillomatosis [8], indicating that patients with a history of this disorder should be considered as candidates for immediate evaluation.

51.2.2 Vocal Fold Polyps

Vocal fold polyps are the most common benign lesions of the larynx, they account for 1.4–2.6% [1, 9] of the total number of ENT outpatients. Polyps can be seen in one or both vocal folds at the same time, they usually are seen at the free edge of the vocal cord. Repetitive vocal trauma, airway infections, allergies, nicotine, gastroesophageal reflux, and anticoagulant medications can be attributed to polyp formation [10]. Laryngeal polyps attributed primarily to gastroesophageal reflux disease (GERD) have been reported [11]. Documented data reports that polyps are usually observed in Middle Ages for both sexes [12–14].

GERD has been reported in up to 80% of pregnancies [15]. It is likely caused by a reduction in lower esophageal sphincter pressure due to an increase in maternal estrogen and progesterone hormones during pregnancy.

There is no evidence specifically linking growth of vocal cord lesions and pregnancy hormones. However, the fact that GERD is seen in most pregnancies and that women in developed countries today postpone childbearing to the age of 30–40 makes us believe that it is likely that a greater number of pregnant women suffering from vocal fold lesions will be seen.

51.2.3 Reinkes's Edema

It represents the edematous swelling of the vocal cord, to be exact the superficial layer of the lamina propria, shows swelling. The etiology is not exactly known [16], but it is supposed that inhaled chemicals (e.g., nicotine), GERD, and hyperfunctional vocal behavior affect Reinke's edema formation [17, 18]. There are no special reports for the progress in pregnancy of this pathology usually seen in 40–60 year-old women. Nevertheless, Köybaşı et al. [19] in their animal study confirmed the presence of increased capillaries and Reinke's edema in the last trimester in pregnant rats. They connect lamina propria thickening to edema and increased GAG. Although they suppose that the increase of GAG may be attributed to the altered sex hormone levels, further investigations are required.

51.2.4 Vocal Fold Cysts

Approximately 14% of nonmalignant vocal cord lesions are classified as vocal fold cysts [20]. Fold cysts in turn are categorized as retention cysts or epidermoid cysts. Retention cysts are formed as inflammatory obstruction of mucous glands in the lamina propria, and they usually occur in occupational groups with high vocal stress [21]. However, epidermoid cysts are mostly congenital or even secondary to vocal trauma.

We know that estrogen has a hypertrophic and proliferative effect on mucosa, and progesterone decreases vascular permeability, giving rise to tissue congestion. However, there is no evidence specifically linking laryngeal pathology and pregnancy. In the literature, symptomatic benign vocal cysts during pregnancy exist in the form of case reports [22].

51.2.5 Vocal Fold Nodules

Vocal fold nodules are among the most common vocal fold pathologies. They are often seen as the result of vocal misuse. These nodules are typically bilateral and symmetrical in the middle third of the vocal fold. Stroboscopic examination shows incomplete glottis closure (classically known as hour-glass closure pattern) [23]. Boys, young women, and teachers are particularly affected [24]. In order to diagnose correctly the vocal nodule, it requires a total evaluation of patient history, voice analysis, laryngoscopic or stroboscopic findings, and histological evidences [25].

51.2.6 Vocal Process Granulomas

These granulomas are categorized as benign chronic inflammatory lesions. They arise in the cartilaginous part of the vocal fold. It is believed they arise after constant mechanical trauma or some kind of inflammation of the posterior glottis. Continual clearing of the throat, coughing, and voice misuse are some examples of constant mechanical trauma, which can damage the epithelium of the vocal process. Repetitive trauma prevents normal healing and leads to reactive overgrowth. As a confirmation to this Thilbeault et al. found evidences of wound-healing overexpression, inflammation, and extracellular matrix remodeling genes in vocal fold granuloma [26]. Other trigger factors include laryngo-pharyngeal reflux [27]. Ylitalo also proposed that in vocal fold granuloma, the initial inflammatory response to traumas is maintained by different factors, namely, GERD and throat clearing [28]. Although this is relatively rare, there are sporadic case reports of granuloma seen during pregnancy [29].

51.2.7 Postintubation Granuloma of the Larynx

Laryngeal granulomas are seen as a result of irritation of the laryngeal structures. This pathology is an uncommon complication of intubation. The patient history is the key of the diagnosis; it differentiates classical contact granulomas from postintubation ones. The modal symptoms are hoarseness, throat clearing, sore throat, and globus sensation. Postintubation granuloma is rare with an incidence of 1/10,000 [30]. Postintubation granulomas are more often seen in women. Even if the patient is pregnant or not in case of a history of tracheal intubation, contact granuloma can be seen. It is known to have a high rate of spontaneous resolution. In case where the expected resolution does not occur, surgical excision is recommended [31, 32].

51.3 Premalignant Lesions of the Larynx During Pregnancy and Postpartum Period

The premalignant laryngeal lesions are very important in ENT practice, since it is assumed that carcinomas often develop from them. As per the definition of the World Health Organization (WHO), premalignant lesions of larynx are "morphological alterations of the mucosa caused by chronic local irritative factors or referable to local expression of generalized illnesses, presenting a higher probability of degeneration into carcinoma with respect to surrounding mucosa" [33].

Clinically identifiable lesions such as erithroplakia, leukoplakia, or erithroleukoplakia may show histological evidences of dysplasia of the laryngeal epithelia.

Vocal fold epithelial lesions are graded according to Lubjana or the WHO grading system [34, 35]. The WHO grading system for vocal cords divides dysplasia into three categories: mild, moderate, and severe dysplasia. Mild dysplasia consists of cytologic and architectural atypia confined to the basal/parabasal layer; moderate dysplasia is characterized by atypical changes progressing into the midspinous layer and severe dysplasia progresses into the upper spinous layer.

The importance of identifying premalignant lesions lies in their ability to predict malignant transformation. Several studies have been done on this subject. Some studies inspecting vocal fold lesions have reported a pathology-independent range of 3.8–11.2% of malignant transformation for all vocal cord lesions and a 10.5–32% malignant transformation rate for lesions with histologic evidence of dysplasia [36–40].

There are no special reports on dysplastic lesions during pregnancy or lactation in the literature. However, we should be conscious that this is a rare condition. Overall cancer cases during pregnancy are uncommon, occurring one out of every thousand pregnancies [41], with laryngeal cancers being even less prevalent. So far, only 11 cases of laryngeal cancer have been reported in the literature [42].

51.4 Management

The surgeon is confronted with many management dilemmas once a pregnant patient is in need of treatment. The following questions should be asked:

- Does the patient show any inspiration difficulty?
- Is the lesion benign, premalignant, or malignant?
- Should the lesion be excised or followed closely?
- If surgery is needed, when is the best time to perform it?

It is obvious that in case of any inspirational difficulty originating from a laryngeal lesion, even if pregnant, patients should undergo surgery. What adds the confusion are the premalignant lesions stabilizing without further progression and not causing obstructive symptoms. Normally, in the presence of widespread leucoplakia, surgeon should perform mapping of the lesion with multiple biopsies. However, in pregnant patients, one can change or postpone this decision depending on the appearance of the lesion, gestational age, or patient's overall general condition. Surgical intervention can be postponed to the postpartum period only if the delay does not worsen the condition. Possibly nonurgent surgery should be delayed until 6 weeks postpartum to make possible resolution of physiological changes in pregnancy [43].

According to American College of Obstetricians and Gynecologists' Committee on obstetric Practice, in spite of the trimester, a pregnant woman should not be denied the chance of surgery. However, it is advisable to perform surgery in the second trimester rather than the third trimester due to the mechanical factors associated with a large uterus and the risk of preterm labor is much higher in the third trimester [44]. Similarly, an overall miscarriage rate of 5.8–10.5% following surgery during the first trimester has been reported [45].

In case surgery is to be done, rapid intravenous induction and intubation, with effective cricoid pressure following a 5 min 100% oxygen, is recommended. The effects of light general anesthesia are associated with catecholamine fluctuation resulting in impaired uteroplacental perfusion, which is pretty more dangerous to fetus. Commonly used anesthetics such as barbiturates, propofol, muscle relaxants, and local anesthetics have been widely used during pregnancy with good safety records [43]. However, it would be advisable to use the lowest effective doses for the shortest time possible, because these drugs cause significant maternal hypotension.

Additionally, whether or not the clinician is planning surgery, antireflux therapy should be prescribed. The initial treatment options should include either antacids or H_2-receptor antagonists such as famotidine or ranitidine. If the patient's symptoms are severe, proton pump inhibitor (PPI) could be started. Except for omeprazole, all PPIs are classified as category B drugs by the Food and Drug Administration (FDA), which means they are safe to use during pregnancy. Omeprazole is currently classified as category C drug.

References

1. Nagata K, et al. Vocal fold polyps and nodules, a 10 year review of 1156 patients. Auris Nasus Larynx (Tokyo). 1983;10(Suppl):S27–35.
2. Sataloff RT. G. Paul Moore lecture. Rational thought: the impact of voice science upon voice care. J Voice. 1995;9(3):21534.
3. Johns MM. Update on the etiology, diagnosis, and treatment of vocal fold nodules, polyps, and cysts. Curr Opin Otolaryngol Head Neck Surg. 2003;11(6):456–61.
4. Roy N, Merrill RM, Gray SD, Smith EM. Voice disorders in the general population: prevalence, risk factors, and occupational impact. Laryngoscope. 2005;115(11):1988–95. https://doi.org/10.1097/01.mlg.0000179174.32345.4.
5. New GB, Erich JB. Benign tumors of the larynx: a study of 722 cases. Arch Otolaryngol. 1938;28:841–910.
6. Derkay CS, Wiatrak B. Recurrent respiratory papillomatosis: a review. Laryngoscope. 2008;118(7):1236–47. https://doi.org/10.1097/MLG.0b013e31816a7135.
7. Essman EJ, Abramson A. Estrogen binding sites on membranes from human laryngeal papilloma. Int J Cancer. 1984;33:33–6.
8. Helmrich G, et al. Fatal laryngeal papillomatosis in pregnancy. Am J Obstet Gynecol. 1992;166:524–5.
9. Sato T, Sumita K. A clinical investigation of vocal fold polyps. Pract Otol (Kyoto). 1965;58:254–9.
10. Martins RH, Defaveri J, Domingues MA, de Albuquerque e Silva R. Vocal polyps: clinical, morphological, and immunohistochemical aspects. J Voice. 2011;25(1):98–106. https://doi.org/10.1016/j.jvoice.2009.05.002.
11. Hassan WA. Laryngeal polyp associated with reflux disease: a case report. J Med Case Rep. 2020;14:2.

12. Kambic V, Randsel Z, Zagri M, Acko M. Vocal cord polyps; incidence, histology and pathogenesis. J Laryngol Otol. 1981;95:609–708.
13. Koike Y. Clinical and histopathological studies on laryngeal polyps. Otologia (Fllklloka). 1968;14:279–305.
14. Yamada K, Muto K, Yoshino K, Miyahara H, Yamada N, Sato T. A clinical study of vocal cord polyps. Pract Otol (Kyoto). 1977;70:43–8.
15. Ali RA, Egan LJ. Gastroesophageal reflux disease in pregnancy. Best Pract Res Clin Gastroenterol. 2007;21(5):793–806.
16. Dworkin JP. Laryngitis: types, causes, and treatments. Otolaryngol Clin North Am. 2008;41(2):419–36, ix. https://doi.org/10.1016/j.otc.2007.11.011.
17. Branski RC, Saltman B, Sulica L, Szeto H, Duflo S, Felsen D, Kraus DH. Cigarette smoke and reactive oxygen species metabolism: implications for the pathophysiology of Reinke's edema. Laryngoscope. 2009;119(10):2014–8. https://doi.org/10.1002/lary.20592.
18. Raabe J, Pascher W. Das Reinke-Ödem: EineUntersuchungzu Fragender Ätiologie, der Prognoseundder Wirksamkeit therapeutischer Interventionen [Reinke's edema: an investigation of questions related to etiology, prognosis and the effectiveness of therapeutic methods]. Laryngorhinootologie. 1999;78(2):97–102. https://doi.org/10.1055/s-2007-996839.
19. Köybaşı Şanal S, Biçer YÖ, Kükner A, Tezcan E. Effect of pregnancy on vocal cord histology: an animal experiment. Balkan Med J. 2016;33:448–52.
20. Bouchayer M, Cornut G. Microsurgery for benign lesions of the vocal folds. Ear Nose Throat J. 1988;67(6):446–9, 452–4, 456-64passim.
21. Bohlender J. Diagnostic and therapeutic pitfalls in benign vocal fold diseases. GMS Curr Top Otorhinolaryngol Head Neck Surg. 2013;12:Doc01, issn:1865-1011.
22. Thomas R et al. Awake videolaryngoscopic intubation in pregnant patient with a large vocal cord lesion. Anaesthesia Cases, 2016-0218. issn:2396-8397.
23. Sataloff RT, Spiegel JR, Hawkshaw MJ. Strobo-video-laryngoscopy: results and clinical value. Ann Otol Rhinol Laryngol. 1991;100(9 Pt 1):725–7.
24. Smolander S, Huttunen K. Voice problems experienced by Finnish comprehensive school teachers and realization of occupational healthcare. Logoped Phoniatr Vocol. 2006;31(4):166–71. https://doi.org/10.1080/14015430600576097.
25. PedersenM MG, lashanJ. Surgical versus non-surgical interventions for vocal cord nodules. Cochrane Database Syst Rev. 2012;6:CD001934. https://doi.org/10.1002/14651858. CD001934.pub2.
26. Thibeaut SL, et al. DNA microarray gene expression analysis of a vocal fold polyp and granuloma. J Speech Lang Hear Res. 2003;46:491–502.
27. Storck C, Brockmann M, Zimmermann E, Nekahm-Heis D, Zorowka PG. Laryngeales Kontaktgranulom. Atiologie, Symptomatik, Diagnoseund Therapie [Laryngealgranuloma. Aetiology, clinical signs, diagnostic procedures, and treatment]. HNO. 2009;57(10):1075–80. https://doi.org/10.1007/s00106-0081778-y.
28. Ylitalo R. Clinical studies of contact granuloma and posterior laryngitis with special regard to esophageopharyngeal reflux. Unpublished doctoral dissertation, Karolinska Institute, Stockholm; 2000.
29. Fukui J, et al. Laryngeal granuloma occurring during pregnancy-a case report. Koutou (The Larynx Japan). 2008;20:129–32. https://doi.org/10.5426/larynx1989.20.2_129.
30. Snow JC, Harano M, Balogh K. Postintubation granuloma of the larynx. Anaesth Analog. 1966;45:425–9.
31. Ylitalo R, Hammarberg B. Voice characteristics, effects of voice therapy, and long-term follow-up of contact granuloma patients. J Voice. 2000;14(4):557–66.
32. Devaney KO, Rinaldo A, Ferlito A. Vocal process granuloma of the larynx—recognition, differential diagnosis and treatment. Oral Oncol. 2005;41(7):666–9.
33. Kramer IR, Lucas RB, Pindborg JJ, et al. Definition of leukoplakia and related lesions: an aid to studies on oral precancer. Oral Surg Oral Med Oral Pathol. 1978;46(4):518–39.
34. Sengiz S, Pabuccuoglu U, Sulen S. Immunohistological comparison of the World Health Organization (WHO) and Ljubljana classifications on the grading of preneoplastic lesions of the larynx. Pathol Res Pract. 2004;200:181–8.

35. World Health Organization Classification of Tumours. Pathology & genetics. Head and neck tumors. International Agency for Research in Cancer (IARC). In: Barnes L, Eveson JW, Reichart P, Sidransky D, editors. Head and neck tumors. Lyon: IARC Press; 2005. p. 177–80.
36. Hellquist H, Cardesa A, Gale N, Kambic V, Michaels L. Criteria for grading in the Ljubljana classification of epithelial hyperplastic laryngeal lesions. A study by members of the working group on epithelial hyperplastic laryngeal lesions of the European Society of Pathology. Histopathology. 1999;34:226–33.
37. Isenberg JS, Crozier DL, Dailey SH. Institutional and comprehensive review of laryngeal leukoplakia. Ann Otol Rhinol Laryngol. 2008;117:74–9.
38. Ricci G, Molini E, Faralli M, Simoncelli C. Retrospective study on precancerous laryngeal lesions: long-term follow-up. Acta Otorhinolaryngol Ital. 2003;23:362–7.
39. Jeannon JP, Soames JV, Aston V, Stafford FW, Wilson JA. Molecular markers in dysplasia of the larynx: expression of cyclin-dependent kinase inhibitors p21, p27 and p53 tumour suppressor gene in predicting cancer risk. Clin Otolaryngol Allied Sci. 2004;29:698–704.
40. Gale N, Kambic V, Michaels L, Cardesa A, Hellquist H, Zidar N, et al. The Ljubljana classification: a practical strategy for the diagnosis of laryngeal precancerous lesions. Adv Anat Pathol. 2000;7:240–51.
41. Pavlidis NA. Coexistence of pregnancy and malignancy. Oncologist. 2002;7:279–87.
42. Pugi J, et al. Supraglottic p16+squamous cell carcinoma during pregnancy: a case report and review of the literature. J Otolaryngol Head Neck Surg. 2019;48:47.
43. Upadya M, Saneesh PJ. Anaesthesia for non-obstetric surgery during pregnancy. Indian J Anaesth. 2016;60:234–41.
44. Fatum M, Rojansky N. Laparoscopic surgery during pregnancy. Obstet Gynecol Surv. 2001;56:50–9.
45. Cohen-Kerem R, Railton C, Oren D, Lishner M, Koren G. Pregnancy outcome following non-obstetric surgical intervention. Am J Surg. 2005;190:467–73.

## Part VI

Head and Neck Neoplasms and Surgery During Pregnancy and the Postpartum Period

Head and Neck Cancer in Pregnancy

52

Rahul Varman, Tam Nguyen, and Yusuf Dundar

52.1 Introduction

Worldwide there are over half a million new cases of head and neck cancer (HNC) diagnosed every year [1]. Cancer during pregnancy is defined as a new cancer diagnosis during pregnancy or in the first year postpartum [2]. Incidence of cancer during pregnancy is around 0.02–0.1% of all pregnancies [3]. The most common invasive cancers arising during pregnancy are breast, skin, hematologic, cervix/uterus, and thyroid [4]. The most common pregnancy HNCs are larynx, melanoma, lymphoma, and oral cavity [5]. Recently, there has been an increase in incidence of head and neck cancers during the past two decades [6]. Tendency for women to delay pregnancy until later reproductive years may account for this increasing trend.

Guidelines exist for management of thyroid cancer in pregnancy; yet, there is limited information on nonthyroid HNC in pregnancy [7]. Challenge in managing head and neck cancer during pregnancy revolves around the balance between maternal and fetal health. Traditional diagnostic and therapeutic methods commonly used in patients with cancer are often contraindicated during pregnancy. Despite this, many advances have been made in terms of cancer treatment and fetal health preservation. Understanding etiologic factors and continued improvement of outcomes for both maternal and fetal health remains a continued medical goal in treating women with HNC during pregnancy.

This chapter aims to review postulated mechanisms, clinical presentations, and management principles of head and neck cancer during pregnancy (Table 52.1).

R. Varman (✉) · T. Nguyen · Y. Dundar
Department of Otolaryngology—Head and Neck Surgery, Texas Tech University,
Health Sciences Center, Lubbock, TX, USA
e-mail: Rahul.Varman@ttuhsc.edu; Tam.Nguyen@ttuhsc.edu; Yusuf.Dundar@ttuhsc.edu

© The Author(s), under exclusive license to Springer Nature
Switzerland AG 2022
C. Cingi et al. (eds.), *ENT Diseases: Diagnosis and Treatment during Pregnancy
and Lactation*, https://doi.org/10.1007/978-3-031-05303-0_52

Table 52.1 Postulated mechanisms and biomolecular factors implicated in head and neck cancer development during pregnancy

Mechanism	Biomolecular factors
Signaling pathway changes	EGFR BCL-XL Placental growth factor (PGF) P53 ERK-MAPK
Immune evasion	Programmed death ligand (PDL) Human leukocyte antigens (HLAs)
Hormone induction	Estrogen Progesterone
Virus induction	HPV E6 protein (target p53) HPV E7 protein (target RB1)

52.1.1 Signaling Pathway Changes

Signaling pathways are a series of chemical reactions in which a group of molecules in a cell work together to control cell function such as cell division or cell death. Signaling pathways play an important role both in fetal development during pregnancy and also in tumor growth. EGFR, which is a growth factor, and BCL-XL an anti-apoptotic protein have both been shown to be upregulated in various HNCs in pregnancy [8]. Studies showed lower number of p53 mutations and CDKN2A deletions in patients with pregnancy-induced HNCs .

Placental growth factor (PGF) is a member of vascular endothelial growth factor (VEGF) that plays a key role in angiogenesis and vasculogenesis particularly during embryo development. Placental trophoblast is a main source of PGF during pregnancy. Recent studies have suggested PGF to play a role in carcinogenesis [9].

52.1.2 Immune Evasion

Pregnancy and cancer are two conditions in which antigenic tissues are tolerated by an intact immune system. Programmed death ligand (PDL-1) is a transmembrane protein speculated to play a major role in suppressing immune system. Studies have shown that levels of PDL-1 are elevated in pregnant women's serum, which may contribute to further suppression of maternal immunity [10]. The expression of PDL-1 in head and neck squamous cell cancer is significantly correlated, and may also play an important therapeutic role of targeted immunotherapy [11].

52.1.3 Hormone Induction

Hormones estrogen and progesterone are made by the placenta during pregnancy to help maintain a healthy pregnancy. These hormones also play a vital role in gene expression involved in a plethora of neoplastic processes. Although it remains a controversial topic, preliminary studies have suggested that estrogen and progesterone receptor expressions are elevated in HNC and may affect the prognosis of the disease [12]. Future studies on estrogen/progesterone receptor expression in HNC in pregnancy could lead to changes in birth control methods.

52.1.4 Virus Induction

HPV-16 and HPV-18 are oncogenic viruses, which have been shown to be increasingly involved in development of HNC. HPV produced oncogenes E6 and E7, which inactivate p53 and Rb tumor suppressors, respectively. In vitro studies have shown that estradiol works synergistically with E7 in inactivation of Rb [13]. Thus, pregnancy-induced estrogen increase may play a role in development of HPV+ HNC during pregnancy.

52.2 Subsites Involved in Head and Neck Cancer in Pregnancy

52.2.1 Nasal and Paranasal Cancer

Nasal cavity and paranasal cancers commonly present older men with common histologic types including squamous cell cancer (SCC) and adenocarcinoma. Risk factors for these cancers such as toxin exposure or woodwork exposure often pose less risk to pregnancy cohort. Clinically cancers of this subsite often present with nasal obstruction or epistaxis, which can often be attributed to pregnancy also. Management of early stages of cancers in this subsite is primarily surgical resection except for small cell carcinoma, lymphoma, and rhabdomyosarcoma. Radiation therapy is limited by orbital and intracranial complications. Advanced stage is managed with multimodal therapy: this includes either primary radiation with surgical salvage or primary surgical excision with postoperative radiation therapy. Case reports of head and neck cancer in this subsite during pregnancy are limited, one of which describes pregnant patient with early stage mucoepidermoid of nasal cavity who was treated with surgical resection and subsequently had uncomplicated birth few months later, and did not require further adjuvant therapy [14].

52.2.2 Nasopharyngeal Cancer

Nasopharyngeal cancer is an uncommon head and neck primary, endemic geographic areas such as Southern China, Southeast Asia, and Norther Africa. Risk factors for cancers in this subsite include genetic predisposition and infection with Epstein-Barr virus. Clinically cancers of this subsite can present with neck mass, unilateral serous otitis media, nasal obstruction, cranial nerve palsies, and epistaxis. Management of early stage in this subsite is often centered around radiotherapy to primary site and bilateral necks. Advanced stage is often managed with chemoradiation followed by adjuvant chemotherapy. There is limited surgical role in management of nasopharyngeal cancers.

Outcomes/Prognosis: A multivariate analysis of head and neck cancer in this subsite during pregnancy found 70% 5-year survival for pregnancy cohort and 78% 5-year survival for the nonpregnant cohort [15].

52.2.3 Oral Cavity Cancer

Oral cavity cancer is the most common head and neck cancer site (excluding non-melanoma skin cancer) and accounts for 33% of all HNCs [16]. Similarly, it is a commonly discovered subsite of HNC during pregnancy. Risk factors for cancers in this subsite are traditionally thought to be due to tobacco and alcohol; however, factors such as marijuana and viral infection are thought to contribute more for the pregnancy subgroup [17]. Clinically cancers of this subsite often present after either patient, dentist, or other care provider notice concerning lesions in oral cavity. Management of early-stage centers around surgical excision of primary tumor while addressing neck at same time. Radiation is less than ideal due to complications arising after radiation to mandible and salivary glands. Advanced stage is often managed with surgical resection and primary reconstruction. Current trends in management of this subsite in pregnancy cohort are similar to nonpregnant cohort with focus on surgical resection. Various case reports and clinical studies describe successful surgical management of oral cavity cancers during pregnancy with good outcomes.

52.2.4 Oropharyngeal Cancer

Oropharyngeal cancer is a common head and neck cancer site and accounts for around 20% of all HNCs [16]. Risk factors include smoking, alcohol, and infection with EBV virus and HPV virus. As mentioned above, oncogenic HPV and estrogen have been thought to play a synergistic role in tumorigenesis during pregnancy. HPV-associated HNSCC can be found in any area of upper aerodigestive tract; however, it occurs most commonly in oropharynx. Current trends suggest that incidence of HPV-positive OPSCC will be greater than the incidence of cervical cancers by the year 2020 [18]. Clinically cancers of this subsite often present with sore throat, dysphagia, odynophagia, neck mass: these are referred to as otalgia, many of which can often be incorrectly attributed to pregnancy. Management of early stage is often single modality resection or primary radiation. Advances in Transoral Robotic Surgery (TORS) have made this approach a strong option for treatment. Advanced stage in this site preferred management is often concurrent chemoradiation, especially if HPV positive. Due to improved prognosis with HPV positivity, recent clinical trials are investigating de-escalation of chemoradiation to decrease side effects. There are limited reports of oropharyngeal cancers and their management during pregnancy.

52.2.5 Laryngeal and Hypopharyngeal Cancers

Laryngeal cancer is the second most common head and neck cancer site (excluding nonmelanoma skin cancer) and accounts for 29% of all HNCs [16]. Hypopharyngeal cancer is less common in the general population, and similarly, literature is limited on HNC in pregnancy affecting this subsite. Risk factors include smoking, alcohol use, radiation exposure, Plummer-Vinson syndrome, exposure to certain metal, wood dust, and asbestos. Clinically cancers in the larynx can present with voice changes, aspiration, referred otalgia, stridor, and hemoptysis. Management of early cancers of the larynx revolves around single modality treatment with options of radiation or surgical resection. Advanced cancers of the larynx are typically managed with multimodal treatment. Occurrence of primary laryngeal cancers during pregnancy remains very rare, and review of case reports suggests often misdiagnosis of hemangioma or papillomatosis in cases where patients present with voice changes during pregnancy. A report of a 33-year-old patient with supraglottic cancer discovered during first trimester who successfully underwent laryngectomy during pregnancy without any complications and subsequently twins were delivered at term without any issues [19].

52.2.6 Salivary Gland Cancers

Salivary gland cancers account for less than 10% of all HNCs [16]. In adult population, Pleomorphic adenoma, mucoepidermoid carcinoma, Warthin tumor, and adenoid cystic carcinoma account for majority of tumors. Acinic cell carcinomas are generally uncommon salivary gland tumors, and unlike other salivary gland tumors tend to show slightly higher incidence in women than in men [20]. Risk factors for salivary gland malignancies include radiation exposure, and certain environmental exposures such as nickel and silica dust. Clinically salivary gland malignancies usually present as a solitary nodule, and can have associated pain, facial nerve paresis, trismus, or neck involvement. Fine-needle aspiration is often used to establish diagnosis with clinically exam CT scan often a good adjunct to counsel on facial nerve risk in this area. Surgical excision is typically the mainstay of parotid malignancies, with certain high-grade histological subtypes benefiting from adjuvant radiation therapy. One case report of 25-year-old pregnant woman who during pregnancy developed Acinic cell carcinoma that was managed with surgical excision, and during a second pregnancy 4 years later had recurrence of same malignancy managed surgical, with chronology raising suspicion of association between pregnancy and pathogenic of acinic cell carcinoma [21].

52.2.7 Nonmelanoma Skin Cancers (NMSCs) and Melanoma

The majority of skin cancers of head and neck are nonmelanoma skin cancers (NMSCs): basal cell carcinoma and squamous cell carcinoma are the most frequent types of NMSCs, with a ratio around 3:1 [22]. Risk factor for pathogenesis of NMSC and Melanoma is cumulative exposure to UV radiation. NMSCs are uncommon during pregnancy, but melanoma is common, forming around 8% of all malignancies during pregnancy, with the peak incidence of malignant melanoma being during reproductive years [23]. Current hypothesis is that estrogen stimulation of melanocytes may preclude to malignant transformation [24]. Clinically melanoma classically presents as a pigmented lesion with characteristic features such as asymmetry, irregular borders, mixed dark colors, wide diameter, and/or evolving features. Notably malignant melanoma is the most common tumor metastasizing to the placenta. Mainstay of management of NMSC and malignant melanoma in pregnant patient remains wide surgical excision with possible neck surgical intervention. Women who had adequate treatment for melanoma should be advised to avoid pregnancy for 2–3 years (5 years, if the patient underwent regional node dissection), because the risk of relapse is highest during this period [5]. Five-year survival was not statistically different between pregnant and nonpregnant cohort with malignant melanoma [25].

52.2.8 Lymphoma

Lymphoma is fifth common subtype of cancer in pregnant patients after breast, melanoma, thyroid, and cervix, with a large subset of patients having associated head and neck involvement. Hodgkin lymphoma is more common than non-Hodgkin lymphoma during pregnancy [26]. Non-Hodgkin lymphoma often presents at early stage, whereas Hodgkin often presents with aggressive advanced disease. Nonspecifisc signs such as fatigue and anemia may be attributed to pregnancy. Ultrasonography and MRI can be safely used in pregnancy as part of imaging workup. Radiation and chemotherapy are mainstays in current guidelines for managing lymphoma. For early stage disease, radiotherapy can often be performed after shielding abdomen. For late stage, current paradigms revolve around termination of pregnancy followed by chemotherapy if early in pregnancy versus initiating chemotherapy if later in pregnancy. Hodgkin disease during pregnancy has better outcomes than those patients with non-Hodgkin lymphoma [27].

52.2.9 Leukemia

Leukemia during pregnancy can often manifest in head and neck as recurrent upper respiratory tract infections or epistaxis. These symptoms and other symptoms can often be overlooked if present during pregnancy. Two primary forms of leukemia are acute and chronic. Treatment of acute leukemia during pregnancy revolves around chemotherapy. Current paradigms leaning toward termination of pregnancy followed by chemotherapy if early pregnancy versus safe use of combination chemotherapy during late pregnancy. Chronic leukemias are rarely diagnosed during pregnancy, and often do not require acute treatments during the pregnancy. Outcomes of leukemias are generally favorable for both mother and fetus [27].

52.3 Management Principles

52.3.1 Goals/Dilemmas

Management of head and neck cancer can be complicated due to balancing levels of fetal and maternal risk from nontreatment or treatment. Generally, current paradigms learn toward maternal survival as primary outcome. If maternal survival is compromised due to condition or treatment, successful postmortem caesarean section of fetus can often be performed in later stages of pregnancy. To facilitate answering difficult questions and decision making in these complex situations, multidisciplinary approach is often used with contributions from various teams including obstetric, surgical, oncology, radiation oncology, and ethics (Table 52.2).

52.3.2 Radiographic Studies

Mainstay of staging head and neck cancers during pregnancy still centers around clinical and radiographic findings. Radiographic studies should focus on characterizing extent of invasion, lymph node involvement, as detecting possible distant metastasis. Primary modalities for diagnostic imaging are computed tomography (CT) and magnetic resonance imaging (MRI). CT threshold of 100 mGy can induce congenital defects, with recommendations being to use less than 50 mGy [28]. MRI has advantage, does not use ionizing radiation, and is therefore safer than CT in this regard.

52.3.3 Treatment Timing

Treatment of head and neck cancer in pregnancy at this time revolves around radiation therapy, chemotherapy, and surgery as with other head and neck cancers in general. Timing of treatments is often a complex decision, which also incorporates patient's preference and subsite involved; however, general principles exist. During first trimester (week 1–week 12), fetus is still forming organs and other structures. This main risk of treatment during this time is teratogenicity associated with certain chemotherapy or anesthetic drugs. Furthermore, stress of interventions has increased

Table 52.2 Examples of difficult questions in managing head and neck cancer in pregnancy

What is best way to evaluate and stage patient with least risk?
Which treatment options are available and best for the mother and fetus?
What is best timing of treatments?
What are treatment outcomes for delayed treatment?
How to balance therapeutic intents with treatment risks?
How to balance and counsel decisions on possible future maternal infertility risks?
If maternal survival expectation is low, what is childcare plan?
When would I recommend elective termination of pregnancy?

Table 52.3 Risks and safest timing of cancer treatment modalities during pregnancy

	Chemotherapy	Radiation therapy	Surgery
General risks	– Teratogenicity – Growth retardation – Preterm labor – Abortion	– Microcephaly – Growth retardation – Mental retardation – Sterility – Childhood malignancy – Abortion	– Generally least toxic to fetus – Anesthesia risks – Standard head/neck surgical risks – Abortion
Safest timing	– 2nd or 3rd trimester	– 2nd or 3rd trimester – Adjuvant commonly after delivery	– 2nd trimester

risk of spontaneous abortion during this time. Second trimester (week 13–week 28) is generally considered safest time for general anesthesia and surgical interventions if being considered. During third trimester (week 28 thru birth), there are various alterations in maternal physiologic parameters including cardiac output, heart rate, and pulmonary function due to increasing size of growing fetus. These factors increase difficulty of providing general anesthesia and surgical intervention during this time has increased risk of premature labor (Table 52.3).

52.3.4 Chemotherapy

Chemotherapy may be a recommended option for treatment of certain head and neck cancers in pregnancy, and is often an adjuvant therapy with definitive therapy often centering around radiation therapy or surgery. When employed on a pregnant patient, generally safer in second or third trimester due to teratogenic effects during first trimester. If advanced/aggressive disease in early pregnancy that may affect maternal survival, current paradigms suggest elective termination of pregnancy prior to chemotherapy use. Also it is important to counsel mother that chemotherapy drugs can be transmitted to infants in breast milk; thus, breast-feeding is contraindicated during chemotherapy [29].

Common chemotherapy agents include cisplatin, doxorubicin, cyclophosphamide, 5-FU, antimetabolites, and alkylating agents. Cisplatin is relatively safe for fetus with adverse effects including hearing loss, and cardiac and cerebral malformations. Antimetabolites and alkylating agents have been shown to have extra teratogenic effects during first trimester. Combination therapy is often synergistic in treating the cancer, but also may similarly confer synergistic negative effects to the fetus. Nonteratogenic adverse effects include reduced birth weight, growth retardations, abortion, and myocardial toxicities.

52.3.5 Radiation Therapy

Radiation therapy is often an option for definitive therapy for head and neck cancers, but as could be expected can pose significant risk to fetal development and safety. Timing, energy, field size, and dispersion are all key factors in determining possible risk to fetus. Radiation therapy for head and neck cancer in pregnancy is most commonly performed after delivery. When decision is made for radiotherapy during pregnancy, energy is often set below 10 Gy for photons to avoid dispersion, and field size is often reduced. Shields placed over abdomen and pelvis are often used to decrease radiation exposure to fetus [30].

Adverse effects with radiation are dose dependent. Doses of less than 0.05 Gy to fetus pose no increased rates of abortion, growth retardation, or congenital malformations [31]. Doses 0.5–2.5 Gy are commonly associated with malformations, with doses to 3.0 Gy often inducing spontaneous abortions. Microcephaly is most common malformation and thought to be due to radiation to glial cells. Mental retardation results from aberrant development of brain cortex. Radiotherapy during early pregnancy can result in temporary growth retardation, which is often permanent if therapy given during late pregnancy. Sterility and increased risk of childhood malignancy are two other commonly discussed risks to fetus with radiotherapy and should be discussed during counseling with patient and family.

52.3.6 Surgery

Surgery remains a durable option in treatment of head and neck cancers in pregnancy due to ability to localize treatment and distance away from developing fetus. General anesthesia agents are generally safe to both mother and fetus. Due to physiologic changes with pregnancy, anesthesia team must be prepared for certain alterations in anesthesia plan for the pregnant patient.

Surgical excision of the cancer is the least toxic treatment option for the developing fetus. As discussed above, subsites with well-documented surgical success in the pregnant population include but are not limited to nasal cavity, oral cavity, larynx, skin, and neck. Multidisciplinary decision making may be needed to discuss subsequent adjuvant therapy.

52.3.7 Elective Termination of Pregnancy

As previously discussed, certain situations portend improved maternal outcomes with elective termination of pregnancy. Again multidisciplinary decision making is important in these situations with final decision by mother and/or family. After termination of pregnancy and stabilization of maternal health, subsequent therapy is often undertaken with goal of minimal time delay. Generally, mothers are able to have subsequent pregnancies, necessitating appropriate counseling of risks of cancer during subsequent pregnancy based on subsite.

52.4 Conclusion

Head and neck cancer during pregnancy experiences increased incidence past two decades. There are limited guidelines on appropriate management of HNC in pregnancy. Challenge remains treating the cancer while preserving fetal health. Clinician should seek to add pregnancy-related factors to foundational expertise to adequately manage these patients. Current treatment options center around chemotherapy, radiation therapy, and surgery. There is a strong necessity for careful counseling and multidisciplinary decision making for the main treatment methods and timing. Continued case reports, basic science studies, and clinical studies will help expand our understanding and optimal management of this unique disease entity.

References

1. Bray F, Ferlay J, Soerjomataram I, Siegel RL, Torre LA, Jemal A. Global cancer statistics 2018: GLOBOCAN estimates of incidence and mortality worldwide for 36 cancers in 185 countries. CA Cancer J Clin. 2018;68(6):394–424.
2. McCormick A, Peterson E. Cancer in pregnancy. Obstet Gynecol Clin. 2018;45(2):187–200.
3. Pentheroudakis G, Pavlidis N. Cancer and pregnancy: poena magna, not anymore. Eur J Cancer. 2006;42(2):126–40.
4. Calsteren KV, Heyns L, Smet FD, Eycken LV, Gziri MM, Gemert WV, et al. Cancer during pregnancy: an analysis of 215 patients emphasizing the obstetrical and the neonatal outcomes. J Clin Oncol. 2010;28(4):683–9.
5. Devaney SL, Devaney KO, Ferlito A, Carbone A, Rinaldo A, Maio M, Friedmann I. Pregnancy and malignant neoplasms of the head and neck. Ann Otol Rhinol Laryngol. 1998;107(11):991–8.
6. Schantz SP, Yu GP. Head and neck cancer incidence trends in young Americans, 1973-1997, with a special analysis for tongue cancer. Arch Otolaryngol Head Neck Surg. 2002;128(3):268–74.
7. Gibelli B, Zamperini P, Proh M, Giugliano G. Management and follow-up of thyroid cancer in pregnant women. Acta Otorhinolaryngol Ital. 2011;31(6):358.
8. Eliassen AM, Hauff SJ, Tang AL, Thomas DH, McHugh JB, Walline HM, et al. Head and neck squamous cell carcinoma in pregnant women. Head Neck. 2013;35(3):335–42.
9. Tae K, El-Naggar AK, Yoo E, Feng L, Lee JJ, Hong WK, et al. Expression of vascular endothelial growth factor and microvessel density in head and neck tumorigenesis. Clin Cancer Res. 2000;6(7):2821–8.
10. Okuyama M, Mezawa H, Kawai T, Urashima M. Elevated soluble PD-L1 in pregnant women's serum suppresses the immune reaction. Front Immunol. 2019;10:86.
11. Chen SW, Li SH, Shi DB, Jiang WM, Song M, Yang AK, et al. Expression of PD-1/PD-L1 in head and neck squamous cell carcinoma and its clinical significance. Int J Biol Markers. 2019;34(4):398–405.
12. Lukits J, Remenar E, Rásó E, Ladányi A, Kásler M, Tímár J. Molecular identification, expression and prognostic role of estrogen-and progesterone receptors in head and neck cancer. Int J Oncol. 2007;30(1):155–60.
13. Chung SH, Shin MK, Korach KS, Lambert PF. Requirement for stromal estrogen receptor alpha in cervical neoplasia. Horm Cancer. 2013;4(1):50–9.
14. Figueiro EA, Horgan RP, Muhanna N, Parrish J, Irish JC, Maxwell CV. Obstetrical outcomes of head and neck (nonthyroid) cancers: a 27-year retrospective series and literature review. Am J Perinatol Rep. 2019;9(1):e15–22.
15. Zhang L, Liu H, Tang LQ, Chen QY, Guo SS, Liu LT, et al. Prognostic effect of pregnancy on young female patients with nasopharyngeal carcinoma: results from a matched cohort analysis. Oncotarget. 2016;7(16):21913.
16. Otterburn D, Saadeh P. Chapter 33. Grabb and Smith's plastic surgery head and neck cancers and salivary gland cancers.
17. Cudney N, Ochs MW, Johnson J, Roccia W, Collins BM, Costello BJ. A unique presentation of a squamous cell carcinoma in a pregnant patient. Quintessence Int. 2010;41(7):581–3.
18. Chaturvedi AK, Engels EA, Anderson WF, Gillison ML. Incidence trends for human papillomavirus-related and-unrelated oral squamous cell carcinomas in the United States. J Clin Oncol. 2008;26(4):612–9.

19. Pytel J, Gerlinger I, Arany A. Twin pregnancy following in vitro fertilisation coinciding with laryngeal cancer. ORL. 1995;57(4):232–4.
20. Sepúlveda I, Frelinghuysen M, Platin E, Spencer ML, Urra A, Ortega P. Acinic cell carcinoma of the parotid gland: a case report and review of the literature. Case Rep Oncol. 2015;8(1):1–8.
21. Al-Zaher NN, Obeid AA. Acinic cell carcinoma in pregnancy: a case report and review of the literature. J Med Case Rep. 2011;5(1):1–4.
22. Ouyang YH. Skin cancer of the head and neck. In: Seminars in plastic surgery, vol. 24, no. 2. New York: Thieme Medical Publishers; 2010. pp. 117–126.
23. Bradley PJ, Raghavan U. Cancers presenting in the head and neck during pregnancy. Curr Opin Otolaryngol Head Neck Surg. 2004;12(2):76–81.
24. De Giorgi V, Gori A, Grazzini M, Rossari S, Scarfi F, Corciova S, Massi D. Estrogens, estrogen receptors and melanoma. Expert Rev Anticancer Ther. 2011;11(5):739–47.
25. O'Meara AT, Cress R, Xing G, Danielsen B, Smith LH. Malignant melanoma in pregnancy: a population-based evaluation. Cancer. 2005;103(6):1217–26.
26. Pohlman B, Macklis RM. Lymphoma and pregnancy. In: Seminars in oncology, vol. 27, no. 6; 2000. pp. 657–666.
27. Gelb AB, van de Rijn M, Warnke RA, Kamel OW. Pregnancy-associated lymphomas: a clinicopathologic study. Cancer. 1996;78(2):304–10.
28. Tremblay E, Thérasse E, Thomassin-Naggara I, Trop I. Quality initiatives: guidelines for use of medical imaging during pregnancy and lactation. Radiographics. 2012;32(3):897–911.
29. Pistilli B, Bellettini G, Giovannetti E, Codacci-Pisanelli G, Azim HA Jr, Benedetti G, Peccatori FA. Chemotherapy, targeted agents, antiemetics and growth-factors in human milk: how should we counsel cancer patients about breastfeeding? Cancer Treat Rev. 2013;39(3):207–11.
30. Podgorsak MB, Meiler RJ, Kowal H, Kishel SP, Orner JB. Technical management of a pregnant patient undergoing radiation therapy to the head and neck. Med Dosim. 1999;24(2):121–8.
31. Williams PM, Fletcher S. Health effects of prenatal radiation exposure. Am Fam Physician. 2010;82(5):488–93.

Atılay Yaylacı, Murat Öztürk, and Tania Sih

53.1 Introduction

A mass in the neck is a common clinical finding encountered in clinical practice. Determining the etiology of a neck mass is not straightforward, owing to developing from a wide array of processes. A neck mass may evolve as an isolated disease, a sign of a systemic disease, or be the only clinically apparent manifestation of malignancy in another part of the head and neck or elsewhere in the body. Therefore, timely diagnosis of a neck mass is paramount, because delayed diagnosis of malignancy worsens prognosis [1].

When clinicians are confronted with a pregnant or lactating woman presenting with a neck mass, they may feel uncomfortable during diagnostic process and implementing treatment due to the concerns regarding both maternal and neonatal morbidities. Although there are guidelines for the evaluation and management of neck mass in adults, albeit they are few in number, none contain any additional specific information concerning pregnancy and the postpartum period. This chapter addresses the diagnosis and management of a neck mass, and the management of benign neck masses with the exception of those deriving from thyroid gland or vascular origin, in pregnancy and the postpartum period. Management of malignant neck masses will not be discussed in this chapter.

A. Yaylacı (✉) · M. Öztürk
Faculty of Medicine, Department of Otorhinolaryngology, Kocaeli University,
Kocaeli, Turkey
e-mail: dratilay@yahoo.com; muratkbb@gmail.com

T. Sih
Medical School University of São Paulo (FMUSP), LIM—Laboratory of Medical
Investigations, São Paulo, Brazil
e-mail: tsih@amcham.com.br

C. Cingi et al. (eds.), *ENT Diseases: Diagnosis and Treatment during Pregnancy
and Lactation*, https://doi.org/10.1007/978-3-031-05303-0_53

53.2　Differential Diagnosis

Neck masses are generally classified into three main categories: inflammatory, congenital, and neoplastic [2]. A basic knowledge of the different pathologies in each category is essential to make an accurate differential diagnosis and to direct adequate diagnostic investigations. As there is no published data, it is impossible to know whether the etiology of the neck masses that occur during pregnancy differs from the normal population in the same age group or whether some neck masses occur more frequently associated with pregnancy. A thorough review of the possible etiology of neck masses goes beyond the scope of this chapter and will not be discussed further.

The age of the patient is the central factor in the etiology of the neck mass, whether the patient is pregnant or not. The age of patient can guide the clinician to further differential considerations, because the relative incidence of some etiologies within a particular age group (<15 years old, 15–40 years old, or >40 years old) is higher than others [3]. Patients younger than 40 years are overwhelmingly diagnosed with benign processes such as inflammatory and congenital lesions [4]. However, patients older than 40 years have a high likelihood of harboring a malignant neoplasm [5]. Gestational age mostly falls into the young adult age group (15–40 years old), so inflammatory masses are expected to be more frequent than those of congenital origin, and congenital masses are more common than neoplastic neck masses. As the age of a pregnant patient increases, the risk for a neoplastic process increases [5]. The majority of malignant masses in adults are attributable to metastasis from head and neck squamous cell carcinoma (HNSCC) [6], but it may also be due to lymphoma, thyroid cancer, salivary gland cancer, skin cancer, or metastasis from distant sites [1]. At this point, it may be worth stating that due to the increasing incidence of human papillomavirus infections and the shifting of the childbearing age with the changing attitudes in women's role in the workplace, we might expect to encounter malignant masses more often in pregnant women [1].

53.3　Diagnostic Tools

53.3.1　History

When evaluating a patient presenting with a neck mass, a thorough gathering of historical information is an important initial step in refining a differential diagnosis. A comprehensive history should include the age, past medical history (upper respiratory infection, dental problem, trauma, exposure to tuberculosis, occupational/sexual history, travel abroad, contact with pets, surgery, irradiation, prior head and neck malignancy), tobacco use, and alcohol abuse [1, 7]. The age is crucial, because the likely diagnosis for any given neck mass is closely related to the patient's age. The mode of onset and duration of the mass, and associated symptoms including sore throat, dysphagia, dysphonia, odynophagia, referred otalgia, nasal obstruction, cranial nerve neuropathies, weight loss, anorexia, malaise, and night sweats, should be sought [8]. If it is possible to narrow the differential diagnosis from history, targeted historical information specific to the possible diagnoses should be further questioned. At this point, it is important to keep in mind that some of these signs and symptoms may either be attributed to pregnancy or disguised by pregnancy. In addition, while assessing the patient's history, anxiety and mood changes due to pregnancy should be taken into consideration.

53.3.2 Physical Examination

Like the historical information, the physical examination also offers valuable information on the prediction of the etiology of neck masses in a pregnant patient. Focusing first on the neck mass itself, a clinician should record information regarding the size, location, mobility, consistency (firm, soft, fluctuant, compressible), and tenderness to palpation [1]. Acute inflammatory masses usually tend to be soft, tender, and mobile [9]. A fluctuant mass can occur with an abscess or a cyst formation [10]. The vertical motion of the mass with swallowing and tongue protrusion is very helpful in distinguishing thyroglossal duct cysts. A pulsatile compressible mass in the region of the carotid bifurcation, which is mobile horizontally but fixed vertically, may indicate a carotid body tumor [3]. However, a firm, painless mass with an irregular surface, fixation to underlying structures or overlying skin is always concerning for malignancy [11]. In addition, multiple interconnected nodes with an elastic, yielding texture are often associated with lymphoma [12].

Identifying the specific location of a neck mass is also important for differential diagnosis. Midline neck masses include thyroglossal duct cyst, dermoid cysts, teratomas, thyroid malignancy, or metastatic lymph nodes from laryngeal malignancy [1]. Branchial cysts, cystic hygromas, thyroid cysts, and parotid cysts tend to occur at specific levels of the lateral neck [12]. The location of the neck mass in a particular lymphatic zone provides a clue to the site of the precipitating infection or the primary source of a malignant neoplasm [5]. The presence of a mass in the supraclavicular fossa provides a strong indication of malignancy and also suggests that the primary lesion will be located at other sites beyond the head and neck [13].

The clinician should also perform a rigorous physical examination of the head and neck. The inspection of the skin over the skull, face, and neck is required for identification of a swelling, ulceration, or pigmented lesion. Endoscopic assessment of the entire mucosa of the upper aerodigestive tract and vocal fold movement should be carried out. Palpation of the floor of mouth, tongue base, salivary, and thyroid glands is mandatory. While concentrating on the head and neck, the clinician should also perform a general physical examination, giving particular attention to the chest and breasts and the axillae [7].

In the workup for possible malignancy (Table 53.1), *a targeted history and physical examination* should be performed first to increase the likelihood of identifying a primary malignancy. Targeted examination should be directed according to the location of the neck mass, by the virtue of the expected lymphatic drainage pattern of HNSCC. A targeted examination of the skin, thyroid, and salivary glands; the

Table 53.1 Medical history, signs and symptoms, and physical findings suggestive of malignancy for a neck mass

History	Signs and symptoms	Physical examination findings
• Age >40 years • Smoking • Alcohol use • Absence of infectious history • Past history of previous head and neck malignancy • Past history of head and neck cutaneous lesions	• A mass that has been present for >2 weeks or uncertain duration • Absence of infectious signs • Hemoptysis • A recent voice change • Dysphagia or odynophagia • Ipsilateral otalgia • A recent hearing loss • Intraoral ulceration • Tonsil asymmetry • Nasal obstruction or epistaxis • Skin lesions • Unexplained weight loss	• Fixed mass • Size >1.5 cm • Firm consistency • Supraclavicular location • Overlying skin ulceration

visualization of the entire upper aerodigestive tract by fiber-optic endoscopy; and otoscopic examination are conducted. The palpation of the tongue base, tonsils, and the floor of mouth should also be performed [1].

53.3.3 Diagnostic Imaging

Depending on the clinical impression of a neck mass from the history and physical examination, appropriate radiographic studies may help to reach a definitive diagnosis. Although it does not always lead to a definitive diagnosis, by narrowing the differential diagnosis, it may direct the clinician to further appropriate interventions. Radiological studies are also needed prior to any attempt at invasive biopsy or surgical intervention [14].

Unfortunately, pregnancy is a challenge for diagnostic imaging due to the potentially deleterious effects of both radiation and contrast material on the fetus. Therefore, when an imaging modality is intended, the benefit of making a significant diagnosis should exceed the risks of the procedure to the mother and fetus [15].

53.3.3.1 Ultrasound Imaging

Given the low risk in pregnancy, the clinician may prefer ultrasonography (USG) as an initial imaging. It is noninvasive and does not use ionizing radiation or contrast medium. USG can accurately differentiate cystic from solid lesions, reactive from metastatic nodes by using nodal size, and high-flow from low-flow vascular malformations. It has a definitive place in the initial assessment of thyroid and salivary gland lesions. Diagnosis of some particular neck masses, such as congenital cysts, hematomas, sialoadenitis from salivary gland calculi, or some benign lesions like lipoma, can easily be made only from ultrasonographic assessment accompanied by historical information and physical examination findings, thereby alleviating the need for further interventions. USG may also recognize paragangliomas, vascular masses, or anomalies, allowing the examiner to avoid an inadvertent biopsy attempt. It is also utilized to select target tissue precisely for fine-needle cytology [12].

However, USG has some downsides. It cannot provide sufficient information on deep-seated lesions. USG is not a substitute for cross-sectional imaging techniques, especially in the evaluation of the possible malignant neck mass, because it does not permit an evaluation of the upper aerodigestive tract and a possible primary lesion. Therefore, USG may not be preferred as an initial imaging study in evaluating patients with a neck mass when the suspicion of malignancy is high. Also, USG is highly operator dependent and does not allow an easy review of the studies by other physicians [12].

53.3.3.2 Computed Tomography and Magnetic Resonance Imaging

Contrast-enhanced computed tomography (CT) or magnetic resonance imaging (MRI) examinations of head and neck should be obtained in patients with a neck mass of uncertain etiology or a neck mass deemed at increased risk for malignancy. Both modalities provide precious information about the mass regarding size, characteristics, localization, extent, and the relationship with other vital structures. These imaging techniques also better ascertain the exact nature of the mass and provide ancillary information, such as evidence of dental disease, salivary calculi, and deeply seated abscess formation [1]. In the presence of metastatic neck mass, imaging can also assist in the detection of the undetectable primary source in the upper aerodigestive tract [5]. In the event of possible future open biopsy, the cross-sectional imaging techniques allow the clinician to better understand the anatomy of the mass and its relation with other structures. This guides the making of decisions concerning both the surgical approach and the risks of potential complications.

Unfortunately, teratogenesis is a major concern in the radiological evaluation of a pregnant patient. However, it is not a major concern after diagnostic CT studies of the head and neck, because the radiation dose is too small to lead to any teratogenic effects [16]. Iodinated intravenous contrast agents are considered category B drugs by the Food and Drug Administration (FDA), which by definition means that there was no risk demonstrated in animal reproductive studies, but no controlled studies in pregnant women have been performed [17]. The use of iodinated contrast in pregnancy carries a low risk of adverse effects and anaphylactic reactions [15], so it should be administered with the usual care [16]. After discussion of the small risk of adverse events with the patient, a CT study with contrast should be performed. This is advised as it is better to obtain diagnostic images with contrast than have to repeat the noncontrast examination because of nondiagnostic images, which would require the repeat to use contrast anyway [16].

MRI has no known biological effects on fetuses, because it inherently does not employ ionizing radiation [18]. The use of gadolinium contrast at any time during pregnancy has been shown to be associated with an increased risk of stillbirth or neonatal death. In addition, there is an increased risk of inflammatory or rheumatological disorders and infiltrative skin conditions from birth. Thus, the use of gadolinium during pregnancy should be avoided if at all possible. Gadolinium is classified as a category C drugs by the FDA and can be used if the potential benefit justifies the potential risk to the fetus. If an MRI study using gadolinium is absolutely essential, the patient must provide informed consent after a discussion of risks and benefits [16]. In lactating mothers, because only a small percentage of iodinated or gadolinium-based contrast is excreted in breast milk and then only a minute fraction entering the infant's gut is absorbed, it is generally considered safe to continue breastfeeding after receiving contrast agents [15].

If the use of contrast is not agreed with pregnant patients, MRI should be preferred, because the diagnostic accuracy of MRI surpasses that of noncontrast CT [15]. For vascular lesions, MR angiograms are an excellent modality for vascular delineation, which obviates the need for contrast injection [19].

53.3.4 Ancillary Testing

In some instances, ancillary testing can lead to diagnosis of a neck mass. The ability of ancillary tests to achieve an accurate diagnosis depends on choosing the relevant tests. It is not advised to try to perform a "neck mass screen" and laboratory investigations should be based on a clinically suspected disease. Some commonly used ancillary tests include complete blood count, C-reactive protein, erythrocyte sedimentation rate, tuberculin test (PPD), antineutrophil antibody, thyroid-stimulating hormone assay, thyroglobulin FNA-needle wash assay, and parathyroid hormone assay. If a particular infection is suspected, such as toxoplasma, brucella, cat-scratch disease, cytomegalovirus, Epstein–Barr virus, or HIV infection, serological testing could be deployed. In the setting of metastatic carcinoma, the submission of some biopsy material may be considered for HPV and p16 status [1].

Ancillary tests may be performed at any time during the workup of a neck mass for patients, regardless of risk status. For patients who are at increased risk of malignancy, ancillary testing must be carried out simultaneously with the malignancy workup to avoid delayed cancer diagnosis [1]. Considering the potential adverse effects of some radiological studies and invasive interventions, ancillary testing may be implemented initially and more frequently to facilitate the diagnosis in pregnant patients.

53.3.5 Biopsy

53.3.5.1 Fine-Needle Aspiration Biopsy

Fine-needle aspiration biopsy (FNAB) is an important diagnostic modality in the evaluation of a neck mass. It is an accurate, cost-effective method, which is performed safely in any trimester during pregnancy [20]. FNAB can be used instead of open biopsy (OB) in most cases, although it is not a substitute for excisional biopsy.

An FNAB is usually indicated when the neck mass is not identified by the historical information and the physical examination; after the failure of an antibiotic trial; or the mass is deemed to indicate an increased risk for malignancy at initial examination [1]. It can be performed with USG guidance, which allows more precise localization and access of deep-seated lesions and collection of an adequate specimen by facilitating directed biopsy of the solid component in cystic or necrotic masses [1, 21]. Besides making the diagnosis with direct smears, FNAB also allows the performance of ancillary tests on the biopsy material, such as immunostaining, microbiological investigations, flow cytometry, or molecular testing [19]. In addition to diagnostic yield, FNAB also helps to determine whether the particular diagnosis warrants further investigations. For example, if the FNAB diagnosis is concordant with an infective or inflammatory process, no further imaging may be required and ancillary testing may be undertaken. Also, the identification of a specific benign lesion, such as lipoma, eliminates further investigation.

FNAB is very sensitive and highly specific for neoplasia. However, it is completely dependent on the skill of the cytopathologist [5]. The sensitivity of FNAB for detecting a malignancy ranges from 77 to 97%, and the specificity ranges from 93 to 100% [22]. The sensitivity for distinguishing benign from malignant salivary gland tumors is approximately 95%. However, its sensitivity for the detection of lymphoma is variable and it does not provide adequate material for subtyping [12].

Due to false-negative and false-positive results, FNAB should always be combined with other diagnostic evidence such as clinical data and imaging results [4]. While an FNAB cytology that is compatible with a benign pathology or negative for malignancy may exclude malignancy in many cases, it may not rule out a cancer diagnosis for a patient with a mass that is clinically suspicious for malignancy [1]. If the validity of the FNAB results is unreliable, OB may be the only definitive diagnostic method [21]. However, before planning an OB, a repeat FNAB is recommended [19]. Inadequate or indeterminate FNAB cytology also warrants the repeating of FNAB. The repeat FNAB may again be conducted under ultrasound guidance, especially if this was not used during the initial FNAB. Core biopsy (CB) may also be an option. A good example of this scenario is cystic neck masses. The overall incidence of malignancy in a given cystic neck mass varies from 4 to 24%, but this jumps to around 80% in patients aged more than 40 years [1]. False-negative rate associated with FNAB cytology is in excess of 50% for cystic lymph node metastasis. Hence, the mass may be erroneously diagnosed as a branchial cleft cyst, thyroglossal duct cyst, thymic cyst, or a thyroid cyst [12]. Therefore, FNAB needs to be repeated, preferably with image guidance.

In general, FNAB is conducted after imaging studies to avoid inadvertent biopsy of a vascular lesion, although some controversy still exists [5]. However, it can also be preferred prior to additional imaging. Performing the FNAB before CT or MR imaging in the pregnant patient, in whom the clinical suspicion for a neoplasm is low and the head and neck examination is negative, may be advisable when further diagnostic workup is undesirable, especially in the overly anxious pregnant patient.

53.3.5.2 Core Biopsy

Core biopsy (CB) is a valuable adjunct to the diagnostic process after an initial inadequate or indeterminate FNAB [1, 19]. It has a high rate of adequacy (95%) and high accuracy; 94% and 96% in detection of neoplasia and malignancy, respectively. CB also has a higher sensitivity than FNAB (92% vs. 74%) for characterizing lymphomas [23]. Navigation-guided CB may be considered for the diagnosis of lesions in difficult-to-reach locations. In the context of these data, a CB may preclude an OB for tissue sampling [24]. It helps to avoid the risks of surgery, especially in pregnant patients.

53.3.5.3 Open Biopsy

Open biopsy for the diagnosis of a neck mass should be avoided whenever possible due to the unwanted consequences such as wound complications, distortion of anatomy, spillage of tumor cells, and interference with subsequent surgical treatment. However, if all efforts including repeated FNAB (or CB), imaging, and examination under anesthesia have failed to yield a diagnosis, yet suspicion for malignancy persists, OB must be considered [1].

OB is performed under general anesthesia due to possible subsequent neck dissection [1]. However, a simple nodal excision under local anesthesia can be sufficient for histologic confirmation and further differentiation if lymphoma is diagnosed and the mass is located in an easily approachable area [3]. In general, OB may entail an excisional biopsy due to concerns regarding tumor seeding. However, excisional biopsy may not be feasible in cases of large or matted masses adherent to vital structures [1]. Therefore, depending on the suspected pathology and location of the neck mass, an incisional biopsy may also be considered.

During the operation, if the mass proves to be metastatic squamous cell carcinoma on frozen examination, a panendoscopy should be carried out [1]. Concomitant definitive neck dissection should be performed when no primary is detected. In cases when diagnosis of adenocarcinoma or lymphoma is made completion of the surgery mandatory, together with further workup and staging procedures prior to further treatment decisions. However, if biopsy results suggest simple inflammation or granuloma, then microbiological investigations are indicated [3]. If frozen section analysis proved the neck mass, with the exception of lymph nodes, benign in nature, and the mass is thought to be easily resected without putting the pregnant women and fetus at risk, the excisional biopsy often proves to be definitive treatment.

53.3.6 Panendoscopy

A panendoscopy under general anesthesia must be carried out if there is a metastatic cervical lymph node in the neck and the primary source is still elusive on imaging or repeat head and neck examination [10]. Panendoscopy involves the visualization of the mucosal surfaces of the upper aerodigestive tract through nasopharyngoscopy, operative laryngoscopy, esophagoscopy, and bronchoscopy [1]. Biopsies should be taken from any obvious lesion or any suspicious area detected by computed tomography [21]. Random biopsies of nonsuspicious normal-appearing mucosa areas are not recommended, as the diagnostic yield is very low [14]. The samples should then be sent for frozen section tissue analysis [21]. If the primary lesion is ascertained, the treatment of the primary and the neck is managed according to the principles of management of cancer in the pregnant patient [5]. If all efforts fail to identify the primary tumor, which occurs in approximately 3% of cases [14], the treatment of an unknown primary malignancy in the head and neck must be conducted.

53.4 Diagnostic Workup

In pregnant and lactating patients who present with a neck mass, potential cervical metastasis of head and neck carcinoma must always be a prime consideration. For this reason, the investigation of a neck mass must rely on excluding malignancy. The presence of metastatic lymphadenopathy in the neck indicates progression of disease, so the main endeavor must determine the primary tumor quickly to institute a timely management of the disease [21]. Unlike those lesions that manifest themselves as malignant cervical lymphadenopathy, several malignant neoplastic masses, such as sarcoma, may occur primarily in the neck [10]. Some persistent neck masses are benign and can be identified based on their clinical features.

Substantially, the diagnosis of a neck mass in pregnant patients is similar to that of nonpregnant patients and the diagnostic workup used in adults with a neck mass can be applied to these patients (Fig. 53.1). However, it can differ in certain points

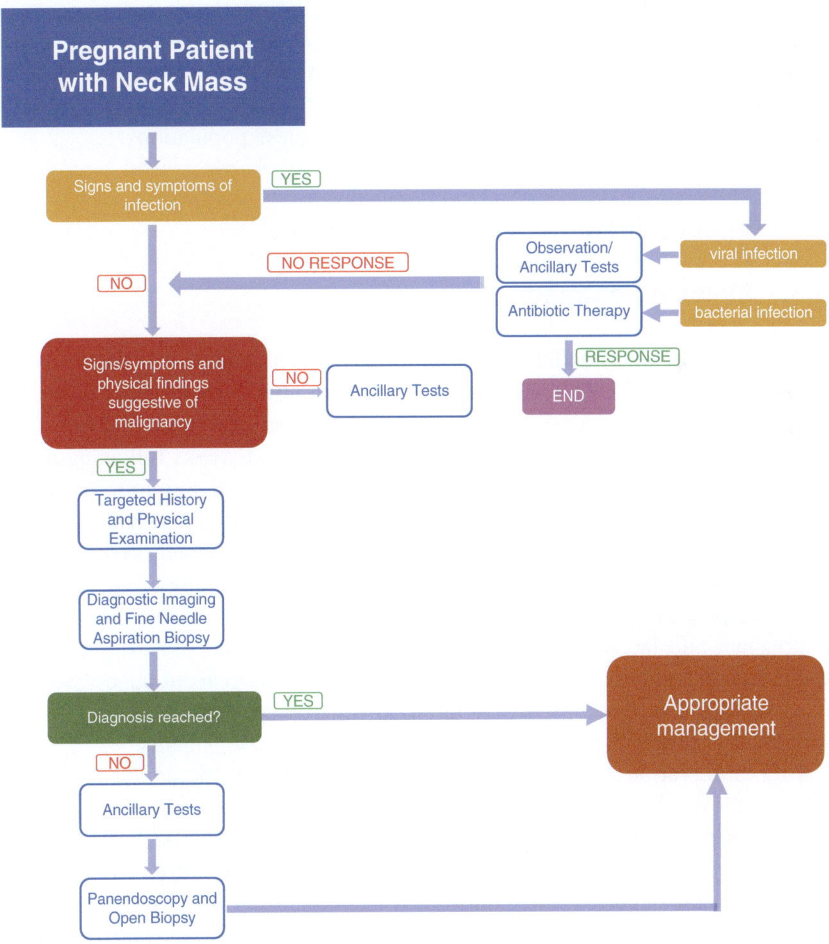

Fig. 53.1 Flowchart for workup of the pregnant patients with a neck mass. (Adopted from reference [1])

on account of some diagnostic modalities that may cause additional harm to mother and the fetus. Diagnostic approaches in breastfeeding women only differ from those used in nonlactating patients due to the possible harm to infant that may be caused by the passing of medications to the breast milk. For this reason, the diagnostic tools utilized in these patients must be chosen carefully to maximize accuracy while minimizing the risk.

The differential diagnosis of neck masses should be conducted in a systematic fashion including a comprehensive history, physical examination, laboratory, and radiological investigations. Throughout the diagnostic process, the clinician should provide information to pregnant and breastfeeding patients about possible diagnoses, explain the necessary diagnostic procedures, and discuss the benefits and possible risks of each for maternal and fetal health. Shared decision making must be conducted among the clinician, the patient, and her obstetrician and written informed consent of the patient must be obtained.

Each case must be evaluated on an individual basis and at each stage of the diagnostic workup. Subsequent investigations should be undertaken according to the results of previous studies until a clear, specific, and definitive diagnosis has been reached. To avoid unnecessary diagnostic investigations that may pose a risk to the pregnant patient and fetus, it is important to focus more on initial diagnostic tools, such as history taking and physical examination, in these populations.

53.5 Management of Benign Neck Masses

53.5.1 Medical Treatment

In pregnancy and breastfeeding age groups, cervical lymphadenitis is the most common neck mass and this typically develops during or after a recent upper respiratory tract infection (URTI). Considering that most URTIs develop from viral infections, lymphadenitis may be observed as it regresses in the 1–2 weeks following resolution of the URTI [25]. For this reason, routine prescription of antibiotics is not recommended for all infectious lymphadenitis. However, if signs and symptoms indicate a bacterial infection, such as rapidly enlarging, fluctuant, asymmetric, or painful lymph nodes, a single course of a broad-spectrum antibiotic that is safe to use during pregnancy and the postpartum period may be reasonable [1]. As noted, for pregnant and lactating patients presenting with lymphadenitis, differentiating viral infection from bacterial infection is more important to avoid unnecessary use of antibiotics. For this purpose, appropriate microbiological, hematological, or serological testing may be implemented more often in these patients.

After observation or antibiotic treatment, the patient should be reassessed. Although the resolution of inflammatory lymphadenopathy may take up to 12 weeks, it is recommended that inflammatory masses should be re-examined within 2 weeks in order not to delay the evaluation for malignancy. In cases where the neck mass resolves over the expected time-course, it is recommended that a further follow-up clinic visit should be undertaken around 2–4 weeks later to assess any recurrence [1].

When a definite cause of lymphadenitis is confirmed, it is treated with specific antimicrobial regimens while taking into account the risks of medication used in pregnant and postpartum patients. Acute infection in salivary glands and congenital lesions are treated with antibiotics. Inflammatory conditions of lymph nodes and salivary glands are managed with appropriate treatment protocols.

53.5.2 Surgical Treatment

Because surgery during pregnancy is complicated by the need to balance the requirements of the patients, surgery is only performed when it is absolutely necessary for the well-being of the mother, fetus, or both. Although no anesthetic agents are teratogens, one should avoid exposure of the developing fetus to perioperative risks such as ionizing radiation, maternal hypoxia or hypercapnia, maternal stress and anxiety, metabolic disturbances such as severe hypoglycemia, and extremes of temperature [26]. The swelling and friability of oropharyngeal tissues, which are most pronounced near the end of pregnancy, can lead to difficulty in ventilation and intubation. Loss of airway control is the most common cause of anesthesia-related maternal mortality [27].

Within the context of these considerations, surgical excision of benign neck masses during pregnancy may be deferred to a time in the postpartum period. At this point, the patients should be informed about the fetal and maternal risks related to the surgery and reassured that these lesions can be followed up, because their treatment is not urgent and they typically have an extremely low risk of malignancy [28]. However, if there is airway compromise, unresponsiveness to antibiotic therapy, or abscess formation, surgery should not be postponed. If abscess formation occurs in the neck, intervention to drain the abscess is warranted. In pregnant patients, type of anesthesia and the approach for abscess drainage should be determined depending on the location and extent of the abscess. If possible, it should be performed with the least invasive approach (e.g., needle aspirations with USG) under local anesthesia, rather than general anesthesia. For any reason, if the surgery is unavoidable but not urgent, whenever possible, the operation should be done in the second trimester, thus avoiding the main period for miscarriage, organogenesis, and teratogenicity, but before the increased risk of preterm labor, which is the most common cause of fetal loss [26].

References

1. Pynnonen MA, Gillespie MB, Roman B, et al. Clinical practice guideline: evaluation of the neck mass in adults. Otolaryngol Head Neck Surg. 2017;157(2_suppl):S1–S30.
2. Balikci HH, Gurdal MM, Ozkul MH, et al. Neck masses: diagnostic analysis of 630 cases in Turkish population. Eur Arch Otorhinolaryngol. 2013;270(11):2953–8.
3. McGuirt WF. The neck mass. Med Clin North Am. 1999;83(1):219–34.
4. Sun GH. Evaluating neck masses in adult and pediatric patients. Medscape. https://www.medscape.com/viewarticle/911554_5. Accessed 11 July 2020.

5. Rosenberg TL, Brown JJ, Jefferson GD. Evaluating the adult patient with a neck mass. Med Clin North Am. 2010;94(5):1017–29.

6. Rosenberg TL. Differential diagnosis of adult neck masses. In: Kountakis SE, editor. Encyclopedia of otolaryngology, head and neck surgery. Berlin: Springer; 2013.

7. Simo R, Jeannon JP. Benign neck disease. In: Watkinson JC, Gilbert RW, editors. Stell & Maran's textbook of head and neck surgery and oncology. London: Hodder Arnold; 2012.

8. Simo R, Leslie A. Differential diagnosis and management of neck lumps. Surgery (Oxford). 2006;24(9):312–22.

9. Thandar MA, Jonas NE. An approach to the neck mass. CME. 2004;22:266–72.

10. Wetmore RF, Potsic WP. Differential diagnosis of neck masses. In: Lesperance MM, Flint PW, editors. Cummings pediatric otolaryngology. Philadelphia: Elsevier Saunders; 2015.

11. Tracy TF Jr, Muratore CS. Management of common head and neck masses. Semin Pediatr Surg. 2007;16(1):3–13.

12. Goffart Y, Hamoir M, Deron P, et al. Management of neck masses in adults. B-ENT. 2005; (suppl 1):133–40.

13. Franzen A, Günzel T, Buchali A, et al. Etiologic and differential diagnostic significance of tumor location in the supraclavicular fossa. Laryngoscope. 2018;128(3):646–50.

14. Maghami E, Ismaila N, Alvarez A, et al. Diagnosis and management of squamous cell carcinoma of unknown primary in the head and neck: ASCO guideline. J Clin Oncol. 2020;38(22):2570–96.

15. Puac P, Rodríguez A, Vallejo C, et al. Safety of contrast material use during pregnancy and lactation. Magn Reson Imaging Clin N Am. 2017;25(4):787–97.

16. Coakley F, Gould R, Hess C, et al. Guidelines for the use of CT and MRI during pregnancy and lactation. https://radiology.ucsf.edu/patient-care/patient-safety/ct-mri-pregnancy. Accessed 11 July 2020.

17. Tirada N, Dreizin D, Khati NJ, et al. Imaging pregnant and lactating patients. Radiographics. 2015;35(6):1751–65.

18. Ray JG, Vermeulen MJ, Bharatha A, et al. Association between MRI exposure during pregnancy and fetal and childhood outcomes. JAMA. 2016;316(9):952–61.

19. Paleri V, Mehanna H. Neck masses. In: Musheer Hussain S, editor. Logan Turner's diseases of the nose, throat and ear head and neck surgery. London: Taylor & Francis Group; 2016.

20. Alexander EK, Pearce EN, Brent GA, et al. 2017 guidelines of the American Thyroid Association for the diagnosis and management of thyroid disease during pregnancy and the postpartum [published correction appears in thyroid. 2017 Sep;27(9):1212]. Thyroid. 2017;27(3):315–89.

21. Gleeson M, Herbert A, Richards A. Management of lateral neck masses in adults. BMJ. 2000;320(7248):1521–4.

22. Haynes J, Arnold KR, Aguirre-Oskins C, et al. Evaluation of neck masses in adults. Am Fam Physician. 2015;91(10):698–706.

23. Novoa E, Gürtler N, Arnoux A, et al. Role of ultrasound-guided core-needle biopsy in the assessment of head and neck lesions: a meta-analysis and systematic review of the literature. Head Neck. 2012;34:1497–503.

24. Kalra A, Prucher GM, Hodges S. The role of core needle biopsies in the management of neck lumps. Ann R Coll Surg Engl. 2019;101(3):193–6.

25. Kamat AR, Schantz SP. Evaluation and management of the solitary neck mass. In: Sclafani AP, editor. Total otolaryngology—head and neck surgery. New York: Thieme Medical Publishers, Inc; 2015.

26. Brodsky JB, Cohen EN, Brown BW, et al. Surgery during pregnancy and fetal outcome. Am J Obstet Gynecol. 1980;138(8):1165–7.

27. Reitman E, Flood P. Anaesthetic considerations for non-obstetric surgery during pregnancy. Br J Anaesth. 2011;107(Suppl 1):i72–8.

28. Z-Coste AH, Lofgren DH, Shermetaro C. Branchial cleft cyst. https://www.ncbi.nlm.nih.gov/books/NBK499914/. Accessed 11 July 2020.

Cough During Pregnancy and Lactation

54

Gökhan Toptaş and Emel Çadallı Tatar

54.1 Introduction

Pregnancy is a complex psychological, biological, and physiological process that affects the expectant mother. Many physiological and hormonal changes occur during pregnancy, which lasts about 40 weeks. These changes might cause various otolaryngologic symptoms and signs; in addition, the management of different respiratory disorders in pregnancy is frequently influenced. Although airway mucosa hyperemia, hypersecretion, and mucosal edema could be seen beginning with the first trimester, these changes particularly maximize during the third trimester. Cough is one of the most frequent pregnant symptoms and should be treated in a multidisciplinary approach. While this treatment is given to pregnant women, special considerations should be made for physiological adaptation to the mother's pregnancy, changes in illness susceptibility, meeting fetal demands, and pharmacological effects on the fetus.

54.2 Anatomical and Physiological Changes in the Respiratory System During Pregnancy

Pregnancy causes significant physical, physiological, and biochemical changes, which have varying effects on various major organs. Changes occur shortly after conception and last during the pregnancy. As it is known, progesterone, estradiol, and cortisol levels increase during pregnancy. Progesterone increases ventilation but

G. Toptaş (✉) · E. Ç. Tatar
Otolaryngology Department, University of Health Sciences, Dışkapı Yıldırım Beyazıt Research and Training Hospital, Ankara, Turkey
e-mail: gogotoptas@hotmail.com; ectatar@gmail.com

© The Author(s), under exclusive license to Springer Nature Switzerland AG 2022
C. Cingi et al. (eds.), *ENT Diseases: Diagnosis and Treatment during Pregnancy and Lactation*, https://doi.org/10.1007/978-3-031-05303-0_54

decreases pulmonary vascular resistance. The response of the β-2 receptor, on the other hand, decreases as well as causes airway inflammation [1]. Additionally, increased mucosal vascularity and edema caused by progesterone-mediated vasodilation can cause rhinitis and epistaxis. Mucosal edema, hyperemia, secretion, and fragility occur in the respiratory tract during pregnancy, particularly in the last trimester. The larynx and trachea are affected by these changes in the upper respiratory tract. Nasal mucosal changes are mainly caused by estrogen. Estrogen induces congestion and hypersecretion, as well as increased tissue hydration and edema. Edema and increased secretion can lead to chronic coughing attacks. These changes in the upper respiratory tract cause pregnant women to mouth breathing [2].

The volume of the lungs changes dramatically during pregnancy. Although the respiratory rate is the same, the tidal volume increases, resulting in a 50% increase in minute ventilation compared to nonpregnant women [3, 4]. The diaphragm rises approximately 4–5 cm from its original position [5]. Hormone-induced relaxation of the ligaments that connect the ribs to the sternum causes the lower ribs to expand outward, increasing chest wall circumference and anteroposterior size. Therefore, pregnant women have become predisposing stress fractures in the ribs, even with minor trauma such as coughing [6, 7].

54.3   Cough

The most common symptom of patients admitted to the hospital is cough. As a result, it is both medically and socially significant [8]. The percentage of patients who come to outpatient clinics with a cough symptom ranges from 3 to 40%. This rate may be higher in pregnant women due to concomitant hormonal factors as increased frequency of reflux and pregnancy-specific rhinitis [8, 9].

Cough is a vagal response that clears foreign material and fluids from the airways [10]. Cough reflexes may be caused by a variety of inflammatory or mechanical changes in the airways, as well as inhalation of thermal and biological irritants, most often from upper airway locations like the larynx, bronchi, and other areas where the proximal airways branch [11]. Coughing is a three-part defensive response that includes (1) an inspiratory phase, (2) a forceful expiratory effort against a closed glottis, and (3) glottis opening followed by fast expiration. Complexity and plasticity characterize the reflex, which is triggered by both chemical and physical stimuli. Receptors on sensory nerves that react to these stimuli are classified as C-fiber receptors, slowly adapting receptors (SARs), or rapidly adapting receptors (RARs) based on their conductive properties [12, 13]. Cough receptors are found in the oropharynx, larynx, carina, external auditory canal, esophagus, diaphragm, and abdominal muscles. Chemical, pharmacological, and mechanical stimuli trigger cough receptors, which are polymodal.

54.3.1 Etiology

Cough may be the first sign of severe respiratory pathology in patients. Cough has a wide range of differential diagnoses, including infectious, inflammatory, and

Table 54.1 Etiology of cough

Pulmonary		Extrapulmonary	
Acute (<8 weeks)	Chronic (>8 weeks)	Acute (<8 weeks)	Chronic (>8 weeks)
Asthma Aspiration Inhalation Intoxication Pneumonia Pulmonary embolism Pneumothorax Pleurisy	Chronic bronchitis Asthma Bronchomalacia Bronchiectasis Cystic fibrosis Lung tumors Infectious diseases Other eosinophilic diseases Cigarette smoking	Infectious disease of the upper airways, mostly viral infection (common cold) Allergic disease Cardiac disease with acute pulmonary congestion	Chronic rhinitis, sinusitis, pharyngitis laryngitis (UACS/postnasal drip) Pregnancy-induced rhinitis Vocal cord dysfunction Obstructive sleep apnea Gastroesophageal reflux disease Drug-induced cough Cigarette smoking

neoplastic illnesses, as well as a variety of pulmonary disorders. For example; bronchopneumonia,, acute-on-chronic bronchitis, asthma, chronic bronchitis, chronic postnasal drip, small cell lung carcinoma, benign tumors, reflux esophagitis, foreign bodies, cardiovascular diseases, irritation of external auditory meatus, as well as in rare cases such as postviral vagal neuropathy [14]. In 88–100% of cases, the cause of cough may be identified, leading to targeted treatments with success rates ranging from 84 to 98% [15]. There are three subtypes of cough: acute; which lasts less than 3 weeks, subacute, which lasts 3–8 weeks, and chronic, which lasts more than 8 weeks. However, the causes of cough can be evaluated basically as acute and chronic (Table 54.1).

54.3.2 Clinical Evaluation

In patients presenting with cough, a detailed history and clinical examination is essential to look for the underlying cause and management of treatment. Some important details about the cough are crucial: for example, abrupt onset would suggest foreign body inhalation, and in gastroesophageal reflux disease (GERD), coughing on phonation or postprandially is common. Aside from its duration, length, and occupational exposure, other pulmonary symptoms, a change in the day, and association with exercise (usually in asthma) are all significant. Especially night coughs have been found to be associated with rhinitis [16]. In addition to cough, the following symptoms should be questioned: For gastroesophageal reflux disease (GERD), metallic taste, heartburn, for "cough syndrome of the upper respiratory tract" discharge, nasal congestion, anosmia, and regular throat clearing, For "sleep apnea syndrome," sleepiness, snoring, and attention problems [17]. Especially in pregnant women and postpartum lactation period, caution should be exercised, because these symptoms will increase. It is important to question about cigarette smoking, asthma, and other atopic conditions in the past or in the family. When asked about a patient's symptoms, they should also be asked how the individual's quality of life is affected. The Leicester Cough Questionnaire is a patient-reported survey that looks at how cough affects quality of life [18]. Another approved questionnaire is the Cough-Specific Quality of Life Questionnaire [19]. Diseases will be explained in subtitles in this chapter of the book due to variations in diagnosis and treatment of a cough during lactation and pregnancy, as well as the prevalence of particular disease subgroups.

54.4 Upper Airway Cough Syndrome

As known upper airway cough syndrome (UACS)—formerly postnasal drip syndrome (PNDS)—is one of the leading causes of chronic cough together with gastroesophageal reflux and asthma in pregnancy. Upper airway cough syndrome refers to chronic cough associated with various upper airway diseases such as chronic allergic rhinitis, chronic nonallergic rhinitis, chronic rhinosinusitis, and pregnancy-induced rhinitis (PIR) [20–22]. Direct nasal mucosa irritation, postnasal drip inflammation in the lower and upper airway inflammation, and cough reflex sensitization are the key mechanisms that cause cough in patients with nasal and sinus diseases [23]. The receptors in the hypopharynx and larynx are believed to be activated by irritant secretion from the paranasal region. These upper airway receptors have been shown to be more responsive in UACS patients than in healthy people [24]. UACS includes all forms of cough, both acute and chronic, caused by upper respiratory tract pathologies. Many studies have shown that UACS, alone or in association with other conditions, is the most common cause of chronic cough [25, 26]. The most common diseases that cause UACS during pregnancy are discussed.

54.5 Pregnancy Rhinitis

The terminology "pregnancy rhinitis" refers to an increase in pregnancy hormones, especially estrogen, in the nasal mucous cycle. Increases in its amount have an adverse effect on mucociliary transport as well as cause nasal congestion and obstruction complaints. Nasal congestion that occurs during the second or third trimester of pregnancy is known as pregnancy-induced rhinitis (PIR) and lasts for 6 weeks or longer with no specific allergic cause, and clears up within 2 weeks of delivery [27]. Along with rhinitis caused by hormonal changes during menstrual periods, puberty, menopausal symptoms, and different endocrine disorders such as acromegaly, PIR is categorized as hormone-induced rhinitis in a different category of nonallergic rhinitis patients [28]. Studies point out that PIR prevalence varies between 9 and 22% during pregnancy [29]. Various studies show that the duration of pregnancy and the severity of nasal obstruction are directly proportional [30]. Increase in nasal symptoms causes chronic postnasal drip and an increase in cough frequency. Pregnancy rhinitis is diagnosed clinically. Congestion is most common in the inferior turbinates on examination. Anterior rhinoscopic findings show watery or viscous clear discharge and inferior turbinates hypertrophy. Endoscopic examination is important in diagnosis for differential diagnosis. Given the limited nature of pregnancy, laboratory testing should be restricted. Pregnant women should avoid using imaging techniques. There have been studies linking PIR, snoring, and OSAS with preeclampsia, gestational hypertension, and intrauterine growth restriction during pregnancy. Aggravation of concomitant asthma and a reduction in life quality are among the complications of pregnancy rhinitis. Mouth breathing due to uncontrolled rhinitis causes dryness in the mouth due to decreased saliva and a decrease in intraoral protection mechanisms, thus increasing the tendency to develop sinusitis. For these reasons, controlling rhinitis during pregnancy both increases the life quality of the mother and reduces the risk of taking additional drugs such as antibiotics and systemic steroids [31]. The first step in the treatment of pregnancy rhinitis is to inform pregnant women about this at their first check-up. General recommendations should be made such as regular exercise, lifting the bed head, and the use of external nasal dilators. Saline irrigation, corticosteroids, intranasal anticholinergic, intranasal decongestants, and oral decongestant drugs could be considered as pharmacological treatments. When used at the recommended dosage, intranasal oxymetazoline can be used safely during pregnancy, since it has no systemic absorption. Oral decongestants can be preferred in cases of severe persistent pregnancy rhinitis, but they should not be used in pregnant women with hypertension. Intranasal corticosteroids, mainly budesonide, beclamatezon, and fluticasone propionate, are used in pregnancy rhinitis. Antihistaminics have not been proven to be effective in the treatment of pregnant rhinitis [32]. The treatment strategy for pregnancy and lactation will be discussed in the treatment subtitle.

54.6 Pregnancy and Allergic Rhinitis

Allergic rhinitis (AR) is a type of persistent nasal mucosa inflammation mediated by immunoglobulin E and triggered by allergens (IgE). The activation of T helper 2 (Th2) cells is involved in the development and maintenance of illness. It affects one out of every six people worldwide. A mix of environmental, genetic, and family susceptibility factors defines the genesis of AR. Seasonal or perennial allergens produce symptoms such as sneezing, rhinorrhea, nasal pruritus, chronic cough, and nasal congestion, which can be persistent or intermittent. In addition to being one of the risk factors for asthma, these symptoms have a negative influence on one's quality of life [33]. In one-third of pregnant women, allergic rhinitis symptoms worsen [34]. Allergic rhinitis and PIR can be easily differentiated with the patient's clinical history. Presence of allergic complaints before pregnancy, history of skin prick test, or the presence of drugs used in the diagnosis of allergic rhinitis helps in making a diagnosis. The main problem during pregnancy is an increase in allergic symptoms, as well as the disease's progression. AR is treated on a symptomatic basis. Environmental management (avoiding allergens), drugs (antihistamines, steroids, anticholinergics, etc.), and immunotherapy are among the treatment options. Despite the success of new antihistamines and local steroids, there are several instances where full symptom relief is not possible. In addition, the use of these medicines in particular patient categories, such as pregnant and lactating women, remains controversial. In the treatment title, the medications will be listed separately.

54.7 Pregnancy and Vasomotor Rhinitis

The symptoms of vasomotor rhinitis are similar to allergic rhinitis, but periodic symptoms are absent and the skin prick test is negative. Etiology of vasomotor rhinitis could be hot-cold exposure, hormonal changes (pregnancy, oral contraceptives containing high estrogen), thyroid pathologies (mixed edema), and medications (antihypertensives (guanethidine-alpha-adrenergic blockade). One of the mechanisms of the disease is increased mucosal parasympathetic involvement, which causes nasal vasodilation, congestion, and secretion. Ipratropium bromide is a nasal spray that is used to treat rhinorrhea. It is an anticholinergic drug (Category B).

54.8 Pregnancy and Gastroesophageal Reflux

Gastroesophageal reflux (GER) is estimated to occur in 30–50% of pregnancies, with the major reason being a decrease in lower esophageal sphincter pressure owing to progesterone surges [35]. According to some studies, this percentage can reach as high as 80%. Pregnancy precipitates GER symptoms, but the symptoms of reflux decrease after birth [36]. Those who had GERD pre-pregnancy are 3.79 times more likely to have GERD during pregnancy [37]. Mechanisms that might cause gastroesophageal cough include the following:

- The lower esophageal afferent neurons are directly affected by the substances or volume of reflux.
- Stimulation of the interconnecting neural pathways between the esophagus and the bronchi leads to an increased cough reflex.
- Coughing causes an increase in gastroesophageal reflux.

The first step should be conservative management by lifestyle and dietary modifications. Elevating the head of the bed, avoiding night feeding, cigarettes and alcohol, and established dietary causes like fatty foods, chocolate, and caffeine are only a few of them [38]. If symptoms in pregnancy are serious enough to require pharmacological treatment, there are a variety of choices currently. Proton pump inhibitors (PPIs), H2-antagonists, and a liquid alginate suspension may be used to treat the condition.

54.9 Asthma in Pregnancy

Bronchial asthma affects 6–12% of pregnant women around the world [39, 40]. Asthma affects pregnancy and leads to severe morbidity for both mother and the baby. It can cause wheezing, shortness of breath, and cough attacks. Severe, untreated asthma is linked to poor prenatal outcomes, such as a higher chance of prematurity, and birth defects or preeclampsia, and other complications [41–43]. Atopy and allergic rhinitis are often associated with asthma. The course of asthma during pregnancy is frequently unclear, with studies finding that about one-third of patients progress, one-third remain the same, and one-third worsen. Some women may experience a postpartum flare-up, even if their symptoms resolve throughout the third trimester of pregnancy. The increased prevalence of GER and pregnant rhinitis, which leads to postnatal drip, are two factors that contribute to the worsening. Establishing the diagnosis of asthma is the first step in treatment. The detection and avoidance of causes is the next step. Smoking should be avoided at all costs. Identification and treatment of GER, allergic rhinitis, and pregnancy rhinitis could be helpful for controlling the symptoms. The goal of asthma treatment is to get as much symptom relief as feasible ("controlled asthma") while using the fewest anti-asthmatic medicines at the lowest dose possible. Drug therapy during pregnancy is exactly the same as nonpregnant individuals. B2-agonists inhalation, oral-intravenous theophyllines, and magnesium sulfate should all be administered as usual. All of the medications mentioned can be used safely during lactation. Asthmatic mothers should be encouraged to breastfeed her baby, because breast-feeding reduces the risk of atopy [1].

54.10 Treatment

Five precaution groups are often used to develop a drug classification system in pregnancy: A, B, C, D, X. The FDA began replacing its old pregnancy classification (A, B, C, D, X) for newly approved drugs in June 2015 in the product information section, with a risk description that is more narrative, clinical factors, and under the pregnancy subsection. Most drugs were approved for cough therapy before this change. Therefore, drugs will be described in the old A through X classifications.

54.10.1 Nasal Saline Irrigation

Nasal irrigation methods should be mentioned as a nonpharmacological option for treating rhinitis and cough during pregnancy. Nasal saline clears the nose of debris and prevents congestion. Nasal lavage with a hypertonic nasal solution can be used to effectively treat pregnant women. According to Garavello et al., nasal irrigations have no obvious negative effects on the fetus [44]. As a result, nasal saline is an excellent first-line treatment.

54.10.2 Intranasal and Oral Decongestants

Oral decongestants that are most often used, such as pseudoephedrine and phenyl-ephrine, carry an FDA class C rating. Because of the possibility of gastroschisis, oral decongestants should be avoided [45]. In addition, an association was discovered between phenylephrine and endocardial cushion defects in the first trimester [46]. Long-acting (oxymetazoline and xylometazoline), intermediate-acting (naphazoline), and short-acting (phenylephrine) are the three types of intranasal decongestants. In a limited number of studies, oxymetazoline was compared to other local decongestants and has been shown that it is safer than the others. Overuse of intranasal decongestants is not recommended after 5 days due to the possibility of rhinitis medicamentosa [32]. There is no particular information about the usage of decongestants when breastfeeding. It is known that pseudoephedrine passes into breast milk.

54.10.3 Corticosteroids

Oral corticosteroids used by mothers during the first trimester have been linked to an increased risk of oral cleft malformations [47]. Systemic corticosteroids can only be used in rare cases during pregnancy to treat allergic rhinitis and asthma. When we look at nasal corticosteroids, budesonide carries an FDA class B rating. Other intranasal steroids are still classified as C, but recent evidence suggests that mometasone and fluticasone are safe to use during pregnancy. Intranasal use of beclomethasone, fluticasone propionate, or mometasone has not been related to any congenital organ malformations. Intranasal triamcinolone, on the other hand, has been linked to a number of respiratory malformations [48]. Although there is no evidence that topical corticosteroids move into breast milk, no substantial changes in breast milk levels or an increase in risk are expected.

54.10.4 Antihistamines

The safety of intranasal histamine during pregnancy is unknown. Chlorpheniramine, loratadine, and cetirizine carry an FDA class B rating. Cetirizine was not linked to a higher incidence of major malformations or a higher risk of teratogenicity [49]. However, mothers who use antihistamines have been associated with retrolental fibroplasia in infants weighing less than 1750 g at birth [50]. The use of antihistamines is not clear in pregnancy rhinitis.

54.10.5 Leukotriene Receptor Antagonists

Montelukast, zafirlukast, and zileuton are examples of leukotriene antagonists. The most researched leukotriene antagonist is montelukast during pregnancy. Montelukast is the most studied leukotriene antagonist. Montelukast carries B FDA pregnancy classification. Montelukast and Zafirlukast have not been associated with an increased risk of significant malformations in human studies [51].

54.10.6 Antitussives

Codeine is a morphine derivative that has a significant cough-inhibiting effect. It has been linked to caesarian birth and postpartum hemorrhage, although it is not teratogenic [52]. The other antitussive used is dextromethorphan. Despite the fact that dextromethorphan is an opium alkaloid, it has no analgesic or respiratory depressant effects at therapeutic dosages, and its dependence and abuse potential is negligible. It has a similar antitussive effect to codeine. If physical measures fail and the dry cough continues, codeine and dextromethorphan may be antitussive for a short period of during pregnancy.

54.10.7 Immunotherapy

Allergy rhinitis, both seasonal and permanent, can be effectively treated with allergen immunotherapy. Immunotherapy can be deemed safe for both the mother and the fetus during pregnancy; nevertheless, due to the risk of anaphylaxis, immunotherapy should not be started during pregnancy. Subcutaneous immunotherapy should not be begun or continued during pregnancy. The authors recommend that individuals who get pregnant and exhibit clinical improvement without systemic responses continue to receive allergy immunotherapy.

References

1. Gaga M, Oikonomidou E, Zervas E, et al. Asthma and pregnancy: interactions and management. Breathe. 2007;3:267–76.
2. Tetikkurt C. Respiratory physiology in pregnancy. Cerrahpaşa J Med. 2000;31:118–22.
3. Tan EK, Tan EL. Alterations in physiology and anatomy during pregnancy. Best Pract Res Clin Obstet Gynaecol. 2013;27(6):791–802. https://doi.org/10.1016/j.bpobgyn.2013.08.001.
4. Alaily AB, Carrol KB. Pulmonary ventilation in pregnancy. Br J Obstet Gynaecol. 1978;85:518–24.
5. Torgersen KL, Curran CA. A systematic approach to the physiologic adaptations of pregnancy. Crit Care Nurs Q. 2006;29(1):2–19. https://doi.org/10.1097/00002727-200601000-00002.
6. Sano A, Tashiro K, Fukuda T. Cough-induced rib fractures. Asian Cardiovasc Thorac Ann. 2015;23:958–60.
7. Baitner AC, Bernstein AD, Jazrawi AJ, et al. Spontaneous rib fracture during pregnancy. A case report and review of the literature. Bull Hosp Jt Dis. 2000;259(3):163–5.
8. Morice A. Chronic cough: epidemiology. Chron Respir Dis. 2008;5(1):43–7. https://doi.org/10.1177/1479972307084252.
9. Irwin RS. Introduction to the diagnosis and management of cough: ACCP evidence-based clinical practice guidelines. Chest. 2006;129(1 Suppl):25–7.
10. Canning BJ. Encoding of the cough reflex. Pulm Pharmacol Ther. 2007;20(4):396–401. https://doi.org/10.1016/j.pupt.2006.12.003.
11. Canning BJ, Mori N, Mazzone SB. Vagal afferent nerves regulating the cough reflex. Respir Physiol Neurobiol. 2006;152:223–42.
12. Schelegle ES, Green JF. An overview of the anatomy and physiology of slowly adapting pulmonary stretch receptors. Respir Physiol. 2001;125:17–31.

13. Sant'Ambrogio F. Nervous receptors in the tracheobronchial tree. Annu Rev Physiol. 1987;49:622–7.
14. Tatar EÇ, Öcal B, Korkmaz H, et al. Postviral vagal neuropathy: what is the role of laryngeal electromyography in improving diagnostic accuracy? J Voice. 2015;29(5):595–9.
15. Irwin RS, Boulet L-P, Cloutier MM, et al. Managing cough as a defense mechanism and as a symptom: a consensus panel report of the American College of Chest Physicians. Chest. 1988;114(Suppl):133–81.
16. Janson C, Chinn S, Jarvis D, et al. Determinants of cough in young adults participating in the European Community Respiratory Health Survey. Eur Respir J. 2001;18(4):647–54. https://doi.org/10.1183/09031936.01.00098701.
17. Sundar KM, Daly SE, Willis AM. A longitudinal study of CPAP therapy for patients with chronic cough and obstructive sleep apnoea. Cough. 2013;9(1):19.
18. Young EC, Smith JA. Quality of life in patients with chronic cough. Ther Adv Respir Dis. 2010;4:49–55.
19. French CT, Irwin RS, Fletcher KE, et al. Evaluation of a cough-specific quality-of-life questionnaire. Chest. 2002;121:1123–31.
20. Irvin RS, French CL, Chang AB, et al. Classification of cough as a symptom in adults and management algorithms. Chest. 2018;153:196–209.
21. Pratter MR. Chronic upper airway cough syndrome secondary to rhinosinus diseases ACCP evidence-based clinical practice guidelines. Chest. 2006;129:63–71.
22. Morice AH, McGarvey L, Pavord I, et al. Recommendations for the management of cough in adults. Thorax. 2006;61(suppl 1):1–24.
23. Lucanska M, Hajtman A, Calkovsky V, et al. Upper airway cough syndrome in pathogenesis of chronic cough. Physiol Res. 2020;69(Suppl 1):35–42. https://doi.org/10.33549/physiolres.934400.
24. Bucca C, Rolla G, Scappaticci E, et al. Extrathoracic and intrathoracic airway responsiveness in sinusitis. J Allergy Clin Immunol. 1995;95(1 Pt 1):52–9. https://doi.org/10.1016/s0091-6749(95)70152-4.
25. Pratter MR, Bartter T, Akers S, et al. An algorithmic approach to chronic cough. Ann Intern Med. 1993;119(10):977–83. https://doi.org/10.7326/0003-4819-119-10-199311150-00003.
26. Smyrnios NA, Irwin RS, Curley FJ, et al. From a prospective study of chronic cough: diagnostic and therapeutic aspects in older adults. Arch Intern Med. 1998;158(11):1222–8. https://doi.org/10.1001/archinte.158.11.1222.
27. Ellegard E, Karlsson G. Nasal congestion during pregnancy. Clin Otolaryngol Allied Sci. 1999;24(4):307–11.
28. Hellings PW, Klimek L, Cingi C, et al. Non-allergic rhinitis: position paper of the European Academy of Allergy and Clinical Immunology. Allergy. 2017;72(11):1657–65.
29. Ellegard E, Hellgren M, Toren K, et al. The incidence of pregnancy rhinitis. Gynecol Obstet Invest. 2000;49(2):98–101.
30. Bende M, Gredmark T. Nasal stuffiness during pregnancy. Laryngoscope. 1999;109:1108–10.
31. Namazy JA, Schatz M. Asthma and rhinitis during pregnancy. Mt Sinai J Med. 2011;78:661–70.
32. Caparroz FA, Gregorio LL, Bongiovanni G, et al. Rhinitis and pregnancy: literature review. Braz J Otorhinolaryngol. 2016;82(1):105–11.
33. Brozek JL, Bousquet J, Agache I, et al. Allergic rhinitis and its impact on asthma (ARIA) guidelines 2016 revision. J Allergy Clin Immunol. 2017;140:950–8.
34. Schatz M, Zeiger R. Allergic disease during pregnancy: current treatment options. J Respir Dis. 1998;19:834–42.
35. Richter JE. Gastroesophageal reflux disease during pregnancy. Gastroenterol Clin North Am. 2003;32(1):235–61.
36. Malfertheiner SF, Malfertheiner MV, Kropf S, et al. A prospective longitudinal cohort study: evolution of GERD symptoms during the course of pregnancy. BMC Gastroenterol. 2012;12:131.
37. Rey E, Rodriguez-Artalejo F, Herraiz MA, et al. Gastroesophageal reflux symptoms during and after pregnancy: a longitudinal study. Am J Gastroenterol. 2007;102:2395–400.

38. Ali RA, Egan LJ. Gastroesophageal reflux disease in pregnancy. Best Pract Res Clin Gastroenterol. 2007;21(5):793–806.
39. Tegethoff M, Olsen J, Schaffner E, et al. Asthma during pregnancy and clinical outcomes in offspring: a national cohort study. Pediatrics. 2013;132(3):483–91.
40. Kwon HL, Triche EW, Belanger K, et al. The epidemiology of asthma during pregnancy: prevalence, diagnosis, and symptoms. Immunol Allergy Clin North Am. 2006;26(1):29–62.
41. Murphy VE, Wang G, Namazy JA, et al. The risk of congenital malformations, perinatal mortality and neonatal hospitalisation among pregnant women with asthma: a systematic review and meta-analysis. BJOG. 2013;120:812–22.
42. Firoozi F, Lemière C, Ducharme FM, et al. Effect of maternal moderate to severe asthma on perinatal outcomes. Respir Med. 2010;104:1278–87.
43. Enriquez R, Griffin MR, Carroll KN, et al. Effect of maternal asthma and asthma control on pregnancy and perinatal outcomes. J Allergy Clin Immunol. 2007;120:625–30.
44. Garavello W, Somigliana E, Acaia B, et al. Nasal lavage in pregnant women with seasonal allergic rhinitis: a randomized study. Int Arch Allergy Immunol. 2010;151:137–41.
45. Torfs CP, Katz EA, Bateson TF, et al. Maternal medications and environmental exposures as risk factors for gastroschisis. Teratology. 1996;54:84–92.
46. Yau WP, Mitchell AA, Lin KJ, et al. Use of decongestants during pregnancy and the risk of birth defects. Am J Epidemiol. 2013;178:198–208.
47. Carmichael SL, Shaw GM. Maternal corticosteroid use and risk of selected congenital anomalies. Am J Med Genet. 1999;86:242–4.
48. Alhussien AH, Alhedaithy RA, Alsaleh SA. Safety of intranasal corticosteroid sprays during pregnancy: an updated review. Eur Arch Otorhinolaryngol. 2018;275(2):325–33.
49. Etwel F, Djokanovic N, Moretti ME, et al. The fetal safety of cetirizine: an observational cohort study and meta-analysis. J Obstet Gynaecol. 2014;34:392–9.
50. Zierler S, Purohit D. Prenatal antihistamine exposure and retrolental fibroplasia. Am J Epidemiol. 1986;123(1):192–6.
51. Bakhireva LN, Jones KL, Schatz M, et al. Safety of leukotriene receptor antagonists in pregnancy. J Allergy Clin Immunol. 2007;119:618–25.
52. Nezvalová-Henriksen K, Spigset O, Nordeng H. Effects of codeine on pregnancy outcome: results from a large population-based cohort study. Eur J Clin Pharmacol. 2011;67:1253–61.

Salivary Gland Infectious and Inflammatory Diseases During Pregnancy and the Postpartum Period

55

Emrah Gülmez, Öner Sakallıoğlu, and Luisa Maria Bellussi

55.1 Introduction

Saliva is a mixture of secretions discharged from the salivary glands into the oral cavity without the addition of pharyngeal, tracheal, and bronchial secretions. There are three pairs of major salivary glands including parotid, submandibular, and sublingual glands, in addition to 700–1000 minor salivary glands in the oral and pharyngeal mucosa.

Pregnancy is a period of numerous metabolic, endocrinological, and physiological changes in the whole body, including the ear, nose, and throat (ENT) region. These changes are mainly caused by hormones such as estrogen and progesterone and affect the physiological and immunological responses in the human body. Elevated serum cortisol levels result in relative gestational immunosuppression that may lead to reactivation of latent viral infections.

The effects of hormonal changes in the ENT region usually disappear with the birth of the infant, while it may persist in some infants. Estrogen and progesterone fluctuation in the third trimester leads to changes in mucosal membranes, particularly in nasal, oral, pharyngeal, and laryngeal membranes.

Saliva is a mixture of secretions discharged from the salivary glands into the oral cavity without the addition of pharyngeal, tracheal, and bronchial secretions. However, the fluids discharged from nasal cavity, pharynx, and oral mucosa drain into oral fluids [1].

E. Gülmez (✉) · Ö. Sakallıoğlu
Department of Otorhinolaryngology, Health Sciences University, Fethi Sekin City Hospital, Elazığ, Turkey
e-mail: emrahgulmez88@gmail.com; onersakallioglu@yahoo.com

L. M. Bellussi
University of Siena—ENT Clinic, Siena, Italy
e-mail: bellussi@unisi.it

C. Cingi et al. (eds.), *ENT Diseases: Diagnosis and Treatment during Pregnancy and Lactation*, https://doi.org/10.1007/978-3-031-05303-0_55

There are three pairs of major salivary glands including parotid, submandibular, and sublingual glands, in addition to 700–1000 minor salivary glands in the oral and pharyngeal mucosa. All of these glands produce serous, mucous, or seromucous secretion depending on their secretory properties. The normal daily production of saliva in a healthy adult varies between 1000 and 1500 cc [1].

Pregnancy is a period of numerous metabolic, endocrinological, and physiological changes in the whole body, including the ear, nose, and throat (ENT) region. These changes are mainly due to the production of hormones such as estrogen and progesterone, as well as placental hormones such as human chorionic gonadotropin (hCG), human placental lactogen (hPL), chorionic somatomammotropin (hCS), human chorionic thyrotropin (hCT), and human chorionic corticotropin (hCC) [2].

The hormonal changes in the body also affect the physiological and immunological responses in the human body. The effects of hormonal changes in the ENT region usually disappear with the birth of the infant, while it may persist in some infants. Estrogen and progesterone fluctuation in the third trimester leads to changes in mucosal membranes, particularly in nasal, oral, pharyngeal, and laryngeal membranes [3, 4].

Hormonal change during pregnancy increases the cardiac output and also leads to increased blood volume as well as inflammation in mucosal membranes. In turn, elevated serum cortisol levels result in relative gestational immunosuppression that may lead to reactivation of latent viral infections [3].

Numerous studies have shown that the oral mucosa is susceptible to the action of sex hormones. In particular, increased progesterone levels may cause bright red gums, bleeding gums, and swollen salivary glands. Therefore, there may be a direct link between oral health and changing hormonal status among women [5, 6].

Reduced saliva pH and flow rate and changes in saliva have been reported during pregnancy [7]. In a study conducted in Brazil, a significant decrease in saliva pH was observed in pregnant women compared to nonpregnant women. Additionally, the level of secretory immunoglobulin A was significantly increased in pregnant women compared to nonpregnant women [8].

55.2 Parotid Gland

Parotid gland is the largest of the salivary glands, lying anterior to the mandible ramus, posterior to the external auditory canal and mastoid process, superior to the zygoma, inferior to the angulus mandible, and medial to the parapharyngeal space. Inside the gland are the facial nerve and its branches, as well as the external carotid artery (ECA) and its branches, v. retromandibularis, and parotid lymphatics. The facial nerve separates the parotid gland into the superficial and deep lobes, although the mentioned separation is not anatomical. In the parotid gland, the facial nerve bifurcates into the temporofacial and cervicofacial divisions. The nerve then divides at the pes anserinus into the five terminal branches: temporal, zygomatic, buccal, marginal mandibular, and cervical. The parotid gland is the only major salivary gland that contains intraglandular lymph nodes [9].

The secretions of the parotid gland reach the oral cavity through the Stensen's duct. This duct traverses the masseter muscle, pierces the buccinator, and then opens out into the oral cavity at the level of the second upper molar.

The parotid gland is supplied by ECA and its branches. These branches synapse and then drain into the external jugular vein. The preganglionic parasympathetic fibers that travel to the parotid gland originate in the inferior salivatory nucleus of the glossopharyngeal nerve. These fibers accompany the glossopharyngeal nerve up to the jugular foramen, leave the nerve in the inferior ganglion, and join the tympanic (Jacobson's) nerve. This nerve forms the tympanic plexus of the middle ear, which gives off the lesser petrosal nerve. The fibers synapse in the otic ganglion, and postganglionic fibers then travel with the auriculotemporal nerve before reaching the parotid gland. Sympathetic fibers originate in the internal carotid plexus. The parotid gland produces serous secretion [10].

55.3 Submandibular Gland

The paired submandibular glands are located beneath the floor of the mouth, lying inferior to the body of the mandible, deep within the anterior part of the submandibular triangle. This triangle is bound by the two bellies of the digastric muscle and the body of the mandible and drains into the oral cavity through Wharton's duct at a location adjacent to the lingual frenulum. Wharton's duct ascends to the floor of the mouth, while the lingual nerve crosses this duct. Submandibular glands are supplied by the facial and lingual nerves. Preganglionic parasympathetic fibers originate in the superior salivatory nucleus and reach the lingual nerve through the chorda tympanic nerve. After synapsing in the submandibular ganglion, they reach the submandibular gland. Sympathetic fibers originate in the internal carotid plexus. Submandibular glands produce serous secretion [11].

55.4 Sublingual Gland

This gland sits on the mylohyoid muscles just beneath the mucosa of the floor of the mouth, adjacent to the lingual frenulum. It drains directly into the floor of the mouth via 10–20 ducts of Rivinus and via a major duct known as Bartholin's duct that drains into the Wharton's duct. The gland produces mucous secretion. Both submandibular and sublingual glands are supplied by the facial and lingual arteries. Its venous drainage is by two vessels: facial vein and sublingual vein [11].

55.5 Physiology

Saliva is a water-soluble composition of various substances with low and high molecular weight. It contains Na+, K+, Ca++, chloride, bicarbonate, urea, uric acid, proteins, lysozymes, IgA, and amylase in certain proportions.

The normal daily production of saliva in a healthy adult varies between 1000 and 1500 cc. The normal saliva flow rate is approximately 0.05–0.3 mL/min, and this rate increases to 0.18–1.7 mL/min when stimulated. Saliva flow rate varies throughout the day, which decreases at night and reaches its lowest circadian level at sleep. At rest, 69% of the saliva is secreted by the submandibular gland, 26% by the parotid gland, and 5% by sublingual glands. When stimulated, the parotid gland provides two-thirds of the salivary output and the minor glands are responsible for 7–8% of this output.

Dehydration, hospitalization, mental stress, emotional disorders, bodily devotion, beta-blockers, radiotherapy, Sjogren's syndrome, chronic infections, and anemia reduce saliva output. On the contrary, stomatitis, smoking, and fruits such as apple and lemon increase saliva output. Decreased salivary flow is considered a predisposing factor for salivary stones.

Main functions of saliva include facilitating food digestion, protecting oral cavity and dental structures, controlling bacteria in the oral cavity, and supporting the immune system [1, 12].

55.6 Patient History and Physical Examination

The onset of the complaint and the relationship between pain and eating should be questioned while taking patient history. On physical examination, palpation of the gland will reveal saliva coming from the orifice of Stensen's or Wharton's duct. Bimanual palpation of the gland and its duct is performed to examine the presence of stiffness, pain, calculi, fluctuation, and mass. In the presence of a mass, its degree of stiffness, presence of pain on palpation, and the state of fixation are assessed. If the available data are not sufficiently informative, radiological and laboratory examinations are performed.

- Recurrent severe attacks → Sialolithiasis or recurrent parotitis.
- Bilateral complaints → Sialadenosis or epidemic parotitis.
- Gender → Sjogren's syndrome is often seen in women.
- Pain, facial paralysis, regional lymph node metastasis, and skin ulcerations → Malignant tumor.
- Adenomas and sialadenosis occur in middle age.
- Incidence of malignant tumor increases with advancing age [13, 14].

55.7 Ultrasonography (USG)

It is helpful in the differentiation of cystic and solid masses and in the imaging of salivary gland calculi. On USG, the ductal system and the deep parotid lobe cannot be evaluated clearly [15].

55.8 Computed Tomography (CT)

It is among the imaging techniques that best distinguish salivary gland tissue from tumors. Its disadvantages include the following: it is a relatively expensive technique, leads to increased exposure to ionizing radiation, and cannot be used in pregnant women [16].

55.9 Magnetic Resonance Imaging (MRI)

It is superior to CT in visualizing soft tissues and it can show even lesions smaller than 2 mm. It cannot be used in patients with a pacemaker and metal clips [17].

55.10 Endemic Parotitis: Viral Parotitis

Swelling, redness, and mild swelling and hyperemia near the orifice of the duct are seen in parotitis. The secretion is not purulent in character. The intake of sour foods increases the pain. There is usually no accompanying fever. Swelling often starts on one side and then starts on the other side within 5 days. Parotitis may be accompanied by the involvement of submandibular and sublingual glands. Parotitis is a generalized viral infection. The causative agent is a neurotropic virus belonging to the paramyxoma group and it may cause an irreversible lesion in the eighth cranial nerve, leading to near-total unilateral deafness. Involvement of the pancreas may result in diabetes, involvement of the testicles and ovaries may lead to infertility, and the involvement of the central nervous system (CNS) may lead to aseptic meningitis. On the third of fourth of the disease, the amount of amylase in blood and urine reaches its maximum level. Treatment in parotitis is symptomatic, often including analgesics and anti-inflammatory drugs to reduce pain and fever. Cytomegalovirus, Coxsackie A, Echovirus, and Influenza virus may cause infections in the salivary glands. Treatment is symptomatic as in parotitis. HIV infection is often accompanied by the involvement of major salivary glands. Serological tests are performed when there is clinical suspicion for HIV [18, 19].

Several prospective epidemiological studies reported no significant increase in the incidence of major congenital anomalies in the infants of women who developed parotitis during pregnancy [20]. Similarly, a retrospective study that evaluated 510 pregnant women infected with parotitis virus during pregnancy reported no significant increase in the incidence of congenital anomalies among the infants. In another study, Ornoy found that parotitis in pregnancy could cause embryonic or fetal death as well as an increased incidence of spontaneous abortion, while it had no significant relationship with fetal congenital anomalies [21, 22].

55.11 Acute Suppurative Sialadenitis

It is a suppurative infection of the salivary gland parenchyma caused by a retrograde bacterial contamination from the oral cavity. It is frequently observed in the parotid gland. *Staphylococcus aureus (S. aureus)* is the most common cause. The salivary gland swells suddenly and is often painful. The infection is accompanied by fever and leukocytosis. If the parotid gland becomes infected, the auricle becomes more prominent. The salivary gland is sensitive on palpation and has a pasty consistency. There may be redness on the skin and if it turns to an abscess, fluctuation can be noticed. Palpation of the duct orifice may reveal purulent discharge coming from the gland. The infection may break out or spread to the external auditory canal via the fissures of Santorini. Patients may have trismus as well.

Patients with restricted oral intake and electrolyte/fluid imbalance in the postoperative period are at risk. Palpation of the parotid gland may reveal purulent discharge coming from the Stensen's duct. Treatment typically includes high-dose parenteral antibiotics effective against bacteria. The fluid/electrolyte imbalance is corrected.

A warm compress is applied on the gland. Sialogogues are recommended to the patient and particular attention is paid to oral hygiene. If there is an abscess, the external incisions are made by preserving the facial nerve [23, 24].

55.12 Sialolithiasis

Most often, only one salivary gland is affected. Submandibular gland is the most commonly involved gland (80%), followed by parotid gland (15%) and other glands (5%). The higher involvement of submandibular gland in sialolithiasis can be explained by the fact that the secretion produced by this gland is more viscous and contains more mucus, the duct of the gland is wide, partially curved, and flows from the bottom to the top, and the duct orifice is narrower than the duct and contains higher amounts of organic matter. Symptoms and complaints become apparent during eating and during periods with an increased number of secretory stimuli. Sudden swelling and severe pain develop under the chin and tongue and in front of and behind the earlobe. Patients with submandibular gland sialolithiasis may present with painful swelling under the chin where the lesion is localized, as well as congestion in the Wharton's duct trace in the floor of the mouth, pain on palpation, hyperemia and congestion depending on the severity of the infection (if present), increased pain and stone stiffness detected on bimanual examination, and mucopurulent secretion in the orifice of the Wharton's duct under the tongue. Almost 70% of submandibular gland calculi are localized to the Wharton's duct. USG can detect the solid mass as well as the width of the duct and the growth of the gland. Endoscopic approach with sialendoscopy is a newly described technique in sialolithiasis. It can be easily performed under local anesthesia and can be used for all gland swelling of unknown cause. Endoscopic intervention depends on the size of the calculi. Almost 97% of the calculi smaller than 3 mm in diameter can be removed with the aid of a wire basket. The calculi localized distal to the Wharton's duct of the submandibular gland can be removed through the oral cavity. The gland is removed in the presence of proximal and parenchymal calculi. In patients with parotid calculi, the calculi located in the Stensen's duct are removed by incisions made in the duct around the papillae. Intraglandular calculi require parotidectomy [23, 25, 26].

55.13 Chronic Recurrent Sialadenitis

It is mostly seen in the parotid gland. Reduction or cessation of saliva secretion is blamed in its pathogenesis. Over time, sialectasis, ductal ectasia, and lymphocyte infiltration occur in the affected salivary gland. Clinically, patients present with recurrent, mildly painful salivary gland swelling. If there are calculi or predisposing factors, they should be promptly treated. In addition to adequate hydration and salivary gland massage, antibiotics are used during acute attacks. In case of insufficient conservative treatment, the gland may need to be removed.

Chronic sclerosing sialadenitis of the submandibular gland (Kuttner tumor): The submandibular gland is hardened and enlarged, making it difficult to distinguish it from a true tumor. Histologically, loss of serous acinar cells, lymphocytic infiltration of interstitial connective tissue, and periductal sclerosis are seen. Therefore, it is considered to be an immunological disease. The salivary gland is removed for treatment, differential diagnosis, and histological examination and thus treated [27, 28].

55.14 Sialadenosis

It is mostly accompanied by recurrent or continuous, bilateral painless swelling of the parotid gland. Painful sialadenosis occurs as a side effect of antihypertensive drugs. It can also be seen in conditions such as diabetes, pregnancy, obesity, hypothyroidism, menopause, adrenal dysfunction, avitaminosis, protein deficiency, hunger strike, and alcoholism. Diagnosis is usually made by a careful history taking, determination of the underlying disease, and the observation of bilateral painless parotid swelling on examination. Treatment is directed at the underlying cause. Parotidectomy can be performed in cases with cosmetic defects caused by parotitis [29, 30].

55.15 Granulomatous Sialadenitis

It may cause a painless swelling in the parotid or submandibular gland. Peri- or intraglandular lymph nodes are the primary site of infection. Infected lymph nodes and salivary glands may need to be removed by preserving the facial nerve. Tuberculosis, actinomycosis, and cat-scratch disease are rare granulomatous diseases [31, 32].

55.16 Sjogren's Syndrome

Xerostomia often manifests as bilateral parotid swelling, keratoconjunctivitis sicca, and connective tissue diseases such as rheumatoid arthritis. Diagnosis is made by histopathological examination of the minor salivary glands in the biopsy of the lower lip. The autoimmune pathological reaction causes atrophy of the salivary gland parenchyma as well as interstitial lymphocytic infiltration and myoepithelial hypertrophy. In some cases, this syndrome may be accompanied by rheumatoid arthritis and multisystemic involvement. There are two types of Sjogren's syndrome: primary Sjogren's syndrome is characterized by xerostomia and xerophthalmia, while secondary Sjogren's syndrome is the condition accompanied by other connective tissue diseases. Ophthalmologic and rheumatologic follow-up along with long-term symptomatic treatment is required [33, 34].

Sjogren's syndrome is likely to worsen during pregnancy and more often in the postpartum period. Pregnancy outcomes in women with Sjogren's syndrome have not been extensively studied. Studies have reported increased rates of spontaneous abortion and associated fetal losses in pregnant women with Sjogren's syndrome. The reasons for this increase have been shown to include older age at the time of conception and low immunological factor mechanisms [35, 36].

Women with Sjogren's syndrome planning to conceive should undergo good counseling regarding all specific risks and complications. The appropriate time for conception should be planned according to contraindicated medications, underlying disease activity, and complications. Ideally, the disease should be controlled 3–6 months before conception [37].

55.17 Points to Consider in Treatment

Penicillins are undoubtedly the most widely prescribed antibiotics in pregnant women. These medications are the oldest known antibiotics. They exert their effect by inhibiting bacterial cell wall synthesis. All penicillin antibiotics are referred to as pregnancy category B [38].

Though not very common, allergic reactions can be seen. Allergic reactions ranging from simple rash to anaphylactic shock may occur. Preterm labor may occur due to excessive histamine release [39].

Since blood volume and glomerular filtration rate increase in pregnant women, plasma levels of antibiotics are reduced significantly compared to nonpregnant women [40].

Cephalosporin antibiotics are the second most widely used antibiotic group in pregnant women, following penicillin antibiotics. Cephalosporins were first discovered in 1940 and are currently grouped into four generations. These antibiotics are referred to as pregnancy category B [41].

Macrolide antibiotics exert bacteriostatic effect by inhibiting the protein synthesis of bacteria. Penicillin antibiotics are the antibiotics of choice in patients with antibiotic allergy [42]. Although erythromycin, roxithromycin, and azithromycin are pregnancy category B, clarithromycin is considered pregnancy category C [43, 44].

Analgesics are the second most widely used medication group during pregnancy and lactation, following vitamins. Paracetamol, nonsteroidal anti-inflammatory drugs (NSAIDs), and some opioids are used by pregnant and breastfeeding women due to acute, chronic, and pregnancy-related pain. Untreated pain can have negative effects on pregnancy. For this reason, after fulfilling certain conditions, pain in pregnant and breastfeeding women should be treated so as to prevent unnecessary pain. In the selection of the analgesic to be used in pregnant women, several factors including pharmacological properties of the drug, duration of treatment, gestation period, and the time of delivery should be considered. In the lactation period, besides pharmacological properties of the drug, factors such as the age of the infant, duration and dose of medication, rate of drug passage from maternal plasma into milk, and breastfeeding time should be taken into consideration. In general, paracetamol, NSAIDs, and opioids are considered safe during pregnancy and lactation when used in appropriate doses and for a short period of time. Aspirin and NSAIDs should be avoided in early pregnancy and in the third trimester. Long-term opioid use is not recommended [45].

Local anesthetics including lidocaine and prilocaine are considered pregnancy category B, while mepivacaine and bupivacaine are considered pregnancy category C. Long-term use of narcotic analgesics in the third trimester leads to neonatal respiratory depression [46].

References

1. Edgar W. Saliva: its secretion, composition and functions. Br Dent J. 1992;172(8):305–12.
2. Bhagat DR, Chowdhary A, Verma S. Physiological changes in ENT during pregnancy. Indian J Otolaryngol Head Neck Surg. 2006;58(3):268–70.
3. Kumar R, Hayhurst KL, Robson AK. Ear, nose, and throat manifestations during pregnancy. Otolaryngol Head Neck Surg. 2011;145(2):188–98.
4. Sherlie VS, Varghese A. ENT changes of pregnancy and its management. Indian J Otolaryngol Head Neck Surg. 2014;66(1):6–9.
5. Ferris G. Alteration in female sex hormones: their effect on oral tissues and dental treatment. Compendium (Newtown, Pa). 1993;14(12):1558–64, 66; quiz 71.
6. Güncü G, Tözüm T, Çaglayan F. Effects of endogenous sex hormones on the periodontium—review of literature. Aust Dent J. 2005;50(3):138–45.
7. Laine M, Tenovuo J, Lehtonen O-P, Ojanotko-Harri A, Vilja P, Tuohimaa P. Pregnancy-related changes in human whole saliva. Arch Oral Biol. 1988;33(12):913–7.
8. Rockenbach MI, Marinho SA, Veeck EB, Lindemann L, Shinkai RS. Salivary flow rate, pH, and concentrations of calcium, phosphate, and sIgA in Brazilian pregnant and non-pregnant women. Head Face Med. 2006;2(1):44.
9. Arıncı K, Elhan A. Anatomi, 1. Cilt, Güneş Kitabevi, ISBN. Ankara; 2006.
10. Moore KL, Dalley AF, Agur AM. Clinically oriented anatomy. Philadelphia: Lippincott Williams & Wilkins; 2013.
11. Snell RS. Clinical anatomy: an illustrated review with questions and explanations. Philadelphia: Lippincott Williams & Wilkins; 2004.

12. Turner B. Mechanisms of fluid secretion by salivary glands. Ann NY Acad Sci. 1993;694:24–35.
13. Kaya S. Tükürük bezi hastalıkları. Ankara: Güneş Tıp Kitabevi; 1997.
14. Byrne MN, Gershon JG, Garvin CF, Gado MH. Preoperative assessment of parotid masses: a comparative evaluation of radiologic techniques to histopathologic diagnosis. Laryngoscope. 1989;99(3):284–92.
15. Salaffi F, Carotti M, Argalia G, Salera D, Giuseppetti G, Grassi W. Usefulness of ultrasonography and color Doppler sonography in the diagnosis of major salivary gland diseases. Reumatismo. 2006;58:138–56.
16. Yousem DM, Kraut MA, Chalian AA. Major salivary gland imaging. Radiology. 2000;216(1):19–29.
17. Shah GV. MR imaging of salivary glands. Magn Reson Imaging Clin N Am. 2002;10(4):631–62.
18. Brook I. Diagnosis and management of parotitis. Arch Otolaryngol Head Neck Surg. 1992;118(5):469–71.
19. Elbadawi LI, Talley P, Rolfes MA, Millman AJ, Reisdorf E, Kramer NA, et al. Non-mumps viral parotitis during the 2014–2015 influenza season in the United States. Clin Infect Dis. 2018;67(4):493–501.
20. Siegel M. Congenital malformations following chickenpox, measles, mumps, and hepatitis: results of a cohort study. JAMA. 1973;226(13):1521–4.
21. Manson MM, Logan WPD, Loy RM. Rubella and other virus infections during pregnancy: a report based on data assembled during 1950-1957 by the medical officers of health of the local authorities of Great Britain. HM Stationery Office; 1960.
22. High P, Handschur E, Eze O, Montana B, Robertson C, Tan C, et al. Update: mumps outbreak-New York and New Jersey, June 2009-January 2010 weekly. Morb Mortal Wkly Rep. 2010;59(5):125–9.
23. Peterson LJ, Hupp T. Contemporary oral and maxillofacial surgery. 4th ed. New York: Mosby; 2003. p. 195–235.
24. Atkinson JC, Wu AJ. Salivary gland dysfunction: causes, symptoms, treatment. J Am Dent Assoc. 1994;125(4):409.
25. Nahlieli O, Baruchin AM. Endoscopic technique for the diagnosis and treatment of obstructive salivary gland diseases. J Oral Maxillofac Surg. 1999;57(12):1394–401.
26. Marchal F, Dulguerov P, Becker M, Barki G, Disant F, Lehmann W. Specificity of parotid sialendoscopy. Laryngoscope. 2001;111(2):264–71.
27. Ahuja A, Richards P, Wong K, King A, Yuen H, Ching A, et al. Kuttner tumour (chronic sclerosing sialadenitis) of the submandibular gland: sonographic appearances. Ultrasound Med Biol. 2003;29(7):913–9.
28. Wang S, Marchal F, Zou Z, Zhou J, Qi S. Classification and management of chronic sialadenitis of the parotid gland. J Oral Rehabil. 2009;36(1):2–8.
29. Coleman H, Altini M, Nayler S, Richards A. Sialadenosis: a presenting sign in bulimia. Head Neck. 1998;20(8):758–62.
30. Pape S, MacLeod R, McLean N, Soames J. Sialadenosis of the salivary glands. Br J Plast Surg. 1995;48(6):419–21.
31. Dangore-Khasbage S, Bhowate RR, Degwekar SS, Bhake AS, Lohe VK. Tuberculosis of parotid gland: a rare clinical entity. Pediatr Dent. 2015;37(1):70–4.
32. Mandel L, Surattanont F. Bilateral parotid swelling: a review. Oral Surg Oral Med Oral Pathol Oral Radiol Endodontol. 2002;93(3):221–37.
33. Andonopoulos A, Drosos A, Skopouli F, Acritidis N, Moutsopoulos H. Secondary Sjögren's syndrome in rheumatoid arthritis. J Rheumatol. 1987;14(6):1098–103.
34. Pijpe J, Kalk W, Van der Wal J, Vissink A, Kluin PM, Roodenburg J, et al. Parotid gland biopsy compared with labial biopsy in the diagnosis of patients with primary Sjögren's syndrome. Rheumatology. 2007;46(2):335–41.
35. Julkunen H, Kaaja R, Kurki P, Palosuo T, Friman C. Fetal outcome in women with primary Sjogren's syndrome: a retrospective case-control study. Obstet Gynecol Surv. 1995;50(11):766–8.

36. Sandhya P, Jeyaseelan L, Scofield RH, Danda D. Clinical characteristics and outcome of primary Sjogren's syndrome: a large Asian Indian cohort. Open Rheumatol J. 2015;9:36.
37. Gupta S, Gupta N. Sjögren syndrome and pregnancy: a literature review. Perm J. 2017;21:16-047.
38. Czeizel AE, Rockenbauer M, Sørensen HT, Olsen J. A population-based case-control teratologic study of ampicillin treatment during pregnancy. Am J Obstet Gynecol. 2001;185(1):140–7.
39. Shepherd GM. Hypersensitivity reactions to drugs: evaluation and management. Mt Sinai J Med. 2003;70(2):113–25.
40. Einarson A, Shuhaiber S, Koren G. Effects of antibacterials on the unborn child. Paediatr Drugs. 2001;3(11):803–16.
41. Christensen B. Which antibiotics are appropriate for treating bacteriuria in pregnancy? J Antimicrob Chemother. 2000;46(suppl_1):29–34.
42. Hedstrom S, Martens MG. Antibiotics in pregnancy. Clin Obstet Gynecol. 1993;36(4):886–92.
43. Einarson A, Phillips E, Mawji F, D'Alimonte D, Schick B, Addis A, et al. A prospective controlled multicentre study of clarithromycin in pregnancy. Am J Perinatol. 1998;15(9):523–5.
44. Garland SM, O'Reilly MA. The risks and benefits of antimicrobial therapy in pregnancy. Drug Saf. 1995;13(3):188–205.
45. Aksu F, Akyüz ME. Gebelik ve Emzirme Döneminde Analjezik Kullanımı (Asetaminofen, Aspirin, Nonsteroid Antiinflamatuar İlaçlar, Opioidler). Türkiye Klinikleri Farmakoloji-Özel Konular. 2018;6(3):86–91.
46. Becker DE, Rosenberg M. Nitrous oxide and the inhalation anesthetics. Anesth Prog. 2008;55(4):124–31.

Başat Fethallah, Nuray Bayar Muluk, and Felicia Manole

56.1   Introduction

Thyroid disorders occur in approximately 5% of pregnant women. Untreated thyroid disease in the mother makes an adverse outcome in pregnancy more likely to occur and may harm the newborn, but treatment can mitigate these consequences. Levothyroxine is frequently used as a treatment for hypothyroidism. In pregnant women, the treatment dose is generally higher than in nonpregnant patients. Hyperthyroid disease in pregnant women is typically treated by means of antithyroid agents, but caution is needed, since methimazole has an association with congenital defects and propylthiouracil raises the risk of toxicity to the liver in the mother. It is advised that pregnant women in the initial trimester be administered propylthiouracil, which can later be converted to methimazole treatment to decrease the likelihood of liver damage. The aim of treating under- or overactivity of the thyroid in pregnant women is to reach a euthyroid state as rapidly as possible and ensure this remains so for the entire pregnancy. Currently, intervention is not recommended in pregnant women suffering from autoimmune thyroiditis nor isolated

B. Fethallah (✉)
Department of Otorhinolaryngology, Samsun Gazi State Hospital, Samsun, Turkey
e-mail: basatf@yahoo.com

N. Bayar Muluk
Department of Otorhinolaryngology, Faculty of Medicine, Kırıkkale University,
Kırıkkale, Turkey
e-mail: nbayarmuluk@yahoo.com

F. Manole
Faculty of Medicine and Pharmacy, Department of Otorhinolaryngology,
University of Oradea, Oradea, Bihor, Romania
e-mail: manole.felicia@gmail.com

C. Cingi et al. (eds.), *ENT Diseases: Diagnosis and Treatment during Pregnancy
and Lactation*, https://doi.org/10.1007/978-3-031-05303-0_56

hypothyroxinemia, provided there are no signs of hypothyroidism. It is usually safe practice to delay treating thyroid nodules or low-grade thyroid carcinoma until the end of pregnancy [1].

56.2 Physiological Changes in the Thyroid Gland in Pregnant Women

The healthy adaptations in thyroid function observed in pregnant women have been extensively studied [2]. Thyroxine-binding globulin levels rise from the beginning of pregnancy until mid-term, in response to an elevation in circulating estrogen. By contrast, thyroid-stimulating hormone concentrations fall initially, since human chorionic gonadotropin exercises a direct stimulatory effect on the thyroid. The thyroid steadily grows in size as the pregnancy progresses and the production of thyroid hormones also goes up. The mother needs greater amounts of dietary iodine because of greater clearance by the kidneys and the demands of the fetus and placenta. In a sense, pregnancy may be considered a form of stress testing for the woman, insofar as a woman whose reserve thyroid capacity is low will be likely to exhibit hypothyroid signs [3].

56.3 Diagnosis

The diagnosis of a thyroid disorder in a pregnant woman is complicated by the fact that pregnancy itself causes changes resembling thyroid disease, for example, gaining weight, feeling excessively tired, and being constipated, which might otherwise indicate an underactive thyroid, or feeling nauseous and wanting to eat more, which may be observed in hyperthyroid individuals [4, 5]. At present, it is recommended that women who are at an elevated risk of thyroid disorders be screened either preconception or during the initial stages of pregnancy by taking a TSH level. If this returns abnormal, further tests are confirmatory of thyroid disease, or allow grading of severity [3, 6]. It is important to note that the reference limits for TSH and free T4 are calculated for nonpregnant individuals and the normal values in pregnancy are known to diverge from these limits due to physiological adaptations [3, 6]. A number of researchers have tried to establish reference ranges for TSH in normal pregnancy at different stages, depending on the trimester and the population involved [7–9]. However, if no such reference range has been calculated, the following values for TSH may be used to diagnose hypothyroidism: >2.5 mIU.L^{-1} up to the end of the 12th week of gestation, and >3.0 mIU.L^{-1} thereafter [3, 6]. The degree to which TSH is raised, as well as the free thyroxine level, may be used to differentiate cases of subclinical from overt hypothyroid disease [3, 6]. The reference range for TSH in pregnant women also extends lower than in nonpregnant individuals; thus, if the nonpregnant reference range is applied to a woman with healthy thyroid function, she may appear to be hyperthyroid on screening, that is, the result will represent a false positive [3]. It may be sensible to repeat a TSH level within a week in a patient where the TSH alone is elevated, or where free thyroxine is low, particularly when only marginally so. This is a helpful practice diagnostically. A study examining cases where the TSH was raised, but free thyroxine levels normal, found that the TSH remained persistently raised in only 56% of pregnant individuals who were tested a second time, 7 days later [10].

The ideal method to quantify free thyroxine levels in pregnant patients utilizes equilibrium dialysis followed by mass spectrometry [11]. Equipment to carry out the assay is not always available, however, and thus, immunoassays are often relied upon, in spite of their tendency to provide an inaccurate measurement of free thyroxine levels because of binding to thyroglobulin [12]. Thyroglobulin is elevated in pregnancy. However, the immunoassay method does at least reflect the overall changes in pregnant women, whereby a rise in the first trimester is followed by falling levels as the pregnancy progresses. Measurements undertaken with a particular type of free thyroxine assay may be compared with each other, but results from different assays cannot be directly compared and thus the laboratory should publish reference intervals that are specific for a particular assay and for a certain stage in the pregnancy [3, 6, 12]. It has been suggested by some experts that the solution to this issue is to measure T4 of both bound and unbound type [6]. This solution suffers from the disadvantage that the T4 reference interval is larger than for free T4, since the levels of thyroglobulin vary, and thus, diagnosis may be complicated, particularly with results just outside the reference range [13]. It is possible to calculate a reference range for T4 in the mid and final trimester by using the reference range in nonpregnant individuals and increasing it by 50% [6]; however, the reference interval for T4 in the first 12 weeks of pregnancy, when thyroglobulin synthesis steps up, has not been established. Accordingly, quantification of free T4 is of greater benefit diagnostically, in distinguishing subclinical from overt thyroid disorders. Nonetheless, the diagnosis and management of thyroid disease in pregnancy is more soundly based on the serum TSH level and the clinical presentation [3, 6].

56.4 Thyroid Nodules and Thyroid Cancer

Thyromegaly occurs in pregnant women, and thus is a potential risk factor in the enlargement of thyroid nodules [3]. At present it is unknown whether diagnosis of thyroid nodules is more common in pregnancy than at other times [3]. In general terms, the way to diagnose a thyroid nodule does not differ according to whether the patient is pregnant or not, with the caveat that radioisotopic scanning is not permissible in a pregnant patient [3, 14]. When a thyroid nodule is noted, the clinician should obtain a thorough history, including family history, and examine the patient physically. Venous blood should be sent for thyroid function tests [3, 14]. Ultrasonic scans of the thyroid possess high accuracy and are of value in pregnant patients for ascertaining the form of the lesion and its growth rate [3]. Biopsy may be safely undertaken using a fine-needle aspirate and its diagnostic efficacy is not affected by pregnancy [3].

The prognosis for pregnant women who have low-grade thyroid neoplasms does not appear to be worsened by delaying treatment until after delivery [3, 14]. Thus, it is reasonable to wait until the end of pregnancy before operating on such patients, albeit the lesion should be followed up ultrasonographically during the pregnancy [3, 14]. Consideration should be given to treating the woman with thyrosuppressive agents, aiming to bring TSH to the level of 0.1–1.5 mIU.L^{-1} [3, 14]. If the lesion is such as to call for operative removal without delay, it is preferable from a safety point of view to operate within the second trimester [3, 14]. In general, nonmalignant nodules of the thyroid do not call for therapy while the patient is pregnant. Treatment may be needed, however, if the nodule compresses other structures or enlarges at an alarming rate [3, 14].

If a pregnant patient has previously had a malignant neoplasm of the thyroid, which is now in remission and is being treated with thyrosuppression, thyrosuppressive treatment should not be discontinued, since there is a benefit to the outcome of pregnancy [3, 15–17]. Thyrosuppressive treatment is guided by the risk that the tumor will persist and the possibility of a recurrent lesion [3]. If the lesion persists, the goal is to maintain TSH at a level under 0.1 mIU.L^{-1}, whereas a level of 0.1–0.5 mIU.L^{-1} is appropriate in a patient where the lesion is remitting but carries a high risk that it may recur. If the lesion is both in remittance and unlikely to recur, the clinician should aim for a level of 0.3–1.5 mIU.L^{-1} [3]. To achieve these treatment objectives, pregnant women with thyroid malignancies generally need to be administered levothyroxine in addition to thyrosuppressive agents; however, the dosage required is less than in a case of primary hypothyroidism [18]. To monitor whether these objectives are being reached, thyroid function tests should be ordered monthly or at six-weekly intervals [1, 3].

56.4.1 Thyroid Nodules

56.4.1.1 Epidemiology

There are a number of studies published in which ultrasonic imaging of the thyroid was used to determine the frequency of nodules in pregnant women [19–23]. Between 3 and 30% of pregnant women were found to have a thyroid nodule, with the lesions becoming more common as age and the number of children increased [20–23]. There have been suggestions that not only does a pregnant state lead to larger nodules, but that it may actually trigger the formation of newly existing nodules. Different studies have reached different conclusions regarding growth of thyroid nodules in pregnancy. One study reported the size doubled [20], whereas a different study [21] noted there was no permanent increase in magnitude. Furthermore, if a woman is found to possess a thyroid nodule during the initial trimester, there is a risk of up to 20% that a further nodule will form by the end of the pregnancy [20, 23].

The malignant potential of pregnancy-associated thyroid nodules is currently not known. Four studies, employing varied methodologies, have been undertaken to answer this question. In the study by Kung AW et al., a prospective methodology was used to follow up 221 pregnant women from South China from the initial trimester onward. In the initial trimester, 15.3% of the women had evidence of thyroid nodules, but this went up to 24.4% when the women were assessed 3 months after delivery. In 34 women, there was at least one thyroid nodule, none of which had malignant neoplastic features [22]. Three other studies, each of which were single center, used a cross-sectional design to evaluate the frequency of cancer in thyroid nodules detected in pregnant women [24–26]. This research reported that between 12 and 43% of nodules were malignant neoplasms. This surprising conclusion should be considered in the light of various biases inherent in the sample selection, namely, the fact that all these cases had been referred to academic centers of expertise in managing thyroid nodules and thus may not be typical of pregnant women with thyroid nodules in general. Accordingly, the incidence of malignancy found in this research is likely to be above that normally expected in pregnant women with thyroid nodular disorders [19].

56.4.1.2 Diagnosis

Just as with any patient presenting with a potential thyroid nodular lesion, a thorough history should be obtained from pregnant patients, followed by examining them physically [27, 28]. Particular details to enquire about include any family history of thyroid malignancy, and whether the patient has been exposed to radiation in the head and neck region, including ionizing radiation. When physically examining a patient, the neck needs to be inspected and palpated with great attention to detail. Venous blood should be sent for estimation of TSH level, although this typically falls within the normal range even when a nodule is present. Where the TSH level is suppressed in patients, the possibility that this is due to thyroid overactivity is usually assessed by a radioisotopic study. This procedure is problematic in a pregnant patient. For one thing, there is a normal fall in TSH during early pregnancy as a result of the rise in beta-human chorionic gonadotropin, since this molecule acts upon the TSH receptor, duplicating the action of TSH. Furthermore, there are concerns that the radionuclides used, that is, Tc-99m pertechnetate or ^{123}I, may be teratogenic. There have been no studies, which explicitly address this issue, but current guidance forbids their use in pregnant women. All radioisotopes have the potential to be teratogenic, since they may either enter the fetal circulation via the placenta or may irradiate the fetus when they accumulate in the mother's urinary bladder or other organs [27, 29]. The recommendation is not routinely to check the baseline levels of thyroglobulin or calcitonin in venous blood [27].

Ultrasonographic imaging of the neck is still the imaging method with the highest accuracy and safety for detection of nodular thyroid disease. It allows assessment of the pattern and distinguishing features of nodes and allows the lymph nodes of the neck to be scanned in pregnant women. There are clinical algorithms available, such as the American Thyroid Association guidelines, TI-RADS, among others, which allow an assessment of the risk of thyroid cancer on the basis of the findings from ultrasonography. The assessment of risk then helps the clinician decide whether to proceed to undertake a biopsy using a fine needle [30, 31].

Aspiration with a fine needle (FNA) is the biopsy method with the highest accuracy and cost-effectiveness to assess thyroid nodules. It is the first-line investigation of a nodule in pregnancy when the TSH is elevated or within the reference range. Up to now, research indicates that FNA benefits from a favorable safety profile and is appropriate throughout pregnancy [32–37]. There do not appear to be any particular cytologically observable effects on thyroid nodules due to pregnancy itself; thus, the standard cytological criteria are applicable [28]. Tan GH et al. undertook a retrospective review of 40 cases where FNA was performed during pregnancy and then histopathology was carried out on a surgically resected specimen later. The cytological and histopathological findings demonstrated a high level of consistency, indicating that pregnancy did not affect the pathological features [24]. This finding indicates also that the patient should be offered the chance to delay FNA until after delivery, as this will not change the outcome. Some experts believe that pregnancy may speed up the development of nodular disorders of the thyroid. It has also been demonstrated that there is a modest benefit from treatment with levothyroxine, resulting in a 20% reduction in size [27, 30, 38]. However, this intervention runs the risk of creating iatrogenic thyrotoxicosis and should therefore not be undertaken. If the cytological appearances from a thyroid nodule in a pregnant patient do not indicate malignancy, management does not differ greatly from the approach in nonpregnant individuals [27, 30]. If cytology indicates an indeterminate result, that is, atypical appearances of unclear etiology, a follicular lesion of uncertain type, potential follicular-type tumor or potentially malignant, the pregnant patient may be followed up in a conservative way until delivery, since most cytological results of this kind are later found to represent benign lesions plus there is an absence of evidence gathered prospectively to favor a more aggressive approach [27]. There is also the problem that the molecular biomarkers recommended to improve risk prediction before surgery in cases where cytology is inconclusive have not undergone validation in samples taken during pregnancy. Theoretically, pregnancy is anticipated to alter RNA transcription in the thyroid and this may impact the validity of diagnostic tests based on RNA synthesis. Tests, which depend on DNA genotyping, should, in theory, be less susceptible to alterations induced by pregnancy [39]. However, the paucity of data on actual use and the possibility of reduced diagnostic utility mean that molecular biomarkers are not suitable for risk stratification of patients with thyroid cytology that is indeterminate [27].

56.4.1.3 Management of Thyroid Nodules in Pregnant Patients

It is estimated that between 5 and 6% of adult females have a thyroid nodule that can be felt on palpation, while with imaging (computed tomography, MRI, or ultrasonography), the presence of a nodule can be detected in approximately 68% of the general adult population [40]. While thyroid nodules occur, whether singly or multiply, with increasing frequency as patients get older, the first presentation of a nodular lesion may occur in young women when they become pregnant. The usual way a nodule is detected is when the neck is palpated. One reason may be that pregnant women have more contact with doctors during pregnancy than at other times. Since the natural history of thyroid nodules involves their slowly enlarging [41, 42], it is reasonable to suppose the majority of nodules were already present before the woman became pregnant. The mean age at which conception occurs in the USA has been going up for the last 40 years, and it has become common for women aged over 30 to attempt to conceive [43]. Given the way thyroid nodules form and the increasing occurrence with age, we may reasonably anticipate that presentations of a thyroid nodule during pregnancy will keep becoming ever more common. This is important to remember, since the reason for assessing thyroid nodules is to identify thyroid malignancy, even though in practice, only around 8–16 in 100 will eventually be shown to be cancerous [40, 44–46].

The endocrine and other physiological adaptations seen in pregnant women appear to have an effect both in terms of triggering nodule formation and in enlarging existing nodules [22, 47]. According to a study undertaken by Kung et al. [22], in which 221 pregnant women were assessed for thyroid nodules throughout their pregnancy, there was an almost 10% increase in patients with a detectable thyroid nodule, from the initial trimester up to the time of delivery. Nonetheless, the majority of nodules detected de novo during the pregnancy were diminutive in size, being under 5 mm in diameter. A different study, undertaken by Karger et al., used a case-control design to examine the frequency of thyroid nodules in parous versus nulliparous patients [47]. This study established that nodular lesions of the thyroid are more common in women who have given birth. A further study [48] examined 26 pregnant women living in an area with low levels of environmental iodine. The researchers discovered that the dimensions of the largest nodules increased by an average of 0.7 mm, but there was no corresponding increase in the volume of the lesions at the level of statistical significance and no new nodules were formed [48]. Even where nodules are newly formed, they may produce no clinically significant changes and thus, the evidence to date does not support routinely screening pregnant women for nodular disease of the thyroid nor repeated follow-up for benign nodular lesions [27, 49].

Assessment of thyroid nodules during pregnancy does not significantly diverge from the procedure adopted at other times [43]. A detailed history should be obtained with a focus on risk factors for thyroid malignancies, such as having been exposed to ionizing radiation as a child, or a family history of thyroid neoplasms. Symptoms that are highly suggestive of malignancy include chronic dysphonia, cervical pain, or cervical lymphadenopathy. When physically examining patients, note the size, location, and characteristics of any nodular lesion. Physical findings strongly suggestive of malignancy include extremely firm (rock hard) nodules, hoarseness, tethering of adjacent structures, and palpable lymph node enlargement, especially when ipsilateral to the nodule only. After assessment in clinic, ultrasonographic assessment is warranted and venous bloods should be obtained for quantification of serum TSH level [49].

Ultrasonographic imaging of the thyroid does not involve exposing the mother or fetus to ionizing radiation and may be safely undertaken in pregnant women. Ultrasound can provide information on where a nodule is and how large, as well as being used to calculate the risk that a nodule represents a malignant neoplasm. The principal characteristics to consider are whether the lesion is solid or contains a cyst, the echogenic quality of the parenchyma, whether the lesion is calcified and if so, how, and if the draining lymph glands demonstrate an increase in size, or exhibit an abnormality. Calcification of the lesion may involve microcalcified foci or a calcified rim. The nodular margins should also be noted. Malignant lesions are most likely to exhibit the following characteristics: markedly hypoechogenic, microfoci of calcification, irregularly shaped outline, or evidence of invasion and abnormal lymph node appearances [50]. Other characteristics are less reliably associated with malignancy. The ultrasonographic appearances and how closely they fit the pattern of a malignant neoplasm are of benefit in calculating cancer risk [30, 51], but suffer from certain limitations linked to inconsistency in reporting appearances [52, 53].

Thyroid function testing is essential in any woman presenting with a thyroid nodule during pregnancy [27], which should include quantification of TSH in serum and should take into account whether the patient is already receiving supplementary thyroid hormone treatment. It is routinely recommended that thyroid hormones, if needed, be supplied in the form of levothyroxine, but there are other forms in which it may be administered, notably as liothyronine or as desiccated thyroid extract. There are two important explanations for an abnormal serum TSH level, which call for different responses. The first possibility is that a thyroid nodule is not under normal physiological control, which may point toward a malignant lesion. However, care must be exercised in reaching this conclusion, since beta-human chorionic gonadotropin in pregnancy normally suppresses TSH levels. Furthermore, the usual next investigation, a radionuclide scan, is contraindicated in pregnancy. The second interpretation may be that the thyroid is underactive; hence, the use of thyroid hormone supplementation, and if this is the case, in the treatment of hypofunction is essential, especially during pregnancy [49].

In patients where there is a nodule but the TSH is not low, the next step to contemplate is fine-needle aspiration biopsy under ultrasonographic guidance (UG-FNA). Before opting for UG-FNA, the most recent guidelines available, the literature on the subject, and the patient's own views must be consulted. Generally speaking, if a nodule, which is solid, has been reported on ultrasonography as at least moderately likely to represent a malignant neoplasm and exceeds 1 cm in diameter, UG-FNA should be performed [30]. However, nodules that appear benign on ultrasonography are unlikely to be malignant and therefore only warrant UG-FNA if they are at least 1.5–2 cm in diameter [30]. Nodules, which only consist of a cystic portion, do not require FNA, since they are not malignant. It is highly unusual for UG-FNA to cause any adverse effects other than slight bruising. On the other hand, the cytological assessment offers a significant advantage by rendering the risk assessment for a thyroid malignancy more accurate [30, 44, 54, 55]. If the aspirated cells are sufficient in number and lack any features associated with malignancy, the specimen will be reported as benign. Where malignant features are seen, the report will state that the cells are malignant. In cases where there are malignant cytological characteristics, but these are inadequate to be sure of a malignant lesion, the report will state that the sample is indeterminate [54, 55]. The usual rate of thyroid FNA aspirates reported as benign is around 70%. Between 5 and 10% of aspirates are reported malignant, while around 5% are inadequate for diagnosis. Nonetheless, there remains a group of aspirates, accounting for between 15 and 30% of those submitted for cytology, in which cytological appearances are reported as indeterminate. In these samples, there is a high percentage, which are eventually shown by histopathology to be malignant neoplasms [55, 56]. However, the test itself can be safely undertaken in a pregnant woman, and lidocaine may be infiltrated subcutaneously if felt necessary [33, 37]. Despite there being no evidence from prospective trials, at present, it appears that there are no pregnancy-related effects to consider when evaluating thyroid FNA samples cytologically [24, 25]. Since the majority of thyroid nodules will predate the pregnancy, even though that is when they are diagnosed, it is reasonable to assume that the cytological characteristics will not differ from those found in nonpregnant patients [57].

How a pregnant patient with a thyroid nodule is managed depends on both ultrasonography and the results of FNA. Generally speaking, thyroid carcinomas detected during pregnancy are relatively indolent [47, 58]. The evidence indicates that these tumors are not associated with adverse pregnancy outcomes [59–62]. It is therefore frequent for clinicians to manage conservatively lesions where the cytology is indeterminate or even frankly malignant. A case-control study undertaken by Moosa and Mazzaferri [59] examined 589 individuals, of which 61 were pregnant, and all of whom had just been given a diagnosis of thyroid carcinoma. Treatment in the pregnant patients began 15 months later than in the nonpregnant controls, but the postponement of treatment was not associated with any additional adverse outcome. A study based on a cancer registry in California, USA, compared outcomes in 595 women who received a diagnosis of thyroid carcinoma either during pregnantcy or within a year of being pregnant with 2270 women of the same age who were not pregnant around the time thyroid carcinoma was diagnosed. There was no difference in mortality between the groups [60].

When FNA results in an indeterminate result, this presents clinicians with difficult choices [30, 63]. Undertaking an operation to remove the nodule for histopathology allows the nature of the lesion to be definitively established, but surgery is always risky in pregnant women. In women who are not pregnant, molecular biomarkers are available to help to clarify the diagnosis in cases of indeterminate cytology [64, 65], but these biomarkers have not been validated for use in pregnant women and are thus not recommended at present. The detection of malignant thyroid neoplasms may be assisted by identification of genetic mutations or deletions in DNA from the lesion. It has been demonstrated in multiple studies that a mutated form of BRAF leads to synthesis of the mutant BRAFV600E protein, which definitively indicates thyroid malignancy. This test is not considered susceptible to change in pregnant patients. Testing for the BRAFV600E protein has a potential role in resolving indeterminate cytology, but it occurs at a relatively low rate in these nodules [66]. In any case, even if BRAFV600E is detected, this finding is not invariably a marker of an aggressive lesion needing urgent surgical excision. Genomic rearrangements involving RET and PTC occur with high specificity in thyroid cancer, but are not commonly detected in FNA samples where cytology is indeterminate. It is also possible to test for mutated versions of other genes present in malignant cells (especially the RAS oncogenes—KRAS, NRAS, and HRAS). However, these may also occur in nonmalignant lesions [67, 68]. There are kits available commercially, which permit the detection of particular oncogenic mutations [69, 70]. Additionally, gene expression profiles may be obtained, a technique that can allow an estimation of the risk of malignancy in nodules of indeterminate significance on cytology. When genes are abnormally expressed, this indicates that cancer cells or the surrounding environment is functioning in a deviant fashion. A gene expression profile kit has now come on the market for clinical use, following stringent testing of its validity, albeit in nonpregnant individuals [71–74]. However, pregnancy-related endocrine alterations potentially influence gene expression. These types of genetic tests in cancer have not undergone validation for use in pregnant patients and because of the incomplete evidence base, it is not advisable to use these tests to resolve an indeterminate cytology result from FNA undertaken while the patient is pregnant [49].

A thyroid nodule of indeterminate status on cytology should not automatically be assumed to represent malignancy, but it is worth bearing in mind that if such a lesion is malignant, they tend to be a more indolent type of thyroid cancer [75]. It is highly unusual for a delay in commencing treatment for a low-grade thyroid neoplasm because of pregnancy to harm the prognosis for the woman, and any decision for surgery needs to consider that surgery itself entails risks and may have complications. At present, the evidence base suggests that treating pregnant women with thyroid nodules conservatively until after they deliver is warranted [49].

56.4.2 Thyroid Carcinoma

56.4.2.1 Differentiated Thyroid Carcinoma (DTC)

If a diagnosis of differentiated thyroid carcinoma (DTC) is made in the first trimester, the lesion should be serially scanned ultrasonographically [27]. The clinician needs to assess the risk of the lesion progressing or recurring and what the likely prognosis is. This topic is covered in Sect. 56.4.2.1.1. The patient should be informed about the risks of surgery, how radionuclide treatment may affect future fertility, and the consequences of suppressing release of TSH. Additionally, the rationale for actively following up the nodule and the optimal point at which to operate should be discussed. At present, the entire evidence base on managing DTC in pregnant women is concerned only with papillary carcinoma [19].

Progression, Risk of Recurrence, and Prognosis

It is still a highly contentious matter what role if any being pregnant may play on the course and outcome of DTC, including the matter of potentially raised risk that the lesion recur. Much of the controversy stems from the paucity of trial evidence to answer these questions and the fact that the evidence base is now quite old, with no RCTs available [19].

There have been a number of studies looking at survival rates (both overall mortality and cancer-related mortality) in women who received a diagnosis of DTC while pregnant or within a year after giving birth versus women with DTC who were not pregnant [59, 61, 62, 76–78]. Four such studies found that survival rates did not differ significantly between groups [59, 61, 62, 76]. Notably, DTC was stage 1 in over 99% of patients in both groups.

The literature confirms that whether surgical intervention occurs while the patient is still pregnant or after delivery does not impact survival rates [59, 61, 76–78]. There have been a half dozen studies using a retrospective design, which were able to show that the progression of DTC was unaffected by pregnancy. This was shown in women who had known DTC and subsequently became pregnant once or multiple times [79–84]. In all these studies, however, the small number of participants, which ranged from 22 to 235 women, imposes limitations on the conclusions reached. However, overall the studies did show that suppression of thyroglobulin synthesis (to a level ranging from below 0.9 ng.mL^{-1} to below 2 ng.mL^{-1}) did not result in recurrent disease, if this was not already detected ultrasonographically before the pregnancy began [82–84]. The study with the highest number of participants was undertaken by Rakhlin et al. and involved 235 women. This studied examined the hypothesis that previous treatment response, as defined by the framework developed in 2015 by the American Thyroid Association, predicts how DTC will develop in a woman who later becomes pregnant. The findings of the authors were that individuals whose tumor had previously responded in an excellent, indeterminate, or biochemically incomplete manner were not at risk of developing a structural thyroid disorder that could be imaged ultrasonographically after the pregnancy reached term. However, women in whom DTC persisted after treatment, when pregnant, had tumors that progressed. However, in only a small number of cases did this result in increased therapeutic input [79]. This result has been replicated in other studies [82, 84].

In the light of the conclusions to the studies cited above, recommendations for how to treat DTC cases in pregnancy may be made as follows: in a woman who had previous DTC, where there was biochemical or structural evidence of incomplete treatment response, ultrasound assessment of the thyroid should be repeated during the pregnancy, alongside serial measurement of thyroglobulin. This is also the recommendation in DTC, which is active or recurrent. In women whose DTC was low grade and in whom the tumor was undetectable by ultrasonography or biochemistry following treatment, there is no indication for repeated measurement of thyroglobulin while the patient is pregnant [27].

Management

Evaluation and Management of Thyroid Cancer During Pregnancy

In the majority of cases where a well-differentiated thyroid carcinoma (WDTC) is either suspected or cytologically confirmed in the first trimester, the tumor requires a baseline evaluation and then follow-up at regular intervals to provide warning that it is becoming less indolent and thus allow surgical intervention even before delivery [30]. If the ultrasound imaging indicates that it is a large nodule, has breached into the trachea or a blood vessel, or has lymphatic spread, surgical intervention may need to be offered. Any operation is best timed to occur in the second trimester, prior to the 24th week of pregnancy. In the majority of cases of WDTC, however, the tumor is unlikely to progress to an important degree before delivery, in which case surgery may be postponed until the end of pregnancy without increasing the risk. The suggestion that surgery may be postponed does not apply in the more unusual categories of thyroid malignant neoplasm, such as medullary, poorly differentiated or anaplastic tumors, or where a WDTC displays aggressive characteristics. In these cases, there are frequently grounds to undertake surgery before delivery can occur and every case must be assessed on its own merits [49].

TSH has a stimulatory effect on thyroid growth; thus, suppression of TSH helps to inhibit the growth of thyroid neoplasms. Where a malignant nodule in a pregnant woman is under conservative management, one strategy is to maintain the circulating level of TSH below 2.0 mU.L^{-1}. Where TSH is just higher than the reference range, it is usually suggested that levothyroxine be initiated, beginning with a dose between 50 and 75 mcg o.d [27]. The TSH level should then be rechecked around 1 month later, the dose of levothyroxine being adjusted until the desired level of TSH suppression is achieved [49].

It is common practice for nonpregnant patients suffering from thyroid cancer of well-differentiated type to receive iodine-131 as a therapeutic adjunct after the main tumor has been resected [30]. This agent is, however, not permissible during pregnancy both because radiation is itself teratogenic and since this radioisotope can easily enter the fetal circulation via the placenta and cause injury to the developing thyroid of the fetus. Thus, in cases where adjunctive radioiodine is required, this should not be commenced until after delivery, and if possible, not until after breast-feeding has finished, since ^{131}I is secreted into breast milk. Cases of WDTC occurring in pregnant women call for conservative management, with watchful waiting and suppression of TSH [49].

56.5   Active Surveillance (Watchful Waiting)

A number of Japanese researchers have been able to demonstrate, using a prospective study design, the appropriateness of watchful waiting as an alternative way to manage thyroid papillary microcarcinomas not exceeding 10 mm diameter, rather than proceeding directly to surgical excision. However, there must be an absence of lymph node involvement on ultrasonic imaging and the lesion must not spread beyond the margins of the thyroid itself [85, 86]. Several researchers in Japan traced the outcomes in 50 pregnant patients with low-risk papillary microcarcinomas who were managed with watchful waiting. This was an extension of earlier research [87, 88]. From this cohort, one patient (2%) had a tumor, which shrank by at least 3 mm, 45 (90%) women had tumors exhibiting stability, and in four patients (8%) alone had the tumor expanded by at least 3 mm. In no patient had the tumor metastasized to the lymphatic system over the course of the pregnancy [87]. Thus, even though a minority of papillary microcarcinomas may expand in pregnant patients, this does not affect an otherwise very favorable prognosis. This result indicates that watchful waiting remains appropriate if the patient becomes pregnant once more, provided disease monitoring remains intense, that is, cervical ultrasonographic assessment should be undertaken at least once in all three trimesters of pregnancy [27].

56.6 Surgery

The conventional approach to treating DTC usually involves surgical excision as the first step. However, in patients who are pregnant, a risk analysis needs to be performed before advocating this step. The potential benefit on the outcome of the tumor needs to be weighed against the risk to the mother and fetus from surgery, including the neonatal period. In patients whose DTC is detected in the first trimester, there should be careful discussion with the patient about the relative advantages of surgery immediately versus after delivery. There have been a few studies, which examined the materno-fetal outcomes of surgical excision of the thyroid during pregnancy. These operations were mostly undertaken within the second trimester, and the total number was small [24, 30, 89–95]. In no patient were any adverse outcomes noted. However, Kuy et al. [96] retrospectively performed a cross-sectional study of a specific population of women who underwent surgical interventions on the thyroid and parathyroid during pregnancy, looking at the outcome from both a clinical and economic perspective. The participants were pregnant women having operations on the thyroid (165 women) or parathyroid (36 women) glands. The Health Care Utilization Project Nationwide Inpatient Sample was used to identify 201 such individuals. Thyroid surgery was undertaken for an indication of malignant neoplasm in 46% of cases. The frequency with which complications occurred in the fetus was 5.5%, while in the mothers, it was 4.5%. Pregnancy was found, by multivariate analysis, to independently predict the risk of endocrine complications or complications in general (odds ratio 2; $p < 0.001$) and lengthier duration of hospitalization (on average by 0.3 days; $p < 0.001$) extended duration of hospital stay after adjustment (by 0.3 days; $p < 0.001$) and greater expense during hospitalization following adjustment ($300, $p < 0.001$) [96]. The endocrine complications consisted of hypoparathyroidism in the mother, hypocalcaemia, tetany, and trauma to the recurrent laryngeal nerve. These findings need to be evaluated cautiously, however, in the light of the differing baseline characteristics between the pregnant women and the other women. This difference was statistically significant. One difference was that the pregnant patients had a greater chance of having been hospitalized in an emergency or other urgent situation, and were more likely to depend on state assistance to fund their treatment. A study conducted since then has compared women who had surgical intervention in the second trimester with women who had their operation within a year after giving birth. There were 24 patients in the former, and 21 patients in the latter group. All had a diagnosis of DTC. The study used a retrospective design and examined both pathological and clinical features of the cases. None of the participants had a spontaneous abortion and no congenital anomalies were noted. The researchers therefore suggest that it is acceptable to carry out thyroid surgery on pregnant women in the second trimester [97].

Generally speaking, where it is necessary to operate on a pregnant woman, the safest time, from the point of view of least risk of spontaneous abortion and premature delivery, is the second trimester [98]. The guidelines at present note three potential indications for thyroid surgery in the middle trimester [27, 30]:

1. The malignant lesion expands significantly in size, that is, the volume goes up by 50% and the lesion measures 20% longer in any two axes.
2. There is cytology confirming that metastasis to the lymphatic system has occurred.
3. Where DTC is graded as advanced and the lesion was noted by the 24th to 26th week of the pregnancy.

Where the lesion fails to show aggressive behavior during pregnancy, surgical excision is best postponed until after the child is born.

56.7　Radioactive Iodine

The ability of iodine-131 to traverse the placental barrier is well known, as well as the tendency for the isotope to accumulate in the thyroid of the fetus when administered to the mother after the twelfth to thirteenth week of pregnancy [99]. When this occurs, the fetus becomes hypothyroid, a condition persisting in the neonatal period. Thus, pregnant women should not be administered this radionuclide.

56.8　Thyroid Hormone Management

The appropriate degree of TSH suppression is calculated on the basis of the likelihood of recurrence, which is correlated with histopathological appearances. The dose is then titrated against therapeutic response [30]. It is especially important to keep TSH below the normal reference interval in cases where the likelihood of recurrent tumor is intermediate or greater, as defined by the 2015 guidelines from the American Thyroid Association and the consensus statement of the European Thyroid Association [30, 100]. There are strong data to show that asymptomatic hyperthyroidism does not cause complications in mothers or their newborns [17]; thus, it is appropriate to aim for the same TSH level whether the patient is pregnant or not, although with the caveat that the level of levothyroxine needed goes up by nearly 30% in pregnant patients [101, 102]. Thyroid function tests need to be instituted regularly to ensure the patient does not become hypothyroid or exhibit symptoms of hyperthyroidism. The TSH level in venous blood needs to be tested once every 4 weeks up to the 16th to 20th week of the pregnancy, after which it should be checked a final time between 26 and 32 weeks gestation [27].

56.9   Tyrosine Kinase Inhibitors (TKIs)

The US FDA and the European Medicines Agency (EMA) has licensed three inhibitors of tyrosine kinase (TKI) for the indication of advanced DTC with metasis formation. These agents are sorafenib, lenvatinib, and cabozantinib. The FDA places these agents in Class D. At present, there has been no research directly concerning teratogenicity in pregnant humans, but evidence from animal models indicates that all the TKIs are teratogenic and toxic to the embryo even at a dose beneath that used in human subjects [103]. The EMA and FDA both advise that TKIs only be used in pregnant women following a thorough risk-benefit analysis, concerning both the mother and fetus. FDA recommendations for sorafenib are to avoid conception and for contraception to be advised to female patients on lenvatinib. There is no specific recommendation by the FDA concerning cabozantinib [103]. It is recommended that any woman who may potentially become pregnant should be started on highly efficacious contraception before starting treatment with any TKI [27].

56.10   Considerations for the Postpartum Period

The assessment and treatment of nodular thyroid lesions in women following delivery does not differ from nonpregnant patients. Where a thyroid malignancy is detected in a woman postpartum, there needs to be a thorough risk-benefit analysis undertaken for the possible therapeutic interventions, whether operative or involving radionuclide administration. Women nursing infants who are diagnosed with a thyroid malignancy require especially careful management. Radioactive ^{131}I must not be used in nursing mothers, since it is secreted into breast milk and has a lengthy half-life of around 8 days. Iodine-123 benefits from a briefer half-life of 13 hours. It can potentially be used in nursing mothers, who will need to use a breast pump for 3–4 days after receiving the dose and safely dispose of the expressed breast milk [27, 104]. If technetium-99m pertechnate is chosen, similar advice applies, with the milk discarded for 24 h [95]. If it is possible, breastfeeding should have ceased 3 months before iodine-131 is administered. Exactly how thyrosuppression affects lactation is an unresolved issue at present [27].

56.11   Preconception Planning and Counselling

Since three quarters of all thyroid neoplasms occur in women, and 36% of thyroid neoplasms occur in women aged under 45, that is, at the period when women are capable of bearing children, family planning is a key issue to consider in treating these lesions [105–107]. One cohort study, which assessed the reproductive history of 18,850 female patients with DTC, based on retrospective review of data from the California Cancer Registry and California Office of State-wide Health Planning and Development database relating to the period 1999–2008, noted that women who had been administered radionuclide treatment (iodine isotopes) for DTC gave birth to their first live child at an older age (median age 34.5 years) than those not administered such treatment (median age 26.1 years) ($p < 0.001$). Even after the potentially confounding factors of tumor type, socioeconomic class, and marital status were controlled for, this age difference was still found in the group aged between 20 and 39 years old ($p < 0.05$). In line with this finding, the birth rate was lower as the woman approached the end of her childbearing years [108]. A study, which looked at a cohort of women in Taiwan, produced similar results [109]. The probable explanation for this delayed birth is that doctors usually caution women against pregnancy in the immediate aftermath of radionuclide therapy or the radioactive isotopes used may also affect reproductive fitness, or both factors operate together. Nonetheless, there is a study indicating that the age at which women first deliver is unaffected by treatment with radionuclides. In the study referred to [110], 53% of the 2360 women who received a diagnosis of DTC when aged between 15 and 39 went on to be administered radioisotopes of iodine. However, the age at first birth did not differ significantly between those who received radionuclide therapy and those who did not [110].

56.12 Management of Pre-existing Thyroid Cancer During Pregnancy

If a woman already has a malignant thyroid neoplasm, it needs to be treated at the earliest and followed up if she conceives. In general, the thyroglobulin (Tg) level in venous blood has the greatest sensitivity of biomarkers to detect recurrence or persistence of the lesion. If a patient has never received radioactive iodine-131, it is difficult to define an exact level signifying that no thyroid malignancy exists; however, provided the mother's circulating level of Tg is not above 2 ng.dL^{-1}, it is unlikely that an active thyroid tumor is present. A Tg level of at least 2 IU.L^{-1}, or one which continually rises [30, 111], should raise the suspicion that the lesion is advancing or has recurred. In approximately 20% of cases of thyroid neoplasia, patients develop immunoglobulins specific for Tg (TgAb). The importance of such antibodies is that they can interfere with assays measuring Tg, rather than their playing a key role in pathogenesis [112], producing a result that underestimates Tg, even a negative result, at least according to the methods most widespread in clinical chemistry laboratories [113, 114]. Thus, prior to measuring Tg levels, the laboratory should screen for anti-Tg immunoglobulins. This is usually done automatically. If the antibody screen is positive, either Tg quantification will not be performed, or an assay of a different type may be employed. However, whenever TgAb is detected, a result for Tg level should be viewed with caution. Indeed, the very existence of TgAb and a rising titer are independently concerning as potential markers of persistence of the thyroid malignancy [30, 115].

In a case where the levels of Tg or TgAb are such as to indicate probable remaining tumor, the first action is a complete physical examination and cervical ultrasonography, with the aim of localizing the lesion. Although other imaging techniques, notably CT, PET, or MRI, do have a role in identifying metastases, their use is problematic in pregnant patients and any decision to undertake such an investigation should be on a case-by-case basis, following a risk-benefit assessment, weighing the probability of detecting metastases calling for immediate treatment against the potential for iatrogenic harm [49].

Replacement of thyroid hormones in pregnancy is a key method of managing pregnant patients following excision of the thyroid. This has two aims: to suppress TSH to a level where it will not stimulate any residual differentiated thyroid carcinoma and to satisfy the alterations in thyroid function needed over the course of the pregnancy [27, 30]. In pregnancy, thyroid hormone levels should normally increase and this naturally places the thyroid under test. Several physiological adaptations contribute to the stress on the thyroid, in particular the increased renal clearance of iodine, a higher degree of thyroid hormones being protein bound in the circulation, due to elevated thyroxine-binding globulin, and the stimulation of the TSH receptor by the rising concentration of human chorionic gonadotropin [27, 116]. Overall, these changes mean that thyroid hormone expression increases by 40% on average in pregnant women [117]. In women whose thyroid is functioning at a reduced rate (which may have necessitated levothyroxine prior to pregnancy) or who have undergone thyroidectomy, the increased synthesis of thyroid hormones cannot be supplied by the thyroid, and, unless external hormones are administered, the mother will become hypothyroid. In this situation, levothyroxine needs to be started or the dose raised to keep TSH at the correct level. There have been detailed studies assessing how the thyroid hormone levels normally rise during pregnancy, a process that starts early in the pregnancy [118]. There is a steady increase in thyroid hormone levels up to the 16th to 20th week of pregnancy, when the level typically peaks. At the midpoint of the pregnancy, the need for raised thyroid hormones ceases rising but remains elevated. After childbirth, the demand for thyroid hormones goes back to the prepregnant state [49].

Any patient presenting with a nodular thyroid or a de novo thyroid malignancy during pregnancy should have their thyroid function tested. If the thyroid is not working correctly, or thyroidectomy is about to be performed, extraneous levothyroxine should be administered to restore thyroid function. If the presentation is before the midpoint in the pregnancy, TSH levels in the mother need to be checked once every 3–4 weeks, up to the 20th week. After week 20, the thyroid hormone requirement is more constant and thus, TSH can be checked every month up to the point that the level falls within the desired range [49].

References

1. Tuija MT. Thyroid disease during pregnancy. Options for management. Expert Rev Endocrinol Metab. 2013;8(6):537–47.
2. Glinoer D, De NP, Bourdoux P, et al. Regulation of maternal thyroid during pregnancy. J Clin Endocrinol Metab. 1990;71(2):276–87.
3. Stagnaro-Green A, Abalovich M, Alexander E, et al. Guidelines of the American Thyroid Association for the diagnosis and management of thyroid disease during pregnancy and postpartum. Thyroid. 2011;21(10):1081–125.
4. Bahn RS, Burch HB, Cooper DS, et al. Hyperthyroidism and other causes of thyrotoxicosis: management guidelines of the American Thyroid Association and American Association of Clinical Endocrinologists. Endocr Pract. 2011;17(3):456–520.

5. Garber JR, Cobin RH, Gharib H, et al. Clinical practice guidelines for hypothyroidism in adults: cosponsored by the American Association of Clinical Endocrinologists and the American Thyroid Association. Thyroid. 2012;22(12):1200–35.

6. De Groot LJ, Abalovich M, Alexander EK, et al. Management of thyroid dysfunction during pregnancy and postpartum: an endocrine society clinical practice guideline. J Clin Endocrinol Metab. 2012;97(8):2543–65.

7. Boas M, Forman JL, Juul A, et al. Narrow intra-individual variation of maternal thyroid function in pregnancy based on a longitudinal study on 132 women. Eur J Endocrinol. 2009;161(6):903–10.

8. Larsson A, Palm M, Hansson LO, Axelsson O. Reference values for clinical chemistry tests during normal pregnancy. BJOG. 2008;115(7):874–81.

9. Männistö T, Surcel HM, Ruokonen A, et al. Early pregnancy reference intervals of thyroid hormone concentrations in a thyroid antibody-negative pregnant population. Thyroid. 2011;21(3):291–8.

10. Yu X, Chen Y, Shan Z, et al. The pattern of thyroid function of subclinical hypothyroid women with levothyroxine treatment during pregnancy. Endocrine. 2013;44(3):710–5. https://doi.org/10.1007/s12020-013-9913-2.

11. Van Houcke SK, Van Uytfanghe K, Shimizu E, et al. IFCC international conventional reference procedure for the measurement of free thyroxine in serum: international federation of clinical chemistry and laboratory medicine (IFCC) working group for standardization of thyroid function tests (WG-STFT) (1). Clin Chem Lab Med. 2011;49(8):1275–81.

12. Sapin R, D'Herbomez M. Free thyroxine measured by equilibrium dialysis and nine immunoassays in sera with various serum thyroxine-binding capacities. Clin Chem. 2003;49(9):1531–5.

13. Midgley JE, Hoermann R. Measurement of total rather than free thyroxine in pregnancy: the diagnostic implications. Thyroid. 2013;23(3):259–61.

14. Cooper DS, Doherty GM, Haugen BR, et al. Revised American thyroid association management guidelines for patients with thyroid nodules and differentiated thyroid cancer. Thyroid. 2009;19(11):1167–214.

15. Männistö T, Vääräsmäki M, Pouta A, et al. Perinatal outcome of children born to mothers with thyroid dysfunction or antibodies: a prospective population-based cohort study. J Clin Endocrinol Metab. 2009;94(3):772–9.

16. Männistö T, Vääräsmäki M, Pouta A, et al. Thyroid dysfunction and autoantibodies during pregnancy as predictive factors of pregnancy complications and maternal morbidity in later life. J Clin Endocrinol Metab. 2010;95(3):1084–94.

17. Casey BM, Dashe JS, Wells CE, et al. Subclinical hyperthyroidism and pregnancy outcomes. Obstet Gynecol. 2006;107(2 Pt 1):337–41.

18. Loh JA, Wartofsky L, Jonklaas J, Burman KD. The magnitude of increased levothyroxine requirements in hypothyroid pregnant women depends upon the etiology of the hypothyroidism. Thyroid. 2009;19(3):269–75.

19. Papaleontiou M, Haymart MR. Thyroid nodules and cancer during pregnancy, post-partum and preconception planning: addressing the uncertainties and challenges. Best Pract Res Clin Endocrinol Metab. 2020;34(4):101363. https://doi.org/10.1016/j.beem.2019.101363. Epub 2019 Nov 22. PMID: 31786102; PMCID: PMC7242146.

20. Glinoer D, Soto MF, Bourdoux P, et al. Pregnancy in patients with mild thyroid abnormalities: maternal and neonatal repercussions. J Clin Endocrinol Metab. 1991;73:421–7.

21. Struve CW, Haupt S, Ohlen S. Influence of frequency of previous pregnancies on the prevalence of thyroid nodules in women without clinical evidence of thyroid disease. Thyroid. 1993;3:7–9.

22. Kung AW, Chau MT, Lao TT, et al. The effect of pregnancy on thyroid nodule formation. J Clin Endocrinol Metab. 2002;87:1010–4.

23. Sahin SB, Ogullar S, Ural UM, et al. Alterations of thyroid volume and nodular size during and after pregnancy in a severe iodine-deficient area. Clin Endocrinol (Oxf). 2014;81:762–8.

24. Tan GH, Gharib H, Goellner JR, et al. Management of thyroid nodules in pregnancy. Arch Intern Med. 1996;156:2317–20.

25. Marley EF, Oertel YC. Fine-needle aspiration of thyroid lesions in 57 pregnant and postpartum women. Diagn Cytopathol. 1997;16:122–5.
26. Rosen IB, Walfish PG, Nikore V. Pregnancy and surgical thyroid disease. Surgery. 1985;98:1135–40.
27. Alexander EK, Pearce EN, Brent GA, et al. 2017 guidelines of the American Thyroid Association for the diagnosis and management of thyroid disease during pregnancy and the postpartum. Thyroid. 2017;27:315–89.
28. Popoveniuc G, Jonklaas J. Thyroid nodules. Med Clin North Am. 2012;96:329–49.
29. IAEA radiation protection of pregnant women in nuclear medicine. 2021. https://www.iaea.org/resources/rpop/health-professionals/nuclear-medicine/pregnant-women.
30. Haugen BR, Alexander EK, Bible KC, et al. 2015 American Thyroid Association management guidelines for adult patients with thyroid nodules and differentiated thyroid cancer: the American Thyroid Association guidelines task force on thyroid nodules and differentiated thyroid cancer. Thyroid. 2016;26:1–133.
31. Tessler FN, Middleton WD, Grant EG. Thyroid imaging reporting and data system (TI-RADS): a user's guide. Radiology. 2018;287:29–36.
32. Papini E, Guglielmi R, Bianchini A, et al. Risk of malignancy in nonpalpable thyroid nodules: predictive value of ultrasound and color-Doppler features. J Clin Endocrinol Metab. 2002;87:1941–6.
33. Belfiore A, La Rosa GL. Fine-needle aspiration biopsy of the thyroid. Endocrinol Metab Clin North Am. 2001;30:361–400.
34. Oertel YC. Fine-needle aspiration and the diagnosis of thyroid cancer. Endocrinol Metab Clin North Am. 1996;25:69–91.
35. Singer PA. Evaluation and management of the solitary thyroid nodule. Otolaryngol Clin North Am. 1996;29:577–91.
36. Choe W, McDougall IR. Thyroid cancer in pregnant women: diagnostic and therapeutic management. Thyroid. 1994;4:433–5.
37. Hamburger JI. Thyroid nodules in pregnancy. Thyroid. 1992;2:165–8.
38. Gharib H, Mazzaferri EL. Thyroxine suppressive therapy in patients with nodular thyroid disease. Ann Intern Med. 1998;128:386–94.
39. Liu JL, Wang TS, Zhao M, et al. A transcriptomic study of maternal thyroid adaptation to pregnancy in rats. Int J Mol Sci. 2015;16:27339–49.
40. Burman KD, Wartofsky L. Clinical practice. Thyroid nodules. N Engl J Med. 2015;373:2347–56.
41. Durante C, Costante G, Lucisano G, et al. The natural history of benign thyroid nodules. JAMA. 2015;313:926–35.
42. Angell TE, Vyas CM, Medici M, et al. Differential growth rates of benign vs. malignant thyroid nodules. J Clin Endocrinol Metab. 2017;102:4642–7.
43. Martin JA, Hamilton BE, Osterman MJK, et al. National vital statistics report; 2015. http://www.cdc.gov/nchs/data/nvsr/nvsr64/nvsr64_01.pdf. Accessed 10 May 2021.
44. Yassa L, Cibas ES, Benson CB, et al. Long-term assessment of a multidisciplinary approach to thyroid nodule diagnostic evaluation. Cancer Cytopathol. 2007;111:508–16.
45. Siegel RL, Miller KD, Jemal A. Cancer statistics, 2018. CA Cancer J Clin. 2018;68:7–30.
46. Brito JP, Morris JC, Montori VM. Thyroid cancer: zealous imaging has increased detection and treatment of low risk tumours. BMJ. 2013;347:f4706.
47. Karger S, Schötz S, Stumvoll M, et al. Impact of pregnancy on prevalence of goitre and nodular thyroid disease in women living in a region of borderline sufficient iodine supply. Horm Metab Res. 2010;42:137–42.
48. Sahin SB, Ogullar S, Ural UM, et al. Alterations of thyroid volume and nodular size during and after pregnancy in a severe iodine-deficient area. Clin Endocrinol. 2014;81:762–8.
49. Angell TE, Alexander EK. Thyroid nodules and thyroid cancer in the pregnant woman. Endocrinol Metab Clin North Am. 2019;48(3):557–67. https://doi.org/10.1016/j.ecl.2019.05.003. Epub 2019 Jun 11. PMID: 31345523.
50. Moon HJ, Sung JM, Kim EK, et al. Diagnostic performance of gray-scale US and elastography in solid thyroid nodules. Radiology. 2012;262:1002–13.

51. Grant EG, Tessler FN, Hoang JK, et al. Thyroid ultrasound reporting lexicon: white paper of the ACR thyroid imaging, reporting and data system (TIRADS) committee. J Am Coll Radiol. 2015;12:1272–9.
52. Hoang JK, Middleton WD, Farjat AE, et al. Interobserver variability of sonographic features used in the American College of Radiology Thyroid Imaging Reporting and Data System. AJR Am J Roentgenol. 2018;211:162–7.
53. Grani G, Lamartina L, Cantisani V, et al. Interobserver agreement of various thyroid imaging reporting and data systems. Endocr Connect. 2018;7:1–7.
54. Cibas ES, Ali SZ. The Bethesda system for reporting thyroid cytopathology. Thyroid. 2009;19:1159–65.
55. Bongiovanni M, Crippa S, Baloch Z, et al. Comparison of 5-tiered and 6-tiered diagnostic systems for the reporting of thyroid cytopathology: a multiinstitutional study. Cancer Cytopathol. 2012;120:117–25.
56. Cibas ES, Ali SZ. The 2017 Bethesda system for reporting thyroid cytopathology. Thyroid. 2017;27:1341–6.
57. Goellner JR, Gharib H, Grant CS, et al. Fine needle aspiration cytology of the thyroid, 1980 to 1986. Acta Cytol. 1987;31:587–90.
58. Rosen IB, Korman M, Walfish PG. Thyroid nodular disease in pregnancy: current diagnosis and management. Clin Obstet Gynecol. 1997;40:81–9.
59. Moosa M, Mazzaferri EL. Outcome of differentiated thyroid cancer diagnosed in pregnant women. J Clin Endocrinol Metab. 1997;82:2862–6.
60. Yasmeen S, Cress R, Romano PS, et al. Thyroid cancer in pregnancy. Int J Gynaecol Obstet. 2005;91:15–20.
61. Herzon FS, Morris DM, Segal MN, et al. Coexistent thyroid cancer and pregnancy. Arch Otolaryngol Head Neck Surg. 1994;120:1191–3.
62. Lee JC, Zhao JT, Clifton-Bligh RJ, et al. Papillary thyroid carcinoma in pregnancy: a variant of the disease? Ann Surg Oncol. 2012;19:4210–6.
63. Durante C, Grani G, Lamartina L, et al. The diagnosis and management of thyroid nodules: a review. JAMA. 2018;319:914–24.
64. Beaudenon-Huibregtse S, Alexander EK, Guttler RB, et al. Centralized molecular testing for oncogenic gene mutations complements the local cytopathologic diagnosis of thyroid nodules. Thyroid. 2014;10:1479–87.
65. Nikiforov YE, Ohori NP, Hodak SP, et al. Impact of mutational testing on the diagnosis and management of patients with cytologically indeterminate thyroid nodules: a prospective analysis of 1056 FNA samples. J Clin Endocrinol Metab. 2011;96:3390–7.
66. Kleiman DA, Sporn MJ, Beninato T, et al. Preoperative BRAF(V600E) mutation screening is unlikely to alter initial surgical treatment of patients with indeterminate thyroid nodules: a prospective case series of 960 patients. Cancer. 2013;119:1495–502.
67. Angell TE. RAS-positive thyroid nodules. Curr Opin Endocrinol Diabetes Obes. 2017;24:372–6.
68. Medici M, Kwong N, Angell TE, et al. The variable phenotype and low-risk nature of RAS-positive thyroid nodules. BMC Med. 2015;13:184–9.
69. Steward DL, Carty SE, Sippel RS, et al. Performance of a multigene genomic classifier in thyroid nodules with indeterminate cytology: a prospective blinded multicenter study. JAMA Oncol. 2019;5(2):204–12. https://doi.org/10.1001/jamaoncol.2018.4616.
70. Labourier E, Shifrin A, Busseniers AE, et al. Molecular testing for miRNA, mRNA, and DNA on fine-needle aspiration improves the preoperative diagnosis of thyroid nodules with indeterminate cytology. J Clin Endocrinol Metab. 2015;100:2743–50.
71. Alexander EK, Kennedy GC, Baloch ZW, et al. Preoperative diagnosis of benign thyroid nodules with indeterminate cytology. N Engl J Med. 2012;367:705–15.
72. Patel KN, Angell TE, Babiarz J, et al. Performance of a genomic sequencing classifier for the preoperative diagnosis of cytologically indeterminate thyroid nodules. JAMA Surg. 2018;153:817–24.
73. Alexander EK, Schorr M, Klopper J, et al. Multicenter clinical experience with the Afirma gene expression classifier. J Clin Endocrinol Metab. 2014;99:119–25.

74. Roth MY, Witt RL, Steward DL. Molecular testing for thyroid nodules: review and current state. Cancer. 2018;124:888–98.
75. Liu X, Medici M, Kwong N, et al. Bethesda categorization of thyroid nodule cytology and prediction of thyroid cancer type and prognosis. Thyroid. 2016;26:256–61.
76. Yasmeen S, Cress R, Romano PS, et al. Thyroid cancer in pregnancy. Int J Gynecol Obstet. 2005;91:15–20.
77. Vannucchi G, Perrino M, Rossi S, et al. Clinical and molecular features of differentiated thyroid cancer diagnosed during pregnancy. Eur J Endocrinol. 2010;162:145–51.
78. Messuti I, Corvisieri S, Bardesono F, et al. Impact of pregnancy on prognosis of differentiated thyroid cancer: clinical and molecular features. Eur J Endocrinol. 2014;170:659–66.
79. Rakhlin L, Fish S, Tuttle RM. Response to therapy status is an excellent predictor of pregnancy-associated structural disease progression in patients previously treated for differentiated thyroid cancer. Thyroid. 2017;27:396–401.
80. Rosvoll RV, Winship T. Thyroid carcinoma and pregnancy. Surg Gynecol Obstet. 1965;121:1039–42.
81. Hill CS Jr, Clark RL, Wolf M. The effect of subsequent pregnancy on patients with thyroid carcinoma. Surg Gynecol Obstet. 1966;122:1219–22.
82. Leboeuf R, Emerick LE, Martorella AJ, et al. Impact of pregnancy on serum thyroglobulin and detection of recurrent disease shortly after delivery in thyroid cancer survivors. Thyroid. 2007;17:543–7.
83. Rosario PW, Barroso AL, Purisch S. The effect of subsequent pregnancy on patients with thyroid carcinoma apparently free of the disease. Thyroid. 2007;17:1175–6.
84. Hirsch D, Levy S, Tsvetov G, et al. Impact of pregnancy on outcome and prognosis of survivors of papillary thyroid cancer. Thyroid. 2010;20:1179–85.
85. Ito Y, Miyauchi A, Kihara M, et al. Patient age is significantly related to the progression of papillary microcarcinoma of the thyroid under observation. Thyroid. 2014;24:27–34.
86. Sugitani I, Toda K, Yamada K, et al. Three distinctly different kinds of papillary thyroid microcarcinoma should be recognized: our treatment strategies and outcomes. World J Surg. 2010;34:1222–31.
87. Ito Y, Miyauchi A, Kudo T, et al. Effects of pregnancy on papillary microcarcinomas of the thyroid re-evaluated in the entire patient series at Kuma hospital. Thyroid. 2016;26:156–60.
88. Shindo H, Amino N, Ito Y, et al. Papillary thyroid microcarcinoma might progress during pregnancy. Thyroid. 2014;24:840–4.
89. Loh KC. Familial nonmedullary thyroid carcinoma: a meta-review of case series. Thyroid. 1997;7:107–13.
90. Tucker MA, Jones PH, Boice JD Jr, et al. Therapeutic radiation at a young age is linked to secondary thyroid cancer. The Late Effects Study Group. Cancer Res. 1991;51:2885–8.
91. Tan GH, Gharib H, Reading CC. Solitary thyroid nodule. Comparison between palpation and ultrasonography. Arch Intern Med. 1995;155:2418–23.
92. Rosen IB, Walfish PG. Pregnancy as a predisposing factor in thyroid neoplasia. Arch Surg. 1986;121:1287–90.
93. Doherty CM, Shindo ML, Rice DH, et al. Management of thyroid nodules during pregnancy. Laryngoscope. 1995;105:251–5.
94. Boucek J, de Haan J, Halaska MJ, et al. Maternal and obstetrical outcome in 35 cases of well-differentiated thyroid carcinoma during pregnancy. Laryngoscope. 2018;128:1493–500.
95. Vini L, Hyer S, Pratt B, et al. Management of differentiated thyroid cancer diagnosed during pregnancy. Eur J Endocrinol. 1999;140:404–6.
96. Kuy S, Roman SA, Desai R, et al. Outcomes following thyroid and parathyroid surgery in pregnant women. Arch Surg. 2009;144:399–406; discussion 406.
97. Uruno T, Shibuya H, Kitagawa W, et al. Optimal timing of surgery for differentiated thyroid cancer in pregnant women. World J Surg. 2014;38:704–8.
98. ACOG clinical guidelines. Nonobstetric surgery during pregnancy. 2018. https://www.acog.org/Clinical-Guidance-and-Publications/Committee-Opinions/Committee-on-Obstetric-Practice/Nonobstetric-Surgery-During-Pregnancy.

99. Gorman CA. Radioiodine and pregnancy. Thyroid. 1999;9:721–6.

100. Pacini F, Schlumberger M, Dralle H, et al. European consensus for the management of patients with differentiated thyroid carcinoma of the follicular epithelium. Eur J Endocrinol. 2006;154:787–803.

101. Alexander EK, Marqusee E, Lawrence J, et al. Timing and magnitude of increases in levo-thyroxine requirements during pregnancy in women with hypothyroidism. N Engl J Med. 2004;351:241–9.

102. Loh JA, Wartofsky L, Jonklaas J, et al. The magnitude of increased levothyroxine require-ments in hypothyroid pregnant women depends upon the etiology of the hypothyroidism. Thyroid. 2009;19:269–75.

103. FDA U.S. Food & Drug Administration. Drug approvals and databases; 2018. https://www.fda.gov/Drugs/InformationonDrugs/default.htm.

104. Howe DB, Beardsley M, Bakhsh S, et al. Model procedure for release of patients or human research subjects administered radioactive materials. Consolidated guidance about materials licenses program-specific guidance about medical use licenses final report US nuclear regula-tory commission Office of nuclear material safety and safeguards 2008;9.

105. American Cancer Society. Key statistics for thyroid cancer; 2018. https://www.cancer.org/cancer/thyroid-cancer/about/keystatistics.html.

106. NIH National Cancer Institute. Surveillance, epidemiology, and end results program. Cancer stat facts: thyroid cancer; 2018. https://seer.cancer.gov/statfacts/html/thyro.html.

107. Haymart MR, Pearce EN. How much should thyroid cancer impact plans for pregnancy? Thyroid. 2017;27:312–4.

108. Wu JX, Young S, Ro K, et al. Reproductive outcomes and nononcologic complications after radioactive iodine ablation for well-differentiated thyroid cancer. Thyroid. 2015;25:133–8.

109. Ko KY, Yen RF, Lin CL, et al. Pregnancy outcome after I-131 therapy for patients with thy-roid cancer: a nationwide population-based cohort study. Medicine. 2016;95:e2685.

110. Anderson C, Engel SM, Weaver MA, et al. Birth rates after radioactive iodine treatment for differentiated thyroid cancer. Int J Cancer. 2017;141:2291–5.

111. Webb RC, Howard RS, Stojadinovic A, et al. The utility of serum thyroglobulin measure-ment at the time of remnant ablation for predicting disease-free status in patients with dif-ferentiated thyroid cancer: a meta-analysis involving 3947 patients. J Clin Endocrinol Metab. 2012;97:2754–63.

112. Latrofa F, Ricci D, Montanelli L, et al. Lymphocytic thyroiditis on histology correlates with serum thyroglobulin autoantibodies in patients with papillary thyroid carcinoma: impact on detection of serum thyroglobulin. J Clin Endocrinol Metab. 2012;97:2380–7.

113. Spencer CA, Takeuchi M, Kazarosyan M, et al. Serum thyroglobulin autoantibodies: preva-lence, influence on serum thyroglobulin measurement, and prognostic significance in patients with differentiated thyroid carcinoma. J Clin Endocrinol Metab. 1998;83:1121–7.

114. Netzel BC, Grebe SK, Carranza Leon BG, et al. Thyroglobulin (Tg) testing revisited: Tg assays, TgAb assays, and correlation of results with clinical outcomes. J Clin Endocrinol Metab. 2015;100:E1074–83.

115. Matrone A, Latrofa F, Torregrossa L, et al. Changing trend of thyroglobulin antibodies in patients with differentiated thyroid cancer treated with total thyroidectomy without 131I ablation. Thyroid. 2018;28:871–9.

116. Korevaar TIM, Medici M, Visser TJ, et al. Thyroid disease in pregnancy: new insights in diagnosis and clinical management. Nat Rev Endocrinol. 2017;13:610–22.

117. Soldin OP. Thyroid function testing in pregnancy and thyroid disease: trimesterspe-cific reference intervals. Ther Drug Monit. 2006;28(1):8–11. https://doi.org/10.1097/01.ftd.0000194498.32398.7b.

118. Alexander EK, Marqusee E, Lawrence J, et al. Timing and magnitude of increases in levo-thyroxine requirements during pregnancy in women with hypothyroidism. N Engl J Med. 2004;351:25–33.

Management of Parathyroid Disorders in Pregnancy and Postpartum Period

57

Bayram Şahin, Ömer Can Topaloğlu, and Sheng-Po Hao

57.1 Introduction

During pregnancy, an average-sized fetus needs 30 g of calcium, 20 g of phosphorus, and 0.8 g of magnesium for the skeletal mineralization and other physiological processes [1, 2]. Maternal physiology adapts itself to meet these mineral and supplementary nutrition needs of the fetus and the newborn during pregnancy and lactation. As a natural consequence of that condition, pregnancy and lactation cause serious changes in the maternal calcium metabolism. Thanks to these activated physiological adaptation mechanisms, calcium and vitamin D needs for the mother do not change during pregnancy and lactation. Most of the calcium in breast milk is provided by increased intestinal absorption and maternal bone resorption. This may lead to a decrease in maternal bone mineral density and an increased risk of fracture in the short term, but not to a negative effect in the long term. Disorders of bone and calcium metabolism are rare in pregnant women, but they may progress more severely when they occur. In such a case, the current process should be evaluated and managed bidirectionally for the health of both mother and fetus.

B. Şahin (✉)
Department of Otorhinolaryngology, Head and Neck Surgery, Kocaeli Health Sciences University, Derince Training and Research Hospital, Kocaeli, Turkey
e-mail: drbayramsahin@gmail.com

Ö. C. Topaloğlu
Department of Endocrinology, Kocaeli Health Sciences University, Derince Training and Research Hospital, Kocaeli, Turkey
e-mail: drhomercan@hotmail.com

S.-P. Hao
Department of Otorhinolaryngology, Shin Kong Wu Ho-Su Memorial Hospital and Fu Jen Catholic University, Taipei, Taiwan
e-mail: shengpo747@gmail.com

C. Cingi et al. (eds.), *ENT Diseases: Diagnosis and Treatment during Pregnancy and Lactation*, https://doi.org/10.1007/978-3-031-05303-0_57

In this section, calcium and parathyroid disorders that may occur during pregnancy and lactation will be examined by reviewing the physiological changes in calcium and mineral metabolism, and information will be given on how to manage these conditions.

57.2 Calcium and Other Minerals, Vitamin D, Parathyroid Hormone (PTH), Calcitonin Physiology in Pregnancy and Lactation

57.2.1 Calcium and Other Minerals

The amount of calcium (30 g) required to meet the mineral needs of the fetal skeleton causes a serious calcium deficit for the mother. Although this amount corresponds to approximately 3% of the total amount of calcium in the mother's skeleton, meeting this need constitutes a problem for the mother. This need is met by resorption from the maternal skeleton and increased calcium absorption from the intestinal system. Except for the pregnancy period, approximately 200 mg of 1000 mg calcium, which enters the intestinal system daily, is absorbed. This amount gradually increases during pregnancy and reaches about 400 mg/day in the third trimester. This increase in calcium absorption is mediated by 1,25-dihydroxy vitamin D (calcitriol).

Total amount of serum calcium consists of ionized (free), complex (with bicarbonate and citrate), and albumin-bound fractions. During pregnancy, serum albumin and hemoglobin values decrease due to hemodilution and albumin level is low until delivery. This decrease in the amount of albumin causes the total serum calcium level to fall well below the normal range, but this is physiologically insignificant. Physiologically important thing is the amount of ionized calcium and this remains unchanged during pregnancy. It is not safe to use the total serum calcium level in the diagnosis and follow-up of hypo- or hypercalcemia during pregnancy due to the physiological decrease. Therefore, ionized calcium should be measured in pregnant women or total serum calcium corrected for albumin should be calculated. During pregnancy, serum phosphorus and magnesium levels remain within the normal limits.

During lactation, total serum calcium corrected for albumin and free calcium level are within the normal limits. During breastfeeding, serum levels of phosphorus increase due to phosphate resorption from the maternal skeleton, renal reabsorption of phosphate, and increased intestinal absorption.

57.2.2 PTH

Data on measuring PTH levels during pregnancy was based on first-generation radioimmunoassay tests, and these tests reported higher PTH values [2]. This is because early generation tests also measured PTH molecules that were biologically inactive. Low serum total calcium and high PTH values caused the suggestion of the concept of physiological secondary hyperparathyroidism during pregnancy. However, this is an erroneous concept and this still can be observed in some sources today [3]. As mentioned before, the decrease in serum calcium results from a decrease in albumin levels, while the ionized calcium level does not change during pregnancy.

More sensitive and accurate results are obtained with two-sided immunoradiometric (IRMA) PTH measurement [4]. Even, newer bio-intact tests do not include PTH fragments (PTH7-84) that accumulate in chronic kidney failure, and therefore, they allow more precise measurements [5]. However, data on the use of these tests during pregnancy are limited.

PTH drops to low-medium levels during the first trimester of pregnancy and returns to the mid-normal range within the next weeks. PTH is at the lower limit of the normal value or undetectable levels in the first few months of breastfeeding when sufficient calcium is consumed. Depending on the completion of lactation, PTH rises and reaches the normal range. Low levels of PTH suggest that PTH is not required for maternal bone mineralization during breastfeeding. This is confirmed by hypoparathyroid and aparathyroid women in whom skeletal and mineral metabolism normalizes during breastfeeding [6].

57.2.3 Vitamin D Metabolism

Maternal physiology adapts to facilitate the transfer of calcium to the fetus and newborn during pregnancy and lactation. PTH-related protein (PTH-rP) levels increase in maternal blood during pregnancy. PTH-rP is produced by fetal parathyroid, placenta, myometrium, and fetal membranes. This protein increases 1-alpha hydroxylase activity in the kidney and placenta, and accordingly, calcitriol synthesis increases. Increase in calcitriol levels causes the level of maternal PTH to decrease [7]. Apart from pregnancy and lactation periods, PTH-rP can usually be detected in the circulation of patients only with malignant hypercalcemia.

The total calcitriol level in pregnancy increases gradually (2–5 times) from the first trimester and remains high until birth. However, the free calcitriol level increases only in the third trimester of pregnancy [8]. However, considering the 20–40% increase in vitamin D–binding protein level and the decrease in the amount of serum albumin during pregnancy, the free calcitriol level increases in all three trimesters compared to normal [9–11]. The calcitriol clearance does not change during pregnancy.

Fetal calcium levels are higher than the maternal level throughout pregnancy, because maternal calcium is transferred to the fetus through active placental transport. Vitamin D level measured from umbilical cord blood was 20% lower than in maternal blood [12]. Hence, vitamin D deficiency is transmitted vertically from mother to baby. Low vitamin D levels make a predisposition to hypocalcemia in the early postnatal period in newborns and rickets in the long term. The level of vitamin D in breast milk is closely related to the levels of vitamin D in maternal blood.

Therefore, babies fed with breast milk are at risk for permanent vitamin D deficiency if the mother has vitamin D deficiency. To prevent this, the American Centers for Disease Control recommends that all nursing mothers receive 400–600 IU of vitamin D daily [13–15].

During breastfeeding, the mother's 25-hydroxy vitamin D stores are thought to be consumed by the newborn, but this is not possible because 25-hydroxy vitamin D cannot pass into breast milk. Although calcitriol can pass into breast milk, it is found in very low concentrations in breast milk, because it is found in large quanties in the maternal circulation only in a short postprandial period. Various clinical studies have shown that there is no significant change in maternal 25-hydroxy vitamin D levels during breastfeeding, even in women with severe vitamin D deficiency [16].

57.2.4 Calcitonin

Serum calcitonin levels increase during pregnancy. It is assumed that the only source for calcitonin is parafollicular C cells located in the thyroid gland. However, it is also synthesized from breast, placenta, and decidual tissues during pregnancy. This extrathyroidal calcitonin synthesis has been demonstrated by studies in total thyroidectomized women who became pregnant. In these women, the level of serum calcitonin, which was undetectable in the prepregnancy period, has been demonstrated to increase to normal values during pregnancy [17]. Increased levels of estrone, estradiol, and estriol during pregnancy can also stimulate the synthesis of calcitonin. In a study conducted in women of reproductive age, serum calcitonin levels have been shown to be 3–5 times higher in those using oral contraceptives or those who were pregnant than those who were not pregnant and not using oral contraceptives [18]. Estrogen replacement therapies (estradiol or synthetic estrogen derivatives) given to women in the postmenopausal period have also been found to increase serum calcitonin levels [19].

It is not known exactly whether calcitonin plays an important role in physiological changes that occur to meet the calcium need in pregnancy. It has been suggested that it protects the maternal skeleton against excessive demineralization in case of increased calcium need in pregnancy, but there are no clinical studies related to this. In studies conducted in pregnant mice without a calcitonin gene, calcium and bone metabolism was found to be normal [20, 21]. To fully understand the role of calcitonin in pregnant women, research should be conducted on pregnant women with mutations in the calcitonin or calcitonin receptor gene.

Calcitonin levels return to normal within the first 6 weeks after birth. It was found that the mice with defective gene encoding calcitonin had bone mineral loss twice than normal during lactation [20]. This finding shows that calcitonin at the physiological level can protect the maternal skeleton from excessive demineralization in breastfeeding. However, it is unknown whether calcitonin plays such a role in human physiology. By calcitonin synthesis from lactating breast tissue, total thyroidectomized women have similar levels of serum calcitonin in lactation with those of women having normal thyroid tissue [17].

57.2.5 Parathyroid Hormone–Related Protein (PTH-rP)

PTH-rP is actually a protein responsible for hypercalcemia that occurs in malignant tumors. Serum levels of PTH-rP increase throughout pregnancy and reach the highest levels in the third trimester. The main source of PTH-rP in pregnancy is maternal breast tissue and placenta. Whether PTH-rP plays any role in maternal physiology is not exactly known, but elevated serum levels stimulate 1-alpha hydroxylase activity in the kidneys and enhance calcitriol synthesis. However, PTH-rP has been shown to be less potent than PTH in stimulating 1-alpha hydroxylase activity [22, 23]. Therefore, it is thought that the increase in PTH-rP during pregnancy contributes to the suppression of PTH levels, although its contribution to calcitriol synthesis is not clear.

PTH-rP levels increase significantly during the lactation period and stimulate calcium resorption from the maternal skeleton and calcium absorption from the kidneys. During lactation, breast tissue acts as an accessory parathyroid gland and PTH-rP is responsible for hyperparathyroidism that occurs in this period. This has been proven in a study in rats with PTH-rP gene ablation [24]. Bone mineral density was found to decrease less in mice treated with gene ablation at the beginning of lactation. In human studies including lactating women, PTH-rP has been shown to correlate positively with ionized calcium and negatively with PTH, and high PTH-rP levels are associated with a greater reduction in bone mineral density [25–27].

57.3 Calcium Absorption and Metabolism in Pregnancy and Lactation

57.3.1 Intestinal Calcium and Phosphate Absorption

Intestinal calcium absorption has been demonstrated to double in an earlier period as 12th week of the pregnancy [2]. This increase in calcium absorption is the main adaptation of mother to meet the fetal calcium need. However, although intestinal calcium absorption increases in the first trimester, the peak in fetal calcium need occurs in the third trimester. It is believed that this allows the maternal skeleton to store calcium before the increased calcium need during pregnancy and lactation. Some studies in rodents have shown that this early increase in intestinal calcium absorption has an important role in increasing bone mineral density [6, 20, 28]. Besides, pregnant women have been shown to have a positive calcium balance in the middle of pregnancy [29]. This is probably related to the increase of intestinal calcium absorption in earlier periods of pregnancy and its effects on skeletal mineralization. The fact that intestinal phosphate absorption doubles during pregnancy has been shown by rodent and other mammalian studies [2]. It probably doubles in human pregnancy, but there are no clinical studies on it [1].

Intestinal calcium absorption, which increases during pregnancy, decreases rapidly during lactation and returns to normal. This also corresponds to the return of calcitriol levels to normal.

57.3.2 Renal Handling

Doubling of intestinal calcium absorption in the first trimester causes three possible scenarios: (1) passage of extra calcium to the fetus, (2) accumulation of extra calcium in the maternal skeleton, and (3) urinary excretion of calcium more than enough. Renal calcium excretion increases until the 12th week of pregnancy and 24-h urine calcium levels increase above normal. Conversely, fasting urine calcium is low or normal. This confirms that hypercalciuria during pregnancy is a result of increased intestinal calcium absorption. During pregnancy, the incidence of kidney stones, secondary to hypercalciuria, has increased. Calcitonin in pharmacological doses increases the excretion of calcium from the kidneys, but it is unknown whether calcitonin, which increases physiologically during pregnancy, has such an effect.

Hypocalciuria during pregnancy has been shown to be associated with low serum calcitriol levels, pregnancy-induced hypertension, and preeclampsia [30–32]. These changes occur secondary to decreased renal function rather than the cause of hypertension. However, dietary calcium supplementation during pregnancy reduces the incidence of preeclampsia. This supports the hypothesis that there is a relationship between calcium metabolism in pregnancy and preeclampsia [2].

In 24 h or less following the termination of pregnancy, renal calcium excretion returns to normal (50 mg) due to the decrease in the glomerular filtration rate. Renal phosphate reabsorption increased in the lactation period. Phosphate, which exceeds the amount required for milk production, is excreted in the urine. Therefore, hyperphosphaturia can also be observed during lactation.

57.3.3 Skeletal Calcium Metabolism

There is no histo-morphometric study evaluating skeletal metabolism in lactating women. Instead, there are cross-sectional and prospective studies evaluating biochemical markers showing bone formation and resorption. However, when evaluating these markers in breastfeeding women, it is necessary to take into account the physiological changes in pregnancy. For example, in contrast to pregnancy, the glomerular filtration rate and fluid volume in the vascular bed decrease in lactation. Bone resorption markers detected in serum and 24-h urine during lactation increase compared to the values in the first trimester of pregnancy. Serum bone formation markers also increase during lactation, but this increase is less than that detected in bone resorption markers. This indicates that bone resorption is more prominent in the lactation process.

The decrease in skeletal mineral density occurring in lactation cannot be suppressed by increased dietary calcium. The size of demineralization occurs in the maternal skeleton and is parallel to the amount of breast milk produced. Bone loss in lactation is due to increased osteoclast number and activity, which are caused by low estrogen levels. This bone loss is faster than those with acute estrogen deficiency observed in the patients under GnRH analog treatment or in women in the early postmenopausal period. Bone loss in lactation corresponds to about 5–10% of skeletal density over a 2–6-month period [7]. This can be explained by the increased PTH-rP levels showing a synergistic effect with estrogen on bone destruction.

In most of the epidemiological studies in pre- and postmenopausal women, previous history of lactation has been shown to have no negative impact on peak bone mass, bone density, and hip fracture risk [7, 33]. Therefore, the decrease in bone mineral density observed in lactation is clinically insignificant in the long term.

57.4 Calcium Disorders During Pregnancy and Lactation

57.4.1 Osteoporosis

Osteoporosis can be defined as a systemic loss in bone tissue that causes an increased risk of fractures, and disruption of bone microarchitecture. The increased risk of fractures in age-related osteoporosis is associated with loss of bone tissue that occurs with age. Besides, the increased bone remodeling with age contributes to the risk of fracture [34]. Pregnancy-related osteoporosis usually occurs during the first pregnancy, and there is no clear relationship between increasing number of parity and an increased risk of osteoporosis [35–38]. Changes in bone mineral metabolism caused by pregnancy can cause excessive skeletal demineralization in some women. In addition, factors such as low dietary calcium intake and vitamin D deficiency may contribute to this situation [35]. Increased bone turnover rate is an independent risk factor for fragility fractures. Therefore, increased bone resorption during pregnancy can also contribute to the risk of fractures.

Typical clinical presentation of osteoporosis associated with pregnancy is the vertebral collapse fracture that occurs due to the selective loss of bone density in the vertebra [39]. Fractures often affect the lower thoracic or lumbar vertebra, causing severe pain in this area. Bone biopsies from pregnant women with collapsed fractures indicate the presence of osteoporosis without osteomalacia, and bone density Z scores are lower than the expected [36–38]. This finding supports that pregnancy causes a significant amount of bone loss in many women. The pain decreases spontaneously in a few weeks in most cases, and bone mineral density becomes normal in the postpartum period. Fractures do not tend to recur in subsequent pregnancies. In a study based on long-term follow-up of women with osteoporosis associated with pregnancy, based on the significant increase in mineral density in the hip and spine in the postpartum period, the researchers concluded that the majority of bone loss occurred due to pregnancy itself [36].

During the lactation period, a decrease in bone mineral density occurs with increased PTH-rP produced from maternal breast tissue and decreased estradiol effect. Therefore, when skeletal resorption is high or the basal bone mass is low, and mineral losses due to lactation cannot be tolerated, lactation-associated osteoporosis may occur. This situation may increase the risk of osteoporotic fracture similar to that of pregnancy. However, it is unknown whether any treatment given to women with increased fracture risk during pregnancy and lactation reduces that risk. There is no definitive evidence to support that dietary calcium supplementation, which is given to minimize calcium loss, can reduce bone loss. Bisphosphonates, which are frequently used in the treatment of osteoporosis in the postmenopausal period, cannot be used in pregnancy due to possible negative effects on the fetal skeleton. Although it has been reported that bisphosphonates, which are accidentally used in short term before conception or shortly after fertilization, did not cause any toxic effect on the embryo, they are contraindicated for use in pregnancy [40].

57.4.2 Hypoparathyroidism

Hypoparathyroidism can be defined as the inability to maintain PTH production, which is necessary to maintain normal serum calcium levels. Low levels of PTH cause hypocalcemia by decreasing intestinal calcium absorption, renal reabsorption of calcium and skeletal resorption. The incidence of hypoparathyroidism during pregnancy is unknown. The most common cause of hypoparathyroidism is the removal or injury of parathyroid glands during thyroid surgery. It may rarely occur due to congenital developmental disorders or autoimmune parathyroid gland damage (autoimmune polyglandular syndrome type 1). The risk of hypoparathyroidism in the normal population varies depending on the type of thyroid pathology, the extent of the surgery, thyroid volume, and the surgeon's experience, but it is reported to be 0.5–6.6% [41].

The diagnosis of hypoparathyroidism is based on clinical history, laboratory tests, and radiological imaging methods. Symptoms of hypocalcaemia usually occur in the form of muscle twitching, numbness, and tingling of the fingers and toes and around the mouth. Some patients may experience carpopedal spasm, laryngeal stridor, and even respiratory distress. On physical examination, occurrence of spasm in the facial muscles when a sharp tap is given over the main trunk of the facial nerve is defined as Chvostek's sign. Although this sign is observed in most patients with hypocalcemia, it should be kept in mind that it can also be observed in normal healthy people. The Trousseau sign is another physical examination finding of hypocalcemia. It is based on the triggering of the carpopedal spasm by reducing the blood flow in the arm with the help of the blood pressure cuff. The cuff pressure should be kept above systolic blood pressure for 2 min before accepting the test as negative.

The diagnosis of hypoparathyroidism is confirmed by low serum calcium and high phosphorus levels. Serum PTH levels are low in primary hypoparathyroidism. In the differential diagnosis, rickets, osteomalacia, and hypomagnesemia should be considered. Bone mineral density may be higher in the patients with hypoparathyroidism compared to those with normal parathyroid function. Dental hypoplasia, defective enamel and root formation, failed tooth eruption also may be encountered. Additionally, osteosclerosis, cortical thickening, or craniofacial abnormalities might be observed in the patients with congenital hypoparathyroidism [42–45].

Hypoparathyroidism during pregnancy is usually seen as a pre-existing condition persisting during pregnancy. Some women have less hypocalcemic symptoms in the early stages of pregnancy, and lesser amount of calcium replacement is required. This can be explained by the limited role of PTH in a pregnant woman and an increase in calcitriol and/or in the absorption of intestinal calcium even in the absence of PTH. However, maternal hypocalcemia should be avoided. Because maternal hypocalcemia is associated with spontaneous abortion, growth and developmental retardation, preterm delivery, intrauterine death, and fetal hyperparathyroidism causing fetal skeletal demineralization and subperiosteal bone resorption [46].

Treatment of hypoparathyroidism during pregnancy is the same as the nonpregnancy period and includes high calcium diet and vitamin D supplementation. The normal calcium supplement during pregnancy is about 1.2 g/day. In the treatment of maternal hypoparathyroidism, it is recommended to give 1–1.5 g of calcium and 0.5–3 μg of calcitriol daily [47]. If calcitriol is used, it should be given in divided doses, because its half-life is shorter than 25(OH)vitamin D. If 25(OH)vitamin D is to be used, it should be given at a dose of 50,000–150,000 IU per week [48]. The main problem in the treatment of hypoparathyroidism is that recurrent hypocalcemia or hypercalcemia episodes. Therefore, serum calcium levels should be checked periodically. In cases of pregnancy-induced hypoparathyroidism, calcium monitoring should be continued during the early postpartum period and lactation, because the calcium and calcitriol need increases temporarily in the first few days following delivery in the hypoparathyroid women [49].

Then, with the initiation of breastfeeding, a significant amount of PTH-rP production occurs from the breast tissue. Some of the produced PTH-rP passes into the maternal circulation and stimulates bone resorption and increases the serum calcium level. This mechanism can temporarily restore bone metabolism and calcium levels during lactation in women with permanent hypoparathyroidism. The need for calcium and calcitriol in women with hypoparathyroidism decreases significantly following the early lactation period. Therefore, if the amount of vitamin D and calcium given is not reduced, hypercalcemia may appear [50, 51]. In the management of hypoparathyroidism during lactation, calcium level corrected by albumin level or free calcium levels should be closely monitored, the doses of calcium and vitamin D given in the treatment should be decreased initially, and then the doses should be increased gradually as breastfeeding decreases.

57.4.3 Hyperparathyroidism

The incidence of primary hyperparathyroidism is estimated to be approximately 0.5% in the normal population [52]. It is quite rare in pregnancy, but there is no clear information about its incidence. The vast majority of reported cases are case reports supported by a review of the literature. As two different large case series evaluating the patients with hyperparathyroidism who were treated surgically are considered, it is seen that only 1% of all parathyroidectomy interventions are performed during pregnancy [53, 54]. As in the general population, the etiological cause is solitary parathyroid adenoma in 80–85% of cases of primary hyperparathyroidism in pregnancy [52, 55]. Diffuse hyperplasia (10–12%), double or triple adenoma (2%), and carcinoma (<1%) are responsible for the remaining 15–20% [56].

Some changes due to pregnancy may mask the laboratory findings of hypercalcemia. These changes can be listed as an increase in glomerular filtration rate, a decrease in serum albumin levels, an increase in intravascular fluid volume and active calcium transport to the fetus. Continuing active calcium transport from mother to fetus at a certain rate (1:1.4) is extremely important for the development of the fetal skeleton. This ratio provides the calcium necessary for the continuation of fetal skeletal maturation without suppressing the fetal parathyroid tissue. Disruption of this rate due to maternal hypercalcemia may lead to suppression of fetal parathyroid tissue and result in neonatal tetany [57].

It has been reported that primary hyperparathyroidism that occurs during pregnancy causes various symptoms that are not specific to hypercalcemia and indistinguishable from those associated with pregnancy [1]. These symptoms can be listed as nausea, vomiting, weight loss, anorexia, headache, and mood changes. However, about 80% of patients are asymptomatic and therefore, diagnosis is usually made incidentally by routine laboratory tests [55]. Increased levels of total serum calcium corrected for albumin or ionized calcium and detectable levels of PTH are diagnostic in most cases. Due to a possible low serum albumin level, total serum calcium level of >9.5 mg/dL in a pregnant woman should be considered suspicious for hypercalcemia and investigated [52].

Hyperparathyroid crisis is an extremely serious complication of primary hyperparathyroidism that can be encountered in pregnancy or the postpartum period. The clinical presentation is characterized by severe nausea and vomiting, fatigue, dehydration, mental status changes, and instability in vital signs. It may even cause a life-threatening situation in some cases. Hypertension is present in most cases, but it must be differentiated from preeclampsia and gestational hypertension. Serum calcium levels are well above normal (>13 mg/dL) in most cases, with hypokalemia and increased serum creatinine levels [52]. If the clinical presentation is not recognized and treated appropriately, it will progress rapidly and may result in coma and death.

Hyperparathyroidism in pregnancy: approximately 80% of fetuses are at risk due to hypercalcemia and possible complications due to this [58]. These complications can be listed as intrauterine growth retardation, preterm delivery, low birth weight, and neonatal hypocalcemic tetany. In infants of mothers with hyperparathyroidism, the frequency of stillbirth and perinatal death was reported as 2%; however, the frequency of neonatal tetany was reported as 15% [59]. The negative effects of hyperparathyroidism in the postnatal period are due to the suppression of fetal and neonatal parathyroid tissues. While this suppression may last up to several months in some cases, it may become permanent in some cases [59–61].

Management of primary hyperparathyroidism during pregnancy can be difficult, because some choices of treatment cannot be used during pregnancy. The treatment to be chosen should be decided by considering the age of the pregnancy, the severity of hypercalcemia, and the balance of benefit/harm. Conservative approaches can be considered in mildly asymptomatic cases due to the low risk of maternal and fetal complications [62, 63]. Surgical treatment is indicated in the presence of symptomatic hypercalcemia. The second trimester is the best time for surgical treatment, since organogenesis in the fetus is completed, it does not carry the risk of preterm delivery, which is possible in the third trimester, and more successful results can be obtained in the second trimester [54, 64, 65].

The effectiveness and reliability of surgical approaches have increased with pre-operative localization studies and minimally invasive surgical techniques. High success and low complication rates are achieved in the vast majority of cases by localization with preoperative neck ultrasonography and intraoperative PTH monitoring. However, since some radiological methods cannot be used during pregnancy, and due to a possibility of a genetic syndrome such as MEN syndromes, especially in young women, exploration of four parathyroid glands with a bilateral surgical approach may be necessary in some cases. Hirsch et al. [62] reported that there was no difference between pregnant women undergoing parathyroidectomy and those observed without surgery in terms of miscarriage or other complications related to pregnancy. In another study, 70 of 109 pregnant women with primary hyperparathyroidism were given medical treatment, while 39 were treated surgically [54]. In the medical treatment group, the neonatal complication rate was 53% and the mortality rate was 16%; however, those were 12.5% and 2.5%, respectively, in the surgical treatment group. For these reasons, surgical treatment in the second trimester remains the most common recommendation for primary hyperparathyroidism [66].

There is no definitive management algorithm for the medical treatment of hyperparathyroidism during pregnancy. In general, it is recommended to ensure adequate hydration, limit calcium intake, and correct electrolyte disturbances. Agents used in the pharmacological treatment of hypercalcemia have not been adequately studied in pregnancy. Therefore, the data on their side effects is insufficient. Calcitonin can be used safely, because it does not pass through the placenta [66]. Oral phosphate therapy (1.5–2.5 g/day) can be used as an effective option to control hypercalcemia, but possible side effects such as diarrhea, hypokalemia, and soft tissue calcification should be considered. Since bisphosphonates have potential toxic effects on the fetal skeleton, they are contraindicated for use in pregnancy. For this reason, they should be preserved for use in the life-threatening hypercalcemic crises [40]. In animal studies with denosumab, an osteoporosis-like clinical presentation was demonstrated in the fetus [67, 68]. It is not recommended for use in human pregnancy, since it can pass through the placenta. Cinacalcet, a calcium-sensing receptor activator used in the treatment of primary and secondary hyperparathyroidism and parathyroid carcinoma in nonpregnant adults, has been tried in pregnancy with hyperparathyroidism [69–72]. However, the calcium-sensing receptor, the target of this drug, is expressed in the placenta and regulates the fetal-placental calcium transfer [73]. For this reason, the use of cinacalcet in pregnancy may cause possible toxic effects on the fetus and newborn.

If the surgical correction of primary hyperparathyroidism is not possible or if it is inappropriate due to possible complications during pregnancy or timing, the treatment will be applied in the postpartum period. Serum calcium levels should be closely monitored in these patients. A hypercalcemic crisis may occur due to the disappearance of placental active calcium transport following birth. It should be noted that if untreated women with primary hyperparathyroidism choose to breastfeed, serum calcium levels may increase more with the effect of PTH-rP secreted by breast tissue.

57.4.4 Vitamin D Insufficiency and Deficiency

Vitamin D insufficiency is defined as 25(OH) vitamin D concentration of 12–20 ng/mL, and vitamin D deficiency as a level of <12 ng/mL [74]. There is no comprehensive clinical study examining the effects of vitamin D deficiency or insufficiency on human pregnancy. The information we have on this subject is based on the data obtained from studies examining vitamin D supplementation, or observational studies and case reports. Vitamin D deficiency in pregnancy and lactation has been reviewed in detail by Barret and McElduff [75]. Vitamin D deficiency in pregnancy is closely related to some problems affecting the mother, fetus, and newborn.

Vitamin D deficiency or insufficiency is not associated with worsening of maternal calcium homeostasis. Maternal hypocalcemia is milder in vitamin D deficiency due to secondary hyperparathyroidism, which increases skeletal resorption and renal reabsorption. However, severe vitamin D deficiency causes maternal hypocalcemia, hypophosphatemia, muscle weakness, myopathy and rickets, or osteomalacia. In addition, vitamin D deficiency has been associated with infertility, decreased in vitro fertilization success, preeclampsia [76], increased insulin resistance and gestational diabetes [77], and increased frequency of cesarean delivery [78].

The amount of vitamin D in breast milk directly correlates with maternal vitamin D levels. Therefore, in the presence of maternal vitamin D deficiency, babies who are only breastfed are particularly at risk. It has been demonstrated that neonatal hypocalcemia and the frequency of associated seizure increase in infants fed with only breast milk [79]. In addition, skeletal developmental disorders including rickets and low bone mineral density, growth and developmental delay are also common. It has also been reported that conditions such as type 1 diabetes, asthma, atopy, schizophrenia, and an increased risk of HIV transmission may be associated with vitamin D deficiency [75]. For these reasons, babies who are only breastfed should take 400 IU vitamin D supplementation daily.

The Institute of Medicine guideline recommends taking 600 IU of vitamin D supplements daily during pregnancy [80]. The upper limit for vitamin D intake is determined as 4000 IU/day. On the other hand, the Endocrine Society indicated that 600 IU of vitamin D should be taken during pregnancy and that a minimum of 1500 IU per day may be required to keep the 25-hydroxy vitamin D level above 30 ng/mL [81]. However, if high doses of vitamin D will be preferred, the possible benefits and harms of the mother and fetus should be considered. The ideal approach should be to maintain an adequate maternal vitamin D level in the pre-pregnancy period and to continue with the recommended daily intake during pregnancy and breastfeeding.

57.5   Conclusion

Physiological adaptive mechanisms in pregnancy and lactation complement the natural regulators of mineral metabolism. Intestinal calcium absorption increases from the early stages of pregnancy to meet the calcium need of the fetus. On the other hand, the source of calcium in breast milk is the resorption from the maternal skeleton and to a lesser extent calcium retention from the kidneys. Giving dietary calcium support in pregnancy increases maternal calcium absorption. However, the effect of calcium supplementation given in the lactation on maternal bone loss is minimal. This temporary loss of bone mass during breastfeeding may threaten skeletal strength and cause fragility fractures in some women. It will take time for bone mineral density to return to normal following the completion of lactation, but this does not cause long-term negative consequences for most women.

References

1. Kovacs CS. Calcium and phosphate metabolism and related disorders during pregnancy and lactation. In: Feingold KR, Anawalt B, Boyce A, et al., editors. Endotext. South Dartmouth: MDText.com; 2000.
2. Kovacs CS. Maternal mineral and bone metabolism during pregnancy, lactation, and post-weaning recovery. Physiol Rev. 2016;96:449–547.
3. Taylor RN, Badell ML. The endocrinology of pregnancy. In: Gardner DG, Shoback DG, editors. Greenspan's basic and clinical endocrinology. 9th ed. New York: Lange Medical Books/ McGraw-Hill; 2011. p. 553–72.
4. Potts JT Jr, Bringhurst FR, Gardella T, Nussbaum S, Segre G, Kronenberg HM. Parathyroid hormone: physiology, chemistry, biosynthesis, secretion, metabolism, and mode of action. In: DeGroot LJ, editor. Endocrinology. Philadelphia: Saunders; 1995. p. 920–66.
5. Tsuchida T, Ishimura E, Hirowatari K, et al. Serum levels of 1–84 and 7–84 parathyroid hormone in predialysis patients with chronic renal failure measured by the intact and bio-PTH assay. Nephron Clin Pract. 2006;102:108–14.
6. Kirby BJ, Ma Y, Martin HM, et al. Upregulation of calcitriol during pregnancy and skeletal recovery after lactation do not require parathyroid hormone. J Bone Miner Res. 2013;28:1987–2000.
7. Kovacs CS, Kronenberg HM. Maternal-fetal calcium and bone metabolism during pregnancy, puerperium, and lactation. Endocr Rev. 1997;18:832–72.

8. Bikle DD, Gee E, Halloran B, et al. Free 1,25-dihydroxyvitamin D levels in serum from normal subjects, pregnant subjects, and subjects with liver disease. J Clin Invest. 1984;74:1966–71.

9. Ardawi MS, Nasrat HA, BA'Aqueel HS. Calcium-regulating hormones and parathyroid hormone-related peptide in normal human pregnancy and postpartum: a longitudinal study. Eur J Endocrinol. 1997;137:402–9.

10. Zhang JY, Lucey AJ, Horgan R, et al. Impact of pregnancy on vitamin D status: a longitudinal study. Br J Nutr. 2014;112:1081–7.

11. Hollis BW, Johnson D, Hulsey TC, et al. Vitamin D supplementation during pregnancy: double-blind, randomized clinical trial of safety and effectiveness. J Bone Miner Res. 2011;26:2341–57.

12. Morley R, Carlin JB, Pasco JA, et al. Maternal 25-hydroxyvitamin D and parathyroid hormone concentrations and offspring birth size. J Clin Endocrinol Metab. 2006;91:906–12.

13. Hollis BW, Wagner CL. Vitamin D requirements during lactation: high-dose maternal supplementation as therapy to prevent hypovitaminosis D for both the mother and the nursing infant. Am J Clin Nutr. 2004;80(6 Suppl):1752–8.

14. Bischoff-Ferrari HA, Willett WC, Orav EJ, et al. A pooled analysis of vitamin D dose requirements for fracture prevention. N Engl J Med. 2012;367:40–9.

15. American Geriatrics Society Work group on Vitamin D Supplementation for Older Adults. Recommendations abstracted from the American Geriatrics Society consensus statement on vitamin D for prevention of falls and their consequences. J Am Geriatr Soc. 2014;62:147–52.

16. Kovacs CS. The role of vitamin D in pregnancy and lactation: insights from animal models and clinical studies. Annu Rev Nutr. 2012;32:97–123.

17. Bucht E, Telenius-Berg M, Lundell G, et al. Immunoextracted calcitonin in milk and plasma from totally thyroidectomized women. Evidence of monomeric calcitonin in plasma during pregnancy and lactation. Acta Endocrinol (Copenh). 1986;113:529–35.

18. Hillyard CJ, Stevenson JC, MacIntyre I. Relative deficiency of plasma-calcitonin in normal women. Lancet. 1978;1:961–2.

19. Stevenson JC, Abeyasekera G, Hillyard CJ, et al. Calcitonin and the calcium-regulating hormones in postmenopausal women: effect of oestrogens. Lancet. 1981;1:693–5.

20. Woodrow JP, Sharpe CJ, Fudge NJ, et al. Calcitonin plays a critical role in regulating skeletal mineral metabolism during lactation. Endocrinology. 2006;147:4010–21.

21. Woodrow JP. Calcitonin modulates skeletal mineral loss during lactation through interactions in mammary tissue and directly though osteoclasts in bone [PhD thesis] [PhD]. St. John's, Newfoundland: Biomedical Sciences, Faculty of Medicine, Memorial University of Newfoundland; 2009.

22. Horwitz MJ, Tedesco MB, Sereika SM, et al. Direct comparison of sustained infusion of human parathyroid hormone-related protein-(136). J Clin Endocrinol Metab. 2003;88:1603–9.

23. Horwitz MJ, Tedesco MB, Sereika SM, et al. Continuous PTH and PTHrP infusion causes suppression of bone formation and discordant effects on 1,25(OH)2 vitamin D. J Bone Miner Res. 2005;20:1792–803.

24. VanHouten JN, Dann P, Stewart AF, et al. Mammary-specific deletion of parathyroid hormone-related protein preserves bone mass during lactation. J Clin Invest. 2003;112:1429–136.

25. Dobnig H, Kainer F, Stepan V, et al. Elevated parathyroid hormone-related peptide levels after human gestation: relationship to changes in bone and mineral metabolism. J Clin Endocrinol Metab. 1995;80:3699–707.

26. Kovacs CS, Chik CL. Hyperprolactinemia caused by lactation and pituitary adenomas is associated with altered serum calcium, phosphate, parathyroid hormone (PTH), and PTH-related peptide levels. J Clin Endocrinol Metab. 1995;80:3036–42.

27. Sowers MF, Hollis BW, Shapiro B, et al. Elevated parathyroid hormone-related peptide associated with lactation and bone density loss. J Am Med Assoc. 1996;276:549–54.

28. Fudge NJ, Kovacs CS. Pregnancy up-regulates intestinal calcium absorption and skeletal mineralization independently of the vitamin D receptor. Endocrinology. 2010;151:886–95.

29. Heaney RP, Skillman TG. Calcium metabolism in normal human pregnancy. J Clin Endocrinol Metab. 1971;33:661–70.

30. Frenkel Y, Barkai G, Mashiach S, et al. Hypocalciuria of preeclampsia is independent of parathyroid hormone level. Obstet Gynecol. 1991;77:689–91.
31. Seely EW, Wood RJ, Brown EM, et al. Lower serum ionized calcium and abnormal calciotropic hormone levels in preeclampsia. J Clin Endocrinol Metab. 1992;74:1436–40.
32. Lalau JD, Jans I, el Esper N, et al. Calcium metabolism, plasma parathyroid hormone, and calcitriol in transient hypertension of pregnancy. Am J Hypertens. 1993;6:522–7.
33. To WW, Wong MW, Leung TW. Relationship between bone mineral density changes in pregnancy and maternal and pregnancy characteristics: a longitudinal study. Acta Obstet Gynecol Scand. 2003;82:820–7.
34. Seeman E, Delmas PD. Bone quality–the material and structural basis of bone strength and fragility. N Engl J Med. 2006;354:2250–61.
35. Kovacs CS, Ralston SH. Presentation and management of osteoporosis presenting in association with pregnancy or lactation. Osteoporos Int. 2015;26:2223–41.
36. Phillips AJ, Ostlere SJ, Smith R. Pregnancy-associated osteoporosis: does the skeleton recover? Osteoporos Int. 2000;11:449–54.
37. Khovidhunkit W, Epstein S. Osteoporosis in pregnancy. Osteoporos Int. 1996;6:345–54.
38. Smith R, Athanasou NA, Ostlere SJ, et al. Pregnancy-associated osteoporosis. Q J Med. 1995;88:865–78.
39. Dunne F, Walters B, Marshall T, et al. Pregnancy associated osteoporosis. Clin Endocrinol. 1993;39:487–90.
40. Levy S, Fayez I, Taguchi N, et al. Pregnancy outcome following in utero exposure to bisphosphonates. Bone. 2009;44:428–30.
41. Shoback D. Clinical practice. Hypoparathyroidism. N Engl J Med. 2008;359:391–403.
42. Goltzman D, Cole DEC. Hypoparathyroidism. In: Favus MJ, editor. Primer on the metabolic bone diseases and disorders of mineral metabolism. 6th ed. Washington: American Society of Bone and Mineral Research; 2006. p. 216.
43. Laway BA, Goswami R, Singh N, et al. Pattern of bone mineral density in patients with sporadic idiopathic hypoparathyroidism. Clin Endocrinol (Oxf). 2006;64:405.
44. Chan FK, Tiu SC, Choi KL, et al. Increased bone mineral density in patients with chronic hypoparathyroidism. J Clin Endocrinol Metab. 2003;88:3155.
45. Kinirons MJ, Glasgow JF. The chronology of dentinal defects related to medical findings in hypoparathyroidism. J Dent. 1985;13:346.
46. Kowacs CS. Calcium and bone metabolism disorders during pregnancy and lactation. Endocrinol Metab Clin North Am. 2011;40:795–826.
47. Cardot-Bauters C. Hypoparathyroidism and pregnancy. Annales D'endocrinologie. 2016;77:172–5.
48. Salle BL, Berthezene F, Glorieux GH. Hypoparathyroidism during pregnancy: treatment with calcitriol. J Clin Endocrinol Metab. 1981;52:810.
49. Sweeney LL, Malabanan AO, Rosen H. Decreased calcitriol requirement during pregnancy and lactation with a window of increased requirement immediately postpartum. Endocr Pract. 2010;16:459–62.
50. Caplan RH, Beguin EA. Hypercalcemia in a calcitriol-treated hypoparathyroid woman during lactation. Obstet Gynecol. 1990;76:485–9.
51. Shomali ME, Ross DS. Hypercalcemia in a woman with hypoparathyroidism associated with increased parathyroid hormone-related protein during lactation. Endocr Pract. 1999;5:198–200.
52. Sullivan SA. Parathyroid diseases. Clin Obstet Gynecol. 2019;62:347–58.
53. Kort KC, Schiller HJ, Numann PJ. Hyperparathyroidism and pregnancy. Am J Surg. 1999;177:66–8.
54. Kelly TR. Primary hyperparathyroidism during pregnancy. Surgery. 1991;110:1028–33.
55. Amaya García M, Acosta Feria M, Soto Moreno A, et al. Primary hyperparathyroidism in pregnancy. Gynecol Endocrinol. 2004;19:111–4.
56. Eigelberger MS, Clark OH. Surgical approaches to primary hyperparathyroidism. Endocrinol Metab Clin North Am. 1995;29:479–502.

57. Kohlmeier L, Marcus R. Calcium disorders of pregnancy. Endocrinol Metab Clin North Am. 1995;24:15–39.

58. Delmonico FL, Neer RM, Cosimi AB. Hyperparathyroidism during pregnancy. Am J Surg. 1976;131:328–37.

59. Shangold MM, Dor N, Welt SI, et al. Hyperparathyroidism and pregnancy: a review. Obstet Gynecol Surv. 1982;37:217–28.

60. Ludwig GD. Hyperparathyroidism in relation to pregnancy. N Engl J Med. 1962;267:637–42.

61. Bruce J, Strong JA. Maternal hyperparathyroidism and parathyroid deficiency in the child, with account of effect of parathyroidectomy on renal function, and of attempt to transplant part of tumor. Q J Med. 1955;24:307–19.

62. Hirsch D, Kopel V, Nadler V, et al. Pregnancy outcomes in women with primary hyperparathyroidism. J Clin Endocrinol Metab. 2015;100:2115–22.

63. Abood A, Vestergaard P. Pregnancy outcomes in women with primary hyperparathyroidism. Eur J Endocrinol. 2014;171:69–76.

64. Kaplan EL, Burrington JD, Klementschitsch P, et al. Primary hyperparathyroidism, pregnancy, and neonatal hypocalcemia. Surgery. 1984;96:717–22.

65. Carella MJ, Gossain VV. Hyperparathyroidism and pregnancy: case report and review. J Gen Intern Med. 1992;7:448–53.

66. Schnatz PF, Curry SL. Primary hyperparathyroidism in pregnancy: evidence-based management. Obstet Gynecol Surv. 2002;57:365–76.

67. Rajala B, Abbasi RA, Hutchinson HT, et al. Acute pancreatitis and primary hyperparathyroidism in pregnancy: treatment of hypercalcemia with magnesium sulfate. Obstet Gynecol. 1987;70:460–2.

68. Dahan M, Chang RJ. Pancreatitis secondary to hyperparathyroidism during pregnancy. Obstet Gynecol. 2001;98:923–5.

69. Horjus C, Groot I, Telting D, et al. Cinacalcet for hyperparathyroidism in pregnancy and puerperium. J Pediatr Endocrinol Metab. 2009;22:741–9.

70. Gonzalo Garcia I, Robles Fradejas M, Martin Macias MLA, et al. Primary hyperparathyroidism in pregnancy treated with cinacalcet: a case report. J Obstet Gynaecol. 2018;38:132–4.

71. Vera L, Oddo S, Di Iorgi N, et al. Primary hyperparathyroidism in pregnancy treated with cinacalcet: a case report and review of the literature. J Med Case Rep. 2016;10:361.

72. Nadarasa K, Bailey M, Chahal H, et al. The use of cinacalcet in pregnancy to treat a complex case of parathyroid carcinoma. Endocrinol Diabetes Metab Case Rep. 2014;2014:140056.

73. Kovacs CS, Ho-Pao CL, Hunzelman JL, et al. Regulation of murine fetal-placental calcium metabolism by the calcium-sensing receptor. J Clin Invest. 1998;101:2812–20.

74. Giustina A, Adler RA, Binkley N, et al. Controversies in vitamin D: summary statement from an international conference. J Clin Endocrinol Metab. 2019;104:234.

75. Barrett H, McElduff A. Vitamin D and pregnancy: an old problem revisited. Best Pract Res Clin Endocrinol Metab. 2010;24:527–39.

76. Haugen M, Brantsaeter AL, Trogstad L, et al. Vitamin D supplementation and reduced risk of preeclampsia in nulliparous women. Epidemiology. 2009;20:720–6.

77. Maghbooli Z, Hossein-Nezhad A, Karimi F, et al. Correlation between vitamin D3 deficiency and insulin resistance in pregnancy. Diabetes Metab Res Rev. 2008;24:27–32.

78. Merewood A, Mehta SD, Chen TC, et al. Association between vitamin D deficiency and primary cesarean section. J Clin Endocrinol Metab. 2009;94:940–5.

79. Robinson PD, Hogler W, Craig ME, et al. The re-emerging burden of rickets: a decade of experience from Sydney. Arch Dis Child. 2006;91:564–8.

80. Ross AC, Manson JE, Abrams SA, et al. The 2011 report on dietary reference intakes for calcium and vitamin D from the Institute of Medicine: what clinicians need to know. J Clin Endocrinol Metab. 2011;96:53–8.

81. Holick MF, Binkley NC, Bischoff-Ferrari HA, et al. Evaluation, treatment, and prevention of vitamin D deficiency: an endocrine society clinical practice guideline. J Clin Endocrinol Metab. 2011;96:3908.

## Part VII

Lower Airway Diseases During Pregnancy and the Postpartum Period

Pulmonary Physiologic Adaptations During Pregnancy

58

Asena Aydin and Sevinc Sarinc Ulasli

58.1 Introduction

Since the beginning of pregnancy, the pregnant woman must adapt to the new process due to the increase in metabolic needs. In this process, the pregnant woman should maintain her needs and meet the needs of the placenta and fetus. Many anatomical and physiological adaptation mechanisms become a part of the continuation of a healthy pregnancy.

Dyspnea, fatigue, lower extremity edema, and bibasilar atelectasis may also occur in normal pregnant women, making it difficult to distinguish pathological conditions. It is essential to know the adaptation mechanisms in a pregnancy period to differentiate which findings are pathological and physiological. In this chapter, physiologic changes in the respiratory system during pregnancy will be discussed emphasizing the differential diagnosis.

A. Aydin (✉)
Department of Chest Diseases, Inegol State Hospital, Bursa, Turkey
e-mail: asena.arisoyaydin@gmail.com

S. S. Ulasli
Department of Chest Diseases, Hacettepe University, School of Medicine, Ankara, Turkey
e-mail: sevincsarinc@gmail.com

C. Cingi et al. (eds.), *ENT Diseases: Diagnosis and Treatment during Pregnancy and Lactation*, https://doi.org/10.1007/978-3-031-05303-0_58

58.2 Anatomic Changes

58.2.1 Upper Airways

During pregnancy, there is increased mucopolysaccharide content in the upper airways due to glandular hyperreactivity. Capillary congestion, edema, and consequently fragility occur with increased secretion in the airways. Thus, the frequency of epistaxis increases, rhinitis gets worse by one to third. In pregnant women who did not have rhinitis before, pregnancy-related rhinitis is seen at a rate of 18–42% [1].

Pregnancy-related rhinitis, an entity different from rhinitis seen in nonpregnant women, is defined as "rhinitis that begins in pregnancy, lasts for at least six weeks, does not show signs of respiratory tract infection, is not due to an allergic etiology, and disappears two weeks after birth." Although it has no proven etiology, studies suggest that it is associated with progesterone, estrogen, placental growth hormone, and prolactin, which increase with pregnancy [2].

Pharyngeal diameter and neck circumference increase due to edema in pregnant women. Hence, Mallampati score increases, and intubation becomes difficult correlated with body weight gain. Since intubation failure is seen ten times more, nasotracheal intubation may need to be performed with an experienced team and a smaller tube [3–5].

58.2.2 Chest Anatomy

In the first trimester, before the uterus is enlarged, collagen loss and flexibility in ligaments and cartilages develop due to increased progesterone and relaxin [6, 7]. As the pregnancy progresses, the diaphragm elevates 2–4 cm because of the enlargement of the uterus. As a result, the subcostal angle widens from 68 to 103°, the thorax diameter widens by ≥ 2 cm, and the chest circumference increases 5–7 cm. The changes return to pre-pregnancy status until 24 weeks of the postpartum period, while the subcostal angle remains 20% of the baseline [1]. Although the diameter of the thorax expands, chest wall compliance decreases due to abdominal pressure. Decreased chest wall compliance and elevated diaphragm cause a decrease in total lung capacity [8].

58.3 Functional Changes

58.3.1 Lung Volumes

Lung reserve volumes decrease because of the elevation of the diaphragm. Expiratory reserve volume (ERV), the additional air volume that can be exhaled after a normal expiration, decreases 15–20% (200–300 mL), and residual volume (RV), the air volume remaining in the lung after ERV, decreases 20–25% (200–400 mL). Functional residual capacity (FRC) is the air volume in the lungs and airways at the end of a normal expiration and decreases by 20–30% (400–700 mL) during pregnancy due to elevation of diaphragm, decreased ERV and RV, and decreased compliance of chest wall. This decrease is more significant in the supine position and during sleep. FRC and RV return to normal limits 48 h after birth. Inspiratory capacity (IC), the air volume that can be inhaled after a normal expiration, increases 5–10% (200–350 mL), and total lung capacity (TLC) decreases by 5% [1]. Despite the decrease in ERV, vital capacity remains constant due to a 30–50% increase in tidal volume.

There is no significant change in spirometric tests during pregnancy. Forced expiratory volume in the first second (FEV1) remains the same, and the FEV1 to forced vital capacity (FVC) ratio does not change [1, 9]. Since there is no problem using spirometry during pregnancy, it should be performed when necessary; abnormal results should be considered pathological and evaluated in terms of the underlying disease.

58.3.2 Oxygen Consumption: Carbon Dioxide Production

During pregnancy, oxygen consumption and carbon dioxide production increase due to the fetus and mother's increased metabolic needs. The volume of maximum oxygen consumption (VO_2max) increases (normal value of VO_2max varies between 34 and 38 mL/kg/min) 20–40% in pregnant women. One-third of this increase is due to the need for the fetus, and the remaining two-third of it is due to the increase in the need for pregnant tissues, especially myocardial and renal tissues. With the increase in oxygen consumption, carbon dioxide production increases by 30% (30–300 mL) [10].

The risk of hypoxia is higher in pregnant women due to the increase in oxygen need and decreased FRC. Since intubation is also difficult due to changes in the upper airway, it is essential to ensure oxygenation of pregnant women who will undergo general anesthesia before intubation [11].

58.3.3 Ventilation

The increase in oxygen consumption and carbon dioxide excretion due to the increase in basal metabolism is balanced with an increase of approximately 50% of the minute ventilation in pregnancy at term. Estrogen and progesterone increase throughout pregnancy and play active roles in increasing ventilation. Progesterone reaches six times more than the levels in the pre-pregnancy period. At the 37th week, the progesterone value reaches 150 nm/mL from its pre-pregnancy value of 25 ng/mL [12].

Progesterone increases the central arterial carbon dioxide pressure ($PaCO_2$) sensitivity, and estrogen increases the number and sensitivity of progesterone receptors in the medulla and hypothalamus. Thus, progesterone directly and estrogen indirectly stimulate the respiratory system. While a 1 mmHg increase in $PaCO_2$ leads to a 1.5 L/min increase in ventilation in nonpregnant women, it causes a 6 L/min increase in pregnant women [10]. Both hormones also increase the sensitivity of peripheral chemoreceptors to hypoxia [13–15].

Progesterone increases minute ventilation and sensitivity to hypercapnia [16]; however, studies showed that estrogen alone is not adequate for these effects.

The ventilation response to hypoxia increases twice during pregnancy [17]. While the respiratory rate does not change, minute ventilation is provided by the increase in tidal volume. A 30–50% increase in tidal volume enables minute ventilation to reach from 6.5 to 10.5 L/min. Thus, arterial oxygen pressure (PaO_2) increases due to the increase in ventilation, despite increased oxygen consumption.

58.3.4 Blood Gases

As a result of the increase in ventilation, PaO_2 increases to 100–105 mmHg, and $PaCO_2$ decreases to 32–34 mmHg levels during pregnancy. Alkalosis is expected with these $PaCO_2$ levels, bicarbonate (HCO_3) excretion increases with renal adaptation, and HCO_3 levels are kept between 15 and 20 mEq/L; thus, the pH is normalized or mild alkalosis is seen [17–19]. For blood gas changes to return to pre-pregnancy levels, at least 1 week should pass after birth.

Fetal $PaCO_2$ is approximately 10 mmHg higher than that of the mother. Low $PaCO_2$ facilitates CO_2 passage from fetus to mother. Also, with the increase of 2,3-diphosphoglycerate in the pregnant woman, the oxygen-hemoglobin dissociation curve shifts to the right, making it easier for the fetus to take oxygen and deliver carbon dioxide [17].

58.3.5 Plasma and Blood Volume Increase

Blood volume increases by 40–50% in pregnant women. The increase in the number and size of fetuses causes the blood volume to increase even more, and it is 20% more in twin pregnancies. This increase begins in the seventh week of pregnancy and lasts until the 32nd week.

In addition to the contribution of estrogen to the increase, an increase in sodium (Na) uptake occurs with a two-fold increase in aldosterone, a 15–30-fold decrease in deoxy-corticosteroid, and an increase in renin and angiotensin. During pregnancy, sodium excretion from the body is increased because of increased progesterone level and glomerular filtration rate (GFR). Thus, approximately 1000 mEq Na excess develops, resulting in a blood volume increase [20–23].

Although blood volume increases to meet the increased metabolic needs, it is also an adaptation developed against blood loss during delivery. Approximately 500–1000 mL blood loss is expected during delivery. For a pregnant woman to develop hypotension and tachycardia due to hemorrhage, nearly 30% of blood volume should be lost. Therefore, pregnant women should be evaluated in terms of replacement without waiting to develop these symptoms [10].

58.3.6 Blood Cell Increase

An increase in prolactin, progesterone, chorionic somatomammotropin, and erythropoietin levels during pregnancy causes a 20% increase in erythrocyte amount compared to nonpregnant women. The increase in erythrocyte production increases the iron requirement to approximately 500 mg during pregnancy. Despite the increase in erythrocyte amount due to the 40–50% increase in the blood volume, the hematocrit decreases dilutional, called the physiological anemia of pregnancy. Iron replacement reduces the depth of anemia [20, 23].

58.3.7 Diffusion Capacity for Carbon Monoxide (DLCO)

Diffusion capacity for carbon monoxide (DLCO) is affected by cardiac output, body position, high altitude, and hemoglobin values. DLCO increases slightly in the first trimester, then decreases to its normal limits by 24–27th weeks. DLCO increases in the supine position in nonpregnant women, explained by the increased venous return. On the contrary, in pregnant women, due to uterine compression in the supine position, venous return decreases, and DLCO does not increase [17].

Although DLCO changes with altitude, it does not differ in the 1st and 2nd trimesters between pregnant and nonpregnant women living at high altitudes; in the 3rd trimester, it is lower in pregnant women [24].

58.3.8 Lung Functions

Muscle strength, measured with maximum trans-diaphragmatic pressure, about 95 cm H_2O, does not change. Increased abdominal pressure with an enlarged uterus decreases chest wall compliance by 35–40% [8]. While chest wall compliance decreases, lung compliance does not change. Since the effect of chest wall compliance is greater than airway resistance, total compliance decreases, and respiratory workload increases.

Closing volume (CV) defines the volume in which the small airways in the lung basal are closed and cannot participate in ventilation; it does not change with pregnancy [25]. Normally closure occurs at a volume between RV and FRC. However, closure may also occur in tidal volume with FRC decrease during pregnancy, especially during delivery [26]. When the closure occurs in tidal volume, ventilation at the base of the lung decreases, and ventilation-perfusion (V/Q) mismatch develops, and the respiratory rate increases [10, 27].

Respiratory muscle strength is preserved during pregnancy. Airway resistance is normal or slightly decreases due to smooth muscle relaxation effects of progesterone.

Changes in pulmonary function tests are depicted in Table 58.1.

Table 58.1 Pulmonary functions during pregnancy

Parameters	Change
Respiratory rate	↑
Tidal volume	↑
Minute ventilation	↑
Chest wall compliance	↓
Forced vital capacity	↔
Forced expiratory volume in the first second	↔
Peak expiratory flow rate	↔
Residual volume	↓
Functional residual capacity	↓
Expiratory reserve volume	↓
Inspiratory capacity	↑
Total lung capacity	↔↓
Respiratory muscle strength	↔
Airway resistance	↔↓
Diffusion capacity for carbon monoxide	↔

58.4 Changes Caused by Exercise in Pregnant Women

The ventilatory effects of pregnancy include changes in diaphragm and chest wall configuration, lung volumes and capacities, and substantial increases in tidal volume (VT), minute ventilation (VE), alveolar ventilation (VA), and the ventilatory equivalents for oxygen (VE/VO$_2$) and carbon dioxide (VE/VCO$_2$) during exercise [28].

Maternal ventilatory reserve is reduced during exercise due to these changes. In this regard, values for VE/VO$_2$ are increased and higher peak values are observed for minute ventilation at maximal exercise in late gestation. As maximum voluntary ventilation is either unchanged or moderately reduced, the capacity to increase minute ventilation in the transition from rest to exercise is reduced [29].

58.5 Changes in Pregnant Women Living at High Altitude

Two percent of the world's population lives at a high altitude, defined as higher than 2500 m. Minute ventilation, FRC, TLC, FVC, FEV1, and DLCO in pregnant women living at high altitudes are higher than those living at sea level. Some adaptation mechanisms are contrary in pregnant women living at high altitudes than pregnant women residing at sea level. In pregnant women living at high altitudes, cardiac output, intravascular blood volume, heart rate decrease, systemic vascular resistance, and hematocrit increase [30, 31].

Intrauterine growth retardation and preeclampsia are more common in pregnant women living at high altitudes. Although a decrease of 100 g in birth weight is expected every 1000 m, this decline is not seen in societies residing at high altitudes for a long time [32, 33].

In pregnancy at high altitudes, adaptation to altitude is achieved with increased ventilation and saturation in the 1st trimester. As the pregnancy progresses, PaO_2, hemoglobin, and DLCO begin to decrease. These changes are not seen in people living at heights for more than three generations [30].

With all these changes, it is expected that dyspnea will be more common in pregnant women residing at high altitudes compared to pregnant women living at sea level [30].

58.6   Sleep-Disordered Breathing During Pregnancy

Sleep-disordered breathing (SDB), which covers a spectrum from snoring to obstructive sleep apnea, usually worsens in pregnancy but may also occur for the first time. Snoring is seen at a rate of 4% in nonpregnant women, while it is seen in about one-fourth of pregnant women in the 3rd trimester. In addition to weight gain, hyperemia in the upper airways, decreased oropharyngeal diameter and FRC, and increased Mallampati score and oxygen consumption are associated with a higher risk of SDB in pregnancy. The clinical worsening of SDB is observed in pregnant women with a diagnosis before pregnancy [34, 35]. Treatment of SDB with continuous positive airway pressure (CPAP) should be encouraged and is safe during pregnancy. Autotitrating CPAP devices are more useful for pregnant women due to weight increase in late gestation.

Contrary to the physiological changes that increase the risk of SDB during pregnancy, the preference of lateral sleeping position during pregnancy is protective against SDB [36].

Due to hormonal changes in pregnant women, a decrease in sleep quality is observed. While estrogen shortens the rapid eye movement (REM) period, progesterone increases non-REM [37].

58.7   Dyspnea

Even if there is no underlying pathology, dyspnea is seen in 70% of pregnant women during pregnancy. Pregnant women with dyspnea have a higher sensitivity to hypoxia and serum CO_2 levels than other pregnant women.

Although it is known that progesterone increases this sensitivity, the high progesterone level cannot be considered as the reason for dyspnea, because its levels are not different in pregnant women with and without dyspnea. Although oxygen consumption, lung capacity, and muscle strength are similar in pregnant women, it is thought that dyspnea seen in some pregnant women is related to respiratory muscles feedback mechanisms.

When dyspnea occurred in pregnant women, it is necessary to differentiate physiological dyspnea from pathological dyspnea. Dyspnea of pregnancy is an isolated symptom, which is not accompanied by other pulmonary and cardiovascular symptoms. Dyspnea of pregnancy initiates in the first or second trimester and gradually worsens through late gestation. Physical and laboratory examinations are within normal limits.

Stage of pregnancy is very important for differential diagnosis of physiologic dyspnea in pregnancy. Differential diagnosis of dyspnea of pregnancy is similar to that in nonpregnant patients in the first half of pregnancy. Pregnancy-related etiologies, like preeclampsia, pulmonary embolism, peripartum cardiomyopathy, pulmonary edema, amniotic fluid embolism, and sepsis, should be noted especially in the third trimester, or postpartum period,

Urgent evaluation is needed if the pregnant woman has sudden onset of dyspnea, hemoptysis, neck or substernal chest pain, heart rate >120 beats/min, respiratory rate >24 breaths/min, pulse oxygen saturation <95%, use of accessory respiratory muscles, difficulty in speaking full sentences, stridor, bronchospasm, asymmetric breath sounds or percussion, diffuse crackles, diaphoresis, cyanosis, depressed or agitated mental status, and oropharyngeal swelling.

58.8 Adaptations Related to Birth

Pregnant women are more resistant to blood loss than nonpregnant women due to increased blood volume during pregnancy. The expected blood loss during standard vaginal delivery is around 500 mL. This amount doubles in cesarean section or twin pregnancy. The fact that the pregnant woman is more resistant should not mean that blood loss during delivery should not be taken seriously; fluid replacement should be performed, and blood replacement should not be delayed in the presence of symptoms such as hypotension or tachycardia [38].

Oxygen consumption increases 40–60% with the birth process. This increase becomes more prominent during contractions [10]. Oxygen demand is provided by increased cardiac output and increased ventilation. With the increase of ventilation, the $PaCO_2$ level decreases; although it differs among pregnant women, it may reach 25 mmHg levels in the first delivery stage. The decrease in $PaCO_2$ continues in each contraction until the cervical dilatation is completed [39].

Cardiac output constantly increases during birth. There is an increase of 15% in the first stage of labor, 30% in the second stage, and 45% in the third stage until the delivery of the baby and placenta. There is an additional 20% increase in cardiac output during uterine contractions as blood passes from the intervillous space to the systemic circulation. The cardiac output increase continues with the contraction of the uterus after birth and the decrease in vena cava pressure. Therefore, the most frequent worsening in pregnant women with underlying heart disease occurs after birth. The cardiac output returns to prenatal levels in 1 h and pre-pregnancy levels in 3–6 months in a healthy woman [5, 38].

The increase in ventilation is seen with the pain, anxiety, and coached breathing of the pregnant women, especially in the second labor phase. It is observed between 7 and 90 L/min, with significant variation among pregnant women. While minute ventilation regresses to its normal level after birth, FRV and RV return to normal limits within 48 h [39].

References

1. Hegewald MJ, Crapo RO. Respiratory physiology in pregnancy. Clin Chest Med. 2011;32:1–13.
2. Ellegård EK. Clinical and pathogenetic characteristics of pregnancy rhinitis. Clin Rev Allergy Immunol. 2004;26:149–59.
3. Pilkington S, Carli F, Dakin MJ, et al. Increase in Mallampati score during pregnancy. Br J Anaesth. 1995;74:638–42.
4. Tao W, Edwards JT, Tu F, Xie Y, Sharma SK. Incidence of unanticipated difficult airway in obstetric patients in a teaching institution. J Anesth. 2012. https://doi.org/10.1007/s00540-012-1338-1. Epub ahead of print. PMID: 22290734.
5. Pancaro C, William RC. Physiologic changes during pregnancy. In: Vacanti C, Segal S, Sikka P, Urman R, editors. Essential clinical anesthesia. Cambridge: Cambridge University Press; 2011. p. 739–43.
6. Goldsmith LT, Weiss G, Steinetz BG. Relaxin and its role in pregnancy. Endocrinol Metab Clin North Am. 1995;24:171–86.
7. LoMauro A, Aliverti A, Frykholm P, et al. Adaptation of lung, chest wall, and respiratory muscles during pregnancy: preparing for birth. J Appl Physiol. 2019;127:1640–50.
8. Marx GF, Murthy PK, Orkin LR. Static compliance before and after vaginal delivery. Br J Anaesth. 1970;42:1100–4.
9. Tan EK, Tan EL. Alterations in physiology and anatomy during pregnancy. Best Pract Res Clin Obstet Gynaecol. 2013;27:791–802.
10. Blackburn ST. Respiratory system. In: Maternal, fetal, neonatal physiology. 5th ed. St. Louis: Elsevier; 2018. p. 297–350.
11. Goodman S. Anesthesia for nonobstetric surgery in the pregnant patient. Semin Perinatol. 2002;26:136–45.
12. LoMauro A, Aliverti A. Respiratory physiology of pregnancy: physiology masterclass. Breathe (Sheff). 2015;11:297–301.
13. Lee SY, Chien DK, Huang CH, Shih SC, Lee WC, Chang WH. Dyspnea in pregnancy. Taiwan J Obstet Gynecol. 2017;56:432–6.
14. Hannhart B, Pickett CK, Moore LG. Effects of estrogen and progesterone on carotid body neural output responsiveness to hypoxia. J Appl Physiol. 1990;68:1909–16.
15. Jensen D, Wolfe LA, Slatkovska L, Webb KA, Davies GA, O'Donnell DE. Effects of human pregnancy on the ventilatory chemoreflex response to carbon dioxide. Am J Physiol Regul Integr Comp Physiol. 2005;288:R1369–75.
16. Zwillich CW, Natalino MR, Sutton FD, Weil JV. Effects of progesterone on chemosensitivity in normal men. J Lab Clin Med. 1978;92:262–9.
17. McCormack MC, Wise RA. Respiratory physiology in pregnancy. In: Bourjeily G, Rosene-Montella K, editors. Pulmonary problems in pregnancy. New York: Humana Press; 2009. p. 19–26.
18. Templeton A, Kelman GR. Maternal blood-gases, PAO_2-PaO_2, physiological shunt and VD/VT in normal pregnancy. Br J Anaesth. 1976;48:1001–4.
19. Prowse CM, Gaensler RA. Respiratory and acid-base changes during pregnancy. Anesthesiology. 1965;26:381–92.
20. O'Day MP. Cardio-respiratory physiological adaptation of pregnancy. Semin Perinatol. 1997;21:268–75.

21. Brown MA, Gallery ED. Volume homeostasis in normal pregnancy and preeclampsia: physiology and clinical implications. Baillieres Clin Obstet Gynaecol. 1994;8:287–310.
22. Thomsen JK, Fogh-Andersen N, Jaszczak P. Atrial natriuretic peptide, blood volume, aldosterone, and sodium excretion during twin pregnancy. Acta Obstet Gynecol Scand. 1994;73:14–20.
23. Ouzounian JG, Elkayam U. Physiologic changes during normal pregnancy and delivery. Cardiol Clin. 2012;30:317–29.
24. McAuliffe F, Kametas N, Rafferty GF, Greenough A, Nicolaides K. Pulmonary diffusing capacity in pregnancy at sea level and at high altitude. Respir Physiol Neurobiol. 2003;134:85–92.
25. Bevan DR, Holdcroft A, Loh L, MacGregor WG, O'Sullivan JC, Sykes MK. Closing volume and pregnancy. Br Med J. 1974;1(5896):13–5.
26. Wise RA, Polito AJ, Krishnan V. Respiratory physiologic changes in pregnancy. Immunol Allergy Clin North Am. 2006;26:1–12.
27. Garrard GS, Littler WA, Redman CW. Closing volume during normal pregnancy. Thorax. 1978;33:488–92.
28. Wolfe LA, Charlesworth SA, Glenn NM, Heenan AP, Davies GA. Effects of pregnancy on maternal work tolerance. Can J Appl Physiol. 2005;30:212–32.
29. McAuley SE, Jensen D, McGrath MJ, Wolfe LA. Effects of human pregnancy and aerobic conditioning on alveolar gas exchange during exercise. Can J Physiol Pharmacol. 2005;83:625–33.
30. McAuliffe F, Kametas N, Krampl E, Ernsting J, Nicolaides K. Blood gases in pregnancy at sea level and at high altitude. BJOG. 2001;108:980–5.
31. Moore LG, Shriver M, Bemis L, Vargas E. An evolutionary model for identifying genetic adaptation to high altitude. In: Roach R, Wagner P, Hackett P, editors. Hypoxia and exercise. New York: Springer; 2007. p. 101–18.
32. Wilson MJ, Lopez M, Vargas M, et al. Greater uterine artery blood flow during pregnancy in multigenerational (Andean) than shorter-term (European) high-altitude residents. Am J Physiol Regul Integr Comp Physiol. 2007;293:R1313–24.
33. Julian CG, Moore LG. Human genetic adaptation to high altitude: evidence from the Andes. Genes (Basel). 2019;10(2):150.
34. Izci B, Vennelle M, Liston WA, Dundas KC, Calder AA, Douglas NJ. Sleep-disordered breathing and upper airway size in pregnancy and post-partum. Eur Respir J. 2006;27:321–7.
35. Pien GW, Fife D, Pack AI, Nkwuo JE, Schwab RJ. Changes in symptoms of sleep-disordered breathing during pregnancy. Sleep. 2005;28:1299–305.
36. Contreras G, Gutiérrez M, Beroíza T, et al. Ventilatory drive and respiratory muscle function in pregnancy. Am Rev Respir Dis. 1991;144:837–41.
37. Bourjeily G, Mohsenin V. Sleep physiology in pregnancy. In: Bourjeily G, Rosene-Montella K, editors. Pulmonary problems in pregnancy. New York: Humana Press; 2009. p. 37–55.
38. Whitty JE, Dombrowski MP. Respiratory diseases in pregnancy. In: Creasy RK, Resnik R, Iams JD, Lockwood CJ, Moore TR, editors. Creasy & Resnik's maternal-fetal medicine, principles and practice. 7th ed. Philadelphia: Saunders; 2014. p. 927–52.
39. Bourjeily G, Ankner G, Mohsenin V. Sleep-disordered breathing in pregnancy. Clin Chest Med. 2011;32:175–89.

Lower Respiratory Infections During Pregnancy

59

Nilüfer Aylin Acet Öztürk and Esra Uzaslan

59.1 Introduction

Physiologic adaptations and changes in immune response during pregnancy may cause an increase for susceptibility to infections. It is hypothesized that specific humoral and cell-mediated response changes, which allow tolerance for fetus, can be an important risk factor for infections in pregnant women [1].

Prevalence of all respiratory tract infections during pregnancy is 9.1% in Hungary [2], while in rural China, prevalence is 38.9%, as per Guo et al. [3]. Radiologically verified pneumonia is seen in 0.08–0.66% of pregnancies in different population-based studies [2, 4, 5]. Pneumonia incidence during pregnancy is calculated as 1.1 per 1000 deliveries in Canada, while pneumonia incidence in the same age group females is calculated as 1.3 per 1000 [6].

Clinical factors evaluated by studies, which are associated with pneumonia during pregnancy, are HIV, asthma, anemia, cocaine use, alcohol abuse, and gestational age [2, 6–10]. Pregnant patients with pneumonia had asthma and anemia more frequently than pregnant women without pneumonia. Although there are conflicting results between studies [11], pneumonia is relatively more frequent in second or third trimester compared to first trimester [6, 9, 11]. The use of steroids for fetal lung maturity and tocolytic agents are related with antepartum pneumonia [12].

Mortality in pregnancy due to pneumonia is significantly reduced after adequate antibiotic treatments [10]. Clinical observations from earlier studies indicated risk of pneumonia complications could be high during pregnancy [9, 10, 13, 14]. However, Jin et al. and Simpson et al. did not find a difference between prognosis in terms of mortality and readmission in 30 days between pregnant and nonpregnant

N. A. Acet Öztürk (✉) · E. Uzaslan
Medical Faculty, Department of Pulmonology, Uludağ University, Bursa, Turkey
e-mail: niluferacet@gmail.com; esra.uzaslan@gmail.com

C. Cingi et al. (eds.), *ENT Diseases: Diagnosis and Treatment during Pregnancy and Lactation*, https://doi.org/10.1007/978-3-031-05303-0_59

women in their studies [1, 15]. Despite being similar in prognosis, significant differences are described for pregnancy outcomes in different studies.

Getahun et al. evaluated acute and chronic respiratory diseases in population-based study including 41,250,539 pregnancies and showed, while acute upper respiratory diseases and acute bronchitis were not associated with increased risk of premature rupture of membranes viral and bacterial pneumonia is associated with increased risk RR: 2.17 [2.06–2.28] of premature rupture of membranes [16]. Pneumonia is also a risk factor for preterm delivery (OR: 5.4 [95% CI: 3.8–7.7], $p < 0.01$) regardless of intrauterine growth restriction (IUGR), severe preeclampsia, and placental abruption [4]. Banhidy et al. also found bronchitis-bronchiolitis and pneumonia to be related with preterm birth (OR: 1.4 [1.1–1.8]) [2].

Romanyuk et al. evaluated 160 pneumonia patients within 181,765 deliveries in Israel [4]. Pneumonia was significantly related with higher labor complications such as malpresentation, placental abruption, prolapse of cord, non-reassuring fetal heart rate patterns, meconium-stained amniotic fluid, low APGAR score at first and fifth minute, and perinatal mortality [4].

Matched case-control study from Taiwan by Chen et al. also identified that pneumonia was a risk factor for adverse pregnancy outcomes such as low APGAR score at fifth minute (OR: 3.86 [95% CI: 1.64–9.06]), preterm birth (OR: 1.71 [95% CI: 1.42–2.05]), low birth weight (OR: 1.73 [95% CI: 1.41–2.12]), preeclampsia/eclampsia (OR: 3.05 [95% CI: 2.01–4.63]), small for gestational age (OR: 1.35 [95% CI: 1.17–1.56]) [5]. Jin et al. calculated relative risk for a small for gestational age birth 1.86 [95% CI: 1.00–3.45] for women with pneumonia during pregnancy (K). Guo et al. also detected a risk increase of low birth weight with respiratory infections (OR: 1.13 [1.01–1.27]) [3].

Factors related with pneumonia were IUGR (OR: 3.7 [95% CI: 2.1–6.6]), severe preeclampsia (OR: 2.6 [95% CI: 1.2–5.7]), previous cesarean section (OR: 2.6 [95% CI: 1.8–3.7]), and placental abruption (OR: 4.2 [95% CI: 1.9–9.1], $p < 0.001$) [4].

Negative effects of respiratory infections during pregnancy are not restricted with adverse pregnancy outcomes. Measured lung compliance in infants drops by 6.5% [95% CI: 1.5–11.3] if mothers of infants experienced respiratory infections during pregnancy. The number of respiratory infections during pregnancy is correlated linearly with lung compliance loss [17].

59.2   Acute Bronchitis

Acute bronchitis is an acute-onset disease that presents with cough and sometimes accompanying sputum symptoms as a result of inflammation of the bronchi. Acute bronchitis is among the most common causes of acute coughs and creates a major clinical burden even though it is mostly a self-limiting disease [18]. Main etiological agents are considered to be viruses. Microbiological tests in general population revealed rhinoviruses, coronaviruses influenza viruses, adenoviruses, parainfluenza viruses, and respiratory syncytial virus as viral pathogens and *S. pneumonia*,

C. pneumonia, B. pertussis, H. influenza, and *M. pneumonia* as bacterial pathogens causing acute bronchitis [19–25].

In the absence of studies addressing management of acute bronchitis in pregnancy, treatment strategies designed for general population are followed [12]. Empiric antibiotic treatment for acute bronchitis without underlying lung disease is not recommended due to limited benefit in studies [25]. Procalcitonin-guided therapy of bronchitis is recommended in general population. Serum procalcitonin levels ≤ 0.25 µg/L upon admission are considered indicative of the absence of bacterial infection therefore a valuable cut-off value for recommendation against use of antibiotics [26]. Macrolides and second- or third-generation cephalosporins are recommended in acute bronchitis requiring antibiotics [25]. Routine use of cough suppressants in order to relieve symptoms is also not recommended due to lack of studies confirming safety of the drugs [12].

Studies about the effect of bronchitis upon pregnancy outcomes are scarce and have conflicting results and are discussed above [2, 16].

59.3 Community-Acquired Pneumonia (CAP)

All patients with suspicion for pneumonia should be evaluated with chest X-ray regardless of pregnancy, because physical examination and clinical symptoms have low sensitivity and specificity for diagnosis [27]. Sputum samples for Gram-stain and culture and urinary samples for serologic antibody/antigen evaluation are recommended in some studies [10]. Potential pathogens in pregnant CAP patients are listed in Table 59.1.

Pneumonia severity indexes designed for general population can be used in pregnant CAP patients for prognosis prediction and need for hospitalization with similar success [28]. Although several clinics have a tendency to hospitalize pregnant patients more often than nonpregnant patients, intensive care unit (ICU) admission criteria are the same in all patients [10]. Maintaining maternal oxygen saturation above 90% is essential, because although fetal hemoglobin has increased oxygen affinity compared to maternal hemoglobin, fetal delivery of oxygen will decrease below that point [29]. Elective delivery can reduce oxygen requirement; however, it does not have an effect on prognosis of pneumonia. Therefore, delivery should be considered only in obstetric indications [30].

Antimicrobial treatment recommendations for different clinical settings are listed in Table 59.2 [31]. However, when empiric treatments are started, local guidelines and local resistance patterns should be also kept in mind. The choice of monotherapy with macrolides should depend on local epidemiology [12]. Appropriate antimicrobial agents for pneumonia during pregnancy are penicillins, cephalosporins, erythromycin, azithromycin, and clarithromycin [12]. Major malformations are not statistically different from expected rate of national data. However, spontaneous abortion rate is reported to be higher with clarithromycin usage in first trimester [32]. Tetracyclines should be avoided in pregnancy due to studies pointing possible depression of bone growth and teeth staining [12]. Quinolones are not

Table 59.1 Pathogens isolated in community-acquired pneumonia [1, 10, 12]

Bacterial pathogens	
Common	**Less common**
Streptococcus pneumonia	*Pseudomonas aeruginosa*
Haemophilus influenzae	*Klebsiella* species
Staphylococcus aureus	*Moraxella catarrhalis*
Chlamidophila pneumonia	*Bordetella pertussis*
Group A β-hemolytic *Streptococci*	*Escherichia coli*
Mycoplasma pneumonia	*Enterobacter* species
Legionella species	*Serratia* species
Viruses	
Common	**Less common**
Influenza	Adenovirus species
Varicella-zoster	Entrovirus
Measles	Epstein-Barr virus
	Cytomegalovirus
	Respiratory syncytial virus
	Parainfluenza virus
	Herpes simplex virus
	Coronaviruses
	Human metapneumovirus
	Hantavirus
Others	
Mycobacterium tuberculosis	*Histoplasma capsulatum*
Mycobacterium avium complex	*Coccidioides immitis*
Pneumocystis jirovecii	*Crypococcus neoformans*
Toxoplasma gondii	*Blastomyces hominis*
Ascaris lumbricoides	*Aspergillus* species
Coxiella burnetti	*Candida* species
Rickettsia ricketsiae	Mucormycotic fungi

recommended in pregnancy. Although exposure to ciprofloxacin was not associated with congenital malformations or spontaneous abortion [33], quinolones have high affinity for bone tissue and may result in arthropathy [12]. Metronidazole exposure and congenital abnormality or low birth weight is not associated in large cohort studies [34, 35].

Prevention of pneumonia can be achieved with vaccination with pneumococcal vaccine in high-risk pregnant patients [12]. Pneumococcal vaccine 13 (PCV13) contains 13 different strains conjugated to inactivated diphtheria toxin resulting in IgG1 immune response. 23-valent polysaccharide pneumococcal vaccine (PPSV23) contains more strains and results in IgG2 immune response. IgG does passively cross placenta, while IgG1 is actively and passively transported through placenta. Therefore, PCV13 provides more protection for neonates [36]. Since safety of PVC13 is not well studied, American College of Obstetrics & Gynecologists [37] guidelines recommend pregnant women with immunocompromising conditions, cerebrospinal fluid leak, asplenism, cochlear implant, and chronic renal, heart, or

Table 59.2 Recommended antimicrobial agents for community-acquired pneumonia [31]

Patient characteristics	Treatment choice	
Otherwise healthy with no recent antimicrobial use	Azithromycin	500 mg × 1, then 250 mg × 1, once daily, orally
Comorbidities or recent antimicrobial use	Azithromycin plus Amoxicillin/ clavulanate	500 mg × 1, then 250 mg × 1, once daily, Orally 875/125 mg, q12 h, orally
Hospital admission, non-ICU	Azithromycin plus Ceftriaxone or Ampicillin	500 mg × 1, then 250 mg × 1, once daily, orally 1–2 gr, once daily, IV 1–2 gr, q6 h, IV
Hospital admission, ICU Without Pseudomonas risk	Azithromycin plus Ceftriaxone or Ampicillin/sulbactam	500 mg × 1, then 250 mg × 1, once daily orally 1–2 gr, once daily, IV 3gr, q6, IV
Hospital admission, ICU With Pseudomonas risk	Azithromycin plus Piperacillin/tazobactam or Cefepime plus Aminoglycoside[a]	500 mg × 1, then 250 mg × 1, once daily orally 3.375 gr, q8, IV 1–2 gr, q8, IV Inhaled/IV

[a] If risk factors for anti-pseudomonal beta-lactam resistance are present

lung failure should be vaccinated with PPSV23. However, if the patient has extremely high risk for infection and benefits of PCV13 vaccination outweigh unknown potential risks for fetus, then the patient can be vaccinated with PCV13 [37]. Holmlund et al. found that maternal vaccination with PPSV23 can decrease infant antibody response to PCV13 vaccination [38]. With that in mind, pregnant patients with low risk for pneumococcal infections should not be vaccinated [36]. McHugh et al. found numerically high rate of preterm births among PPSV23 vaccinated pregnant women thus raised questions of safety [39].

59.4 Influenza Pneumonia

Influenza has a self-limiting nature and is characterized with fever, myalgia, cough, rhinorrhea, and extreme malaise [10]. Influenza virus infection is common during pregnancy and while mortality is lower than previous epidemics, hospital admission rates are still high in pregnant women [12]. During 2009 influenza A pandemic, 22.6% of infected pregnant women were admitted to ICU and 6% of the hospitalized pregnant patients died. Severity of illness was higher in pregnant women in their third trimester [40]. Case fatality in pregnant women infected with H1N1 is shown to be higher compared to general population in low income countries but similar in countries like Canada and Lithuania [41–43]. In a recent meta-analysis evaluating 186,656 patients, pregnancy was associated with 6.8 [6.0–7.6] times higher risk for hospitalization but lower risk of ICU admission and mortality was not associated with pregnancy status [44]. Pregnancy increases risk of complications associated with influenza [45]. Influenza-related morbidity is higher in pregnant women especially during third trimester compared to nonpregnant women, 10.5 of 10,000 versus 1.9 of 10,000 [46].

Murine and mouse models of maternal infection suggest histopathological changes in brain and behavioral alterations in offsprings might appear despite placental transmission of influenza virus [47, 48] MacKenzie et al. could not find any association between congenital malformations and influenza infection in their review of literature [49]. However, Silasi et al. found an association between spontaneous abortion and preterm birth with influenza infection [50]. McNeal et al. evaluated hospital admission for respiratory illness during influenza season in a 13-year time interval in Nova Scotia. Hospitalized pregnant patients delivered infants small for gestational age (RR: 1.66) and lower birth weight [51].

Treatment and prophylaxis options for influenza treatment are M2 ion channel inhibitors (amantadine and rimantadine) and neuraminidase inhibitors (zanamivir and oseltamivir). Case studies identified a relationship of risk of cardiac anomalies and tibial hemimelia with amantadine treatment during pregnancy [52, 53]. Oseltamivir use during pregnancy evaluated from postmarketing safety data including 2926 pregnant women indicated spontaneous or therapeutic abortion, preterm delivery, and birth defect rates were not different from general population rates [54]. Also comparative study of 33 exposed and 674 unexposed pregnant women showed no relation between pregnancy loss, preterm birth, neonatal pathology, and oseltamivir use [55].

Meta-analysis proved seasonal influenza vaccination is protective (RR: 0.3 [0.26–0.71]) against laboratory confirmed influenza infection [56]. Inactivated vaccine is recommended for pregnant women and women planning on being pregnant [57], while attenuated vaccine is recommended postpartum [58].

59.5 COVID-19

Coronavirus disease 2019 (COVID-19) is caused by novel SARS-CoV-2 virus [59]. Data from previous influenza pandemics suggest pregnant women might have an increased risk of infection and mortality due to COVID-19 [60]. Normal gestation is characterized by activation of all renin-angiotensin-aldosterone system and in relation upregulation of ACE2. Because SARS-CoV-2 is binding ACE2, pregnancy might be a risk factor for infection. It is also hypothesized that due to nature of immune response during first and third trimester of pregnancy, these trimesters might be at higher risk for exaggerated immune response and cytokine storm. Vertical transmission of virus through placenta is not yet proven, but even without virus transmission, inflammation can affect developing fetus [61].

There are still relatively few studies upon COVID-19 disease and pregnancy. Meta-analysis conducted by Gao et al. revealed that pregnant women experienced less fever and cough symptoms than nonpregnant women [61]. Pregnant COVID-19 patients presented with fever (51%), cough (31%), lymphopenia (49%) and most of the patients showed positive thorax CT findings (71%). Interestingly Khalil et al. found that only 11% of the infected pregnant women showed symptoms of COVID-19 disease [62]. Cohort study from USA revealed that pregnancy was related with 5.4 times higher risk for hospitalization, 1.5 times higher risk for ICU admission [63]. The incidence of severe cases was 12%, while adverse pregnancy outcomes were frequent; incidence of preterm labor was 23%, incidence of fetal distress was 29%, and incidence of neonatal asphyxia or neonatal death was 9% [61].

Treatment of pregnant patients varies between institutes. Clinical trials for major treatment options for COVID-19 such as remdesivir, lopinavir/ritonavir, and interferon are still ongoing but pregnant women are excluded from these studies. Safety studies about azithromycin use during pregnancy have conflicting results. There are studies reporting increased risk of fetal malformations and pyloric stenosis in contrast with studies reporting no adverse effect. Colchicine was related with increased preterm birth rate and lower birth-weight but was not related with major congenital anomalies. Chloroquine and hydroxychloroquine did not show relation with poor pregnancy outcomes. Lopinavir/ritonavir is the most widely used treatment for HIV in pregnant women and studies reported similar pregnancy outcomes with general population. Interferon β has no adverse effect upon fetus, since it does not cross placental barrier. Tocilizumab use in pregnancy is not recommended due to insufficient data. Favipiravir inhibits RNA polymerase enzyme and is approved in China and Japan. However, there is a warning of teratogenic risk derived from an animal study, but there are no safety studies on humans [64]. Systemic corticosteroids are used in pregnant women for lung development in preterm birth; however, there are no studies evaluating corticosteroid treatment in pregnant COVID-19 patients. It is reasonable to use corticosteroids in accordance with pregnancy conditions and maternal illness severity [65].

In conclusion, physiological and immunological changes create vulnerability to infections during pregnancy. It is a delicate balance for clinicians to diagnose and treat pregnant women without harming fetus. Immunization of women with planned pregnancy is at most important for infectious disease prevention and therefore must be encouraged.

Acknowledgments *This chapter of the book is dedicated to all mothers who are concerned about protecting the health of their unborn babies while fighting against infections during their pregnancy.*

References

1. Sheffield JS, Cunningham FG. Community-acquired pneumonia in pregnancy. Obstet Gynecol. 2009;114(4):915–22. https://doi.org/10.1097/AOG.0b013e3181b8e76d. PMID: 19888052.
2. Bánhidy F, Acs N, Puhó EH, Czeizel AE. Maternal acute respiratory infectious diseases during pregnancy and birth outcomes. Eur J Epidemiol. 2008;23(1):29–35. https://doi.org/10.1007/s10654-007-9206-2. Epub 2007 Nov 20. PMID: 18027089.

3. Guo L, Qu P, Zhang R, Zhao D, Wang H, Liu R, Mi B, Yan H, Dang S. Propensity score-matched analysis on the association between pregnancy infections and adverse birth outcomes in rural northwestern China. Sci Rep. 2018;8(1):5154. https://doi.org/10.1038/s41598-018-23306-5. PMID: 29581446; PMCID: PMC5979963.

4. Romanyuk V, Raichel L, Sergienko R, Sheiner E. Pneumonia during pregnancy: radiological characteristics, predisposing factors and pregnancy outcomes. J Matern Fetal Neonatal Med. 2011;24(1):113–7. https://doi.org/10.3109/14767051003678275.

5. Chen YH, Keller J, Wang IT, Lin CC, Lin HC. Pneumonia and pregnancy outcomes: a nationwide population-based study. Am J Obstet Gynecol. 2012;207(4):288.e1–7. https://doi.org/10.1016/j.ajog.2012.08.023. Epub 2012 Aug 17. PMID: 23021691; PMCID: PMC7093888.

6. Shariatzadeh MR, Marrie TJ. Pneumonia during pregnancy. Am J Med. 2006;119(10):872–6. https://doi.org/10.1016/j.amjmed.2006.01.014. PMID: 17000219.

7. Benedetti TJ, Valle R, Ledger WJ. Antepartum pneumonia in pregnancy. Am J Obstet Gynecol. 1982;144(4):413–7. https://doi.org/10.1016/0002-9378(82)90246-0. PMID: 7124859.

8. Richey SD, Roberts SW, Ramin KD, Ramin SM, Cunningham FG. Pneumonia complicating pregnancy. Obstet Gynecol. 1994;84(4):525–8. PMID: 8090388.

9. Munn MB, Groome LJ, Atterbury JL, Baker SL, Hoff C. Pneumonia as a complication of pregnancy. J Matern Fetal Med. 1999;8(4):151–4. https://doi.org/10.1002/(SICI)1520-6661 (199907/08)8:4<151::AID-MFM2>3.0.CO;2-H.

10. Goodnight WH, Soper DE. Pneumonia in pregnancy. Crit Care Med. 2005;33(10 Suppl):S390–7. https://doi.org/10.1097/01.ccm.0000182483.24836.66. PMID: 16215363.

11. Jin Y, Carriere KC, Marrie TJ, Predy G, Johnson DH. The effects of community-acquired pneumonia during pregnancy ending with a live birth. Am J Obstet Gynecol. 2003;188(3):800–6. https://doi.org/10.1067/mob.2003.175. PMID: 12634660.

12. Lim WS, Macfarlane JT, Colthorpe CL. Treatment of community-acquired lower respiratory tract infections during pregnancy. Am J Respir Med. 2003;2:221–33.

13. Madinger NE, Greenspoon JS, Ellrodt AG. Pneumonia during pregnancy: has modern technology improved maternal and fetal outcome? Am J Obstet Gynecol. 1989;161:657–62.

14. Jenkins TM, Troiano NH, Graves CR, et al. Mechanical ventilation in an obstetric population: characteristics and delivery rates. Am J Obstet Gynecol. 2003;188(2):549–52.

15. Simpson JC, Macfarlane JT, Watson J, et al. A national confidential enquiry into community acquired pneumonia deaths in young adults in England and Wales. Thorax. 2000;55:1040–5. https://doi.org/10.1136/thorax.55.12.1040.

16. Getahun D, Ananth CV, Oyelese Y, Peltier MR, Smulian JC, Vintzileos AM. Acute and chronic respiratory diseases in pregnancy: associations with spontaneous premature rupture of membranes. J Matern Fetal Neonatal Med. 2007;20(9):669–75. https://doi.org/10.1080/14767050701516063. PMID: 17701667.

17. Van Putte-Katier N, Uiterwaal CS, De Jong BM, Kimpen JL, Verheij TJ, Van Der Ent CK, Whistler Study Group. The influence of maternal respiratory infections during pregnancy on infant lung function. Pediatr Pulmonol. 2007;42(10):945–51. https://doi.org/10.1002/ppul.20688.

18. Macfarlane J. Lower respiratory tract infection and pneumonia in the community. Semin Respir Infect. 1999;14:151–62.

19. Macfarlane J, Holmes W, Gard P, et al. Prospective study of the incidence, aetiology and outcome of adult lower respiratory tract illness in the community. Thorax. 2001;56:109–14. https://doi.org/10.1136/thorax.56.2.109.

20. Macfarlane JT, Colville A, Guion A, et al. Prospective study of aetiology and outcome of adult lower-respiratory-tract infections in the community. Lancet. 1993;341:511–4. https://doi.org/10.1016/0140-6736(93)90275-L.

21. Nicholson KG, Kent J, Hammersley V, et al. Risk factors for lower respiratory complications of rhinovirus infections in elderly people living in the community: prospective cohort study. BMJ. 1996;313:1119–23. https://doi.org/10.1136/bmj.313.7065.1119.

22. Boldy DA, Skidmore SJ, Ayres JG. Acute bronchitis in the community: clinical features, infective factors, changes in pulmonary function and bronchial reactivity to histamine. Respir Med. 1990;84:377–85. https://doi.org/10.1016/S0954-6111(08)80072-8.

23. Woodhead MA, Macfarlane JT, McCracken JS, et al. Prospective study of the aetiology and outcome of pneumonia in the community. Lancet. 1987;I:671–4. https://doi.org/10.1016/S0140-6736(87)90430-2.

24. Lim WS, Macfarlane JT, Boswell TC, et al. Study of community acquired pneumonia aetiology (SCAPA) in adults admitted to hospital: implications for management guidelines. Thorax. 2001;56:296–301. https://doi.org/10.1136/thorax.56.4.296.

25. Flaherty KR, Saint S, Fendrick AM, Martinez FJ. The spectrum of acute bronchitis. Using baseline factors to guide empirical therapy. Postgrad Med. 2001;109(2):39–47. https://doi.org/10.3810/pgm.2001.02.859.

26. Schuetz P, Bolliger R, Merker M, Christ-Crain M, Stolz D, Tamm M, Luyt CE, Wolff M, Schroeder S, Nobre V, Reinhart K, Branche A, Damas P, Nijsten M, Deliberato RO, Verduri A, Beghé B, Cao B, Shehabi Y, Jensen JS, Beishuizen A, de Jong E, Briel M, Welte T, Mueller B. Procalcitonin-guided antibiotic therapy algorithms for different types of acute respiratory infections based on previous trials. Expert Rev Anti Infect Ther. 2018;16(7):555–64. https://doi.org/10.1080/14787210.2018.1496331.

27. Kasper DL, Braunwald E, Fauci AS, et al., editors. Harrison's principles of internal medicine. 16th ed. New York: McGraw-Hill; 2005.

28. Yost NP, Bloom SL, Richey SD, et al. An appraisal of treatment guidelines for antepartum community acquired pneumonia. Am J Obstet Gynecol. 2000;183:131–5.

29. Maccato M. Respiratory insufficiency due to pneumonia in pregnancy. Obstet Gynecol Clin North Am. 1991;18:289–99.

30. Tomlinson MW, Caruthers TJ, Whitty JE, et al. Does delivery improve maternal condition in the respiratory-compromised gravida? Obstet Gynecol. 1998;91:108–11.

31. Rac H, Gould AP, Eiland LS, Griffin B, McLaughlin M, Stover KR, Bland CM, Bookstaver PB. Common bacterial and viral infections: review of management in the pregnant patient. Ann Pharmacother. 2019;53(6):639–51. https://doi.org/10.1177/1060028018817935.

32. Einarson A, Phillips E, Mawji F, et al. A prospective controlled multicentre study of clarithromycin in pregnancy. Am J Perinatol. 1998;15:523–5. https://doi.org/10.1055/s-2007-994053.

33. NHS Northern Yorkshire Regional Drug Therapeutics Centre. The National Teratology Information Service. Toxbase. 2000. Antibiotics: use in pregnancy.

34. Piper JM, Mitchel EF, Ray WA. Prenatal use of metronidazole and birth defects: no association. Obstet Gynecol. 1993;82:348–52.

35. Czeizel AE, Rockenbauer M. A population based case-control teratologic study of oral metronidazole treatment during pregnancy. Br J Obstet Gynaecol. 1998;105:322–7. https://doi.org/10.1111/j.1471-0528.1998.tb10094.x.

36. Moumne O, Duff P. Treatment and prevention of pneumococcal infection. Clin Obstet Gynecol. 2019;62(4):781–9. https://doi.org/10.1097/GRF.0000000000000451. PMID: 31008732.

37. ACOG technical bulletin. Pulmonary disease in pregnancy. Number 224—June 1996. American College of Obstetricians and Gynecologists. Int J Gynaecol Obstet. 1996;54(2):187–96. PMID: 9236324.

38. Holmlund E, Nohynek H, Quiambao B, et al. Mother-infant vaccination with pneumococcal polysaccharide vaccine: persistence of maternal antibodies and responses of infants to vaccination. Vaccine. 2011;29:4565–75.

39. McHugh L, Binks M, Ware RS, Snelling T, Nelson S, Nelson J, Dunbar M, Mulholland EK, Andrews RM. Birth outcomes in Aboriginal mother-infant pairs from the Northern Territory, Australia, who received 23-valent polysaccharide pneumococcal vaccination during pregnancy, 2006-2011: the PneuMum randomised controlled trial. Aust N Z J Obstet Gynaecol. 2020;60(1):82–7. https://doi.org/10.1111/ajo.13002.

40. Siston AM, Rasmussen SA, Honein MA, et al. Pandemic 2009 influenza A (H1N1) virus illness among pregnant women in the United States. J Am Med Assoc. 2010;303(15):1517–25.

41. Pramanick A, Rathore S, Peter JV, Moorthy M, Lionel J. Pandemic (H1N1) 2009 virus infection during pregnancy in South India. Int J Gynecol Obstet. 2011;113(1):32–5.
42. Rolland-Harris E, Vachon J, Kropp R, et al. Hospitalization of pregnant women with pandemic A (H1N1) 2009 influenza in Canada. Epidemiol Infect. 2012;140:1316–27.
43. Mickiene A, Daniusevičiute L, Vanagaite N, et al. Hospitalized adult patients with 2009 pandemic influenza a (H1N1) in Kaunas, Lithuania. Medicina. 2011;47(1):11–8.
44. Mertz D, Lo CK, Lytvyn L, Ortiz JR, Loeb M, Flurisk-Investigators. Pregnancy as a risk factor for severe influenza infection: an individual participant data meta-analysis. BMC Infect Dis. 2019;19(1):683. https://doi.org/10.1186/s12879-019-4318-3.
45. Kort BA, Cefalo RC, Baker VV. Fatal influenza A pneumonia in pregnancy. Am J Perinatol. 1986;3:179–82.
46. Neuzil KM, Reed GW, Mitchel EF, et al. Impact of influenza on acute cardiopulmonary hospitalizations in pregnant women. Am J Epidemiol. 1998;148:1094–102.
47. Fatemi SHEJ, Kanodia R, Kist D, Emamian ES, Patterson PH, et al. Prenatal viral infection leads to pyramidal cell atrophy and macrocephaly in adulthood: implications for genesis of autism and schizophrenia. Cell Mol Neurobiol. 2002;22:25–33.
48. Shi LFS, Sidwell RW, Patterson PH. Maternal influenza infection causes marked behavioral and pharmacological changes in the offspring. J Neurosci. 2003;23:297–302.
49. MacKenzie JS, Houghton M. Influenza infections during pregnancy: association with congenital malformations and with subsequent neoplasms in children, and potential hazards of live virus vaccines. Bacteriol Rev. 1974;38:356–70.
50. Silasi M, Cardenas I, Kwon JY, Racicot K, Aldo P, Mor G. Viral infections during pregnancy. Am J Reprod Immunol. 2015;73:199–213. https://doi.org/10.1111/aji.12355.
51. McNeil SA, Dodds LA, Fell DB, Allen VM, Halperin BA, Steinhoff MC, MacDonald NE. Effect of respiratory hospitalization during pregnancy on infant outcomes. Am J Obstet Gynecol. 2011;204(6 Suppl 1):S54–7. https://doi.org/10.1016/j.ajog.2011.04.031. Epub 2011 Apr 24. PMID: 21640231.
52. Levy M, Pastuszak A, Koren G. Fetal outcome following intrauterine amantadine exposure. Reprod Toxicol. 1991;5:79–81.
53. Rosa F. Amantadine pregnancy experience. Reprod Toxicol. 1994;8:531.
54. Wollenhaupt M, Chandrasekaran A, Tomianovic D. The safety of oseltamivir in pregnancy: an updated review of post-marketing data. Pharmacoepidemiol Drug Saf. 2014;23(10):1035–42. https://doi.org/10.1002/pds.3673.
55. Beau AB, Hurault-Delarue C, Vial T, Montastruc JL, Damase-Michel C, Lacroix I. Safety of oseltamivir during pregnancy: a comparative study using the EFEMERIS database. BJOG. 2014;121(7):895–900. https://doi.org/10.1111/1471-0528.12617. Epub 2014 Feb 11. PMID: 24512604.
56. Quach THT, Mallis NA, Cordero JF. Influenza vaccine efficacy and effectiveness in pregnant women: systematic review and meta-analysis. Matern Child Health J. 2020;24(2):229–40. https://doi.org/10.1007/s10995-019-02844-y. PMID: 31865602.
57. Committee on Obstetric Practice and Immunization Expert Work Group; Centers for Disease Control and Prevention's Advisory Committee on Immunization, United States; American College of Obstetricians and Gynecologists. Committee opinion no. 608: influenza vaccination during pregnancy. Obstet Gynecol. 2014;124:648–51. https://doi.org/10.1097/01.AOG.0000453599.11566.11.
58. ACOG Committee opinion no. 732: influenza vaccination during pregnancy. Obstet Gynecol. 2018;131:e109–e114. https://doi.org/10.1097/AOG.0000000000002588.
59. WHO. Novel coronavirus—China. 2020. https://www.who.int/csr/don/12-january-2020-novel-coronavirus-china/en/.
60. Narang K, Enninga EAL, Gunaratne MDSK, Ibirogba ER, Trad ATA, Elrefaei A, Theiler RN, Ruano R, Szymanski LM, Chakraborty R, Garovic VD. SARS-CoV-2 infection and COVID-19 during pregnancy: a multidisciplinary review. Mayo Clin Proc. 2020;95(8):1750–65. https://doi.org/10.1016/j.mayocp.2020.05.011.

61. Gao YJ, Ye L, Zhang JS, Yin YX, Liu M, Yu HB, Zhou R. Clinical features and outcomes of pregnant women with COVID-19: a systematic review and meta-analysis. BMC Infect Dis. 2020;20(1):564. https://doi.org/10.1186/s12879-020-05274-2.
62. Khalil A, Hill R, Ladhani S, Pattisson K, O'Brien P. SARS-CoV-2 in pregnancy: symptomatic pregnant women are only the tip of the iceberg. Am J Obstet Gynecol. 2020;223(2):296–7. https://doi.org/10.1016/j.ajog.2020.05.005.
63. Ellington S, Strid P, Tong VT, Woodworth K, Galang RR, Zambrano LD, Nahabedian J, Anderson K, Gilboa SM. Characteristics of women of reproductive age with laboratory-confirmed SARS-CoV-2 infection by pregnancy status—United States, January 22-June 7, 2020. MMWR Morb Mortal Wkly Rep. 2020;69:769–75. https://doi.org/10.15585/mmwr.mm6925a1.
64. Louchet M, Sibiude J, Peytavin G, Picone O, Tréluyer JM, Mandelbrot L. Placental transfer and safety in pregnancy of medications under investigation to treat coronavirus disease 2019. Am J Obstet Gynecol MFM. 2020;2(3):100159. https://doi.org/10.1016/j.ajogmf.2020.100159.
65. Wastnedge EAN, Reynolds RM, van Boeckel SR, Stock SJ, Denison FC, Maybin JA, Critchley HOD. Pregnancy and COVID-19. Physiol Rev. 2021;101(1):303–18. https://doi.org/10.1152/physrev.00024.2020.

Bronchitis During Pregnancy and in the Postpartum Period

Melike Aloğlu and Fusun Yıldız

60.1 Introduction

Acute bronchitis is a condition involving inflammation of the large airways within the lung and is self-limiting [1]. Its annual prevalence in adults is approximately 5%. A bacterial cause for acute bronchitis is unusual, and, in fact, 95% of cases in otherwise healthy adults are due to viruses. The majority of cases, as with viral diseases of the airways in general, are observed during the influenza season [2].

In pregnancy, there are a number of mechanical, biochemical, hemodynamic, and immunological alterations, which progress over the course of gestation, becoming readily apparent during the third trimester. Normally, during a pregnancy, there is an increasing proinflammatory response of the innate immune system, termed the "controlled systemic inflammatory state." While the selective suppression of Th1 cell-mediated immunity does protect the fetus from the mother's cytotoxic T lymphocyte activity, it is also predictable that it may weaken maternal responses to infection [3].

The frequency and course of airway infections during pregnancy resemble those seen in nonpregnant individuals [1]. However, both due to concerns about the course of the pregnancy and to the outcome for both the mother and fetus, bronchitis is a condition requiring a sensitive approach, from the point of view of the mother and the treating physician alike.

M. Aloğlu (✉)
Department of Pulmonology, Ankara Atatürk Hospital for Chest Diseases and Chest Surgery, Ankara, Turkey
e-mail: drmelikeb@gmail.com

F. Yıldız
Department of Pulmonology, Cyprus International University, Nicosia, Cyprus
e-mail: fusun.yildiz@gmail.com

C. Cingi et al. (eds.), *ENT Diseases: Diagnosis and Treatment during Pregnancy and Lactation*, https://doi.org/10.1007/978-3-031-05303-0_60

60.2 Symptoms and Clinical Findings

Clinically, acute bronchitis presents as coughing, weakness, shortness of breath, and wheezing. The principal symptom, however, is a cough, which may be dry or productive. Symptoms such as rhinorrhea, a sore throat, mild fever, myalgia, and weakness, as seen in upper respiratory tract infections, are common in the prodrome [2].

In a study of 155 pregnant women suffering from an acute respiratory tract infection carried out in Texas, USA, symptoms indicative of a lower respiratory tract infection were observed in the following order of frequency: nasal discharge (90%), shortness of breath (83%), coughing (76%), sore throat (72%), chest pain (41%), and wheeze (41%) [4].

On physical examination, rales (from pooled secretions) and wheezing were auscultated. The presence of fine crackles or rhonchi should raise a suspicion of pneumonia. Tachycardia may be noted secondary to dehydration in a viral illness or due to pyrexia.

There are no specific findings on thoracic imaging. Chest X-ray is typically of normal appearances; however, the interstitial markings may be more visible than usual due to thickening of the bronchial wall. The American College of Chest Physicians (ACCP) only recommends the use of chest radiography where there is tachycardia (>100 bpm), a respiratory rate above 24 min^{-1}, a body temperature exceeding 38 °C, and fremitus or increased vocal resonance (aegophony) are noted.

In the presence of pyrexia, a full blood count and blood biochemical investigations may be requested. These tests may show a slight rise in white blood cells and alterations in biochemical parameters linked to dehydration.

Unless there are strong suspicions of a bacterial infection, microbiological tests are not cost-effective [2].

60.3 Microbiological Factors

The main pathogens responsible for lower respiratory tract infections (LRTI) other than pneumonia are all viral. The commonly isolated pathogens are rhinovirus, coronavirus, influenza virus, parainfluenza virus, adenovirus, and respiratory syncytial virus (RSV).

The essential role of *Mycoplasma pneumoniae*, *Chlamydia pneumoniae*, and *Streptococcus pneumoniae* is unclear; however, in certain studies, they were implicated in less than 6% of cases of LRTI [1].

In their study concerning respiratory tract infections published in 2020, Kolosov et al. found that an infection occurred within the first trimester in 21% of cases, and in 40% of cases in the second and third trimesters. *Streptococcus viridans* was cultured in 40% of specimens taken from infected pregnant women, *Steptococcus pneumoniae* in 21%, *Neisseria* spp. in 40%, and *Staphylococcus epidermidis* in 4%. In 43% of patients, at least two different pathogens were detected. From the same study, the rates of detection of viral pathogens were as follows: influenza A (2%), parainfluenza virus (12%), rhinovirus (8%), and adenovirus (17%) [5].

60.4   Maternal Consequences

Although there is no apparent increase in the incidence of influenza virus infections in pregnant women (i.e., it remains between 1 and 21%), due to the suppression of cellular immunity and other physiological adaptations, the infection may be noted to be more severe and, if pneumonia subsequently develops, it may cause greater morbidity and mortality, particularly in the later stages of pregnancy [3]. In a study published by Schanzer in 2007 [6], the rate of hospitalization among otherwise healthy pregnant women due to influenza was 104 in 100,000, thus an 18-fold increase in the rate seen in nonpregnant, otherwise healthy individuals.

The rate of hospital admission for influenza infection in pregnant women with comorbidities is higher than in those who are not pregnant [7], being particularly high in pregnant women suffering from cardiopulmonary disorders. The frequency of hospital admission in healthy pregnant women during the third trimester was found to be similar to that seen in high-risk individuals, where it may reach 250 in 100,000 [8].

During the H1N1 Influenza A Pandemic, although pregnant women made up only 1% of the population, they accounted for 5% of the deaths. These deaths occurred at different rates, depending on the trimester, with 7.1% occurring in the first, 26.8% in the second, and 64.3% in the third trimester. In all three trimesters, there was a relationship between not starting antiviral therapy and suffering complications, particularly in the early stages of infection, that is, between the onset of symptoms and 48 h later [9].

Falsey et al. found that RSV infection, which is another factor in cases of acute bronchitis, is seen in 4– 10% of adults, including pregnant women. They observed that 85% of patients were symptomatic, 16% developed a need to be admitted to hospital, and 4% died [10]. In Wheeler's published case series [11], 2 out of 3 pregnant women who had an RSV infection ended up requiring intensive care unit (ICU) admission.

RSV and influenza infections affect pregnant and postpartum women more severely than the healthy general population, in a similar way to patients who are immunocompromised. By contrast, there was no difference in the severity of illness between pregnant or postpartum women compared to a healthy population when the agent of acute bronchitis was a different pathogen, the human metapneumovirus (HMPV) [10–12].

60.5   Consequences for the Fetus or Neonate

A study, which investigated possible connections between placental abruption and acute upper respiratory tract infection (URTI), viral or bacterial pneumonia, acute bronchitis or bronchiolitis, chronic bronchitis or asthma, found no association between the conditions. In the same study, when the pregnant women were grouped by race, an increased risk of *abruptio placentae* was demonstrated in cases of acute URTI, pneumonia, and acute bronchitis. This risk is relatively higher in caucasian women [13].

A study carried out in Hungary established that out of a sample of 38,151 newborns, 3455 mothers suffered with a respiratory tract infection of some sort, ranging from sinusitis to pneumonia. It was found that the severe infections on this spectrum, such as bronchitis, bronchiolitis, and pneumonia, had an associated risk of preterm birth that was 1.4-fold increased [14].

Studies carried out in the USA during the 2009 H1N1 pandemic revealed that although influenza infection may result in spontaneous abortion or preterm delivery, there was a low risk of vertical transmission to the fetus. However, it was found that the children of mothers exposed during pregnancy to influenza A were at an increased risk of developing schizophrenia and bipolar disorder in the long term [9]. In animal models where there was exposure during pregnancy to live virus, bacterial endotoxins, or viral mimics, it has been shown that development of the fetal brain may be affected by proinflammatory cytokines and the pyrexia response and this may be what is happening to create a risk factor for schizophrenia [15].

Influenza-like illness (ILI) in pregnancy is associated with a five-fold increased risk of morbidity and mortality. During the 2009 pandemic in America, the rate of preterm delivery rose from 7 in 1000 to 39 in 1000, while stillbirths rose from 6 in 1000 to 27 in 1000. Also during the same pandemic, the frequency of giving birth to a child of low birth weight (LBW) by mothers who were positive on PCR testing for H1N1 was higher than in mothers with influenza-like illnesses who tested PCR negative for H1N1 [16]. It was observed, during the same pandemic, that there was a five-fold increase in perinatal mortality in those who contracted influenza during pregnancy and a three-fold increase in preterm births [17].

There is limited evidence available about the ability of the influenza A virus to cross the placental barrier. It was shown in the 2009 pandemic that the fetal trophoblast can be infected and that the development of chorionic villitis can increase the risk of maternal and fetal deaths. Vertical viral transmission via the placenta has been described in sporadic cases [16].

One study included 3693 women and examined another agent causing viral bronchitis, human metapneumovirus (HMPV). Of the 55 women who were infected with HMPV, 25 were pregnant. When pregnant or postpartum women were compared with those who were neither pregnant nor postpartum, no difference was noted in the severity of the HMPV infection, but women who suffered from a pyrexial illness linked to HMPV infection were found to be at risk of having a low birthweight child ($p = 0.031$) [12].

In a study dating from 1993 to 2004, which examined the relationship between acute and chronic airway infections and premature rupture of the membranes (PROM), no significant association was established between being ill with acute bronchitis while pregnant and PROM [18].

In a Chinese-hospital-based case-control study of URTI or influenza in pregnant mothers, it was found the children were at an elevated risk of developing congenital cardiac disease, in particular ventricular septal defects (VSDs). It was also found there was a possibly raised risk for Tetralogy of Fallot (TOF) in these patients [19].

While respiratory syncytial virus (RSV) infection is rarely severe, a cohort study carried out in Nepal established there was a relationship between RSV and preterm delivery and low birth weight babies [16]. In a similar fashion, a rhinovirus infection causing pyrexia was found to be associated with a 1.6 fold increased risk of a low birth weight baby [20].

While influenza A has the largest effect on morbidity among viral infections in pregnant mothers, coronaviruses can also lead to similar consequences. The coronaviruses responsible for SARS and MERS have been found to be associated with spontaneous abortion, fetal growth retardation, and both maternal and neonatal mortalities [16].

In a study of 185 pregnant women who tested PCR positive for the newly recognized SARS-CoV-2 coronavirus, among the live births, 18.6% required neonatal intensive care unit admission, low birth weight affected 10.3%, pneumonia was found in 6.2%, 1.3% of neonates were positive on PCR for SARS-CoV-2 ($n = 2$), and neonatal death occurred in 0.69% ($n = 1$) [21]. A Texan study [22] found that early neonatal infection with SARS-CoV-2 occurred at a rate of 3%, but there were no significant differences in hospitalization or placental anomaly when comparisons were made with women without COVID and nonpregnant women [22].

60.6 Treatment and Prophylaxis

When a decision is to be taken on the use of antimicrobials in pregnancy, several factors need to be borne in mind, specifically: the severity of the maternal infection; the potential consequences of failure to treat infection in the mother; the effects of pregnancy on the pharmacokinetics of the drug; and any potential toxic effects of medication on the fetus.

Given that acute bronchitis is principally due to viral pathogens and is a self-limiting illness, the approach in pregnant patients is similar to that taken in nonpregnant individuals, that is, mostly supportive treatment. Where medication is to be prescribed, a number of general principles should be taken into considerations, namely, the stage of the pregnancy, avoiding the use of newly introduced pharmacological agents, using the lowest effective dose, keeping the course duration as brief as possible, and, wherever feasible, adopting monotherapy.

The most common request for medication from pregnant women is due to a cough; however, it is known that the risk of a major malformation in the baby is increased by the use of dextromethorphan, which is an ingredient in the majority of antitussive preparations [1].

Among the alternative treatment options for pyrexia and myalgia, the COX-2 inhibitors do have the potential to dampen down inflammation and reduce the severity of the illness, but they can cause preterm delivery and musculoskeletal defects; so, other nonsteroidal anti-inflammatory drugs (NSAIDs) are recommended [16]. Prenatal use of paracetamol (acetaminophen) is not associated with any birth defects, but is a risk factor for the development of childhood asthma (odds ratio: 1.26–1.35) [23, 24]. Nevertheless, it may be used as a safer choice in symptomatic treatment.

60.7 Antibacterial Therapy

Since the frequency of bacterial involvement in cases of acute bronchitis is low, generally, there is no call for the use of antibiotic therapy. In a Cochrane review involving 750 patients with acute bronchitis aged 8 years or older, the risk of discovering a cough and abnormal lung findings was lower in those taking antibacterial therapy. However, no difference was observed in nocturnal cough, productive cough, or limitations on activity. Indeed, there was a significantly higher risk of nausea, vomiting, headache, skin rash, and vaginitis in those taking antibiotics [25]. However, occasionally, antibiotics may be prescribed where there is a bacterial superinfection on top of the viral infection, or where the aim is to take advantage of an anti-inflammatory effect. It has been noted that 19–44% of pregnant women are prescribed antibiotics for some kind of infection [26].

In a Hungarian study, there were 308 women treated during pregnancy with a cephalosporin, and in a control group, 440 pregnant women plus 16 pregnant women from the general population were treated with similar antibiotics. The conclusion from this study was that there was no teratogenic effect from cephalexin, cefaclor, or ceftibutin [27].

Furthermore, in a study on macrolides prescribed on an occasional basis to benefit from their anti-inflammatory effects, no increased risk of congenital malformations was found with the newer macrolides (clarithromycin, azithromycin, and roxithromycin) in the first trimester compared to erythromycin. Macrolides can be used as the first choice in patients with penicillin allergy in the treatment of Gram-negative URTIs, LRTIs, soft tissue infections, and *Helicobacter pylori* peptic ulcer as the main indication [28].

In a study conducted between 2014 and 2018 involving 20 pregnant women who took antibiotics for a variety of infections, it was found that the infants of women using cefprozil, azithromycin, co-amoxiclav, benzathine benzylpenicillin G, or sulbactam-ampicillin were all healthy [29]. There is also a publication [30], which states that the use of ampicillin in the 2nd and 3rd trimesters leads to an increased prevalence of cleft palate.

Penicillin is safe and the antibiotic of first choice during pregnancy, provided there is no allergy. Another group of first-line antibiotics are the cephalosporins. Aminoglycosides should be avoided due to the risk of nephrotoxicity and ototoxicity, but can be used for life-threatening Gram-negative infections and where the safer antibiotics usually recommended do not work. Lincosamides should be used only when use of penicillin, cephalosporin, and erythromycin does not result in eradication of the infection [31].

Alongside the teratogenic effects of antibiotic use during pregnancy, another potential consequence is neonatal antibiotic resistance. In a multicenter study involving six hospitals in which 8476 pregnant women were followed up, the diagnosis of sepsis was mentioned in 96 newborn infants out of a total 8593 live births, and ampicillin resistance was detected in 45% of the pathogens cultured from these patients. Ampicillin resistance was found to be significantly associated with preterm birth, as well as antepartum/intrapartum or any prenatal antibiotic exposure ($p < 0.05$) [32].

In addition, it has been shown that infants exposed during pregnancy to antibiotics have a 1.66-fold increased risk of developing atopic dermatitis within the first year of life and a 3.01-fold increased risk of a food allergy [33].

A cohort study, conducted in Canada in 2017, examined major congenital malformations detected within the first year of life among 13,938 live births following maternal use of antibiotics in the first trimester. Clindamycin was associated with increased musculoskeletal malformations and with ventricular or atrial septal defects (VSD-ASD). An increase in circulatory system and cardiac malformations and the risk of VSD-ASD were detected with doxycycline. Following the use of quinolone, moxifloxacin, ofloxacin, macrolides, erythromycin, and phenoxymethylpenicillin, defects were detected in a single case. In the same study, congenital defects were not observed with the use of amoxicillin, cephalosporins, or nitrofurantoin [34].

No relationship was found between the use of antibiotics during pregnancy and the risk of developing cerebral palsy (CP) or epilepsy in infants, but the risk of developing CP and epilepsy was found to be 1.78 times higher with macrolide exposure than with penicillin exposure [26].

Sarkar's 2006 study reported on outcomes following the use of azithromycin in 123 pregnant women with an average course of 5 days. There were 113 live births in total, 6 spontaneous abortions, 3 fetal deaths, and 1 therapeutic abortion. No developmental anomaly occurred and the risk of a major malformation compared to the background risk (1–3%) was not raised. The author suggested that the single dose was especially advantageous and, because of the brief duration of use for acute bronchitis, this agent could be reliably recommended during pregnancy [35].

Based on the poor outcomes observed in animal studies, it is recommended to avoid the use of fluoroquinolones and tetracyclines during pregnancy due to possible side effects on fetal cartilage, bone, and teeth, but there are also publications stating that their use is safe [36, 37]. In a study concerning quinolones published in Germany in 2014, the babies of 949 pregnant women who used quinolone in the first trimester, and those of 3796 pregnant women who did not use it, were evaluated. There was no increase in the risk of major congenital defects and spontaneous abortion with the use of quinolone, but an increase in the risk of developing major congenital defects was observed with moxifloxacin, albeit this result did not reach statistical significance [38].

60.8 Antiviral Therapy

In viral infections of the respiratory tract, antiviral treatment is typically not called for; however, antiviral treatment can be given in immunocompromised individuals, elderly and pregnant women, since RSV and, even more so, influenza infections can become severe and result in serious morbidity and mortality.

Although the principal way to treat RSV infection is by supportive therapy, ribavirin, a nucleoside analog, may be administered in immunocompromised patients.

However, the use of ribavirin is contraindicated in pregnancy due to its teratogenic effects [11].

M2 ion channel inhibitors from among the adamantane derivatives, as well as neuraminidase inhibitor antivirals, are used against influenza virus in the general population. Adamantane group drugs such as amantadine and rimantadine are only effective against influenza A virus and have been found in animal studies to be embryotoxic. Many congenital anomalies, including cardiac anomalies, have been detected following exposure to amantadine and rimantadine; therefore, its use in pregnancy is not recommended [39–41]. Neuraminidase inhibitors are effective against both influenza A and influenza B viruses and are used in all adults, including during pregnancy. Despite the intensive use of oseltamivir in the 2009 H1N1 pandemic, no adverse events associated with it were observed. Neuraminidase inhibitors are known to reduce symptom duration, illness severity, and viral shedding, provided they are initiated within 48 h of symptomatic onset. A significant relationship was established between oseltamivir therapy and reduced admission to ICU, decreased reliance on mechanical ventilation, and fewer deaths among pregnant women admitted to hospital during the 2009 pandemic. In H1N1 influenza A viral infections, initiation of antiviral therapy early in pregnancy resulted in significant decreases in preterm labor, ICU admission, and maternal mortality [42].

In one of the studies undertaken on the effects of oseltamivir is pregnancy, a risk of late transient hypoglycemia was noted. In numerous other studies, there were no findings indicating either a negative pregnancy outcome or an increased risk of anomaly in the infant [43]. The Infectious Diseases Society of America (IDSA) 2018 guidelines recommend commencing antiviral treatment (oseltamivir) as soon as possible if a suspected or confirmed influenza virus infection develops during pregnancy or within 2 weeks postpartum. Since the increased renal filtration and secretion that occurs during pregnancy results in a reduced systemic exposure to oseltamivir carboxylate, the risk of dose-related adverse events is lower, and accordingly, administration of higher doses may be considered if needed. It has been demonstrated in numerous studies that oseltamivir produces no adverse effects on infants; hence, it is safe to use oseltamivir in the postpartum period, and stopping breastfeeding while using oseltamivir is not required [44].

60.9 Prophylactic Vaccination

In 2004, the American Society of Obstetrics and Gynecology and, in 2008, the Canadian National Advisory Committee on Immunization (NACI) recommended influenza vaccination for all pregnant women [3].

Influenza vaccination protects not only the mother but also the fetus from the negative effects of influenza. The American Centers for Disease Control and Prevention (CDC) and the World Health Organization (WHO) recommend influenza vaccination for women planning a pregnancy or actually pregnant during the winter/peak influenza season [42].

In a review published in 2015, it was shown that vaccinating mothers against influenza does not increase the risk of preterm birth [45]. In a review published in 2018, it was found that the risk of laboratory-proven influenza infection decreased in babies aged 6 months or younger whose mothers received influenza vaccination while pregnant [46]. In a meta-analysis published in 2019, it was reported that while pregnant women can be vaccinated against influenza in any trimester, immunoglobulin titers measured from cord or neonatal blood samples were 1.5–2 times higher when vaccination was performed in the later trimesters [47].

Influenza vaccine has not been found to have any long-term adverse effects on infants. In a retrospective cohort study conducted in Canada, when the data concerned with 104,249 live births were examined, it was found that 31,295 (30%) had been vaccinated against pandemic H1N1. The offspring of these pregnant women were followed up for 5 years, with no pediatric adverse outcomes recorded over the 5 years of follow-up [48].

Influenza vaccination in all three trimesters of pregnancy is safe for the mother, the course of the pregnancy, and the fetus/neonate, and is recommended [47].

References

1. Lim WS, Macfarlane JT, Colthorpe CL. Treatment of community-acquired lower respiratory tract infections during pregnancy. Am J Respir Med. 2003;2(3):221–33. https://doi.org/10.1007/BF03256651. PMID: 14720004; PMCID: PMC7100023.
2. Singh A, Avula A, Zahn E. Acute bronchitis. In: StatPearls [Internet]. Treasure Island: StatPearls Publishing; 2020. PMID: 28846312.
3. Skowronski DM, De Serres G. Is routine influenza immunization warranted in early pregnancy? Vaccine. 2009;27(35):4754–70. https://doi.org/10.1016/j.vaccine.2009.03.079.
4. Hause AM, Avadhanula V, Maccato ML, Pinell PM, Bond N, Santarcangelo P, Ferlic-Stark L, Munoz FM, Piedra PA. A cross-sectional surveillance study of the frequency and etiology of acute respiratory illness among pregnant women. J Infect Dis. 2018;218(4):528–35. https://doi.org/10.1093/infdis/jiy167. PMID: 29741642; PMCID: PMC7107407.
5. Kolosov VP, Andrievskaya IA, Zhukovets IV, Talchenkova TV, Bereza KV, Abuldinov AS. Features of acute respiratory viral infections in pregnant women. Eur Respir J. 2020;56(suppl 64):2384. https://doi.org/10.1183/13993003.congress-2020.2384.
6. Schanzer DL, Langley JM, Tam TWS. Influenza-attributed hospitalization rates among pregnant women in Canada 1994–2000. JOGC. 2007;29:622–9.
7. Dodds L, McNeil SA, Fell SB, Allen VM, Coombs A, Scott J, et al. Impact of influenza exposure on rates of hospital admissions and physician visits because of respiratory illness among pregnant women. CMAJ. 2007;176:463–8.
8. Munoz FM, Greisinger AJ, Wehmanen OA, Mouzoon ME, Hoyle JC, Smith FA, Glezen WP. Safety of influenza vaccination during pregnancy. Am J Obstet Gynecol. 2005;192(4):1098–106. https://doi.org/10.1016/j.ajog.2004.12.019. PMID: 15846187.
9. Siston AM, Rasmussen SA, Honein MA, et al. Pandemic 2009 influenza A(H1N1) virus illness among pregnant women in the United States. JAMA. 2010;303(15):1517–25.
10. Falsey AR, Hennessey PA, Formica MA, Cox C, Walsh EE. Respiratory syncytial virus infection in elderly and high-risk adults. N Engl J Med. 2005;352(17):1749–59. PMID: 15858184.
11. Wheeler SM, Dotters-Katz S, Heine RP, Grotegut CA, Swamy GK. Maternal effects of respiratory syncytial virus infection during pregnancy. Emerg Infect Dis. 2015;21(11):1951–5. https://doi.org/10.3201/eid2111.150497. PMID: 26485575.

12. Lenahan JL, Englund JA, Katz J, Kuypers J, Wald A, Magaret A, Tielsch JM, Khatry SK, LeClerq SC, Shrestha L, Steinhoff MC, Chu HY. Human Metapneumovirus and other respiratory viral infections during pregnancy and birth, Nepal. Emerg Infect Dis. 2017;23(8):1341–9. https://doi.org/10.3201/eid2308.161358. PMID: 28726613; PMCID: PMC5547777.

13. Getahun D, Ananth CV, Peltier MR, Smulian JC, Vintzileos AM. Acute and chronic respiratory diseases in pregnancy: associations with placental abruption. Am J Obstet Gynecol. 2006;195(4):1180–4.

14. Acs N, Bánhidy F, Puhó EH, Czeizel AE. Acute respiratory infections during pregnancy and congenital abnormalities: a population-based case-control study. Congenit Anom (Kyoto). 2006;46(2):86–96. https://doi.org/10.1111/j.1741-4520.2006.00108.x. PMID: 16732767.

15. Boksa P, Luheshi GN. On the use of animal modeling to study maternal infection during pregnancy and prenatal cytokine exposure as risk factors for schizophrenia. Clin Neurosci Res. 2003;3(4–5):339–46.

16. Littauer EQ, Skountzou I. Hormonal regulation of physiology, innate immunity and antibody response to H1N1 influenza virus infection during pregnancy. Front Immunol. 2018;(9):2455. https://doi.org/10.3389/fimmu.2018.02455. PMID: 30420854; PMCID: PMC6215819.

17. Lim BH, Mahmood TA. Influenza A H1N1 2009 (Swine Flu) and pregnancy. J Obstet Gynaecol India. 2011;61(4):386–93. https://doi.org/10.1007/s13224-011-0055-2. Epub 2011 Sep 23. PMID: 22851818; PMCID: PMC3295877.

18. Getahun D, Ananth CV, Oyelese Y, Peltier MR, Smulian JC, Vintzileos AM. Acute and chronic respiratory diseases in pregnancy: associations with spontaneous premature rupture of membranes. J Matern Fetal Neonatal Med. 2007;20(9):669–75. https://doi.org/10.1080/14767050701516063. PMID: 17701667.

19. Xia YQ, Zhao KN, Zhao AD, Zhu JZ, Hong HF, Wang YL, Li SH. Associations of maternal upper respiratory tract infection/influenza during early pregnancy with congenital heart disease in offspring: evidence from a case-control study and meta-analysis. BMC Cardiovasc Disord. 2019;19(1):277. https://doi.org/10.1186/s12872-019-1206-0. PMID: 31791237; PMCID: PMC6889668.

20. Philpott EK, Englund JA, Katz J, Tielsch J, Khatry S, LeClerq SC, Shrestha L, Kuypers J, Magaret AS, Steinhoff MC, Chu HY. Febrile rhinovirus illness during pregnancy is associated with low birth weight in Nepal. Open Forum Infect Dis. 2017;4(2):ofx073. https://doi.org/10.1093/ofid/ofx073. Erratum in: Open Forum Infect Dis. 2018 Jan 30;5(1):ofx182. PMID: 28584855; PMCID: PMC5450902.

21. Narang K, Enninga EAL, Gunaratne MDSK, et al. SARS-CoV-2 infection and COVID-19 during pregnancy: a multidisciplinary review. Mayo Clin Proc. 2020;95(8):1750–65. https://doi.org/10.1016/j.mayocp.2020.05.011.

22. Adhikari EH, Moreno W, Zofkie AC, MacDonald L, McIntire DD, Collins RRJ, Spong CY. Pregnancy outcomes among women with and without severe acute respiratory syndrome coronavirus 2 infection. JAMA Netw Open. 2020;3(11):e2029256. https://doi.org/10.1001/jamanetworkopen.2020.29256. PMID: 33211113; PMCID: PMC7677755.

23. Sordillo JE, Scirica CV, Rifas-Shiman SL, Gillman MW, Bunyavanich S, Camargo CA, Weiss ST, Gold DR, Litonjua AA. Prenatal and infant exposure to acetaminophen and ibuprofen and the risk for wheeze and asthma in children. J Allergy Clin Immunol. 2014;4596(2):297–585, ISSN 0091-6749. https://doi.org/10.1016/j.jaci.2014.07.065.

24. Andersen AB, Farkas DK, Mehnert F, Ehrenstein V, Erichsen R. Use of prescription paracetamol during pregnancy and risk of asthma in children: a population-based Danish cohort study. Clin Epidemiol. 2012;4:33–40. https://doi.org/10.2147/CLEP.S28312. Epub 2012 Feb 1. PMID: 22355259; PMCID: PMC4614522.

25. Smucny J, Fahey T, Becker L, Glazier R. Antibiotics for acute bronchitis. Cochrane Database Syst Rev. 2004;(4):CD000245. https://doi.org/10.1002/14651858.CD000245.pub2. Update in: Cochrane Database Syst Rev. 2014;3:CD000245. PMID: 15494994.

26. Meeraus WH, Petersen I, Gilbert R. Association between antibiotic prescribing in pregnancy and cerebral palsy or epilepsy in children born at term: a cohort study using the health

improvement network. PLoS One. 2015;10(3):e0122034. Published 2015 Mar 25. https://doi.org/10.1371/journal.pone.0122034.

27. Czeizel AE, Rockenbauer M, Sørensen HT, Olsen J. Use of cephalosporins during pregnancy and in the presence of congenital abnormalities: a population-based, case-control study. Am J Obstet Gynecol. 2001;184(6):1289–96.

28. Bar-Oz B, Diav-Citrin O, Shechtman S, Tellem R, Arnon J, Francetic I, Berkovitch M, Ornoy A. Pregnancy outcome after gestational exposure to the new macrolides: a prospective multicenter observational study. Eur J Obstet Gynecol Reprod Biol. 2008;141(1):31–4. https://doi.org/10.1016/j.ejogrb.2008.07.008. Epub 2008 Aug 29. PMID: 18760873.

29. Aykan D, Ergun Y. Maternal antibiotic exposure and fetal outcomes: is there evidence for teratogenicity? Ann Med Res. 2019;26:646–52. https://doi.org/10.5455/annalsmedres.2018.12.279.

30. Czeizel AE, Rockenbauer M, Sørensen HT, Olsen J. A population-based case-control teratologic study of ampicillin treatment during pregnancy. Am J Obstet Gynecol. 2001;185(1):140–7.

31. Mylonas I. Antibiotic chemotherapy during pregnancy and lactation period: aspects for consideration. Arch Gynecol Obstet. 2011;283:7–18. https://doi.org/10.1007/s00404-010-1646-3.

32. Mercer BM, Carr TL, Beazley DD, Crouse DT, Sibai BM. Antibiotic use in pregnancy and drug-resistant infant sepsis. Am J Obstet Gynecol. 1999;181(4):816–21. https://doi.org/10.1016/s0002-9378(99)70307-8. PMID: 10521735.

33. Metzler S, Frei R, Schmaußer-Hechfellner E, von Mutius E, Pekkanen J, Karvonen AM, Kirjavainen PV, Dalphin JC, Divaret-Chauveau A, Riedler J, Lauener R, Roduit C, PASTURE/EFRAIM Study Group. Association between antibiotic treatment during pregnancy and infancy and the development of allergic diseases. Pediatr Allergy Immunol. 2019;30(4):423–33. https://doi.org/10.1111/pai.13039. Epub 2019 Mar 5. PMID: 30734960.

34. Muanda FT, Sheehy O, Bérard A. Use of antibiotics during pregnancy and the risk of major congenital malformations: a population based cohort study. Br J Clin Pharmacol. 2017;83(11):2557–71. https://doi.org/10.1111/bcp.13364. Epub 2017 Aug 11. PMID: 28722171; PMCID: PMC5651310.

35. Sarkar M, Woodland C, Koren G, Einarson AR. Pregnancy outcome following gestational exposure to azithromycin. BMC Pregnancy Childbirth. 2006;(6):18. https://doi.org/10.1186/1471-2393-6-18. PMID: 16734900; PMCID: PMC1481555.

36. Linseman DA, Hampton LA, Branstetter DG. Quinolone-induced arthropathy in the neonatal mouse. Morphological analysis of articular lesions produced by pipemidic acid and ciprofloxacin. Fundam Appl Toxicol. 1995;28:59–64.

37. Bar-Oz B, Moretti ME, Boskovic R, et al. The safety of quinolones—a meta-analysis of pregnancy outcomes. Eur J Obstet Gynecol Reprod Biol. 2009;143:75–8.

38. Padberg S, Wacker E, Meister R, et al. Observational cohort study of pregnancy outcome after first-trimester exposure to fluoroquinolones. Antimicrob Agents Chemother. 2014;58:4392–8.

39. Rosa F. Amantadine pregnancy experience [letter]. Reprod Toxicol. 1994;8:531.

40. Nora JJ, Nora AH, Way GL. Cardiovascular maldevelopment associated with maternal exposure to amantadine [letter]. Lancet. 1975;II:607.

41. Pandit PB, Chitayat D, Jefferies AL, et al. Tibial hemimelia and tetralogy of Fallot associated with first trimester exposure to amantadine. Reprod Toxicol. 1994;8:89–92.

42. Louis M, Oyiengo DO, Bourjeily G. Pulmonary disorders in pregnancy. In: Rosene-Montella K, editor. Medical management of the pregnant patient. New York: Springer; 2015. https://doi.org/10.1007/978-1-4614-1244-1_11.

43. Padberg S. Anti-infective agents. In: Drugs during pregnancy and lactation; 2015. pp. 115–176. doi:https://doi.org/10.1016/B978-0-12-408078-2.00007-X.

44. Uyeki T, Bernstein H, Bradley J, Englund J, File T, Fry A, Gravenstein S, Hayden F, Harper S, Hirshon J, Ison M, Johnston B, Knight S, Mcgeer A, Riley L, Wolfe C, Alexander P, Pavia A. Clinical practice guidelines by the Infectious Diseases Society of America: 2018 update on diagnosis, treatment, chemoprophylaxis, and institutional outbreak management of seasonal influenza. Clin Infect Dis. 2019;68:895–902. https://doi.org/10.1093/cid/ciy874.

45. Nunes MC, Madhi SA. Review on the effects of influenza vaccination during pregnancy on preterm births. Hum Vaccin Immunother. 2015;11(11):2538–48. https://doi.org/10.108 0/21645515.2015.1059976. Epub 2015 Aug 12. PMID: 26267701; PMCID: PMC4685674.
46. Nunes MC, Madhi SA. Influenza vaccination during pregnancy for prevention of influenza confirmed illness in the infants: a systematic review and meta-analysis. Hum Vaccin Immunother. 2018;14(3):758–66. https://doi.org/10.1080/21645515.2017.1345385. Epub 2017 Oct 18. PMID: 28708952; PMCID: PMC5861794.
47. Cuningham W, Geard N, Fielding JE, Braat S, Madhi SA, Nunes MC, Christian LM, Lin SY, Lee CN, Yamaguchi K, Bisgaard H, Chawes B, Chao AS, Blanchard-Rohner G, Schlaudecker EP, Fisher BM, McVernon J, Moss R. Optimal timing of influenza vaccine during pregnancy: a systematic review and meta-analysis. Influenza Other Respir Viruses. 2019;13(5):438–52. https://doi.org/10.1111/irv.12649. Epub 2019 Jun 5. PMID: 31165580; PMCID: PMC6692549.
48. Walsh Laura K, Jessy D, Linda D, Steven H, Kumanan W, Benchimol EI, et al. Health outcomes of young children born to mothers who received 2009 pandemic H1N1 influenza vaccination during pregnancy: retrospective cohort study. BMJ. 2019;366:l4151.

Bacterial Pneumonia During Pregnancy

61

Şule Gül, Mehmet Atilla Uysal, and Derya Kocakaya

61.1 Introduction

Pneumonia is a significant cause of morbidity and mortality worldwide. Some physiological and immunological changes that develop during pregnancy may facilitate the development of pneumonia. Bacterial agents take first place among the microorganisms that cause pneumonia both for community-acquired pneumonia (CAP) and hospital-acquired pneumonia (HAP). Although treatment of bacterial pneumonia does not differ for pregnancy, antibiotics that are not suitable for use during pregnancy should be kept in mind while deciding the appropriate treatment. In the follow-up, both mother and fetus should be followed closely, and follow-up should be planned with a multidisciplinary approach. Because bacterial pneumonia in pregnancy is a significant cause of morbidity and mortality due to the complications it may cause, it is essential to pay attention to preventive measures, especially during pregnancy.

Pneumonia is a disease characterized by inflammation in the lung parenchyma and inflammatory infiltration in the alveolar area due to infectious or noninfectious causes. Infectious causes include bacteria, viruses, and fungi. The most common noninfectious causes are food or liquid aspiration, acid-alkali substance inhalation, or radiation [1, 2].

Ş. Gül (✉) · M. A. Uysal
Ministry of Health, Yedikule Chest Diseases and Thoracic Surgery Training and Research Hospital, Istanbul, Turkey
e-mail: suleeyhan@gmail.com; dratilla@yahoo.com

D. Kocakaya
Medical Faculty, Department of Pulmonology, Istanbul, Turkey
e-mail: drderyagun@gmail.com

C. Cingi et al. (eds.), *ENT Diseases: Diagnosis and Treatment during Pregnancy and Lactation*, https://doi.org/10.1007/978-3-031-05303-0_61

According to the World Health Organization (WHO) data, lower respiratory tract infections are the fourth most common causes of death, and they killed 2.6 million people in 2019 [3].

The incidence of pneumonia during pregnancy varies between 0.7 and 2.7 per 1000, and this rate is similar to the pneumonia rates seen in the nonpregnant population. However, having pneumonia during pregnancy leads to many maternal complications. Pneumonia is the most common cause of fatal nonobstetric infection in pregnant women [4, 5] and observed more frequently in the later weeks of pregnancy, especially in the second and third trimesters [5, 6].

Some physiological changes in the respiratory tract and immune system during pregnancy may facilitate the development of pneumonia. These changes are discussed in detail below and summarized in Table 61.1.

- **Changes in the upper respiratory tract:** Mucosal edema, hyperemia, capillary congestion, and fragility begin in the first trimester and gradually increase toward the third trimester. The increase in estrogen can cause changes in the nasal mucosa and bleeding [7].
- **Changes in the chest:** The subcostal angle widens due to the relaxin secretion during pregnancy and other hormonal changes. The diaphragm rises by 4–5 cm as the pregnancy progresses and the chest wall circumference may increase up to 5–7 cm, and the anteroposterior diameter may increase up to 2 cm. This may cause difficulty in removal of the secretions of the pregnant woman [7–9].
- **Changes in lung volumes and function:** Progesterone increases the amount of air breathed in and out by directly stimulating the respiratory center in the

Table 61.1 Physiological changes and conditions that increase risk of pneumonia in pregnancy

Physiopathological changes	• Mucosal edema, congestion, and increased fragility • Diaphragm elevation and increased chest diameter • Increased oxygen demand and minute ventilation • Reduction in pulmonary resistance
Immunological changes	• Decreased cellular immune response • Decrease in the number of T helper 1 cells • Decrease in proinflammatory cytokines and increase in anti-inflammatory cytokines • Decreased lymphokine response to alloantigens
Other changes	• Decreased lower esophageal sphincter tone • Physiological anemia
Habits and diseases of the pregnant person	• Lung and heart diseases • Liver diseases • Smoking • Substance use • Immunosuppressive illness or drug use
Factors related to pregnancy and childbirth	• Use of steroids for fetal maturation • Use of tocolytic drugs to induce labor • Abruptio placenta • Using sedation, anesthesia/analgesia for labor

medulla oblongata. Therefore, a 30–50% increase occurs in tidal volume (TV) as well as 15–20% (300–500 mL) decrease in functional residual capacity (FRC) with increased minute ventilation and rise of diaphragm. Despite changes in TV and FRC, spirometric measurements remain normal in pregnancy. Therefore, changes in spirometry should not be attributed to pregnancy and should be investigated for underlying diseases. In addition, the presence of tachypnea should be considered, since an increase in respiratory rate is not expected despite the increase in minute ventilation in normal pregnancies [7, 8]. An increase in minute ventilation leads to an increase in the partial pressure of oxygen (PaO_2) in arterial blood and a decrease in the partial pressure of carbon dioxide ($PaCO_2$). The perception of dyspnea due to respiratory alkalosis deepens. The increase in hemoglobin and PaO_2 during pregnancy meets the excess O_2 consumption needed due to pregnancy. Even if the amount of hemoglobin increases, the increase in blood volume leads to physiological anemia. Excess progesterone secretion causes a decrease in pulmonary resistance. All these physiological and respiratory changes reduce tolerance to hypoxia in pregnancy and make it difficult to compensate for the respiratory disease response [7, 10, 11].

- Immunological changes: Estriol (E3), the main estrogen secreted during pregnancy, causes a decrease in $CD4^+$, $CD8^+$ T cells. Progesterone causes $CD4^+$ T cells to switch toward T helper type 2 (Th2) cells. Th2/Th1 cell ratio increases as 4/1, and accordingly, anti-inflammatory cytokine release such as interleukin (IL)-4, IL-5, IL-10 increases, while the release of proinflammatory cytokines interferon-gamma (IFN-γ), IL-2, and tumor necrosis factor-alpha (TNF-α) decreases [11, 12]. In addition, progesterone, human chorionic gonadotropin, alpha-fetoprotein, and cortisol released during pregnancy suppress the cellular immune system [9]. With these immunological mechanisms, the fetus is placed and attached to the uterus, but the susceptibility to bacterial and viral infections increases.
- Other changes: Lower esophageal sphincter pressure decreases with the effect of progesterone, intra-abdominal pressure increases with the growing uterus, and the risk of aspiration pneumonia increases [13]. Advanced gestational age and the presence of anemia observed during pregnancy also pose a risk for developing pneumonia [14].

Apart from these physiological changes, some diseases and conditions in pregnant women are also contributing to the risk of pneumonia. Presence of lung, heart, and liver diseases; smoking; presence of a disease-causing immunosuppression; and use of immunosuppressive drugs have been shown in studies to increase the risk of pneumonia. Administration of corticosteroids for fetal lung maturation and the use of tocolytic drugs to trigger labor also increase the risk of pneumonia [9, 13].

Bacterial pneumonia in pregnancy can be divided into community-acquired and hospital-acquired pneumonia as in nonpregnant individuals.

61.2 Community-Acquired Pneumonia in Pregnancy

Community-acquired pneumonia (CAP) occurs mostly via inhalation or aspiration of nasopharyngeal secretions in otherwise healthy individuals, causing direct lung injury and interstitial inflammation. But rarely the hematogenous spread can cause CAP [11].

Even with further developments, the detection rate of the causative agent in CAP remains around 40–60%. In adults, bacteria are the main cause of CAP by 60–80% of cases, while 10–20% are caused by atypical pathogens, and 10–15% by viruses [13]. Since only bacterial causes will be mentioned in this section, the agents that most commonly cause bacterial pneumonia in pregnancy are summarized in Table 61.2 [11].

Streptococcus pneumoniae is the most common bacterial agent of CAP in pregnant women as in the whole society. However, with the widespread application of the conjugated pneumococcal vaccine in recent years, its incidence has decreased. However, the prevalence of β-lactamase-producing species is increasing worldwide [10]. Apart from this, *Staphylococcus aureus* infections can be seen after *Haemophilus influenzae* and especially after viral influenza infection. *Mycoplasma pneumoniae*, *Chlamydia pneumoniae*, and *Legionella* species can be seen among atypical agents, similar to nonpregnant individuals [8]. In CAP, Gram-negative pathogens (*E. coli*, *Enterobacter* species, etc.) are more common in patients with underlying diseases such as bronchiectasis and chronic obstructive pulmonary disease (COPD), diabetes, and a history of hospitalization [1].

61.2.1 Clinical Properties and Physical Examination

The clinical picture due to pneumonia in pregnant women is similar to that of non-pregnant individuals. In infection with typical bacterial agents, the symptoms begin acutely. The most common complaints are fever, chills, productive cough, and pleuritic chest pain. Cough is seen in more than 90% of patients, while dyspnea and sputum production are seen in about 60% [10, 11]. In the presence of pneumonia with atypical agents, the complaints have a subacute onset. Body temperature is usually

Table 61.2 Bacterial pathogens causing community-acquired pneumonia in pregnancy

Common	• *Streptococcus pneumoniae*
	• *Mycoplasma pneumoniae*
	• *Haemophilus influenzae*
	• *Staphylococcus aureus*
	• *Chlamydia pneumoniae* and *chlamydia psittaci*
Rare	• *Pseudomonas aeruginosa*
	• *Legionella* species
	• *Klebsiella* species
	• *Moraxella catarrhalis*
	• *Bordetella pertussis*
	• *Escherichia coli (E.coli)*
	• *Enterobacter* species and *Serratia* species

subfebrile, and complaints such as muscle pain, headache, and abdominal pain are in the foreground. The cough is usually dry. Although dyspnea in pregnancy may be confused with physiological dyspnea, cough is not a pregnancy-related symptom, and further investigation should be performed in the presence of cough [1, 15].

On physical examination, tachypnea, cyanosis, use of auxiliary respiratory muscles, and sternal retraction are signs of respiratory failure. Dullness to percussion may be a sign of consolidation. Inspiratory rales, bronchial breath sounds, or decreased breath sounds can be heard supporting the diagnosis. Although the sensitivity of physical examination alone is low, it has an important part of the diagnostic approach together with clinical properties, laboratory findings, and imaging [11, 13].

61.2.2 Laboratory Findings and Imaging

A complete blood count, biochemical tests for liver and renal functions, blood glucose level, and electrolytes should be performed. Assessment of oxygenation with pulse oximetry or arterial blood gas analysis should be checked in every pregnant patient with pneumonia. The condition of the fetus should be checked with an electronic fetal monitor. In microbiology, sputum gram stain and culture and urinary antigen may be requested if necessary. Although positivity is very rarely detected, blood cultures can also be taken in cases with severe pneumonia [4].

Postero-anterior (PA) chest X-ray should be taken in every pregnant patient with suspected pneumonia. The unit of dose absorbed by radiological imaging is expressed as "rad" or "gray" (Gy). In general, radiation dose below 50 mGy does not cause fetal anomalies or spontaneous abortion. The dose taken with a PA chest X-ray is less than 0.003 mGy. The highest dose taken is 34 mGy with computed tomography (CT) angiography. Dose exposures above 100 mGy may cause fetal abnormalities or abortion [13, 16].

The most common radiological findings in pneumonia with typical bacterial agents are lobar consolidation, bronchopneumonia, cavitation, and pleural effusion. The lobe/segment is kept homogeneous; the typical finding is air bronchograms (Fig. 61.1a, b). In bronchopneumonia, patchy infiltrates in both lungs do not show

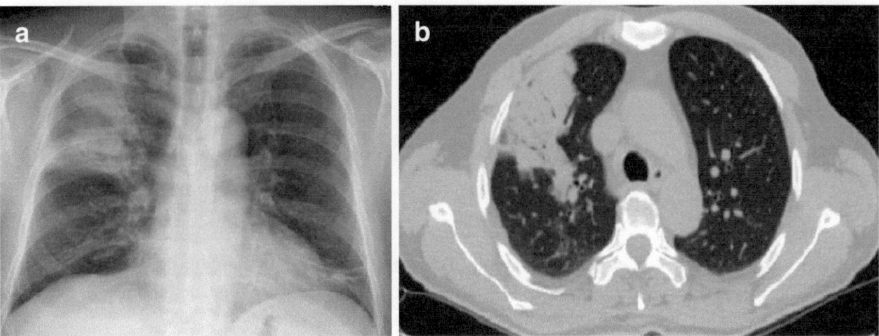

Fig. 61.1 Postero-anterior chest X-ray of a patient with (**a**) right upper lobe pneumonia, consolidation with air bronchograms (**b**) computed tomography images

lobe/segment distinction (Fig. 61.2). While *Streptococcus pneumoniae* and *Klebsiella* species usually cause lobar pneumonia, *Staphylococcus aureus*, *Haemophilus influenza*, and *Pseudomonas aeruginosa* show involvement as bronchopneumonia [1].

Atypical pathogens cause interstitial pneumonia in the form of reticulonodular images that do not show lobe/segment separation. Ground-glass areas or intermittent patchy consolidations may be seen in some atypical infections, such as *Mycoplasma* (Fig. 61.3). *Legionella* can cause both interstitial and lobar pneumonia.

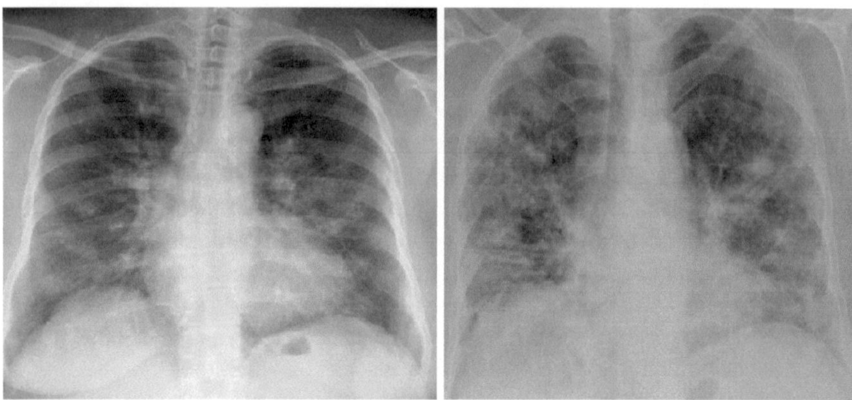

Fig. 61.2 Examples of bronchopneumonia with bilateral patchy infiltrates on postero-anterior chest X-rays

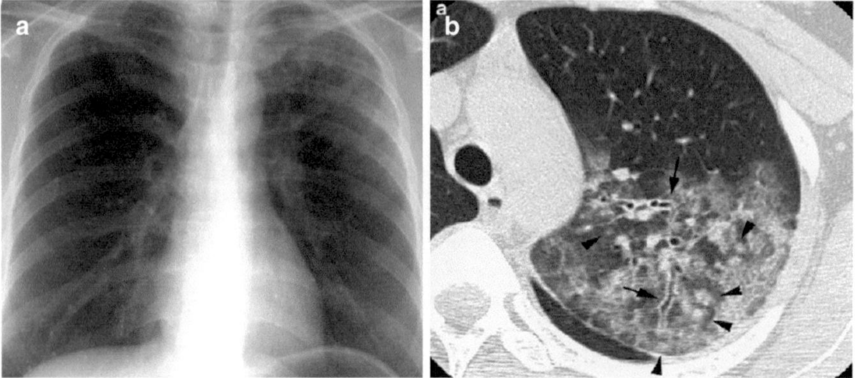

Fig. 61.3 *Mycoplasma pneumonia* case with infiltration in the left upper zone in (**a**): the postero-anterior chest X-ray and (**b**) ground glass opacities, bronchial wall thickening, and nodularities in the left upper lobe posterior segment on computed tomography images [17]

61.2.3 Treatment and Follow-Up

Deciding where to treat the patient is an important point after the diagnosis of CAP in pregnancy. Pregnant women who have no underlying health problems and have normal vital signs and laboratory values can receive outpatient treatment if close follow-up is possible. However, pregnant women with pneumonia who have underlying chronic diseases such as asthma, COPD, diabetes, cardiac disease, kidney failure, and who have complicating factors for severe pneumonia (Table 61.3) should be treated in hospital [11, 18, 19].

Conditions that pose a risk for the development of pneumonia with specific bacterial pathogens [1] are listed below:

- Penicillin-resistant pneumococci: Age > 65 years old, use of beta-lactam antibiotics in the last 3 months, alcoholism, immunosuppressive conditions, multiple comorbid diseases, contact with a nursery child.
- *Pseudomonas aeruginosa*: Structural lung disease (bronchiectasis, cystic fibrosis, advanced COPD), steroid use and history of aspiration, malnutrition, previous use of broad-spectrum antibiotics.
- *Legionella pneumophilia*: recent travel with accommodation, staying in a hotel, office environment, changes in home plumbing, smoking history, presence of malignancy, steroid use.
- Gram-negative enteric bacteria: Alcohol use, living in a nursing home, concomitant cardiopulmonary disease, multiple comorbidities, recent antibiotic use
- Anaerobic bacteria: Alcohol intake, periodontal disease/poor oral hygiene, suspected aspiration (epilepsy, alcohol addiction, coma, etc.), substance abuse, obstructive bronchial pathologies.
- *Haemophilus influenzae*: History of smoking, COPD.
- *Staphylococcus aureus*: Living in a nursing home, recent flu, intravenous substance abuse.

After deciding where the patient will receive the treatment, empirical antibiotic therapy should be started immediately. It is recommended to start the treatment in

Table 61.3 Complicating factors for severe community-acquired pneumonia [18]

- Respiratory rate $\geq$ 30 breaths/minute
- PAO_2/FiO_2 (fractional inspired oxygen) $\leq$ 250
- Multilobar infiltrates
- Pulmonary cavitation
- Confusion/disorientation
- Uremia (blood urea nitrogen level $\geq$ 20 mg/dl
- Leukopenia (white blood cell count <4000 cells/mm^3—Due to infection alone/not chemotherapy induced)
- Thrombocytopenia (platelet count <100,000/mm^3)
- Hypothermia (<36°C) or hyperthermia (>39°C)
- Hypotension (requiring aggressive fluid resuscitation)
- Multiorgan dysfunction and septic shock

Table 61.4 Infectious Diseases Society of America and American Thoracic Society Treatment strategies for community-acquired pneumonia [18]

Outpatient treatment (No comorbidities or risk factors for specific pathogens)	Amoxicillin 500 mg-1gr three times daily OR Doxycycline 100 mg two times daily OR Azithromycin 500 mg once day on the first day, then 250 mg once daily OR Clarithromycin 500 mg twice daily
Outpatient treatment (with comorbidities)	Combination therapy with amoxicillin/clavulanate or cephalosporin[a] and macrolide or doxycycline[b] OR Monotherapy with respiratory fluoroquinolone[c]
Inpatient treatment (without complicating factors)	β lactam[d] + macrolide[e] combination OR Respiratory fluoroquionolone alone[c]
Inpatient treatment (without complicating factors)	β lactam[d] + macrolide[e] OR β lactam[d] + respiratory fluoroquinolone[c]

[a] Amoxicillin/clavulanate 500 mg/125 mg three times daily, amoxicillin/clavulanate 875 mg/125 mg twice daily, 2000 mg/125 mg twice daily, cefpodoxime 200 mg twice daily, or cefuroxime 500 mg twice daily

[b] Azithromycin 500 mg on first day then 250 mg daily, clarithromycin 500 mg twice daily, or doxycycline 100 mg twice daily

[c] Levofloxacin 750 mg daily, moxifloxacin 400 mg daily

[d] Ampicillin-sulbactam 1.5–3 g every 6 h, cefotaxime 1–2 g every 8 h, ceftriaxone 1–2 g every 24 h or ceftaroline 600 mg every 12 h

[e] Azithromycin 500 mg daily, clarithromycin 500 mg twice daily

the first 4 h, within 8 h at least, because studies have found that the starting time of antibiotics is associated with mortality. There is no established guideline for the use of antibiotics in CAP in pregnant women. The treatment scheme that ATS considers appropriate for outpatient and hospital treatment in CAP is summarized in Table 61.4. Treatment of pneumonia with specific bacterial pathogens should be treated with patient-specific assessment.

In this table, which is given for nonpregnant patients in the treatment of CAP, there are points to be considered for pregnant women. Although there was no objection to the use of macrolide antibiotics in pregnant women in previous publications, recent publications showed that macrolides are associated with spontaneous abortions and malformations in the baby, especially in the first trimester of pregnancy. Although azithromycin and clarithromycin are considered safer than other macrolides, some animal experiments have provided evidence that they have teratogenic effects. In studies, it has been observed that the penicillin group is safer than macrolides in pregnant women [20, 21].

Since fluoroquinolones were found to cause fetal arthropathy and malformation in animal experiments, their use was risky. There are conflicting results in this regard. In addition to studies showing that fluoroquinolones pose a risk for abortion, especially in the first trimester, some meta-analyses published in recent years have not found a relationship between fluoroquinolones and low birth weight, fetal malformation, and miscarriage. Even though it has been stated that fluoroquinolones should not be used, especially in the first trimester, they should only be used in other periods when necessary, and dose adjustment should be made if necessary [20, 22, 23]. In addition, since it has been shown that quinolones accumulate in the bone tissue of adolescents and children and cause arthralgia and tendonitis, their use is not recommended for those under the age of 18 and pregnant women [15]. It was stated that the American Food and Drug Administration (FDA) category should be considered for all drugs both during pregnancy and lactation [24].

In addition to antibiotic treatment, oxygenation and fetal follow-up should be done regularly in pregnant women. Since the affinity of fetal hemoglobin to oxygen is higher than that of adult hemoglobin, the fetus is more resistant to low oxygen in the maternal blood. However, when maternal oxygen saturation falls below 90%, the oxygen supply to the fetus decreases [4]. When maternal saturation begins to fall below 95%, an arterial blood gas evaluation should be performed. PaO_2 should be ≥ 70 mmHg to ensure adequate oxygenation of the placenta. Respiratory failure in pneumonia is due to intrapulmonary shunt rather than hypoventilation, so respiratory physiotherapy and noninvasive mechanical ventilation can be applied to prevent alveolar collapse and reduce alveolar-arterial oxygen gradient in pregnant women with respiratory failure [13].

After the treatment is started, clinical improvement is usually observed within 48–72 h. Antibiotic changes should not be made in the first 72 h without significant clinical deterioration. Fever response should be obtained in 2–4 days, cough resolves in 7–10 days. Radiological recovery may take up to 6 weeks. A minimum of 5 days of treatment should be given in uncomplicated CAP [11]. If the causative agent is isolated, treatment can be given for 7–10 days in pneumococcal pneumonia, 14–21 days in Legionella pneumonia, 10–14 days if an atypical agent is considered, at least 2–3 weeks in severe pneumonia, and 4–6 weeks in the presence of an abscess [1].

Despite treatment, respiratory failure may develop in 10% of pregnant women. Indications for admission to intensive care unit and intubation are similar to non-pregnant individuals: inadequate oxygenation ($PaO_2 < 60$ mmHg or oxygen saturation $< 85\%$ with 60% FiO_2), insufficient ventilation ($PaCO_2 > 50$ mmHg), sepsis requiring invasive hemodynamic monitoring, and unresolved metabolic acidosis. Elective delivery may improve the respiratory status of the pregnant women, but there is not enough data on this subject [4].

61.2.4 Complications

In the follow-up of CAP, some pulmonary complications may develop as well as maternal or fetal complications.

Pulmonary complications can be listed as follows:

- Parapneumonic effusion.
- Lung abscess, necrosis (Fig. 61.4).
- Pneumocele, pneumothorax.
- Bronchopleural fistula.
- Hilar and mediastinal lymphadenopathy.
- Adult respiratory distress syndrome (ARDS).
- Bronchiectasis, fibrotic sequelae changes.

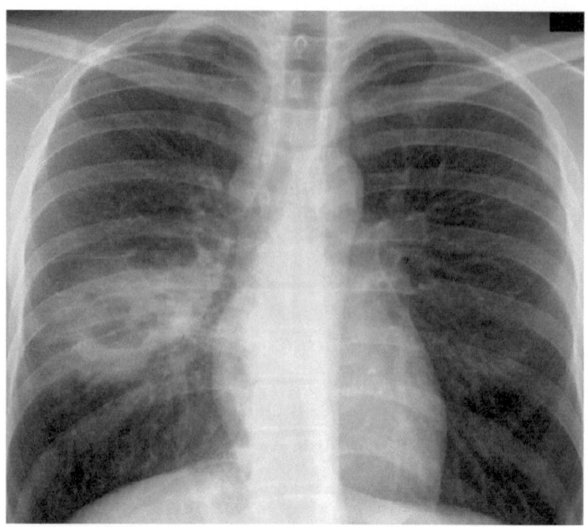

Fig. 61.4 Lung abscess in the lower zone of the right lung

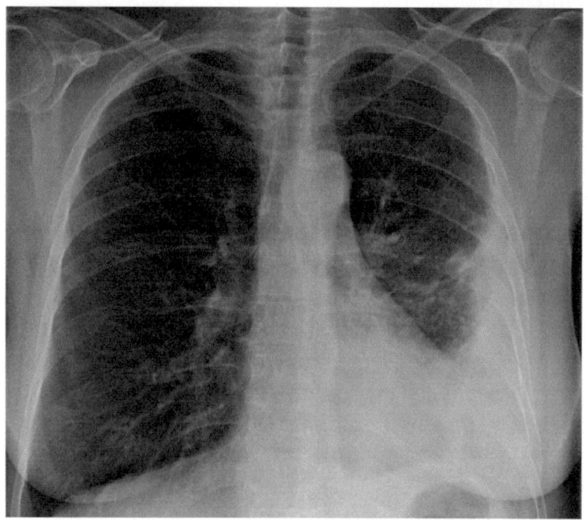

Fig. 61.5 Parapneumonic effusion in the lower zone of the left lung

Parapneumonic effusion (PPE) is the most common and most important complication of pneumonia. It has been shown that PPE can develop in 57% of hospitalized pneumonia patients (Fig. 61.5). It mainly develops due to late initiation of treatment or lack of appropriate antibiotic selection. There may be delays in diagnosing pneumonia in pregnant women, mainly due to the absence of radiological imaging or its rejection by the patient. The approach to PPE in pregnancy is similar to nonpregnant individuals. A combination of second- or third-generation cephalosporin and macrolide is recommended for treatment selection. In case of complicated PPE or empyema, it can be safely drained. Although there are limited data on the use of fibrinolytic agents, teratogenicity and serious fetal or maternal side effects, primarily related to the use of streptokinase, have not been observed [25].

In the case of pneumonia in pregnancy, especially in the presence of hypoxia, the risk of maternal/fetal complications increases. Although the mechanism is not known, it is thought that the placenta is affected by the infection and the intrauterine spread of the infection through the placenta causes complications. There was no difference in complication risk between bacterial and viral agents. It has been determined that having pneumonia, especially in the first trimester, increases the risk more. In many studies, it has been shown that having pneumonia during pregnancy is associated with intrauterine growth retardation, cesarean delivery, low birth weight, and low Apgar score [6, 26]. It has been found that preterm delivery is 44% more common in the presence of pneumonia and is more common in pregnant women with comorbid diseases [11]. Maternal and fetal complications that can be seen due to pneumonia in pregnancy can be listed as follows:

- Preeclampsia/eclampsia.
- Obligation to have a cesarean delivery.
- Intrauterine growth retardation.
- Low birth weight.
- Preterm birth.
- Abruptio placenta/placenta previa.
- Complications such as low Apgar score.

61.2.5 Prevention

To prevent pneumococcal pneumonia, vaccination is recommended for pregnant women with comorbid conditions such as Human Immunodeficiency Virus infection, asthma, diabetes, chronic kidney disease, and heart disease. Pre-pregnancy vaccination is recommended whenever possible. There are two types of pneumococcal vaccines: conjugated pneumococcal vaccine (PCV) (13-valent) and pneumococcal polysaccharide vaccine (PPPSV23) (23-valent). A 23-valent-pneumococcal vaccine is recommended for pregnant women. It has been shown that the vaccine is 60–70% protective, especially in pregnant women with comorbid diseases. In addition, quitting smoking and preventing second hand smoking, adequate nutrition, adequate hydration and rest, and avoiding crowded environments during flu seasons can be specified as other protective measures [2, 13].

61.3 Hospital-Acquired Pneumonia in Pregnancy

The approach to hospital-acquired pneumonia (HAP) in pregnancy is similar to that of nonpregnant population. In addition, the risk of aspiration increases in pregnant women due to low gastric sphincter tone delayed gastric emptying and uterine compression, and the risk of aspiration pneumonia increases even more, especially in cases where anesthesia is required [9].

The definitions in HAP [27] that should be known first are as follows:

- **Hospital-acquired pneumonia:** Pneumonia that occurs 48 h after hospitalization or develops within the first 48 h after discharge in a patient known to have no pneumonia at the time of hospitalization.
- **Ventilator-associated pneumonia (VAP):** Pneumonia that develops 48 h after intubation in a patient who is not known to have pneumonia during intubation.

HAP accounts for approximately 15% of hospital-acquired infections. A quarter of HAPs are intensive care unit related, and 90% of them develop while the patient is on a mechanical ventilator. VAP is seen in 9–27% of all intubated patients. The mortality rate due to HAP is in the range of 30–70%. The mortality rate from HAP in intensive care unit is 20% [27, 28].

61.3.1 Etiopathogenesis

HAP can develop by inhalation, aspiration of microorganisms colonized in the oropharyngeal region, or hematogenous spread. On the other hand, contamination by medical devices, invasive procedures, and poor hand hygiene of healthcare professionals also pose exogenous risk for HAP [13]. It has been mentioned before that the risk of aspiration increases with specific mechanisms in pregnancy. In HAP and VAP, conditions such as interventional procedures applied to the respiratory and gastrointestinal system, invasive mechanical ventilation, low cuff pressure of the intubation tube, and use of infected nebulizer devices further increase microaspiration risk.

The causative agents are usually bacteria. The most common bacterial agents are Gram-negative bacteria. The causative agent in HAP is a Gram-negative pathogen in 55–85% of cases, Gram-positive ones in 20–30%, and polymicrobial infection in 40–60% of cases [1]. Multidrug-resistant bacteria (MDR) and non–multidrug resistant bacteria that are frequently seen as causative pathogen in HAP are summarized in Table 61.5 [13].

Table 61.5 Bacterial agents in hospital-acquired pneumonia [13]

Multidrug-resistant bacteria	Non–multidrug-resistant bacteria
• *Acinetobacter baumannii-calcoaceticus complex* • *Pseudomonas aeruginosa* • *Klebsiella pneumoniae* (extended-spectrum beta-lactamase (ESBL) and/or carbapenemase producing) • *Escherichia coli* and other *Enterobacteriaceae* (ESBL and/or carbapenemase producing) • *Stenotrophomonas maltophilia* • Methicillin-resistant *Staphylococcus aureus* (MRSA)	• *Streptococcus pneumonia* • *Haemophilus influenza* • *Enterobacteriaceae* members (*Escherichia coli, Klebsiella pneumoniae, Proteus* species, *Serratia marcescens*) • *Methicillin-susceptible Staphylococcus aureus* (MSSA) • *Legionella pneumophilia*

Table 61.6 Risk factors for multidrug-resistant pathogens [29]

Risk factors for multidrug-resistant VAP	• History of intravenous antibiotic use in the last 90 days • Concurrent septic shock with VAP • Having ARDS before VAP • History of hospitalization for ≥5 days before VAP • Need of acute renal replacement therapy before VAP
Risk factors for multidrug-resistant HAP	• History of parenteral antibiotic use in the last 90 days
Risk factors for HAP/VAP caused by MRSA	• History of parenteral antibiotic use in the last 90 days
Risk factors for HAP/VAP caused by MDR *Pseudomonas* species	• History of parenteral antibiotic use in the last 90 days

VAP ventilator-associated pneumonia, *ARDS* acute respiratory distress syndrome, *HAP* hospital-acquired pneumonia, *MRSA* methicillin-resistant *Staphylococcus aureus*

Some conditions may pose a risk for developing MDR bacteria and pneumonia in HAP and VAP. These factors have been updated in the 2016 Infectious Diseases Society of America (IDSA) and American Thoracic Society (ATS) guideline and summarized in Table 61.6 [29]. Appropriate empirical antibiotic therapy should be initiated by evaluating the patient's risk factors, and the possible factors that can affect the management of HAP in pregnant women should be kept in mind, such as respiratory diseases, gynecological factors, anesthesia, and intensive care and pediatric care.

61.3.2 Diagnosis

Diagnosis in HAP begins with clinical suspicion. The clinical, radiological, and microbiological results facilitate the diagnosis. In the presence of at least two of the following factors, together with new or progressive infiltrate on the chest X-ray, the diagnosis of HAP can be made, and treatment can be started [27].

1. Hypo/hyperthermia (fever >38 °C or <36 °C).
2. Leukopenia (<4000/mm^3) or leukocytosis (>12,000/mm^3).
3. Purulent sputum or tracheal secretion.
4. Decreased oxygenation.

Microbiological sampling must be done for the isolation of the agent. With the sampling taken from the respiratory tract, the diagnosis can be made in 70% of the patients with high suspicion. If necessary, blood cultures and serological tests can also be performed [28]. Procalcitonin can be used as a biomarker, but it will not be beneficial to use C-reactive protein (CRP) and erythrocyte sedimentation rate (ESR), since they may also increase in pregnancy [13].

61.3.3 Treatment

Treatment of hospital-acquired pneumonia in pregnant women is similar to that of nonpregnant patients. The point to be considered is to avoid unsuitable antibiotics use in pregnancy and switch to oral therapy quickly when an adequate clinical response is obtained. Similar to nonpregnant patients, it is necessary to decide which empirical treatment will be given first. Here, the resistant microorganism profile of the hospital and the intensive care unit, the risk factors of the patient for multidrug-resistant pathogens, the history of hospitalization, and previously used antibiotics gain importance.

The treatment algorithm suggested by IDSA/ATS in HAP is summarized in Table 61.7.

Table 61.7 IDSA/ATS Recommendations for Treatment of HAP [29]

No mortality risk[a] and no MRSA risk	Piperacillin-tazobactam 4.5 g IV for four times daily OR Cefepime 2 g IV for three times daily OR Levofloxacin[b] 750 mg IV once daily OR Imipenem 500 mg IV for four times daily Meropenem 1 g IV for three times daily
No mortality risk[a] but increased MRSA risk	Piperacillin-tazobactam 4.5 g IV for four times daily OR Cefepime or ceftazidime 2 g IV for three times daily OR Levofloxacin[b] 750 mg IV once daily OR Imipenem 500 mg IV for four times daily OR Meropenem 1 g IV for three times daily OR Aztreonam 2 g IV for three times daily + Vancomycin 15 mg/kg IV for 2–3 times daily OR Linezolid 600 mg IV for two times daily
High-risk of mortality[a] or a history of intravenous antibiotic use in the past 90 days	Piperacillin-tazobactam 4.5 g IV for four times daily OR Cefepime or ceftazidime 2 g IV for three times daily OR Levofloxacin[b] 750 mg IV once daily OR Imipenem 500 mg IV for four times daily Meropenem 1 g IV for three times daily OR Amikacin 15–20 mg/kg IV daily OR Gentamicin[b] 5–7 mg/kg IV daily OR Tobramycin[b] 5–7 mg/kg IV daily OR Aztreonam 2 g IV for three times daily + Vancomycin 15 mg/kg IV for 2–3 times daily OR Linezolid 600 mg IV for two times daily

IDSA Infectious Diseases Society of America, *ATS* American Thoracic Society, *MRSA* methicillin-resistant *Staphylococcus aureus*, *IV* intravenous, *MSSA* methicillin-susceptible *Staphylococcus aureus*
[a] Mortality risk: the need for ventilatory support due to pneumonia or septic shock
[b] Quinolones and aminoglycosides are not recommended during pregnancy

If the patient is at risk of multidrug-resistant *Pseudomonas* infection, dual antipseudomonal antibiotics are recommended, but neither drug should be in the beta-lactam group. Linezolid or vancomycin should be added to the treatment if the patient has a risk of MRSA or if there is a risk of MRSA in addition to the risk of *Pseudomonas*. If a specific organism is detected in the culture results while the patient's empirical treatment continues, the treatment should be tailored accordingly. If *Acinetobacter* species growth occurs in the culture, carbapenem or ampicillin-sulbactam can be preferred depending on the sensitivity [13].

The duration of treatment should be at least 7 days, similar to patients who are not pregnant. If an MDR organism is detected, treatment should be completed for at least 14 days. In follow-up, procalcitonin levels can be used together with clinical findings [29]. After the adequate clinical response, switch to oral treatment should be done as soon as possible. Attention should be paid to the fact that the agents chosen in oral therapy has a similar antimicrobial effect to the drugs used in intravenous therapy and their use in pregnancy.

61.4 Conclusion

The approach to community-acquired and hospital-acquired pneumonia caused by bacterial agents during pregnancy is similar to that of nonpregnant patients. The risk of pneumonia increases with the physiological and immunological mechanisms that occur during pregnancy. An increase in morbidity and mortality can be observed along with many complications related to pneumonia. Therefore, it is essential to comply with preventive measures. In treatment, due to antibiotics that are not suitable for use in pregnancy, antibiotic selection should be considered, and follow-up should be carried out multidisciplinary.

References

1. Şen N, Özhan MH. Pnömoni. Tüsad Eğitim Kitapları Serisi; 2017
2. Salmon B, Bruick-Sorge C. Pneumonia in pregnant women. AWHONN Lifelines. 2003;7:48–52. https://doi.org/10.1177/1091592303251728.
3. https://www.who.int/news-room/fact-sheets/detail/the-top-10-causes-of-death.
4. Goodnight WH, Soper DE. Pneumonia in pregnancy. Crit Care Med. 2005;33(10 Suppl):S390–7. https://doi.org/10.1097/01.CCM.0000182483.24836.66.
5. Tang P, Wang J, Song Y. Characteristics and pregnancy outcomes of patients with severe pneumonia complicating pregnancy: a retrospective study of 12 cases and a literature review. BMC Pregnancy Childbirth. 2018;18:1–6. https://doi.org/10.1186/s12884-018-2070-0.
6. Chen YH, Keller J, Te WI, et al. Pneumonia and pregnancy outcomes: a nationwide population-based study. Am J Obstet Gynecol. 2012;207:288.e1–7. https://doi.org/10.1016/j.ajog.2012.08.023.
7. Bobrowski RA. Pulmonary physiology in pregnancy. Clin Obstet Gynecol. 2010;53:285–300. https://doi.org/10.1097/GRF.0b013e3181e04776.
8. Mehta N, Chen K, Hardy E, Powrie R. Respiratory disease in pregnancy. Best Pract Res Clin Obstetr Gynaecol. 2015;29:598–611. https://doi.org/10.1016/j.bpobgyn.2015.04.005.
9. Lim WS. Respiratory diseases in pregnancy.2: pneumonia and pregnancy. Thorax. 2001;56:398–405. https://doi.org/10.1136/thorax.56.5.398.

10. Laibl V, Sheffield J. The management of respiratory infections during pregnancy. Immunol Allergy Clin N Am. 2006;26:155–72. https://doi.org/10.1016/j.iac.2005.11.003.

11. Sheffield JS. Obstet Gynecol. Community-acquired pneumonia in pregnancy. 2009;114:915–22. https://doi.org/10.1097/AOG.0b013e3181b8e76d.

12. Mathad JS, Gupta A. Pulmonary infections in pregnancy. Semin Respir Crit Care Med. 2017;38:174–84. https://doi.org/10.1055/s-0037-1602375.

13. Yorgancıoğlu A, Topçu F, Ocaklı B Gebelik ve akciğer; 2019

14. Shariatzadeh MR, Marrie TJ. Pneumonia during pregnancy. Am J Med. 2006;119:872–6. https://doi.org/10.1016/j.amjmed.2006.01.014.

15. Lim WS, Macfarlane JT, Colthorpe CL. Treatment of community-acquired lower respiratory tract infections during pregnancy. Am J Respir Med. 2003;2:221–33. https://doi.org/10.1007/BF03256651.

16. Rocha APC, Carmo RL, Melo RFQ, et al. Imaging evaluation of nonobstetric conditions during pregnancy: what every radiologist should know. Radiol Bras. 2020;53:185–94. https://doi.org/10.1590/0100-3984.2019.0059.

17. Tanaka N, Emoto T, Suda H, et al. Community-acquired pneumonia: a correlative study between chest radiographic and HRCT findings. Jpn J Radiol. 2015;33:317–28. https://doi.org/10.1007/s11604-015-0420-7.

18. Metlay JP, Waterer GW, Long AC, et al. Diagnosis and treatment of adults with community-acquired pneumonia. Am J Respir Crit Care Med. 2019;200:E45–67. https://doi.org/10.1164/rccm.201908-1581ST.

19. Houck PM, Bratzler DW, Nsa W, et al. Timing of antibiotic administration and outcomes for medicare patients hospitalized with community-acquired pneumonia. Arch Intern Med. 2004;164:637–44. https://doi.org/10.1001/archinte.164.6.637.

20. Muanda FT, Sheehy O, Berard A. Use of antibiotics during pregnancy and risk of spontaneous abortion. CMAJ. 2017;189:E625–33. https://doi.org/10.1503/cmaj.161020.

21. Fan H, Gilbert R, O'Callaghan F, Li L. Associations between macrolide antibiotics prescribing during pregnancy and adverse child outcomes in the UK: population based cohort study. BMJ. 2020;368 https://doi.org/10.1136/bmj.m331.

22. Ziv A, Masarwa R, Perlman A, et al. Pregnancy outcomes following exposure to quinolone antibiotics – a systematic review and meta-analysis. Pharm Res. 2018;35:1–9. https://doi.org/10.1007/s11095-018-2383-8.

23. Yefet E, Schwartz N, Chazan B, et al. The safety of quinolones and fluoroquinolones in pregnancy: a meta-analysis. BJOG Int J Obstet Gynaecol. 2018;125(1069–1076) https://doi.org/10.1111/1471-0528.15119.

24. Nahum GG, Uhl K, Kennedy DL. Antibiotic use in pregnancy and lactation: what is and is not known about teratogenic and toxic risks. Obstet Gynecol. 2006;107(5):1120–38. https://doi.org/10.1097/01.AOG.0000216197.26783.b5.

25. Dikensoy E, Dikensoy Ö, Light RW. Management of parapneumonic effusion in pregnant women. Tuberkuloz ve Torak's. 2018;66:64–7. https://doi.org/10.5578/tt.66557.

26. Romanyuk V, Raichel L, Sergienko R, Sheiner E. Pneumonia during pregnancy: radiological characteristics, predisposing factors and pregnancy outcomes. J Matern Fetal Neonatal Med. 2011;24:113–7. https://doi.org/10.3109/14767051003678275.

27. American Thoracic Society; Infectious Diseases Society of America. Guidelines for the management of adults with hospital-acquired, ventilator-associated, and healthcare-associated pneumonia. Am J Respir Crit Care Med. 2005;171:388–416. https://doi.org/10.1164/rccm.200405-644ST.

28. Leone M, Bouadma L, Bouhemad B, et al. Hospital-acquired pneumonia in ICU. Anaesth Crit Care Pain Med. 2018;37:83–98. https://doi.org/10.1016/j.accpm.2017.11.006.

29. Kalil AC, Metersky ML, Klompas M, et al. Management of Adults with Hospital-acquired and Ventilator-associated Pneumonia: 2016 Clinical Practice Guidelines by the Infectious Diseases Society of America and the American Thoracic Society. Clin Infect Dis. 2016;63:e61–e111. https://doi.org/10.1093/cid/ciw353.

Nevra Güllü Arslan, Gaye Ulubay, and Szymon Skoczyński

62.1 Introduction

Pregnancy is a condition that can affect all organ systems differently by creating anatomical, physiological, and biochemical changes and cause susceptibility to infections. The suspicion of pneumonia is postponed by the patients and physicians due to avoid both the radiation that may be needed to be exposed for diagnosis and drugs' teratogenic effects.

Pneumonia is the most common cause of fatal nonobstetric infection in pregnant patients [1]. Risk factors such as cesarean section and delivery that develop in the peripartum period may increase hospital admissions because of pneumonia in the postpartum period [2]. Besides the development of pneumonia during pregnancy may cause complications in delivery [3]. It has been reported that pneumonia during pregnancy may be associated with placental abruption, eclampsia, premature birth, intrauterine growth retardation, and even maternal death [4].

While the incidence of antepartum pneumonia was found to be 0.5–1.5 per 1000 pregnancies in the United States [5], the annual incidence was 0.7% in a study conducted in East Asia [6]. However, since most of the reviews are case reports, an exact incidence cannot be given.

N. G. Arslan (✉)
Department of Pulmonology, Samsun Training and Research Hospital, Samsun, Turkey
e-mail: nevragullu@gmail.com

G. Ulubay
Faculty of Medicine, Department of Chest Diseases, Baskent University, Ankara, Turkey
e-mail: gayeulubay@yahoo.com

S. Skoczyński
Department of Pneumonology, Faculty of Medical Sciences in Katowice, Medical University of Silesia, Katowice, Poland
e-mail: simon.mds@poczta.fm

813

C. Cingi et al. (eds.), *ENT Diseases: Diagnosis and Treatment during Pregnancy and Lactation*, https://doi.org/10.1007/978-3-031-05303-0_62

In studies, mostly retrospective, investigating the incidence of pneumonia in pregnant women, it was found that the incidence and mortality rate of community-acquired pneumonia (CAP) is not very different compared to non-pregnant young adults [7]. However, the effect of pneumonia on the fetus is more pronounced. Preterm labor can develop before 34 weeks in 43% of mothers with pneumonia. This may be due to prostaglandin production or the host's inflammatory response to infection. Also, birth weights of babies born to mothers with pneumonia were significantly low, associated with preterm birth [8]. As there are studies reporting that the risk of pneumonia is lowest in the first trimester and is often between 24 and 31 weeks [9], there are also different reports declare that first trimester pneumonia with no adequate treatment, was more common (93.6% in 1462 pregnant women with pneumonia) because they were not aware of their pregnancy.

Pneumonia may also occur in the postpartum period. In this period, the most common reason for hospital admissions is infectious conditions. The most common nonobstetric causes are gall bladder infections and then pneumonia. Pneumonia is seen two times more frequently in those who give birth by cesarean section, depending on the discomfort caused by the abdominal incision and the underlying medical condition that causes cesarean section [2].

62.2 Pneumonia During Pregnancy

62.2.1 Pathophysiology and Risk Factors

The first change occur during pregnancy is on cellular immunity to protect the fetus from the mother. Especially in the second and third trimesters, lymphocyte proliferation, natural killer (NK) cells, circulating T-helper cells, and lymphocyte cytotoxic activity decrease [10, 11]. Besides hormones such as progesterone, human chorionic gonadotropin, alpha-fetoprotein, and cortisol, which are dominant during pregnancy, inhibit cell-derived immunity [12]; edema and congestion may occur in the respiratory mucosa by increased progesterone.

Anatomically, the diaphragm's elevation and the thoracic cavity deformation may cause problems for the mother to cleanse her secretions. A decrease in functional residual capacity (10–25%), an increase in oxygen demand (20%), and an increase in lung fluid can also increase the lungs' sensitivity to infections during pregnancy. Raised possibility of aspiration due to increased intra-abdominal pressure during delivery and losing the cough reflex for 4–5 h due to spinal anesthesia poses the lung infection risk in the postpartum period. Increasing the gastric pH of cesarean patients has recently decreased this risk.

Also underlying conditions, such as smoking, asthma, lung diseases, such as cystic fibrosis or HIV infection, being on immunosuppressive therapy, recent influenza infection, and placental abruption, increase the risk of pneumonia in pregnancy puerperium. Advanced gestational age is also accepted as an independent risk factor [13].

A case-control study was conducted with 358 pregnant patients; anemia and low serum albumin levels were associated with severe CAP [14]. In a national survey conducted on 1462 pregnant women, a significant relationship was found between having pneumonia and low birth weight, preterm labor, need for cesarean section, low Apgar score, typical gestational age, and preeclampsia/eclampsia [15]. In the same study, when etiological factors were examined, no difference was observed between viral and bacterial agents. It has been reported in different tasks that the use of antepartum corticosteroids given to increase lung maturity in premature babies is a risk factor for maternal pneumonia [8, 16], and it was also mentioned that the tocolytic agents used increase the risk of pneumonia by increasing pulmonary edema [16]. Hypoxia, which occurs in severe pneumonia, affects the placenta's oxygenation, causing it to secrete antiangiogenic and proinflammatory factors and increase the risk of preeclampsia/eclampsia due to endothelial dysfunction and hypertension in the mother [17].

62.2.2 Diagnosis

The diagnosis of pneumonia is difficult from the symptomatic stage, because respiratory symptoms may occur for different reasons from the beginning of pregnancy. Dyspnea is seen in 50% of women in the 19th week of pregnancy and increases to 76% at the 31st week [18]. Medical conditions such as asthma, pulmonary embolism, and amniotic fluid embolism or only uterine enlargement can cause dyspnea, but it can be differentiated from these medical conditions as it occurs from the early stages of pregnancy and rarely occurs at rest. However, cough is not a common symptom, except because of atelectasis in the lower lobes in the later stages of pregnancy, and requires investigation. Again, the disease can manifest itself with symptoms such as fever and weakness.

While the maternal radiation dose obtained with standard posterior-anterior chest radiography is 5–30 mRad, the fetus is exposed to 100 times less (300 μRad) [19]. In radiologic differential diagnosis, noncardiogenic pulmonary edema related with preeclampsia/eclampsia, pulmonary edema due to tocolytic agents, aspiration pneumonia, or rarely observed pulmonary metastasis of choriocarcinoma can be listed. If the abdomen or pelvis is not being imaged, such as in chest CT, there is no risk to the baby from radiation. The amount of radiation used in normal CT imaging has never been shown to cause harm to fetus. CT should be the initial diagnostic imaging modality for suspected pulmonary embolism. The fetal radiation dose from CT pulmonary angiography is substantially less than that from ventilation perfusion scintigraphy in all trimesters. Iodinated contrast can cross placenta, enter the fetal circulation, and pass directly into the amniotic fluid. Standard recommendation is that lactating women who receive intravascular iodinated contrast or gadolinium should discontinue breast-feeding for 24 h.

To all suspicious patients, saturation control, routine blood biochemistry, and cell count are recommended. Since blood cultures may give false-positive results, they should only be taken from seriously ill patients who have not used antibiotics before. Sputum examination and culture should be investigated if a resistant agent is suspected or there is no response to empirical therapy. Routine serological analysis is not recommended in pregnant CAP patients. However, if there is a severe CAP chart, urine *Legionella* and pneumococcal antigen may be requested, and induced sputum should be considered to isolate the etiologic agent.

62.2.3 Etiology

Data on pneumonia rates in pregnant women are limited, since they are primarily based on routine blood and sputum samples obtained from retrospective studies. Diagnostic tests are still not recommended routinely, because it may vary according to the way it is taken (sputum, blood, bronchial lavage), the use of antibiotics, serology, and antigen detection [20]. According to many case reports or case series, agents, which are difficult to detect on routine sputum analyses like *mumps, infectious mononucleosis, swine influenza, Influenza A* (including H1N11), *Staphylococcus aureus* (including methicillin-resistant forms), *Legionella, Varicella, Chlamydophila pneumoniae, coccidioidomycosis*, and other fungal agents, may cause CAP during pregnancy [21–23]. Chen et al. [15] has been reported that the pneumonia complications do not differ in viral and bacterial infections. However, it is known that conditions due to some agents have a more severe course, primarily due to changes in pregnant patients' cellular immunity (Table 62.1).

Chickenpox can be seen in 1 out of 10,000 births during pregnancy and can cause both mother and fetus complications. Pneumonia risk may increase up to 9% [25].

Influenza A is another agent that can cause an epidemic in pregnant women and progress with high mortality. While the maternal mortality rate increased up to 50% in the pandemics in 1918 and 1957, with the H1N1 epidemic that emerged most

Table 62.1 Etiological agents (Adopted from [24])

Bacteriological analysis of pregnant women with pneumonia (in the order of frequency)
1. *Streptococcus pneumoniae* (including drug-resistant streptococcus pneumonia)
2. *Hemophilus influenzae*
3. No pathogens identified
4. Atypical pneumonia agents: • *Legionella* species (especially in severe pneumonia)   • *Mycoplasma pneumoniae*   • *Chlamydophila pneumoniae*
5. Viral agents   • Influenza A   • Varicella
6. *Staphylococcus aureus* (also methicillin-resistant strains)
7. *Pseudomonas* aeruginosa (bronchiectasis, cystic fibrosis)
8. Aspiration
9. Fungi   • Coccidioidomycosis
10. *Pneumocystis jiroveci* (HIV infection)

recently in 2009, complications that increase morbidity and mortality in pregnant women and seriously affect both mother and fetus have emerged. Mortality developed significantly in the third trimester; premature birth, the urgent need for cesarean section, fetal distress, fetal deaths were occurred.

Another virus with a severe course during pregnancy was the coronavirus that caused severe acute respiratory syndrome (SARS). In a series of 12 patients examined, half of the patients needed intensive care, 1/3 of them required a mechanical ventilator, 7 of them were infected in the first trimester, complications such as spontaneous abortion, low gestational age, and preterm delivery have been observed, and maternal mortality was determined as 25% [26].

Antibiotic resistance can be observed in 40% of *S pneumoniae* infections. It has been reported that there is resistance against it especially if there is an antibiotic usage in the last 3 months [27]. Although infections caused by community-acquired strains of methicillin-resistant *S. aureus* (MRSA) usually occur in the skin and soft tissue, it has been reported that they may rarely cause bilateral necrotizing pneumonia, especially after influenza infections [28].

Again due to aspiration of oropharyngeal fluid or gastric content during delivery, primarily anaerobic or Gram-negative agents may cause infection in pneumonia.

62.2.4 Clinical Course

Symptoms of pregnant pneumonia patients are not different from those of nonpregnant adults. Dyspnea, cough, fever, sputum, pleuritic chest pain, nausea, and vomiting can be observed, but the important thing is recognizing the severe disease.

Pneumonia severity index (PSI) is used in adults to predict the severity of the disease, to foresee about hospital or intensive care admission by using the patient's age, underlying systemic disease, laboratory and clinical findings, but pregnant women were not included in this evaluation. When Shariatzadeh and Marrie [29] applied this index to same aged patients and pregnant women, they found that all pregnant patients were included in the low-risk group, but they needed two times more hospitalization than the control group. Again in a study of Yoast et al. [9], when evaluated according to PSI in pregnant women, 2/3 of the patients should be transferred to home, but with such an approach, 10 out of 79 patients can apply complications that require readmission to the hospital. Therefore, it should be kept in mind that PSI may be insufficient in evaluating the patient's severity in pregnant patients who come with CAP. While deciding on intensive care admission, it should not be ignored that this group of patients was more prone to hypoxia and especially in cases of infection such as varicella-zoster intensive care follow-up may be required because of progressive disease. During the H1N1 epidemic, it was reported that pregnant patients had four times more hospitalizations and intensive care hospitalizations than the average population. The risk of death was higher than seasonal flu [30, 31].

62.2.5 Bacterial Pneumonia

Development of pneumonia in pregnant women provides susceptibility to conditions such as preterm labor, preterm labor, and pulmonary edema. Pregnancy-related physiological changes make the patient more susceptible to hypoxia and tachypnea (respiratory alkalosis resulting from decreasing uterine blood flow). Keeping the maternal saturation > 95% and PO2 > 70 is essential for the placenta's fetal face.

In the treatment of mild symptomatic community-acquired pneumonia in pregnant women, azithromycin is recommended in addition to amoxicillin or amoxicillin/clavulanate. Clindamycin can be used in the patient group with B-lactam allergy. In cases requiring hospitalization but without a severe course, anti-pneumococcal beta-lactam (ceftriaxone, cefotaxime, ampicillin-sulbactam) in addition to azithromycin (in countries with known macrolide resistance >25%) should be preferred. Clindamycin-azithromycin combination can be used in patients with cephalosporin allergy. However, the combination of vancomycin (for MRSA and *S. pneumonia*), azithromycin, aztreonam is recommended in patients with severe pneumonia with this allergy. Fluoroquinolones (risk of fetal arthropathy and malformation), clarithromycin (increased risk of miscarriage, preliminary human study), tetracycline are drugs that should not be used in pregnancy. In cases where tetracycline must be used (e.g., Rocky-mountain fever), doxycycline is considered a more suitable choice, although there is not enough data [32].

62.2.6 Viral Pneumonia

62.2.6.1 Influenza Virus

Influenza A group is the most common type of infection in humans from the influenza virus family, which has three different antigen types. Neuzil et al. [33] have reported that pregnant women are affected by influenza more than nonpregnant women and especially in pregnancies with underground asthma and advanced age, acute cardiopulmonary disease in the third trimester that requires hospitalization has been reported more frequently. Mertz et al. agree that pregnant women are more affected from influenza pneumonia than the general population or fertile women [34]; but contrary to many studies, they declare that pregnant women are not more likely to have a severe course of death. They thought that results in previous studies were related to selecting the patient group, who had a more severe disease because of having some risk factors and who were admitted to the hospital. It has also been reported that epidemic influenza infections have a more severe course than sporadic ones [35].

In the update [36] made by WHO in 2012, priority was given to a group, pregnant women, for vaccination for the first time. The reasons for this decision are studies, which are reporting a high risk of influenza in pregnant women, the possibility of protecting infants with placental antibody passage, and safety and efficiency of vaccine.

While maternal mortality was high in influenza outbreaks in the early 1900s, this increase stopped in 1958. However, this situation has changed with the H1N1 epidemic that occurred in 2009–2010. According to the US Centers for Disease Control (CDC) report [37], death occurred in 5% of 509 pregnant women hospitalized. Starting antiviral therapy 4 days later than the symptom onset increased the risk of entering the intensive care unit, and a worse prognosis was observed. The most common comorbidity in this group is obesity and asthma, and it has been stated that the risk of death is higher in 2nd- and third-trimester pregnant women.

Symptoms are not different in pregnant patients; there is an incubation period of 1–4 days. It may occur with fever, myalgia, cough, headache, and appetite loss. Bacterial or viral agent pneumonia should be considered, especially if symptoms last more than 5 days in this group of patients. If bacterial superinfection is suspected, empirical antibacterial therapy for *S. aureus* strains, including *H influenza, pneumococcus, MRSA*, and antiviral treatment, should be initiated from the first stage disease. The CDC recommends that antiviral treatment be taken as soon as symptoms begin in pregnant patients. Agents such as amantadine and rimantadine provide a decrease in symptoms when given for the first 48 h. Still, they are only effective for Influenza A. Oseltamivir and Zanamivir effectively influence Influenza A and B. It can be used both for prevention in risky pregnancies and for treatment in complicated cases.

Although there are many publications about Oseltamivir and Amantadine's teratogenicity, a final result has not been obtained. Because despite these doubts, much better results have been obtained with the use of these drugs singly or in combination in the first 2 days since 2009 [37]. Oseltamivir was detected at a rate of 1% of the serum level in breast milk. Zanamivir did not affect lactation in mice. Although prophylactic treatment of antivirals can be started after contact with virus, the primary method of protection is vaccination. It is recommended that every woman who is pregnant during the influenza season should be vaccinated. The same approach applies to the H1N1 vaccine. The inactivated vaccine is used for this group. While vaccination can be done in any pregnancy period, there are opinions that it should be avoided in the first trimester if possible [38].

62.2.6.2 Varicella

Varicella infestation is more common in the pregnant group than nonpregnant patients, and it has a severe and complicated course. Varicella vaccine is contraindicated in pregnant women as it is a live vaccine. Although pneumonia is the most severe complication, congenital disabilities can also be observed. Studies are reporting 35–40% mortality in pregnant patients [21, 25]. A study in which 46 patients, who were followed up for varicella pneumonia in Spain and two, were pregnant was evaluated; it was reported that 24% needed intensive care, but no deaths occurred [39]. All patients with varicella pneumonia require hospitalization; mortality is 25% in the group that needs mechanical ventilation.

Varicella-zoster causes self-limiting and mild varicella disease in children, while 10% of adults have a primary infection risk. While this risk is 4–6.8% in pregnant women, infection occurs at a rate of 70% after close and intensive contact [40].

Pregnancy is a risk factor in terms of complication of primary infection with pneumonia [41]. T-cell function abnormalities during pregnancy and increased corticosteroid levels in the circulation increase virulence. The difficulty of pneumonia and a more severe course are frequently observed in pregnant women with last trimester disease.

The virus has an incubation period of 10 days to 3 weeks. The virus enters the circulation 24–48 h before the onset of the mother's rash, and 24% of the fetus becomes transplacentally infected during this period. This situation results in 1.2% congenital malformation [42].

Pneumonia complaints such as fever, rash, and malaise occur 2–5 days after the onset. Cough, chest pain, shortness of breath, sometimes hemoptysis, and oral mucosal ulcers can be seen. While pneumonia can be asymptomatic, it can also progress to respiratory failure [43]. Radiologically; if it does not progress to acute lung damage or respiratory loss within 14 days, lesions in the form of interstitial, diffuse, or nodular infiltrates can be observed [42]. The more skin lesions, the more widespread infiltration is expected. Varicella pneumonia may cause sequelae as diffuse pulmonary calcification in the late period [44].

Varicella, which has an intrauterine effect of 10–20% on the fetus, classically occurs in 3 patterns. The first is "varicella embryopathy" caused by maternal disease before 20 weeks; the second is "congenital varicella" that develops between 20 weeks and birth. And finally, "neonatal varicella" arising from active lesions present at birth [45]. Varicella embryopathy can be seen until the 26th week; it can progress with skin scars, central nervous system involvement, skeletal lesions, and extremity hypoplasia. The most extensive series defined for congenital varicella is a 13-year study in which 1373 varicella-infected pregnant women were examined [45]. The infection was passed on from the mother to the fetus, when the innocent fetus was 13–20-week old, causing fetal anomaly. This anomaly can range from superficial skin lesions to severe multiorgan failure. Therefore, it has been stated that although the use of prophylactic immunoglobulin does not reduce the incidence of embryopathy to pregnant women who have not had varicella infection or immunization before, it may minimize fetal disease if the mother is given before infected [45]. The aim of giving immun prophylaxis to a seronegative pregnant woman after contact is to protect the mother from the disease, not the fetus. Gaymard et al. [46] recommended performing serology control and using immunoglobulin or valaciclovir in case of seronegativity, for a pregnant woman who comes into contact with a suspected case, or regardless of virology especially in the first trimester, starting valaciclovir after contact with the definitive case.

Acyclovir, a DNA polymerase inhibitor, should be initiated in all patients. No increase was observed in the number and pattern of postpartum defects in pregnant women exposed to this drug [47–49]. However, there is no evidence that it changes the course of the disease. Haake et al. [25] reported that the treatment initiated within the first 36 h after the contact decreased the hospital period, decreased the average fever, increased oxygenation, and less respiratory distress developed. The recommended dose is 7.5 mg/kg (3–18 mg/kg) every 8 h. It was mentioned in some small series that low-dose steroids could be added to the treatment [21].

62.2.6.3   Coronavirus Infections

Coronaviruses are pathogens classified in the Coronavirida family, primarily targeting the human respiratory system [50]. The coronavirus outbreaks so far: Severe Acute Respiratory Syndrome (SARS–CoV) [51] in 2003, Middle East Respiratory Syndrome (MERS–CoV) [52] in 2012, and SARS-CoV-2 (COVID-19) [53]. These started as a respiratory tract infection and led to severe respiratory failure, severe pneumonia, and death, which are common to all of them. These effects in the pregnant population increase obstetric and neonatal adverse risks and cause severe respiratory disease [54].

As a result of physiological changes in pregnant women, it has been shown that SARS-CoV and MERS-CoV infections have a more complicated course in pregnant women [55].

COVID-19 and other corona infections are often observed before 37 weeks. Complications such as preeclampsia, preterm labor, premature rupture of membranes, fetal growth retardation, and miscarriage may develop. Many CoV-infected pregnant women require intensive care follow-up, severe respiratory failure, and death [56]. The most common cause of such cases is MERS-CoV. Cesarean section is needed in three-quarters of pregnant women. Fetal distress and neonatal asphyxia are the most common complications in newborns.

Common symptoms in all pregnant women infected with coronavirus: fever, weakness, cough, and myalgia [57]. The high postpartum fever may occur because of burnout-related immunity decrease, blood loss, genital anatomic change, sweating during delivery, and postpartum lactation. However, once fever develops, the clinician should not ignore mastitis, urinary tract infection, cold, and reproductive system infection. Gastrointestinal system complaints such as diarrhea and abdominal pain can be seen in all Coronavirus infections. More than half of the pregnant patients can be treated with antivirals and antibiotics. Gestational diabetes (9.6%) and hypertension (8.5%) are the most common diseases seen together [56]. Laboratory findings such as leukocytopenia and lymphocytopenia can be used to differentiate from bacterial infections. Liu et al. [58] drew attention because leukocytosis, lymphopenia, neutrophil dominance, and normal initial average body temperature are more prominent in COVID-19-positive pregnant women than nonpregnant female patients.

The most common CT findings in pregnant patients with COVID-19 and non-COVID-19 pneumonia are ground glass (57.9%) and bilateral involvement (65.8%) [56] (Figs. 62.1 and 62.2). However, the ground-glass appearance is detected less frequently than in nonpregnant patients [58] due to cell infiltration and interstitial thickening, cell exudation, and hyaline membrane formation. The most commonly used agents in the treatment of antiviral and bacterial superinfections are hydroxychloroquine (79.7%), ribavirin (65.2%), oseltamivir (56.5%), azithromycin (35%), and oxygen therapy.

There is no exact data on the intrauterine transmission of SARS-CoV-2, MERS-CoV, and SARS-CoV. There was no PCR positivity investigated in amniotic fluid, vaginal fluid during delivery, cord blood, umbilical core, fetal membrane, placenta, and neonatal nasopharyngeal/throat swabs [59–61]. The reason for this may be a

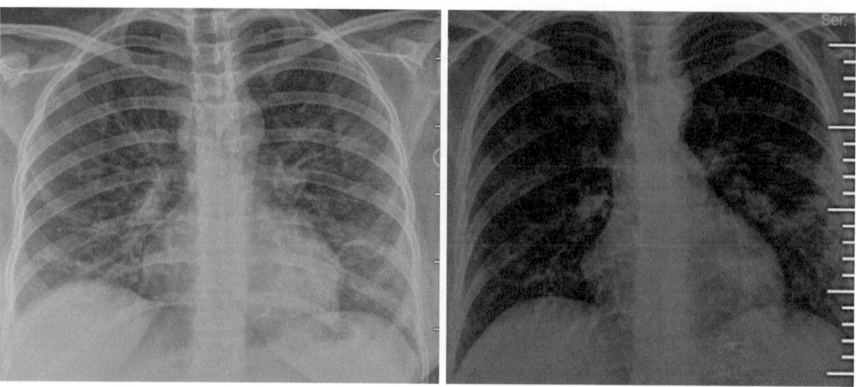

Fig. 62.1 Posterior anterior lung X-ray of two pregnant women infected with COVID-19

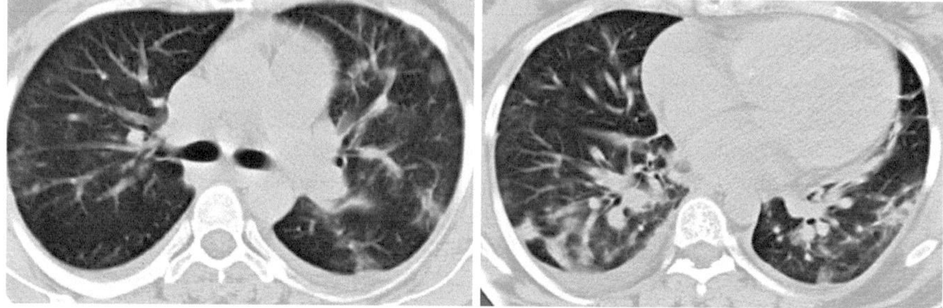

Fig. 62.2 Computed tomography images of a pregnant woman infected with COVID-19; ground glass opacities, pleural effusion, consolidation, interseptal thickening

deficient expression of angio converting enzyme 2 (ACE2) in maternal-fetal interface cells [62]. Adequate protection and isolation measures should be taken during and after birth to prevent transmission to the baby.

In a study examining pregnant women infected with _SARS-CoV_, it was stated that babies born from infected mothers were PCR negative, spontaneous abortion was observed in 3 of 7 pregnant women who were infected in the first trimester, and 4 of 5 pregnant women who were infected after 24 weeks had preterm delivery and intrauterine growth retardation despite recovery before birth [26]. Stockman et al. reported that in a patient who was positive for SARS-CoV antibody at the time of delivery, cord blood and placenta were seronegative and also antibodies were negative in breast milk at postpartum 12–30 days [63]. Studies are expressing that the combination of lopinavir/ritonavir and ribavirin may be effective in treatment [64].

Infection with _MERS-CoV_ may show a clinical course ranging from an asymptomatic chart to multiple organ failure, septic shock, and death. Mortality has been reported as approximately 36% for MERS and about 10% for SARS [65]. In a study examining pregnant women infected with MERS-CoV [66], five pregnant women were admitted to intensive care, one patient had a 34-week preterm delivery, and one infant died 4 h after birth. However, a MERS-CoV-positive patient who was admitted with acute vaginal bleeding and the absence of virus on the baby has been an example that the disease can be passed on without contamination [67]. Studies suggest the combination of interferon + ribavirin + LPV/r in the treatment of MERS [68].

Liu et al. [58] reported that some of the 15 pregnant women infected with *COVID-19* recovered despite not receiving antiviral treatment, and there was no postpartum progression in tomography images and symptoms. No difference was observed between COVID-19-positive and COVID-19-negative pregnant women regarding birth weight, fetal distress, neonatal asphyxia, and preterm labor [69]. Besides Zhu et al. [70] reported that six of ten fetuses born from COVID-19-positive mothers had Pediatric Critical Illness Score (PCIS) index below 90, and perinatal infection might be associated with preterm labor liver dysfunction, thrombocytopenia, fetal-respiratory distress, and death. According to WHO's guide on March 13, 2020, there is no specific treatment recommended for COVID-19-positive pregnant women. Data are showing that chloroquine and remdesevir inhibit the replication of SARS-CoV-2 in cell cultures [71]. However, reports have been made regarding the adverse effect of chloroquine on fetal development. Therefore, Zhou et al. stated that hydroxychloroquine is a safer option in pregnant women [72].

62.2.7 Fungal Pneumonia

Factors such as *Cryptococcus neoformans, Histoplasma capsulatum, Sporothrix schenkii, Blastomyces dermatitidis*, and *Coccidioides immitis* may rarely cause pneumonia during pregnancy [73]. In the pregnancies of healthy women, these infections are usually overcome without treatment. However, they may progress as disseminated diseases, especially in the third trimester and pregnant women with HIV infection [74].

Coccidioidomycosis (CM) is a fungal infection that can be seen endemically in some parts of America and Africa and can be complicated, especially in pregnant women. Flu-like symptoms can occur in different clinics, such as weight loss, erythema nodosum, or pneumonia. The last trimester of pregnancy is a risky period, especially for disseminated disease. Lung involvement may be in the form of pleural effusion, military infiltration, or cavity. The presence of erythema nodosum may be a sign that the disease will be mild [74]. In disseminating illness or pneumonia, treatment with intravenous *Amphotericin-B* is recommended, and oral *Fluconazole* maintenance is recommended in the postpartum period [74]. While in nonmeningeal infections, first-trimester Ampho-B, second-third trimester itraconazole/fluconazole (400 mg/day) is recommended, in meningeal infections, Ampho-B intrathecal is recommended in first-trimester [75].

Other fungal infections are rarely seen during pregnancy, so the effect of pregnancy on these infections or the presence of infection on pregnancy is not apparent [76]. IDSA does not have a specific treatment recommendation for Aspergillosis in pregnant women. The recommended treatment for Cryptococcus, Histoplasmosis, Blastomyces, Sporotrichosis (cold application is recommended for skin lesions), and invasive Candidiasis in all trimesters is Ampho-B [75].

Fluconazole dose more than 300 mg is accepted to be teratogenic and contraindicated during pregnancy by the FDA; however, a single dose of 300 mg in the absence of a topical agent after the first trimester was considered not to increase the risk of congenital disorders. Voriconazole has been recognized in category D by the FDA for its embryotoxic/teratogenic effects in animal experiments. Unless there is a disease threatening the mother's life, its use in pregnancy is not recommended. On the other hand, Amphotericin B was accepted as category B by the FDA, and it was stated that it was the safest antifungal to be used in pregnancy [77].

62.2.8 Pneumonia in HIV Patients

Pregnancy theoretically increases HIV-related immunosuppression, leading to increased respiratory tract infections and maternal and fetal mortalities [78]. Besides the vertical transition is an important problem for the newborn. Antiretroviral therapy decreases the risk of disease by increasing the CD4 + cell count. Although early initiation of this treatment and reducing the last trimester viral load reduces the risk of vertical transmission, the long-term effects of use from the first trimester are still unclear. While *Efavirenz* is not recommended in the first trimester due to its impact on gestation, *Reltagravir* can be used in exceptional cases during pregnancy. Among the protease inhibitors, *Lopinavir* and *Ritonavir* are the most commonly used agents [79].

Bacterial respiratory infections are the most common respiratory complication in HIV patients due to the low CD4 cell count. Especially *Pneumocystis jiroveci (PCP)* is a severe source of infection for both mother and fetus. In a study examining 22 pregnant women who were PCP positive during pregnancy, in 59% of patients needing a mechanical ventilator, 50% of maternal deaths, five intrauterine, and four neonatal deaths were reported [80]. Women infected with PCP should receive *trimethoprim-sulfa (TMP-SMX)* treatment, and steroids should be added to the treatment when oxygen is needed. These patients should be followed up in terms of preterm labor; babies of pregnant women who have received TMP-SMX should be monitored for hyperbilirubinemia and kernicterus. In terms of PCP prophylaxis, when the CD4 cell count of HIV + pregnant women fall below 200, TMP-SMX should be started, but aerosol *Pentamidine* without systemic absorption should be preferred, since it may have teratogenic effects in the first trimester [3].

62.3 Future Directions for CAP in Pregnancies

Lung ultrasound could be a safe and repeatable imaging tool avoiding X-ray exposure to detect respiratory diseases in pregnancy. Ultrasound can be performed directly at the bedside by a single operator. Although CT represents the gold standard to assess lung involvement in patients with suspected COVID-19, there is a need for rapid assessment of the maternal lung. Chinese Critical Care Ultrasound Study Group and Italian Academy of Thoracic Ultrasound suggested lung ultrasound as an accurate tool to detect lung involvement in COVID-19 [81]. According to these suggestions, characteristic findings are (1) thickening of the pleural line with pleural line irregularity, (2) B lines in a variety of patterns including focal, multifocal, and confluent, (3) consolidations in a variety of patterns including multifocal small, non-translobar, and translobar with occasional mobile air bronchograms, (4) appearance of A lines during recovery phase, and (5) pleural effusions are uncommon [82].

62.4 Postpartum Pneumonia

The loss of the placenta, which is the center of the immune changes in postpartum pregnancy, creates a new immunophysiological situation. Having a normal immunity can take up to 1 year after birth [83]. The cytotoxicity effect of NK cells, which are in a suppressed state during pregnancy, returns to normal after 6 months [84].

The study by Maureen et al. in which they examined the immunity changes in the postpartum period reported that cellular immunity stimulated with IFNγ and IL-2 may be low until the postpartum third month, TNF-α may also show a similar pattern, and that CRP and IL-6 may be elevated in the early postpartum period [85].

The cellular immune response, which is in a suppressed state during pregnancy, can emerge as the clinical manifestation of latent infections called "immune reconstitution inflammatory syndrome" in the puerperal period and may progress to ARDS [86]. It has been frequently observed in HIV-positive patients after the initiation of antiretroviral therapy, and it was stated that it could progress fatally if left without treatment [87]. Treatment benefits from steroids.

Despite many advances in diagnosis, medical management, and antimicrobial therapy, sepsis is one of the most important maternal mortality causes in the puerperal period. Community-acquired pneumonia is also among the causes of sepsis. There is no significant difference in etiology than the nonpregnant population (*Streptococcus pneumoniae, Hemophilus influenzae, Mycoplasma pneumoniae, Legionella, Chlamydia pneumoniae*). Pregnant or postpartum (2 weeks postpartum) infected women with influenza are at risk for bacterial pneumonia [88].

Besides aspiration of gastric contents due to increased intra-abdominal pressure during delivery and loosening of the gastroesophageal junction, insufficient hunger in emergency cesarean section may lead to a chemical pneumonia picture. Aspiration pneumonia findings are not different from classical pneumonia. Radiologically the presence of multifocal infiltration in the lung's dependent areas, expectoration of the stomach contents by coughing, rales in the physical examination, and low fever are findings in favor of aspiration. Two phases occur depending on the amount, pH, and particle size of the aspirated content. While acute bronchospasm and intense cough are observed in the first phase, inflammation, increased capillary permeability, atelectasis due to surfactant loss, pulmonary infiltrate, and hypoxemia can be observed in the second phase after 6–12 h. The diagnosis is made when no other reason to explain these clinical findings can be found and anamnesis. Some cases may progress to lung abscess [89] or ARDS [90] (Tables 62.2, 62.3 and 62.4).

Table 62.2 Pregnancy and postpartum period community-acquired pneumonia diagnostic protocols

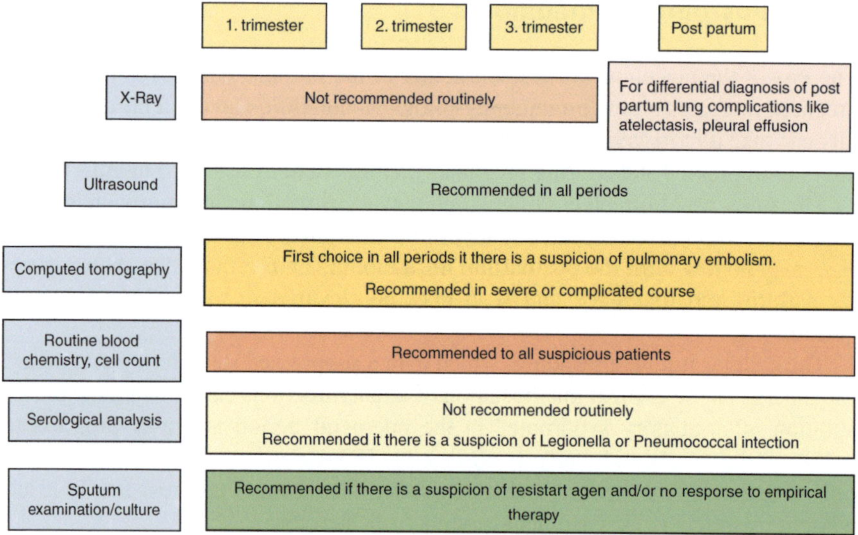

Table 62.3 Pregnancy period CAP diagnostic and treatment protocols

Pregnant women with CAP symptoms

↓

Physical examination, anamnesis, contact inquiry

↓

Routine blood chemistry, cell count

↓

X-ray(?), Ultrasonography (if avaible), Computed tomography (severe and complicated course)

→ Suspicion of complicated or severe course of CAP

↓

Serological analyses or sputum examination/culture

<u>Empirical treatment</u>

Bacterial pneumonia → *Amoxicillin or amoxicillin/clavulanate +/- azithromycin*

OR

Clindamycin (β-lactam allergy) +/- azithromycin

<u>Severe course or complicated bacterial pneumonia</u>

Anti pseudomonal β-lactam + azithromycin

OR in case of β-lactam allergy

Vancomycin + Azithromycin + Aztreonam

Influenza → *Amantadine* (Influenza A)

Oseltamivir/ Zanamivir (Influenza A/B, complicated course)

*Vaccinations during influenza season

Varicella → *Immunprophylaxis* (seronegative pregnant woman after contact)

→ *Valaciclovir* (seronegative pregnant woman after contact with a suspected case)

→ *Acyclovir* (in 36 hours after contact)

SARS → *Lopinavir Rizonavir (LPV/r)* OR *Ribavirin*

MERS-CoV → *Interferon + Ribavirin + LPV/r*

COVID 19 → *Remdesevir* OR *Hydroxychloroquine* (no specific treatment according WHO)

Fungal infectios → *Amphotericin B*

Flucanozole (maintenance therapy)

PCP (HIV+ patients) → *TMP-SMX*

Table 62.4 Pregnancy and postpartum period CAP treatment agents

Drug classification	Pregnancy usage safety	Suggestions
Antibacterial agents		
• Penicillins	• Category B	• Safe to take while breastfeeding
• Cephalosporins	• Category B	• Safe to take while breastfeeding
• Macrolides	• Category B	• Azithromicin and Aztreonam as combination treatment in severe patient. Exposure to macrolides via breastmilk may be associated with pyloric stenosis. Clarithromycin is safer because of low levels in breastmilk
• Quinolons	• Category C	
• Tetracyclines	• Category D	• Arthralgia and tendonitis reported in adults but none in human pregnancy. Ciprofloxacin level is low in breastmilk
• Clindamycin	• Category B	• Avoid, especially at or after 12 weeks, because of skin lesions on the fetus. Doxycycline may be preferable. Short-term use is acceptable in nursing mothers
		• In case of β-lactam allergy. Has the potential to cause adverse effects on the breastfed infant's gastrointestinal flora
Antiviral agents		
• Acyclovir	• Category B	• 7.5 mg/kg 3 times a day, reliable during both pregnancy and lactation
• Oseltamivir	• Category C	• %1 passes to breastmilk, for patients with definite diagnosis of influenza A/B and COVID-19, 2 × 75 mg/ day
• Favipiravir	• Category D	
• Lopinavir (200 mg)- ritonavir(50 mg)	• Category C • Category D	• In case of severe COVID-19 pneumonia, 2 × 1600 mg first day, 2 × 600 mg maintenance, total 5 days. No report about breastmilk
• Ribavirin	• Category C • Category C	• 2 × 2 po, 10–14 days, does not increase congenital malformation risk, may increase preterm delivery. Appears in breastmilk and serum of breastmilk infants
• Amantadine		• No reports of congenital malformations until this time. Breastmilk level is lower than doses received by infants treated for RSV
• Zanamavir		• Possible association with cleft palate. No report about breastmilk
		• May be preferable instead of amantadine. No report about breastmilk
Antifungal agents		
• Amphoterecin B	• Category B	• For all trimesters, intrathecal recommended for meningeal infections of first trimester. Acceptable to use in nursing women
• Topical nystatin	• Category A	• 150 mg/day, category D for 400–600 mg/day dosage, can be used for maintenance therapy of Amfo-B in postpartum period
• Ketoconazole	• Category C	
• Fluconazole	• Category C	
• Itraconazole	• Category C	• No report about breastmilk
• Voriconazole	• Category D	• Excreted in breast milk, should not be used by nursing women
• Terbinafin	• Category B	
• Caspofungin	• Category C	• No report about breastmilk

References

1. Kaunitz AM, Hughes JM, Grimes DA, et al. Causes of maternal mortality in the United States. Obstet Gynecol. 1985;65(5):605–12.
2. Belfort MA, Clark SL, Saade GR, et al. Hospital readmission after delivery: evidence for an increased incidence of nonurogenital infection in the immediate postpartum period. Am J Obstet Gynecol. 2010;202(1):35.e1–7.
3. Brito V, Niederman MS. Pneumonia complicating pregnancy. Clin Chest Med. 2011;32(1):121–32, ix
4. Frye D, Clark SL, Piacenza D, Shay-Zapien G. Pulmonary complications in pregnancy: considerations for care. J Perinat Neonatal Nurs. 2011;25:235–44.
5. Sheffield JS, Cunningham FG. Community-acquired pneumonia in pregnancy. Obstet Gynecol. 2009;114:915–22.
6. Chen YH, Keller J, Wang IT, Lin CC, Lin HC. Pneumonia and pregnancy outcomes: a nationwide population-based study. Am J Obstet Gynecol. 2012;207(288):e1–7.
7. Lim WS, Macfarlane JT, Colthorpe CL. Pneumonia and pregnancy. Thorax. 2001;56:398–405.
8. Munn MB, Groome LJ, Atterbury JL, et al. Pneumonia as a complication of pregnancy. J Matern Fetal Med. 1999;8:151–4.
9. Yost NP, Bloom SL, Richey SD, et al. An appraisal of treatment guidelines for antepartum community-acquired pneumonia. Am J Obstet Gynecol. 2000;183:131–5.
10. Baley JE, Schacter BZ. Mechanisms of diminished natural killer cell activity in pregnant women and neonates. J Immunol. 1985;134:3042–8.
11. Sidama V, Pacini F, Yang SL, et al. Decreased levels of helper T cells: a possible cause of immunodeficiency in pregnancy. N Engl J Med. 1982;307:352–6.
12. Lederman MM. Cell-mediated immunity and pregnancy. Chest. 1984;86:6–9S.
13. Graves CR. Pneumonia in pregnancy. Clin Obstet Gynecol. 2010;53:329–36.
14. He Y, Li M, Mai C, Chen L, Zhang X, Zhou J. Anemia and low albumin levels are associated with severe community-acquired pneumonia in pregnancy: a case-control study Tohoku. J Exp Med. 2019;248:297–305.
15. Chen Y-H, Keller J, Wang I-T, et al. Pneumonia and pregnancy outcomes: a nationwide population-based study. Am J Obstet Gynecol. 2012;207(288):e1–7.
16. Rotmensch S, Vishnu TH, Celentano C, et al. Maternal infectious morbidity following multiple courses of betamethasone. J Infect. 1999;39:49–54.
17. Sava RI, March KL, Pepine CJ. Hypertension in pregnancy: taking cues from pathophysiology for clinical practice. Clin Cardiol. 2018;41:220–7.
18. Milne JA, Howie AD, Pack AI. Dyspnoea during normal pregnancy. Br J Obstet Gynaecol. 1978;85:260–3.
19. Diethelm L, Xu H. Diagnostic imaging of the lung during pregnancy. Clin Obstet Gynecol. 1996;39:36–55.
20. Mandell LA, Wunderink RG, Anzueto A, et al. Infectious diseases society of America/American thoracic society consensus guidelines on the management of community-acquired pneumonia in adults. Clin Infect Dis. 2007;44:S27–72.
21. Goodnight WH, Soper DE. Pneumonia in pregnancy. Crit Care Med. 2005;33:S390–7.
22. Catanzaro A. Pulmonary mycosis in pregnant women. Chest. 1984;86:14S–9S.
23. Stein SJ, Greenspoon JS. Rubeola during pregnancy. Obstet Gynecol. 1991;78:925–9.
24. Khan S, Niederman MS. Pneumonia in the pregnant patient. Pulmonary problems in pregnancy. New York (NY): Humana Press; 2009. p. 177–96.
25. Haake DA, Zakowski PC, Haake DL, et al. Early treatment with acyclovir for varicella pneumonia in otherwise healthy adults: retrospective controlled study and review. Rev Infect Dis. 1990;12:788–98.
26. Wong SF, Chow KM, Leung TN, et al. pregnancy and perinatal outcomes of women with SARS. Am J Obstet Gynecol 2004;191:292-297.

27. Vanderkooi OG, Low DE, Green K, et al. Predicting antimicrobial resistance in invasive pneumococcal infections. Clin Infect Dis. 2005;40:1288–97.
28. Micek ST, Dunne M, Kollef MH. Pleuropulmonary complications of Panton-valentine leukocidin-positive community-acquired methicillin-resistant Staphylococcus aureus: importance of treatment with antimicrobials inhibiting exotoxin production. Chest. 2005;128:2732–8.
29. Shariatzadeh MR, Marrie TJ. Pneumonia during pregnancy. Am J Med. 2006;119:872–6.
30. Louie JK, Acosta M, Jamieson DJ, et al. Severe 2009 H1N1 influenza in pregnant and postpartum women in California. N Engl J Med. 2010;362:27–35.
31. Callaghan WM, Chu SY, Jamieson DJ. Deaths from seasonal influenza among pregnant women in the pneumonia complicating pregnancy 131 United States, 1998–2005. Obstet Gynecol. 2010;115:919–23.
32. Larson L, File TM Jr. Treatment of respiratory infections in pregnant women. 2020.
33. Neuzil KM, Reed GW, Mitchel EF, et al. Impact of influenza on acute cardiopulmonary hospitalizations in pregnant women. Am J Epidemiol. 1998;148:1094–102.
34. Mertz D, et al. Pregnancy as a risk factor for severe outcomes from influenza virus infection: a systematic review and meta-analysis of observational studies. Vaccine. 2017;35:521–8.
35. Laibl VR, Sheffield JS. Influenza and pneumonia in pregnancy. Clin Perinatol. 2005;32:727–38.
36. World Health Organization. Vaccines against influenza. WHO position paper – November 2012; 2012. Accessed 11 Jan 2016.
37. Siston AM, Rasmussen SA, Honein MA, et al. Pandemic 2009 influenza A(H1N1) virus illness among pregnant women in the United States. JAMA. 2010;303:1517–25.
38. Harper SA, Fukuda K, Uyeki TM, et al. Prevention and control of influenza. Recommendations of the advisory committee on immunization practices. MMWR Recomm Rep. 2004;53:1–40.
39. China E, Ballester I, Betlloch I, et al. Varicella-zoster virus pneumonia in an adult population: has mortality decreased? Scand J Infect Dis. 2010;42:215–21.
40. Sauerbrei A, Sonntag S, Wutzler P. Prevalence of varicella zoster in pregnant patients. Zentralbl Gynakol. 1990;112:223–6.
41. Ellis M, Neal K, Webb A. Is smoking a risk factor for pneumonia in adults with chickenpox? BMJ. 1986;294:1002.
42. Cox SM, Cunningham FG, Luby J. Management of varicella pneumonia complicating pregnancy. Am J Perinatol. 1990;7:300–1.
43. Harris RE, Rhoades ER. Varicella pneumonia complicating pregnancy: report of a case and review of the literature. Obstet Gynecol. 1965;25:734–40.
44. Eder SE, Apuzzio JJ, Weiss G. Varicella pneumonia during pregnancy: treatment of two cases with acyclovir. Am J Perinatol. 1988;5:16–8.
45. Katz VL, Kuller JA, McMahon MJ, et al. Varicella during pregnancy: maternal and fetal effects. West J Med. 1995;163:446–50.
46. Gaymard A, Maxime Pichon M, Bal A, Massoud M, Buenerd A, Massardier J. How to manage chickenpox during pregnancy: case reports. Ann Biol Clin (Paris). 2018;76(6):669–74. https://doi.org/10.1684/ABC.2018.1385.
47. Centers for Disease Control. Pregnancy outcomes following systemic prenatal acyclovir exposure- June 1, 1984–June 30, 1993. MMWR. 1993;42:806–9.
48. Andrews EB, Yankasas BC, Cordero JF, et al. Acyclovir in pregnancy registry: six years experience. Obstet Gynecol. 1992;79:7–13.
49. Stone KM, Reiff-Eldridge R, White AD, et al. Pregnancy outcomes following systemic prenatal acyclovir exposure: Conclusions from the international acyclovir pregnancy registry, 1984–1999. Birth Defects Res A Clin Mol Teratol. 2004;70:201–7.
50. Poon LC, Yang H, Lee JC, Copel JA, Leung TY, Zhang Y, et al. ISUOG InterimGuidance on 2019 novel coronavirus infection during pregnancy and puerperium: information for healthcare professionals. Ultrasound Obstet Gynecol. 2020;55(6):848–62. https://doi.org/10.1002/uog.22013.

51. Lau SK, Woo PC, Li KS, Huang Y, Tsoi H-W, Wong BH, et al. Severe acute respiratory syndrome coronavirus-like virus in Chinese horseshoe bats. Proc Natl Acad Sci. 2005;102(39):14040–5.
52. Zaki AM, Van Boheemen S, Bestebroer TM, Osterhaus AD, Fouchier RA. Isolation of a novel coronavirus from a man with pneumonia in Saudi Arabia. N Engl J Med. 2012;367(19):1814–20.
53. Organization WH. WHO director-general's opening remarks at the media briefing on covid-19–11 March 2020.
54. Perlman S. Another decade, another coronavirus. Mass Medical Soc. 2020;
55. Schwartz DA, Graham AL. Potential maternal and infant outcomes from (Wuhan) coronavirus 2019-nCoV infecting pregnant women: lessons from SARS, MERS, and other human coronavirus infections. Viruses. 2020;12(2):194.
56. Diriba K, Awulachew E, Getu E. The effect of coronavirus infection (SARS-CoV-2, MERS-CoV, and SARS-CoV) during pregnancy and the possibility of vertical maternal-fetal transmission: a systematic review and meta-analysis. Eur J Med Res. 2020;25:39.
57. Chen N, Zhou M, Dong X, Qu J, Gong F, Han Y, et al. Epidemiological and clinical characteristics of 99 cases of 2019 novel coronavirus pneumonia in Wuhan, China: a descriptive study. Lancet. 2020;395(10223):507–13.
58. Liu H, Liu F, Li J, Zhang T, Wang D, Lan W. Clinical and CT imaging features of the COVID-19 pneumonia: focus on pregnant women and children. J Infect. 2020;80(5):e7–e13.
59. Chen H, Guo J, Wang C, Luo F, Yu X, Zhang W, et al. Clinical characteristics and intrauterine vertical transmission potential of COVID-19 infection in nine pregnant women: a retrospective review of medical records. Lancet. 2020;395(10226):809–15.
60. Haddad LB, Jamieson DJ, Rasmussen SA. Pregnant women and the Ebola crisis. N Engl J Med. 2018;379(26):2492–3.
61. Murphy S. Newborn baby tests positive for coronavirus in London. The Guardian. 2020;
62. Li M, Chen L, Zhang J, Xiong C, Li X. The SARS-CoV-2 receptor ACE2 expression of the maternal-fetal interface and fetal organs by single-cell transcriptome study. PLoS One. 2020;15(4):e0230295. https://doi.org/10.1371/journal.pone.0230295.
63. Stockman LJ, Lowther SA, Coy K, Saw J, Parashar UD. SARS during pregnancy, United States. Emerg Infect Dis. 2004;10(9):1689–90.
64. Yao TT., Dan J Qian, Wen-Yan, Zhu ZY, Wang GQ A systematic review of lopinavir therapy for SARS coronavirus and MERS coronavirus A possible reference for coronavirus disease-19 treatment option J Med Virol 2020;92(6):556–563. DOI: https://doi.org/10.1002/jmv.25729.
65. de Wit E, van Doremalen N, Falzarano D, Munster VJ. SARS and MERS: recent insights into emerging coronaviruses. Nat Rev Microbiol. 2016;14(8):523–34.
66. Assiri A, Abedi GR, Al Masri M, Bin Saeed A, Gerber SI, Watson JT. Middle East respiratory syndrome coronavirus infection during pregnancy: a report of 5 cases from Saudi Arabia. Clin Infect Dis. 2016;63(7):951–3.
67. Jeong SY, Sung SI, Sung JH, et al. MERS-CoV infection in a pregnant woman in Korea. J Korean Med Sci. 2017;32(10):1717–20.
68. Chong YP, Song JY, Seo YB, Choi JP, Shin HS, Rapid Response Team. Antiviral treatment guidelines for Middle East respiratory syndrome. Infect Chemother. 2015;47(3):212–22.
69. Zhang L, Jiang Y, Wei M, et al. Analysis of the pregnancy outcomes in pregnant women with COVID-19 in Hubei Province. Zhonghua Fu Chan Ke Za Zhi. 2020;55:E009.
70. Zhu H, Wang L, Fang C, et al. Clinical analysis of 10 neonates born to mothers with 2019-nCoV pneumonia. Transl Pediatr. 2020;9(1):51–60.
71. Wang M, Cao R, Zhang L, et al. Remdesivir and chloroquine effectively inhibit the recently emerged novel coronavirus (2019-nCoV) in vitro. Cell Res. 2020;30(3):269–71.
72. Zhou D, Dai SM, Tong Q. COVID-19: a recommendation to examine the effect of hydroxychloroquine in preventing infection and progression. J Antimicrob Chemother. 2020;75(7):1667–70. https://doi.org/10.1093/jac/dkaa114.
73. Ramsey PS, Ramin KD. Pneumonia in pregnancy: medical complications of pregnancy. Obstet Gynecol Clin N Am. 2001;28:553e69.
74. Spinello I, Johnson R, Baqui S. Coccidioidomycosis and pregnancy. Ann NY Acad Sci. 2007;1111:358e64.

75. Bercovitch RS, Catanzaro A, Schwartz BS, et al. Coccidioidomycosis during pregnancy: a review and recommendations for management. Clin Infect Dis. 2011;53:363–8.

76. Rodrigues JM, Niederman MS. Pneumonia complicating pregnancy. Clin Chest Med. 1992;13:679e91.

77. Pilmis B, Jullien V, Sobel J, Lecuit M, Lortholary O, Charlier C. Antifungal drugs during pregnancy: an updated review. J Antimicrob Chemother. 2015;70:14–22. https://doi.org/10.1093/jac/dku355.

78. Kumar RM, Uduman SA, Khurrana AK. Impact of pregnancy on maternal AIDS. J Reprod Med. 1997;42:429e34.

79. Senise J, Bonafé S, Castelo A, The management of HIV-infected pregnant women Curr Opin Obstet Gynecol 2012 Dec;24(6):395–401.

80. Ahmad H, Mehta NJ, Manikal VM, et al. Pneumocystis carinii pneumonia in pregnancy. Chest. 2001;120:666e71.

81. Buonsenso D, Raffaelli F, Tamburrini E, et al. Clinical role of lung ultrasound for diagnosis and monitoring of COVID-19 pneumonia in pregnant women. Ultrasound Obstet Gynecol. 2020 Jul;56(1):106–9. https://doi.org/10.1002/uog.22055.

82. Peng QY, Wang XT, Zhang LN, Chinese Critical Care Ultrasound Study Group (CCUSG). Findings of lung ultrasonography of novel corona virus pneumonia during the 2019–2020 epidemic. Intensive Care Med. 2020;12:1–2.

83. Watanabe M, Iwatani Y, Kaneda T, Hidaka Y, Mitsuda N, Morimoto Y, Amino N. Changes in T, B, and NK lymphocyte subsets during and after normal pregnancy. Am J Reprod Immunol. 1989;1997(37):368–77.

84. Groer MW, El-Badri N, Djeu J, Williams SN, Kane B, Szekeres K. Suppression of natural killer cell cytotoxicity in postpartum women: time course and potential mechanisms. Biol Res Nurs. 2014;16(3):320–6.

85. Groer ME, Jevitt C, Ji M. Immune changes and dysphoric moods across the postpartum. Am J Reprod Immunol. 2015;73(3):193–8.

86. Viruez-Soto JA, Ibáñez-Velasco BR, Bailey-Rojas FB, Zavala-Barrios B, Briones-Garduño JC. Díaz de León-Ponce MA Acute respiratory distress syndrome in puerperium. Rev Mex Anest. 2016;39:227–31.

87. Mok HP, Hart E, Venkatesan P. Early development of immune reconstitution inflammatory syndrome related to Pneumocystis pneumonia after antiretroviral therapy. Int J STD AIDS. 2014;25(5):373–7. https://doi.org/10.1177/0956462413506888.

88. Metersky ML, Masterton RG, Lode H, File TM, Babinchak T. Epidemiology, microbiology, and treatment considerations for bacterial pneumonia complicating influenza. Int J Infect Dis. 2012;16(5):e321–31.

89. Raghavendran K, Nemzek J, Napolitano LM, Knight PR. Aspirationinduced lung injury. Crit Care Med. 2011;39(4):818–26.

90. Duarte AG. ARDS in pregnancy. Clin Obstet Gynecol. 2014;57:862.

Tuberculosis During Pregnancy

Fatma Tokgoz Akyil and Kamil Janeczek

63.1   Introduction

Tuberculosis (TB) is one of the leading causes of death worldwide and the most common cause of death from a single infectious agent. TB is caused by the droplet transmission of *Mycobacterium tuberculosis* (*M. tuberculosis*) bacilli, which sick people shed into the air. About a quarter of the world's population is considered to be infected with *M. tuberculosis* bacillus, and approximately 10 million (8.9–11 million) people were infected with TB in 2019. Although TB is a preventable and treatable disease, it caused 1.2 million deaths in HIV (human immunodeficiency virus) negative individuals and 208,000 deaths in HIV-positive individuals in 2019 [1].

Women constitute 35% of reported TB patients, but it is thought that female patient identification or reporting is lacking [2]. According to 2013 data, 3.3 million female TB patients and 510,000 TB-related deaths were recorded in women [3]. In women, the frequency of TB disease increases during pregnancy [4]. Although new data are not available in recent years, 216,500 pregnant TB patients were reported in 2011, half of whom were from Africa. TB disease can cause undesirable consequences for both the mother and the infant during pregnancy, birth, and postpartum [5]. All over the world, significant progress has been made in maternal health in recent decades, and maternal deaths have decreased from approximately 485,000 to

F. T. Akyil (✉)
Ministry of Health, Yedikule Chest Diseases and Thoracic Surgery Training and Research Hospital, Istanbul, Turkey
e-mail: fatmatokgoz86@gmail.com

K. Janeczek
Department of Pulmonary Diseases and Children Rheumatology, Medical University of Lublin, Lublin, Poland
e-mail: kamiljaneczek@umlub.pl

C. Cingi et al. (eds.), *ENT Diseases: Diagnosis and Treatment during Pregnancy and Lactation*, https://doi.org/10.1007/978-3-031-05303-0_63

295,000 from 2000 to 2017 [6]. On the other hand, 28% of recorded deaths are caused by non-obstetric etiology, including TB [7].

In this chapter, we plan to discuss the effects of pregnancy on TB and its impact on pregnancy.

63.2   Effects of Pregnancy on Tuberculosis

Historically, it was thought that TB had a positive effect on pregnancy but afterward a negative impact. In studies involving many patients, the results that TB did not progress differently during pregnancy gained weight. It was noted that 7% of 250 female pregnant patients in the pretreatment period went with progressive disease, and 8% showed progression in the first year following pregnancy [8]. These findings were also supported in subsequent studies and pregnant and nonpregnant women; It has been found that the course of TB disease and the frequency of extrapulmonary disease are similar [9]. However, in regression analyzes, the incidence of TB was found to be higher in the 6 months following pregnancy [10].

However, the issue is still under investigation, and there is no clear consensus. A progressive decrease occurs in tumor necrosis factor-alpha (TNF-a) levels during pregnancy [11]. In a recent analysis conducted in Sweden, TB was recorded in 553 of 649,342 women between the ages of 15 and 49 who gave birth between 2005 and 2013, 85 of them during pregnancy and 79 at 6 months postpartum. It has been argued that TB is higher during pregnancy and postpartum, and that risky patients can be screened [12].

63.3   Effects of Tuberculosis on Pregnancy

TB can occur in women of reproductive age at any stage, including fertility, pregnancy, and postpartum. The effect of TB may vary from many factors such as the severity of the disease, its prevalence, a gestational week at the time of diagnosis, concurrent HIV infection, TB drug susceptibility tests, and treatments.

Reproductive or genital TB is known to be a significant cause of infertility or ectopic pregnancy. Even after TB treatment, natural pregnancy may not occur, and in vitro fertilization may be required [13, 14]. When TB in pregnancy is diagnosed early and treated appropriately, no adverse effects are expected during pregnancy [15, 16]. The risk of spontaneous abortion, low weight gain, preterm labor, and neonatal death may increase [17, 18]. TB increases the risk of perinatal death in pregnancy six times, and the risk of low birth weight and prematurity in newborns increases 2–3 times [19–21].

It has been reported that the probability of oligoamniosis and premature rupture of membranes is higher, and the mean birth weight is lower in 30 pregnant patients diagnosed with extrapulmonary TB between 2008 and 2017 in India compared to healthy pregnant women. In this series, 22 of the pregnant women were under extrapulmonary TB treatment before pregnancy, 8 of them were diagnosed during pregnancy, and all of them were treated with isoniazid, rifampicin (RIF), pyrazinamide (PZA), and ethambutol regimen for 2 months, and with isoniazid and RIF for 4 months [22].

As supported by current studies, maternal TB causes an increase in the risk of mortality, miscarriage, stillbirth, preterm birth, and low birth weight and can have adverse effects on both maternal and infant. Negative outcomes are higher in pregnant women diagnosed in the last trimester. In HIV-positive pregnant women, both the risk of severe TB disease and side effects increase [23].

WHO recommends a systematic evaluation of active TB in pregnant women in populations with a population TB prevalence higher than 100/100,000 [24].

63.4 Tuberculosis and Newborn

The most common way of transmission in infants is through maternal droplet transmission. A rare route is a congenital or neonatal transmission. In this case, the mortality is approximately 50%. Congenital TB can occur with maternal TB endometritis or by transmitting hematogenously disseminated TB infection to the fetus through the umbilical vein or the aspiration of infected amniotic fluid [25]. Congenital TB is very rare, and less than 200 cases have been reported in the literature [26].

In congenital TB, the primary focus develops in the liver due to the involvement of the periportal lymph nodes. More than 80% of primary infections in adults occur in the lungs. Unlike adults, TB bacillus infects the lungs secondarily in newborns.

Unlike adults, neonatal TB develops in the liver. Showing primary hepatic complex or classified granuloma histopathologically by percutaneous liver biopsy in the first week in the newborn, detecting TB bacilli in the placenta, or proving the presence of genital TB in the mother is necessary for final diagnosis [27]. Although tuberculin skin test (TCT) results negative in infants, it should be kept in mind that interferon-gamma release tests (IGRAs) may be positive. HIV test, lumbar puncture, acid-resistant bacillus (ARB) staining in blood, respiratory tract, and placental materials, and histopathological evaluation of the placenta should be performed in those with congenital TB possibility [28].

63.5 Latent Tuberculosis Infection and Treatment in Pregnancy

Although screening for latent TB infection (LTBI) in pregnancy is not routinely recommended, screening for LTBI is recommended in the presence of HIV infection or other conditions that cause immunosuppression. If possible, it is more appropriate to do this screening before pregnancy, when the pregnancy is planned.

In the American Thoracic Society (ATS) guidelines, when LTBI is detected in pregnant women, considering the risk of hepatotoxicity, it is recommended that the treatment be postponed until after delivery. Delaying LTBI treatment is not recommended in HIV-positive pregnant women with a history of close contact with a TB patient [29]. When INH is used in pregnant and lactating women, pyridoxine

(25 mg/day) should be routinely added to the treatment. In addition, it is recommended that infants use pyridoxine supplementation since approximately 20% of the INH used by the mother passes into breast milk [30, 31].

Treatment options when LTBI is detected in an HIV-negative pregnant woman [32] are as follows:

(a) Isoniazid (INH) (5 mg/kg/day, max 300 mg) for 9 months.
(b) INH at a dose of 15 mg/kg 2 days a week for 9 months with directly observed therapy.
(c) Rifampin (600 mg/day for 4 months) in those who have contact with patients with INH resistance or who have INH toxicity [33].

63.6 Clinical Findings and Diagnosis of Active Tuberculosis in Pregnancy

TB symptoms may be perceived as pregnancy-related symptoms during pregnancy and may delay the diagnosis of TB. Pregnant women diagnosed with TB may be asymptomatic and without complaints. If the diagnosis is made late or not diagnosed, it may lead to congenital infection in the infant [9].

Pulmonary TB is rarer during pregnancy and constitutes 90% of patients with pulmonary TB. TB findings are similar in pregnant and nonpregnant women. While the most common symptoms of pulmonary TB in pregnant women are cough, weight loss, fever, weakness, and fatigue, up to 20% of patients may be asymptomatic at the time of diagnosis [9]. Symptoms such as weakness and fatigue in pregnant women can be attributed to pregnancy, and weight loss may be more challenging to understand. The possibility of TB should be kept in mind, especially in patients with suspected TB exposure and in pregnant women with a history of traveling to regions with high TB incidence.

TCT or interferon-gamma release tests (IGRAs) can be used for diagnosis. The responses of these tests are not expected to change during pregnancy, but the test may be harmful in approximately one-fourth of patients with active TB [34]. In about half of HIV patients, TCT may be negative regardless of pregnancy [35]. Therefore, the place of TCT and IGST tests in the diagnosis of TB is limited. Positive results only support the diagnosis of TB, and adverse effects are not sufficient to exclude a diagnosis of active TB. The use of these tests in immigrants from high prevalence countries, intravenous drug abusers, populations at risk for HIV infection, or HIV-positive patients is supported [35]. WHO has proposed a simple algorithm based on four symptoms in HIV patients. He suggested that active TB can be excluded in the absence of cough, fever, weight loss, and night sweats, and it was found that the diagnoses excluded in this way were 99% accurate [36].

When TB is suspected in anamnesis and/or during physical examination findings of the pregnant patient, laboratory tests, then a chest X-ray may be taken after the 12th week of pregnancy, if possible, with preservation of the abdomen sputum examinations for microbiological detection of M.

63.7 Active Tuberculosis Treatment in Pregnancy

When active TB is not treated during pregnancy, it may have more severe consequences than the possible harms of anti-tuberculous therapy for both mother and fetus [37]. When TB is detected in pregnant women, treatment should be started without delay.

WHO recommends using a standard four-drug regimen without making any specific changes in pregnant women diagnosed with drug-sensitive TB [38].

The nonresistant TB treatment regimen is established in pregnant women with INH, rifampin, and ethambutol. The first 2 months of INH, rifampin, and ethambutol treatment are completed in 9 months, with 7 months of INH and rifampin regimen. Ethambutol can be discontinued after 1 month if it is sensitive to INH and rifampin [25]. In the United States, as a general approach, PZA treatment is not recommended in pregnant women at the initial stage. Still, it is recommended to add PZA when HIV-positive patients, extrapulmonary TB, and diffuse TB are detected. This approach to PZA is due to the lack of sufficient evidence regarding its safety in pregnant women [39].

The duration of treatment is 6 months if PZA is used and 9 months if it is not used. All first-line drugs can be used in breastfeeding [40]. In the USA, the preferred regimen for empirical treatment of drug-susceptible active TB during pregnancy is INH, rifampin, and EMB administered for 2 months, followed by a total of 9 months of treatment for 7 months [25]. INH, rifampin, and EMB are generally considered acceptable for use in pregnancy.

In patients who are pregnant under TB treatment, the treatment should be continued without interruption. If necessary, the treatment regimen should be replaced with a regimen suitable for pregnancy.

Patients should be evaluated at least monthly to optimize adherence and to assess drug toxicity [39].

INH can cross the placenta but is safe in all trimesters. There is a risk of hepatitis and peripheral neurotoxicity in the peripartum period in INH use [39]. Pyridoxine should be used in pregnant and lactating women using INH [30, 31].

Rifampicin (RIF): Although it has been reported to be associated with neonatal hemorrhage [33, 39], it is generally considered safe. Vitamin K (10 mg/day) supplementation may be recommended in pregnant women using RIF in the last 4–8 weeks of pregnancy. Rifabutin can be used in patients who are HIV positive and under antiretroviral therapy.

Ethambutol was also not associated with an increased risk when used at the appropriate dose.

Pyrazinamide (PZA): WHO has suggested that PZA can be used routinely, but its routine use was not recommended in the United States due to insufficient evidence. Many international organizations recommend its use, including the International Association of TB and Lung Diseases (IUATLD), the British Thoracic Society, the ATS, and India's Revised National Tuberculosis Control Program. It is especially recommended in pregnant women with TB meningitis, HIV-positive patients, and suspected drug resistance [41, 42].

Since it has been shown that streptomycin in pregnant women may cause sensorineural hearing loss in infants, it should not be used [41].

Liver function tests, HIV, hepatitis B, and C tests are recommended before starting treatment. The risk of hepatitis, especially from isoniazid, increases during pregnancy [43]. Close follow-up is required in terms of hepatotoxicity. The risk of hepatotoxicity is especially highest during pregnancy and postpartum at 3 months [44]. After the treatment is started, it is recommended that the patients be reevaluated with laboratory tests at least once a month by questioning the drug's side effects in detail [45].

Since the risk of hemolytic anemia in the newborn may increase due to RIF crossing the placenta after delivery, routine vitamin K supplementation is recommended for infants [43].

63.8 Multidrug-Resistant Tuberculosis (MDR-TB) in Pregnancy

Information on the regimen to be established when resistance to first-line drugs is detected is limited. Since the prognosis of multidrug-resistant tuberculosis (MDR-TB) patients may be worse, treatment should be started without delay. It is generally accepted to use similar treatment with nonpregnant women [46]. While there are opinions recommending termination of pregnancy, pregnancies successfully terminated with appropriate regimens have also been reported [25, 47].

Currently, WHO recommends establishing an individualized regimen containing at least four drugs with an acceptable safety profile and low teratogenic risk [48].

Although there is no randomized controlled study on PZA, it is accepted that it can be used when it is difficult to establish a drug regimen [49].

There was no significant teratogenic effect with para-aminosalicylic acid used in combination with INH in pregnant women. The use of ethionamide and prothionamide in pregnant women is not considered safe since teratogenic effects on the central nervous system have been detected [50].

The general approach is to avoid aminoglycosides because of the risk of ototoxicity and fetal malformation and not to use ethionamide and prothionamide because of their potential teratogenic effects [51]. For these reasons, pregnant women are not suitable for MDR-TB shortened 9–11 months treatment [24].

Delaminid is not recommended because it has been shown to have a teratogenic effect in animal studies [52]. It may also be necessary to use drugs such as cycloserine, ofloxacin, amikacin, kanamycin, capreomycin, and ethionamide, whose safety in pregnancy has not been proven [33]. Bedaquiline has not shown any effect in animal studies [52]. In animal studies, bedaquiline and delaminid were also found to be excreted in milk [52].

Pregnancy may be detected in a patient under MDR-TB treatment, or a pregnant woman may be diagnosed with MDR-TB. In the literature, pregnancy termination rates are not high in both cases, and there is no clear recommendation on this issue. There are cases where maternal and fetal death were reported and cases whose pregnancy was successfully terminated with close follow-up and appropriate treatment [53–56].

A recent study has been published on 108 pregnant women who were started on MDR-TB treatment in South Africa between 2013 and 2017. It has been reported that 72 (67%) patients resulted in the cure or completion of therapy, and 91% of 109 babies were born alive in an average of 38 months. There were 57 (52%) pregnancies resulting in an infant with a birth weight of more than 2500 g and an infant living longer than 28 days when the birth occurred at 37 weeks and later. HIV-positive patients have a higher risk. Preterm birth was found in 28 infants, low birth weight in 33, a congenital anomaly in 4, fetal death in 4, and stillbirth in 6 infants. The study concluded that bedaquiline, as a frequently used drug, did not affect pregnancy outcomes, but it could be associated with low birth weight, and it was emphasized that further studies are needed [57].

63.9 Conclusion

As a result, pregnancy, and TB is an issue that has risks for both mother and baby, the dynamics of treatment has not been fully clarified, and there are points where sufficient reliable evidence and guidelines are not clear at many points. It is crucial to rapidly evaluate risky pregnant women regarding TB, initiate appropriate treatment without delay, and follow-up the patients closely.

References

1. WHO. Global Tuberculosis Report 2020. Geneva: World Health Organization; 2020. Licence: CC BY-NC-SA 3.0 IGO. https://apps.who.int/iris/bitstream/handle/10665/336069/9789240013131-eng.pdf. Accessed 26 Mar 2021.
2. Hertz D, Schneider B. Sex differences in tuberculosis. Semin Immunopathol. 2019;41(2):225–37.
3. World Health Organization. Global tuberculosis report 2014. Geneva; 2014.
4. Vasakova M. Challenges of antituberculosis treatment in patients with difficult clinical conditions. Clin Respir J. 2015;9(2):143–52.
5. Sugarman J, Colvin C, Moran AC, et al. Tuberculosis in pregnancy: an estimate of the global burden of disease. Lancet Glob Health. 2014;2(12):e710–6.
6. Trends in maternal mortality 2000 to 2017: estimates by WHO, UNICEF, UNFPA. World Bank Group and the United Nations Population Division. Geneva: World Health Organization; 2019. Licence: CC BY-NC-SA 3.0 IGO
7. Say L, Chou D, Gemmill A, et al. Global causes of maternal death: a WHO systematic analysis. Lancet Global Health. 2014;2:e323–e33.
8. Hedvall E. Pregnancy and tuberculosis. Acta Med Scand Suppl. 1953;286:1–101.
9. Gould JM, Aronoff SC. 2016. Tuberculosis and pregnancy—maternal, fetal, and neonatal considerations Microbiol Spectrum 4(6):TNMI7-0016-2016. doi:https://doi.org/10.1128/microbiolspec.TNMI7-0016-2016.
10. Zenner D, Kruijshaar ME, Andrews N, Abubakar I. Risk of tuberculosis in pregnancy: a national, primary care-based cohort and self-controlled case series study. Am J Respir Crit Care Med. 2012;185:779–84.

11. Kraus TA, Engel SM, Sperling RS, et al. Characterizing the pregnancy immune phenotype: results of the viral immunity and pregnancy (VIP) study. J Clin Immunol. 2012;32:300–11.

12. Jonsson J, Kühlmann-Berenzon S, Berggren I, et al. Increased risk of active tuberculosis during pregnancy and postpartum: a register-based cohort study in Sweden. Eur Respir J. 2020;55:1901886.

13. Mondal SK, Dutta TK. A ten year clinicopathological study of female genital tuberculosis and impact on fertility. J Nepal Med Assoc. 2009;48:52–7.

14. Bapna N, Swarankarm M, Kotia N. Genital tuberculosis and its consequences on subsequent fertility. J Obstet Gynaecol India. 2005;55:534–7.

15. Schaefer G, Zervoudakis IA, Fuchs FF, David S. Pregnancy and pulmonary tuberculosis. Obstet Gynecol. 1975;46(6):706–15.

16. Mehta BR. Pregnancy and tuberculosis. Dis Chest. 1961;39:505–11.

17. Ormerod P. Tuberculosis in pregnancy and the puerperium. Thorax. 2001;56(6):494–9.

18. Kishan J, Sailaja, Kaur S. Tuberculosis and pregnancy. In: Proceedings of the National Conference on Pulmonary diseases (NAPCON '01), Mumbai, Maharashtra; 2001.

19. Jana N, Vasishta K, Jindal SK, Khunnu B, Ghosh K. Perinatal outcome in pregnancies complicated by pulmonary tuberculosis. Int J Gynaecol Obstet. 1994;44:119–24.

20. Figueroa-Damián R, Arredondo-García JL. Neonatal outcome of children born to women with tuberculosis. Arch Med Res. 2001;32:66–9.

21. Lin HC, Lin HC, Chen SF. Increased risk of low birth weight and small for gestational age infants among women with tuberculosis. BJOG. 2010;117:585–90.

22. Yadav V, Sharma JB, Kachhawa G, Kulshrestha V, Mahey R, Kumari R, Kriplani A. Obstetrical and perinatal outcome in pregnant women with extrapulmonary tuberculosis. Indian J Tuberc. 2019;66(1):158–62. https://doi.org/10.1016/j.ijtb.2018.10.010.

23. Snow KJ, Bekker A, Huang GK, Graham SM. Tuberculosis in pregnant women and neonates: a meta-review of current evidence. Paediatr Respir Rev. 2020;36:27–32. https://doi.org/10.1016/j.prrv.2020.02.001.

24. World Health Organization. WHO recommendations on antenatal care for a positive pregnancy experience. World Health Organization; 2016.

25. Starke JR. Tuberculosis in childhood and pregnancy. In: Friedman LN, editor. Tuberculosis: current concepts and treatment. Boca Raton, FL: CRC Press; 2000.

26. Peng W, Yang J, Liu E. Analysis of 170 cases of congenital TB reported in the literature between 1946 and 2009. Pediatr Pulmonol. 2011;46(12):1215–24.

27. Cantwell MR, Shehab ZM, Costello AM. Brief report: congenital tuberculosis. N Engl J Med. 1994;330(15):1051–4.

28. Arslan E, Görkem Ü. Tuberculosis during pregnancy. Bozok Med J. 2020;10(1):264–71.

29. American Thoracic Society. American Thoracic Society. Medical Section of the American Lung Association: treatment of tuberculosis and tuberculosis infection in adults and children. Am Rev Respir Dis. 1986;134:355–63.

30. American Thoracic Society. Targeted tuberculin testing and treatment of latent tuberculosis infection. MMWR Recommend Rep. 2000;49(RR-6):1–51.

31. Centers for Disease Control and Prevention. Latent TB infection: a guide for primary healthcare providers. Atlanta, GA: US Department of Health and Human Services; 2016.

32. WHO. Tuberculosis Global Fact. World Health Organisation; 2010/2011.

33. Snider DJ. Pregnancy and tuberculosis. Chest. 1984;86(3 Suppl):10S–3S.

34. Huebner RE, Schein MF, Bass JB Jr. The tuberculin skin test. Clin Infect Dis. 1993;17:968–75.

35. Centers for Disease Control. Screening for tuberculosis and tuberculous infection in high-risk populations. Recommendations of the Advisory Committee for Elimination of Tuberculosis. MMWR Recommend Rep. 1990;39(RR-8):1–7.

36. Gupta A, Chandrasekhar A, Gupte N, Patil S, Bhosale R, Sambarey P, Ghorpade S, Nayak U, Garda L, Sastry J, Bharadwaj R, Bollinger RC, Byramjee Jeejeebhoy Medical College–Johns Hopkins University Study Group. Symptom screening among HIV-infected pregnant women is acceptable and has a high negative predictive value; 2011.

37. Carter EJ, Mates S. Tuberculosis during pregnancy. The Rhode Island experience, 1987 to 1991. Chest. 1994;106(5):1466–70.
38. World Health Organization. Compendium of WHO guidelines and associated standards: ensuring optimum delivery of the cascade of care for patients with tuberculosis; 2018.
39. Snider DE, Layde PM, Johnson MW, Lyle MA. Treatment of tuberculosis during pregnancy. Am Rev Respir Dis. 1980;122(1):65–79.
40. Centers for Disease Control and Prevention. Treatment of tuberculosis, American Thoracic Society. CDC and Infectious Diseases Society of America. MMWR Recommend Rep. 2003;52(RR-11):1–77.
41. Anderson GD. Tuberculosis in pregnancy. Semin Perinatol. 1997;21(4):328–35.
42. Management, Control and Prevention of Tuberculosis; Guidelinesfor Health Care Providers (2002–2005), Department of Human Services, Victoria, Australia; 2002.
43. Nhan-Chang CL, Jones TB. Tuberculosis in pregnancy. Clin Obstet Gynecol. 2010;53(2):311–21.
44. Knight M, Kurinczuk JJ, Nelson-Piercy C, Spark P, Brocklehurst P. Tuberculosis in pregnancy in the UK. BJOG. 2009;116(4):584–8.
45. Marks SM, Mase SR, Morris SB. Systematic review, meta-analysis, and cost-effectiveness of treatment of latent tuberculosis to reduce progression to multidrug-resistant tuberculosis. Clin Infect Dis. 2017;64(12):1670–7.
46. Sobhy S, Babiker Z, Zamora J, Khan KS, Kunst H. Maternal and perinatal mortality and morbidity associated with tuberculosis during pregnancy and the postpartum period: a systematic review and meta-analysis. BJOG. 2017;124(5):727–33.
47. Vallejo JG, Starke JR. Tuberculosis and pregnancy. Clin Chest Med. 1992;13(4):693–707.
48. Gupta A, Hughes MD, Garcia-Prats AJ, McIntire K, Hesseling AC. Inclusion of key populations in clinical trials of new antituberculosis treatments: current barriers and recommendations for pregnant and lactating women, children, and HIV-infected persons. PLoS Med. 2019;16:e1002882.
49. Falzon D, Schünemann HJ, Harausz E, González-Angulo L, Lienhardt C, Jaramillo E, et al. World Health Organization treatment guidelines for drug-resistant tuberculosis, 2016 update. Eur Respir J. 2017;49(3):1602308.
50. Schardein JL. Chemically induced birth defects. 3rd ed. New York, NY: Marcel Dekker; 2000.
51. Gupta A, Mathad JS, Abdel-Rahman SM, et al. Toward earlier inclusion of pregnant and postpartum women in tuberculosis drug trials: consensus statements from an international expert panel. Indian J Surg. 2016;62(6):761–9.
52. Esmail A, Sabur NF, Okpechi I, Dheda K. Management of drug-resistant tuberculosis in special sub-populations including those with HIV co-infection, pregnancy, diabetes, organ-specific dysfunction, and in the critically ill. J Thorac Dis. 2018;10(5):3102–18.
53. Palacios E, Dallman R, Muñoz M, Hurtado R, Chalco K, Guerra D, et al. Drug- resistant tuberculosis and pregnancy: treatment outcomes of 38 cases in Lima. Peru Clin Infect Dis. 2009;48(10):1413–9.
54. Tabarsi P, Moradi A, Baghaei P, Marjani M, Shamaei M, Mansouri N, et al. Standardised second-line treatment of multidrug-resistant tuberculosis during pregnancy. Int J Tuberc Lung Dis. 2011;15(4):547–50.
55. De Oliveira HB, Mateus SHR. Characterization of multidrug-resistant tuberculosis during pregnancy in Campinas, State of Sao Paulo, Brazil, from 1995 to 2007. Rev Soc Bras Med Trop. 2011;44(5):627–30.
56. Khan M, Pillay T, Moodley J, Ramjee A, Padayatchi N. Pregnancies complicated by multidrug-resistant tuberculosis and HIV co-infection in Durban, South Africa. Int J Tuberc Lung Dis. 2007;11(6):706–8.
57. Loveday M, Hughes J, Sunkari B, Master I, Huang S, Reddy T, Chotoo S, Green N, Seddon JA. Maternal and infant outcomes among pregnant women treated for multidrug/rifampicin-resistant tuberculosis in South Africa. Clin Infect Dis. 2021;72(7):1158–68.

Pulmonary Embolism During Pregnancy and the Postpartum Period

64

Ozlem Sengoren Dikis and Sevinc Sarinc Ulasli

64.1 Introduction

Pregnancy and the postpartum period are known risk factors for venous thromboembolism (VTE) [1]. In pregnancy, VTE can be observed as lower extremity deep vein thrombosis (DVT) alone, as well as together with pulmonary embolism (PE). The incidence rate of VTE is 4–50 times higher in pregnant women compared to non-pregnant women of the same age [2]. The risk increases especially in the postpartum period [3]. Over the last 15 years, there has been a 4.6-fold increase in the number of pulmonary thromboembolism (PTE) patients [4]. The most important causes of this increase can be listed as fast-food nutritional habit, obesity, prolongation of human lifetime and technological improvements in diagnostic processes. Physiological causes that increase the probability of VTE development during pregnancy and in the postpartum period are: (1) Thrombocyte activation, reduced fibrinolytic and protein S activities, (2) Relaxation effect of progesterone secretion on venous smooth muscles during pregnancy, (3) Estrogen causing an increase in levels of procoagulant factors [5–8], (4) Decrease of anticoagulant factors—protein S and antithrombin levels—via estrogen, (5) Compression effect of the uterus during pregnancy on the iliac vein and inferior vena cava, (6) Vascular intimal injury due to surgical applications such as cesarean, forceps and vacuum, (7) Stasis due to immobility during pregnancy and the postpartum period, (8) Genetic factors such as deficiencies of protein S, Protein C and antithrombin leading to thrombophilia, (9) Maternal age of

O. S. Dikis (✉)
Department of Chest Diseases, School of Medicine, Mugla Sitki Kocman University, Mugla, Turkey
e-mail: ozlemsengoren@hotmail.com

S. S. Ulasli
Department of Chest Diseases, School of Medicine, Hacettepe University, Ankara, Turkey
e-mail: sevincsarinc@gmail.com

C. Cingi et al. (eds.), *ENT Diseases: Diagnosis and Treatment during Pregnancy and Lactation*, https://doi.org/10.1007/978-3-031-05303-0_64

843

Table 64.1 Risk factors for pulmonary embolism in pregnancy and the postpartum period

Preexisting factors
Prior VTE
Obesity
Medical comorbidities (e.g. cancer, sickle cell disease, systemic lupus erythematosus)
Genetic risk factors (e.g. protein C deficiency, protein S deficiency, AT III deficiency)
Thrombophilia (e.g. antiphospholipid syndrome)
Age > 35 years
Smoking
Varicose veins
Obstetric factors
In vitro fertilization
Stillbirth
Pre-eclampsia
Postpartum haemorrhage
Caesarean section
Multiple pregnancies
Prolonged labor
Preterm birth

35 years and above, (10) VTE history prior to the pregnancy, (11) Obesity (BMI $\geq$ 30 kg/m^2), heart disease, sickle cell disease and systemic lupus erythematosus, and (12) Multiparas and delivery by caesarean section [9, 10].

Risk factors for VTE in pregnancy and the postpartum period are depicted in Table 64.1.

Pregnancy physiological processes and comorbid thrombophilia create a tendency to PE, whereas physiological changes in pregnancy develop symptoms similar to PE and this causes difficulty in diagnosis. While dyspnea, tachypnea, tachycardia and leg swelling are common symptoms during pregnancy, especially an abnormal increase of dyspnea and comorbid DVT symptoms are important clues for PE. The most common symptoms are dyspnea, pleuritic chest pain and cough [5]. VTE accounts for 1.1 deaths per 100,000 deliveries and 9% of all maternal deaths in the United States [11]. Diagnosis and treatment of thromboembolism is vital due to its high prevalence during pregnancy and the postpartum period and the severity of its outcomes.

64.2 Diagnosis of PE

It is usually difficult to diagnose PE during pregnancy. Major difficulties are: confusion of PE symptoms with pregnancy symptoms and especially concern of the patient and the clinician about the ionizing radiation that the fetus would receive. Hemodynamic changes observed in pregnancy lead to common symptoms and results, such as dyspnea (70%), tachypnea, tachycardia and leg swelling. Complaints of dyspnea increase gradually as the pregnancy progresses. Especially DVT symptoms, such as abnormal increase of dyspnea, and pain, swelling, tenderness, warmth and/or erythema in the lower extremity are important clues for PE. Similar to other patient populations, primarily it is essential to have clinical suspicion in order to make a thromboembolic disease diagnosis during pregnancy. Thus, if one or more symptoms of acute pleuritic chest pain, hemoptysis and dyspnea are observed in the pregnant woman [5], a distinctive diagnosis must be made in terms of the clinical probability of PTE.

Wells and Geneva Criteria, clinical probability scoring methods, are not validated to be used in pregnancy, according to the American Thoracic Society and Thoracic Radiology Practice Guideline published in 2011 [12], whereas in the study published by Cutts et al. in 2014, evaluating 183 patients retrospectively, the sensitivity and negative predictive value of the modified Wells criteria have been found to be close to 100% [6].

Therefore, randomized controlled studies are needed to provide a validated clinical probability scoring system to identify the PTE clinical probability in pregnancy.

64.2.1 Laboratory Tests

64.2.1.1 D-Dimer

D-dimer, the fibrinogen degradation product, is physiologically high during pregnancy. Moreover, it is indicated that D-dimer levels can be positive in 50% of patients during the first 20 weeks of pregnancy [13]. Hence, a negative D-dimer level can be used to exclude PE in patients within this period, whereas in the following weeks, D-dimer level increases gradually and returns to normal in the 4–6th postpartum week. In a prospective study performed with eighty-nine pregnant women, D-dimer levels differentiated by pregnancy trimester and by higher cutoff values have been detected in patients with thromboembolic disease [7]. However, wide-range prospective studies are needed for these values to be used for early diagnosis in pregnancy.

In recently published guidelines of the ESC, evidence category 2a was specified, according to which D-dimer measurements and clinical prediction rules exclude PE during pregnancy and the postpartum period [8].

64.2.1.2 Arterial Blood Gas Analysis

Respiratory alkalosis is a common finding in pregnancy and PE. Therefore, this finding is not diagnostic for pregnant women with suspected PE.

Since partial oxygen pressure (PaO2) may be lower in the supine position during the third trimester of pregnancy, arterial blood must be drawn from the patient in an upright position. In pregnant women associated with hypoxemia, chest radiography must be obtained by protecting the abdomen with a lead apron. In the presence of a normal chest radiography, further examinations must be performed for PE after excluding other pathologies (pulmonary edema, cardiomegaly, pneumothorax, pneumonia, etc.).

64.2.2 Compression Ultrasound (CUS)

If leg symptoms (e.g. pain, swelling, erythema in the legs) coexist with high D-dimer level in a pregnant woman, proximal vein compression ultrasound (CUS) has high sensitivity (95%) and specificity (>95%) [14]. CUS is the first examination to be performed for proximal vein thrombosis [15].

Detection of proximal DVT is sufficient for initiation of anticoagulant therapy and thoracic imaging is not necessary. However, in case of negative ultrasound, further diagnostic procedures must be performed if a clinical suspicion of PE persists [15].

64.2.3 Echocardiography

Echocardiography is not routine in diagnostic procedure for suspected PE pregnant women. Echocardiography can be used in exclusion of cardiomyopathy associated with pregnancy valvular heart disease, idiopathic pulmonary hypertension or in evaluation of right ventricular size. Especially, right ventricular failure findings in echocardiography of pregnant women with acute dyspnea indicate most probably a diagnosis of PE.

64.2.4 Imaging

Radiologic imaging is the most valuable method for the final diagnosis of PE. Here, the most important factor for clinicians' hesitation in radiologic diagnostic techniques is the radiation dose to which the fetus would be exposed. Fetal and maternal radiation doses have been updated in the last guidelines of the ESC (Table 64.2) [8]. The National Council of Radiation Protection and Measurements have specified the dose that can lead to radiation-associated anomalies for the fetus as <50 mGy [16]. Lung scintigraphy can be preferred to CT to avoid high-dose maternal radiation and especially the carcinogenic risk in breast [17]. The diagnostic value of scintigraphy and CT is similar in pregnancy, and the results of normal perfusion scintigraphy and negative CT are considered to be closely reliable [18]. However, conventional pulmonary angiography must not be implemented during pregnancy due to the risk of high-dose fetal radiation exposure (2.2–3.7 mSV) [16].

64.2.4.1 Chest X-Ray

Chest X-ray results are not specific and sensitive for PE. Chest X-ray is usually normal in PE suspected pregnant women, whereas the presence of abnormal findings among the main chest X-ray findings of PE, such as Westermark sign (focal peripheral oligemia and hyperlucency), Hampton hump (pleural-based, usually triangular or wedge-shaped peripheral consolidation), Fleischner sign (dilation of

Table 64.2 Estimated radiation doses of imaging tests for PE diagnosis

Test	Estimated fetal radiation exposure (mSV)	Estimated maternal radiation exposure to breast tissue (mSV)
Chest X-ray	<0.01	0.01
Perfusion lung scan with technetium-99 m-labeled albumin		
– Low dose: ~40 MBq	0.11–0.20	0.28–0.50
– High dose: ~200 MBq	0.20–0.60	1.2
Ventilation lung scan	0.10–0.30	<0.01
Computed tomography pulmonary angiography	0.24–0.66	10–70

central pulmonary artery due to pulmonary hypertension or distension caused by embolism), knuckle sign (abrupt tapering or cutoff of a pulmonary artery), linear atelectasis in lower lobes, elevated diaphragm and pleural effusion [19–23] may indicate PE.

64.2.4.2 MR Pulmonary Angiography (MRPA)

There are not enough studies to determine the sensitivity and specificity of MR pulmonary angiography in PE diagnosis in pregnant women. Even though a fetal teratogenic effect of gadolinium has not been observed, it is classified as a category C agent by the US Food and Drug Administration since its long-term and high-dose exposure teratogenic effects have been demonstrated in animals [24].

64.2.4.3 Computed Tomography Pulmonary Angiography (CTPA) and Perfusion Scan

According to the diagnostic algorithm of the American Thoracic Society/Society of Thoracic Radiology [25, 26] in case the chest X-ray is normal in PE suspected pregnant women without DVT symptoms or those who are CUS negative, lung scintigraphy must be the first choice. If the chest X-ray is abnormal or scintigraphy is not diagnostic (low/intermediate probability perfusion defects), then computed tomography pulmonary angiography (CTPA) is recommended. In case of a technically insufficient CTPA, the CTPA must be repeated or CUS must be performed. No further process needs to be done in case of negative CTPA. The diagnostic algorithm of PE during pregnancy and the postpartum period is outlined in Fig. 64.1.

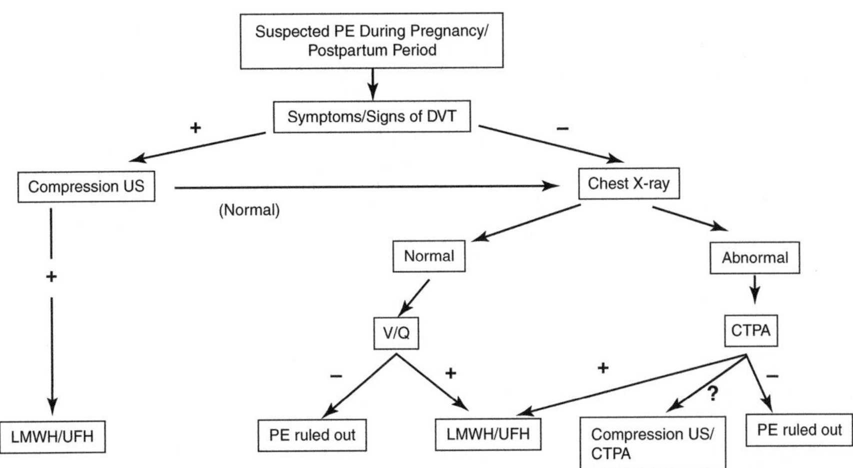

Fig. 64.1 Diagnostic algorithm of PE during pregnancy and the postpartum 6-week period. (Adopted from Reference [26]). *CTPA* computed tomography pulmonary angiography, *DVT* deep venous thrombosis, *LMWH* low molecular weight heparin, *PE* pulmonary embolism, *V/Q* ventilation perfusion scan, *UFH* unfractionated heparin, *US* ultrasound

64.3　Treatment

Anticoagulant therapy must be started immediately if PE is suspected in a pregnant woman, and this treatment must be sustained till the diagnosis is excluded. For PE treatment and prophylaxis in pregnant women, unfractionated heparin (UFH) or low molecular weight heparin (LMWH) are used, which do not cross the placenta and which do not cause fetal hemorrhage or malformation, in contrast to Vitamin K antagonists, Warfarin and new oral anticoagulants (NOACs).

There has been no randomized study conducted to identify the therapeutic range of LMWH in pregnancy, and the existing study results are not consistent [27, 28].

Even though it is assumed that measurement of plasma anti-activated factor X activity (anti-Xa) can be clinically useful in the determination of LMWH dose, the American College of Chest Physicians does not make a recommendation about anti-Xa follow-up due to insufficient data [29]. Anti-activated factor X activity measurements can be performed for LMWH dose adjustment of pregnant women in particular cases, such as renal failure, recurrent PE and extremely low or high body weight [30, 31]. Therefore, similar dosing to non-pregnant patients, either with o.d. or b.i.d. regimens based on early pregnancy weight, can be initiated for PE treatment during pregnancy [32].

Fondaparinux, despite its minor transplacental passage, can be recommended to pregnant PE patients with allergy to LMWH, heparin-induced thrombocytopenia or who experience side effects [33]. Fondaparinux is not recommended for breastfeeding mothers.

If spontaneous delivery is planned for the pregnant woman under LMWH therapy, delivery action must be planned and completed in a multidisciplinary approach against the risk of bleeding. In case regional anesthesia will be applied, heparin must be discontinued 24 h before the delivery. If there is no bleeding 12 h after the caesarean section or 6 h after the normal vaginal delivery, heparin must be restarted. Anticoagulant therapy should be planned to last for a minimum of 3 months in total and must continue for at least >6 weeks following delivery since the postpartum period constitutes the highest risk period for PE recurrence. Warfarin can be used in the postpartum period and in breastfeeding mothers. Use of NOACs is not recommended in pregnant and breastfeeding women [34].

There are not enough studies researching the efficiency and reliability of thrombolytic therapy in pregnant women. Even though thrombolytic therapy is not recommended in pregnant women, it must be used in case of high-risk, life-threatening PE. In the ESC guideline, tissue-plasminogen activator (tPA) is recommended as a thrombolytic agent to be used in acute PE during pregnancy [35]Considering studies demonstrating that t-PA is as efficient at the standard dose and at the same time more reliable in terms of bleeding in life threatening—high-risk PE pregnant women [36, 37], the patient can be evaluated in terms of reduced dose rt-PA (0.6 mg/kg, maximum 50 mg/2 h infusion) implementation.

Thrombolytic therapy and surgical embolectomy are recommended for high-risk PE pregnant women [8].

Even though there are a limited number of studies on the use of vena cava filters in pregnant women, it has been indicated that they have similar indications as for non-pregnant PE patients [8].

Last but not least, the effects of thromboprophylaxis during pregnancy and the early postnatal period on the risk of venous thromboembolic disease and adverse effects in women at increased risk of VTE have been assessed in a recent metanalysis [38]. The evidence was found to be uncertain on the benefit or harm of VTE thromboprophylaxis in women during pregnancy and the early postnatal period at increased risk of VTE after analysis of twenty-nine trials (involving 3839 women), including heparin (LMWH and UFH), hydroxyethyl starch (HES) and compression stockings or device interventions. Therefore, further randomized trials with large sample sizes are needed to conclude on the effects of currently used interventions to prevent VTE in women during pregnancy and the postpartum period.

64.4 Amniotic Fluid Embolism

Non-thrombotic PE is defined as the embolization of non-thrombotic material originating from many different cell types as well as non-biologic or foreign materials to the pulmonary vasculature. Amniotic fluid embolism (AFE) is a rare condition characterized by unexplained sudden cardiovascular or respiratory deterioration presenting with mental status changes, central nervous system irritability and a cutaneous rash, and accompanied by disseminated intravascular coagulation during pregnancy or after delivery. Previously, amniotic fluid embolism (AFE) was thought to occur during normal labor via uterine vein tears or during cesarean section due to the entrance of amniotic fluid into the maternal circulation. However, an immunological origin has been postulated as an underlying mechanism due to the absence of mechanical obstruction of pulmonary blood flow in AFE [39]. Pre-existing cardiac, cerebrovascular and renal disorders, placenta previa, polyhydramnios, stillbirth, chorioamnionitis, hypertensive disorders, instrumental delivery and caesarean section are suggested as risk factors for AFE [8].

AFE remains a rare occurrence with an incidence of approximately 2–7/100,000 births and a mortality rate of 0.5–6 deaths per 100,000 deliveries [40–42].

Bilateral homogeneous opacities suggestive of pulmonary edema can be found on chest X-ray and diffuse bilateral ground glass opacities are observed on thorax computed tomography scan.

Management of AFE is supported by the treatment of bleeding and coagulopathy [8].

References

1. Marik PE, Plante LA. Venous thromboembolic disease and pregnancy. N Engl J Med. 2008;359(19):2025–33.
2. Stone SE, Morris TA. Pulmonary embolism during and after pregnancy. Crit Care Med. 2005;33(10 Suppl):S294–300.

3. Bates SM, Greer IA, Hirsh J, Ginsberg JS. Use of antithrombotic agents during pregnancy: the seventh ACCP conference on antithrombotic and thrombolytic therapy. Chest. 2004;126:627–44.
4. Royal College of Obstetricians and Gynecologists. Reducing the risk of venous thromboembolism during pregnancy and the puerperium. Green-top Guideline 2015; No. 37a.
5. Gherman RB, Goodwin TM, Leung B, Byrne JD, Hethumumi R, Montoro M. Incidence, clinical characteristics, and timing of objectively diagnosed venous thromboembolism during pregnancy. Obstet Gynecol. 1999;94:730–4.
6. Cutts BA, Tran HA, Merriman E, Nandurkar D, Soo G, Dasgupta D, et al. The utility of the Wells clinical prediction model and ventilation-perfusion scanning for pulmonary embolism diagnosis in pregnancy. Blood Coagul Fibrinolysis. 2014;25:375–8.
7. Kovac M, Mikovic Z, Rakicevic L, Srzentic S, Mandic V, Djordjevic V, et al. The use of D-dimer with new cutoff can be useful in diagnosis of venous thromboembolism in pregnancy. Eur J Obstet Gynecol Reprod Biol. 2010;148(1):27–30.
8. Konstantinides SV, Meyer G, Becattini C, Bueno H, Geersing GJ, Harjola VP, et al. 2019 ESC guidelines for the diagnosis and management of acute pulmonary embolism developed in collaboration with the European Respiratory Society (ERS): the task force for the diagnosis and management of acute pulmonary embolism of the European Society of Cardiology (ESC). Eur Respir J. 2019;54:1901647.
9. Tanaka H, Tanaka K, Katsuragi S, Hayata E, Nakata M, Hasegawa J, Sekizawa A, Ishiwata I, Ikeda T. Pulmonary thromboembolism during pregnancy and puerperium: comparison of survival and death cases. J Obstet Gynaecol Res. 2021;47(4):1312–21. https://doi.org/10.1111/jog.14687. Epub 2021 Feb 1
10. Battinelli EM, Marshall A, Connors JM. The role of thrombophilia in pregnancy. Thrombosis. 2013;2013:516420.
11. Thromboembolism in Pregnancy. Practice Bulletin No. 123. American College of Obstetricians and Gynecologists. Obstet Gynecol. 2011;118:718–29.
12. Leung AN, Bull TM, Jaeschke R, Lockwood CJ, Boiselle PM, Hurwitz LM, et al. An official American Thoracic Society/Society of Thoracic Radiology clinical practice guideline: evaluation of suspected pulmonary embolism in pregnancy. Am J Respir Crit Care Med. 2011;184(10):1200–8.
13. Chabloz P, Reber G, Boehlen F, Hohlfeld P, de Moerloose P. TAFI antigen and D-dimer levels during normal pregnancy and at delivery. Br J Haematol. 2001;115:150–2.
14. Polak JF, Wilkinson DL. Ultrasonographic diagnosis of symptomatic deep venous thrombosis in pregnancy. Am J Obstet Gynecol. 1991;165(3):625–9.
15. Leung AN, Bull TM, Jaeschke R, Lockwood CJ, Boiselle PM, Hurwitz LM, et al. An Official American Thoracic Society/Society of Thoracic Radiology Clinical Practice guideline:evaluation of suspected pulmonary embolism in pregnancy. Am J Respir Crit Care Med. 2011;184:1200–8. https://doi.org/10.1164/rccm.201108-1575ST.
16. McCollough CH, Schueler BA, Atwell TD, Braun NN, Regner DM, Brown DL, LeRoy AJ. AJ. Radiation exposure and pregnancy: when should we be concerned? Radiographics. 2007;27(4):909–17.; discussion 917-8. https://doi.org/10.1148/rg.274065149. PMID: 17620458.
17. Chen MM, Coakley FV, Kaimal A, Laros RK Jr. Guidelines for computed tomography and magnetic resonance imaging use during pregnancy and lactation. Obstet Gynecol. 2008;112(2 Pt 1):333–40. https://doi.org/10.1097/AOG.0b013e318180a505. PMID: 18669732
18. Ridge CA, McDermott S, Freyne BJ, Brennan DJ, Collins CD, Skehan SJ. Pulmonary embolism in pregnancy: comparison of pulmonary CT angiography and lung scintigraphy. AJR Am J Roentgenol. 2009;193:1223–7.
19. Worsley DF, Alavi A, Aronchick JM, Chen JT, Greenspan RH, Ravin CE. Chest radiographic findings in patients with acute pulmonary embolism: observations from the PIOPED study. Radiology. 1993;189:133–6.
20. Han D, Lee KS, Franquet T, Müller NL, Kim TS, Kim H, et al. Thrombotic and nonthrombotic pulmonary arterial embolism: spectrum of imaging findings. Radiographics. 2003;23:1521–39.

21. Kluetz PG, White CS. Acute pulmonary embolism: imaging in the emergency department. Radiol Clin N Am. 2006;44:259–71.
22. Elliott CG, Goldhaber SZ, Visani L, DeRosa M. Chest radiographs in acute pulmonary embolism. Results from the international cooperative pulmonary embolism registry. Chest. 2000;118:33–8.
23. Stein PD, Athanasoulis C, Greenspan RH, Henry JW. Relation of plain chest radiographic findings to pulmonary arterial pressure and arterial blood oxygen levels in patients with acute pulmonary embolism. Am J Cardiol. 1992;69:394–6.
24. Food and Drug Administration, HHS. Content and format of labeling for human prescription drug and biological products; requirements for pregnancy and lactation labeling. Final rule. Fed Regist. 2014;79(233):72063–103.
25. Leung AN, Bull TM, Jaeschke R, Lockwood CJ, Boiselle PM, Hurwitz LM, et al. An Official American Thoracic Society/Society of Thoracic Radiology Clinical Practice guideline: evaluation of suspected pulmonary embolism in pregnancy. Am J Respir Crit Care Med. 2011;184:1200–8. https://doi.org/10.1164/rccm.201108-1575ST.
26. Leung AN, Bull TM, Jaeschke R, Lockwood CJ, Boiselle PM, Hurwitz LM, et al. American Thoracic Society documents: an official American Thoracic Society/Society of Thoracic Radiology Clinical Practice Guideline—Evaluation of suspected pulmonary embolism in pregnancy. Radiology. 2012;262:635–46. https://doi.org/10.1148/radiol.11114045.
27. Crowther MA, Spitzer K, Julian J, Ginsberg J, Johnston M, Crowther R, et al. Pharmacokinetic profile of a lowmolecular weight heparin (reviparin) in pregnant patients. A prospective cohort study. Thromb Res. 2000;98:133–8.
28. Smith MP, Norris LA, Steer PJ, Savidge GF, Bonnar J. Tinzaparin sodium for thrombosis treatment and prevention during pregnancy. Am J Obstet Gynecol. 2004;190:495–501.
29. Bates SM, Greer IA, Middeldorp S, Veenstra DL, Prabulos AM, Vandvik PO. VTE, thrombophilia, antithrombotic therapy, and pregnancy: antithrombotic therapy and prevention of thrombosis, 9th ed: American College of Chest Physicians Evidence-Based Clinical Practice Guidelines. Chest. 2012;141(Suppl 2):e691–736. https://doi.org/10.1378/chest.11-2300.
30. Baglin T, Barrowcliffe TW, Cohen A, Greaves M. British Committee for Standards in Haematology Guidelines on the use and monitoring of heparin. Br J Haematol. 2006;133:19.
31. Greer I, Hunt BJ. Low molecular weight heparin in pregnancy: current issues. Br J Haematol. 2005;128:593–601.
32. Greer IA. Prevention and mangement of venous thromboembolism in pregnancy. Clin Chest Med. 2003;24:123–37.
33. Dempfle CE. Minor transplacental passage of fondaparinux in vivo. N Engl J Med. 2004;350:1914–5.
34. Cohen H, Arachchillage DR, Middeldorp S, Beyer-Westendorf J, Abdul-Kadir R. Management of direct oral anticoagulants in women of childbearing potential: guidance from the SSC of the ISTH. J Thromb Haemost. 2016;14:1673–6.
35. Konstantinides SV, Torbicki A, Agnelli G, Danchin N, Fitzmaurice D, Galiè N, et al. ESC guidelines on the diagnosis and management of acute pulmonary embolism. Eur Heart J. 2014;35:3033–69, 3069a–3069k. https://doi.org/10.1093/eurheartj/ehu283.
36. Zhang Z, Zhai Z, Liang L, Dai H, Huang K, Lu W, et al. Lower dosage of recombinant tissue-type plasminogen activator (rt-PA) in the treatment of acute pulmonary embolism: a systematic review and metaanalysis. Thromb Res. 2014;133:357–63.
37. Meyer G, Vicaut E, Danays T, Agnelli G, Becattini C, Beyer-Westendorf J, et al. Fibrinolysis for patients with intermediaterisk pulmonary embolism. N Engl J Med. 2014;370:1402–11. https://doi.org/10.1056/NEJMoa1302097.
38. Middleton P, Shepherd E, Gomersall JC. Venous thromboembolism prophylaxis for women at risk during pregnancy and the early postnatal period. Cochrane Database Syst Rev. 2021;3:CD001689. https://doi.org/10.1002/14651858.CD001689.pub4.
39. McCabe BE, Veselis CA, Goykhman I, Hochhold J, Eisenberg D, Son H. Beyond pulmonary embolism; nonthrombotic pulmonary embolism as diagnostic challenges. Curr Probl

Diagn Radiol. 2019;48(4):387–92. https://doi.org/10.1067/j.cpradiol.2018.07.007. Epub 2018 Aug 17
40. Fitzpatrick KE, Tuffnell D, Kurinczuk JJ, Knight M. Incidence, risk factors, management and outcomes of amniotic-fluid embolism: a population-based cohort and nested case-control study. BJOG. 2016;123:100–9.
41. Society for Maternal-Fetal Medicine, Pacheco LD, Saade G, Hankins GD, Clark SL. Amniotic fluid embolism: diagnosis and management. Am J Obstet Gynecol. 2016;215:B16–24.
42. Clark SL, Romero R, Dildy GA, et al. Proposed diagnostic criteria for the case definition of amniotic fluid embolism in research studies. Am J Obstet Gynecol. 2016;215:408–12.

Asthma During Pregnancy and Lactation

65

Özge Oral Tapan and Sebahat Genç

65.1 Introduction

Asthma is one of the most common medical conditions encountered during pregnancy, occurring in 3–8% of pregnant women [1–3]. Pregnancy may also be associated with changes in the course of asthma that were previously present, and asthma may affect pregnancy outcomes.

The principles of pharmacologic therapy for asthma during pregnancy are similar to those in nonpregnant patients. When considering the use of asthma medications in a pregnant woman or anticipates pregnancy, concerns about the potential risks of asthma medication are generally outweighed by the possible adverse effects of untreated asthma.

The management of asthma in pregnancy, including the safety data for specific asthma medications, general management, and recommended pharmacotherapy for acute and chronic asthma in pregnancy, is reviewed under this topic.

65.2 Respiratory Physiology During Pregnancy

Throughout pregnancy, spirometry remains within normal limits, with forced vital capacity (FVC), forced expiratory volume in 1 s (FEV1), and PEF not changing or modestly increasing with unaltered FEV1/FVC index [4–9].

Conversely, lung volumes undergo significant changes: Expiratory reserve volume (ERV) gradually decreases during the second half of pregnancy (reduction of 8–40% at term) because residual volume reduces (by 7–22%). Functional residual

Ö. O. Tapan (✉) · S. Genç
Medical Faculty, Department of Pulmonology, Muğla Sıtkı Koçman University,
Muğla, Turkey
e-mail: ozgeoral@mu.edu.tr; sebahatgenc@mu.edu.tr

C. Cingi et al. (eds.), *ENT Diseases: Diagnosis and Treatment during Pregnancy and Lactation*, https://doi.org/10.1007/978-3-031-05303-0_65

capacity (FRC) then decreases (by 9.5–25%) while inspiratory capacity increases at the same rate to maintain stable [4–6].

Respiratory resistance increases while respiratory conductance decreases during pregnancy. Total pulmonary and airway resistances tend to decrease in late pregnancy due to hormonally induced relaxation of tracheobronchial tree smooth muscles [4, 5, 8].

Pulmonary static and dynamic compliance, diffusing capacity, and static lung recoil pressure does not change during pregnancy [4, 5, 10].

The respiratory function does not differ between singleton and twin pregnancies [7]. Although spirometry is minimally affected by a pregnancy, some pulmonary function test measurements change during pregnancy. Vital capacity (VC) and total lung capacity (TLC) are usually preserved during pregnancy due to increased mobility and flaring of the ribs and unimpaired diaphragmatic excursion. However, TLC may decrease slightly in the last trimester. In contrast, residual volume (RV) and FRC usually decrease during gestation due to diaphragm elevation from the enlarging uterus.

As in nonpregnant patients, the diagnosis of asthma can be confirmed by demonstrating reversible airflow limitation before and after bronchodilator inhalation or before and after initiation of empiric treatment for asthma. Bronchoprovocation challenge is generally avoided during pregnancy, so limited data are available about maternal airway hyperresponsiveness during pregnancy [11].

Minute ventilation increases during pregnancy, presumably due to increased circulating levels of progesterone [12]. The increase in minute ventilation, which exceeds metabolic demands, lowers alveolar and arterial tension of carbon dioxide ($PaCO_2$) while simultaneously increasing alveolar and arterial oxygen tension (PAO_2 and PaO_2). The resulting respiratory alkalosis induces secondary compensation through renal loss of bicarbonate. Thus, normal blood gases during pregnancy reveal a higher PaO_2 (100–106 mmHg (13.1–14.1 kPa)) and a lower $PaCO_2$ (28–30 mmHg (3.72–3.99 kPa)) than in the nonpregnant state, typically accompanied by a slightly alkalotic pH.

During an acute asthma exacerbation, any associated changes in blood gases are superimposed on the "normal" respiratory alkalosis of pregnancy. Thus, a $PaCO_2 > 35$ mmHg (4.66 kPa) or a $PaO_2 < 70$ mmHg (9.31 kPa) associated with acute asthma represent a more severe compromise during pregnancy than in the nongravid state.

Arterial oxygen tension PaO_2 in the fetus is only about one-third to one-fourth of the PaO_2 in the adult [13]. The fetus thrives typically at this low oxygen level due to several compensations, such as fetal hemoglobin and changes in the oxyhemoglobin dissociation curve. However, fetal oxygenation may be threatened in many ways that are potentially relevant to gestational asthma. First, maternal hypoxemia directly reduces the oxygen supply to the fetus. Second, hypocapnia and/or alkalosis may cause fetal hypoxia, although the exact mechanism is unclear. Finally, a reduction in uterine blood flow (potentially due to exogenous or endogenous vasoconstrictors, dehydration, hypotension, or significant maternal alkalosis) may compromise fetal oxygenation. It appears that the fetus can compensate for hypoxemia in some ways, including redistribution of circulation to vital organs, decreased gross body movements, and increased tissue oxygen extraction. The exact level and duration of fetal hypoxemia that exceed these compensatory mechanisms are not defined in humans. A typical response to chronic hypoxia is deferment of growth needs in favor of vital functions, resulting in a small gestational age fetus.

65.3 Effects of Pregnancy on Asthma

The clinical effect of pregnancy on asthma is variable [13–16]. This was illustrated by a prospective study that followed 366 pregnancies in 330 asthmatic women [17]. Asthma worsened during pregnancy in 35%, improved in 28%, and was unchanged in 33%; 4% were uncertain about a change. Most studies suggest that asthma severity before pregnancy predicts asthma severity during pregnancy [15–18]. The following additional trends were noted among 330 pregnant women with asthma [17]:

- In women who improved, the improvement was gradual as the pregnancy progressed.
- In women whose asthma worsened, the increase in symptoms was most prominent between weeks 29 and 36 of gestation, although other studies have reported increased asthma exacerbations in weeks 14–24 [18].
- Asthma was generally less severe during the last 4 weeks of pregnancy.
- Substantial asthma symptoms were uncommon during labor and delivery.
- The course of asthma in successive pregnancies in an individual patient tended to be similar.

Asthma exacerbations occur in 20–36% of pregnant asthmatic patients [17, 18]. Being overweight or obese [19] and excessive first-trimester weight gain [20] have been identified as risk factors for asthma exacerbations during pregnancy. Other studies have shown that asthma exacerbations are more common and more severe in women who smoke during pregnancy [21] and that maternal anxiety increases the risk of asthma exacerbations [22]. These exacerbations are not uniformly distributed throughout pregnancy. In one observational study that followed 504 pregnant asthmatic patients, exacerbations occurred most frequently during weeks 17 through 24 of pregnancy [18]. A similar observational study of 146 patients revealed a peak incidence of severe asthma exacerbations during weeks 14 through 24 of pregnancy and a peak incidence of mild asthma exacerbations during weeks 25 through 32 [18].

The reason for the unequal distribution of asthma exacerbations throughout gestation is unclear. However, it has been demonstrated that many women decrease or stop taking their asthma medication shortly after becoming aware of the pregnancy [18, 22–24], which can lead to subsequent deterioration in asthma control. In particular, inadequate use of inhaled glucocorticoids may increase the risk of an asthma exacerbation [14, 18]. In one of the prospective studies mentioned above, only 4% of women taking inhaled glucocorticoids continuously from the start of pregnancy developed an acute attack, compared with 17% of women who were not [18].

65.4 Maintaining Asthma Control

The two primary goals of asthma management are prevention of acute exacerbations and optimization of ongoing asthma control. These are not changed in pregnancy settings and should serve to maximize both maternal and fetal health [3]. While the use of any medication during pregnancy raises concerns about potential adverse effects on the mother or fetus, the benefit of active treatment to maintain asthma control and prevent exacerbations outweighs the potential risks of routinely used asthma medications.

65.4.1 Pharmacological Therapy

The general principles of pharmacologic therapy for asthma during pregnancy are similar to those in nonpregnant patients. They involve a step-wise approach to achieve and maintain asthma control, as recommended by national and international guidelines (Table 65.1).

Current guidelines emphasize the following points [18, 25–27]:

- All patients should have access to an inhaler for quick relief of asthma symptoms. Choices include a short-acting beta-agonist (e.g., albuterol) or a combination inhaler with formoterol and a low-dose inhaled glucocorticoid (e.g., formoterol-budesonide).
- For patients with mild persistent or more severe asthma, inhaled glucocorticoids reduce exacerbations during pregnancy, and cessation of inhaled glucocorticoids

Table 65.1 Asthma medications and safety categories that can be used during pregnancy

Medicine	Security category of the drug
Salbutamol	C
Terbutaline	C
Albuterol	C
Formoterol	C
Salmeterol	C
Beclomethasone	C
Budesonide	B
Fluticasone	C
Mometasone	C
Triamcinolone	C
Ciclesonide	C
Flunisolide	C
Systemic corticosteroids	C
Salmeterol/fluticasone C	C
Montelukast	B
Theophylline	C
Anti IgE (Omalizumab)	B

during pregnancy increases the risk of an exacerbation. Budesonide has been the preferred inhaled glucocorticoid for use during pregnancy, as more published gestational human data are available for that medication [28, 29]. However, other inhaled glucocorticoids could be continued if the patient was well-controlled on one of these medications before pregnancy. More recent data for fluticasone have been reassuring regarding low birth weight (<2500 g), small for gestational age (<10th percentile for babies of same gestational age), preterm birth (<37 weeks) [30], and major congenital malformations [31].

- Salmeterol has been recommended as the inhaled long-acting beta-agonist of choice in the United States due to the longer duration of clinical experience with this agent compared with formoterol. However, retrospective cohort studies provide reassuring data for both salmeterol and formoterol [30, 32].
- Montelukast could be considered an alternative but not preferred therapy for mild persistent asthma or add-on therapy to inhaled glucocorticoids, especially for patients who have shown a uniquely favorable response before pregnancy. More pregnancy data are available for montelukast than zafirlukast.

The short-acting, beta-2 adrenergic bronchodilators (SABAs) are used to provide quick relief of asthma symptoms and appear to be relatively safe during pregnancy. However, some case-control studies have suggested a slight increase in the risk of specific infant abnormalities, as noted by the following reports:

A small increased risk of gastroschisis was reported among infants exposed in utero to bronchodilators [33].

In a case-control study using European registry data, gastroschisis (odds ratio [OR] 1.89, 95% CI 1.12–3.20) and cleft palate (OR 1.63, 95% CI 1.05–2.52) were associated with a greater likelihood of first trimester beta-agonist exposure [34].

An association with cardiac defects was noted in a cohort study that examined the effect of exposure to bronchodilator therapy during pregnancy [33].

A case-control study reported a 30% increased risk (OR 1.3, 95% CI 1.1–1.5) of autism spectrum disorder in children exposed to maternal beta-2 adrenergic receptor agonist drugs during gestation [35].

One problem with assessing the consequences of bronchodilator use in pregnancy is confounding introduced by indication; SABA use is a marker for poorly controlled asthma and more frequent exacerbations, which may independently contribute to the development of congenital anomalies [36]. Furthermore, some studies only have access to data about prescriptions filled and not the frequency of actual use [37]. Even if the statistical associations for relative risk are valid, the anomalies mentioned above are infrequent. Therefore, the absolute increase in risk is minimal and, as noted earlier, less than the risk of poorly controlled maternal asthma.

Clinical experience with inhalation of the long-acting, selective beta-2 adrenergic bronchodilators (LABAs) during pregnancy is less extensive than with the SABAs (Table 65.1). Salmeterol is not expected to increase the risk of congenital anomalies, based on data from animal studies and limited human experience [38]. Animal studies are also reassuring for formoterol, although data from human pregnancies are limited [39, 40]. A retrospective database study showed that salmeterol and formoterol do not increase the risk of delivering low birth weight, small for gestational age, or preterm infants [30, 32]. Given these findings, a continuation of a LABA during pregnancy is reasonable if a LABA has been needed (in combination with an inhaled glucocorticoid) to achieve asthma control before pregnancy [18, 26].

Human safety data for newer LABAs, such as indacaterol, olodaterol, and vilanterol, are lacking. Some adverse effects were noted in animal studies of olodaterol but are not reported with indacaterol or vilanterol. Of these agents, the only one available in an inhaled glucocorticoid combination inhaler is vilanterol, which is available with fluticasone furoate.

When comparing a combination LABA plus inhaled glucocorticoid versus monotherapy with a higher dose of the inhaled glucocorticoid, the risk of congenital malformations appears similar. In a study of 1302 pregnant women with asthma, the OR for a major congenital malformation (MCM) was not increased (OR 1.1, 95% CI 0.6–1.9) when a LABA plus low dose inhaled glucocorticoid was compared with a medium dose inhaled glucocorticoid or when a LABA plus medium-dose inhaled glucocorticoid was compared with a high-dose inhaled glucocorticoid (OR 1.2, 95% CI 0.5–2.7) [41].

Systemic glucocorticoids have been used relatively extensively during pregnancy to treat asthma exacerbations and rarely control severe asthma. For each pregnant woman, the potential risks of gestational oral glucocorticoids must be balanced against the risks to the mother or infant of inadequately treated asthma. As the dangers of severe uncontrolled asthma include maternal or fetal mortality, these risks are more significant than the potential risk of systemic glucocorticoids. Thus, oral glucocorticoids should be used during pregnancy when indicated to manage severe asthma [27, 42].

Several potential areas of concern have been raised with systemic glucocorticoids: congenital malformations (primarily cleft palate), preeclampsia, gestational diabetes, low birth weight, and neonatal adrenal insufficiency. Among the studies in which systemic glucocorticoids were used for the management of asthma during pregnancy [29, 30, 33, 35, 43, 44], some showed a slightly increased risk of prematurity and a somewhat higher risk of low birth weight (<2500 g) [33, 43, 44].

Data from animal studies in several species suggest that high dose systemic glucocorticoids may lead to cleft palate. Human studies are less concerning, but a possible effect cannot be dismissed. Palatal closure is usually complete by the 12th week of pregnancy, so that the potential risk would be limited to administration during the first trimester. The risk of cleft lip/palate with systemic glucocorticoid use is discussed separately.

A large, prospective cohort study of 2123 pregnant women with asthma recruited from 16 centers in the United States in the period from December 1994 to February 2000 found that oral glucocorticoid use was significantly associated with preterm birth (before 37 weeks of gestation, OR 1.54, 95% CI 1.02–2.33) and low birth weight (<2500 g, OR 1.80, 95% CI 1.13–2.88) [43]. Increased prematurity and/or lower birth weights have been noted in other studies as well [29, 33, 44–49]. The authors did not evaluate the relationship between these effects and the dose or duration of therapy.

An increased risk of preeclampsia has been associated with oral glucocorticoid use in several studies [43, 50, 51]. Neonatal adrenal insufficiency following maternal glucocorticoid administration is distinctly unusual, probably because the nonhalogenated glucocorticoids are metabolized mainly to inactive metabolites by the placenta [47]. Gestational diabetes and hypertension are additional potential maternal complications of systemic glucocorticoid administration [50].

However, it remains possible that the consequences of severe uncontrolled asthma caused some or all of these reported adverse effects, given that asthma symptoms were powerful enough to require oral glucocorticoids.

In contrast with oral/systemic glucocorticoids, the safety data on inhaled glucocorticoids are reassuring [47–50, 52–58]. Budesonide, beclomethasone, and fluticasone are preferred among the inhaled glucocorticoids as more safety information is available for these agents [3, 18]. However, if the patient's asthma was already well-controlled on an alternate agent (e.g., ciclesonide, mometasone) before pregnancy, there is no need to change therapy.

In a population-based study using the United Kingdom's Clinical Practice Research Datalink, the risk of MCM was assessed among 5362 pregnancies with inhaled glucocorticoid exposure during the first trimester and known fetal outcomes at 1 year of age [31]. Eighty-nine MCMs were identified following exposure to non-fluticasone-inhaled glucocorticoids and 42 following exposure to fluticasone propionate (overall 2.4%). When fluticasone was compared with other inhaled glucocorticoids, the adjusted OR for MCM was 1.1 (95% CI 0.5–2.3), suggesting no increase in risk with fluticasone.

In a retrospective database study, the ORs of low birth weight, preterm, or small for gestational age were not significantly different in infants from 3190 mothers exposed to fluticasone propionate than 608 mothers exposed to budesonide [30].

A separate study of 13,280 pregnancies in women with asthma confirmed that low to moderate doses of inhaled glucocorticoids was NOT associated with an increased risk of congenital malformations. However, the use of high doses (>1000 mcg/day) during the first trimester was associated with a 63% increase in the risk of all congenital malformations [48]. The strength of this observation is limited because the study was underpowered to assess the risk of specific malformations, such as cleft palate, which has been associated with maternal use of systemic glucocorticoids. In addition, the authors could not exclude the possibility that greater asthma severity contributed to the overall increased risk of malformations. Benefit-risk considerations favor using high dose inhaled glucocorticoids over a lower amount when needed for asthma control to avoid the use of systemic oral glucocorticoids, with the potential risks listed above.

Two randomized trials support the efficacy and safety of inhaled glucocorticoids during pregnancy. One study assessed 84 pregnant women managed with or without inhaled beclomethasone after discharge following an asthma hospitalization during pregnancy [59]. This medication significantly decreased the rate of readmission for asthma (12% versus 33%), and no adverse events or outcomes were reported. A subsequent study compared inhaled beclomethasone to theophylline to manage moderate asthma during pregnancy [54]. Although exacerbation rates were similar in the two groups, pulmonary function was better in the beclomethasone group, and fewer patients in the beclomethasone group discontinued therapy due to side effects.

Muscarinic antagonists (also known as anticholinergic agents), such as ipratropium, glycopyrrolate, and tiotropium, are not generally used as primary therapy for asthma. However, questions may arise about their safety during pregnancy.

The minimal chronotropic effect of inhaled ipratropium in the mother suggests that the inhaled preparation should have negligible chronotropic effects on the fetus. Gestational animal studies are also reassuring for ipratropium [50]. Consequently, inhaled ipratropium, which is sometimes used for quick relief of asthma symptoms during an exacerbation, is felt to be safe for intermittent use during pregnancy [27].

The inhaled long-acting muscarinic antagonist (LAMA), tiotropium, is approved by the US Food and Drug Administration (FDA) for asthma but is usually reserved for patients with moderate-to-severe asthma, which is not controlled a LABA-inhaled glucocorticoid combination. The safety of inhaled tiotropium during pregnancy is uncertain as adverse effects were reported with high doses in animal studies, and human fetal outcomes have not been reported [18]. Other LAMAs (e.g., aclidinium, glycopyrrolate, and umeclidinium) are not approved for use in asthma, although it is reasonable to assume that they would have similar effects.

Montelukast and zafirlukast (leukotriene receptor antagonists) and zileuton (a 5-lipoxygenase inhibitor) affect leukotriene synthesis or action. We suggest using montelukast in preference to zileuton. We would reserve these agents for add-on therapy to inhaled glucocorticoids, especially in patients who had an excellent response to this medication before pregnancy [27].

The first prospective, controlled study of leukotriene receptor antagonists in pregnancy followed 96 women taking these medications, 122 women taking SABAs only, and 346 women without asthma. No increase in significant congenital disabilities or adverse outcomes was detected in the offspring of patients receiving these medications [54]. A subsequent study with a similar design described 180 montelukast-exposed pregnancies compared to 180 disease-matched controls and 180 pregnancies in non-asthmatic women. In this study, montelukast did not appear to increase the baseline rate of major malformations, although lower birth weights were seen in both asthmatic groups [58]. More extensive studies are needed to detect small increases in adverse pregnancy outcomes or rare congenital disabilities.

A large retrospective insurance claims cohort analysis compared the incidences of selected congenital malformations in infants of mothers exposed to montelukast ($n = 1535$), inhaled corticosteroids ($n = 3918$), other asthma medications ($n = 8834$), and controls with no asthma medications or asthma diagnoses ($n = 38,828$) [60]. No significant differences between groups were observed.

No teratogenicity was observed with montelukast given to rats or rabbits at doses greater than 300 times the maximum human daily oral dose on an mg/m^2 basis [61, 62]. Human studies are reassuring, although the numbers of pregnant women included are small.

In contrast, adverse events were noted in animal reproduction studies of zileuton, and adequate studies of zileuton in pregnant women are lacking [63].

The initiation of subcutaneous or sublingual allergen immunotherapy is not recommended during pregnancy due to the potential harm to the fetus should a systemic allergic reaction occur [43, 64]. However, patients who tolerate maintenance immunotherapy (or at least a substantial dosage) and derive benefit may continue it. Immunotherapy during pregnancy is discussed in more detail separately.

Omalizumab is a humanized, recombinant IgG1; monoclonal anti-immunoglobulin E antibody approved for add-on therapy in patients with moderate to severe asthma inadequately controlled despite appropriate use of inhaled glucocorticoids. Studies of the safety of omalizumab in pregnancy are limited, although available data are reassuring. Immunoglobulin G molecules, such as omalizumab, are known to cross the placenta.

A prospective observational registry study reported pregnancy outcomes of 250 pregnant women exposed to omalizumab [65]. The incidences of prematurity (15%), small for gestational age (9.7%), and MCMs were not substantially different from outcomes reported in other studies of women with more severe asthma. The initiation of omalizumab during pregnancy is not recommended. However, if a woman becomes pregnant while receiving omalizumab, it is suggested that therapy can be continued if the benefits are estimated to outweigh the potential harms. The anti-interleukin (IL)-5 antibody preparations, benralizumab, mepolizumab, and reslizumab, are approved by the FDA for add-on maintenance therapy in patients with severe eosinophilic asthma. The use of these agents in severe asthma is discussed separately. Monoclonal antibodies, including benralizumab, mepolizumab, and reslizumab, are likely to cross the placenta in increasing amounts as pregnancy progresses [66, 67].

Methylxanthines and cromoglycates are rarely used to manage asthma due to the availability of alternative agents with greater effectiveness and ease of use. The clinical use of methylxanthines (theophylline, aminophylline) during pregnancy is limited because of the potential for altered metabolism during pregnancy, the need for drug level monitoring, and the potential for fetal tachycardia and irritability at the time of delivery. Moreover, inhaled glucocorticoids are more effective than theophylline for persistent asthma in nonpregnant patients and at least as effective as theophylline, with fewer side effects in pregnant women [54]. Extensive clinical experience suggests that theophylline does not increase the risk of fetal anomalies [3, 68]. Methylxanthines binding to albumin and hepatic clearance is altered during pregnancy, necessitating careful assessment of serum levels and adjustments to dosing throughout pregnancy. Like the beta-2 adrenergic agonists, theophylline can inhibit uterine muscle contraction in vitro, but this effect is not clinically significant. Methylxanthines are transferred across the placenta, leading to theophylline concentrations in neonatal and cord blood similar to those in maternal blood [69]. Transient tachycardia and irritability have been reported in some neonates of mothers receiving methylxanthines.

The availability of the cromolyn sodium and nedocromil is limited and varies from one country to another. Animal and limited human data on use during pregnancy ($n = 318$) have not demonstrated an increase in fetal malformations or other adverse effects with cromolyn sodium [29, 35]. The one study that reported an increase in musculoskeletal abnormalities with maternal use of chromones had a tiny number of exposures ($n = 5$), limiting the strength of the observation [34].

The categorization of drugs used in pregnancy was made by the FDA (ABCDX) in 1979 [33, 66]. In 2015, it was further developed and changed with the Pregnancy and Lactation Labeling Rule (PLLR) system. This system is grouped into (1) pregnancy, childbirth, (2) lactation, and (3) men and women of reproductive potential and includes risk, clinical practice, and backup data for each drug. It is thought that the transition to this system will take some time.

65.4.2 Non-pharmacologic Treatments

The primary non-pharmacologic interventions to maintain asthma control during pregnancy are patient education, avoidance of irritants (e.g., cigarette smoke), and management of allergenic triggers of asthma.

The principles of patient education are generally similar for pregnant and non-pregnant patients with asthma. Important issues include early recognition of signs and symptoms of an asthma exacerbation, avoidance of precipitating factors, correct use of medications, and developing a treatment plan for acute exacerbations.

65.4.2.1 Patient Education

The primary issues specific to pregnancy are education about the interrelationships between asthma and pregnancy and the safety of asthma medications during pregnancy. The clinician should clearly explain that it is safer for pregnant women with asthma to take asthma medications than to have ongoing symptoms or exacerbations of asthma [26, 36, 70]. Women should be reassured that safe and adequate asthma treatment is possible during pregnancy and that reasonable asthma control can help minimize the risk of complications [3].

65.4.2.2 Smoking Cessation

The pregnant asthmatic mother must discontinue smoking during pregnancy [63]. First, smoking may predispose the patient to asthma exacerbations, bronchitis, or sinusitis, necessitating an increased need for medication [21]. Second, cigarette smoking is associated with numerous adverse pregnancy outcomes, including spontaneous pregnancy loss, placental abruption, preterm premature rupture of membranes (PPROM), placenta previa, preterm labor and delivery, low birth weight, and ectopic pregnancy. The risks associated with maternal smoking during pregnancy and methods to enable smoking cessation are discussed separately.

65.4.2.3 Control of Environmental Triggers

Control of environmental triggers is an essential component of asthma management during pregnancy as it helps reduce the need for pharmacologic intervention. This includes avoiding exposure to allergens and nonspecific airway irritants, such as tobacco smoke, dust, and environmental pollutants. Particular allergens of concern are dander from pets and antigens from household dust mites.

Careful follow-up by clinicians experienced in managing asthma is essential. The optimal frequency of asthma evaluations is not known; generally, the frequency is determined based on the prepregnancy degree of asthma control. In an observational study, visits every 4 weeks improved adherence to controller medication and asthma control [59]. All pregnant patients should have ready access to their clinician should their symptoms change or increase. It is also essential that effective communication exists among the clinician managing asthma, the patient, and the obstetrician.

Asthmatic symptoms are often most remarkable at night, leading to nocturnal awakening or symptoms when waking up in the morning. During times of worsening symptoms, the functional assessment may provide a more accurate reflection of the patient's condition than spirometric measurements at the clinician's office.

Diminished pulmonary function during pregnancy is associated with adverse perinatal outcomes [30, 70]; it is, therefore, essential to monitor pulmonary function in patients with asthma.

Although monitoring pulmonary function using spirometry can be helpful, measurement of PEF or FEV1 using a portable device offers the advantages of less expense and greater ease of serial measurements at home. The frequency of size should be individualized; patients with more severe asthma may need to measure their PEF twice a day: upon awakening and approximately 12 h later.

An additional issue for pregnant women with asthma is the difficulty differentiating symptoms due to asthma exacerbation from the normal sensation of dyspnea experienced during pregnancy. The presence of cough and wheezing suggests asthma. Objective information can also be obtained by measuring the PEF or FEV1; reductions in either suggest an asthma exacerbation.

65.4.3 Acute Exacerbations

Acute asthma exacerbations are common during pregnancy and increase the risk of preeclampsia, gestational diabetes, placental abruption, and placenta previa [29, 49, 71]. The recommended pharmacotherapy of acute asthma during pregnancy does not differ substantially from the management in nonpregnant patients [30].

65.5 Maternal and Fetal Monitoring

For acute asthma exacerbations that require emergency department management or hospitalization, fetal monitoring may be indicated in addition to routine monitoring for asthma [72]. Early consultation with the obstetrics service for co-management is appropriate.

65.5.1 Maternal Monitoring

Continuous measurement of oxygen saturation by pulse oximetry (SpO_2) is prudent, aiming for a $SpO_2 \geq 95\%$. Measurement of expiratory airflow with a peak flow meter (or spirometer) is the best method for objective assessment of the severity of an asthma attack. Peak flow measurements can also be used to monitor a patient's response to treatment and as a predictive marker for the possibility of hypercapnia. Average values for PEF are not significantly altered by pregnancy.

The changes in blood gases that occur secondary to acute asthma during pregnancy are superimposed on pregnancy's "normal" respiratory alkalosis. Thus, an arterial carbon dioxide tension ($PaCO_2$) >35 mmHg or an arterial oxygen tension (PaO_2) <70 mmHg associated with acute asthma represents a more severe compromise during pregnancy than in the nongravid state.

A chest radiograph is not indicated for most asthma exacerbations and is reserved for patients with suspected pneumonia, pneumothorax, or impending or actual respiratory failure.

65.5.2 Fetal Monitoring

Fetal heart rate monitoring is the best available method for determining whether the fetus is adequately oxygenated. After 23–24 weeks of gestation, noninvasive fetal heart rate monitoring is appropriate during asthma exacerbations requiring emergency department treatment or hospitalization. The fetal heart rate tracing should be evaluated by a clinician experienced in fetal heart rate assessment.

65.6 Supportive Care

65.6.1 Maternal Positioning

In general, pregnant patients with acute asthma should rest in a seated or lateral position, rather than supine, particularly in the third trimester, to avoid aortocaval compression by the gravid uterus.

65.6.2 Hydration

Intravenous fluids are not necessary unless the patient is unable to maintain oral hydration.

Supplemental oxygen:

Supplemental oxygen (initially 3–4 L/min by nasal cannula) should be administered, adjusting the fraction of inspired oxygen (FiO_2) to maintain a PaO_2 of at least 70 mmHg and/or SpO_2 of 95% or greater [27].

65.6.3 Medications

The recommended agents for managing acute asthma exacerbations in pregnant patients are the same as for asthma exacerbations in nonpregnant adults and adolescents. These agents include inhaled short-acting beta-agonists, inhaled ipratropium, oral or intravenous glucocorticoids, and, if appropriate, intravenous magnesium sulfate.

65.6.4 Respiratory Infections

Most respiratory infections that trigger asthma exacerbation are viral rather than bacterial and do not require antibiotic therapy [25]. However, testing for and treating influenza may be appropriate, depending on the time of year and symptom pattern.

65.6.5 Peripartum Care

A few issues are relevant to the peripartum management of the asthmatic patient and her baby [27]:

- Oxytocin is the drug of choice for induction of labor and control of postpartum hemorrhage [73].
- Analogs of prostaglandin F2-alpha (e.g., carboprost) can cause bronchoconstriction [74, 75] and should not be used for termination of pregnancy, cervical ripening, induction of labor, or control of uterine bleeding [76].
- Prostaglandin E2 (dinoprostone, in gel or suppository form) and prostaglandin E1 (misoprostol) are considered safer analogs if prostaglandin treatment is required due to their bronchodilatory effects [72].
- For peripartum pain control, morphine and meperidine should be avoided, if possible, since they can induce histamine release, especially from skin mast cells. However, evidence of acute bronchoconstriction caused by these agents is lacking. Butorphanol or fentanyl may be appropriate alternatives.
- Epidural anesthesia is preferred for the asthmatic patient who opts for pain control during labor. It reduces oxygen consumption and minute ventilation in the first and second stages of work and usually can provide adequate anesthesia if cesarean delivery becomes necessary.
- If general anesthesia is required, ketamine and halogenated anesthetics are preferred because they may have a bronchodilatory effect.
- Isolated case reports have described bronchoconstriction following the use of ergot derivatives in the peripartum care of patients with asthma [27]; this may be an idiosyncratic reaction.
- If high doses of SABA have been given during labor and delivery, blood glucose levels should be monitored in the baby (especially if preterm) for the first 24 h.

65.7   Lactation and Asthma

- Changes in the course of asthma during pregnancy usually return to the prenatal state within 3 months of delivery [26].
- It is okay to use all treatments, including systemic steroids, used to treat asthma during the lactation period [33].
- The passage of drugs used as inhalers into breast milk is negligible [77, 78].

- Less than 1% of the theophylline dose, which is used systemically, passes into breast milk, and there is no harm in using it [79]. Less than 1% of the Montelukast dose was detected in breast milk [80]. Similarly, only 0.1% of orally or intravenously administered systemic steroids are found in breast milk, and its use during lactation is okay [81].
- The harmful effects of asthma medications used by breastfeeding mothers on the baby have not been shown. For all these reasons, postpartum asthmatic mothers should be encouraged to breastfeed their babies, and especially to breastfeed [26].

As a result; Keeping in mind that pregnancy is a physiological event, it should be left to its natural course as much as possible.

The biggest mistakes to be made;

- To evaluate the asthma weight more minor than it is and better control it,
- Continuing the treatment with only rescue treatments and not using control treatments,
- Preferring systemic steroids instead of increasing steps in maintenance treatment, when necessary,
- Not using a written plan,
- Not being under the control of an expert in difficult situations,
- Not to quit smoking,
- Not getting the flu vaccine,
- Ignoring the pregnancy drug categories of the drugs to be used used [26, 30].

65.7.1 Drug Use in Lactation

The asthmatic mother should be encouraged to breastfeed her baby because the risk of developing the atopic disease in the baby of an asthmatic mother is 1/10. If the parents are atopic, this rate reaches 1/3. Breastfeeding reduces the risk of atopy [63]. All inhaled drugs, oral steroids, antihistamines, cromolyn, and methylxanthines can be used safely during lactation [63, 82].

References

1. Kwon HL, Belanger K, Bracken MB. Asthma prevalence among pregnant and childbearing-aged women in the United States: estimates from national health surveys. Ann Epidemiol. 2003;13:317.
2. Van Zutphen AR, Bell EM, Browne ML, et al. Maternal asthma medication use during pregnancy and risk of congenital heart defects. Birth Defects Res A Clin Mol Teratol. 2015;103:951.
3. Namaz J, Schatz M. The treatment of allergic respiratory disease during pregnancy. J Investig Allergol Clin Immunol. 2016;26:1.
4. Weinberger SE, Weiss ST, Cohen WR, et al. Pregnancy and the lung. Am Rev Respir Dis. 1980;121:559–81.

5. Jensen D, Webb KA, Davies GA, et al. Mechanical ventilatory constraints during incremental cycle exercise in human pregnancy: implications for respiratory sensation. J Physiol. 2008;586:4735–50.
6. Jensen D, Duffin J, Lam YM, et al. Physiological mechanisms of hyperventilation during human pregnancy. Respir Physiol Neurobiol. 2008;161:76–86.
7. McAuliffe F, Kametas N, Costello J, et al. Respiratory function in singleton and twin pregnancy. BLOG. 2002;109:765–9.
8. Kolarzyk E, Szot WM, Lyszczarz J. Lung function and breathing regulation parameters during pregnancy. Arch Gynecol Obstet. 2005;272:53–8.
9. Grindheim G, Toska K, Estensen ME, et al. Changes in pulmonary function during pregnancy: a longitudinal cohort study. BLOG. 2012;119:94–101.
10. Contreras G, Gutiérrez M, Beroíza T, et al. Ventilatory drive and respiratory muscle function in pregnancy. Am Rev Respir Dis. 1991;144:837–41.
11. Management of Asthma During Pregnancy: Report of the Working Group on Asthma and Pregnancy NIH Publication No. 93–3279. Bethesda, MD: National Asthma Education Program; National Institutes of Health; 1993.
12. Wise RA, Polito AJ, Krishnan V. Respiratory physiologic changes in pregnancy. Immunol Allergy Clin N Am. 2006;26:1.
13. Cousins L. Fetal oxygenation, assessment of fetal Well-being, and obstetric management of the pregnant patient with asthma. J Allergy Clin Immunol. 1999;103:S343.
14. Murphy VE, Gibson PG, Smith R, Clifton VL. Asthma during pregnancy: mechanisms and treatment implications. Eur Respir J. 2005;25:731.
15. Nelson-Piercy C. Asthma in pregnancy. Thorax. 2001;56:325.
16. Gluck JC. The change of asthma course during pregnancy. Clin Rev Allergy Immunol. 2004;26:171.
17. Schatz M, Dombrowski MP, Wise R, et al. Asthma morbidity during pregnancy can be predicted by severity classification. J Allergy Clin Immunol. 2003;112:283.
18. Murphy VE, Gibson P, Talbot PI, Clifton VL. Severe asthma exacerbations during pregnancy. Obstet Gynecol. 2005;106:1046.
19. Murphy VE, Jensen ME, Powell H, Gibson PG. Influence of maternal body mass index and macrophage activation on asthma exacerbations in pregnancy. J Allergy Clin Immunol Pract. 2017;5:981.
20. Ali Z, Nilas L, Ulrik CS. Excessive gestational weight gain in the first trimester is a risk factor for exacerbation of asthma during pregnancy: a prospective study of 1283 pregnancies. J Allergy Clin Immunol. 2018;141:761.
21. Murphy VE, Clifton VL, Gibson PG. The effect of cigarette smoking on asthma control during exacerbations in pregnant women. Thorax. 2010;65:739.
22. Powell H, McCaffery K, Murphy VE, et al. Psychosocial variables are related to future exacerbation risk and perinatal outcomes in pregnant women with asthma. J Asthma. 2013;50:383.
23. Enriquez R, Wu P, Griffin MR, et al. Cessation of asthma medication in early pregnancy. Am J Obstet Gynecol. 2006;195:149.
24. Sawicki E, Stewart K, Wong S, et al. Management of asthma by pregnant women attending an Australian maternity hospital. Aust N Z J Obstet Gynaecol. 2012;52:183.
25. Lim AS, Stewart K, Abramson MJ, et al. Asthma during pregnancy: the experiences, concerns and views of pregnant women with asthma. J Asthma. 2012;49:474.
26. Zetstra-van der Woude PA, Vroegop JS, Bos HJ, de Jong-van den Berg LT. A population analysis of prescriptions for asthma medications during pregnancy. J Allergy Clin Immunol. 2013;131:711.
27. National Asthma Education and Prevention Program: Expert panel report III: Guidelines for diagnosing and managing asthma. Bethesda, MD: National Heart, Lung, and Blood Institute. (NIH publication no. 08–4051); 2007. www.nhlbi.nih.gov/guidelines/asthma/asthgdln.htm. Accessed 1 Mar 2021.
28. Global Initiative for Asthma (GINA). Global strategy for asthma management and prevention. www.ginasthma.org. Accessed 1 Mar 2021.

29. Middleton PG, Gade EJ, Aguilera C, et al. ERS/TSANZ task force statement on the management of reproduction and pregnancy in women with airways diseases. Eur Respir J. 2020;55(2):1901208.
30. National Heart, Lung, and Blood Institute, National Asthma Education and Prevention Program Asthma and Pregnancy Working Group. NAEPP expert panel report. Managing asthma during pregnancy: recommendations for the pharmacologic treatment-2004 update. J Allergy Clin Immunol. 2005;115:34.
31. Källén B, Rydhstroem H, Aberg A. Congenital malformations after the use of inhaled budesonide in early pregnancy. Obstet Gynecol. 1999;93:392.
32. Ericson A, Kallen B. Use of drugs during pregnancy—unique Swedish registration method can be improved. Infor Swedish Med Prod Agency. 1999;1:9.
33. Cossette B, Beauchesne MF, Forget A, et al. Relative perinatal safety of salmeterol vs formoterol and fluticasone vs budesonide use during pregnancy. Ann Allergy Asthma Immunol. 2014;112:459.
34. Charlton RA, Snowball JM, Nightingale AL, Davis KJ. Safety of fluticasone propionate prescribed for asthma during pregnancy: a UK population-based cohort study. J Allergy Clin Immunol Pract. 2015;3:772.
35. Cossette B, Forget A, Beauchesne MF, et al. Impact of maternal use of asthma-controller therapy on perinatal outcomes. Thorax. 2013;68:724.
36. Lin S, Munsie JP, Herdt-Losavio ML, et al. Maternal asthma medication use and the risk of gastroschisis. Am J Epidemiol. 2008;168:73.
37. Garner E, Hansen AV, Morris J, et al. Use of asthma medication during pregnancy and risk of specific congenital anomalies: a European case-malformed control study. J Allergy Clin Immunol. 2015;136:1496.
38. Källén B, Olausson PO. Use of anti-asthmatic drugs during pregnancy. 3. Congenital malformations in the infants. Eur J Clin Pharmacol. 2007;63:383.
39. Gaya NB, Lee BK, Burstyn I, et al. In utero exposure to β-2-adrenergic receptor agonist drugs and risk for autism spectrum disorders. Pediatrics. 2016;137:e20151316.
40. Blais L, Forget A. Asthma exacerbations during the first trimester of pregnancy and the risk of congenital malformations among asthmatic women. J Allergy Clin Immunol. 2008;121:1379.
41. http://www.reprotox.org/Members/AgentDetail.aspx?a=3721. Accessed 1 Mar 2021.
42. http://www.reprotox.org/Members/AgentDetail.aspx?a=4360. Accessed 1 Mar 2021.
43. Wilton LV, Shakir SA. A post-marketing surveillance study of formoterol (Foradil): its use in general practice in England. Drug Saf. 2002;25:213.
44. Elton S, Forget A, Beauchesne MF, Blais L. Risk of congenital malformations for asthmatic pregnant women using a long-acting β2-agonist and inhaled corticosteroid combination versus higher-dose inhaled corticosteroid monotherapy. J Allergy Clin Immunol. 2015;135:123.
45. Dombrowski MP, Schatz M. ACOG Committee on Practice Bulletins-Obstetrics. ACOG practice bulletin: clinical management guidelines for obstetrician-gynecologists number 90, February 2008: asthma in pregnancy. Obstet Gynecol. 2008;111:457. Reaffirmed 2019
46. Schatz M, Dombrowski MP, Wise R, et al. The relationship of asthma medication use to perinatal outcomes. J Allergy Clin Immunol. 2004;113:1040.
47. Bracken MB, Triche EW, Belanger K, et al. Asthma symptoms, severity, and drug therapy: a prospective study of effects on 2205 pregnancies. Obstet Gynecol. 2003;102:739.
48. Schatz M. The efficacy and safety of asthma medications during pregnancy. Semin Perinatol. 2001;25:145.
49. Bakhireva LN, Jones KL, Schatz M, et al. Asthma medication use in pregnancy and fetal growth. J Allergy Clin Immunol. 2005;116:503.
50. Fitzsimons R, Greenberger PA, Patterson R. Outcome of pregnancy in women requiring corticosteroids for severe asthma. J Allergy Clin Immunol. 1986;78:349.
51. Schatz M, Patterson R, Zeitz S, et al. Corticosteroid therapy for the pregnant asthmatic patient. JAMA. 1975;233:804.
52. Park-Wyllie L, Mazzotta P, Pastuszak A, et al. Birth defects after maternal exposure to corticosteroids: prospective cohort study and meta-analysis of epidemiological studies. Teratology. 2000;62:385.

53. Gur C, Diav-Citrin O, Shechtman S, et al. Pregnancy outcome after first trimester exposure to corticosteroids: a prospective controlled study. Reprod Toxicol. 2004;18:93.
54. Perlow JH, Montgomery D, Morgan MA, et al. Severity of asthma and perinatal outcome. Am J Obstet Gynecol. 1992;167:963.
55. Reinisch JM, Simon NG, Karow WG, Gandelman R. Prenatal exposure to prednisone in humans and animals retards intrauterine growth. Science. 1978;202:436.
56. Namaz JA, Murphy VE, Powell H, et al. Effects of asthma severity, exacerbations and oral corticosteroids on perinatal outcomes. Eur Respir J. 2013;41:1082.
57. Stenius-Aarniala B, Piirilä P, Teramo K. Asthma and pregnancy: a prospective study of 198 pregnancies. Thorax. 1988;43:12.
58. Martel MJ, Rey E, Beauchesne MF, et al. Use of inhaled corticosteroids during pregnancy and risk of pregnancy-induced hypertension: nested case-control study. BMJ. 2005;330:230.
59. Schatz M, Hoffman, et al. Asthma and allergic diseases during pregnancy. In: Adkinson NF, Yunginger JW, Busse WW, et al., editors. Middleton's allergy: principles and practice. 6th ed. St. Louis, MO: Mosby; 2003. p. 1303.
60. Norjavaara E, de Verdier MG. Normal pregnancy outcomes in a population-based study including 2,968 pregnant women exposed to budesonide. J Allergy Clin Immunol. 2003;111:736.
61. Greenberger PA, Patterson R. Beclomethasone diproprionate for severe asthma during pregnancy. Ann Intern Med. 1983;98:478.
62. Dombrowski MP, Brown CL, Berry SM. Preliminary experience with triamcinolone acetonide during pregnancy. J Matern Fetal Med. 1996;5:310.
63. Dombrowski MP, Schatz M, Wise R, et al. Randomized trial of inhaled beclomethasone dipropionate versus theophylline for moderate asthma during pregnancy. Am J Obstet Gynecol. 2004;190:737.
64. Dombrowski M, Thom E, McNellis D. Maternal-fetal medicine units (MFMU) studies of inhaled corticosteroids during pregnancy. J Allergy Clin Immunol. 1999;103:S356.
65. Blais L, Beauchesne MF, Rey E, et al. Use of inhaled corticosteroids during the first trimester of pregnancy and the risk of congenital malformations among women with asthma. Thorax. 2007;62:320.
66. Blais L, Beauchesne MF, Lemière C, Elftouh N. High doses of inhaled corticosteroids during the first trimester of pregnancy and congenital malformations. J Allergy Clin Immunol. 2009;124:1229.
67. Breton MC, Beauchesne MF, Lemière C, et al. Risk of perinatal mortality associated with inhaled corticosteroid use for the treatment of asthma during pregnancy. J Allergy Clin Immunol. 2010;126:772.
68. Hodyl NA, Stark MJ, Osei-Kumah A, et al. Fetal glucocorticoid-regulated pathways are not affected by inhaled corticosteroid use for asthma during pregnancy. Am J Respir Crit Care Med. 2011;183:716.
69. Tegethoff M, Greene N, Olsen J, et al. Inhaled glucocorticoids during pregnancy and offspring pediatric diseases: a national cohort study. Am J Respir Crit Care Med. 2012;185:557.
70. Wendel PJ, Ramin SM, Barnett-Hamm C, et al. Asthma treatment in pregnancy: a randomized controlled study. Am J Obstet Gynecol. 1996;175:150.
71. National Asthma Education and Prevention Program Expert Panel Executive Summary Report: Guidelines for the Diagnosis and Management of Asthma - Update on Selected Topics 2002. National Institutes of Health, National Heart, Lung, and Blood Institute, Publication No. 02–5075; 2002. www.nhlbi.nih.gov/guidelines/asthma/asthgdln.pdf. Accessed 1 Mar 2021.
72. Bakhireva LN, Jones KL, Schatz M, et al. Safety of leukotriene receptor antagonists in pregnancy. J Allergy Clin Immunol. 2007;119:618.
73. Sarkar M, Koren G, Kalra S, et al. Montelukast use during pregnancy: a multicentre, prospective, comparative study of infant outcomes. Eur J Clin Pharmacol. 2009;65:1259.
74. Nelsen LM, Shields KE, Cunningham ML, et al. Congenital malformations among infants born to women receiving montelukast, inhaled corticosteroids, and other asthma medications. J Allergy Clin Immunol. 2012;129:251.
75. Reprotox. http://www.reprotox.org/Members/AgentDetail.aspx?a=4087. Accessed 1 Mar 2021.

76. Reprotox. http://www.reprotox.org/Members/AgentDetail.aspx?a=3993. Accessed 1 Mar 2021.
77. Reprotox. http://www.reprotox.org/Members/AgentDetail.aspx?a=3722. Accessed 1 Mar 2021.
78. Bucher HU, Gautschi K. Detection of caffeine, theophylline and theobromine in the umbilical cord blood and breast milk. Helv Paediatr Acta. 1985;40:163.
79. Namaz JA, Blais L, Andrews EB, et al. Pregnancy outcomes in the omalizumab pregnancy registry and a disease-matched comparator cohort. J Allergy Clin Immunol. 2020;145:528.
80. US Food and Drug Administration. Reslizumab (Cinqair) prescribing information. http://www.cinqair.com/pdf/PrescribingInformation.pdf. Accessed 1 Mar 2021.
81. US Food and Drug Administration. Mepolizumab prescribing information. https://www.gsk-source.com/pharma/content/dam/GlaxoSmithKline/US/en/Prescribing_Information/Nucala/pdf/NUCALA-PI-PIL.PDF. Accessed 1 Mar 2021.
82. Bain E, Pierides KL, Clifton VL, et al. Interventions for managing asthma in pregnancy. Cochrane Database Syst Rev. 2014;2014(10):CD010660.

Restrictive Lung Diseases in Pregnancy

66

Baris Demirkol and Erdogan Cetinkaya

66.1 Introduction

"Restrictive lung disease" refers to a range of conditions that may occur within the lung itself, the pleura or outside the lung proper and which all share the common features of placing limits on the ability of the lung to expand, leading to restricted pulmonary volume, greater exertion needed to breathe and insufficient ventilation, with or without inadequate oxygenation. In pregnant women, there are a number of anatomical and physiological adaptations that take place, which also affect the respiratory system. One such physiological adaptation is a decrease in pulmonary volume [1], coupled with a greater need for breathing. Women who already suffer from a restrictive lung disease may find that pregnancy imposes a further strain on the respiratory system [2]. However, such cases are not particularly common, given that restrictive lung disease usually develops at a later stage in life than childbearing [3]. In the majority of pregnant women, the reserve capacity of the respiratory system offsets the effects of this strain on ventilation, and no harm is done to the feto-maternal unit. For pregnancy to come to a safe conclusion, a woman should usually have an FVC of at least 1 L or 50% of the predicted value. In certain cases, a pregnancy may still succeed with very marked pulmonary restriction, but women with such conditions should be advised against becoming pregnant and if this does occur, may need to consider a termination of pregnancy [4].

B. Demirkol (✉)
Department of Pulmonology, Basaksehir Cam and Sakura City Hospital, University of Health Sciences, Istanbul, Turkey
e-mail: barisdemirkol34@gmail.com

E. Cetinkaya
Department of Pulmonology, Yedikule Chest Diseases and Thoracic Surgery Training and Research Hospital, University of Health Sciences, Istanbul, Turkey
e-mail: erdogancetinkaya1962@gmail.com

C. Cingi et al. (eds.), *ENT Diseases: Diagnosis and Treatment during Pregnancy and Lactation*, https://doi.org/10.1007/978-3-031-05303-0_66

66.2 Diffuse Parenchymal Lung Diseases

There are numerous, quite different disorders affecting the parenchyma of the lung, all of which feature inflammation and pulmonary fibrosis. One group consists of diffuse pulmonary parenchymal disorders or interstitial lung diseases (ILDs). ILDs are of two types: those with an established aetiology and idiopathic disorders of unknown cause [5] (Table 66.1).

Various measures of pulmonary function are reduced in cases of ILD, including TLC (total lung capacity), FRC (functional residual capacity), RV (residual volume), FEV$_1$ (forced expiratory volume in 1 s) and FVC (forced vital capacity).

Table 66.1 Diffuse parenchymal lung diseases

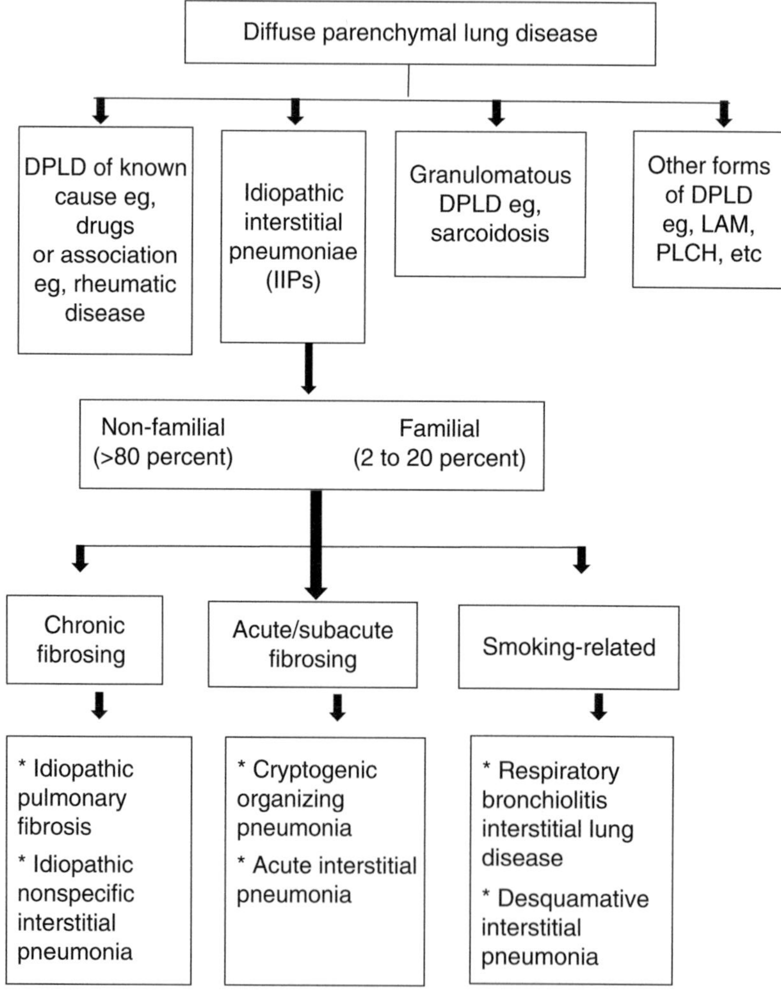

DPLD diffuse parenchymal lung disease, *IIP* idiopathic interstitial pneumonia, *LAM* lymphangioleiomyomatosis, *PLCH* pulmonary Langerhans cell histiocytosis/histiocytosis X

Since the reduction affects both FEV_1 and FVC, the ratio of FEV_1 to FVC may remain the same, or even rise. The expiratory reserve volume (ERV) goes down from the midpoint of pregnancy onwards and is between 8 and 40% below the usual volume at the time of delivery. This is caused by a fall of between 7 and 22% in RV. FRC goes down by between 9.5 and 25%, with a compensatory rise in inspiratory capacity, allowing the TLC to remain the same. A number of lung parameters are unaffected by pregnancy, notably the static and dynamic compliance of the lung, the diffusion capacity and the pulmonary recoil pressure at rest [6–10]. If a woman with ILD falls pregnant and lung function is being evaluated, the results should be interpreted with these normal alterations kept in mind.

The majority of ILDs only rarely present as a problem in pregnant women, because few are observed in women young enough to bear children. Nonetheless, there are certain ILDs that are associated with a younger age at onset, and the age at which pregnancy occurs is rising in many global regions. The evidence base for treatment ILDs in pregnancy and the likely prognosis consists of a number of small case series. What is clear, however, is that if the severity of ILD is mild, pregnant women mostly do not experience ILD-related complications [3, 11].

66.2.1 Drug-Induced Lung Diseases in Pregnancy

The evidence base for **drug-induced** ILD at the time of conception or pregnancy so far consists only of case reports. There are reports that ILD may be triggered by drugs used in fertility medicine during in vitro fertilisation. In between 0.1 and 0.2% of fertility treatment cycles, inducing egg release artificially may result in ovarian hyperstimulation syndrome. Ovarian hyperstimulation syndrome is of high severity in between 1 case in 200 and 1 in 20. In such patients, fluid builds up in the abdominal cavity or the pleural cavity and tends to cause a pleural effusion. Reports indicate that acute respiratory distress syndrome is observed in 2.4% of patients, particularly following large fluid intake. It is also frequent to note pulmonary infiltrative foci dispersed in the lung, which often occurs in conjunction with a raised diaphragm, pleural effusion and atelectasis [12]. When progesterone is given intramuscularly, there is an associated risk of acute eosinophilic pneumonia. Failure to diagnose this condition in a timely manner may lead to loss of life [13]. The use of nitrofurantoin, commonly employed to treat infections of the urinary tract in pregnant women, may produce a toxic effect on the lungs, both acutely and chronically. Whilst this adverse effect is uncommon, amongst cases of ILD related to drug use, it is one of the most frequent [14, 15]. The clinical picture may involve pyrexia, chills, coughing, pain in the chest related to the pleura and dyspnoea. It is known that nitrofurantoin has an association with interstitial pneumonia (which may be acute or chronic), alveolar haemorrhage, pulmonary oedema of non-cardiac origin, ARDS, bronchoconstriction and pleural effusion, with or without an anaphylactic reaction [16]. The principal way to treat this is to stop the drug. If the effects are of high severity, steroid treatment may be required [17].

66.2.2 Connective Tissue Disease-Related Interstitial Lung Disease in Pregnancy

The overall prevalence of autoimmune disease in females is between 6 and 10 times higher than in males. The peak onset occurs at childbearing age. Accordingly, patients with autoimmune disorders may be frequently encountered amongst pregnant women [18]. Most autoimmune conditions are more prevalent in women than men. Reasons put forward to explain this female predilection have included endocrine changes in women, which may be exogenous when triggered by oral hormonal contraceptives, or endogenous, such as related to the menstrual cycle or the changes associated with being pregnant. Other potential factors to consider are the different genetic make-up of males and females, which may be directly due to the differences in the sex chromosomes, or indirectly due to microchimerism. Men and women also have different lifestyles, based on gender roles [19]. Given the rarity of the majority of autoimmune diseases, it is no great surprise that prospective evidence related to rheumatological disorders in pregnant women is not very substantial.

One of the autoimmune disorders which do occur relatively frequently in women of reproductive age is systemic lupus erythematosus (SLE). It has been estimated that 4500 pregnancies occur amongst female patients with SLE in the US annually [20, 21]. Comparable estimates are not available for Europe as a whole, but there is a pregnancy register for Germany, Rhekiss, in which there are recorded in excess of 100 pregnancies amongst women with SLE between 2015 and 2017 [22]. The adverse outcomes that may occur in such cases include a higher risk of spontaneous abortion, intrauterine growth restriction (IUGR), premature delivery, hypertension of various causes, death of the foetus and lupus in the newborn [23–27]. When the disorder affects the lung, the most frequent presentation involves disease of the pleura. Chronic disease affecting the pulmonary interstitium is seldom seen. Pregnancy carries a slight increase in risk that active disease may worsen [28], whilst pneumonitis secondary to SLE may be noted after delivery [29]. The extra-pulmonary manifestations of SLE are potentially more grave in pregnant women, such as thrombosis secondary to antiphospholipid antibody production, declining kidney function and a higher frequency of pre-eclampsia [30]. Following delivery, lupus pneumonitis is especially likely to occur. This condition presents with an abrupt onset of shortness of breath, pyrexia and decreased oxygen saturation. X-rays show opacities of the alveoli on lung films. Whilst administration of corticosteroids typically improves the situation, acute lupus pneumonitis has the potential to cause the patient's death. There is bleeding from the alveoli in fewer than 2 in 100 cases of SLE, but this is a particular concern in young female patients [29]. In such a situation, the first-line agents employed are steroids at high dose, sometimes in combination with immunosuppressant medications.

Female patients with SLE require contraceptive advice to prevent an unwanted pregnancy. It is common practice to advise women with SLE not to use oral contraceptives containing oestrogen. However, if a woman has SLE that remains stable and there are no antiphospholipid antibodies, it is safe for her to use a combined oral contraceptive preparation. Nonetheless, the prohibition on oestrogen-based agents applies to any woman with antiphospholipid antibodies, whether or not antiphospholipid syndrome has been conclusively proven, as well as to those in whom thrombotic risks are present.

Female SLE patients who have pulmonary hypertension (a tension of greater than 25 mmHg whilst resting), advanced stage cardiac failure, restrictive lung disease of high severity with an FVC below 1 L or chronic kidney failure where the creatinine level is above 2.8 mg/dL, should not allow themselves to become pregnant [24]. A well-integrated multidisciplinary team is the best way to ensure a favourable pregnancy outcome. This approach involves a pregnancy risk analysis and assignment of a category of risk before conception occurs and an individualised treatment and follow-up plan thereafter.

Rheumatoid arthritis (RA), which has a global prevalence of between 1 in 200 and 1 in 100 of the general population, is a disorder characterised by chronic inflammation [31]. It is frequent for the disorder to have pulmonary manifestations, which vary considerably, from involvement of the airways and pleura to bronchiectatic lesions, nodule formation, proneness to infection and toxicity from medications [32–34]. ILD is seen in 10% or more of sufferers of RA [35, 36]. The most usual histological appearances do not differ from those seen in usual interstitial pneumonia. A longstanding observation is that at least 70% of women with RA have fewer symptoms from the disorder in the middle and last trimester of pregnancy [37]. The sole disorder of connective tissue for which such an improvement has been reported in the literature is RA [38]. However, there are also reports from a number of studies indicating that RA has associated risks of low birth weight [39], pre-eclampsia and the requirement for caesarean delivery [40, 41].

The most appropriate way to educate RA patients about risks involved in pregnancy and to prevent inadvertent foetal exposure to potential teratogens is to ensure that RA is thoroughly assessed and women are offered pregnancy counselling prior to conception (Table 66.2) [42].

In the past, female patients suffering from systemic sclerosis (SSc) were advised to avoid pregnancy as such pregnancies were considered highly risky [43]. More recently, studies indicate that the risks may not be as extreme as previously thought, albeit definite risks are still acknowledged. There is an elevated risk of disorders causing hypertension in pregnant patients, such as pre-eclampsia, as well as risks of IUGR and prolonged hospitalisation [44]. SSc involving the respiratory tract

Table 66.2 Approach to drugs and biological agents in pregnant women with RA

Insufficient data on the safety	Safe to take during pregnancy	Contraindicated medications
Anti-TNF İnfliximab Etanercept Adalimumab Cyclosporine A Rituximab Tocilizumab Anakinra	NSAIDs (generally considered safe until week 20; from 20 weeks on, NSAIDs should be avoided) Glucocorticoids (caution at high doses) Sulfasalazine Azathioprine Hydroxychloroquine	Methotrexate Leflunomide Cyclophosphamide

frequently leads to ILD and raised blood pressure within the pulmonary artery. These two complications account for most of the associated fatalities [45]. However, usually SSc exhibits stability in pregnant patients. Successful outcomes from pregnancy are seen in some patients with SSc, but their risk of premature birth, low neonatal weight and IUGR is elevated compared to other women and, in cases where the disorder has led to organ impairment of high severity, women should be warned that pregnancy may present an unreasonable risk [44, 46–49].

One study involving 17 pregnancies in women with SSc of high severity (5 of whom had ILD) employed a prospective methodology. Three women delivered prematurely, although none of the neonates involved died. These three individuals had an FVC under 65% of the normal value. Another woman went on to need a termination of pregnancy. She developed acute respiratory failure and died. Another individual suffering from ILD, whose FVC was under 55%, needed to have a termination of pregnancy before the end of the initial trimester [46]. It is potentially safe to employ hydroxychloroquine and corticosteroids (low doses) if acute renal failure develops, even in pregnant patients. Since ACE (angiotensin-converting enzyme) inhibitors are of much greater benefit in such situations than other blood pressure agents, they may be employed, even though they are potentially teratogenic and may make the kidneys fail at birth. Whilst the woman is pregnant or nursing her infant, it is unsafe to use penicillamine, cyclophosphamide or methotrexate; however, azathioprine is acceptable. There exists a solitary case report in the literature detailing the successful outcome of pregnancy in a woman who was being administered cyclosporine A at a low dose [50].

Polymyositis and dermatomyositis occur with a relatively high frequency in females of reproductive age. They may occur in association with ILD. The outcome of pregnancy depends on the respiratory manifestations, overall activity of the disorder and degree of muscular weakness [51]. It has been established that these disorders do not lead to a worse prognosis for the mother or foetus and indeed the condition generally improves whilst the mother is pregnant, although worsening often follows after delivery has occurred. No link has been established between becoming pregnant and the onset of myositis [52].

66.2.3 Idiopathic Interstitial Pneumonitis in Pregnancy

Idiopathic pulmonary fibrosis (IPF) is a disorder of the lung characterised by chronic, gradually worsening fibrosis. This disorder is the most frequently occurring idiopathic cause of interstitial pneumonia. It has a male predilection and seldom occurs in individuals before the age of 50 years. The median age of patients diagnosed is approximately 65 [53–55]. There are several case reports detailing the course of illness in pregnancy, with a variety of outcomes. In one patient, the pregnancy led to maternal death. In another, a termination of pregnancy was performed. Two cases, however, led to a successful outcome, albeit in one case the mother had to be artificially ventilated [56–58]. Nintedanib may not be commenced until after a negative pregnancy test. Women on this agent should avoid pregnancy, including for a minimum of 3 months after the agent stops [59]. At the moment, there is a lack of evidence to indicate the risks in pregnancy of major congenital anomalies or spontaneous abortion in pregnant women taking pirfenidone.

Cryptogenic organising pneumonia (COP) was previously designated by the term BOOP (bronchiolitis obliterans organising pneumonia). It is an organising pneumonia of unknown aetiology. The disease is diffuse, being found throughout the pulmonary interstitium, the distal bronchioles, respiratory bronchioles, alveolar ducts and the walls of the alveoli themselves [60]. Reports of COP occurring during pregnancy are rare. There is a single case report concerning a pregnant woman aged 27 and HIV+, who used illicit cocaine and whose breathing became acutely distressed at the 13th week of her pregnancy. Histopathology indicated COP. The administration of steroids led her to gradually improve; however, the foetal membranes ruptured prematurely during the 34th week [61]. A different case report gives an account of a pregnant female patient who also developed acutely distressed breathing and in whom surgical pathology revealed an organising pneumonia. This patient had a raised eosinophil level in the circulation as well as in the alveoli [62]. In this case, the condition initially failed to improve with corticosteroid administration. The foetus died in utero, but the maternal pulmonary condition then improved swiftly.

66.2.4 Granulomatous Diffuse Parenchymal Lung Diseases in Pregnancy

Sarcoidosis is a disease involving the formation of granulomas within multiple body systems. Its cause has not been established. The frequency in pregnant women is between 1 in 1500 and 1 in 2000 [63–66]. Most female sarcoidosis patients already have pulmonary involvement by the time they are 40 years old, whilst other organs are more variably involved, such as the eyes, skin, joints, nervous system or elsewhere [64, 67]. Generally, the condition is treated with corticosteroids, although this may sometimes be supplemented with immunosuppressants, such as methotrexate (contraindicated in pregnant women), azathioprine or cyclosporine. Köcher et al. undertook a cohort study that involved 764 singleton pregnancies. There was a 60% greater likelihood of pre-eclampsia occurring in first-time mothers with sarcoidosis. The risk for premature delivery went up by 30% (RR 1.3; 95% CI 1.0–1.8) in maternal sarcoidosis. However, there was no elevation in the risk of congenital defects [68]. Sarcoidosis does not appear to cause adverse pregnancy outcomes, albeit IUGR has been noted in some cases [69]. The majority of the studies conducted on sarcoidosis in pregnant women conclude that the disease has no association with adverse outcomes in pregnancy, despite the fact that it is a multi-system disorder [70–75].

66.2.5 Other Forms of Diffuse Parenchymal Lung Diseases in Pregnancy

Lymphangioleiomyomatosis (LAM) is a rare disorder. It virtually always occurs in women of childbearing age. Those afflicted experience progressive shortness of breath and serial CT imaging reveals ongoing cyst formation. The age range associated with LAM means that pregnancy is likely in these patients. Two case series involving large numbers of LAM patients have been reported [76, 77]. The condition was identified 20% of the time in patients who were pregnant. There was a definite deterioration in the condition in 14% of pregnant patients. The guidelines produced by the European Respiratory Society (ERS) indicate that LAM occurring during pregnancy leads to an elevated risk of pneumo- or chylothorax, haemorrhage from an angiomyolipoma and an increase in the rate at which pulmonary function deteriorates. The ERS states that the advice offered about pregnancy should be individually tailored, but women with severe LAM should be advised not to risk a pregnancy [78]. A further matter to consider is the safety of sirolimus prior to conception and during the actual pregnancy.

A study by Shen L et al. [79] involved 30 women (34 pregnancies), who had been diagnosed with LAM. Pregnancy only led to a successful outcome in under a third (10 out of 34, 29.4%) of cases. These same individuals had given birth to a live infant in 20 out of 32 (62.5%) pregnancies prior to the condition being detected. The foetus was spontaneously aborted in 6 pregnancies. In 5 of these 6 instances, the mother was taking sirolimus whilst pregnant. Some 18 women (52.9%) requested the termination of pregnancy after learning they had LAM. On the other hand, 6 women taking sirolimus prior to conception gave birth to fully healthy infants [79]. Another study examined 230 women on a disease register for LAM. Two-thirds of these women had been pregnant. A live infant was produced in 66.9% of cases. Miscarriage occurred in 16.7% of pregnancies, a termination was carried out in 15.0% and 1.4% ended in stillbirth [80]. A recently published study that investigated lung function and pulmonary cyst formation prior to and following pregnancy, and involving 16 individuals with LAM, noted that lung function deteriorated after pregnancy [81].

Acute eosinophilic pneumonia (AEP) is characterised by a swiftly progressive acute respiratory failure in individuals with no prior disease. It is an eosinophilic-type pneumonia. There are a number of case reports and some case series involving few patients reported in which a woman developed acute eosinophilic pneumonitis after receiving an intramuscular injection of progesterone as part of assisted conception. This injection was given to boost luteal phase support needed following in vitro fertilisation. One possible explanation for this is that the patients were hypersensitive to sesame oil, which may be included in pharmaceutical preparations [82]. The use of steroids is efficacious in these cases [83]. Administration of progesterone vaginally also prevents AEP occurring [13]. In one of these individuals, the resulting infant was delivered at 34 weeks due to the foetus becoming distressed [84].

66.3   Diseases of the Chest Wall in Pregnancy

The wall of the thorax has a crucial role in how breathing works, assisting the bulk movement of air into and out of the chest and hence the respiratory alveoli. Thus, disorders which compromise the thoracic wall may interfere with the action of breathing and impair respiratory function, even to the point of respiratory failure.

Disorders which affect the thoracic walls produce deformity that destroys the symmetry of the thoracic cage. This then restricts ventilation-associated movement and results in a lower TLC and a reduction in the FRC. Deformation of the chest wall results in less efficient action by the respiratory muscles, which are now sub-optimally placed on the curve indicating tension vs muscle length [85]. Furthermore, the lung and walls of the chest demonstrate less dynamic compliance and this adds to the exertion needed to accomplish ventilation. Patients tend to adapt to this situation by breathing more shallowly but faster than usual, which makes breathing less tiring. Unfortunately, this compensatory action only adds to the percentage of lung consisting of dead space and results in the alveoli being under-ventilated [86].

As pregnancy advances, the uterus grows larger and larger, which raises the intra-abdominal pressure. This actually makes it easier for the diaphragm to contract and relax, raising the thoracic cage and letting it recoil [87]. Nonetheless, where the chest wall movement is restricted in some way, due to neuromuscular conditions or disorders of the wall itself, the negative pressure within the thorax may cause the cage to move in a paradoxical fashion. The increasing volume occupied by the uterus means the thorax also changes shape, the subcostal angle becomes considerably wider (1.5×) and the width of the inferior thorax grows as a result of the ligaments becoming more lax in response to a high circulating progesterone level. The diaphragm becomes more sharply curved and rises higher [88]. The zone of apposition increases in size and the diaphragm sits 4–5 cm higher than in the non-pregnant state as a result of the upwards pressure exerted by the abdomen [89]. This elevation of the diaphragm mimics the restrictions to thoracic mobility which occur in disorders affecting the thoracic wall and in neuromuscular diseases. The FRC of the lungs goes down in pregnancy by approximately 18% [90].

Conditions which affect the thoracic wall include defects present at birth or developing during childhood, kyphosis and scoliosis, ankylosing spondylitis and injury (whether accidental or of iatrogenic origin). Examples of the latter two are flail chest and post-thoracoplasty. Extremely overweight individuals may also develop problems with the thoracic wall.

Kyphotic defects bend the spine in the anteroposterior plane. A slightly kyphotic chest has no pathological significance. Scoliotic defects result in the spine curving to one side or both. The Cobb angle of curvature is used to grade how severe a kyphotic or scoliotic defect is. It is calculated by measuring the angle between the vertebrae at each end of the main defective area.

If the Cobb angle exceeds 100 degrees, respiratory problems become likely, even to the extent of respiratory failure [91]. Kyphoscoliotic defects result in restrictive type impairment of pulmonary function. The TLC and VC both go down, but the RV is less affected. This means that the ratio of RV to TLC rises.

It is unusual for pregnant women to suffer from kyphoscoliosis. Indeed, the frequency of this condition has been calculated to lie between 0.02 and 0.7% in pregnancy. Kyphoscoliosis of a severity sufficient to interfere with normal pregnancy occurs in only 0.072% of cases [92]. Chopra et al. studied 46,828 women who had a pregnancy between 1998 and 2009 [93]. Of these pregnancies, 34 occurred in 22 women with kyphoscoliosis. In this case series, although the rate of caesarean section rose due to malpresentation or other obstetric reasons, there was no reported increase in maternal morbidity or mortality.

Pregnancy does not need to be advised against in female patients suffering from kyphoscoliotic conditions [94]. One case series of 5 pregnant women whose kyphoscoliotic lesions were of high severity, with a VC that was between only 20 and 58% of normal, revealed that the FVC worsened very slightly over the course of the pregnancy and may even have improved in some individuals [3]. Physicians, however, should be aware that hypercapnic respiratory failure may develop. To enable early warning about such a contingency, patients should be screened for hypoventilation occurring at night [95]. Women use a large volume of oxygen and exert themselves significantly during labour and delivery, so this period may present increased risk that respiratory failure develop. If a woman gets symptoms related to hypoventilation at night or respiratory failure begins whilst pregnant, nocturnal nasal intermittent positive pressure ventilation (NIPPV) may be required [96]. The use of NIPPV in particular cases, where a pregnant woman has kyphoscoliosis and pulmonary function is significantly impaired, renders the situation safer for both mother and foetus. The rationale for use of NIPPV is to halt any decline in respiratory function and to stop the development of cardiorespiratory failure [97].

It is common for physicians to advise women whose muscles of respiration are severely compromised, and when VC is no higher than 60% of the healthy level, not to allow conception to occur. Such patients are frequently warned that pregnancy may cause respiratory problems and might result in tracheostomy and the need for invasive artificial ventilation [98].

66.4 Neuromuscular Disorders in Pregnancy

There are multiple neuromuscular disorders (NMDs) that may begin during pregnancy or already exist in pregnant patients, of which a percentage are immunological or involve inflammation. These last may worsen, improve or remain unchanged by the effects of being pregnant. Some of the different categories of NMDs seen are neuropathies (with a focus or generalised), diseases of the neuromuscular junction, muscular diseases (both inherited and acquired), channelopathies, motor neuropathies and diseases affecting the autonomic nervous system [99–101].

The muscles involved in respiration may be affected by NMDs, which may then cause respiratory failure to develop. Individuals who have NMDs that are chronic or which advance swiftly suffer most of the associated morbidity from, and the majority of deaths are related to, respiratory failure (Table 66.3) [102, 103]. The mechanisms by which this situation develops are weaker muscular pull in the inspiratory

Table 66.3 Factors to consider in pregnant NMD patients

Neuromuscular diseases affecting respiratory system		
Neuropathic disease	Disorders of the neuromuscular junction	Myopathies
Motor neuron disease • Amyotrophic lateral sclerosis • Poliomyelitis, post-polio syndrome • Spinal muscular atrophy • Paralytic rabies Peripheral neuropathies • Guillain–Barré syndrome, chronic inflammatory demyelinating polyneuropathy • Critical illness polyneuropathy • Unilateral or bilateral diaphragm paralysis • Charcot–Marie–tooth disease	Myasthenia gravis, congenital myasthenic syndrome, Lambert–Eaton myasthenic syndrome Botulism, poisoning with curare and organophosphate	Acquired myopathies • Polymyositis, dermatomyositis • Critical illness myopathy Inherited myopathies Progressive muscular dystrophy • Duchenne muscular dystrophy • Becker muscular dystrophy • Facioscapulohumeral muscular dystrophy • Limb-girdle muscular dystrophy • Myotonic dystrophy Congenital myopathies • Nemaline myopathy, core diseases, myotubular myopathy Congenital muscular dystrophy • Ullrich congenital muscular dystrophy, Emery–Dreifuss muscular dystrophy, merosin-deficient congenital muscular dystrophy, merosin-positive congenital muscular dystrophy, rigid spine muscular dystrophy Metabolic myopathies • Mitochondrial myopathy, glycogen storage disease type 2

phase, which causes alveolar hypoventilation and less powerful expiration, which means secretions within the airways tend to pool. This situation predisposes the individual to chronic respiratory insufficiency and may cause the patient's life to be endangered (Table 66.4) [103].

Individuals with NMDs experience a stepwise deterioration in vital capacity and exert themselves to a greater extent to be able to breathe. These effects arise from the muscles responsible for inspiration being weakened and the fact that the pulmonary tissues and chest wall are less compliant, which adds to the elastic load they need to overcome. In response to the strain of exerting themselves to breathe, patients may breathe more rapidly, taking lesser deep breaths each time. Over the longer term, this leads to persistent microatelectasis and less compliance of the respiratory tract structures [104–108]. Since these individuals are not very active, it may be a long term before shortness of breath becomes clinically apparent. Thus, physicians must undertake pulmonary function testing and myography on a serial basis from the beginning. These two investigations provide the best quality prognostic information [109, 110]. One of the key parameters to consider is how quickly the FVC worsens over time. VC should be measured with the patient both sitting up and lying down. Furthermore, the contractile strength of the muscles of respiration

Table 66.4 Signs and symptoms of respiratory failure

Symptoms	Clinical signs	Laboratory data
Progressive, asymmetric weakness Fatigue Dyspnoea Dysphagia Dysphonia Non-productive cough İnsomnia	Stridor Tachycardia Tachypnoea Bradypnea Cyanosis Cough after swallowing Abdominal paradox Staccato speech Reduced physical capacity Orthopnoea Recurrent pulmonary infections	$VC \leq 15$ mL·kg^{-1}, $VC \leq 1$ L or 50% drop from value in stable state, or >20% drop from sitting to supine position MIP ≤ 30 cmH$_2$O MEP ≤ 40 cmH$_2$O Nocturnal desaturation $Pa,CO_2 > 45$ mmHg

VC vital capacity, *MIP* maximum inspiratory pressure, *MEP* maximum expiratory pressure, *Pa,CO$_2$* arterial carbon dioxide tension

may be followed up over time by repeating evaluation of the maximal inspiratory and expiratory pressures (MIP and MEP).

When a female patient who is suffering from an NMD, whether it is heritable or acquired, becomes pregnant, there are several difficulties that may arise, such as generalised weakness becoming more severe, the respiratory muscles becoming weaker and the potential for medications used in NMDs to cause teratogenicity. There are a variety of comorbidities associated with specific NMDs, and these may be affected by being pregnant. Examples include cardiac involvement in spinocerebellar ataxia or spinal muscular atrophy, or the involvement of multiple organ systems in mitochondrial myopathies [100]. The progress of a disease may be altered by pregnancy, as occurs in myasthenia gravis, a condition where the effect is somewhat heterogeneous, with 41% of pregnant patients becoming more severely affected whilst pregnant, 29% experiencing improvement and 30% experiencing no discernible alteration, according to a case series involving many patients dating from 1999 [111, 112]. NMDs tend to worsen in the initial trimester of pregnancy, as well as following delivery. The degree to which the disorder appeared under control before pregnancy has poor predictive value in estimating the effect of pregnancy. The condition always has the potential to become more severe. Terminating a pregnancy, however, does not lead to an improvement in the NMD [113]. Considered over the long term, nonetheless, past pregnancies do not lead to worse outcomes in NMDs [112].

Traditional advice for female patients suffering from NMDs was to avoid pregnancy altogether. More recently, advances in medicine have seen the emergence of case reports where women with NMDs have successfully delivered healthy infants, which has led other patients to wish to achieve parenthood. The fact that a patient's respiratory reserve is extremely low does not absolutely preclude the possibility of a successful pregnancy, as has been seen in certain patients, whose vital capacity was extremely low, even only 8% of the expected value, but who still managed to deliver a healthy child [112].

If the muscles of respiration are weak, then hypoventilation may result, a feature that NMDs have in common with kyphoscoliotic disorders, as described above. The likelihood that hypercapnic respiratory failure will develop needs to be borne in mind. If this occurs, non-invasive ventilatory techniques may be called for during sleep, and possibly at other times, too. In pregnant women whose muscles are especially weak, obstetric intervention in the form of a forceps or ventouse (vacuum suction) delivery may be necessary. Obstetricians should be careful about the use of intravenous magnesium sulphate in NMD patients with pre-eclampsia, since this agent also interferes with neuromuscular function [114]. The mechanism by which this side effect occurs is through inhibition of calcium entry into the neuronal bouton, which then stops the release of acetylcholine into the synapse. This may prevent the nervous signal to the muscle being acted upon. This interaction is of special significance in pregnant women who have myasthenia gravis.

Even though pregnancy in patients with NMDs presents many problems to patients and their physicians, in the majority of cases, the pregnancy has a positive outcome. It is often the case that the requirements of the foetus and the mother need to be balanced during the pregnancy itself and at the time of delivery. This is a feature common to complex pregnancies in general. To achieve the best outcome, the patient should be under the care of a multidisciplinary team, the membership of which should consist of colleagues from obstetrics, neurology, neonatology, clinical genetics, anaesthesia, respiratory medicine and the related nursing and midwifery teams (see Table 66.3) [115].

References

1. Elkus R, Popovich J Jr. Respiratory physiology in pregnancy. Clin Chest Med. 1992;13(4):555–65.
2. Rees GB, Broughton Pipkin F, Symonds EM, Patrick JM. A longitudinal study of respiratory changes in normal human pregnancy with cross-sectional data on subjects with pregnancy induced hypertension. Am J Obstet Gynecol. 1990;162(3):826–30.
3. Lapinsky SE, Tram C, Mehta S, Maxwell CV. Restrictive lung disease in pregnancy. Chest. 2014;145:394–8.
4. King TE Jr. Restrictive lung disease in pregnancy. Clin Chest Med. 1992;13(4):607–22.
5. King TE Jr. Approach to the adult with interstitial lung disease: Clinical evaluation; 2021. www.uptodate.com. Accessed 1 May 2021.
6. Weinberger SE, Weiss ST, Cohen WR, et al. Pregnancy and the lung. Am Rev Respir Dis. 1980;121:559–81.
7. Contreras G, Gutiérrez M, Beroíza T, et al. Ventilatory drive and respiratory muscle function in pregnancy. Am Rev Respir Dis. 1991;144:837–41.
8. Gilroy RJ, Mangura BT, Lavietes MH. Rib cage and abdominal volume displacements during breathing in pregnancy. Am Rev Respir Dis. 1988;137:668–72.
9. Jensen D, Webb KA, Davies GA, et al. Mechanical ventilatory constraints during incremental cycle exercise in human pregnancy: implications for respiratory sensation. J Physiol. 2008;586:4735–50.
10. McAuliffe F, Kametas N, Costello J, et al. Respiratory function in singleton and twin pregnancy. BJOG. 2002;109:765–9.

11. Boggess KA, Easterling TR, Raghu G. Management and outcome of pregnant women with interstitial and restrictive lung disease. Am J Obstet Gynecol. 1995;173:1007–14.

12. Abramov Y, Elchalal U, Schenker JG. Pulmonary manifestations of severe ovarian hyperstimulation syndrome: a multicenter study. Fertil Steril. 1999;71(4):645–51.

13. Bouckaert Y, Robert F, Englert Y, et al. Acute eosinophilic pneumonia associated with intramuscular administration of progesterone as luteal phase support after IVF: case report. Hum Reprod. 2004;19(8):1806–10.

14. Gopal M, Northington G, Arya L. Clinical symptoms predictive of recurrent urinary tract infections. Am J Obstet Gynecol. 2007;197(74):e1–4.

15. Gupta K, Hooton TM, Naber KG, Wullt B, Colgan R, Miller LG, et al. International clinical practice guidelines for the treatment of acute uncomplicated cystitis and pyelonephritis in women: a 2010 update by the Infectious Diseases Society of America and the European Society for Microbiology and Infectious Diseases. Clin Infect Dis. 2011;52:e103–20.

16. Camus P. The drug-induced respiratory disease website. www.pneumotox.com. Accessed 1 May 2021.

17. Boggess KA, Benedetti TJ. Raghu G nitrofurantoin-induced pulmonary toxicity during pregnancy: a report of a case and review of the literature. Obstet Gynecol Surv. 1996;51(6):367–70.

18. Peaceman A, Ramsey-Goldman R. Autoimmune connective tissue disease in pregnancy. Glob Libr Women's Med. 2008; ISSN: 1756–2228; https://doi.org/10.3843/GLOWM.10167.

19. Olivier JE, Silman AJ. Why are women predisposed to autoimmune rheumatic diseases? Arthritis Res Ther. 2009;11(5):252–60.

20. Clowse ME, Jamison M, Myers E, et al. A national study of the complications of lupus in pregnancy. Am J Obstet Gynecol. 2008;199(2):127.e1–6.

21. Chakravarty EF, Nelson L, Krishnan E. Obstetric hospitalizations in the United States for women with systemic lupus erythematosus and rheumatoid arthritis. Arthr Rheum. 2006;54(3):899–907.

22. Strangfeld A, Bungartz C, Weiß A, et al. Pregnancy course and outcome in SLE patients compared to patients with other connective tissue and inflammatory rheumatic diseases – data from a prospective cohort study. Ann Rheum Dis. Poster Presentation THU0261. 2017;76(2).

23. Østensen M, Cetin I. Autoimmune connective tissue diseases. Best Pract Res Clin Obstet Gynaecol. 2015;29(5):658–70.

24. Marden W, Littlejohn EA, Somers EC. Pregnancy and autoimmune connective tissue diseases. Best Pract Res Clin Rheumatol. 2016;30(1):63–80.

25. Perricone C, De Carolis C, Perricone R. Pregnancy and autoimmunity: a common problem. Best Pract Res Clin Rheumatol. 2012;26(1):47–60.

26. Buyon JP, Kim MY, Guerra MM, Laskin CA, Petri M, Lockshin MD, et al. Predictors of pregnancy outcomes in patients with lupus: a cohort study. Ann Intern Med. 2015;163(3):153–63.

27. Andreoli L, Bertsias G, Agmon Levin N, Brown S, Cervera R, Costedoat-Chalumeau N, et al. EULAR recommendations for women's health and the management of family planning, assisted reproduction, pregnancy and menopause in patients with SLE and/or antiphospholipid syndrome. Ann Rheum Dis. 2017;76(3):476–85.

28. Ruiz-Irastorza G, Lima F, Alves J, et al. Increased rate of lupus flare during pregnancy and the puerperium: a prospective study of 78 pregnancies. Br J Rheumatol. 1996;35:133–8.

29. Murin S, Wiedemann HP, Matthay RA. Pulmonary manifestations of systemic lupus erythematosus. Clin Chest Med. 1998;19:641–65.

30. Knight CL, Nelson-Piercy C. Management of systemic lupus erythematosus during pregnancy: challenges and solutions. Open Access Rheumatol. 2017;9:37–53.

31. Smolen JS, Aletaha D, McInnes IB. Rheumatoid arthritis. Lancet. 2016;388:2023–38.

32. Prete M, Racanelli V, Digiglio L, Vacca A, Dammacco F, Perosa F. Extra-articular manifestations of rheumatoid arthritis: an update. Autoimmun Rev. 2011;11:123–31.

33. Yunt ZX, Solomon JJ. Lung disease in rheumatoid arthritis. Rheum Dis Clin N Am. 2015;41:225–36.

34. Esposito AJ, Chu SG, Madan R, Doyle TJ, Dellaripa PF. Thoracic manifestations of rheumatoid arthritis. Clin Chest Med. 2019;40:545–60.
35. Olson AL, Swigris JJ, Sprunger DB, et al. Rheumatoid arthritis-interstitial lung disease-associated mortality. Am J Respir Crit Care Med. 2010;183:372–8.
36. Tanaka N, Kim JS, Newell JD, et al. Rheumatoid arthritis-related lung diseases: CT findings. Radiology. 2004;232(1):81–91.
37. Nelson JL, Ostensen M. Pregnancy and rheumatoid arthritis. Rheum Dis Clin N Am. 1997;23(1):195–212.
38. Silman A, Kay A, Brennan P. Timing of pregnancy in relation to the onset of rheumatoid arthritis. Arthritis Rheum. 1992;35:152.
39. Bowden AP, Barrett JH, Fallow W, et al. Women with inflammatory polyarthritis have babies of lower birth weight. J Rheumatol. 2001;28(2):355–9.
40. Skomsvoll JF, Ostensen M, Irgens LM, et al. Pregnancy complications and delivery practice in women with connective tissue disease and inflammatory rheumatic disease in Norway. Acta Obstet Gynecol Scand. 2000;79(6):490–5.
41. Skomsvoll JF, Baste V, Irgens LM, et al. The recurrence risk of adverse outcome in the second pregnancy in women with rheumatic disease. Obstet Gynecol. 2002;100(6):1196–202.
42. Bermas BL. Rheumatoid arthritis and pregnancy; 2021. www.uptodate.com. Accessed 1 May 2021.
43. Cook WA. Letter: Raynaud phenomenon in pregnancy. JAMA. 1976;235:145–6.
44. Chakravarty EF, Khanna D, Chung L. Pregnancy outcomes in systemic sclerosis, primary pulmonary hypertension, and sickle cell disease. Obstet Gynecol. 2008;111:927–34.
45. Tyndall AJ, Bannert B, Vonk M, et al. Causes and risk factors for death in systemic sclerosis: a study from the EULAR scleroderma trials and research (EUSTAR) database. Ann Rheum Dis. 2010;69(10):1809–15.
46. Steen VD, Medsger TA. Fertility and pregnancy outcome in women with systemic sclerosis. Arthritis Rheum. 1999;42:763–8.
47. Taraborelli M, Ramoni V, Brucato A, et al. Brief report: successful pregnancies but a higher risk of preterm births in patients with systemic sclerosis: an Italian multicenter study. Arthritis Rheum. 2012;64:1970–7.
48. ARA Subcommittee. Preliminary criteria for the classification of systemic sclerosis (scleroderma). Subcommittee for scleroderma criteria of the American rheumatism association diagnostic and therapeutic criteria committee. Arthritis Rheum. 1980;23:581–90.
49. LeRoy EC, Medsger J. Criteria for the classification of early systemic sclerosis. J Rheumatol. 2001;28:1573–6.
50. Basso M, Ghio M, Filaci G, et al. A case of successful pregnancy in a woman with systemic sclerosis treated with cyclosporin. Rheumatology (Oxford). 2004;43(10):1310–1.
51. Ishii N, Ono H, Kawaguchi T, et al. Dermatomyositis and pregnancy: case report and review of the literature. Dermatologica. 1991;183:146–9.
52. Pinal-Fernandez I, Selva-O'Callaghan A, Fernandez-Codina A, et al. 'Pregnancy in adult-onset idiopathic inflammatory myopathy': report from a cohort of myositis patients from a single center. Semin Arthritis Rheum. 2014;44:234–40.
53. Raghu G, Collard HR, Egan JJ, et al. For the ATS/ERS/JRS/ALAT committee on idiopathic pulmonary fibrosis study group. An official ATS/ERS/JRS/ALAT statement: idiopathic pulmonary fibrosis: evidence-based guidelines for diagnosis and management. Am J Respir Crit Care Med. 2011;183:788–824.
54. American Thoracic Society. Idiopathic pulmonary fibrosis: diagnosis and treatment. International consensus statement. American thoracic society (ATS), and the European Respiratory Society (ERS). Am J Respir Crit Care Med. 2000;161:646–64.
55. Raghu G, Weycker D, Edelsberg J, Bradford WZ, Oster G. Incidence and prevalence of idiopathic pulmonary fibrosis. Am J Respir Crit Care Med. 2006;174:810–6.
56. Hassan W, Darwish A. Idiopathic pulmonary fibrosis and pregnancy: a case controlled study. [abstract]. Eur Respir J. 2009;36:100s.

57. Sholapurkar SL, Vasishta K, Dhall GI, et al. Idiopathic pulmonary fibrosis (IPF) necessitating therapeutic midtrimester abortion: a case report. Asia Oceania J Obstet Gynaecol. 1991;17(4):303–6.
58. Sharma CP, Aggarwal AN, Vashisht K, et al. Successful outcome of pregnancy in idiopathic pulmonary fibrosis. J Assoc Physicians India. 2002;50:1446–8.
59. Ofev (nintedanib) capsules [prescribing information]. Ridgefield, CT: Boehringer Ingelheim Pharmaceuticals, Inc; October 2014.
60. Cordier JF. Cryptogenic organising pneumonia. Eur Respir J. 2006;28:422.
61. Ghidini A, Mariani E, Patregnani C, et al. Bronchiolitis obliterans organizing pneumonia in pregnancy. Obstet Gynecol. 1999;94(5 Pt 2):843.
62. Adoun M, Ferrand E, Hira M, et al. Un cas atypique de pneumopathie organise'e cryptoge'nique au cours d'une grossesse. Rev Mal Respir. 2002;19(5 Pt 1):638–40. [in French]
63. Bhide A, Shehata HA. Respiratory disease in pregnancy. Curr Obstet Gynaecol. 2004;14:175–82.
64. Cunningham FG, Leveno KJ, Bloom SL, Hauth JC, Rouse DJ, Spong CY. Chapter 46. Pulmonary disorders. In: Cunningham FG, Leveno KJ, Bloom SL, Hauth JC, Rouse DJ, Spong CY, editors. Williams obstetrics. 23rd ed. New York: McGraw-Hill; 2010.
65. de Regt RH. Sarcoidosis and pregnancy. Obstet Gynecol. 1987;70:369–72.
66. Oberstein EM, Marder A, Pitts S, Glassberg MK. Pulmonary complications in pregnancy: emboli and other diseases. J Resp Dis. 2002;23:175–81.
67. Cohen R, Talwar A, Efferen LS. Exacerbation of underlying pulmonary disease in pregnancy. Crit Care Clin. 2004;20:713–30.
68. Köcher L, et al. Maternal and fetal outcomes in sarcoidosis pregnancy: a Swedish population-based cohort study. Eur Respir J. 2019;54:OA5156. https://doi.org/10.1183/13993003.congress-2019.OA5156.
69. Cipriani A, Casara D, Di VG, et al. Sarcoidosis and pregnancy. Sarcoidosis. 1991;8:183–5.
70. Freymond N, Cottin V, Cordier JF. Infiltrative lung diseases in pregnancy. Clin Chest Med. 2011;32:133–46.
71. Ishizuka T, Iizuka K, Aoki H, Utsugi M, Shimizu Y, Hisada T, et al. A patient with pulmonary sarcoidosis, who experienced remission and relapse through two deliveries. Jpn J Chest Dis. 2005;64:449–55.
72. Miloskovic V. Sarcoidosis in pregnancy – diagnostic, prognostic and therapeutic problems. Med Pregl. 2005;58(Suppl 1):51–4.
73. Sugishita K, Togashi Y, Aizawa A, Asakawa M, Usui S, Ito N, et al. Postpartum complete atrioventricular block due to cardiac sarcoidosis: steroid therapy without permanent pacemaker. Int Heart J. 2008;49:377–84.
74. Vannozzi G, Tozzi A, Chibbaro G, Mello G, Ponzalli M. Hepatic and mesenteric sarcoidosis without thoracic involvement: a case of severe noncirrhotic portal hypertension and successful pregnancy. Eur J Gastroen Hepatol. 2008;20:1032–5.
75. Wallmuller C, Domanovits H, Mayr FB, Laggner AN. Cardiac arrest in a 35-year-old pregnant woman with sarcoidosis. Resuscitation. 2012;83:e151–e2.
76. Urban T, Lazor R, Lacronique J, et al. Pulmonary lymphangioleiomyomatosis. A study of 69 patients. Medicine (Baltimore). 1999;78(5):321–37.
77. Johnson SR, Tattersfield AE. Clinical experience of lymphangioleiomyomatosis in the UK. Thorax. 2000;55(12):1052–7.
78. Johnson SR, Cordier JF, Lazor R, Cottin V, Costabel U, Harari S, et al. Euro pean respiratory society guidelines for the diagnosis and management of lymphangioleiomyomatosis. Eur Respir J. 2010;35(1):14–26.
79. Shen L, et al. Pregnancy after the diagnosis of lymphangioleiomyomatosis (LAM). Orphanet J Rare Dis. 2021;16:133.
80. Ryu JH, Moss J, Beck GJ, Lee JC, Brown KK, Chapman JT, et al. The NHLBI lymphangioleiomyomatosis registry: characteristics of 230 patients at enrollment. Am J Respir Crit Care Med. 2006;173(1):105–11.

81. Taveira-DaSilva AM, Johnson SR, Julien-Williams P, Johnson J, Stylianou M, Moss J. Pregnancy in lymphangioleiomyomatosis: clinical and lung func tion outcomes in two national cohorts. Thorax. 2020;75(10):904–7.
82. Phy JL, Weiss WT, Weiler CR, Damario MA. Hypersensitivity to progesterone-in-oil after in vitro fertilization and embryo transfer. Fertil Steril. 2003;80:1272–5.
83. Veysman B, Vlahos I, Oshva L. Pneumonitis and eosinophilia after in vitro fertilization treatment. Ann Emerg Med. 2006;47:472–5.
84. Kotani Y, Shiota M, Umemoto M, et al. Emergency cesarean section as a result of acute eosinophilic pneumonia during pregnancy. Tohoku J Exp Med. 2009;219(3):251–5.
85. Pehrsson K, Bake B, Larsson S, et al. Lung function in adult idiopathic scoliosis: 20 year follow up. Thorax. 1991;46:474–8.
86. Kafer E. Idiopatic scoliosis. Gas exchange and the age dependence of arterial blood gases. J Clin Invest. 1976;58:825–33.
87. Gilroy RJ, Mangura BT, Lavietes MH. Rib cage and abdominal volume displacements during pregnancy. Am Rev Respir Dis. 1988;137:668–72.
88. Weinberg SE, Weiss ST, Cohen WR, et al. Pregnancy and the lung: state of the art. Am Rev Respir Dis. 1980;121:559–81.
89. Shneerson JM. Pregnancy in neuromuscular and skeletal disorders. Monaldi Arch Chest Dis. 1994;49:227–30.
90. Cugell DW, Frank NR, Gaensler EA. Pulmonary function in pregnancy. Serial observations in normal women. Am Rev Tuberc. 1953;67:568–72.
91. Pehrsson K, Bake B, Larsson S, Nachemson A. Lung function in adult idiopathic scoliosis: a 20 year follow up. Thorax. 1991;46(7):474–8.
92. To W, Wong M. Kyphoscoliosis complicating pregnancy. Int J Gynecol Obstet. 1999;55(2):123–8.
93. Chopra S, Adhikari K, Agarwaln SV, Sikka P. Kyphoscoliosis complicating pregnancy, maternal and neonatal outcome. Arch Gynecol Obstet. 2011;284(2):295–7. https://doi.org/10.1007/s00404-010-1638-3. Epub 2010 Aug 14
94. Bhardwaj A, Nagandla K. Musculoskeletal symptoms and orthopaedic complications in pregnancy: pathophysiology, diagnostic approaches and modern management. Postgrad Med J. 2014;90(1066):450–60.
95. Sawicka EH, Branthwaite MA. Respiration during sleep in kyphoscoliosis. Thorax. 1987;42:801–8.
96. Restrick LJ, Clapp BR, Mikelsons C, Wedzicha JA. Nasal ventilation in pregnancy treatment of nocturnal hypoventilation in a patient with kyphoscoliosis. Eur Respir J. 1997;10(11):2657–8.
97. Kahler CM, Hogl B, Habeler R, Brezinka C, Hamacher J, Dienstl A, Prior C. Management of respiratory deterioration in apregnant patient by non-invasive positive pressure ventilation. Wien Klin Wochenschr. 2002;114:874–7.
98. Yim R, Kirschner K, Murphy E, et al. Successful pregnancy in a patient with spinal muscular atrophy and severe kyphodcoliosis. Am J Phys Med Rehabil. 2003;82:222–5.
99. Sax TW, Rosenbaum RB. Neuromuscular disorders in pregnancy. Muscle Nerve. 2006;34:559–71.
100. Guidon AC, Massey EW. Neuromuscular disorders in pregnancy. Neurol Clin. 2012;30:889–911.
101. Edmundson C, Guidon AC. Neuromuscular disorders in pregnancy. Semin Neurol. 2017;37:643–52.
102. Finder JD, Brinkrant D, Carl J, et al. Respiratory care of the patient with Duchenne muscular dystrophy. ATS consensus statement. Am J Respir Crit Care Med. 2004;170:456–65.
103. Ambrosino N, Carpenè N, Gherardi M. Chronic respiratory care for neuromuscular diseases in adults. Eur Respir J. 2009;34:444–51.
104. Gozal D. Pulmonary manifestations of neuromuscular disease with special reference to Duchenne muscular dystrophy and spinal muscular atrophy. Pediatr Pulmonol. 2000;29:141–50.

105. Bach JR. Progressive neuromuscular and degenerative diseases. In: Ambrosino N, Goldstein RS, editors. Ventilatory support for chronic respiratory failure. New York: Informa Healthcare Pub; 2008. p. 445–55.
106. Vitacca M, Clini E, Facchetti D, et al. Breathing pattern and respiratory mechanics in patients with amyotrophic lateral sclerosis. Eur Respir J. 1997;10:1614–21.
107. Polkey MI, Lyall RA, Moxham J, et al. Respiratory aspects of neurological disease. J Neurol Neurosurg Psychiatry. 1999;66:5–15.
108. Polkey MI, Lyall RA, Green M, et al. Expiratory muscle function in amyotrophic lateral sclerosis. Am J Respir Crit Care Med. 1998;158:734–41.
109. Toussaint M, Steens M, Soudon P. Lung function accurately predicts hypercapnia in patients with Duchenne muscular dystrophy. Chest. 2007;131:368–75.
110. Phillips MF, Quinlivan RCM, Edwards RHT, et al. Changes in spirometry over time as a prognostic marker in patients with Duchenne muscular dystrophy. Am J Respir Crit Care Med. 2001;164:2191–4.
111. Ciafaloni E, Massey J. Myasthenia gravis and pregnancy. Neurol Clin. 2004;22:771.
112. Batocchi AP, Majolini L, Evoli A, et al. Course and treatment of myasthenia gravis during pregnancy. Neurology. 1999;52(3):447–52.
113. Varner M. Myasthenia gravis and pregnancy. Clin Obstet Gynecol. 2013;56(2):372–81.
114. Bashuk RG, Krendel DA. Myasthenia gravis presenting as weakness after magnesium administration. Muscle Nerve. 1990;13:708–12.
115. Norwood F, Rudnik-Schöneborn S. 179th ENMC international workshop: pregnancy in women with neuromuscular disorders 5–7 November 2010, Naarden, The Netherlands. Neuromuscul Disord. 2012;22(02):183–90.

Part VIII

Miscellaneous Topics

Complementary Medicine Products for Use in Pregnancy and the Postpartum Period

67

Atakan Özturan, Sevilay Aynacı, and Özlem Naciye Şahin

67.1 Introduction

The utilisation of complementary and alternative medical (CAM) products during pregnancy has been addressed by a number of reviews of the scientific literature, although these are limited in extent [1–3]. There are also published recommendations on how healthcare practitioners can use these products in pregnant patients [1, 4]. The literature reviews published so far, however, have focused more on the results themselves than on critiquing the methodological approach and examining the significance of the results claimed. The few reviews that are authored by health professionals show that CAM techniques, especially herbalism, chiropraxy, acupuncture or acupressure, massage, homoeopathy and aromatherapy enjoy widespread use and support amongst those working in maternity settings [5].

According to Mohamed et al., some 56.2% of pregnant women considered CAM approaches to possess greater efficacy than conventional medicine, whilst 62.7% thought that both CAM and conventional medicine were equally efficacious [6, 7].

Eisenberg's research [8] established that the rate of use of any CAM product for any indication amongst women was 48.9%. Some 32% of males and females who responded to a survey claimed they made use of a CAM therapeutic technique in addition to seeking advice from a conventional doctor, but under 40% of such individuals had informed their doctor about the use of the CAM therapy. An implication

A. Özturan (✉) · S. Aynacı
Department of Otorhynolaryngology, Eskisehir City Hospital, Eskisehir, Turkey
e-mail: atakanozturan@gmail.com; aynacisevilay@gmail.com

Ö. N. Şahin
Faculty of Medicine, Department of Pediatrics, Acıbadem Mehmet Ali Aydınlar University, İstanbul, Turkey
e-mail: ozlemnaciyeatansahin@yahoo.com

C. Cingi et al. (eds.), *ENT Diseases: Diagnosis and Treatment during Pregnancy and Lactation*, https://doi.org/10.1007/978-3-031-05303-0_67

of the absence of disclosure is that the likelihood of drug interactions being predicted or diagnosed is lower [9].

There are a variety of reasons for the growing popularity of CAM therapies, as investigated by Tiran and Mack [10]. They note that CAM tends to view the patient more holistically, gives greater autonomy to the patients, a more real sense of being viewed as an individual, and practitioners generally offer longer appointments to their clients. Reasons for patients to prefer CAM include the desire not to leave any stone unturned in the search for a cure, the perception that side effects are less severe, that the professional environment in which CAM therapy is provided is less directive and gives greater choice to patients, and that practitioners of CAM have a deeper involvement with the patient and a more holistic view [11, 12]. Astin [12] noted that it was more likely that CAM treatments would be sought by individuals with a higher level of education and concerns about their health, but dissatisfaction with conventional medicine was not associated with higher utilisation of CAM. Both Eisenberg and Astin noted in their sample of respondents that anxiety and depressive symptoms were some of the most frequent reasons for individuals to seek out CAM.

67.2 Complementary and Herbal Medicine

The use of phytotherapy goes back millennia. There is evidence to show that Hippocrates (fifth century BCE) and Galen (second century CE), working in the Greek herbalist tradition, employed *Hypericum perforatum* for a number of different indications [14].

The following herbs and dietary supplements enjoy widespread use in CAM [15]:

Black bugbane (*Actaea racemosa*). *The term Cimicifuga racemosa is a synonym.*
German chamomile (*Matricaria recutita*).
Capsicum pepper, cayenne (*Capsicum frutescens, Capsicum annuum*).
Coenzyme Q10 (*Ubiquinol, Ubiquinone, Ubidecarenone*).
Small Cranberry (*Vaccinium macrocarpon, Vaccinium oxycoccos*).
Creatine.
DHEA (Dehydroepiandrosterone).
Narrow-leaved purple coneflower (*Echinacea angustifolia*).
Evening primrose oil (*Oenothera biennis*).
Feverfew (*Tanacetum parthenium*).
Fish oil.
Flax, flaxseed oil, linseed (*Linum usitatissimum*).
Garlic (*Allium sativum*).
Ginkgo biloba.
Ginseng (*Panax quinquefolius, Panax ginseng, Eleutherococcus senticosus*).
Glucosamine and chondroitin.
Green tea (*Camellia sinensis*).
Hawthorn (*Crataegus monogyna*).

Horse chestnut seed extract (*Aesculus hippocastanum*).
Kava kava (*Piper methysticum*).
Melatonin.
Mary thistle (*Silymarin, Silybum marianum*).
Omega-3 fatty acids.
Probiotics.
S-adenosylmethionine (SAMe).
Saw palmetto (*Serenoa repens*).
St. John's wort (*H. perforatum*).
Turmeric (curcumin, *Curcuma longa*).
Valerian *(Valeriana officinalis)*.

A survey conducted by telephone across the whole USA which investigated utilisation of CAM therapies [16] ascertained that herbal medicines were employed by 2.5% of the sample. A later survey showed that this rate had risen by just under five times, such that 12.1% of adults in the US stated that they had taken a herbal preparation over the preceding 12 months [17]. The Dietary Supplement Health and Education Act (DSHEA) was passed by the US Congress in 1994, which may be a reason why the figure had risen so sharply. Under this legislation, there is no requirement for producers of herbal medicines to prove they are safe or even effective before offering them for sale [15].

A survey, again in the USA, found a usage rate amongst adults of natural medicines (a category encompassing herbal medicines as well as other naturally occurring organic substances, such as glucosamine sulphate (extracted from the skeletons of crustaceans) or fish oils) of 17.7% [1]. The National Health Interview Survey noted that ten substances accounted for the most frequently consumed natural medicines or supplements [15]. Fish oils were used by 7.8% of US adults, whilst 2.6% made use of either glucosamine or chondroitin. Some 1.6% of US adults consume pro- or pre-biotics, whilst 1.3% make use of melatonin and the same proportion uses Co-enzyme Q-10. Meanwhile, 9 in 1000 adults use echinacea and 8 take cranberry (ditto garlic). Ginseng and Ginkgo biloba were both in use by 0.7% of those surveyed.

67.2.1 Traditional Chinese Medicine

There are a number of different herbs prescribed by practitioners of traditional Chinese medicine to alleviate the symptoms of depression. This philosophy posits the existence of seven varying emotional states: joy, anger, worry, thoughtfulness, melancholy, fear and terror. Chinese medicine considers all such emotions healthy except where they are felt without an external trigger of the kind usually associated with that feeling [18]. In the Chinese system, disorders of affect begin in particular organs and affect how those organs work. Three of the seven basic emotions in this system fit more closely with Western conceptions of depressive illness, namely worry, anger and melancholy. The organs linked to these feelings are the heart, spleen and liver [18].

The conventional approach in Chinese herbal medicine is to make use of herbs in combination. This approach is the same in a depressed patient. The patent medicines which are sourced from China to be used in traditional Chinese medicine suffer from the drawback that they are frequently contaminated with other substances. There are several companies situated in Western countries that also produce preparations intended for use in traditional Chinese medicine. These companies state that their products are guaranteed not to be contaminated [9].

67.2.2 Omega-3 Dietary Supplements

Fish and oil made from fish are rich in polyunsaturated fatty acids, as are some other foodstuffs. These acids are frequently taken in the form of supplements to the diet. Research indicates that consumption of omega-3 polyunsaturated fatty acids offers benefits to patients suffering from depressive illness [19]. Evidence from a study utilising an ecological design points to a role for docosahexaenoic acid (DHA) in the pathogenesis of postnatal depression. Hibbeln [20], using reports gathered from 23 different countries, looked at the frequency of postnatal depression in women in different countries and compared this with the level of DHA in breast milk, together with the level of dietary consumption of seafood.

67.2.3 Quality and Efficacy

The existing regulatory framework within which herbal medicines are manufactured is insufficient to ensure that the products currently on the market in the USA and other countries are of consistent quality. This inconsistency in manufacturing has potential impacts on how efficacious and safe a product is likely to be, and thus imposes limits on how much they can be relied upon clinically [15].

67.2.3.1 Quality

There are numerous factors which influence the eventual quality of herbal products by affecting how consistent and standardised products derived from plants actually are [15].

In the case of a number of herbal preparations in frequent medicinal use, the ingredients are sourced from a group of closely related species. For example, echinacea is often used to treat and guard against coryza. The source of these preparations is three species within the genus *Echinacea*: *E. purpurea*, *E. pallida* and *E. angustifolia*. It has not been fully established how extracts of these different species differ pharmacologically. Another issue is the potential for particular plant species to be wrongly identified and incorrectly labelled, which has resulted in severe harm on occasion [21].

Even within a species, different regions of the plant may produce different pharmacological effects. Echinacea preparations differ in terms of the proportion between the various parts of the plant used (roots vs stem etc). It has not been established how the different portions of the plant differ. Another issue arises if parts of the plant that are not the usual constituents of a preparation are also added to it [22].

67.2.3.2 Efficacy

Research dating from before the year 2000, mostly undertaken in Europe, had claimed clinical efficacy for some frequently used herbal preparations, in particular echinacea for infections of the upper respiratory tract, *S. repens* for non-malignant enlargement of the prostate, ginkgo for dementia and *H. perforatum* for depressive disorders. Despite these claims, research carried out since 2000, in which greater experimental rigour was applied (sufficient power, double-blinding and placebo control, plus standardisation of the preparations used) have failed to replicate the finding of efficacy [15].

Nonetheless, there are a number of herbal medicines and nutritional supplements that have been subject to controlled trials, and some of these have produced promising results in terms of therapeutic benefit. Now, further, methodologically sound trials with standardisation are called for. Healthcare professionals who recommend particular preparations or products need to be aware of any quality issues in the evidence indicating how safe and efficacious particular products are [15]. The following have so far shown promising results:

- Products made from soy (*Glycine max*) targeting hypercholesterolaemia.
- Products containing ginger (*Zingiber officinale*) to suppress nausea and vomiting, as may occur post-surgery, following chemotherapy, travel sickness and as morning sickness. Most trials have found that ginger has greater efficacy than placebo. However, there are insufficient data to be sure how safe ginger products are in pregnant women.
- Probiotic-containing preparations used to treat disorders of the gut, such as ulcerative colitis, pouchitis, diarrhoea secondary to infection and irritable bowel syndrome.
- Nutritional supplements rich in omega-3 fatty acids, e.g. eicosapentaenoic acid (EPA) and docosahexaenoic acid (DHA) may lessen the risk of developing circulatory disorders.

67.3 Complementary Medicine in Pregnancy and Lactation

According to the World Health Organisation, CAM is a "broad set of health care practices that are not part of that country's own tradition and are not integrated into the dominant health care system" [13]. CAM is a widely based umbrella term, covering such disparate entities as acupuncture, aromatherapy, herbalism and homoeopathy [23]. The literature on the prevalence of CAM treatments suffers from a number of limitations, particularly inconsistency in the use of the term CAM, biases and the existence of confounders. However, research from all over the globe indicates that women are frequent users of CAM therapies, with between 56 and 88%

of women in the UK reporting use [24], a prevalence of above 50% in women in Australia who were in middle or old age [25] and more than 90% of women in Canada who had already undergone menopause [26]. Despite this high usage, CAM generally differs from conventional pharmaceutical approaches in lacking robust evidence for efficacy, effectiveness or safety [27, 28]. This lack of evidence is problematic to healthcare professionals, who might wish to recommend CAM therapies, especially so in pregnant women, where there is a potential for teratogenic toxicity [5, 29].

67.3.1 Pregnancy and Nursing

There is a paucity of research concentrating on the safety aspects of herbal preparations when administered to pregnant or lactating women. Since there is such a slender evidence base for use in pregnancy and lactation, and given the persistent concerns about quality control in herbal medicines, it is usually best to avoid recommending such products to any woman planning a pregnancy, currently pregnant or breastfeeding [15].

67.3.2 Infants and Children

It is necessary to caution the parents or guardians of children of all ages that herbal medicinal preparations have generally been poorly studied in patients during childhood. Furthermore, there are problems deciding on suitable dosages for children. Children are even more likely to be affected by product contamination than adults and this is a longstanding issue with herbal medicines [15].

There is increasing awareness worldwide that pregnant and breastfeeding women are making use of CAM therapies. A study involving several different countries (23 in total) noted that the countries where the most women in this category relied on herbal remedies were Russia (69.0%), Australia (43.8%) and Poland (49.8%) [30]. One study from Indianapolis (USA) examined the use of medicinal herbs by women of Hispanic origin. The population was surveyed at a particular point in time, when it was discovered that 14.2% used herbal medicines while pregnant, and 13.0% used this type of product when lactating [31]. Research from the UK into CAM noted that some 5.1% of pregnant women were taking dietary supplements, 34.9% vitamins and 5.4% herbal medicines. The study authors also noted that 35% of the patients utilising a CAM product had consulted an individual practising CAM professionally [32]. CAM has also been found to be popular in poorer countries, with 12% of pregnant women based in Nairobi, Kenya, reporting use of herbal preparations. This figure was 52.4% in the Tumpat area of Malaysia [33, 34]. The issue of the unknown teratogenic effect of herbal medicines in pregnancy and the potential harms from transfer in breast milk are often discussed. There is a dearth of research into the effects of CAM remedies on the foetus and on the nursing infant [35–38].

References

1. Adams J, Lui CW, Sibbritt D, Broom A, Wardle J, Homer C, Beck S. Women's use of complementary and alternative medicine during pregnancy: a critical review of the literature. Birth. 2009;36(3):237–45. https://doi.org/10.1111/j.1523-536X.2009.00328.x.
2. Hall HG, Griffiths DL, McKenna LG. The use of complementary and alternative medicine by pregnant women: a literature review. Midwifery. 2011;27(6):817–24. https://doi.org/10.1016/j.midw.2010.08.007. Epub 2011 Jan 17. PMID: 21247674
3. Steel A, Adams J, Sibbritt D. Complementary and alternative medicine in pregnancy: a systematic review. J Austral Tradit Med Soc. 2012;17(4):205.
4. Hall HG, McKenna LG, Griffiths DL. Midwives' support for complementary and alternative medicine: a literature review. Women Birth. 2012;25(1):4–12. https://doi.org/10.1016/j.wombi.2010.12.005. Epub 2011 Jan 13. PMID: 21236745
5. Pallivalappila AR, Stewart D, Shetty A, Pande B, McLay JS. Complementary and alternative medicines use during pregnancy: a systematic review of pregnant women and healthcare professional views and experiences. Evid Based Complement Alternat Med. 2013;2013:205639.
6. Lapi F, Vannacci A, Moschini M, Cipollini F, Morsuillo M, Gallo E, Banchelli G, Cecchi E, Di Pirro M, Giovannini MG, Cariglia MT, Gori L, Firenzuoli F, Mugelli A. Use, attitudes and knowledge of complementary and alternative drugs (CADs) among pregnant women: a preliminary survey in Tuscany. Evid Based Complement Alternat Med. 2010;7(4):477–86. https://doi.org/10.1093/ecam/nen031. Epub 2008 May 7. PMID: 18955336; PMCID: PMC2892351
7. Mohamed H, Abdin J, Al KD. Knowledge, attitude and practice of complementary and alternative medicine (CAM) among pregnant women: a preliminary survey in Qatar. Middle East J Fam Med. 2010;7(10):5–14.
8. Eisenberg DM, Davis RB, Ettner SL, Appel MS, Wilkey S, Van Rompay M, et al. Trends in alternative medicine use in the United States, 1990-1997: results of a follow-up national survey. JAMA. 1998;280:1569–75.
9. Weier KM, Beal MW. Complementary therapies as adjuncts in the treatment of postpartum depression. J Midwifery Womens Health. 2004;49(2). https://www.medscape.com/viewarticle/471895_4. Accessed 1 Apr 2021.
10. Tiran D, Mack S, editors. Complementary therapies for pregnancy and childbirth. New York, NY: Bailliére Tindall; 2000.
11. Ernst E, Rand JI, Stevinson C. Complementary therapies for depression: an overview. Arch Gen Psychiatry. 1998;55:1026–32.
12. Astin JA. Why patients use alternative medicine: results of a national study. JAMA. 1998;279:1548–53.
13. World Health Organisation. Traditional medicines: definitions; 2013. http://www.who.int/medicines/areas/traditional/definitions/en/index.html.
14. Bilia AR, Gallori S, Vincieri FF. St. John's wort and depression: efficacy, safety and tolerability-an update. Life Sci. 2002;70:3077.
15. Saper RB. Overview of herbal medicine and dietary supplements. Elmore JG, Seres D, Kunins L, editors. UpToDate. Last updated: Jan 04, 2021.
16. Eisenberg DM, Kessler RC, Foster C, et al. Unconventional medicine in the United States. Prevalence, costs, and patterns of use. N Engl J Med. 1993;328:246.
17. Eisenberg DM, Davis RB, Ettner SL, et al. Trends in alternative medicine use in the United States, 1990-1997: results of a follow-up national survey. JAMA. 1998;280:1569.
18. Gaeddert A. Can Chinese herbs help clients with depression? Townsend letter for Doctors and Patients; 2001, April 26.
19. Severus WE, Littman AB, Stoll AL. Omega-3 fatty acids, homocystiene, and the increased risk of cardiovascular mortality in major depression. Harvard Rev Psychiatry. 2001;9:280–93.
20. Hibbeln JR. Seafood consumption, the DHA content of mothers' milk and prevalence rates of postpartum depression: a cross-national, ecological analysis. J Affect Disord. 2002;69:15–29.
21. Ernst E. Harmless herbs? A review of the recent literature. Am J Med. 1998;104:170.

22. Choffnes D. Nature's pharmacopeia: a world of medicinal plants. New York: Columbia University Press; 2016.
23. Ernst E, Pittler MH, Wider B. The desktop guide to complementary and alternative medicine. Amsterdam: Mosby Elsevier; 2006.
24. Hunt KJ, Coelho HF, Wider B, Perry R, Hung SK, Terry R, Ernst E. Complementary and alternative medicine use in England: results from a national survey. Int J Clin Pract. 2010;64(11):1496–502. https://doi.org/10.1111/j.1742-1241.2010.02484.x. PMID: 20698902
25. Sarris J, Robins Wahlin TB, Goncalves DC, Byrne GJ. Comparative use of complementary medicine, allied health, and manual therapies by middle-aged and older Australian women. J Women Aging. 2010;22(4):273–82. https://doi.org/10.1080/08952841.2010.518876. PMID: 20967681
26. Lunny CA, Fraser SN. The use of complementary and alternative medicines among a sample of Canadian menopausal-aged women. J Midwifery Womens Health. 2010;55(4):335–43.
27. Broussard CS, Louik C, Honein MA, Mitchell AA, National Birth Defects Prevention Study. Herbal use before and during pregnancy. Am J Obstet Gynecol. 2010;202(5):443.e1–6. https://doi.org/10.1016/j.ajog.2009.10.865. Epub 2009 Dec 29. PMID: 20035911
28. Fugh-Berman A, Kronenberg F. Complementary and alternative medicine (CAM) in reproductive-age women: a review of randomized controlled trials. Reprod Toxicol. 2003;17(2):137–52. https://doi.org/10.1016/s0890-6238(02)00128-4. PMID: 12642146
29. Marcus DM, Snodgrass WR. Do no harm: avoidance of herbal medicines during pregnancy. Obstet Gynecol. 2005;105(5 Pt 1):1119–22. https://doi.org/10.1097/01.AOG.0000158858.79134.ea. PMID: 15863553
30. Kennedy DA, Lupattelli A, Koren G, Nordeng H. Herbal medicine use in pregnancy: results of a multinational study. BMC Complement Altern Med. 2013;13:355. http://www.biomedcentral.com/1472-6882/13/355
31. Kochhar K, Saywell RM Jr, Zollinger TW, Mandzuk CA, Haas DM, Howell LK, et al. Herbal remedy use among Hispanic women during pregnancy and while breastfeeding: are physicians informed? Hispanic Health Care Int. 2010;8:93–106. https://doi.org/10.1891/1540-4153.8.2.93.
32. Hall HR, Jolly K. Women's use of complementary and alternative medicines during pregnancy: a cross-sectional study. Midwifery. 2014;30:499–505. https://doi.org/10.1016/j.midw.2013.06.001.
33. Rahman AA, Daud WNW, Sulaiman SA, Ahmad Z, Hamid AM. The impact of knowledge and sociodemographic factors on the dangerous use of herbal medicines during pregnancy in Tumpat district. Intern Med J. 2008;15:209–12.
34. Mothupi MC. Use of herbal medicine during pregnancy among women with access to public healthcare in Nairobi, Kenya: a cross-sectional survey. BMC Complement Altern Med. 2014;14:432. https://doi.org/10.1186/1472-6882-14-432.
35. Mills E, Dugoua J-J, Perri D, Koren G. Herbal medicines in pregnancy and lactation: an evidence-based approach. London/New York: Taylor & Francis; 2006.
36. Dugoua J-J. Herbal medicines and pregnancy. J Popul Ther Clin Pharmacol. 2010;17:e370–e8.
37. Amer MR, Cipriano GC, Venci JV, Gandhi MA. Safety of popular herbal supplements in lactating women. J Hum Lact. 2015;31:348–53.
38. Barnes LAJ, Barclay L, McCaffery K, Aslani P. Complementary medicine products used in pregnancy and lactation and an examination of the information sources accessed pertaining to maternal health literacy: a systematic review of qualitative studies. BMC Complement Altern Med. 2018;18(1):229. https://doi.org/10.1186/s12906-018-2283-9. PMID: 30064415; PMCID: PMC6069845

Afflictions of Postpartum Mental Health

Leman İnanç and Ümit Başar Semiz

68.1 Introduction

Problems of mental health associated with puerperium are well known since antiquity. Hippocrates had documented a case of postpartum delirium circa 400 BC in a mother giving birth to twins [1].

According to the report conducted by World Health Organization [2] approximately 13% of women who have just given birth worldwide experience a diverse range of mental disorders. All women are vulnerable to severe mental disorders during the postnatal period compared to any other period of their life [3].

In modern times, the diagnostic manuals DSM-5 [4] and ICD-10 [5] do not have separate criteria distinguishing postpartum mental disorders from those that are not associated with giving birth although they both have additional specifiers for postpartum onset [6].

Some studies show that rates of psychiatric admission seem to be increased particularly during the first 2 weeks to the first month after childbirth [7, 8] and psychiatric admissions seem to remain elevated above general population during the 2-year late postpartum period [7, 9].

The mildest and most common postpartum affliction is a mood change that occurs after giving birth, and is usually called postpartum blues, baby blues, or motherhood blues [10]. A more severe form is the postpartum depression that affects

L. İnanç (✉)
Faculty of Medicine, Department of Psychiatry, İzmir Bakırçay University, İzmir, Turkey
e-mail: leman.inanc@bakircay.edu.tr

Ü. B. Semiz
Faculty of Humanities and Social Sciences, Department of Psychology, İstanbul Sabahattin Zaim University, Istanbul, Turkey
e-mail: umit.semiz@izu.edu.tr

C. Cingi et al. (eds.), *ENT Diseases: Diagnosis and Treatment during Pregnancy and Lactation*, https://doi.org/10.1007/978-3-031-05303-0_68

a smaller proportion of mothers [10–12]. Postpartum depression is usually coupled with anxiety symptoms and is distinguished from postpartum anxiety that does not carry depressive symptoms [13]. Postpartum depression can be worsened by a psychotic component and hence a distinction is made for non-psychotic postpartum depression [14]. Postpartum psychosis can manifest as a postpartum mania too [15]. Postpartum psychosis is a serious condition that is a leading cause of mother and infant death as a result of suicide and infanticide [15, 16]. Postpartum anxiety on the other hand can be seen together with obsessive compulsive disorder (OCD) symptoms that lead to postpartum OCD diagnosis [17].

Postpartum mental disorders have a significant effect on the mother-infant relationship [18]. They all worsen the bond between mother and child and lower the quality of infant care as well as mother's self-care [18, 19]. Hence interventions, prevention strategies, therapies, and treatments are all important in restoring this bond, which is important for the attachment style that the infant is going to develop.

Cultural and evolutionary perspectives have also been proposed to explain postpartum mental health issues. Evolutionary perspectives tend to emphasize the cost of infant care and the tradeoff between quantity and quality of children suggesting that postpartum mental health issues lower the fertility when the quality of support is lacking [20]. In case of the postpartum OCD, there seems to be an evolutionary advantage of maternal obsessions [21]. Cultural perspectives on the other hand point out that mental disorders like postpartum depression are experienced differently in different cultures. Since the postpartum depression assessment was developed in the western societies it is argued that it cannot catch the different somatizations experienced for example by Japanese mothers who are culturally less reluctant to show emotion, which is reflected in the lower cutoff value in the Japanese version of the Edinburgh Postnatal Depression Scale [10].

It is worth mentioning that different cultures have different cultural rituals dealing with mother and child care. It has been hypothesized that those rituals act as preventing measures protecting and supporting the mother during the postpartum period [2]. An example for this is the "lohusa" period in the Turkish culture that lasts about 6 weeks and entails special care for the mother. Similar rituals exist in other cultures too.

68.2 Postpartum Blues

68.2.1 Clinical Characteristics

Postpartum blues is the most commonly observed, self-limited [22] puerperal mood disturbance [10]. DSM-IV describes postpartum blues as a mild and temporary form of depression [23]. It is characterized by mild symptoms of fluctuating mood and emotions, tearfulness [22], and general anxiety often accompanied by irritability and sleep disturbances [10]. Other names for postpartum blues are baby blues or maternity blues. It peaks 3–68 days after the delivery of the baby and coincides with the start of the lactation, which suggests that the hormonal changes are to blame for this condition [24, 25].

68.2.2 Epidemiology

The prevalence of postpartum blues has been reported to be present in between 50 and 75% of all mothers giving birth [26, 27]. Left untreated 20% of mothers develop into a full-blown depression [2]. It has been suggested that postpartum blues is one of the most important predictors for postpartum depression [10].

68.2.3 Assessment

An assessment instrument for evaluation of the postpartum blues is the Stein's Blues Scale [28], which is a 13-item self-rating questionnaire. The total sum is used for evaluation and the possible range of scores is going from 0 to 26. A score of 8 or more indicates presence of postpartum blues in the patient.

68.2.4 Risk Factors

There is a hypothesis that pregnancy induced hypertension and methyldopa used to treat it, which can cause postpartum mood disorders [29]. It is suggested that maternity blues may be related to insufficient maternal care in childhood and to poor family support during pregnancy [30]. The exact cause of postpartum blues is not known, but various risk factors include hormonal changes, sociocultural factors, economic problems, and relationship conflicts [31]. According to a study by Manjunath et al., previous psychiatric illness, abortion, and obstetric complications did not have significant association with postpartum blues [32].

68.2.5 Etiology

It has been suggested that sudden hormonal changes after birth are to blame for baby blues. There is a 100-fold increase in estrogen during pregnancy. This falls suddenly after giving birth [33]. A study by Sacher et al. implicates the sudden drop of estrogen and subsequent increase in MAO-A peaking on fourth or fifth day after birth [34]. MAO-A is known to degrade neurotransmitter hence rapidly depleting them. Some studies have also proposed that there is not a clear correlation between the levels of estrogen, progesterone, prolactin, follicle-stimulating or luteinizing hormones, thyroid hormones, levels of electrolytes, cyclic adenosine monophosphate, monoamines, monoamine oxidases and clinical features of postpartum blues [35].

68.2.6 Prognosis

Postpartum blues do not necessitate treatment and usually resolves within 2 weeks but it can turn into depression in mothers who are at risk for postpartum depression [36]. Educating women about postpartum blues near term and providing information about the depressive state that may develop are important interventions [22].

68.2.7 Differential Diagnosis

Postpartum blues is a depressive mood disorder that does not meet the criteria for depression. The screening for depression can be made using the Edinburgh Postnatal Depression Scale [37].

68.3 Postpartum Depression

68.3.1 Clinical Characteristics

Postpartum depression is defined in DSM 5 as a major depressive episode that starts during the pregnancy or in the first 4 weeks after the delivery [4]. Many studies expand this period to include the first year and even the second year after parturition [7, 38, 39]. Postpartum depression (PPD) is one of the most common, disabling mental health disorder faced by postnatal women [11]. It presents with emotional lability, dysphoria, feelings of guilt, low self-worth, sleep troubles, confusion, and suicide ideation [25]. Mothers with postpartum depression are less involved with the infant and show less emotional attachment and fewer caregiving behaviors [18, 39].

68.3.2 Epidemiology

The prevalence of postpartum depression in new mothers is estimated to be between 10–28%, mostly favoring a figure closer to 10% [40, 41] and if severe requires hospitalization [7]. A study by Sun et al. in China estimates a higher percentage of around 25% hypothesizing that the special circumstances of the child planning policies in China are to blame for the higher than average rate [11].

68.3.3 Assessment

The screening for postpartum depression can be done using the Edinburgh Postnatal Depression Scale [37], which is a self-reporting instrument containing 10 Likert type questions rated from 0 to 3. The range of possible scores is from 0 to 30. The cutoff value for western cultures is between 12 and 13. The Japanese adaptation of the test has a cutoff value between 8 and 9 [42]. A total higher than the cutoff value is considered as a possible postpartum depression. Beck Depression Inventory can be further used to measure the severity of the depression [43]. It is a self-reporting multiple-choice questionnaire that has 21 items each scored from 0 to 3. The total indicates the severity of the depression. However, it should be kept in mind that several items in BDI measure somatic symptoms that are normal during puerperium [44].

68.3.4 Risk Factors

Having had postpartum blues is a risk factor for developing postpartum depression as well as having a history of depression before gestation or having a history of depression in the family [10, 45]. Other risk factors include young maternal age, low socio-economic status [46, 47], low level of social support, marital instability, and children with health problems [45]. Being at advanced maternal age [48], obstetric complications during pregnancy [11, 49], and history of childhood sexual abuse associated with depression in the postpartum [50] also increase the risk of postpartum depression.

68.3.5 Differential Diagnosis

Postpartum anemia should be ruled out [51]. Similarly, diseases of the thyroid gland should be considered [52].

68.3.6 Treatment and Prevention

Mothers at risk for postpartum depression can be supported with health professional home visits and cognitive behavioral therapy or psychotherapy [11, 33, 53]. These preventative measures increase the perceived social support and help mothers cope. Selective serotonin reuptake inhibitors (SSRI) seem to have little or no teratogenic effect and their short-term effect on the infants does not seem to be detrimental however the long-term effects are not known and thus they have to be used carefully [54]. They also pass into mother's milk although at a much lower rate than through the placenta. Two SSRIs with short half-life and low passage into milk are paroxetine and sertraline [55]. Risk of admission for psychosis culminated during the second week after childbirth, and admission rates for nonpsychotic depression were highest during the first week of postpartum period [7].

68.4 Postpartum Anxiety and OCD (Obsessive Compulsive Disorder)

68.4.1 Clinical Characteristics

Women are affected by anxiety disorders which worsen or emerge during and after pregnancy. Anxiety in pregnancy is normal as pregnancy is a signifier of major life changes like entrance into motherhood. In the postpartum period, the increased responsibilities of the new mothers and concerns about the care of the baby increase the likelihood of anxiety disorders [13]. Histories of miscarriages is also a factor making woman prone to anxiety [56]. It is highly comorbid with depression and hence has been mostly researched in the context of postpartum depression [13, 53]. However, anxiety does not always manifest together with depression. Anxiety in the postpartum period also seems to be distinct from generalized anxiety disorder (GAD) as it is mostly related to the motherhood and infant-related issues [13]. Some studies have called this pregnancy-related anxiety [13, 57]. Typical issues would be mother's body image, health of the infant, and fear of giving birth (tokophobia) [57]. 75% of women who developed postpartum anxiety, reported feeling anger, fear, or lack of control during childbirth [9].

During the course of obsessive-compulsive disorder, mothers often experience negative thoughts about the baby, accompanied by feelings of shame and guilt over not being able to care or respond appropriately to her infant. Mothers often reported that family members cannot understand the illness and that this was detrimental to their recovery [58, 59]. Those mothers that had OCD before the pregnancy typically report worsening symptoms [59, 60]. However, a lot of mothers report OCD symptoms for the first time in the postpartum period [61]. Just like in the postpartum anxiety, the target of compulsions and obsessions is pregnancy-related. Obsessions of mothers involve intrusive and inappropriate thoughts and images that concern the infant. Typically, they are about cleanliness, infant's health, and fear of harming the baby. Compulsions are typically frequent checks on the baby's health an example being waking the baby at night to check whether it is breathing or not [33]. If anxiety symptoms persist for a prolonged period, they can lead to functional impairment and other negative impact on mother's and infant's life [62]. When anxiety and OCD severity reach a level at which mother's functioning is impaired, a medical intervention is necessary. Adverse outcomes of preexisting anxiety disorder can cause some health problems in a long term such as preterm delivery, mother-baby attachment issues, and abnormal child development [63].

Anxiety and OCD can also affect the mother-infant relationships negatively. Anxious mothers show exaggerated behaviors when dealing with the infant. Those with obsessive thoughts may avoid interacting with the child if they have an obsessive fear of harming the child. A typical case would be a mother asking the father to bathe the baby as she has the fear of drowning it [33, 61, 64]. Avoidance is here used as a coping mechanism however if the baby's father is not available the baby would not receive the necessary care. Mother's functioning as a caregiver for the infant is thus impaired. There have been studies that suggest that anxiety in mother leads to delayed mental development in the infant [65].

68.4.2 Epidemiology

The prevalence of postpartum anxiety has been estimated to be between 20 and 25% [66]. Prevalence of OCD during pregnancy has been estimated to be 2.1% [67]. Postpartum the estimated prevalence rises to 2.4% [67, 68]. Viswasam et al. reported that 39% of pregnant women experience new onset of OCD with worsening compulsivity in the postpartum period. These findings suggest that pregnancy may be a specific risk factor for the occurrence and/or exacerbation of OCD [63].

68.4.3 Assessment

Beck Anxiety Inventory can be used to measure the anxiety in expectant mothers but there are other pregnancy-related anxiety measuring instruments such as: Cambridge Worry Scale, Perinatal Anxiety Screening Scale, Pregnancy Anxiety Scale, Prenatal Distress Questionnaire, Pregnancy Related Anxiety Questionnaire, Pregnancy Related Thoughts, Pregnancy Specific Anxiety Scale [13]. There is also the Wijma Delivery Expectancy/Experience Questionnaire to assess fear of giving birth (tokophobia) [13]. Perinatal Obsessive-Compulsive Scale is an instrument that can be used to screen mothers for OCD. It has 23 items evaluating both thoughts and behaviors. A score of 9 or higher indicates the presence of OCD in postpartum mothers [69].

68.4.4 Risk Factors

There are many factors that increase the mother's anxiety symptoms and anxiety disorders in the postpartum period. Mother's and baby's health, breastfeeding problems, financial problems, lack of social support are risk factors that increase the likelihood of anxiety disorder. High-risk pregnancies lead to a higher risk for postpartum anxiety too [13]. An estimate by Fairbrother et al. puts high-risk pregnancies to be more than 5.2 times more likely to get postpartum anxiety than normal pregnancies [70]. High-risk pregnancies can be due to obesity, advanced maternal age, history of miscarriages, preeclampsia, pregestational diabetes, or other reasons. A comprehensive literature search was performed on a wide range of databases by Leach et al. about the anxiety disorders during perinatal period (pregnancy and first 12 months after birth). Prominent risk factors for anxiety disorders include socioeconomic problems, preexisting mental disorders, adverse circumstances around the pregnancy and birth, and poor couple relationship quality [71].

68.4.5 Prognosis

A Croatian study by Rados et al. measured state anxiety during pregnancy, 2 days postpartum, and 6 weeks postpartum using State-Trait Anxiety Inventory. They found that 10% of the mothers who did not have anxiety during pregnancy show anxiety 2 days postpartum. While a lot of the mothers with new-onset anxiety get better 6 weeks postpartum the total rate of mothers who show new-onset anxiety remains constant at 10% as other mothers without prior anxiety develop postpartum anxiety. Meanwhile, 65% of the mothers who had anxiety during pregnancy get better 2 days postpartum although 30% of them relapse 6 weeks postpartum. Meanwhile 40% of the mothers who had anxiety during the pregnancy and 2 days postpartum get better 6 weeks postpartum [72].

68.4.6 Differential Diagnosis

Chronic patterns of obsessive thoughts and compulsion point to OCD.

68.4.7 Treatment and Prevention

SSRIs and clomipramine could be used. CBT and exposure therapy may also help the patient [61].

68.5 Postpartum Psychosis

68.5.1 Clinical Characteristics

Postpartum psychosis is the most rare and severe type of postnatal mental health disorder with sudden onset and symptoms presenting as early as 2–3 days after childbirth [3]. It has been suggested that postpartum psychosis is on the spectrum of bipolar disorders [73, 74]. Postpartum psychosis usually starts within several weeks of the delivery [20, 74]. DSM-5 has a specifier if the onset is within 4 weeks of the delivery [4]. DSM-II had postpartum psychosis as a last resort diagnosis, which was removed in DSM-IV [75]. Patients present with an acute manic episode or psychotic depression [15]. The patient presents with paranoid, grandiose, bizarre delusions, mood swings, confused thinking, and disorganized behavior [73, 76]. The main symptom is that the patients have lost contact with reality. There may be delusions and hallucinations. It has been reported that in postpartum psychosis compared to regular psychosis the incidence of bizarre behavior as well as non-auditory hallucinations is higher [75, 77]. There may also be delirium-like symptoms, disorientation, and confusion [15]. Altruistic delusions of suicide or infanticide to save the child from "fate worse than death" have been reported [77].

68.5.2 Epidemiology

The estimates are that the prevalence of postpartum psychosis is from 1 to 2 of every 1000 births [78, 79].

68.5.3 Risk Factors

Women with bipolar disorder are at increased risk of postpartum psychosis [80]. Major risk factors include history of bipolar disorder, having had postpartum psychosis in previous pregnancies, family history of a psychotic illness like schizophrenia or bipolar disorder [75]. Primiparity, advanced maternal age, and a mood disorder during pregnancy are also risk factors for postpartum psychosis [75]. Risk factors related to postpartum psychosis include younger age [81], low socioeconomic status [81, 82], having obstetric complications [81], primiparity [38, 83], immunological factors [75, 84, 85], and sustained sleep loss during delivery and the early postpartum [75, 80, 86].

68.5.4 Prognosis

It is a psychiatric emergency condition presenting with a risk to mother's and infant's life [77]. Approximately 17% of new mothers with bipolar disorder are admitted for psychiatric treatment in the early postpartum [87].

68.5.5 Differential Diagnosis

An organic illness as well as possible drug abuse should be ruled out. The patient's urine can be checked for cannabis use that could trigger psychotic symptoms [77]. Cocaine use can also cause paranoid delusions. History of drug abuse should also be considered as psychosis may be a result of the drug withdrawal [15]. Physical illnesses that can present with psychosis could be: febrile infections, Sheehan's syndrome, urea cycle disorder [88], and some autoimmune disorders like Graves' Disease [89]. Full blood and metabolic panel is advisable. The B12 levels, thyroid functions, electrolyte, and ammonia levels should be checked [77, 90]. Full neurological evaluation is also necessary. There are reports of cases of encephalitis that present as atypical postpartum psychosis [84, 91]. Lumbar puncture and EEG as well as head imaging could be requested [77].

68.5.6 Treatment and Prevention

Antidepressants for psychotic depression, neuroleptics, mood stabilizers, and ECT can be used to treat postpartum psychosis [92]. Lithium can be used in the cases of mania. If lithium or diazepam is used the infant should not be breastfed. Lithium also should not be used during the pregnancy as it is teratogenic. Atypical antipsychotics like olanzapine and quetiapine are better tolerated. Breastfed babies should be monitored for failure to gain weight, difficulties in feeding, and sedation. All of the above could be signs of drug toxicity [77]. Sleep improving interventions are important [86]. Possible such interventions are finding a doula or having the partner bottle feed the baby during the night.

References

1. Hippocrates. Of the Epidemics, Book II, Translated by Francis Adams. http://classics.mit.edu/Hippocrates/epidemics.2.ii.html. Accessed 16 Mar 2021.
2. World Health Organization. Maternal mental health & child health and development. Department of Mental Health and Substance Abuse. Geneva: WHO; 2008.

3. Plunkett C, Peters S, Wieck A, Wittkowski A. A qualitative investigation in the role of the baby in recovery from postpartum psychosis. Clin Psychol Psychother. 2017;24(5):1099–108.

4. American Psychiatric Association. Diagnostic and statistical manual of mental disorders. 5th ed). DSM-5. Arlington, VA: American Psychiatric Association; 2013.

5. World Health Organization (WHO). The ICD-10 classification of mental and behavioural disorders. Geneva: World Health Organization; 1993.

6. Di Florio A, Meltzer-Brody S. Is postpartum depression a distinct disorder? Curr Psychiatry Rep. 2015;17(10):1–6.

7. Martin JL, McLean G, Cantwell R, Smith DJ. Admission to psychiatric hospital in the early and late postpartum periods: Scottish national linkage study. BMJ Open. 2016;6(1)

8. Munk-Olsen T, Laursen TM, Mendelson T, Pedersen CB, Mors O, Mortensen PB. Risks and predictors of readmission for a mental disorder during the postpartum period. Arch Gen Psychiatry. 2009;66(2):189–95.

9. Polachek IS, Fung K, Vigod SN. First lifetime psychiatric admission in the postpartum period: a population-based comparison to women with prior psychiatric admission. Gen Hosp Psychiatry. 2016;40:25–32.

10. Watanabe M, Wada K, Sakata Y, Aratake Y, Kato N, Ohta H, Tanaka K. Maternity blues as predictor of postpartum depression: a prospective cohort study among Japanese women. J Psychosom Obstet Gynecol. 2008;29(3):211–7.

11. Sun M, Tang S, Chen J, Li Y, Bai W, Plummer V, Lam L, Qin C, Cross WM. A study protocol of mobile phone app-based cognitive behaviour training for the prevention of postpartum depression among high-risk mothers. BMC Public Health. 2019;19(1):710.

12. Bina R. Predictors of postpartum depression service use: a theory-informed, integrative systematic review. Women Birth. 2020;33(1):24–32.

13. Araji S, Griffin A, Dixon L, Spencer SK, Peavie C, Wallace K. An overview of maternal anxiety during pregnancy and the post-partum period. J Ment Health Clin Psychol. 2020;4(4)

14. Miller LJ. Postpartum depression. JAMA. 2002;287(6):762–5.

15. Bergink V, Rasgon N, Wisner KL. Postpartum psychosis: madness, mania, and melancholia in motherhood. Am J Psychiatr. 2016;173(12):1179–88.

16. Stewart G. Puerperal psychosis: a brief review and unusual case report. Malawi Med J. 2019;31(2):161–3.

17. Sharma V, Sommerdyk C. Obsessive–compulsive disorder in the postpartum period: diagnosis, differential diagnosis and management. Womens Health. 2015;11(4):543–52.

18. Heinisch C, Galeris MG, Gabler S, Simen S, Junge-Hoffmeister J, Fößel J, Spangler G. Mothers with postpartum psychiatric disorders: proposal for an adapted method to assess maternal sensitivity in interaction with the child. Front Psych. 2019;10:471.

19. Matthies LM, Müller M, Doster A, Sohn C, Wallwiener M, Reck C, Wallwiener S. Maternal–fetal attachment protects against postpartum anxiety: the mediating role of postpartum bonding and partnership satisfaction. Arch Gynecol Obstet. 2020;301(1):107–17.

20. Jones I, Smith S. Puerperal psychosis: identifying and caring for women at risk. Adv Psychiatr Treat. 2009;15(6):411–8.

21. Starcevic V, Eslick GD, Viswasam K, Berle D. Symptoms of obsessive-compulsive disorder during pregnancy and the postpartum period: a systematic review and meta-analysis. Psychiatry Q. 2020;91:965–81.

22. Gale S, Harlow BL. Postpartum mood disorders: a review of clinical and epidemiological factors. J Psychosom Obstet Gynecol. 2003;24(4):257–66.

23. American Psychiatric Association. Diagnostic and statistical manual of mental disorders IV. Washington, DC: American Medical Association; 1994.

24. Bloch M, Schmidt PJ, Danaceau M, Murphy J, Nieman L, Rubinow DR. Effects of gonadal steroids in women with a history of postpartum depression. Am J Psychiatr. 2000;157(6):924–30.

25. Kołomańska-Bogucka D, Mazur-Bialy AI. Physical activity and the occurrence of postnatal depression—a systematic review. Medicina. 2019;55(9):560.

26. Faisal-Cury A, Menezes PR, Tedesco JJA, Kahalle S, Zugaib M. Maternity "blues": prevalence and risk factors. Span J Psychol. 2008;11(2):593–9.

27. Rai S, Pathak A, Sharma I. Postpartum psychiatric disorders: early diagnosis and management. Indian J Psychiatry. 2015;57(2):216.

28. Stein GS. The pattern of mental change and body weight change in the first post-partum week. J Psychosom Res. 1980;24(3–4):165–71.

29. Wiciński M, Malinowski B, Puk O, Socha M, Słupski M. Methyldopa as an inductor of postpartum depression and maternal blues: a review. Biomed Pharmacother. 2020;127:110–96.

30. Murata A, Nadaoka T, Morioka Y, Oiji A, Saito H. Prevalence and background factors of maternity blues. Gynecol Obstet Investig. 1998;46(2):99–104.

31. Alvarado-Esquivel C, Sifuentes-Alvarez A, Salas-Martinez C, Martínez-García S. Validation of the Edinburgh postpartum depression scale in a population of puerperal women in Mexico. Clin Pract Epidemiol Ment Health. 2006;29(2):23.

32. Manjunath NG, Venkatesh G, Rajanna. Postpartum blue is common in socially and economically insecure mothers. Indian J Community Med. 2011;36(3):231–3.

33. O'Hara MW, Wisner KL. Perinatal mental illness: definition, description and aetiology. Best Pract Res Clin Obstet Gynaecol. 2014;28(1):3–12.

34. Sacher J, Wilson AA, Houle S, Rusjan P, Hassan S, Bloomfield PM, Stewart DE, Meyer JH. Elevated brain monoamine oxidase A binding in the early postpartum period. Arch Gen Psychiatry. 2010;67(5):468–74.

35. Robinson GE, Stewart DE. Postpartum psychiatric disorders. Can Med Assoc J. 1986;134(1):31.

36. Fossey L, Papiernik E, Bydlowski M. Postpartum blues: a clinical syndrome and predictor of postnatal depression? J Psychosom Obstet Gynecol. 1997;18(1):17–21.

37. Cox JL, Holden JM, Sagovsky R. Detection of postnatal depression: development of the 10-item Edinburgh postnatal depression scale. Br J Psychiatry. 1987;150(6):782–6.

38. Di Florio A, Jones L, Forty L, Gordon-Smith K, Robertson Blackmore E, Heron J, Craddock N, Jones I. Mood disorders and parity-A clue to the aetiology of the postpartum trigger. J Affect Disord. 2014;152–154:334–9.

39. Seth S, Lewis AJ, Galbally M. Perinatal maternal depression and cortisol function in pregnancy and the postpartum period: a systematic literature review. BMC Pregnancy Childbirth. 2016;16(1):1–19.

40. Seyfried LS, Marcus SM. Postpartum mood disorders. Int Rev Psychiatry. 2003;15:231–42.

41. Ryan D, Kostaras X. Psychiatric disorders in the postpartum period. B C Med J. 2005;47(2):100.

42. Takehara K, Tachibana Y, Yoshida K, Mori R, Kakee N, Kubo T. Prevalence trends of pre- and postnatal depression in Japanese women: a population-based longitudinal study. J Affect Disord. 2018;225:389–94.

43. Beck AT, Steer RA, Brown G. Beck depression inventory–II. Psychol Assess. 1996.

44. Noble RE. Depression in women. Metabolism. 2005;54(5):49–52.

45. Howard LM, Molyneaux E, Dennis CL, Rochat T, Stein A, Milgrom J. Non psychotic mental disorders in the perinatal period. Lancet. 2014;384(9956):1775–88.

46. Goyal D, Gay C, Lee KA. How much does low socioeconomic status increase the risk of prenatal and postpartum depressive symptoms in first-time mothers? Women's Health Issues. 2010;20(2):96–104.

47. Fisher J, Mello MCD, Patel V, Rahman A, Tran T, Holton S, Holmes W. Prevalence and determinants of common perinatal mental disorders in women in low-and lower-middle-income countries: a systematic review. Bull World Health Organ. 2012;90:139–49.

48. Kang C, Gao YQ, Song L, Pang RY, Wang Y. The influence of the new fertility policy on size and structure of maternity in obstetric and gynecologic hospitals. Popul Res. 2015;39(6):85–93.

49. Koutra K, Vassilaki M, Georgiou V, Koutis A, Bitsios P, Kogevinas M, Chatzi L. Pregnancy, perinatal and postpartum complications as determinants of postpartum depression: the Rhea mother–child cohort in Crete, Greece. Epidemiol Psychiatr Sci. 2018;27(3):244.

50. Dennis CL, Vigod S. The relationship between postpartum depression, domestic violence, childhood violence, and substance use: epidemiologic study of a large community sample. Violence Women. 2013;19:503–17.

51. Corwin EJ, Murray-Kolb LE, Beard JL. Low hemoglobin level is a risk factor for postpartum depression. J Nutr. 2003;133(12):4139–42.

52. Dowlati Y, Meyer JH. Promising leads and pitfalls: a review of dietary supplements and hormone treatments to prevent postpartum blues and postpartum depression. Arch Womens Ment Health. 2021;24(3):381–9.
53. Shulman B, Dueck R, Ryan D, Breau G, Sadowski I, Misri S. Feasibility of a mindfulness-based cognitive therapy group intervention as an adjunctive treatment for postpartum depression and anxiety. J Affect Disord. 2018;235:61–7.
54. Wisner KL, Perel JM, Findling RL. Antidepressant treatment during breast-feeding. Am J Psychiatry. 1996;153(9):1132–7.
55. Sriraman NK, Melvin K, Meltzer-Brody S, Academy of Breastfeeding Medicine. ABM clinical protocol# 18: use of antidepressants in breastfeeding mothers. Breastfeed Med. 2015;10(6):290–9.
56. Martini J, Asselmann E, Einsle F, Strehle J, Wittchen HU. A prospective-longitudinal study on the association of anxiety disorders prior to pregnancy and pregnancy-and child-related fears. J Anxiety Disord. 2016;40:58–66.
57. Huizink AC, Mulder EJ, de Medina PGR, Visser GH, Buitelaar JK. Is pregnancy anxiety a distinctive syndrome? Early Hum Dev. 2004;79(2):81–91.
58. Miller ES, Chu C, Gollan J, Gossett DR. Obsessive-compulsive symptoms during the postpartum period. A prospective cohort. J Reprod Med. 2013;58(3–4):115–22.
59. Zambaldi CF, Cantilino A, Montenegro AC, Paes JA, de Albuquerque TLC, Sougey EB. Postpartum obsessive-compulsive disorder: prevalence and clinical characteristics. Compr Psychiatry. 2009;50(6):503–9.
60. Labad J, Menchón JM, Alonso P, Segalàs C, Jiménez S, Vallejo J. Female reproductive cycle and obsessive-compulsive disorder. J Clin Psychiatry. 2005;66(4):428–35.
61. Brandes M, Soares CN, Cohen LS. Postpartum onset obsessive-compulsive disorder: diagnosis and management. Arch Womens Ment Health. 2004;7(2):99–110.
62. Furtado M, Chow CH, Owais S, Frey BN, Van Lieshout RJ. Risk factors of new onset anxiety and anxiety exacerbation in the perinatal period: a systematic review and meta-analysis. J Affect Disord. 2018;238:626–35.
63. Viswasam K, Eslick GD, Starcevic V. Prevalence, onset and course of anxiety disorders during pregnancy: a systematic review and meta analysis. J Affect Disord. 2019;255:27–40.
64. Wisner KL, Peindl KS, Hanusa BH. Obsessions and compulsions in women with postpartum depression. J Clin Psychiatry. 1999;60(3):176–80.
65. Polte C, Junge C, von Soest T, Seidler A, Eberhard-Gran M, Garthus-Niegel S. Impact of maternal perinatal anxiety on social-emotional development of 2-year-olds, a prospective study of Norwegian mothers and their offspring. Matern Child Health J. 2019;23(3):386–96.
66. Lonstein JS. Regulation of anxiety during the postpartum period. Front Neuroendocrinol. 2007;28(2–3):115–41.
67. Fairbrother N, Janssen P, Antony MM, Tucker E, Young AH. Perinatal anxiety disorder prevalence and incidence. J Affect Disord. 2016;200:148–55.
68. Russell EJ, Fawcett JM, Mazmanian D. Focus on Women's mental health meta-analysis. J Clin Psychiatry. 2013;74(4):377–85.
69. Lord C, Rieder A, Hall GB, Soares CN, Steiner M. Piloting the perinatal obsessive-compulsive scale (POCS): development and validation. J Anxiety Disord. 2011;25(8):1079–84.
70. Fairbrother N, Young AH, Zhang A, Janssen P, Antony MM. The prevalence and incidence of perinatal anxiety disorders among women experiencing a medically complicated pregnancy. Arch Womens Ment Health. 2017;20(2):311–9.
71. Leach LS, Poyser C, Fairweather-Schmidt K. Maternal perinatal anxiety: a review of prevalence and correlates. Clin Psychol. 2017;21(1):4–19.
72. Nakić Radoš S, Tadinac M, Herman R. Anxiety during pregnancy and postpartum: course, predictors and comorbidity with postpartum depression. Acta Clin Croat. 2018;57(1):39–51.
73. Sit D, Rothschild AJ, Wisner KL. A review of postpartum psychosis. J Women's Health. 2006;15(4):352–68.
74. Di Florio A, Smith S, Jones IR. Postpartum psychosis. Obstetric Gynaecol. 2013;15(3):145–50.

75. Jones I, Chandra PS, Dazzan P, Howard LM. Bipolar disorder, affective psychosis, and schizophrenia in pregnancy and the post-partum period. Lancet. 2014;384(9956):1789–99.
76. Heron J, McGuinness M, Blackmore ER, Craddock N, Jones I. Early postpartum symptoms in puerperal psychosis. BJOG Int J Obstet Gynaecol. 2008;115(3):348–53.
77. Lisette RC, Crystal C. Psychiatric emergencies in pregnancy and postpartum. Clin Obstet Gynecol. 2018;61(3):615.
78. Halbreich U. Postpartum disorders: multiple interacting underlying mechanisms and risk factors. J Affect Disord. 2005;88:1–7.
79. Munk-Olsen T, Laursen TM, Pedersen CB, Mors O, Mortensen PB. New parents and mental disorders: a population-based register study. JAMA. 2006;296(21):2582–9.
80. Perry A, Gordon-Smith K, Di Florio A, Forty L, Craddock N, Jones L, Jones I. Adverse childhood life events and postpartum psychosis in bipolar disorder. J Affect Disord. 2016;205:69–72.
81. Upadhyaya SK, Sharma A, Raval CM. Postpartum psychosis: risk factors identification. N Am J Med Sci. 2014;6(6):274–7.
82. Nager A, Johansson LM, Sundquist K. Neighbourhood socioeconomic environment and risk of postpartum psychosis. Arch Womens Ment Health. 2006;9:81–6.
83. Blackmore ER, Jones I, Doshi M, Haque S, Holder R, Brockington I, Craddock N. Obstetric variables associated with bipolar affective puerperal psychosis. Br J Psychiatry. 2006;188(1):32–6.
84. Berginklitis V, Armangue T, Titulaer MJ, Markx S, Dalmau J, Kushner SA. Autoimmune encephalitis in postpartum psychosis. Am J Psychiatr. 2015;172(9):901–8.
85. Davies W. Understanding the pathophysiology of postpartum psychosis: challenges and new approaches. World J Psychiatry. 2017;7(2):77–88.
86. Sharma V, Mazmanian D. Sleep loss and postpartum psychosis. Bipolar Disord. 2003;5(2):98–105.
87. Wesseloo R, Kamperman AM, Munk-Olsen T, Pop VJM, Kushner SA, Berginklitis V. Risk of postpartum relapse in bipolar disorder and postpartum psychosis: a systematic review and metaanalysis. Am J Psychiatry. 2016;173:117–27.
88. Fassier T, Guffon N, Acquaviva C, D'Amato T, Durand DV, Domenech P. Misdiagnosed postpartum psychosis revealing a late-onset urea cycle disorder. Am J Psychiatr. 2011;168(6):576–80.
89. Dahale AB, Chandra PS, Sherine L, Thippeswamy H, Desai G, Reddy D. Postpartum psychosis in a woman with Graves' disease: a case report. Gen Hosp Psychiatry. 2014;36(6):761–77.
90. Tinkelman A, Hill EA, Deligiannidis KM. Management of new onset psychosis in the postpartum period. J Clin Psychiatry. 2017;78(9):1423–4.
91. Reddy MSS, Thippeswamy H, Ganjekar S, Nagappa M, Mahadevan A, Arvinda HR, Chandra PS, Taly AB. Anti-NMDA receptor encephalitis presenting as postpartum psychosis—a clinical description and review. Arch Womens Ment Health. 2018;21(4):465–9.
92. Focht A, Kellner CH. Electroconvulsive therapy (ECT) in the treatment of postpartum psychosis. J ECT. 2012;28(1):31–3.

Filler and Neurotoxin Injections During Pregnancy and the Postpartum Period

69

Fevzi Meşe, Nuray Bayar Muluk, and Cemal Cingi

69.1 Introduction

Women usually strive to be more beautiful at every period in their lives. Pregnancy and the postpartum period are times when women often believe that their beauty decreases. At such times, they fear they have become ugly and may aim to look more beautiful by seeking minor cosmetic procedures on their faces. This section will deal with neurotoxin and surface filling applications during pregnancy.

69.1.1 Fillers

The initial filler to enter the market in the first half of the 1970s was bovine collagen. It could be injected into the face to replace lost volume. Since that time, numerous products to augment the soft tissues have become available [1]. Over the last 10 years, both the volume of new products licensed for this indication and the number of individuals requesting these enhancements have experienced an

F. Meşe (✉)
Department of Otorhynolaryngology, Private Batman World Hospital, Batman, Turkey
e-mail: feyzimese@gmail.com

N. Bayar Muluk
Department of Otorhinolaryngology, Faculty of Medicine, Kırıkkale University, Kırıkkale, Turkey
e-mail: nbayarmuluk@yahoo.com

C. Cingi
Department of Otorhinolaryngology, Faculty of Medicine, Eskişehir Osmangazi University, Eskişehir, Turkey
e-mail: cemal@ogu.edu.tr

913

C. Cingi et al. (eds.), *ENT Diseases: Diagnosis and Treatment during Pregnancy and Lactation*, https://doi.org/10.1007/978-3-031-05303-0_69

unprecedented increase. For example, in the USA alone, doctors and nurse practitioners carried out some two million procedures for facial augmentation in 2012 [2, 3]. The type of filling agent most favoured by American practitioners is hyaluronic acid (HA), employed in 87% of the total procedures performed where fillers are involved. The use of HA as a filler has grown by 38% since 2004 [2]. On a global scale, too, HA is the filler enjoying the highest level of use [4, 5]. There are, however, significant differences between the fillers on the market, and no one product can claim to be ideal. Indeed, the variety of desired outcomes and expectations from different patients means a range of fillers needs to be considered when planning a procedure [6–8].

The rhytides, folds, and lines that indicate ageing in the face may be treated by injection of soft tissue filling agents. The facial regions where fillers are often used include the frons, glabella, nasolabial folds, and lips. Scars secondary to acne and lipoatrophy seen in HIV+ patients may deform the facial contours and call for particular fillers in their treatment. Alongside their licensed indications, many practitioners have begun to suggest ways in which these agents may be employed "off-label."

The treatment consists of an injection of a filling substance into the wrinkled area. This is typically HA, but may be collagen or fat. The injected filler gives the skin a smoother contour and takes away the impression of an undesirable wrinkle or hollow. Fillers fall into a number of different types [9]. Certain fillers consist in large part of HA. HA is a naturally occurring molecule found within the human body and is incorporated into the deeper levels of the skin. Fillers containing HA have two key advantages: they persist for more time than collagenous fillers and allow for some correction if the first attempt does not produce the intended result [9]. To remedy a misplaced filler, the enzyme hyaluronidase may be injected in the same area [10]. This enzyme breaks down the HA filler and allows it to be absorbed, reversing the effect.

Another popular type of filler is made of collagen. Collagen is the key structural protein in skin. Its gradual breakdown contributes significantly to ageing [11]. Loss of the collagenous structure makes skin appear laxer. Another option is to use fat as filler. Fat may be transplanted, either autologously or heterologously [12].

The use of fillers is contraindicated if the patient has a known hypersensitivity or a previous severe allergic reaction or anaphylaxis to a component used within the filler, or has a haemostatic disorder. To give a specific example, there is a contraindication to the use of Hylan B gel in patients with an allergy to eggs or products derived from birds. Likewise, the HA fillers produced by recombinant bacteria must not be injected into any patient who is hypersensitive to proteins expressed by Gram-positive bacteria. Cutaneous testing is required before using fillers derived from bovine materials, such as bovine collagen or Bellafill [7].

The use of fillers is also relatively contraindicated in patients who have recently taken agents that influence coagulation and haemostasis, notably aspirin, the non-steroidal anti-inflammatory drugs (NSAIDs), or certain herbal preparations [7].

The following are amongst the fillers in most frequent use [13, 14]:

- Hylaform (manufactured by Genzyme). This product contains HA extracted from the dermis on the combs of male cockerels. The concentration of HA is 5.5 mg/mL, it has a particle size of 500 μm, and there is 20% cross-linkage. It is licensed in the US to treat facial wrinkles and folds, including nasolabial folds, of at least moderate severity.
- Restylane/Restylane-L (manufactured by Galderma). This product contains HA obtained from genetically modified *Streptococcus equi* bacteria. Cross-linkage is with butanediol diglycidyl ether (BDDE). This non-animal stabilised hyaluronic acid (NASHA) is in suspension in phosphate-buffered saline at pH 7 and at a concentration of 20 mg/mL. The particle size is 400 μm. HA has 1% cross-linkage. Lidocaine 0.3% is incorporated into Restylane-L. It is licensed in the US to treat facial wrinkles and folds, including nasolabial folds, of at least moderate severity.
- Perlane/Perlane-L (manufactured by Galderma). This product contains HA obtained from genetically modified *Streptococcus equi* bacteria. Cross-linkage is with BDDE. This NASHA is in suspension in phosphate-buffered saline at pH 7 and at a concentration of 20 mg/mL. The particle size is between 940 and 1090 μm. Lidocaine 0.3% is incorporated. It is licensed in the US to treat facial wrinkles and folds, including nasolabial folds, of at least moderate severity.
- Juvéderm XC (manufactured by Allergan). This product contains HA obtained from genetically modified *Streptococcus equi* bacteria. Cross-linkage is with BDDE. It is manufactured as a homogenised gel with a concentration of 24 mg/mL. It is licensed in the US to treat facial wrinkles and folds, including nasolabial folds, of at least moderate severity.
- Juvéderm Voluma XC (manufactured by Allergan). This product contains HA obtained from genetically modified *Streptococcus equi* bacteria. Cross-linkage is with BDDE. It is manufactured as a homogenised gel with a concentration of 24 mg/mL. This production has a greater degree of cross-linkage. It is licensed in the US for use in adults no younger than 21 with volume loss in the malar region due to ageing. The filler is deeply injected.
- Prevelle Silk (manufactured by Mentor). This product contains HA obtained from genetically modified *Streptococcus equi* bacteria and comes in the form of a homogenised gel. It is licensed in the US to treat facial wrinkles and folds, including nasolabial folds, of at least moderate severity.
- Belotero Balance (manufactured by Merz). This product contains HA obtained from genetically modified *Streptococcus equi* bacteria and comes in the form of a homogenised gel. It is licensed in the US to treat facial wrinkles and folds of at least moderate severity.
- Radiesse (manufactured by Merz). This product comprises microspheres of between 25- and 45-microns diameter in suspension in a gelatinous mixture of sterile water, glycerin and sodium carboxymethylcellulose. It is licensed in the

US for treatment of lipoatrophy in HIV+ patients and to treat facial wrinkles and folds, including nasolabial folds, of at least moderate severity.

- Sculptra (manufactured by Galderma). This product contains a mixture of poly-L-lactic acid, mannitol, and sodium carboxymethylcellulose. It is licensed in the US for treatment of lipoatrophy in HIV+ patients.
- Bellafill (previously marketed as ArteFill; manufactured by Suneva Medical). This product consists of microspherical polymethylacrylate with a diameter of between 30 and 50 microns. It is licensed in the US to treat nasolabial folds and scarring secondary to acne [15].

69.2 Fillers in Pregnancy

The complete lack of scientific testing of the use of fillers during pregnancy has left an unfortunate gap in knowledge about safety in pregnant patients. Although there are reports concerning the use of botulinum toxin in pregnant patients, there are no such reports in the literature concerning fillers. Despite these limitations in the evidence base, majority of clinicians concur that the use of filler probably carries little risk to the foetus as the injected substance remains localised and systemic penetration is probably minimal. There is some potential for risk where fillers have an incorporated local anaesthetic. The most frequently employed agent of this kind is lidocaine [16]. Lidocaine has been separately categorised under the FDA scheme as a category B agent, indicating probable safety when used in pregnant patients. It is also worth considering that the dose of local anaesthetic found in fillers is considerably below the upper safety margin established for lidocaine [12].

According to Lee et al. [17], it is impossible to comment authoritatively on how safe the majority of aesthetic procedures, such as chemical peels, injected substances, fillers, and laser treatments actually are in pregnant women. There is an extensive evidence base indicating that use of onabotulinum toxin by neurology specialists is safe in pregnancy, albeit there are sporadic accounts of spontaneous abortions in women who have previously miscarried. There are plentiful data showing that it is safe to undertake carbon dioxide laser ablation of genital warts in pregnant women.

Lee et al. conclude by recommending that any elective aesthetic procedure not occur until following delivery, given the lack of data from controlled trials examining how safe particular interventions are during pregnancy and the postpartum period [17].

69.3 Neurotoxins

The source of botulinum toxin type A (BTX-A) is the *Clostridium botulinum* bacterium. It is extracted and then purified. There are many different ways this agent can be used therapeutically, such as to treat spasmodic torticollis, focal spasticity, squint, achalasia, spasm of the eyelids, excessive sweating, migraine, and tension headache

[18]. Many skin specialists and cosmetic surgeons favour the use of this neurotoxin to cause a non-permanent paralysis of muscles in the face and thereby reduce the appearance of rhytides [19, 20].

The molecular mass of botulinum toxin is 150 kDa, meaning it is considered large [20]. Intramuscular injection within the recommended dosage interval is not anticipated to result in leakage into the circulation [22]. Accordingly, BTX-A is unlikely to be able to cross into the foetal circulation. Pregnant rabbits injected with intravenous doses of high lethality did not have detectable amounts of botulinum toxin in either the placenta or the foetal circulation [21]. Nonetheless, where rabbits received injections of BTX-A at doses of 0.125 U/kg and 0.5 U/kg daily, and 2 U/kg, 4 U/kg, and 6 U/kg on a daily basis, congenital anomalies and spontaneous abortions were noted to occur [20]. This result was not replicated in pregnant mice, however [20].

69.4 Neurotoxin Injections in Pregnant Women

69.4.1 Experimental Reports

The *C. botulinum* bacterium synthesises botulinum toxin A in the form of a single linear polypeptide with a molecular mass of 150 kDa [22]. There are a limited number of studies available where BTX-A was administered to an animal during pregnancy. From the data gathered, BTX-A does not appear to transfer to the foetus, which may be a result of its large molecular mass. In a particular experiment, a dose of high lethality was administered to pregnant rabbits, after which the concentration in various body fluids was measured [23]. BTX-A levels were below the limit of detection in placental and foetal tissues at the time the rabbits died [23]. The level below which no teratogenic effect is observable in the period of organogenesis (NOEL = no observed effect level) as determined in mice and rats is 4 U.kg^{-1}. Scaling this up for a female adult human weighing 60 kg gives a dose of 240 U. When the dose to which the animals were exposed reached 8 or 16 U.kg^{-1}, there was a reduction in the body mass of the foetus and ossification was delayed. This second effect was possibly transient [24]. In comparison with single massive dose exposure, chronic (daily) exposure to smaller amounts (0.125 U.kg^{-1} between the eighth and 18th day of gestation or 2 U.kg^{-1} on the sixth and 13th day) resulted in toxicity of a severe degree in the mother, miscarriage, and foetal anomalies [24, 25].

69.4.2 Human Reports

Since BTX-A is employed in such a wide variety of medical (for relief of dystonia, muscular spasm, migraine, and tension headache) and cosmetic applications, not to mention numerous other off-label indications, it seems likely that cases of inadvertent maternofoetal exposure to BTX-A will accumulate as time passes. Furthermore, there may well be instances where a condition treated with BTX-A, e.g. hemifacial spasm, becomes more severe whilst a woman is pregnant and calls for use of the agent [26]. For BTX-A to have an effect on the uterine muscle, or to cross the placental barrier, it would need to be transported from far away, i.e. from the site of injection, whether intramuscular or subcutaneous. There are reports in which a technique, such as single fibre electromyography, has found that BTX-A has been transported to a remote site, such as reaching the arm following injection into the muscles of the face [27]. This appears more likely with a raised dose [28]. Although the agent was detected, there do not appear to be any clinically noted effects, such as muscular weakness [27–29].

Instances of women who suffer from botulism, not related to treatment with BTX-A, during pregnancy have frequently been reported. In one case, the mother underwent total paralysis and was placed on a ventilator. Despite the maternal condition, the foetus remained moving as normal at 5 months and the pregnancy ended normally with a vaginal delivery at the expected date [30]. In some other cases, delivery occurred either as expected or somewhat early [31–34].

In two cases in which the infant was delivered prematurely, clinical signs of botulism were entirely absent in the children and botulinum toxin was below the level of detection by serology [31, 32]. There is a possibility that BTX-A may have a therapeutic use as a tocolytic in foetal surgical procedures, since it has been noted that BTX-A suppresses contractility of the myometrium in vitro and this action can be subsequently reversed [35].

Some researchers report that BTX-A is not detected in structures adjacent but separate from the site of injection. When rabbits had BTX-A injected into the blephara, this agent reached an undetectable level in the eye and when the rat gastrocnemius muscle was injected, muscles on the opposite side also had undetectable levels of BTX-A [35]. In a different experiment utilising an electromyographic technique, BTX-A injected into the vastus lateralis of humans did not lead to increased nerve fibres density remotely, nor remodelling at a subclinical level [36].

Morgan et al. [25] concluded that, whilst the evidence had limitations, there was no certain indication that injecting mothers with BTX-A resulted in foetal injury. Nevertheless, in line with the licensed indication, they advise against injecting women during pregnancy, at least until greater evidence accumulates. Since there is also a lack of data about the level of BTX-A in breast milk, lactating women should also not be administered BTX-A. In cases where there is a strong clinical need for BTX-A and the patient provides consent after being fully informed of the potential risks, then off-label prescription becomes the responsibility of the prescribing neurologist and the patient.

The published literature about the effects of botulin toxin on pregnant women consists of a few case reports and one survey [37–51]. There are reports detailing seven instances where a woman in the second or last trimester of pregnancy has contracted botulism [37–43]. In none of these cases were congenital anomalies noted, nor were there features of botulism in the newborn. In one woman, the degree of paralysis was so profound that the only observable movement occurred when the foetus moved [39]. Botulin toxin was undetectable serologically in the two infants tested [37, 43]. A study gathered 28 cases where a pregnant woman had been exposed to BTX-A therapeutically, in 18 or more of which, the exposure was within the initial trimester. These pregnancies had the following outcomes: 25 normal deliveries of a living infant, 1 termination of pregnancy and 2 miscarriages [31–36]. The two women who miscarried had done so previously. Three further reports are available concerning cases where a woman in the initial trimester of pregnancy was administered BTX-A for cosmetic reasons. The outcome of pregnancy was recorded as normal in two cases, but not stated in the third [37, 38].

According to Tan et al. [19], provided BTX-A is administered with a correct technique, systemic overspill should not occur. Thus, since this agent acts only within a confined area of the body and given the absence of evidence for harm, it might be expected that BTX-A could be safely given to pregnant women. Nonetheless, currently the slender evidence base means that the risk to both the mother and unborn child should be weighed carefully against anticipated benefit when advising a pregnant woman about receiving BTX-A therapy [19].

69.5 Neurotoxins During Postpartum Period

There is no published evidence in existence regarding therapeutic use of botulinum toxin A in lactating women. Nonetheless, since this agent is below the level of detection in the systemic circulation after intramuscular injection, it is improbable that it will be present in breast milk. Furthermore, breastfeeding appears protective against botulism [52]. There is a case of an infant who was nursing whilst the mother suffered from botulism, but no toxin was detectable in breast milk or in the infant's circulation. The doses of botulin toxin administered therapeutically are an order of magnitude below the level at which botulism occurs, thus, even where an infant does ingest the toxin via breast milk, it is likely to be at a level insufficient to harm the infant [53–55].

A breastfeeding mother who ate fermented salmon eggs was found to have botulinum toxin present in serum and in her stools. This patient was administered 2 vials containing trivalent botulism antitoxin, by an intramuscular and intravenous route. Breast milk was tested 3 days following the onset of symptoms and 4 h post antitoxin administration and was found to contain neither *C. botulinum* nor the toxin [56].

In the same case, the infant was also tested for both toxin and C. botulinum. Blood and stool had undetectable levels of toxin and the stools did not contain evidence of *C. botulinum*.

References

1. Chacon AH. Fillers in dermatology: from past to present. Cutis. 2015;96(5):E17–9.
2. ASAPS website. http://www.surgery.org/sites/default/files/ASAPS-2012-Stats.pdf.
3. ASPS Website. http://www.plasticsurgery.org/.
4. Buck DW 2nd, Alam M, Kim JY. Injectable fillers for facial rejuvenation: a review. J Plast Reconstr Aesthet Surg. 2009;62(1):11–8. (Medline).

5. Walker K, Pellegrini MV. Hyaluronic acid. 2018. (Medline). (Full Text).

6. Choi MS. Basic rheology of dermal filler. Arch Plast Surg. 2020;47(4):301–4.

7. Winkler AA. Injection facial fillers. In: Meyers AD (Ed). Medscape. Updated: Aug 13, 2020. https://emedicine.medscape.com/article/1574158-overview#a2. Accessed 1 Apr 2021.

8. Alam M, Gladstone H, Kramer EM, Murphy JP Jr, Nouri K, Neuhaus IM. ASDS guidelines of care: injectable fillers. Dermatol Surg. 2008 Jun;34(Suppl 1):S115–48.

9. Sator PG. Skin treatments and dermatological procedures to promote youthful skin. Clin Interv Aging. 2006;1(1):51–6. PMID: 18047257

10. Dong J, Gantz M, Goldenberg G. Efficacy and safety of new dermal fillers. Cutis. 2016;98(5):309–13. PMID: 28040813

11. Tobin DJ. Introduction to skin aging. J Tissue Viability. 2017;26(1):37–46. PMID: 27020864

12. Trivedi M, Murase J. Botox and Dermal Fillers During Pregnancy. Learnskin. https://www.learnskin.com/articles/facial-rejuvenation-in-pregnancy. Accessed 1 Apr 2021.

13. Eppley BL, Dadvand B. Injectable soft-tissue fillers: clinical overview. Plast Reconstr Surg. 2006;118(4):98e–106e.

14. Johl SS, Burgett RA. Dermal filler agents: a practical review. Curr Opin Ophthalmol. 2006 Oct;17(5):471–9.

15. FDA approves first dermal filler to treat acne scarring. Medscape Jan 6 2015.

16. Trivedi MK, Kroumpouzos G, Murase JE. A review of the safety of cosmetic procedures during pregnancy and lactation. Int J Womens Dermatol. 2017;3(1):6–10. PMID: 28492048

17. Lee KC, Korgavkar K, Dufresne RG Jr, Higgins HW 2nd. Safety of cosmetic dermatologic procedures during pregnancy. Dermatol Surg. 2013;39(11):1573–86. https://doi.org/10.1111/dsu.12322. Epub 2013 Oct 29. PMID: 24164677

18. Botox (product monograph). Irvine, CA: Allergan Inc.; 2011.

19. Tan M, Kim E, Koren G, Bozzo P. Botulinum toxin type A in pregnancy. Can Fam Physician. 2013;59(11):1183–4. PMID: 24235190; PMCID: PMC3828093

20. Botox cosmetic (product monograph). Irvine, CA: Allergan Inc.; 2011.

21. Hildebrand GJ, Lamanna C, Heckly RJ. Distribution and particle size of type a botulinum toxin in body fluids of intravenously injected rabbits. Proc Soc Exp Biol Med. 1961;107(284):284–9.

22. Simpson LL. Molecular pharmacology of botulinum toxin and tetanus toxin. Ann Rev Pharmacol Toxicol. 1986;26:427–53.

23. Hildebrand GJ, Lamana C, Heckly RJ. Distribution and particle and particle size of type A botulinum toxin in body fluids of intravenously injected rabbits. Proc Soc Exp Biol Med. 1961;107:284–9.

24. Allergan Pharmaceuticals BOTOX package insert, July 2004.

25. Morgan JC, Iyer SS, Moser ET, Singer C, Sethi KD. Botulinum toxin a during pregnancy: a survey of treating physicians. J Neurol Neurosurg Psychiatry. 2006;77(1):117–9. https://doi.org/10.1136/jnnp.2005.063792. PMID: 16361610; PMCID: PMC2117417

26. Cersósimo MG, Bertoti A, Roca CU, et al. Botulinum toxin in a case of hemimasticatory spasm with severe worsening during pregnancy. Clin Neuropharmacol. 2004;27:6–8.

27. Sanders DB, Massey EW, Buckley EG. Botulinum toxin for blepharospasm: single-fiber EMG studies. Neurology. 1986;36:545–7.

28. Lange DJ, Brin MF, Warner CL, et al. Distant effects of local injection of botulinum toxin. Muscle Nerve. 1987;10:552–5.

29. Lange DJ, Rubin M, Greene PE, et al. Distant effects of locally injected botulinum toxin: a double-blind study of single fiber EMG changes. Muscle Nerve. 1991;14:672–5.

30. Polo JM, Martin J, Berciano J. Botulism and pregnancy. Lancet. 1996;348:195.

31. Type A botulism—Idaho, Oregon, 1973. MMWR Morb Mortal Wkly Rep. 1973;22:218.

32. St. Clair EH, DiLiberti JH, O'Brien ML. Observations of an infant born to a mother with botulism. J Pediatr. 1975;87:658.

33. Wound botulism—California, 1995, MMWR Morb Mortal Wkly Rep. 1995;44:889–92.

34. Robin L, Herman D, Redett R. Botulism in a pregnant women. N Engl J Med. 1996;335:823–4.

35. Garza JJ, Downard CD, Clayton N, et al. Clostridium botulinum toxin inhibits myometrial activity in vitro: possible application on the prevention of preterm labor after fetal surgery. J Pediatr Surg. 2003;38:511–3.

36. Fertl E, Schnider P, Schneider B, et al. Remote effects of chronic botulinum toxin treatment: electrophysiologic results do not indicate subclinical remodeling of noninjected muscles. Eur Neurol. 2000;44:139–43.
37. St Clair EH, DiLiberti JH, O'Brien ML. Observations of an infant born to a mother with botulism (letter). J Pediatr. 1975;87(4):658.
38. Centers for Disease Control and Prevention Wound botulism—California, 1995. MMWR Morb Mortal Wkly Rep. 1995;44(48):889–92.
39. Polo JM, Martin J, Berciano J. Botulism and pregnancy. Lancet. 1996;348(9021):195.
40. Robin L, Herman D, Redett R. Botulism in a pregnant woman. N Engl J Med. 1996;335(11):823–4.
41. Morrison GA, Lang C, Huda S. Botulism in a pregnant intravenous drug abuser. Anaesthesia. 2006;61(1):57–60.
42. Magri K, Bresson V, Barbier C. Botulisme et grossesse. J Gynecol Obstet Biol Reprod (Paris). 2006;35(6):624–6.
43. Centers for Disease Control and Prevention type A botulism—Oregon. MMWR. 1973;22(26):218–23.
44. Newman WJ, Davis TL, Padaliya BB, Covington CD, Gill CE, Abramovitch AI, et al. Botulinum toxin type A therapy during pregnancy. Mov Disord. 2004;19(11):1384–5.
45. Bodkin CL, Maurer KB, Wszolek ZK. Botulinum toxin type A therapy during pregnancy. Mov Disord. 2005;20(8):1081–2.
46. Morgan JC, Iyer SS, Moser ET, Singer C, Sethi KD. Botulism toxin A during pregnancy: a survey of treating physicians. J Neurol Neurosurg Psychiatry. 2006;77(1):117–9.
47. Wataganara T, Leelakusolvong S, Sunsaneevithayakul P, Vantanasiri C. Treatment of severe achalasia during pregnancy with esophagoscopic injection of botulinum toxin A: a case report. J Perinatol. 2009;29(9):637–9.
48. Li Yim JF, Weir CR. Botulinum toxin and pregnancy—a cautionary tale. Strabismus. 2010;18(2):65–6.
49. Aranda MA, Herranz A, del Val J, Bellido S, García-Ruiz P. Botulinum toxin A during pregnancy, still a debate. Eur J Neurol. 2012;19(8):e81–2.
50. De Oliveira ME. Botulinum toxin and pregnancy. Skinmed. 2006;5(6):308.
51. Kuczkowski KM. Anesthetic implications of botulinum toxin type A (Botox) injections for the treatment of 'the aging face' in the parturient. Acta Anaesthesiol Scand. 2007;51(4):515–6.
52. Arnon SS, Damus K, Thompson B, et al. Protective role of human milk against sudden death from infant botulism. J Pediatr. 1982;100:568–73.
53. Butler DC, Heller MM, Murase JE. Safety of dermatologic medications in pregnancy and lactation: part II. Lactation J Am Acad Dermatol. 2014;70(417):e1–10.
54. Lee KC, Korgavkar K, Dufresne RG Jr, et al. Safety of cosmetic dermatologic procedures during pregnancy. Dermatol Surg. 2013;39:1573–86.
55. Drugs and Lactation Database (LactMed) (Internet). Bethesda (MD): National Library of Medicine (US); 2006. OnabotulinumtoxinA. 2020 Sep 21. PMID: 33017114.
56. Middaugh J. Botulism and breast milk. N Engl J Med. 1978;298:343.

Female Voice During Pregnancy and Postpartum Period

70

Ilter Denizoglu and Ibrahim Cukurova

70.1 Introduction

The endocrine system is a complex feedback process and hormones communicate signals with receptors located in target organs. The squamous epithelium of the vocal fold mucosa and cervix have been found to give similar responses to sex hormones [1]. This is possibly because both types of tissues have estrogen, progesterone and androgen receptors. The larynx, in this sense, is highly responsive, especially to sex hormones (estrogen, progesterone and androgens) [2]. As a major target organ, larynx—and its functional output voice—is affected by hormonal changes [3, 4, 6]. Hormonal equilibrium problems will inevitably deteriorate the biomechanical properties of the vocal fold tissue and result in irregularities in the oscillatory patterns of the vocal fold mucosa [7].

Estrogen, secreted by the ovaries, has a proliferative effect on the mucosa, in advance, decreased desquamation and epithelial thickening [8]. It increases the secretion of mucus from glandular cells and prepares the tissue that enables the progesterone to be effective. In the larynx, estrogens cause a thickening of the vocal fold mucosa (especially in the superficial layer of lamina propria) which results in greater vibratory amplitude and deepen the vocal timbre. It

I. Denizoglu (✉)
Vocology Centre, Izmir, Turkey
e-mail: ilterdenizoglu@gmail.com

I. Cukurova
Section of Otorhinolaryngology, Tepecik Training and Research Hospital,
İzmir Faculty of Medicine, University of Health Sciences, Izmir, Turkey
e-mail: Cukurova57@gmail.com

C. Cingi et al. (eds.), *ENT Diseases: Diagnosis and Treatment during Pregnancy and Lactation*, https://doi.org/10.1007/978-3-031-05303-0_70

923

also increases the oxygenation of the vocal fold tissue and capillary permeability. Mucosa becomes moistened and lubricated which, in turn, results in decreased shear stress and lowered phonation threshold pressure. Overall, estrogen seems to have positive effects on the functional characteristics of the voice organ [9].

Progesterone is principally secreted by the corpus luteum of the ovaries approximately between 15–55 years of age and its main function is to prepare the uterus for gestation. It is also secreted from placenta during pregnancy [10]. Progesterone decreases the capillary permeability and creates an imbalance in the distribution of interstitial fluid. This results in a diffuse tissue edema due to restriction of the capillaries from draining tissues and prevents interstitial fluid from vascular reuptake. This is not the same regarding the thickening of the superficial layer of the lamina propria by estrogen. Progesterone also thickens and decreases the secretions of the mucous glands above and below the vocal folds. Similar to estrogen, progesterone causes the shedding of surface cells of the vocal folds [9].

Androgens are normally secreted in small amounts from the female ovaries and adrenal glands. However, if the amount increases pathologically, vocal masculinization (reduced fundamental frequency and deepening of voice timbre) may be seen. Regarding the muscle strength, pulmonary functions and connective tissue health, normal levels of androgens in females may have a supportive effect by strengthening the vocal muscles and keeping the vocal mucosa at a certain thickness.

Sex hormones have a fluctuating balance between puberty and menopause. Physiologically, the menstrual cycle is interrupted by pregnancy. Sex hormone-associated syndromes involving larynx in females are related to three important hormonal periods: menstruation (laryngopathia premenstrualis), pregnancy (laryngopathia gravidarum) and menopause (menopausal vocal syndrome).

70.2 Voice in Menstrual Period

Sex hormones show prominent changes during menstrual cycle; in the follicular phase, estrogens increase and progesterone decreases, and in the luteal phase, progesterone may show a gradual increase with a decrease in estrogen. The effects of hormonal fluctuations on phonation are not homogenous, but are especially prevalent in female singers [11]. It is an interesting finding that voice quality is found to be in its best level in the ovulatory phase and worst in the premenstrual phase [3] which may be related to the expression of fertility. The laryngopathia premenstrualis may be seen up to 40% of women [12]. However, for those who are not professional voice performers, the findings may be ignored and a clinical referral may not be needed. On the other hand, it can have career-threatening consequences for a singer.

Premenstrual voice problems are caused by high levels of estrogens (edema in follicular phase) and progesterone (dryness in luteal phase). Estrogens are high in the first half of the female menstrual cycle which creates an ideal environment for vocal fold vibration (well-lubricated and less epithelial desquamation). The estrogen effect also increases the capillary permeability leading to a fluid shift into the interstitial compartment making the vocal fold mass more pliable and supple, which is biomechanically ideal for vibration. In the second half of the menstruation cycle, progesterone levels increase and this results in epithelial desquamation, mucosal dryness and thickness.

Biomechanically, due to decreased capillary permeability (prevention of the excess interstitial fluid into circulation) vocal fold edema may affect vocal range (loss of high pitches, decreased habitual fundamental frequency) [4]. Clinical examination may not reveal prominent visual changes, though, glottic closure pattern may give clues about the biomechanical-acoustical consequences of the anatomical changes on vibrating tissues. In order to compensate the decrease in the fundamental frequency, glottic closure pattern may be changed by muscular reorganization. Occasionally, this compensatory behavioral change is seen as a posterior glottic gap. Voice therapy is the treatment of choice in this case which aims to prevent and rehabilitate the malregulative process (Fig. 70.1) [13]. This is especially important in female singers who have increased hormonal imbalances. They may experience problems in vocal performance 5–6 days before and a few days after the menses which may require a related performance schedule (approximately between the fourth and 24th days of menstrual cycle).

Because of the increased bleeding risk, professional voice performers may need to avoid increased mechanical impact on vocal folds (i.e. high-pitched forte singing) [14, 15]. Laryngostroboscopic examination may reveal reduced vibratory amplitude, edema, venous dilatation and glottic gap, to some extent due to muscular hypotonicity [16, 17] The vocal fatigue in the premenstrual period may be the result of the reduced muscular tonus.

Management of voice disorders in the menstrual period starts with counseling. Hydration, modified voice rest and avoiding vocal abuse and misuse are other preventive measures. Semi-occluded vocal tract (SOVT) exercises may be used for

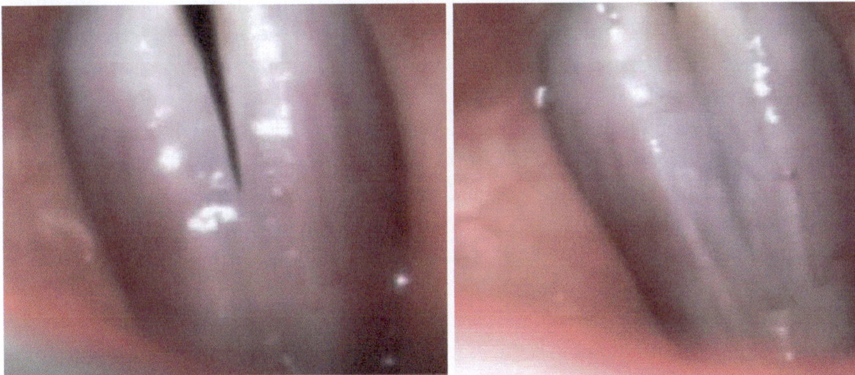

Fig. 70.1 The posterior glottic gap before (left) and after (right) voice therapy

proper glottic closure and massage effect. Multivitamins, phlebotonics and anti-edematous drugs have also been suggested for symptomatic treatment [1].

70.3   Voice in Pregnancy

Pregnancy is a special period that physiologically pauses the hormonal cycle and also eliminates the vocal changes due to menstrual period [7]. During pregnancy, the sex hormones directly affect mucosa, muscle, bone tissues, genital tract and cerebral cortex. The rapid hormonal changes that occur during pregnancy also manifest themselves in the larynx, which is a major target organ for sex hormones [18]. Therefore, changes related to voice are common during pregnancy and instead of cyclic changes, the pregnant women experience a continuous vocal process throughout pregnancy. Most of them disappear during the early postpartum period without referring to the voice clinic, [19] however, these changes may be permanent in some cases [20].

Due to pregnancy-related vomiting (morning sickness) in the first trimester, the larynx is exposed to a serious attack of acid and gastric enzymes. High progesterone levels reduce the tonus of the lower esophageal sphincter, the motility of the stomach increases and the possibility of laryngopharyngeal reflux increases with the effect of the gradually increasing intraabdominal pressure after the second trimester [21].

Most prominent voice changes during pregnancy are expected in the third trimester because of the hormonal, metabolic and mechanical effects. Especially, the progesterone levels are high and progesterone effects are dominant. The physiological consequences increase the phonation threshold pressure and collision threshold pressure levels [22, 23]. This is possibly because of the increased tissue viscosity and mucus thickness. The acoustic output of this situation may manifest itself in a decrease in vocal brightness and maximum phonation time [19, 22]. Although acoustic analysis may not reveal prominent changes, voice handicap index has been shown to deteriorate significantly in the third trimester [19].

In the third trimester, the application of the abdominodiaphragmatic breathing technique becomes difficult due to excessive tension in the abdominal muscles, and during this period, professional voice performers are deprived of support, also known as appoggio [24].

It may be recommended to restrict or temporarily suspend the stage performances, especially in the last stages of pregnancy. Of course, this situation may vary from person to person (uterus size and position, maternal body structure, weight gain, reflux level etc.). Sometimes professional stage performance in the middle of the second trimester may be adversely affected, while in some, stage performance can be sustained with waist restrictions until the last weeks before birth. It has been postulated [25] that a professional vocal performer can sing even better into the seventh month of pregnancy with nicely plump and well-lubricated vocal folds affected by sex hormones.

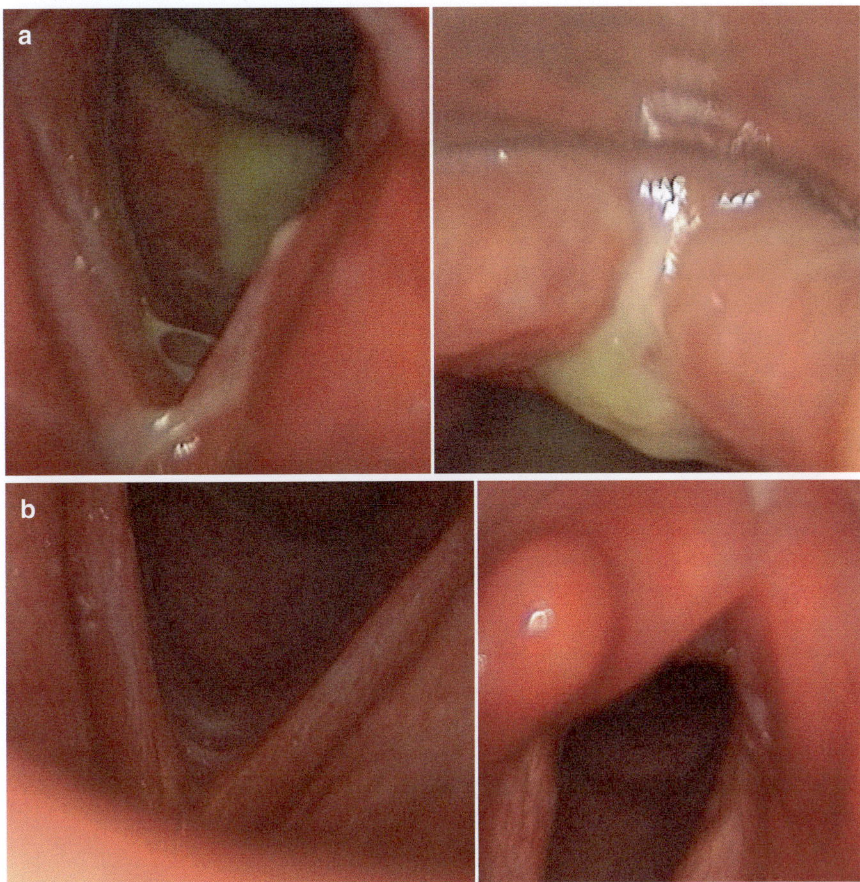

Fig. 70.2 (**a**) Laryngeal changes in the last trimester: Subglottic edema, vocal fold hyperemia and crusting (left) and interarytenoid edema and crusting (right). (**b**) Laryngeal recovery in the early postpartum period: Vocal fold mucosa (left) and interarytenoid region (right)

It is important to continue the daily vocal exercise program both to protect the sportive vocal endurance and to compensate for edema and other structural changes in the vocal fold mucosa. In this period, SOVT exercises with low back pressure in mid-low vocal range can be applied. In addition to the massage effect, these exercises are aimed to prevent malregulative glottic closure patterns [13].

Laryngopathia gravidarum is an uncommon voice disorder that occurs during pregnancy. It is more common in pregnant women with preeclampsia [26–28]. Clinical manifestations are related to laryngeal mucosal edema, dryness and even crusting which may impair vocal vibratory dynamics [29]. Although physiopathological mechanisms are not understood well, edema of the superficial layer of the lamina propria is the possible explanation for the voice changes due to preeclampsia. Increased risk of laryngopharyngeal reflux may worsen the symptoms, especially in the last trimester (Fig. 70.2a).

In fact, laryngopathia gravidarum can also be expressed as excessive changes that occur during pregnancy that do not require a clinical referral and recover in the early postpartum period (Fig. 70.2b). Rarely, severe respiratory tract obstruction may occur requiring a tracheotomy [30].

70.4 Voice in Postpartum Period

Breastfeeding increases the levels of oxytocin and prolactin, and inhibits the release of sex hormones. If breastfeeding is continued like a pacifier after milk intake ends, estrogen and progesterone levels drop too low, causing amenorrhea and a hormonal situation similar to that of menopause (mucosal dryness and atrophy) may occur [21]. However, this situation returns to normal when breastfeeding does not take long and menstruation starts again. Exclusive breastfeeding is recommended [31] in the first 6 months of life followed by continued breastfeeding as complementary foods are introduced for another 6 months (or longer as mutually desired by mother and infant). So, due to the fact that the breastfeeding period continues for an average of 12 months and the initiation of foods other than breast milk over time, vocal disorders (mucosal atrophy and dryness) experienced in menopause are rarely encountered in the postpartum period.

70.5 Voice in Postmenopausal Period

In the postmenopausal period, a relative increase of testosterone and decrease in estrogens and progesterone levels may lead to vocal fatigue, loss of high pitches and deepening of the voice [3, 5]. Mucosal atrophy and reduced glandular cells may impair vibratory mechanics, and muscular atrophy may cause reduced glottal impact and bowing. Hormone replacement therapy is a rational choice in management of menopausal voice syndrome in order to preserve loudness and pitch but systemic side effects are to be concerned. Voice lift surgery can also be a treatment of choice in selected patients by injection medialization (fat, fascia, collagen, hydroxyapatite) or thyroplasty. Voice therapy may be a powerful tool in order to increase the phonatory efficiency. Especially, the SOVT exercises can be used for increasing the strength of the vocal muscles within the scope of exercise physiology and principles of physiotherapy (overload, progression and adaptation). In advance, mucosal response to training through cellular mechanotransduction seems to be an effective factor in voice therapy [32].

70.6 Conclusion

The larynx is a major target for the sex hormones. Voice changes affect especially the female professional voice performers in the fluctuations of sex hormones during puberty, menstruation, pregnancy, lactation and menopause periods. Diagnosis and management of voice problems during these periods require multidimensional thinking and strategical approach. Coinciding pathologies such as laryngopharyngeal reflux, morning sickness, excessive breastfeeding, preeclampsia etc. are ought to be concerned.

References

1. Abitbol J, Abitbol P, Abitbol B. Sex hormones and the female voice. J Voice. 1999;13(3):424–46.
2. Voelter C, Kleinsasser N, Joa P, Nowack I, Martinez R, Hagen R, Voelker HU. Hormone receptors in the human vocal fold. Eur Arch Otorhinolaryngol. 2008;265(10):1239–44.
3. Raj A, Gupta B, Chowdhury A, Chadha S. A study of voice changes in various phases of menstrual cycle and in postmenopausal women. J Voice. 2010;24(3):363–8.
4. D'haeseleer E, Depypere H, Claeys S, Borsel JV, Van Lierde K. The menopause and the female larynx, clinical aspects and therapeutic options: a literature review. Maturitas. 2009;64(1):27–32.
5. D'haeseleer E, Depypere H, Claeys S, Baudonck N, Van Lierde K. The impact of hormone therapy on vocal quality in postmenopausal women. J Voice. 2012;26(5):671.e1–7.
6. Damste PH. Virilization of the voice due to anabolic steroids. Folia Phoniatr (Basel). 1964;16:10–8.
7. Lã FMB, Ledger WL, Davidson JW, Howard DM, Jones GL. The effects of a third generation combined oral contraceptive pill on the classical singing voice. J Voice. 2007;21(6):754–61.
8. Amir O, Biron-Shental T. The impact of hormonal fluctuations on female vocal folds. Curr Opin Otolaryngol Head Neck Surg. 2004;12(3):180.
9. Abitbol J. Odyssey of the voice. San Diego, CA: Plural Publishing; 2006.
10. Henderson VW. Progesterone and human cognition. Climacteric. 2018;21(4):333–40.
11. Nawka T, Wirth G. Stimmstörungen. 5th ed. Köln: Deutscher Ärzte-Verlag GmbH; 2008.
12. Lacina O. Der Einfluss der Menstruation auf die Stimme der Sangerinnen. Folia Phoniatr. 1968;20:13–24.
13. Denizoglu I. Textbook of clinical vocology (in Turkish). Ankara: Karaca Publishing; 2020.
14. Chernobelsky SI. A study of menses-related changes to the larynx in singers with voice abuse. Folia Phoniatr Logop. 2002;54(1):2–7.
15. Davis CB, Davis ML. The effects of premenstrual syndrome (PMS) on the female singer. J Voice. 1993;7(4):337–53.
16. Chae SW, Choi G, Kang HJ, Choi JO, Jin SM. Clinical analysis of voice change as a parameter of premenstrual syndrome. J Voice. 2001;15(2):278–83.
17. Barillari MR, Volpe U, Innaro N, Barillari U. Is menstrual dysphonia associated with greater disability and lower quality of life? J Voice. 2016;30(1):88–92.
18. Hamdan A, Mahfoud L, Sibai A, Seoud M. Effect of pregnancy on the speaking voice. J Voice. 2009;23(4):490–3.
19. Saltürk Z, Kumral TL, Bekiten G, Atar Y, Ataç E, Aydoğdu I, Yıldırım G, Kılıç A, Uyar Y. Objective and subjective aspects of voice in pregnancy. J Voice. 2015;30(1):70–3.
20. Deuster CV. Irreversible Stimmstörung in der Schwangersheft. HNO. 1977;25:430–2.
21. Sataloff RT. Clinical assessment of voice. 2nd ed. San Diego, CA: Plural Publishing; 2017.
22. Lã FMB, Sundberg J. Pregnancy and the singing voice: reports from a case study. J Voice. 2002;26(4):431–9.

23. Hancock AB, Gross HE. Acoustic and aerodynamic measures of the voice during pregnancy. J Voice. 2014;29(1):53–8.

24. Cassiraga VL, Castellano AV, Abasolo J, Abin EN, Izbizky GH. Pregnancy and voice: changes during the third trimester. J Voice. 2012;26(5):584–6.

25. Abitbol J. The female voice. San Diego, CA: Plural Publishing; 2019.

26. Bhatia PL, Singh MS, Jha BK. Laryngopathia gravidarum. Ear Nose Throat J. 1981;60:408–12.

27. Hoing R, Seitzer D. Clinical aspects of laryngopathia gravidarum. Laryngol Rhinol Otol (Stuttg). 1988;67(11):564–6.

28. Brimacombe J. Acute pharyngolaryngeal oedema and pre-eclamptic toxaemia. Anaesth Intensive Care. 1992;20(1):97–8.

29. Moses RL, Paige T, Cavalli G, Broker B, Malhotra R, Shrager D, Atkins J, Keane W. Laryngotracheobronchitis in pregnancy and its clinical implications. Otolaryngol Head Neck Surg. 1997;116(3):401–3.

30. Laitinen K. Life-threatening laryngeal edema in a pregnant woman previously treated for thyroid carcinoma. Obstet Gynecol. 1991;78(5 pt 2):937–8.

31. AAP (American Academy of Pediatrics). Section on breastfeeding, breastfeeding and the use of human milk. Pediatrics. 2012;129(3):e827–41.

32. Lenell C, Sandage MJ, Johnson AM. A tutorial of the effects of sex hormones on laryngeal senescence and neuromuscular response to exercise. J Speech Lang Hear Res. 2019;62(3):602–10.

Nutritional Approaches to Decrease Allergy Outcomes in the Offspring of Allergic Mothers

Gülce Cingi and İrem Kaya Cebioğlu

71.1 Introduction

Sufficiency of nutrition in terms of macro and micronutrients is crucial during the period of pregnancy and lactation to shape not only the health of the mother but also the health and development of the baby and may predispose future health problems for the baby. The ideal behavior of feeding infants during the first 6 months is exclusive breastfeeding, it is an essential source of energy and nutrients and protects against gastrointestinal and other infections [1]. Strong immune and digestive systems are considered to develop in breastfeeding infants because of the growth of positive bacteria in the gut that provides a healthy microbial population [1]. Nutritional intakes should be planned by a dietitian considering the body mass index (BMI), ethnicity, food selection according to culture, ability to reach food, and the socioeconomic status of the patient [2].

71.2 Energy Requirement

During pregnancy, overall calorie intake should rise by approximately 300 kcal/day. This figure is based on an estimate of 80,000 calories required to sustain a full-term pregnancy, and it takes into consideration not just the requirements of the increased

G. Cingi (✉)
Private Nutrition and Dietetics Clinic, Istanbul, Turkey
e-mail: gulcecingi@gmail.com

İ. K. Cebioğlu
Faculty of Health Sciences, Department of Nutrition and Dietetics, Yeditepe University, Istanbul, Turkey
e-mail: irem.cebioglu@yeditepe.edu.tr

C. Cingi et al. (eds.), *ENT Diseases: Diagnosis and Treatment during Pregnancy and Lactation*, https://doi.org/10.1007/978-3-031-05303-0_71

metabolism of mother and fetal, but also the fetal and placental development [2]. Throughout the second trimester, the daily recommended intake (DRI) for energy increases by just 340 kcal per day, while in the third trimester, it increases by 452 kcal daily. Considering individual variances in energy expenditure and basal metabolic rate, the range of appropriate energy consumption varies substantially if maternal weight gain is within desired range or when the breastfed infant is gaining the appropriate amount of weight [1, 2]. The extra calorie recommendation for lactating women was set as approximately 500 calories, this value was determined by the average amount of milk produced per day [3].

71.3 Macronutrients

71.3.1 Protein

The increased protein intake is essential to be able to maintain maternal and fetal tissues synthesis during pregnancy. The protein need rises gradually during the period of pregnancy, peaking in the third trimester. Since the protein requirement is increased compared to a normal individual, it is recommended to consume about 60 g of protein per day. For non-pregnant women 0.8 g/kg/day is consumed daily however in pregnancy protein intake can be up to 1.1 g/kg/day as needs increase [1, 2]. Protein intake should be increased by at least 25 g per day for each additional fetus in both pregnancy and lactation [2, 4]. Protein deficit during pregnancy may have negative outcomes, such as fetal development deficits. In addition, the fact that protein is necessary for the production of neurotransmitters and hormones increases its importance even more.

71.3.2 Carbohydrates

The recommended daily allowance (RDA) for carbohydrates rises modestly aiding in the maintenance of normal blood glucose levels and the avoidance of ketosis. Carbohydrates must account for 45–64% of daily calories, while intentive carbohydrate selection is required to ensure that all of the necessary nutrients are met throughout pregnancy and lactation. Complex carbohydrates from whole grains, vegetables, and fruits should be prioritized above simple sugars, such as refined liquid sugars, either from natural juices or artificially made drinks.

71.3.3 Fiber

The greater sources of fiber including whole-grain bread, cereals, leafy green vegetables, and fresh or dried fruits should be consumed in sufficient amounts daily to supply minerals, vitamins, and fiber needs. The DRI for fiber during pregnancy is 14 g/day per 1000 kcal consumed. If this amount is fulfilled, it will also greatly help the management of constipation, which is commonly seen in the pregnancy period.

71.3.4 Lipids

Similar to nonpregnant women, total fat consumption should account for 20% to 35% of daily calories. The fat content of the diet should be determined by the amount of energy required for optimal growth. The need for guidelines reporting the consumption of omega-6 PUFA (linoleic acid) and omega-3 PUFA (alpha-linolenic acid) is slightly higher [1, 5]. Although it is not a DRI, a daily intake of 200 mg of docosahexaenoic acid (DHA) is recommended, and this can be met by the consumption of fish once or twice a week [1, 5]. Pregnant women must consume seafood like salmon, sardines, and anchovies, which are low in mercury and high in omega-3 fatty acids. However, shark, swordfish, tilefish, and king mackerel are high in mercury and should be avoided during pregnancy. According to existing data, fish-oil supplementation does not provide equal beneficial effects as eating the actual fish [6].

71.4 Micronutrients

71.4.1 Vitamins and Minerals

The optimum progression of pregnancy and lactation requires all vitamins and minerals. Although not all vitamins and minerals, the need for most of them is increased. Prenatal multivitamins are recommended in the pre-conception and the pregnancy period to meet this requirement and minimize any deficiencies. In absence of vitamin or mineral insufficiency or a limited diet, nutritional supplements are not required for the mother [1]. The woman should be given all the nutrients she requires, including a range of meals that are sufficient in calories. However, many physicians urge that prenatal vitamin/mineral supplements be continued to be used throughout the breastfeeding period [7] (AAP 2012). The composition of milk depends on the nutrition of a mother. For example, the content of fatty acids, the concentration of selenium, iodine, and some of the B vitamins in a mother's milk reflect her food consumption [1] (Table 71.1).

Folic acid is the synthetic version of folate. Vitamin B, that occurs naturally, is included in most vitamin supplements and fortified foods. Citrus fruits, dark-green leafy vegetables, nuts, and liver are high in folate, while bread, cereal, and pasta are typically fortified. Because of the rapidly proliferating cells associated with fetal development, folate needs to rise throughout pregnancy. Folic acid supplements are recommended by The U.S. Preventive Services Task Force (USPSTF) to be administered 400–800 mcg before conception in order to decrease the risk for neural tube defects [1, 2, 9].

Cobalamin is utilized in enzyme reactions and is an essential vitamin for growth and development, as well as immunological function [10]. Because vitamin B12 is only naturally available in foods derived from animals, vegetarians, particularly vegans, are at risk of dietary deficiency and should prefer supplements of foods fortified with B12. Insufficient levels of folate and B12 can harm an infant's cognitive and motor development, while also increasing the risk of neural tube defects and fetal growth problems [1].

Table 71.1 Recommended daily dietary allowances for pregnant and lactating women

Nutrient	Nonpregnant	Pregnant	Lactation
Vitamin A (mg/d)	700	770	1300
Vitamin D (mg/d)	5	15	15
Vitamin E (mg/d)	15	15	19
Vitamin K (mg/d)	90	90	90
Folate (mg/d)	400	600	500
Niacin (mg/d)	14	18	17
Riboflavin (mg/d)	1.1	1.4	1.6
Thiamine (mg/d)	1.1	1.4	1.4
Vitamin B_6 (mg/d)	1.3	1.9	2
Vitamin B_{12} (mg/d)	2.4	2.6	2.8
Vitamin C (mg/d)	75	85	120
Calcium (mg/d)	1000	1000	1000
Iron (mg/d)	18	27	9
Phosphorus (mg/d)	700	700	700
Selenium (mg/d)	55	60	70
Zinc (mg/d)	8	11	12

Applies to women >18 years
Data from: [2, 8]

Vitamin A is vital for cellular differentiation, ocular development, immunological function, lung development, and maturity, including gene expression, during stages of fast growth [1, 10]. Extreme dosages of vitamin A (>10,000 IU/d) have been linked to cranial-facial (face, palate, ears) and cardiac birth abnormalities. Supplementation is generally not essential and is frequently confined to 5000 IU/day [1]. The form of vitamin A associated with teratogenic outcomes, however, is the retinol form, not the carotenoid form found in foods like carrots [2].

Vitamin D is one of the fat-soluble vitamins which is mostly available in fortified milk or juices and some breakfast cereals, although it may also be found naturally in eggs, salmon, and other fatty fish. The active form of vitamin D is 1,25-dihydroxyvitamin D which stimulates calcium absorption from the intestines, allowing proper bone mineralization and development. Vitamin D demands do not rise throughout pregnancy, according to the IOM, and daily doses of 600 IU (15 mcg) are adequate for bone health [1]. Supplements (1000–2000 IU per day) might be administered if vitamin D insufficiency is identified during pregnancy [1]. The optimal 25(OH)D blood levels during pregnancy are unknown, but they must be at least 20 ng/ml (50 nmol/L) to maintain bone health [1, 11]. Other experts recommend minimum levels of 32 ng/ml (80 nmol/L) during pregnancy, however levels over 70 nmol/L have been associated with an elevated risk of growth limitation and infant eczema [1, 12]. AAP advises that all infants get vitamin D 400 IU (10 mcg) as daily supplementation starting from birth, which will make it easy for infants to obtain sufficient vitamin D.

During pregnancy, the RDA for iron greatly increases. A pregnant woman's usual requirements are increased by 17 mg per day; typical absorption from a regular diet is 1–2 mg per day, and 3–5 mg daily if the diet incorporates high-iron items

[13]. If the serum ferritin level is less than 20 mcg/L in the first trimester, supplementation may be required [13]. Since women mostly do not have enough iron reserves to meet the metabolic needs of pregnancy, iron supplementation (typically in the form of a ferrous salt) is frequently given, though the quantity of elemental iron in each formulation differs [14]. Due to considerable heme concentration, red meats are the finest suppliers of iron, and several organ meats may have even greater quantities. However, due to the high amount of vitamin A found in liver and liver products, it is necessary to limit the amount of these products consumed in the first trimester [1]. Vegetable sources of iron, which solely comprise nonheme iron, are less readily absorbed. Vegetarian women should pay particular attention to their iron intake and strive to keep their hematocrit from dropping so low that cannot be recovered [1].

71.5 How to Prevent or Decrease Atopic Outcomes of the Offspring During Pregnancy and Lactation

The prevalence of allergies is seen to be increased greatly worldwide over the years, particularly in the Western countries including Europe, United States, and Australia. There is evidence that the main causes affecting the future development of allergic and atopic diseases include factors encountered during fetal life and early life, epigenetic changes [15], and many environmental causes [16, 17]. Allergy is an excessive reaction to an external antigen irrespective of its cause. Atopy is an excessive immunological response mediated by IgE thus all atopic diseases are type I disorders of hypersensitivity [18].

Atopy affects a large part of the overall population in developed nations, generally approximated at 10–30% [19]. Around 80% of atopic people have an allergy background in the family, compared to approximately 20% of the population on average. There's just 50% conformity among monozygotic twins [19]. The sensitivity to atopic diseases is hereditary, however, there is evidence of numerous genes with modest effects rather than of one or two causal predominant genes [19, 20]. The population of 10–12% of the United States has allergic rhinitis [19]. Atopy is an immunological response to a variety of antigens and allergenic substances, resulting in the differentiation of CD4+ Th2 and overproduction of immunoglobulin E (IgE) [19]. The clinical outcome is that hypersensitivity responses become more common. Among the most common symptoms of atopy, followed by food allergy and atopic dermatitis are allergic bronchial asthma and allergic rhinitis; urticaria, allergic conjunctivitis, angioedema, IgE-mediated medication allergy, and anaphylactic shock also encompass other illnesses classified as atopic [19]. If an individual has atopic disease, there is a high probability of one or more other atopic diseases including atopic dermatitis, allergic rhinoconjunctivitis, hay fever, asthma, and food allergy [21]. The atopy etiology is not clear. Epidemiological studies show precisely that genetic variables may have an essential role in controlling the atopic tendency, the overall IgE synthesis, and the development of particular epitopic IgE antibodies. The propensity for overproduction of IgE is influenced by the inheritance of more than one gene, and this can run in families, as evidenced by the autosomal transmission of allergy [19, 22]. A theory has been proposed to explain the development of atopy, suggesting that T helper cells and T suppressor lymphocytes can be abnormally regulated to aid in plasmic cell IgE production [19, 23, 24].

Developing a primary preventative approach is important for the prevention of allergies. Among environmental reasons, one of the most prominent factors in terms of modifiability is diet. The proposal that early prevention has a key opportunity has aroused attention on the potential of dietary measures for mothers of offspring who have a higher risk for atopy thus, it could be targeted as an early approach for food allergy prevention [25].

Pregnancy is a highly anabolic physiological condition that requires a special diet with adequate amounts of micronutrients, trace elements, and vitamins [26]. Essential nutrients are passed by the placenta from the mother throughout her gestation in the fetal circulation [27]. Because prenatal life is a key era for the formation of an immune system, the significance of intrauterine exposure in allergic disease etiology has been studied in several studies [28]. As a result, dietary variables related to allergic diseases probably start to have an impact on utero. In various trials, asthma and allergic conditions have been beneficially affected by ingestion of specific foods and dietary groups by pregnant women [26, 29–31]. In recent decades, it has been observed that nutrition in the world has changed, especially in western societies. Modified, processed foods and foods with prolonged storage are often consumed, such as soft drinks, fast foods, with high saturated fat, trans fat, and industrial sugar content and low antioxidant, vitamin, and mineral content thus usually poor in nutritional value [32]. This direction of diet change led to an increase in omega 6 and a decrease in the amount of omega 3 intakes and it was seen that this situation has the potential to increase the prevalence of asthma by increasing the production of prostaglandin E2 (PGE2) [32, 33]. T-helper (Th) 1 is suppressed by PGE2, and Th2 is increased, thereby decreasing the IFN gamma. Th2 is linked to asthma and atopic diseases with an increase in the IgE isotype switch [32]. Considering these situations, the contribution of the dietary intake of the mother during pregnancy is changing the possibility of the baby developing allergic diseases in the future has been examined in many studies and it has been concluded that the mother's diet can shape the atopic outcomes of the baby to a certain extent.

## 71.6	Nutritional Approach in Lactation and Pregnancy to Reduce Allergic Outcomes

Maternal nutrition during pregnancy and lactation can be modified to some extent in order to reduce the likelihood of genetically predisposed infants having atopic diseases. During pregnancy, the atopic mother must be fed in a balanced and nutritious manner in terms of micro and macronutrients. The inclusion of vegetables, fruits, seafood, and vitamin D sources in a balanced diet during pregnancy and lactation by atopic mothers contributes to adequate vitamin and mineral intake, thus, an improved immune system of the infant and a lower incidence of allergies, but margarine, nuts, vegetable oils, fast food, and soft drinks cause an increased incidence of atopy [34]. A diet with high content of Omega-6 fatty acids but poor in omega-3 fatty acids may stimulate the T-helper type 2 (Th2) cytokine production thus promoting atopic responses [35]. A systematic review by the European Academy of Allergy and Clinical Immunology found thirty-eight papers that have an association between maternal diet throughout pregnancy and eczema outcomes in the offspring [36]. Studies showed a significantly lowered incidence of childhood eczema with maternal consumption of beta-carotene, vitamin E, zinc, calcium, magnesium, and copper throughout pregnancy considering vitamins and minerals. Increased dermatitis risk was related to fast foods, shellfish, alcohol, and meat (not specified) [36]. Several RCTs tested the time impact of dietary restriction of common allergen foods on families which have atopic disease history during pregnancy and lactation however, there is presently inadequate evidence of substantial impacts on prevention of atopic illness in infants by maternal diet limitations [34, 36] Vitamin D is a multi-role hormone involving immunoregulation. Association of low vitamin D status as a risk factor for the development of atopy, including food allergy, is growing interest [37]. Researches have shown links between cow's milk consumption and lowered atopy [34]. However as cow's milk is enriched by vitamin D in some areas, these relationships may indirectly reflect vitamin D intakes and positive outcomes could be attributed to vitamin D. However, an RCT assessing the efficacy of vitamin D complementation revealed no difference in wheezing, allergy, lung function, and allergic inflammation between kids in the supplemented and non-supplemented subgroups [38].

A healthy diet and adequate vitamin C intake are shown to increase the amount of vitamin C in breast milk, resulting in a lower incidence of eczema in infants up to 1-year-old [39]. Intake of $n-6$ PUFA (LA), which has been believed to be closely linked to the increasing frequency and incidence of atopic diseases in childhood, grew throughout the later portion of the twentieth century [33, 40]. The sources of long-chain $n-3$ PUFAs include fish and fish oils, and these fatty acids are used to counteract the impact of $n-6$ PUFAs. Therefore, $n-3$ PUFAs are deemed to prevent atopic sensitization and clinical symptoms [41]. PUFAs ensure that membrane protein function, membrane fluidity, cell signaling, gene expression, and cellular function remain in favorable environments [41]. It is therefore apparent that during pregnancy and breastfeeding, fish oil supplementation leads to a higher status of $n-3$ PUFAs for the offspring. The supply of early fish oil is linked to immunological cord blood alterations and these may remain. On the flip side, a diet high in $n-3$ PUFAs may affect the Th cell balance by limiting Th2 cell differentiation and thereby preventing allergy progression [35]. A study revealed that reduced consumption of fish raised the risk of respiratory symptoms (current wheeze) by 21% in comparison with greater intakes [42]. Studies show that the therapeutic effects of early fish oil administration include reduced sensitivity to common food allergens and reduced prevalence and severity of atopic dermatitis in the first year of life, with potential persistence into adolescents with reduced eczema, hay fever, and asthma [41]. however future studies are needed. Study investigations demonstrated a lowered risk of linked childhood eczema with maternal fish consumption during the period of pregnancy (high omega-3) and dermatitis and study reports saw a lowered risk for childhood asthma [26, 34, 36]. The systematic review based on RCTs evaluated the influence of the supplementation of omega-3 fatty acid just in pregnancies and showed that omega-3 fatty acid consumption, based on pooled estimations, significantly decreases the allergic sensitivity to eggs and peanuts in the children [43]. In another study, it was concluded that the child's consumption of fish is more important than maternal fish consumption in order to prevent eczema in the offspring [31].

Breastfeeding duration of at least 4 months has been shown to prevent or postpone atopic dermatitis, cow's milk allergy, and wheezing during early childhood compared to feeding with the formula of intact cow's milk protein [44]. Also, comparative tests of different hydrolyzed formulations showed that the same protecting effect does not exist in all formulas. In preventing atopic diseases, extensively hydrolyzed formulas can be more efficient than partly hydrolyzed. More study is also required to evaluate if the advantages continue to late childhood and adolescence [44]. Although solid foods should not be added to infant nutrition before 4–6 months, there is no convincing proof at present that postponing their implementation after that time has important preventive effects on the development of atopic diseases, whether breast milk or cow milk formula are fed to children. Such as the introduction of extremely allergenic foods such as fish, eggs, and meals that contain peanuts protein is delayed [44].

The placental membrane was demonstrated to transfer heavy metals, including selenium [45, 46]. Heavy metals such as selenium, usually taken with the consumption of food, have been proposed to decrease the likelihood of developing allergies and asthma [47, 48]. However, there is little information on this issue. Research had shown an adverse link between the high level of maternal plasma selenium levels during pregnancy and the likelihood of the kid wheezing 1–3 years of age [49]. During pregnancy, the incidence of asthma, allergic rhinitis, or atopic dermatitis was not related to maternal plasma selenium [48, 49]. However, a comparative study by Shaheen et al. [50] had seen no relationship between prenatal and postnatal atopic dermatitis exposure to high selenium levels, according to the mixed results more research is needed on selenium consumption and atopic outcomes.

Probiotics are living bacteria with different health advantages promoted by yeasts. They are frequently added to yogurts or supplemented with meals and are usually regarded as "good" bacteria. When disorders occur, probiotics are considered to help restore the normal balance of bacteria in the stomach and intestines. Some data suggest that probiotics in some conditions can be useful, such as helping avoid diarrhea in the use of antibiotics and reducing some symptoms of irritable bowel syndrome (IBS) [51–53]. There is also evidence regarding the effects of probiotic consumption in the prevention of allergic diseases. The intestinal microbiota is in an eubiotic condition in a healthy state, contrarily, allergic diseases including eczema, asthma, and food allergy have been related to gut dysbiosis [54–58]. Allergic diseases have revealed a decreased microbial diversity in newborn microbiota prior to the actual development of atopic disorders, including less Lactobacilli and Bifidobacteria [54]. Increasing interest was noted in the management of microbiota by prebiotics, probiotics, or synbiotics to re-establish the microbial balance in the prevention of atopic diseases [54]. Clear evidence of probiotics, but modest evidence of prenatal supplements to support this preventative impact on eczema in high-risk children also the optimum prebiotic or probiotic strain, dose, duration, and timing is unclear [54]. In particular, there was a greater advantage of a combined pre and post-natal intervention, however, it remained unfulfilled to define optimum intervention period during gestation, timing, and length for post-natal intervention, as well as the appropriate target group [36, 59–61]. A recent meta-analysis on the effects of probiotic consumption on eczema onset in children during pregnancy has found that supplementation of lactobacilli throughout pregnancy averts atopic dermatitis in children between 2 and 7 years of age but not a mixture of different bacterial strains [25, 62]. However, this effect wasn't seen on food allergies for both mixed probiotics or only Lactobacillus GG supplementation during pregnancy [63–65].

71.7 The Mediterranean Diet

The established dietary patterns in the Mediterranean region gave the name to the Mediterranean Diet (MedDiet) [66]. It includes a high amount of fruit and vegetable intake, whole-grain cereals and breads, vegetables and nuts, low to moderate intakes of dairy products and eggs; alcohol, poultry, and meat are consumed in restricted amounts [32, 66]. The MedDiet is rich in antioxidants, carbohydrates, and fibers, and is low in saturated fatty acids. The amount of $n-3$ polyunsaturated fatty acids (PUFAs) and monounsaturated fatty acids are also high, largely obtained from olive oil and fish [32, 67]. Research has proven the advantages of Mediterranean dietary interventions not only providing for primer and seconder prevention of cardiovascular diseases, but also managing, type 2 diabetes, obesity, metabolic syndrome, neurodegenerative diseases, or cancer [66, 68, 69]. Adopting Mediterranean dietary patterns has also been seen to be related to lower risk for allergic outcomes and higher atopy risk eating patterns that include vegetable oils, margarine, nuts, and fast foods [34]. The Mediterranean diet content is rich in antioxidants, monounsaturated fatty acids, vitamin D, phenolic acids, and phytic acid from whole grains. Also, vitamins C and E, carotenoids, selenium, and flavonoids are plentiful in fruit, vegetable, and legumes [32, 67]. Olive oil is also a key component of MedDiet for cooking and dressing salads [32, 66]. Oleic acid, phenol derivatives (hydroxytyrosol, tyrosol, ligstroside, and oleuropein), and squalene, which have all been proven to be significant antioxidant ingredients, are the major active components of olive oil [32]. One study showed that the mother's olive oil use in pregnancies, but not MedDiet, remained a protective factor for wheezing during the first year of her childhood after multivariate analysis [70]. Therefore, greater adherence to MedDiet or olive oil appears fair to believe that it can have a preventive impact on childhood asthma and allergic disorders. This diet's capacity to prevent oxidative stress might influence the development of asthma but does not seem to affect allergic rhinitis, eczema, or atopy [32, 71]. Finally, investigations of mother adapting to MedDiet during pregnancy demonstrated a protective impact only during the first year of the offspring, however, the progress of atopic diseases in later years of life were not clear on asthma/wheeze symptoms [32].

References

1. Mahan L, Stumpt SRJ. Krause's food & nutrition care process, vol. 14. 14th ed. Pain Medicine (United States); 2017.
2. Kominiarek MA, Rajan P. Nutrition recommendations in pregnancy and lactation. Med Clin N Am. 2016;100:1199–215.
3. Centers for Disease Prevention and Control (CDC). Maternal Diet [Internet]; 2020. https://www.cdc.gov/breastfeeding/breastfeeding-special-circumstances/diet-and-micronutrients/maternal-diet.html
4. Goodnight W, Newman R. Optimal nutrition for improved twin pregnancy outcome. Obstet Gynecol. 2009;114:1121–34.
5. Koletzko B, Cetin I, Thomas Brenna J, Alvino G, von Berlepsch J, Biesalski HK, et al. Dietary fat intakes for pregnant and lactating women. Br J Nutr. 2007;98(5):873–7.
6. Zibaeenezhad MJ, Ghavipisheh M, Attar A, Aslani A. Comparison of the effect of omega-3 supplements and fresh fish on lipid profile: a randomized, open-labeled trial. Nutr Diabetes [Internet]. 2017;7(12):1–8. https://doi.org/10.1038/s41387-017-0007-8.
7. Eidelman AI, Schanler RJ. Breastfeeding and the use of human milk. Pediatrics. 2012;129:496–506.
8. Institute of Medicine. Dietary reference intakes: the essential guide to nutrient requirements (2006). The National Academies Press; 2006.
9. (CDC): Centers for Disease Control and Prevention. Folic Acid; 2021.
10. Wu G, Imhoff-Kunsch B, Girard AW. Biological mechanisms for nutritional regulation of maternal health and fetal development. Paediatr Perinat Epidemiol. 2012;26 Suppl 1:4–26.
11. ACOG Committee Opinion No. 495: vitamin D: screening and supplementation during pregnancy. Obstet Gynecol. 2011;118:197–8.
12. Brannon PM, Picciano MF. Vitamin D in pregnancy and lactation in humans. Annu Rev Nutr. 2011;31:89–115.
13. Lee AI, Okam MM. Anemia in pregnancy. Hematol Oncol Clin North Am. 2011;25:241–59.
14. Office of Dietary Supplements (ODS) NI of H (NIH). Dietary Supplement Fact Sheet: Iron [Internet]; 2014. http://ods.od.nih.gov/factsheets/Iron-HealthProfessional.
15. Bollati V, Baccarelli A. Environmental epigenetics. Heredity. 2010;105:105–12.
16. Baïz N, Dargent-Molina P, Wark JD, Souberbielle JC, Annesi-Maesano I. Cord serum 25-hydroxyvitamin D and risk of early childhood transient wheezing and atopic dermatitis. J Allergy Clin Immunol. 2014;133(1):147–53.
17. Gillman MW. Developmental origins of health and disease. N Engl J Med. 2005;353(17):1848–50.
18. Peter J. Delves MM. Overview of allergic and atopic disorders [internet]; 2020. https://www.msdmanuals.com/professional/immunology-allergic-disorders/allergic,-autoimmune,-and-other-hypersensitivity-disorders/overview-of-allergic-and-atopic-disorders
19. Justiz Vaillant AA, Modi P, Jan A. Atopy. Updated 2022 May 1. In: StatPearls [Internet]. Treasure Island (FL): StatPearls Publishing; 2022 Jan. Available from: https://www.ncbi.nlm.nih.gov/books/NBK542187/. Accessed online at May 27, 2022.
20. Huang JL. Asthma severity and genetics in Taiwan. J Microbiol Immunol Infect. 2005;38:158–63.
21. Thomsen SF. Epidemiology and natural history of atopic diseases. Eur Clin Respir J. 2015;24:2.
22. Qi S, Liu G, Dong X, Huang N, Li W, Chen H. Microarray data analysis to identify differentially expressed genes and biological pathways associated with asthma. Exp Ther Med. 2018;16(3):1613–20.

23. Hemler JA, Phillips EJ, Mallal SA, Kendall PL. The evolving story of human leukocyte antigen and the immunogenetics of peanut allergy. Ann Allergy Asthma Immunol. 2015;115(6):471–6.
24. Kim JH, Lee SY, Kang MJ, Yoon J, Jung S, Cho HJ, et al. Association of genetic polymorphisms with atopic dermatitis, clinical severity and total IgE: a replication and extended study. Allergy Asthma Immunol Res. 2018;10(4):397–405.
25. Luengo O, Song Y. The potential of maternal dietary modification for prevention of food allergy. J Allergy Ther. 2013:S3.
26. Baïz N, Just J, Chastang J, Forhan A, De Lauzon-Guillain B, Magnier AM, et al. Maternal diet before and during pregnancy and risk of asthma and allergic rhinitis in children. Allergy Asthma Clin Immunol. 2019;15:40.
27. Harding JE. The nutritional basis of the fetal origins of adult disease. Int J Epidemiol. 2001;30(1):15–23.
28. Prescott SL. Early origins of allergic disease: a review of processes and influences during early immune development. Curr Opin Allergy Clin Immunol. 2003;3(2):125–32.
29. Chatzi L, Kogevinas M. Prenatal and childhood Mediterranean diet and the development of asthma and allergies in children. Public Health Nutr. 2009;12(9A):1629–34.
30. Willers SM, Wijga AH, Brunekreef B, Kerkhof M, Gerritsen J, Hoekstra MO, et al. Maternal food consumption during pregnancy and the longitudinal development of childhood asthma. Am J Respir Crit Care Med. 2008;178(2):124–31.
31. Øien T, Storrø O, Johnsen R. Do early intake of fish and fish oil protect against eczema and doctor-diagnosed asthma at 2 years of age? A cohort study. J Epidemiol Community Health. 2010;64(2):124–9.
32. Castro-Rodriguez JA, Garcia-Marcos L. What are the effects of a mediterranean diet on allergies and asthma in children? Front Pediatrics. 2017;5:72.
33. Black PN, Sharpe S. Dietary fat and asthma: is there a connection? Eur Respir J. 1997;10(1):6–12.
34. Netting MJ, Middleton PF, Makrides M. Does maternal diet during pregnancy and lactation affect outcomes in offspring? A systematic review of food-based approaches. Nutrition. 2014;30:1225–41.
35. Palmer DJ, Sullivan T, Gold MS, Prescott SL, Heddle R, Gibson RA, et al. Effect of n-3 long chain polyunsaturated fatty acid supplementation in pregnancy on infants' allergies in first year of life: randomised controlled trial. BMJ. 2012;344:e184.
36. Venter C, Agostoni C, Arshad SH, Ben-Abdallah M, Du Toit G, Fleischer DM, et al. Dietary factors during pregnancy and atopic outcomes in childhood: a systematic review from the European academy of allergy and clinical immunology. Pediatr Allergy Immunol. 2020;31(8):889–912.
37. Vuillermin PJ, Ponsonby AL, Kemp AS, Allen KJ. Potential links between the emerging risk factors for food allergy and vitamin D status. Clin Exp Allergy. 2013;43:599–607.
38. Goldring ST, Griffiths CJ, Martineau AR, Robinson S, Yu C, Poulton S, et al. Prenatal vitamin D supplementation and child respiratory health: a randomised controlled trial. PLoS One. 2013;8(6):e66627.
39. Hoppu U, Rinne M, Salo-Väänänen P, Lampi AM, Piironen V, Isolauri E. Vitamin C in breast milk may reduce the risk of atopy in the infant. Eur J Clin Nutr. 2005;59(1):123–8.
40. Hodge L, Peat JK, Salome C. Increased consumption of polyunsaturated oils may be a cause of increased prevalence of childhood asthma. Aust NZ J Med. 1994;24(6):727.
41. Kremmyda LS, Vlachava M, Noakes PS, Diaper ND, Miles EA, Calder PC. Atopy risk in infants and children in relation to early exposure to fish, oily fish, or long-chain omega-3 fatty acids: a systematic review. Clin Rev Allergy Immunol. 2011;41:36–66.
42. Antova T, Pattenden S, Nikiforov B, Leonardi GS, Boeva B, Fletcher T, et al. Nutrition and respiratory health in children in six central and eastern European countries. Thorax. 2003;58(3):231–6.
43. Vahdaninia M, Mackenzie H, Dean T, Helps S. ω-3 LCPUFA supplementation during pregnancy and risk of allergic outcomes or sensitization in offspring: a systematic review and meta-analysis. Ann Allergy Asthma Immunol. 2019;122(3):302–13.
44. Greer FR, Sicherer SH, Burks AW, Baker RD, Bhatia JJS, Daniels SR, et al. Effects of early nutritional interventions on the development of atopic disease in infants and children: the role

of maternal dietary restriction, breastfeeding, timing of introduction of complementary foods, and hydrolyzed formulas. Pediatrics. 2008;121(1):183–91.

45. Barceloux DG. Selenium. J Toxicol Clin Toxicol. 1999;37(2):145–72.

46. Rudge CV, Röllin HB, Nogueira CM, Thomassen Y, Rudge MC, Odland JO. The placenta as a barrier for toxic and essential elements in paired maternal and cord blood samples of south African delivering women. J Environ Monit. 2009;11(7):1322–30.

47. Devereux G, McNeill G, Newman G, Turner S, Craig L, Martindale S, et al. Early childhood wheezing symptoms in relation to plasma selenium in pregnant mothers and neonates. Clin Exp Allergy. 2007;37(7):1000–8.

48. Thomson CD, Wickens K, Miller J, Ingham T, Lampshire P, Epton MJ, et al. Selenium status and allergic disease in a cohort of New Zealand children. Clin Exp Allergy. 2012;42(4):560–7.

49. Baïz N, Chastang J, Ibanez G, Annesi-Maesano I. Prenatal exposure to selenium may protect against wheezing in children by the age of 3: immunity. Inflamm Dis. 2017;5(1):37–44.

50. Shaheen SO, Newson RB, Henderson AJ, Emmett PM, Sherriff A, Cooke M. Umbilical cord trace elements and minerals and risk of early childhood wheezing and eczema. Eur Respir J. 2004;24(2):292–7.

51. Catinean A, Neag AM, Nita A, Buzea M, Buzoianu AD. Bacillus spp. spores-a promising treatment option for patients with irritable bowel syndrome. Nutrients. 2019;11(9):1–10.

52. Pedersen N, Andersen NN, Végh Z, Jensen L, Ankersen DV, Felding M, et al. Ehealth: low FODMAP diet vs lactobacillus rhamnosus GG in irritable bowel syndrome. World J Gastroenterol. 2014;20(43):16215–26.

53. Herndon CC, Wang YP, Lu CL. Targeting the gut microbiota for the treatment of irritable bowel syndrome. Kaohsiung J Med Sci. 2020;36(3):160–70.

54. Sestito S, D'Auria E, Baldassarre ME, Salvatore S, Tallarico V, Stefanelli E, et al. The role of prebiotics and probiotics in prevention of allergic diseases in infants, vol. 8. Front Pediatr; 2020;8:583946.

55. Abrahamsson TR, Jakobsson HE, Andersson AF, Björkstén B, Engstrand L, Jenmalm MC. Low gut microbiota diversity in early infancy precedes asthma at school age. Clin Exp Allergy. 2014;44(6):842–50.

56. Abrahamsson TR, Jakobsson HE, Andersson AF, Björkstén B, Engstrand L, Jenmalm MC. Low diversity of the gut microbiota in infants with atopic eczema. J Allergy Clin Immunol. 2012;129(2):434–40.

57. Ling Z, Li Z, Liu X, Cheng Y, Luo Y, Tong X, et al. Altered fecal microbiota composition associated with food allergy in infants. Appl Environ Microbiol. 2014;80(8):2546–54.

58. Bisgaard H, Li N, Bonnelykke K, Chawes BLK, Skov T, Paludan-Müller G, et al. Reduced diversity of the intestinal microbiota during infancy is associated with increased risk of allergic disease at school age. J Allergy Clin Immunol. 2011;128(3):646–52.e1–5.

59. Muraro A, Halken S, Arshad SH, Beyer K, Dubois AEJ, Du Toit G, et al. EAACI food allergy and anaphylaxis guidelines. Primary prevention of food allergy. Allergy Eur J Allergy Clin Immunol. 2014;69(5):590–601.

60. Azad MB, Coneys GJ, Kozyrskyj Prof AL, Field Prof CJ, Ramsey Prof CD, Becker AB, et al. Probiotic supplementation during pregnancy or infancy for the prevention of asthma and wheeze: systematic review and meta-analysis. BMJ. 2013;347:f6471.

61. Cuello-Garcia CA, Brozek JL, Fiocchi A, Pawankar R, Yepes-Nuñez JJ, Terracciano L, et al. Probiotics for the prevention of allergy: a systematic review and meta-analysis of randomized controlled trials. J Allergy Clin Immunol. 2015;136(4):952–61.

62. Doege K, Grajecki D, Zyriax BC, Detinkina E, Zu Eulenburg C, Buhling KJ. Impact of maternal supplementation with probiotics during pregnancy on atopic eczema in childhood-a meta-analysis. Br J Nutr. 2012;107(1):1–6.

63. Niers L, Martín R, Rijkers G, Sengers F, Timmerman H, Van Uden N, et al. The effects of selected probiotic strains on the development of eczema (the PandA study). Allergy Eur. J Allergy Clin Immunol. 2009;64(9):1349–58.

64. Boyle RJ, Ismail IH, Kivivuori S, Licciardi PV, Robins-Browne RM, Mah LJ, et al. Lactobacillus GG treatment during pregnancy for the prevention of eczema: a randomized controlled trial. Allergy Eur. J Allergy Clin Immunol. 2011;66(4):509–16.
65. Ou CY, Kuo HC, Wang L, Hsu TY, Chuang H, Liu CA, et al. Prenatal and postnatal probiotics reduces maternal but not childhood allergic diseases: a randomized, double-blind, placebo-controlled trial. Clin Exp Allergy. 2012;42(9):1386–96.
66. Lăcătuşu CM, Grigorescu ED, Floria M, Onofriescu A, Mihai BM. The mediterranean diet: from an environment-driven food culture to an emerging medical prescription. Int J Environ Res Public Health. 2019;16(6):942.
67. Trichopoulou A, Lagiou P. Healthy traditional Mediterranean diet: an expression of culture, history, and lifestyle. Nutr Rev. 1997;55(11 Pt 1):383–9.
68. Gotsis E, Anagnostis P, Mariolis A, Vlachou A, Katsiki N, Karagiannis A. Health benefits of the Mediterranean diet. Angiology. 2015;66(4):304–18.
69. Sofi F, Macchi C, Abbate R, Gensini GF, Casini A. Mediterranean diet and health. Biofactors. 2013;39(4):335–42.
70. Castro-Rodriguez JA, Garcia-Marcos L, Sanchez-Solis M, Pérez-Fernández V, Martinez-Torres A, Mallol J. Olive oil during pregnancy is associated with reduced wheezing during the first year of life of the offspring. Pediatr Pulmonol. 2010;45(4):395–402.
71. Vardavas CI, Papadaki A, Saris WHM, Kafatos AG. Does adherence to the Mediterranean diet modify the impact of smoking on health? Public Health. 2009;123:459–60.

Management of Vascular Lesions During Pregnancy and Postpartum Period

Alper Dilci, Mustafa Acar, and Marwan Al Qunaee

72.1 Introduction

During pregnancy, immunologic, endocrine, metabolic, vascular changes may lead to physiologic and pathologic changes in skin and mucosal surfaces. It is a highly dynamic process and significant alterations occur to the cardiovascular system to ensure adequate uteroplacental circulation for fetal growth and development. These changes are believed to be mediated by elevated levels of estrogen and progesterone. In addition, Relaxin a peptide hormone produced by the corpus luteum that reaches peak levels in the first trimester may also have a significant endothelium-dependent vasodilator role in pregnancy. Along with the marked vasodilation, the cardiac output and heart rate also increased [1].

Consequently, pregnancy may have marked adverse effects through initiating the process of developing vascular malformations or worsening the symptoms in patients with underlying vascular malformations. In either situation, it can result in serious complications.

A. Dilci (✉)
Division of Otorhinolaryngology, Head and Neck Surgery, Usak University Faculty of Medicine, Usak, Turkey
e-mail: alperdilci@yahoo.com

M. Acar
The Acar Ear, Nose, and Throat Diseases and Surgery Clinic, Eskişehir, Turkey
e-mail: drmustafaacar@hotmail.com

M. Al Qunaee
Division of Otolaryngology, Head and Neck Surgery, Saint Paul's Sinus Center, University of British Columbia, Vancouver, BC, Canada
e-mail: marwanalqunaee@gmail.com

C. Cingi et al. (eds.), *ENT Diseases: Diagnosis and Treatment during Pregnancy and Lactation*, https://doi.org/10.1007/978-3-031-05303-0_72

Changes that occur during pregnancy will progressively resolve at the postpartum period due to a decrease in hormone levels. Urgent treatment protocols should be applied if a severe complication of these lesions occurs. In this section, vascular lesions located in the head and neck area and management strategies in pregnancy and postpartum period are described briefly.

Vascular anomalies consist of vascular malformations and tumors and are frequently encountered in the head and neck region and are presented in about 4–5% in pediatric group [2, 3]. These anomalies include various malformations of vascularities ranging from capillary anomalies to complex vascular lesions. In the characteristics of these lesions, different presentations, growth behaviours, and treatment modalities could be observed. Proper, accurate and early diagnosis is very important and helpful because observation and treatment periods could be prolonged [4].

International Society for the Study of Vascular Anomalies (ISSVA) described the classification system, which is most commonly used today. It is a detailed classification system based on Mullikan and Glowacki's early studies [2]. Vascular anomalies are evaluated in two main groups: vascular tumors and vascular malformations according to these schemes (Table 72.1).

72.2 Vascular Tumors

72.2.1 Infantile Hemangioma

Infantile hemangioma (IH) is a benign proliferation of blood vessels that occurs in approximately 5% of the newborn population, with a reported incidence as high as 10% in the first year of life, making it one of the most common tumors of infancy.

Table 72.1 International Society for the Study of Vascular Anomalies classification of vascular anomalies (https://www.issva.org/UserFiles/file/ISSVA-Classification-2018.pdf)

Vascular tumors	Vascular malformations
Benign	*Slow flow malformations*
Infantile hemangioma	Capillary (port-wine stain, telangiectasia, angiokeratoma)
Congenital hemangioma	
Tufted angioma	Venous (common sporadic venous malformation, lymphatic malformation, familial cutaneous and mucosal venous malformation)
Spindle cell hemangioma	
Pyogenic granuloma (also known as lobular capillary hemangioma)	
Locally aggressive	*Fast flow malformations*
Kaposiform hemangioendothelioma	Arterial malformation
Hemangioendothelioma	Arteriovenous malformation
Papillary intralymphatic angioendothelioma	Arteriovenous fistula
Malign	*Complex combined vascular malformations*
Angiosarcoma	Capillary venous malformation
Epithelioid hemangioma	Capillary lymphatic malformation
	Lymphovenous malformation

These lesions are presented approximately 60% in the head and neck region. It will rapidly grow in size (proliferative phase), then become smaller (involution phase) over time [5, 6]. No first onset case has been reported in adults and relapse of the proliferation phase has not been observed.

Histologically, IHs consist of proliferated immature endothelial cells and disorganized vessels. GLUT-1 is positively detected in up to 97% of patients and can be used as a specific marker for IH. This specificity is very useful in the differential diagnosis of such lesions. A biopsy can be performed on suspected lesions and an accurate diagnosis can be achieved by examining the presence of this marker [7].

IHs can be classified as focal, multifocal, segmental, and indeterminate. There is single localized lesion in focal type, multiple lesions are present in multifocal type and there are diffuse plaques in segmental type. Extra imaging techniques are required for more than 5 lesions. Hepatic hemangiomas that can lead to serious and life-threatening bleeding can be diagnosed by this way. Segmental hemangiomas are located in the cranial nerve dermatomes, most often in the trigeminal nerve pathway. They may accompany with malformations of posterior fossa, cardiovascular anomalies, and anomalies of eye (PHACE syndrome). The incidence of subglottic hemangiomas is increased in these patients.

IHs can also be classified according to their thickness: superficial, deep, and compound. Superficial hemangiomas are in the classic bright-red color like strawberry appearance. Deep IHs are presented like a subcutaneous mass under the skin. Compound type IHs show features of both types. Deeply located IHs may appear darker red or purple in color.

Typical characteristic of IH is rapid growth phase followed by involution phase. These lesions are usually not presented at birth, but these lesions occur in the first few months of life. Rapid growth, ulceration, bleeding, and cosmetic deformities may be observed in the first age. Rapid growth pattern up to 80% of potential size can be observed at age 1. The involution phase can continue for years and is usually completed by the age of 10. At the end of the involution phase, aberrant vessels, fibrofatty tissues, and telangiectasias may remain, and these lesions may require treatment.

Propranolol, a nonselective adrenergic blocker, is used as the first-line treatment for IHs. With this treatment, decrease in size and discoloration of lesion from bright red to gray are observed. Early treatment is important for IHs located in the subglottic region, eye, or areas that may cause cosmetic deformities [8]. Diagnosis should be clarified by performing GLUT-1 examination for a resistant lesion to treatment [9].

Subglottic IH is characterized by airway obstruction and stridor symptoms presented in the first years of life. Early diagnosis with laryngoscopy or bronchoscopy is very crucial. These lesions are mostly located unilaterally and posterolateral of the airway. Propranolol therapy with intubation, tracheostomy, endoscopic laser resection, and open surgery is the main treatment options for subglottic IHs with respiratory distress [10]. If medical treatment is contraindicated or fails to produce an adequate effect, other treatment options should be considered, including intralesional corticosteroid injection, CO_2 laser ablation, and surgical resection. The treatment preference will be determined by the experience of the surgeon.

Corticosteroids are the other option in the treatment protocol and may be administered systemically, intralesionally, or topically. Steroids show similiar effects with propranolol however systemic steroids can have more potential side effects than propranolol. But, intralesional and topical use of steroids are effective and safe treatment options for IHs. If the lesion does not respond to corticosteroids or propranolol, vincristine or IFN-α-2b can be evaluated by clinician [11].

Surgical excision of lesion should be considered when there is threat to life or function, complicated course, failure of pharmacotherapy, cosmetic revision of scars after lesion involution, atypical growth, or emotional burden. Approximately 50% of IHs are treated surgically. Lesions that cause destruction of surrounding tissue and cosmetic deformity due to the rapid growth should be treated without delay. Surgical resection or pulsed dye laser treatment may be required for the residual tissues after the involution period. It is important to treat the lesion in the early period when it is small and has not spread to surrounding tissues.

Intrinsic defects or somatic endothelial mutation and extrinsic factors are the main theories due to the origin of this lesion [12]. The placental theory is one of the major theories. Due to this idea, a fetal placental progenitor is the cell type of origin. IHs are detected more frequently in babies of mothers who underwent transcervical chorionic villus sampling [13]. Theoretically, it is thought that placental cells shedding into the maternal bloodstream or placental angioblasts shedding into the fetal circulation during transcervical chorionic villus sampling may cause the formation of IH. Lu Y et al. presented a case of a 26-year-old woman with multiple infantile hemangioma-like lesions with 5-week history after therapeutic abortion by dilatation and curettage. In this case, placental cells incidentally found in maternal circulation may cause hemangioma-like lesions in maternal body.

IHs are not observed during pregnancy or postpartum period. These types of hemangiomas have involution period and these lesions regress in maximum 10 years. The hemangiomatic lesions observed in adults are typically congenital hemangiomas (CHs). During pregnancy, CHs typically do not cause serious complications and usually wait and see regimen is suitable.

72.2.2 Congenital Hemangioma

CHs are similar to IHs. CH clinically presents as fully developed lesions at birth which either rapidly involutes or no involution can be observed. CH is further subcategorized into rapidly involuting CH (RICH) and non-involuting CHs (NICHs). RICH undergoes a rapid regression phase and completely disappears by 12–18 months of age. In some newborns, cardiac failure may be observed due to high flow. NICH does not show a regression phase, may grow proportionately with the growth of the child, and can be mistaken for vascular malformations [14]. Hormonal changes, infection, and trauma can cause lesions to grow and become symptomatic.

Researches have suggested a possible role for estrogen as a mediator for vascular proliferation and hemangioma formation. However, the mechanism is not fully understood [15]. Since most of the IHs are involuted, they are not encountered during pregnancy. Non-regressive hemangiomas can still grow with the effect of estrogen during pregnancy. These lesions usually consist of aberrant vessels with fibrofatty tissue so complications are not observed during pregnancy. With the rapid decline of estrogen after pregnancy, the lesion will also be regressed. Lesions not involutes after pregnancy can be treated in accordance with the usual treatment protocols for hemangiomas.

Hemangiomas in the head and neck generally do not cause complications. Epistaxis or bleeding in the mucosal surfaces can be observed due to possible effects of estrogen. Local treatment protocols aim to control bleeding can be applied. Small resectable lesions can be treated with local surgeries or waited for possible regression after pregnancy.

72.2.3 Tufted Angioma

Tufted angiomas are rare lesions characterized by red and violet plaques. These lesions generally may invade the border of dermis and are seen mainly in the trunk and extremities in the first 5 years of life. Adult forms are commonly seen in the oral mucosa and head and neck region [16]. The differential diagnosis should be made from kaposi sarcoma and angiosarcoma. Lesions that do not cause cosmetic deformity can be followed up without any treatment. Complete surgical excision is recommended for a small lesion. Topical rapamycin, cryotherapy, electron beam radiation, and pulsed dye laser may be applied [17].

The pathogenesis of tufted angioma is unclear and may be associated with some vascular growth factors. Pregnancy could be a predisposing factor for vascular proliferation, indicating estrogen promoting its development. Estrogen is a vasoactive hormone that promotes vasomotor instability and increases cutaneous blood flow, venous distensibility, and vascular permeability and fragility. Progesterone has been shown to have vasodilatory and.

vasoconstrictive effects on skin vessels. Biopsy can be performed under local anesthesia during pregnancy. If pathological diagnosis confirmed as tufted angioma, observation is the best suggestion for pregnant patient. If there is bleeding or other complication occurs, local surgical interventions can be suitable.

72.2.4 Spindle Cell Hemangioma

Spindle cell hemangioma can present a small nodule with a red or brown color. The diameter of lesion ranges from a few milimeter to centimeter. They are generally presented as a solitary lesion or bundle of lesions. The most common treatment is surgical excision. It is very rare lesion and it was not reported in pregnant cases.

72.2.5 Epithelioid Hemangioma

Epithelioid hemangiomas are commonly presented as single or multiple vascular nodules. These lesions grow slowly, bleed easily and can itch. It is most common in adults and it is localized mostly in pre-auricular area in the head and neck region [18].

Local surgical interventions may be used for controlling these lesions during pregnancy. It is commonly observed if there are no complications during the pregnancy period.

72.2.6 Pyogenic Granuloma

Pyogenic granulomas, also known as lobular capillary hemangiomas, commonly present as a angiomatous pedunculated polyps that frequently bleed spontaneously. The term pyogenic granuloma is considered by many as a misnomer due to the fact that the lesion is not associated with any purulence and is not currently thought to be of bacterial origin [19, 20]. The common occurrence of this lesion during pregnancy makes this lesion being called as pregnancy tumor [21]. The most common site is the anterior maxillary gingiva. When seen in pregnancy, the lips, tongue, and buccal mucosa are common sites. These lesions are often seen after trauma, infection, burns, and during pregnancy [22]. It is commonly localized in the gingiva and nasal cavity of the woman in the first trimester of pregnancy. Its incidence is between 2% and 5%. As the hormone levels decrease after labor, the lesions regress and disappear [23].

Treatment considerations during pregnancy are very important. Management should be based on the patient's condition and should range from oral hygiene and supportive therapy to control bleeding, medications accelerating fetal lung maturity, and termination of pregnancy to save patient's life. Curettage, shave excision and laser phototherapy, or full-thickness excision are the main treatment options for this lesion. The management of this lesion during pregnancy is complex. The size of the lesion, bleeding potential, the trimester of pregnancy, the gestational age of the fetus and the results of the possible surgery should be evaluated. Hanick et al. presented a laryngeal pyogenic granuloma that causes bleeding and airway obstruction. Urgent surgery was applied to their patient in the third trimester according to reduce the risk of teratogenicity and premature labor [24].

Pyogenic granuloma is associated with the use of oral contraceptives in addition to its relevance during pregnancy [25]. This suggests that this lesion may be estrogen or progesterone sensitive [21]. These circulating hormones promote possible endothelial and vascular growth important for formation of pyogenic granuloma. Poor oral hygiene and local bacterial biofilms may be a precipitating factor for oral lesions.

Although regression of the lesion after childbirth is observed, surgical resection may still be required in the postpartum period in some cases for lesions that fail to resolve. Most lesions are followed without treatment during pregnancy. However, if a lesion requiring surgery is encountered, the entire lesion must be removed. Otherwise, the lesion may grow again with the effect of hormones during pregnancy. Promising results have been reported for various new treatment strategies (e.g., laser therapy, alitretinoin gel, and sclerosing agents) [25]. Corticosteroids may be used as a medical treatment during pregnancy but propranolol should not be used because of the possible side effects to baby.

72.2.7 Kaposiform Hemangioendothelioma

Kaposiform hemangioendotheliomas are rare and aggressive vascular tumors. Growing hemangiomatous lesion accompanied with thrombocytopenia and pain is defined as Kassabach—Meritt phenomenon. The most common location of the lesion is extremities, approximately 20% of lesion may be located in the head and neck region. It is commonly managed with multimodal protocols consisting of propranolol, steroids, and chemotherapeutic agents. mTOR inhibitors such as everolimus and sirolimus are successful clinically in some regimens [26]. Retiform hemangioendothelioma, polymorphous hemangioendothelioma, and papillary intralymphatic angioendothelioma (PILA) are the other several types of hemangioendotheliomas but these types are very rarely observed.

72.2.8 Kaposi Sarcoma

It is a mesenchymal tumor arising from lymphatic endothelial cells. It is associated with AIDS and HHV—8 plays an important role in the pathogenesis of kaposi sarcoma and immune dysregulation. There are four main variants: classical, endemic, iatrogenic (posttransplant), and AIDS-related. Prognosis of iatrogenic and AIDS-related types are much worse and commonly disseminate to whole body. Oral and laryngeal-pharyngeal mucosal cutaneous lesions are the most common presentation of the KS in the head and neck area.

Some trials have shown that human chorionic gonadotropin has an antiproliferative effect on KS. However, due to the fetal toxicity of anti-KS treatments, close monitoring of the mother and monitoring of skin lesions are crucial [27].

72.2.9 Angiosarcoma

Angiosarcomas are rare tumors accounting for less than 1% of all sarcomas. Overall survival is approximately 6–16 months and recurrence or metastatic lesions could be seen. Angiosarcoma can be seen at any age, most commonly between the ages of 60 and 70 [28]. Approximately half of them are seen in the head and neck region. It mostly metastasizes to the lungs and bones by hematogenous spread. Radiotherapy and chronic lymphedema are the most common risk factors.

The most effective treatment is the complete surgical removal of the tumor but adequate.

surgical margins are often very difficult to secure. Scholsem M. et al. presented a 36-week uncomplicated pregnancy with a temporal bone angiosarcoma. In this case, they preferred to wait for labor for managing the treatment. After labor, chemoradiation and surgery were done, but she died of metastatic disease 26 months after diagnosis [29]. Samadian M, et al. also presented a 20th week of pregnant case with an angiosarcoma of the skull. They operated the patient and they terminated the pregnancy after surgery and pathological confimation for chemotherapy regimen [30].

72.2.10 Epithelioid Hemangioendothelioma

Epithelioid hemangioendothelioma is a rarely seen tumor. Lungs, liver, and bones are the most common affected areas. They can be located in the head and neck area also.

Moran et al. presented a 25-year-old pregnant woman with epithelioid hemangioendothelioma in the oral cavity. They described an enlarging mass located in the junction of hard and soft palate. After completion of pregnancy wide surgical resection was performed in this case. Clinical course of this lesion is between the hemangioma and angiosarcoma. Wide local excision is considered but recurrence may be seen [31].

72.2.11 Angiofibroma

Angiofibromas are uncommon and constitute <1% of all head and neck tumors. It is a benign vascular tumor; it is exclusively presented in adolescent males and has local agressive and destructive pattern. The site of origin of this tumor is thought to arise from nasopharynx, near the superior margin of the sphenopalatine foramen or in the recess behind the sphenopalatine ganglion in the pterygopalatine fossa.

The pathogenesis of this lesion remains uncertain and unclear. The predilection of juvenile angiofibroma (JNA) for young adolescent males led to a suggested interrelationship between hormones and JNA. These tumors consist of irregular vascular tissue with single epithelial layer; it results in severe bleeding. Clinically, it usually presents with unilateral nasal obstruction, epistaxis, and nasopharyngeal mass. Angiofibroma was not to be mentioned and detailed in this section, since it is considered exclusive for males.

72.2.12 Paraganglioma

Paragangliomas are rarely seen neuroendoocrine neoplasms differentiated from neural crest and are often seen in the head and neck region. It is frequently presented around the carotid arteries, jugular bulbus, vagal nerve, and tympanic plexus. They are tumors with firm and consistent chief cells surrounded by sustentacular cells and divided by a fibrovascular stroma. Average growth rate of tumor is about 1 mm per year [32].

Paragangliomas can be metabolically active by releasing vasoactive substances such as catecholamines and dopamine. Excessive sweating, hypertension, tachycardia, nervousness, and weight loss are the main symptoms associated with catecholamine secretions. Urinary metanephrine, urinary vanilylmandelic acid levels, and serum catecholamine levels are useful for evaluating these patients.

Several reports have described an association between pheochromocytoma and both familial and nonfamilial paragangliomas. Paragangliomas may be presented in patients with familial multiple endocrine neoplasia, MEN2A, and MEN2B.

Malignant paragangliomas are rarely seen, and the diagnosis can be mentioned only if there is proven metastatic disease. Non-malignant paragangliomas may be observed with regional lymph nodes and it is not enough to confirm it is malignant. Both CT and MRI can commonly useful for the diagnosis of paraganglioma. Angiography is crucial for detection of vascular supply of tumor and is important for preoperative embolization.

Paragangliomas are highly vascular tumors and neural involvement, invading to the skull base and intracranial invasion can be seen. These properties contribute to the challenging nature of effectively treating these tumors. Evolution of skull base surgery, embolization protocols, and vascular bypass procedures result in surgery for mainstay treatment for these tumors. However, the outcome is dependent on many factors that might influence the ideal result of complete tumor removal. In older patients, possible neural or vascular deficits after surgery cause serious morbidities. Wait and scan management can be advisable because of slow-growing patterns of this tumor. Major contraindications for surgery due to high risk of morbidities are intracranial invasion, skull base destruction, old age of the patient, medical comorbidities, and multiple paragangliomas. Preoperative angiography and combined endovascular embolization and subsequent surgery have major advantages for treatment. Tumor edema can occur due to the embolization, and short-term steroid treatment is the best option for facilitating the tumor dissection.

Radiotherapy may be used for advanced and unresectable paragangliomas. It is useful also in elderly patients. Stereotactic radiosurgery offers a targeted, short-term, high-dose treatment option with minor complications. Multiple trials have reported the success of this approach in providing good local control.

Its occurrence during pregnancy is uncommon, and diagnosis may be confounded by gestation-related hypertensive disorders. During pregnancy, catecholamine secreted neck paragangliomas may be rarely seen. Catecholamine secretion may be increased during pregnancy. It has been suggested that surgical resection is reasonable if the diagnosis is confirmed and the tumour identified before 24 weeks of gestation. Otherwise, it may be preferable to allow the pregnancy to progress under adequate alpha- and beta-blockade until fetal maturity is reached. After completion of pregnancy, usual treatment protocols for paragangliomas can be used.

Carotid body tumor: The carotid body is located in posteromedial side of the carotid bifurcation. As the tumor enlarges, it tends to widen the carotid bifurcation and it pushes the internal carotid artery (ICA) to the posterolaterally. The tumor can extend superiorly to the base of the skull and may invade lower cranial nerves.

The most common age of presentation for carotid body tumors is approximately between 40 and 50 years with female predominancy. Superior of the carotid bifurcation under the SCM muscle is the most common site of the tumor. They are vertically fixed and laterally mobile and may be pulsatile with palpation. Carotid body tumors are very slow-growing tumors; it can take from months to years for the patient to seek medical treatment. Open or incisional biopsy is contraindicated because of hemorrhage; fine needle aspiration biopsy may be applied if there is a suspicion on diagnosis. Carotid body tumors are exposed through a transverse or oblique incision along the anterior sternocleidomastoid muscle. Subadventitial dissection should be applied for adequate tumor removal [33].

72.2.13 Tympanic Paraganglioma

They usually present in the ear and its related portions. Middle ear cavity, mastoid air cells, and jugular bulb are the most effected areas. It tends to spread along in multiple directions like deep portions of temporal bone, skull base, and posterior cranial fossa. It can extend intracranially via internal auditory canal and labyrinth. Tympanic paragangliomas are slow-growing tumors like other paragangliomas.

Tympanic paragangliomas occur most commonly in females in the sixth decade. Most common symptoms are conductive hearing loss, pulsatile tinnitus, and a red-blue mass behind the tympanic membrane. If tympanic perforation occurs, vascular polypoid lesion in the external ear can be seen. Invasion of ossicles produces conductive hearing loss and vestibular involvement produces sensorineural hearing loss, tinnitus, and vertigo.

Small tumors confined to the middle ear can be operated transcanally and there is no need for preoperative embolization to these lesions. Postauricular, transmastoid with fascial recess approach, transcervial, cervicomastoid, and infratemporal fossa aproaches provide exposure to tumor resection if tumor extends beyond the middle ear borders.

72.2.14 Jugular Paraganglioma

Jugular paragangliomas are more commonly presented in females in the fifth and sixth decade. It may invade the middle ear, internal jugular vein, and skull base. Tumors invading the middle ear show similar symptoms like tympanic paragangliomas. Lower cranial nerve (VII-XII) invasions are common. Facial paralysis, tongue disorders due to hypoglossal nerve palsy, hoarseness, regurgitation, dysphagia, or shoulder weakness or drop are common symptoms due to this invasion of cranial nerves by the tumor [34].

72.2.15 Vagal Paraganglioma

Vagal paragangliomas are rarely observed and constitute about 5% of all head and neck paragangliomas. They present as an ovoid or spindle-shaped asymptomatic neck mass located in the upper neck.

Ganglion nodosum is one of the commonest arising point of the tumor. They have diffuse pattern within the nerve compared to other paragangliomas. Therefore, vagus nerve may be sacrificied during the surgery to achieve the complete tumor resection. Poststyloid parapharyngeal area or skull base invasion could be observed. Early involvement of the internal jugular vein and lower cranial nerves may be seen due to invasion of jugular foramen.

Patients may have cranial neuropathies at the diagnosis. Unilateral vocal cord paralysis, hoarseness, dysphagia, nasal regurgitation, atrophy of the half of the tongue, shoulder weakness, and Horner syndrome are the main symptoms. Hearing loss and pulsatile tinnitus may be observed due to the temporal bone extension. The progression of symptoms is often helpful in differentiating vagal paragangliomas from other head and neck paragangliomas.

A combined cervicomastoid approach to the skull base is best option for safe and wide exposure to tumor. Vagal nerve sacrification are commonly observed; so surgery should not be considered in most of the cases.

72.2.16 Hemangiopericytoma

Hemangiopericytoma is a rare tumor that originates from the pericytes or Zimmerman cells surrounding vessels. Nearly 10–25% of hemangiopericytomas occur in the head and neck, and 5% of tumors present within the paranasal sinuses and nasal cavity.The clinical characteristic is variable; it may act as a slowly growing tumor to local destructive tumor in the head and neck region. It is difficult to distinguish the clinical behaviour of these tumors, so close and long-term follow-up is crucial.

For decreasing tumor vascularity and size preoperatively, embolization may be suggested. The main treatment of hemangiopericytomas is wide surgical excision. Lateral rhinotomy, midfacial degloving, craniofacial resection, or endoscopic surgery are the main surgical approaches. Close follow-up and surgical resection after completion of pregnancy is the best treatment option for these lesions.

72.2.17 Vascular Malformations

Vascular malformations arise from an error in morphogenesis in any combination of arterial, venous, and lymphatic vascular networks. These vascular anomalies present at birth, grow proportionally to the size of the child, and do not exhibit any tendency to involute spontaneously. Trauma, puberty, and pregnancy can also cause accelerated growth. The great majority of congenital vascular malformations are recognizable in childhood.

72.2.18 Capillary Malformation

When capillary malformations (CMs) present on cutaneous or mucosal surfaces they are commonly known as port-wine stains or nevus flammeus. These lesions are are the most common congenital vascular malformations. They present initially as flat and bright pink, red, or violaceous lesion affect the face (90%), followed by the neck, trunk, leg, arm, and hand. Most of the times CMs occur as a sporadic unifocal lesions; however, in some instances they can be part of an underlying syndrome such as in Sturge-Weber syndrome where CMs are associated with CNS and/or ocular anomalies. The gold standard therapy is still the pulsed dye laser treatment for cosmetic purposes. Surgical management can be helpful in patients with soft tissue or bony hypertrophy.

Pregnancy may promote the progression of port wine stain. The blood volume in women during pregnancy is significantly higher than normal, and blood stagnation may exist in the deformed blood vessels, resulting in further expansion of the affected blood vessels. Estrogen is vasoactive and has vasodilating effects, possibly resulting in endothelial dilation through various mechanisms that cause progression of these lesions.

Sometimes pyogenic granulomas occur within a port-wine stain without trauma. These lesions may be a priming lesion for pyogenic granuloma during pregnancy. Priming mechanisms may include the circulatory changes or the hormonal changes of pregnancy.

72.2.19 Venous Malformation

Venous malformations (VM) are the other common type of vascular malformation, previously termed as cavernous hemangioma. VM results from errors in vascular morphogenesis. They may be presented at birth or may present as late as adulthood.

Blue or purplish compressible masses on the skin is the typical characteristic of the lesion. VMs can occasionally be completely intraosseous and the mandible is the most common bone location. They are sensitive to changes in venous flow such as Valsalva or ipsilateral jugular vein compression [35]. One of the most common and specific feature for diffenrential diagnosis is the phleboliths. Thrombosis of the lesion may occur and phleboliths may be palpated as very firm nodules. Due to venous stasis or thrombus, pain is the other symptom of this lesion [36].

VMs are made up of aberrant vessels and venous niduses. These vessels are tortuous, consisting of disorganized smooth muscles and thin walls with lack of internal elastic membranes.

Sclerotherapy, surgery, or laser therapy are the main treatment options for VMs. A single procedure is enough for small and well-contained lesions to achieve complete cure. For large VMs, complete excision is difficult and risky additionally recurrence is common for large lesions. Depth of the lesion, proximity to vital structures, and presence of mucosal involvement are important parameters for deciding the treatment protocol. Sclerotherapy typically involves an alcohol-based agent (sodium tetradecyl sulfate, ethanolamine) injected into the malformation with the help of fluoroscopy. Two sessions are usually enough for routine sclerotherapy, with most patients requiring up to maximum 4 sessions and interval between sessions is mostly between 3 and 12 months [37].

Some lesions are separated from surrounding tissues with definitive borders and surgical removal is safe and easy. Surgery is difficult and risky for lesions that have invaded tissues and lesions with poorly defined borders. Large lesions located in the parotid and massateric region should be approached very carefully. There may be some connections with the dural venous system and internal jugular vein. These types of lesions are often in close relationship with facial nerve. For large and invasive cases, reduction in the lesion instead of complete excision may be considered to prevent complications [38].

During pregnancy, VM may progress with the effect of estrogen and progesterone. These hormones are vasoactive and vasadilatator so some changes of characteristics of these lesions may be observed. Close follow-up and observation are the best treatment option for these lesions.

72.2.20 Lymphatic Malformation

Lymphatic malformation (LM) results from some problems during the development of the lymphatic system embryologically. LMs are often diagnosed before age 2 and prenatal diagnosis are possible. Airway obstruction after birth can be occured due to large macrocystic lesions [39]. LMs are branched into macrocystic (bigger than 2 cm), microcystic (smaller than 2 cm), or mixed. Histologically, all LMs are consisting of heterogenous irregular thin-walled ectatic vessels [40].

Lesions located in the head and neck region require treatment due to deformity and psychosocial difficulties. It is problematic due to its progression over time and the possibility of recurrence. Infection, bleeding within the lesion, upper respiratory tract infections, and hormonal changes due to puberty may cause acute growth in the lesion.

A staging system (de Serres classification) is useful for LMs: stage I, unilateral infrahyoid; stage II, unilateral suprahyoid; stage III, unilateral infrahyoid and suprahyoid; and stage IV, bilateral suprahyoid. Higher stage diseases usually require complex treatment strategies due to possibilit of functional impairment. In general, low-grade and laterally located lesions carry better prognosis than high-grade lesions and medially located [41].

The treatment of LMs should be designed due to the patient's lesion characteristics and associated functional impairment. Sclerotherapy and surgery, with conservative management measures are the main treatment models. There is no statistically significant difference between surgery and sclerotherapy in the results of treatment [42]. In conservative management, LMs will continue to enlarge over time and integration and expansion into normal tissues are observed. Inflammatory episodes can occur, and antibiotics and steroids can be used.

In the sclerotherapy method, lesion is aspirated, and a sclerosing agent is injected, which will cause an inflammatory response in the cyst under ultrasound guidance. The walls of the cysts become sclerosed and the lymphatic fluid cannot be filled with lymphatic fluid and the cyst can not expand. Ethanol, sotradecol, or doxycycline and bleomycine are the most common agents for sclerotherapy. Multiple treatment sessions are often required. Swelling, overlying skin tear, pain, airway obstruction, cranial nerves neuropathies, and prolonged swelling are the most common complications after a session [43].

Surgery is the best treatment option for focal and macrocystic lesions. In surgical treatment, eradication of the disease and protecting the normal tissue as much as possible are more important and balance should be maintained. Debulking surgery is enough for large LMs instead of total removal surgery if there is a risk for neurovascularities. However, for prevention of recurrence complete resection surgery is important [44]. Local resection, CO_2 laser, and coblation are other therapy options for supercial lesions.

LMs in pregnancy have been reported and have even been noted to change in appearance and size presumably secondary to the hematologic and hormonal changes that accompany pregnancy. Galili Y et al. presented a nasopharyngeal lymphatic malformation in pregnant patient. During pregnancy the lesion progressed, airway and swallowing problems occurred.

In this pregnant woman with potential airway obstruction treatment was urgent and surgical intervention was applied [45]. However, Mestak O et al. presented a case with a severe recurrent lympahtic malformation. After contraception use and pregnancy, they observed moderated regression of lymphatic malformation. Effect of contraception and hormonal changes during pregnancy resulted in decreased production and accumulation of lymph in the lymphatic malformation may be the underlying mechanism of this regression [46].

72.2.21 Arteriovenous Malformation

AVMs are rarely observed lesions and they are risky and challenging types of vascular lesions [47]. Aberrant AV connections with high flow stream are found in this lesion and capillary bed are bypassed. More vessels may be recruited over time and it may invade and destroy adjacent tissue. AV fistula is also high flow lesion but recruiting of vessels is the main differentiating characteristic of this lesion. Head and neck region is the most common site extracranially.

AVMs can be evalauted in two major branches: focal or diffuse. If there is a single arterial feeder with a clear bordered nidus, this type of AVM is focal type. It usually presents as a soft tissue mass with discrete borders. The prognosis of focal AVMs is better due to the ability of complete excision. Diffuse AVMs are invasive types and destroy tissue boundaries. It usually recurs after surgical or embolization therapy.

Many AVMs are often presented after 40 years of age. Surgery, trauma, and pregnancy can cause the formation of AVMs and congenital types can be diagnosed also. Bleeding, skin ulceration, and pulsatile nodule are the main symptoms. Arterial steal, venous congestion, and high output cardiac failure can be observed also. AVMs are sensitive to hormonal changes and can show rapid growth during puberty. Trauma and hormonal changes are the main growth triggers. AVMs are pulsatile, warm, and may have a thrill; these symptoms are potential distinguisher from other vascular lesions clinically. Intermittent or rapid expansion due to hormonal changes is also characteristic. There have been no reported cases of spontaneous regression of AVMs.

Magnetic resonance angiography and CT angiography are very useful imaging techniques for diagnosis and treatment planning. Arterial flow voids are typical for AVMs and it will be seen on MRI.

Combination of embolization and surgery is the mainstay of treatment option of AVMs. Ethanol, polyvinyl alcohol, coils, and Onyx are the main embolizing agents. Surgery should be applied after 24–48 h after embolization however recurrence rates are high. Surgical therapy is effective and best treatment option for small and focal lesions. Superselective preoperative embolization can help to the surgey via defining the borders of lesion with decreasing the blood flow. Diffuse and large lesions have a high rate of recurrence. Staged and multiple surgeries or complex tissue flap reconstruction techniques may be useful for large and diffuse lesions.

The main goal of surgery is complete resection of the AVM. Incomplete or partial resections of AVMs will eventually expand and become a problem. Surgery is the best option for cure in small and focal lesions. For controlling diffuse lesions surgery is still the best chance however recurrence rates are quite high up to 93% in diffuse AVMs.

The pathogenesis of AVM is unclear, they tend to grow during pregnancy, likely attributable to both hemodynamic and hormonal factors. The lesions are likely to bleed, and their accelerated growth during pregnancy may lead to ulceration, rupture, and/or hemorrhage. An otolaryngology and/or vascular surgery consultation is essential early in pregnancy to evaluate the lesions and to determine if devascularization (or removal) of the AVM is necessary [48].

Pregnancy appears to increase the risk of bleeding from AVM. Maternal mortality, associated with untreated AVM, is reported to be 33%. Enlarging of lesion may be observed due to infection, trauma, and hormonal changes such as during pregnancy and adolescence. Heart failure may occur in documented cases of AVM in pregnancy, and the exact mechanism is often unclear. Coexistence of pregnancy and AVM may increase the cardiac output to the advanced levels. Many AVMs show spontaneous postpartum regression; changes of levels of hormones in pregnancy with causing venodilation may be responsible of progression of AVM. The increase of progesterone may cause severe morbidity and mortality in both mother and baby by causing dilatation and rupture of vasculars of AVM. If possible, treatment should be postponed to the postpartum period. Treatments in the literature aim to stabilize the AVM by decreasing the hormone levels and to reach delivery [49].

References

1. Fisher C, Maclean M, Morecroft I, Seed A, et al. Is the pregnancy hormone relaxin also a vasodilator peptide secreted by the heart? Circulation. 2002;106(3):292–5.
2. Mulliken J, Glowacki J. Hemangiomas and vascular malformations in infants and children: a classification based on endothelial characteristics. Plast Reconstr Surg. 1982;69(3):412–20.

3. Eivazi B, Werner J. Management of vascular malformations and hemangiomas of the head and neck-an update. Curr Opin Otolaryngol Head Neck Surg. 2013;21(2):157–63.
4. Hoff SR, Rastatter JC, Richter GT. Head and neck vascular lesions. Otolaryngol Clin N Am. 2015;48(1):29–45.
5. Kohout MP, Hansen M, Pribaz J, et al. Arteriovenous malformations of the head and neck: natural history and management. Plast Reconstr Surg. 1998;102:643–54.
6. Hartzell L, Buckmiller L. Current management of infantile hemangiomas and their common associated conditions. Otolaryngol Clin N Am. 2012;45:545–56.
7. Badi A, Kerschner J, North P, et al. Histopathologic and immunophenotypic profile of subglottic hemangioma: multicenter study. Int J Pediatr Otorhinolaryngol. 2009;73(9):1187–91.
8. Bauman N, McCarter R, Guzzetta P, et al. Propranolol vs prednisolone for symptomatic proliferating infantile hemangiomas: a randomized clinical trial. JAMA Otolaryngol Head Neck Surg. 2014;140(4):323.
9. Drolet B, Frommelt P, Chamlin S, et al. Initiation and use of propranolol for infantile hemangioma: report of a consensus conference. Pediatrics. 2013;131(1):128–40.
10. Bajaj Y, Kapoor K, Ifeacho S, et al. Great Ormond street hospital treatment guidelines for use of propranolol in infantile isolated subglottic haemangioma. J Laryngol Otol. 2013;127(3):295–8.
11. Zheng JW, Zhou Q, Yang XJ, Wang YA, Fan XD, Zhou GY, et al. Treatment guideline for hemangiomas and vascular malformations of the head and neck. Head Neck. 2010;32:1088–98.
12. Bauland CG, Smit JM, Bartelink LR, Zondervan HA, Spauwen PH. Hemangioma in the newborn: increased incidence after chorionic villus sampling. Prenatal Diagn. 2010;30:913–7.
13. Lo K, Mihm M, Fay A. Current theories on the pathogenesis of infantile hemangioma. Semin Ophthalmol. 2009;24:172–7.
14. Brahmbhatt AN, Skalski KA, Bhatt AA. Vascular lesions of the head and neck: an update on classification and imaging review. Insights Imaging. 2020;11(1):19.
15. Sun ZY, Yang L, Yi CG, et al. Possibilities and potential roles of estrogen in the pathogenesis of proliferation hemangiomas formation. Med Hypothesis. 2008;71:286–92.
16. Kim YH, Lee GH, Lee SH, Cho JH. An acquired tufted angioma of the nasal cavity. Auris Nasus Larynx. 2013;40:581–58.
17. Pietroletti R, Leardi S, Simi M. Perianal acquired tufted angioma associated with pregnancy: case report. Tech Coloproctol. 2002;6(2):117–9.
18. Al-Muharraqi MA, Faqi MK, Uddin F, Ladak K, Darwish A. Angiolymphoid hyperplasia with eosinophilia (epithelioid hemangioma) of the face: an unusual presentation. Int J Surg Case Rep. 2011;2:258–60.
19. Kamal R, Dahiya P, Puri A. Oral pyogenic granuloma: various concepts of etiopathogenesis. J Oral Maxillofac Pathol. 2012;16:79–82.
20. Rachappa MM, Triveni MN. Capillary hemangioma or pyogenic granuloma: a diagnostic dilemma. Contemp Clin Dent. 2010;1:119–22.
21. Jones JE, Nguyen A, Tabaee A. Pyogenic granuloma (pregnancy tumor) of the nasal cavity. A case report. J Reprod Med. 2000;45:749–53.
22. Demir Y, Demir S, Aktepe F. Cutaneous lobular capillary hemangioma induced by pregnancy. J Cutan Pathol. 2004;31:77–80.
23. Choudhary S, MacKinnon CA, Morrissey GP, Tan ST. A case of giant nasal pyogenic granuloma gravidarum. J Craniofac Surg. 2005;16:319–21.
24. Hanick AL, Meleca JB, Billings SD, Bryson PC. Pyogenic granuloma of the larynx: arare cause of hemoptysis. Am J Otolaryngol. 2019;40:331–3.
25. Zarrinneshan AA, Zapanta PE, Wall SJ. Nasal pyogenic granuloma. Otolaryngol Head Neck Surg. 2007;136:130–1.
26. Chinello M, Di Carlo D, Olivieri F, et al. Successful management of kaposiform hemangioendothelioma with long-term sirolimus treatment: a case report and review of the literature. Mediterr J Hematol Infect Dis. 2018;10:e043.
27. Curtiss P, Strazzulla LC, Friedman-Kien AE. An update on Kaposi's sarcoma: epidemiology, pathogenesis and treatment. Dermatol Ther. 2016;6:465–70.

28. Young RJ, Brown NJ, Reed MW, Hughes D, Woll PJ. Angiosarcoma. Lancet Oncol. 2010;11:983–91.
29. Scholsem M, Raket D, Flandroy P, Sciot R, Deprez M. Primary temporal bone angiosarcoma: a case report. J Neuro-Oncol. 2005;75(2):121–5.
30. Samadian M, Rakhshan M, Haddadian K, Rezaei O, Zamani SAM, Khormae F. Angiosarcoma of skull in a pregnant woman: case report and review of literature. Turk Neurosurg. 2012;22(1):113–5.
31. Moran WJ, Dobleman TJ, Bostwick DG. Epithelioid hemangioendothelioma of the palate. Laryngoscope. 1987;97(11):1299–302.
32. Jansen JC, van den Berg R, Kuiper A, van der Mey AG, Zwinderman AH, Cornelisse CJ. Estimation of growth rate in patients with head and neck paragangliomas influences the treatment proposal. Cancer. 2000;88:2811–6.
33. Wang SJ, Wang MB, Barauskas TM, Calcaterra TC. Surgical management of carotid body tumors. Otolaryngol Head Neck Surg. 2000;123:202–6.
34. Foote RL, Pollock BE, Gorman DA, et al. Glomus jugulare tumor: tumor control and complications after stereotactic radiosurgery. Head Neck. 2002;24:332–9.
35. Richter G, Braswell L. Management of venous malformations. Facial Plast Surg. 2012;28(6):603–10.
36. Glade R, Richter G, James C, et al. Diagnosis and management of pediatric cervicofacialvenous malformations: retrospective review from a vascular anomalies center. Laryngoscope. 2010;120(2):229–35.
37. Gurgacz S, Zamora L, Scott A. Percutaneous sclerotherapy for vascular malformations: a systematic review. Ann Vasc Surg. 2014;28(5):1335–49.
38. Colletti G, Colombo V, Mattassi R, et al. The strangling technique to treat large cervicofacial venous malformations: a preliminary report. Head Neck. 2013;36(10):E94–8.
39. Manning S, Perkins J. Lymphatic malformations. Curr Opin Otolaryngol Head Neck Surg. 2013;21(6):571–5.
40. Perkins J, Manning S, Tempero R, et al. Lymphatic malformations: current cellular and clinical investigations. Otolaryngol Head Neck Surg. 2010;142(6):789–94.
41. De Serres L, Sie K, Richardson M. Lymphatic malformations of the head and neck. Arch Otolaryngol Head Neck Surg. 1995;121(5):577–82.
42. Balakrishnan K, Menezes M, Chen B, et al. Primary surgery vs primary sclerotherapy for head and neck lymphatic malformations. JAMA Otolaryngol Head Neck Surg. 2014;140(1):41–5.
43. Adams M, Saltzman B, Perkins J. Head and neck lymphatic malformation treatment. Otolaryngol Head Neck Surg. 2012;147(4):627–39.
44. Buckmiller L, Richter G, Suen J. Diagnosis and management of hemangiomas and vascular malformations of the head and neck. Oral Dis. 2010;16(5):405–18.
45. Galili Y, Lytle M, Amandeep K, Bartolomei J, Ge L, Carlan SJ, Madruga M. Lymphatic malformation of the nasopharynx in a young pregnant female: a case report. Am J Case Rep. 2019;20:868–71.
46. Mestak O, Mestak J, Pokorna K, Bruna J, Sukop A. Unusual regression of severe recurrent lymphatic malformation of a face after contraception and pregnancy. Gynecol Endocrinol. 2012;28(10):764–6.
47. Richter G, Suen J. Clinical course of arteriovenous malformations of the head and neck: a case series. Otolaryngol Head Neck Surg. 2010;142(2):184–90.
48. Diep J, Dandu K, Xiong M, Shulman SM, Gonzalez-Fiol AJ. Airway arteriovenous malformation in pregnancy. Can J Anesth. 2017;64:1071–2.
49. Martines F, Immordino V. Arteriovenous malformation of the base of tongue in pregnancy: case report. Acta Otorhinolaryngol Ital. 2019;29:274–8.

General Principles of Ent Surgery in Pregnancy

Ömer Bayir, Latif Akan, and Hakan Korkmaz

73.1 Introduction

Women's hormonal systems are unique because of the cyclical changes observed during pregnancy, the menstrual cycle, and menopause. During these periods, physiological changes arise in the body depending on the varying levels of estrogen and progesterone hormones [1, 2]. Every organ system is affected by the metabolic, endocrinological, and physiological changes that occur during pregnancy. As a result, various symptoms may arise. For this reason, otolaryngologists and head and neck surgeons need to master the physiological changes occurring in pregnancy and the associated symptoms. On the other hand, diagnosing diseases may become more complicated due to nonspecific symptoms [1, 2].

When surgery is planned for pregnant patients, the timing of the surgery, the anesthesia method to be applied, and early postoperative follow-up are highly important. The main reason is that any intervention made to the mother can also affect the baby [3, 4]. For this reason, anesthesia methods and anesthetic agents should be carefully selected during interventions. Since alterations in the hemodynamic status of the pregnant woman during the operation are important, they should be carefully monitored. Due to the physiological changes during pregnancy, it is essential to be more cautious about some issues during general anesthesia:

- The complicated hemodynamic alterations take place during pregnancy due to increased blood volume, increased heart rate, and cardiac output, and on the other hand, supine position hypotension caused by aortic and vena caval compression of the enlarged uterus.

Ö. Bayir (✉) · L. Akan · H. Korkmaz
Department of Otolaryngology Head and Neck Surgery, Dışkapı Yıldırım Beyazıt Training and Research Hospital, University of Health Sciences Turkey, Ankara, Turkey
e-mail: bayiromer@hotmail.com; akanlatif@gmail.com; mhkorkmaz@hotmail.com

C. Cingi et al. (eds.), *ENT Diseases: Diagnosis and Treatment during Pregnancy and Lactation*, https://doi.org/10.1007/978-3-031-05303-0_73

- Decreased functional residual capacity due to elevated diaphragm may cause hypoperfusion of mother and fetus.
- Gastric emptying is slower owing to the compression of the enlarged uterus on the stomach and reduced smooth muscle contractions due to the high progesterone levels. Gastrin levels are high during pregnancy, which augments stomach acid production. Therefore, special precautions should be taken to prevent aspiration during anesthesia for pregnant women [3–6].

The era of pregnancy in which the surgery was performed is also a risk factor. Elective surgeries should not be performed principally during pregnancy. If the surgery is necessary, the second trimester should be chosen as a general rule. Since the first trimester is the period of organogenesis, miscarriage rates and malformation risks are relatively high. Surgery in the third trimester has a risk of causing preterm labor. Ideally, the treatment plan can be administered under general or regional anesthesia in a way that is safe for the mother and minimizes harm to the fetus [3–6].

Due to the limited number of cases and insufficient studies in the literature, there are no guidelines for the treatment protocol of most diseases, and the treatment method is created specifically for the patient. For this reason, a coordinated and multidisciplinary approach of the departments related to the disease, including obstetrics, surgery, anesthesia, neonatology, and radiology is mandatory for the procedures to be performed during pregnancy.

As the authors of this chapter, we have preferred to describe the procedures that can be performed regarding Ear Nose Throat, and Head and Neck Surgery during pregnancy by dividing them into sections.

73.2 Rhinology

Physiological alterations in pregnancy cause mucosal edema as a result of increased interstitial fluid volume, increased blood volume, increased vascularity, and overactivity of the parasympathetic system. Nasal patency has been shown to decrease during pregnancy with anterior rhinoscopy, and nasal tests such as peak inspiratory and expiratory nasal flow and saccharin tests [1, 2].

Nasal congestion or rhinitis that develops during pregnancy is known as 'pregnancy rhinitis.' This condition occurs in 5–32% of pregnant women. It occurs at the end of the first trimester and may persist until birth or several weeks later. On clinical examination, the edematous nasal mucosa can be seen [1, 2].

Rhinology-related elective surgeries should not be performed during pregnancy; if a surgical procedure is required, the second trimester should be selected. On the other hand, there are some complicated situations that should be intervened.

73.2.1 Epistaxis

Although epistaxis is common during pregnancy, large volume epistaxis is rare. In addition to the hormonal changes, pregnancy-associated coagulopathies such as pregnancy thrombocytopenia, idiopathic thrombocytopenic purpura, HELLP syndrome, and coagulopathy caused by vitamin K deficiency associated with hyperemesis gravidarum can occur. The management of epistaxis in pregnancy becomes more complicated due to absolute or relative contraindications. Otolaryngology surgeons need to be aware of which options can be used safely and effectively. Most bleedings can be treated with simple interventions [7].

Among the local treatment options, materials such as silver nitrate, paraffin gauze, absorbable hemostatic gelatin sponge, bio-resorbable and bio-fragmentable nasal packing materials, and electrocautery are suitable as the first step. Although there is no definite contraindication for posterior packing, it should be kept in mind that it may cause hypoxemia. Hemostatic matrix materials are not recommended due to inadequate evidence for use in pregnancy. However, considering the topical use of these materials in some case reports, especially in patients who are not suitable for surgery, and due to the low theoretical risk of harming the fetus, particularly in the third trimester, it may be thought that the benefits of their use may outweigh the risks. The problems associated with cocaine use are well known, so nasal preparations, especially cocaine-based, should be avoided in pregnancy. Strip gauze soaked with bismuth iodoform paraffin paste (BIPP) is contraindicated in pregnancy. Surgical treatments (such as vascular ligation) may come to the forefront when these interventions are unsuccessful. Here, in addition to the risks of general anesthesia, nasal usage of local anesthetics and topical vasoconstrictors should be used cautiously because of the risk of systemic absorption which may cause a decrease in uterine blood supply [7]. Radiological embolization may be teratogenic for pregnant women in the first trimester due to the administration of contrast material. However, it can be considered in cases where surgery cannot be performed and if the mother's life is at risk.

73.2.1.1 Granuloma Gravidarum

Nasal granuloma gravidarum is a rare, rapidly growing, hemorrhagic benign lesion that is histologically similar to a pyogenic granuloma or lobular type capillary hemangioma. These are hormone-dependent lesions and usually regress after pregnancy, but can cause significant epistaxis. It can be treated with surgical excision in cases where epistaxis and obstruction symptoms are evident or there is a possible risk of malignancy [8, 9].

73.2.1.2 Complications of Sinusitis

In pregnancy, a relationship was found between mucosal edema and rhinitis, but no relationship was determined between pregnancy and sinusitis. The partial similarities between the nonspecific findings of rhinitis and the symptoms of sinusitis in pregnancy and the fact that the findings suggestive of sinusitis complications may be related to pregnancy-specific conditions make the diagnosis difficult (worsening of diabetic retinopathy, visual effects of pregnancy-induced coagulopathy, and the central and visual effects of preeclampsia/eclampsia, etc.) [1, 2].

When orbital or intracranial complications of sinusitis are suspected, magnetic resonance imaging (MRI) should be preferred instead of computed tomography (CT) to prevent radiation exposure to the fetus as a radiological imaging method [10]. While making treatment plans, whether to be treated conservatively or surgically, which antibiotic regimen to choose, other treatment options, and the timing of all these should be considered. Considering that delays in surgery in the presence of orbital or intracranial complications may cause irreversible blindness, permanent neurological damage, and even death, appropriate treatment should be performed in the presence of surgical indications, such as in nonpregnant patients [10–12].

Although there are limited reports on the treatment of brain abscess, which is a very advanced complication of sinusitis, craniotomy is safe and effective in pregnancy. Given the risk posed by increased intracranial pressure, the timing of delivery is also important in this situation. In some cases, clinicians opted for an early cesarean section due to increased intracranial pressure during delivery and concerns about spontaneous vaginal delivery. On the other hand, although there is little data to guide, vaginal delivery has been performed safely in patients with non-sinogenic brain abscess and increased intracranial pressure due to noninfectious reasons. As a result, issues related to delivery route and timing should be based on individual clinical factors and a multidisciplinary approach should be approached [11–13].

73.3 Otology–Neurotology

Estrogen α and β receptors have been reported to have a unique distribution in the auditory pathways and fluid and electrolyte regulatory regions. Due to this fact, low-frequency sensory hearing loss and tolerance problems that mimic cochlear pathology may occur during pregnancy, but this situation returns to normal in the postpartum period. On the other hand, eustachian tube dysfunction is estimated to affect 5–30% of pregnant women and there may be variabilities in terms of its symptoms [1, 2].

As a general principle, elective surgeries should not be performed primarily during pregnancy. There is limited data in the literature on otological surgeries during pregnancy. Doyle et al. reported in 1993 that in two pregnant women with acoustic neuroma, any complications did not develop after surgery [14]. According to the results of the acoustic neuroma case series of Gaughan et al., it was recommended that uncomplicated cases should be treated after pregnancy [15]. Jacob et al. reported a case of chronic otitis media with intracranial complications at the 35th week of pregnancy. In this case, considering that there may be some negative effects on the fetus due to long-term general anesthesia, and due to the forthcoming term, the delivery was first performed by cesarean section. After that, while under anesthesia, abscess drainage and mastoidectomy were performed in the same session and no complications developed [16].

In the light of these limited data, it is recommended that complicated otitis cases be treated as nonpregnant patients and elective surgeries should be postponed after delivery.

73.4 Larynx

Laryngeal symptoms, acute or chronic, may occur as a result of physiological changes in the larynx during pregnancy. Pregnant women may present with dyspnea, hoarseness, sore throat, and odynophagia. In the laryngeal examination, edema may be observed especially on the aryepiglottic folds, arytenoids, and vocal cords [1, 2]. Due to the symptoms that develop after these physiological changes, it becomes difficult to diagnose other diseases affecting the airway. This becomes even more complicated, especially in slowly progressing situations. As a general principle, elective surgeries should not be performed primarily during pregnancy. However, hypoxemia potentially may occur when pregnancy-related changes are added, particularly in cases that narrow the airway can be harmful to both the mother and the fetus, and planning should be performed considering these factors [17, 18].

73.4.1 Hemangioma

About 80% of hemangiomas occur in women, and 50% of all hemangiomas are located in the head and neck region. Although cavernous hemangiomas of the larynx are rare, they are more common especially in women during pregnancy. These may occur in less than 5% of all pregnant women, and their development or enlargement may be associated with the increased estrogen levels during pregnancy. Pre-existing hemangiomas can also enlarge during pregnancy. These symptoms are much more pronounced in the third trimester and regress after delivery but do not recover completely. Therefore, it may require treatment in the postpartum period. In some cases, tracheostomy may be needed to provide airway during pregnancy [2].

73.4.2 Idiopathic Subglottic Stenosis

Since idiopathic subglottic stenosis (ISGS) is relatively indeterminate and slowly progressive, the disease may first be misdiagnosed as asthma or bronchiolitis, and the actual diagnosis and treatment are often delayed. In a survey of more than 400 women with ISGS, it was seen that 5.8% were diagnosed during pregnancy. The treatment protocol is not clear due to the lack of sufficient studies in the literature. Treatment options include follow-up, bougie or balloon dilation, cricotracheal resection, and tracheostomy. It is known that inadequate oxygenation during pregnancy, such as ISGS, may cause ischemic placental complications including pre-eclampsia and intrauterine growth retardation, and treatment should be performed to prevent their occurrence. In the treatment approach, treatments that are likely to cause uterine contractions and premature delivery, or cause maternal hypoxia or acidosis should be avoided. To diminish the risk of these complications, it is vital to choose a treatment modality that is effective in maintaining the airway and oxygenation, yet is minimally invasive, simple, rapid, and minimizes maternal and fetal stress. Although dilatation is generally preferred in the literature since it is a minimally invasive and rapid method in ISGS patients, but a surgical procedure may be required over again after pregnancy. On the other hand, it should not be forgotten that there may be situations where the airway needs urgent interventions in these patients. In some cases, an early cesarean section may be required [17, 18].

73.4.3 Cord Vocal Paralysis

While unilateral vocal cord paralysis causes voice disorders, bilateral paralysis results in breathing difficulties. While the most common cause of bilateral vocal cord paralysis (BVCP) is due to thyroidectomy surgery, rare causes include trauma, neurological diseases, and malignancies. The incidence of BVCP after thyroidectomy is not very rare and can sometimes be severe enough to necessitate emergency tracheotomy. Some patients can by some means tolerate the condition and have a chronic respiratory problem. In a 23-week pregnant patient who developed BCVP after thyroidectomy 2 years ago, due to the augmented symptoms, Korkmaz et al. improved airway patency with suture arytenoid laterofixation. However, due to the development of laryngeal edema, tracheotomy was performed on the second day after the operation. Decannulation was performed during the sixth month after normal delivery at term [19]. As in this case, with the emergence of symptoms during pregnancy in BVCP, as in ISGS, an urgent diagnosis should be performed and emergency airway surgery may be required.

73.5 Approach to Head Neck Tumors

Head and neck tumors (HNT) in pregnancy are rare and can be difficult to diagnose as symptoms may be nonspecific. A multidisciplinary approach of medical oncology, surgery, and radiation oncology teams as well as obstetrics, anesthesia, and neonatology departments are critical for the treatment plan. The aim is to accurately diagnose, stage, and plan treatments for HNT during pregnancy while seeking to ensure optimum maternal and neonatal outcomes [3, 5, 6, 20].

The most common invasive malignancies diagnosed during pregnancy are breast cancer, melanoma, hematological, cervix/uterine, and thyroid malignancies. Guidelines are available for the management of thyroid cancer in pregnancy. In contrast, there is limited information about non-thyroid HNT in pregnancy. When planning surgery as a treatment for HNT complicated by pregnancy, it is important to consider the gestational age, type of general anesthesia, and the type of procedure planned. In addition, pregnancy has a considerable impact on anatomical, endocrinological, and systemic functions. The operation should be performed in the second trimester when possible, in malignant tumors of the head and neck region that can be cured only by surgery. Since the first trimester is the period of organogenesis, spontaneous abortion rates are relatively high, after operations. Surgery in the third trimester has a risk of causing preterm labor. It is thought that the effects of anesthesia and surgery, such as low birth weight and mortality, may be caused by the situation that required the procedure rather than the anesthetic agent used [3–6, 20]. In the presence of malignancy that will adversely affect the survival of the mother and require adjuvant treatments such as chemotherapy and radiotherapy, the fetus may need to be evacuated.

However, preferring between maternal advantage and potential fetal harm should not be merely a medical decision. Individualized treatment is an opportunity.

Comprehensive information and appropriate support should be provided to the patients and their families so that they can fully participate in the decision-making process. Patient care can be improved if surgery is performed in a specialized obstetrics center where oncological treatment can be managed together with the obstetric aspects [21, 22].

73.5.1 Oral Cavity Cancers

There are no international guidelines for the treatment of oral cavity cancers during pregnancy. Yokoshima et al. reported the outcomes of surgical treatment of tongue cancers during pregnancy, and suggested that if the optimal treatment would not be provided, it may result in a worse prognosis. In another study, the standard treatment was not applied to six patients with tongue cancer, and disease progression was observed in three of the cases, and two died in a short time. Previous studies in the literature prove that pregnant women with tongue cancer should be treated as nonpregnant patients and suggest that following the standard surgical procedure in tongue cancer may be the most appropriate treatment to ensure maternal and infant wellbeing [21, 22].

73.5.2 Nasal Cavity Cancers

Although nasal cavity tumors are mostly seen in elderly men, some cases diagnosed during pregnancy have been reported in the literature. For example, in a case, nasal cavity mucoepidermoid carcinoma was diagnosed at the 13th week of pregnancy that was treated by maxillectomy, and a cesarean delivery was performed at term without the need for adjuvant chemotherapy/radiotherapy in the postpartum period. In the light of this information, physical examination or definitive surgery can be performed under general anesthesia if it is indicated, regardless of the trimester of pregnancy, and it is another approach to treat pregnant patients like nonpregnant ones [6].

73.5.3 Larynx Cancers

Although larynx cancer is a relatively rare disease, it is the most common HNT in most countries (excluding skin and thyroid cancers). Depending on the factors such as the stage and histological type of the disease, and age, general health status, and preference of the patient, the treatment preference may be surgery, radiotherapy, or a combination of these [3].

In 1980, Ferlito and Nicolai reported a case of laryngeal squamous cell carcinoma in a pregnant woman who presented with progressive hoarseness and diagnosed in the second trimester. The patient underwent laryngectomy and radical neck dissection after term delivery [23]. In 1995, Pytel et al. reported a case of a

33-year-old woman carrying a twin pregnancy with supraglottic laryngeal cancer detected in the first trimester. This patient underwent an uncomplicated supraglottic laryngectomy during pregnancy without any recurrence, and the twins were born at term [24]. In another publication, survival of pregnant and nonpregnant women with a comparable type of laryngeal cancer with appropriate treatment was almost similar. At this point, early cesarean delivery, therapeutic abortion, and all other options should be considered and the treatment plan should be tailored by informing the patient. In cases of delaying or rejecting treatment in some social situations, adequate information should be provided about the progression of the disease and hypoxemia that may develop due to respiratory distress [3, 20].

Generally, early-stage laryngeal cancers can be treated with transoral or open surgeries, with safe oncological results. However, it should be considered that patients with extralaryngeal extension and regional metastases can receive adjuvant treatments in addition to surgery, and fetal evacuation or preterm delivery should be regarded. The most appropriate treatment options should be determined together with the patient by evaluating the risks.

73.6 Thyroid and Parathyroid Surgery

73.6.1 Thyroid Surgery

Thyroid cancer is the most common endocrine malignancy. Although it is seen in all adult age groups, women are affected 2–4 times more than men. The highest incidence in women is reported between the ages of 30 and 50, and diagnosis in pregnancy is not uncommon. Among all cancers diagnosed during pregnancy, thyroid cancer occurs in 6–10% and is one of the most common cancers [4, 25, 26].

Although the incidence of thyroid nodules in pregnant women is below 10%, the risk of malignancy in these nodules has been reported to be between 15 and 50%. It has been reported that solitary thyroid nodules detected during pregnancy are approximately three times more likely to be malignant compared to a nonpregnant woman of the same age [21]. On the other hand, the effects of pregnancy on thyroid cancer are still controversial. In a few studies, pregnancy was identified as an unfavorable prognostic factor. In contrast, larger population-based studies did not show that pregnancy has an adverse effect on the prognosis of differentiated thyroid cancers (DTC). Even though the approach to the thyroid nodules in pregnant women is similar to that of nonpregnant women, nuclear medicine examinations should be avoided in hyperfunctioning thyroid nodules [4, 25, 26].

The American Thyroid Association (ATA) recommends ultrasound (US) for the evaluation of thyroid nodules, also during pregnancy. In the presence of a nodule in the US, the features of this nodule should be evaluated, and if it is benign, the patient should be followed up with the US. Fine needle aspiration biopsy (FNAB) should be performed if US has some features such as microcalcification, hypoechoic pattern, vascular staining, irregularly circumscribed nodules, elastogram elevation, and pathological lymph node. In addition, in nodules that grow rapidly or cause compression symptoms, even if it has benign features on US, FNAB should be performed. It has been stated that FNAB can be applied safely throughout the entire pregnancy and does not pose a maternal or fetal risk [27, 28].

According to ATA guidelines, studies in the literature suggest that maternal and neonatal complications should be evaluated and papillary thyroid cancers detected in early pregnancy should be followed sonographically before recommending an operation during pregnancy, since delaying surgery until postpartum in DTC does not cause a worse prognosis. It recommends considering surgery during pregnancy if it enlarges significantly before the 24th–26th gestational weeks or if cytologically malignant cervical lymph nodes are present. However, it has been suggested that if the disease remains stable in mid-pregnancy or is diagnosed in the second half of pregnancy, surgery can be postponed until postpartum [27, 28].

The ATA strongly recommends that for pregnant women with cytologically indeterminate (AUS/FLUS, SFN, or SUSP) nodules in the absence of cytologically malignant lymph nodes or other signs of metastatic disease, they do not routinely require surgery during pregnancy. On the other hand, if there is clinical suspicion of aggressive behavior in cytologically ambiguous nodules during pregnancy, surgery is recommended, albeit weakly [27, 28]. The effects of pregnancy on women with newly diagnosed medullary carcinoma or anaplastic cancer are unknown. However, a delay in treatment can adversely affect the outcomes. Therefore, considering surgery after assessing all clinical factors is strongly recommended [27, 28].

Although the approach to the nodules detected during pregnancy is controversial, the treatment plan should be evaluated together with the patient's clinical characteristics and decided together with the patient. In a study conducted in Japan, 24 of 45 DTC patients were operated during pregnancy (19 in the second trimester) and 21 after delivery, with similar recurrence rates and no pregnancy loss or birth defects. The authors concluded that although thyroidectomy can be performed safely in the second trimester, surgery is recommended after delivery in most patients with nonaggressive DTC [29]. In a previous study, conducted by Cunningham and Slaughter surgical exploration is recommended if thyroid malignancy is suspected in the first or second trimesters, and after delivery if diagnosed in the third trimester [30].

Herzon et al. stated that surgical treatment can be postponed until delivery in pregnant women with DTC [31]. In the light of this information, although it is affirmed that there is no change in the natural course and prognosis of the disease when the surgical treatment of DTC is postponed until post-pregnancy, it should be performed in the second trimester if possible to minimize complications for both mother and fetus when surgery is indicated or desired during pregnancy. It is recommended that the surgery should be done by an experienced surgeon [4, 25, 26]. On the other hand, the risk of maternal hypothyroidism and hypoparathyroidism after thyroidectomy should also be considered. Of course, radioiodine therapy should be delayed until after delivery (6 months if possible) to avoid undesirable effects on the fetus [25, 26].

73.6.2 Parathyroid Surgery

There are 2 methods in the treatment of primary hyperparathyroidism in pregnancy. The first one can be managed conservatively with oral or intravenous dehydration, a low calcium diet, and vitamin D supplementation, with or without forced diuresis [3]. Other treatment options, such as calcitonine and cinacalcet, are not used in pregnancy due to limited safety data. The use of bisphosphonate therapies should be avoided because of the risk of adverse effects on fetal skeletal development. The parathyroidectomy is the second definitive treatment of primary hyperparathyroidism and is recommended during pregnancy, especially in patients with previous pregnancy loss, and when serum calcium is higher than 2.75 mmol/L. Surgery is preferably performed in the second trimester because of the continuing organogenesis in the first trimester and the risk of preterm labor in the third trimester. However, if all efforts in medical treatment fail or if maternal and/or fetal complications occur, emergency parathyroidectomy is recommended regardless of the gestational age of the fetus [32].

Recent retrospective data have shown that patients treated with parathyroidectomy have lower rates of preeclampsia and preterm labor compared to the patients treated medically [32]. Ideally, the treatment plan can be implemented in a way that is safe for the mother and minimizes harm to the fetus.

References

1. Sherlie VS, Varghese A. ENT changes of pregnancy and its management. Indian J Otolaryngol Head Neck Surg. 2014;66(1):6–9.
2. Bhagat DR, Chowdhary A, Verma S. Physiological changes in ENT during pregnancy. Indian J Otolaryngol Head Neck Surg. 2006;58(3):268–70.
3. Bradley PJ, Ullas R. Cancers presenting in the head and neck during pregnancy. Curr Opin Otolaryngol Head Neck Surg. 2004;12(2):76–81.
4. Bayır Ö, Polat R, Saylam G, et al. Gebelikte diferansiye tiroid kanseri cerrahisi ve anestezi ilkeleri: Üç olgu sunumu. Kulak Burun Bogaz Ihtis Derg. 2015;25(6):350–6.
5. Atabo A, Bradley PJ. Management principles of head and neck cancers during pregnancy: a review and case series. Oral Oncol. 2008;44(3):236–41.
6. Figueiró-Filho EA, Horgan RP, Muhanna N, et al. Obstetrical outcomes of head and neck (non-thyroid) cancers: a 27-year retrospective series and literature review. AJP Rep. 2019;9(1):e15.
7. Crunkhorn R E M, Mitchell-Innes A, Muzaffar J (2014) Torrential epistaxis in the third trimester: a management conundrum. BMJ Case Rep. 2014:bcr2014203892
8. Delbrouck C, Chamiec M, Hassid S, et al. Lobular capillary haemangioma of the nasal cavity during pregnancy. J Laryngol Otol. 2011;125(9):973.
9. Yusof JM, Abd Halim A, Hamizan AKW. Severe epistaxis in pregnancy due to nasal pyogenic granuloma: a case report. J Taibah Univ Med Sci. 2020;15(4):334–7.
10. Ismi O, Vayisoglu Y, Dinc E, et al. Central retinal artery occlusion and irreversible blindness due to paranasal sinus infection in a pregnant woman. Journal of Craniofacial Surgery. 2014;25(6):e557–9.
11. Domville-Lewis C, Friedland PL, Santa Maria PL. Pott's puffy tumour and intracranial complications of frontal sinusitis in pregnancy. J Laryngol Otol. 2013;127(S1):S35.
12. Cosar M, Hatiboglu MA, Cosar E, et al. Intracranial mucocele in pregnancy. J Clin Neurosci. 2007;14(10):1000–3.

13. Wax JR, Blackstone J, Mancall A, et al. Sinogenic brain abscess complicating pregnancy. Am J Obstet Gynecol. 2004;191(5):1711–2.
14. Doyle KJ, Luxford WM. Acoustic neuroma in pregnancy. Am J Otol. 1994;15(1):111–3.
15. Gaughan RK, Harner SG. Acoustic neuroma and pregnancy. Am J Otol. 1993;14(1):88–91.
16. Jacob CE, Kurien M, Varghese AM, et al. Treatment of otogenic brain abscess in pregnancy. Otol Neurotol. 2009;30(5):602–3.
17. Damrose EJ, Manson L, Nekhendzy V, et al. Management of subglottic stenosis in pregnancy using advanced apnoeic ventilatory techniques. J Laryngol Otol. 2019;133(5):399–403.
18. McCrary H, Torrecillas V, Conley M, et al. Idiopathic subglottic stenosis during pregnancy: a support group survey. Ann Otol Rhinol Laryngol. 2021;130(2):188–94.
19. Korkmaz MH, Bayır Ö, Tatar EÇ, et al. Glottic airway gain after 'suture arytenoid laterofixation' in bilateral vocal cord paralysis. Acta Otolaryngol. 2015;135(9):931–6.
20. Devaney SL, Devaney KO, Ferlito A, et al. Pregnancy and malignant neoplasms of the head and neck. Ann Otol Rhinol Laryngol. 1998;107(11):991–8.
21. Yokoshima K, Nakamizo M, Sakanushi A, et al. Surgical management of tongue cancer during pregnancy. Auris Nasus Larynx. 2012;39(4):428–30.
22. Tagliabue M, Elrefaey SH, Peccatori F, et al. Tongue cancer during pregnancy: surgery and more, a multidisciplinary challenge. Crit Rev Oncol Hematol. 2016;98:1–11.
23. Ferlito A, Nicolai P. Laryngeal cancer in pregnancy. Acta Otorhinolaryngol Belg. 1980;34(6):706–9.
24. Pytel J, Gerlinger I, Arany A. Twin pregnancy following in vitro fertilisation coinciding with laryngeal cancer. ORL. 1995;57(4):232–4.
25. Varghese SS, Varghese A, Ayshford C. Differentiated thyroid cancer and pregnancy. Indian J Surg. 2014;76(4):293–6.
26. Boucek J, de Haan J, Halaska MJ, et al. Maternal and obstetrical outcome in 35 cases of well-differentiated thyroid carcinoma during pregnancy. Laryngoscope. 2018;128(6):1493–500.
27. Stagnaro-Green A, Abalovich M, Alexander E, et al. Guidelines of the American Thyroid Association for the diagnosis and management of thyroid disease during pregnancy and postpartum. Thyroid. 2011;21(10):1081–125.
28. Alexander EK, Pearce EN, Brent GA, et al. Guidelines of the American Thyroid Association for the Diagnosis and Management of Thyroid Disease During Pregnancy and the Postpartum. Thyroid. 2017;27(3):315–89.
29. Uruno T, Shibuya H, Kitagawa W, et al. Optimal timing of surgery for differentiated thyroid cancer in pregnant women. World J Surg. 2014;38(3):704–8.
30. Cunningham MP, Slaughter DP. Surgical treatment of disease of the thyroid gland in pregnancy. Surg Gynecol Obstet. 1970;131(3):486–8.
31. Herzon FS, Morris DM, Segal MN, et al. Coexistent thyroid cancer and pregnancy. Archiv Otolaryngol Head Neck Surg. 1994;120(11):1191–3.
32. McCarthy A, Howarth S, Khoo S, et al. Management of primary hyperparathyroidism in pregnancy: a case series. Endocrinol Diabetes Metab Case Rep. 2019;16(1):19–0039.

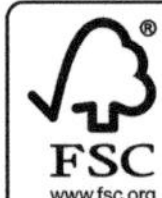

MIX
Papier aus verantwortungsvollen Quellen
Paper from responsible sources
FSC® C105338

If you have any concerns about our products,
you can contact us on
ProductSafety@springernature.com

In case Publisher is established outside the EU,
the EU authorized representative is:
Springer Nature Customer Service Center GmbH
Europaplatz 3, 69115 Heidelberg, Germany

Printed by Libri Plureos GmbH
in Hamburg, Germany